Immunology of
Infectious Diseases

Immunology of Infectious Diseases

Edited by

STEFAN H. E. KAUFMANN
Max Planck Institute for Infection Biology, Berlin, Germany

ALAN SHER
Laboratory of Parasitic Diseases, National Institute of Allergy and Infectious Diseases,
National Institutes of Health, Bethesda, Maryland

RAFI AHMED
Emory Vaccine Center, Emory University School of Medicine,
Atlanta, Georgia

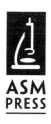

ASM
PRESS

Washington, D.C.

Address editorial correspondence to ASM Press, 1752 N Street NW, Washington, DC 20036-2904, USA

Send orders to ASM Press, P.O. Box 605, Herndon, VA 20172, USA
Phone: (800) 546-2416; (703) 661-1593
Fax: (703) 661-1501
E-mail: books@asmusa.org
Online: www.asmpress.org

Library of Congress Cataloging-in-Publication Data

Immunology of infectious diseases / edited by Stefan H. E. Kaufmann, Alan
Sher, Rafi Ahmed.
    p. cm.
  Includes bibliographical references and index.
  ISBN 1-55581-214-7
  1. Immune response. 2. Communicable diseases—Immunological aspects. I. Kaufmann, S. H. E.
  (Stefan H. E.) II. Sher, Alan. III. Ahmed, Rafi.
QR186.I46835 2002
616.9′0479—dc21   00-069980

10 9 8 7 6 5 4 3 2 1

Cover figure: Human herpesvirus 6 maturing from an infected T-lymphoblastic cell line (pseudocolorized electron micrograph). Courtesy of Volker Brinkmann.

CONTENTS

CONTRIBUTORS

Laurent Abel
Laboratory of Human Genetics of Infectious
Diseases, Necker Medical School, 75015 Paris,
France

Rafi Ahmed
Emory Vaccine Center and Department of
Microbiology and Immunology, Emory University
School of Medicine, Atlanta, GA 30322

Charles M. Bangham
Department of Immunology, Imperial College
School of Medicine at St. Mary's, Norfolk Place,
London W2 1PG, United Kingdom

Jack R. Bennink
Laboratory of Viral Diseases, National Institutes of
Allergy and Infectious Diseases, Bethesda,
MD 20892-0440

Christine A. Biron
Department of Molecular Microbiology and
Immunology, Division of Biology and Medicine,
Brown University, Providence, RI 02912

Michel Brahic
Unité des Virus Lents, CNRS URA 1930, Institut
Pasteur, 28 rue du Dr Roux, 75724 Paris, France

Michael S. Brehm
Department of Pathology, University of
Massachusetts Medical School, Worcester,
MA 01655

Gordon D. Brown
Sir William Dunn School of Pathology, University
of Oxford, South Parks Rd., Oxford OX1 3RE,
United Kingdom

Jean-François Bureau
Unité des Virus Lents, CNRS URA 1930, Institut
Pasteur, 28 rue du Dr Roux, 75724 Paris, France

Arturo Casadevall
Albert Einstein College of Medicine, 1300 Morris
Park Ave., Bronx, NY 10461

Jean-Laurent Casanova
Laboratory of Human Genetics of Infectious
Diseases, Necker Medical School, 75015 Paris,
France

Helen L. Collins
Department of Immunology, Max Planck Institute
for Infection Biology, 10117 Berlin, Germany

Marc Dalod
Department of Molecular Microbiology and
Immunology, Division of Biology and Medicine,
Brown University, Providence, RI 02912

Mark Feinberg
Departments of Medicine and of Microbiology and
Immunology, Emory University School of Medicine
and Emory Vaccine Research Center, Atlanta,
GA 30329

Deborah J. Fowell
Center for Vaccine Biology and Immunology,
University of Rochester Medical Center, 601
Elmwood Ave., Box 69, Rochester, NY 14642

Gabriel Gachelin
Unité de Biologie Moléculaire du Gène, Institut
Pasteur, 28 rue du Dr Roux, 75724 Paris, France

Thomas Ganz
Departments of Medicine and Pathology, UCLA
School of Medicine, Los Angeles, CA 90095-1690

Werner Goebel
Lehrstuhl für Mikrobiologie, Biozentrum,
Am Hubland, 97074 Würzburg, Germany

Siamon Gordon
Sir William Dunn School of Pathology, University of Oxford, South Parks Rd., Oxford OX1 3RE, United Kingdom

Richard K. Grencis
Immunology Group, School of Biological Sciences, University of Manchester, Manchester, United Kingdom

Philippe Gros
Centre for the Study of Host Resistance, Department of Biochemistry, McGill University, Montréal, Québec H3G 1Y6, Canada

Amy C. Herring
Pulmonary Division, Department of Internal Medicine, University of Michigan Medical Center, Ann Arbor, MI 48109

Gary B. Huffnagle
Pulmonary Division, University of Michigan Medical Center, Ann Arbor, MI 48109

Austin L. Hughes
Department of Biological Sciences, University of South Carolina, Columbia, SC 29208

Christopher A. Hunter
Department of Pathobiology, School of Veterinary Medicine, University of Pennsylvania, 3800 Spruce St., Philadelphia, PA 19104

David C. Johnson
Department of Molecular Microbiology and Immunology, Oregon Health Sciences University, Portland, OR 97201

Stefan H. E. Kaufmann
Department of Immunology, Max Planck Institute for Infection Biology, 10117 Berlin, Germany

Jean-Pierre Kraehenbuhl
Swiss Institute for Experimental Cancer Research, Institute of Biochemistry, University of Lausanne, CH-1066 Epalinges, Switzerland

Michael Kuhn
Lehrstuhl für Mikrobiologie, Biozentrum, Am Hubland, 97074 Würzburg, Germany

Dominic Kwiatkowski
Molecular Infectious Diseases Group, Institute of Molecular Medicine, John Radcliffe Hospital, Oxford OX3 9DS, United Kingdom

J. Gibson Lanier
Emory Vaccine Center and Department of Microbiology and Immunology, Emory University School of Medicine, Atlanta, GA 30322

Robert I. Lehrer
Department of Medicine, UCLA School of Medicine, Los Angeles, CA 90095-1690

John M. Mansfield
Department of Bacteriology, University of Wisconsin—Madison, Madison, WI 53706

Grant McFadden
Department of Microbiology and Immunology, The University of Western Ontario and The John P. Robarts Research Institute, London, Ontario N6G 2V4, Canada

John D. McKinney
The Rockefeller University, 1230 York Ave., New York, NY 10021

Robert Modlin
Division of Dermatology and Department of Microbiology and Immunology, UCLA School of Medicine, Los Angeles, CA 90095

Tim R. Mosmann
Center for Vaccine Biology and Immunology, University of Rochester Medical Center, 601 Elmwood Ave., Box 609, Rochester, NY 14642

Ernesto J. Muñoz-Elías
The Rockefeller University, 1230 York Ave., New York, NY 10021

Marian R. Neutra
Department of Pediatrics, Harvard Medical School, GI Cell Biology Laboratory, Children's Hospital, Boston, MA 02115

Shawn P. O'Neil
Division of Microbiology and Immunology, Yerkes Research Center, Emory University School of Medicine, Atlanta, GA 30329

Martin Olivier
Infectious Diseases Unit, CHUL, Laval University, Sainte-Foy, Quebec G1V 4G2, Canada

Eric Pamer
Infectious Disease Service, Laboratory of Antimicrobial Immunity, Memorial Sloan-Kettering Cancer Center, New York, NY 10021

Edward J. Pearce
Department of Microbiology and Immunology,
College of Veterinary Medicine, Cornell University,
Ithaca, NY 14853

Dana J. Philpott
Unité de Pathogénie Microbienne Moléculaire,
INSERM U 389, Institut Pasteur, 25-28 Rue du
Docteur Roux, 75724 Paris, France

Brian D. Robertson
Department of Infectious Diseases and
Microbiology, Faculty of Medicine, Imperial
College, London W2 1PG, United Kingdom

Luigina Romani
Microbiology Section, Department of Experimental
Medicine and Biochemical Sciences, School of
Medicine, University of Perugia, Via del Giochetto,
06122 Perugia, Italy

Thais P. Salazar-Mather
Department of Molecular Microbiology and
Immunology, Division of Biology and Medicine,
Brown University, Providence, RI 02912

Philippe J. Sansonetti
Unité de Pathogénie Microbienne Moléculaire,
INSERM U 389, Institut Pasteur, 25-28 Rue du
Docteur Roux, 75724 Paris, France

Erwin Schurr
Centre for the Study of Host Resistance,
Departments of Medicine and Human Genetics,
McGill University, and McGill University Health
Centre Research Institute, Montréal General
Hospital, Montréal, Québec H3G 1A4, Canada

Phillip Scott
Department of Pathobiology, School of Veterinary
Medicine, University of Pennsylvania, 3800 Spruce
St., Philadelphia, PA 19104

Nilufer P. Seth
Department of Cancer Immunology and AIDS,
Dana-Farber Cancer Institute and Harvard Medical
School, Boston, MA 02115

Alan Sher
Laboratory of Parasitic Diseases, NIAID, NIH,
Building 4, Room 126, Bethesda, MD 20892-0425

Wun-Ju Shieh
Infectious Disease Pathology Activity, Division of
Viral and Rickettsial Diseases, National Center for
Infectious Diseases, Centers for Disease Control and
Prevention, 1600 Clifton Rd., N.E., Mail Stop
G-32, Atlanta, GA 30333

Guido Silvestri
Departments of Medicine and of Microbiology and
Immunology, Emory University School of Medicine
and Emory Vaccine Research Center, Atlanta,
GA 30329

Steffen Stenger
Institut für Klinische Mikrobiologie, Immunologie,
und Hygiene, Friedrich-Alexander Universität
Erlangen-Nürnberg, D-91054 Erlangen, Germany

Eva Szomolanyi-Tsuda
Department of Pathology, University of
Massachusetts Medical School, Worcester,
MA 01655

Rick L. Tarleton
Department of Cellular Biology, University of
Georgia, Athens, GA 30602

Emil R. Unanue
Department of Pathology and Immunology,
Washington University School of Medicine,
St. Louis, MO 63110

Raymond M. Welsh
Department of Pathology, University of
Massachusetts Medical School, Worcester,
MA 01655

Kai W. Wucherpfennig
Department of Cancer Immunology and AIDS,
Dana-Farber Cancer Institute and Harvard Medical
School, Boston, MA 02115

Thomas A. Wynn
Immunobiology Section, Laboratory of Parasitic
Diseases, National Institutes of Health, Bldg. 4, Rm.
126, Bethesda, MD 20892

Jonathan W. Yewdell
Laboratory of Viral Diseases, National Institute of
Allergy and Infectious Diseases, Bethesda,
MD 20892-0440

Douglas Young
Department of Infectious Diseases and
Microbiology, Faculty of Medicine, Imperial
College, London W2 1PG, United Kingdom

Sherif R. Zaki
Infectious Disease Pathology, National Center for
Infectious Diseases, Centers for Disease Control and
Prevention, 1600 Clifton Rd., N.E., Mail Stop
G-32, Atlanta, GA 30345

PREFACE

Excellent textbooks and review volumes on immunology, virology, parasitology, medical microbiology, and infectious diseases abound. So what gap is this book aiming to fill?

Although microbiology and immunology can look back to common beginnings 120 years ago, the fields parted ways toward the end of the 20th century and have been marching to different drums. This separation had its logic at that time. It was realized that immunology encompasses more than antimicrobial defense, and medical microbiology became more and more fascinating as our understanding of the etiologic agents of diseases increased as well as the advent of chemotherapy. This is the reason that infectious diseases were often being viewed from the microbes' *or* the host's perspective. Such a singular view tends to emphasize unique microbial or immune aspects instead of focusing on the true cross talk between the pathogen and the host. We therefore asked a team of experts with a true interest in the immunology of infectious diseases to review not the monologues of,

but the dialogue between, pathogens and the host immune system. Instead of covering an exhaustive number of diseases, we placed emphasis on the general mechanisms underlying immune responses to infectious diseases. We hope this textbook fills a gap and helps to reestablish a deeper relationship between immunology and medical microbiology.

We express our deep appreciation and thanks to the editorial staff of ASM, in particular Greg Payne and Susan Birch. We also cordially thank our associates Caitlin McCoull, Lucia Lom-Terborg, and Vivian Kirkwood for their secretarial and administrative support. Last but not least, we are grateful to our colleagues for their efforts and valuable time. By contributing to this textbook, they have generously shared their extraordinary expertise.

Stefan H. E. Kaufmann
Alan Sher
Rafi Ahmed

Immunology of Infectious Diseases
Edited by S. H. E. Kaufmann, A. Sher, and R. Ahmed
© 2002 ASM Press, Washington, D.C.

Introduction

Stefan H. E. Kaufmann, Alan Sher, and Rafi Ahmed

The concept behind this book is to examine different aspects of the host response to the plethora of infectious agents. Although we appreciate that infection is an encounter between microbe and host, this book will emphasize the host side of the interaction. We adhere to the idea that the strategies of immune defense and pathogen survival coevolved in a dynamic process. This process led simultaneously to the development of novel survival mechanisms and virulence factors in microbial pathogens and to distinct host defense mechanisms for counteracting pathogen survival. At its most polarized level, this coevolution occurred in the form of a gene-by-gene counteraction. More frequently, however, it proceeded such that a pattern of virulence factors was matched by a pattern of host defense mechanisms. In this struggle between pathogen and host, the immune system assumed responsibility for the control of the invader. Although microbes and host immune systems rely on different basic mechanisms, the outcome of their combat is delicately balanced; pathogens have not fully succeeded in controlling "us," and we have not fully succeeded in controlling "them."

In essence, pathogens rely on rapid variability. In an attempt to directly compete with this strategy, the immune system uses recombination to produce an immense array of specific receptors, thus combining exclusive specificity with broad coverage. Aside from this, the immune system has succeeded in forming one more weapon through the development of specific memory, which allows more efficacious combat on subsequent encounters with the pathogen. Obviously, specific memory also forms the basis for vaccination, which was developed by humans using a totally different part of their bodies, namely, the intellect.

What has been said so far about host resistance relates mostly to the so-called acquired immune response, which develops slowly but is highly efficient once fully activated and is thus responsible for the eradication of most pathogens. Combined with appropriate control mechanisms, its unique specificity guarantees that the highly aggressive acquired immune response does not cause too much harm to the host itself. However, acquired immunity is not without drawbacks in the fight against microbial invaders. In particular, the primary response develops slowly and is unable to immediately control fast-replicating microbes. Hence, an additional mechanism that is capable of combating invading pathogens must be available without delay. This response must be short-lived and tightly regulated in order to avoid any exaggerated effects on the host. This is the domain of the innate immune system, a fact that was largely ignored by basic immunologists although regarded as essential by those interested in infectious diseases. Without doubt, the innate immune system is phylogenetically much older than the acquired immune system. While its generally unsophisticated response was useful in protecting species with high reproduction rates, it was insufficient for the higher vertebrates, including humans. These species needed to exploit somatic recombination to overcome the dangers inherent in low reproduction rates.

Our attitude toward the innate immune systems has changed with the awareness that it is not only a rapid response mechanism but also a critical switchboard determining the type of acquired immune response that evolves. Although the innate immune system does not distinguish between different microbial pathogens, it is vital that it distinguish foreign invaders from the host's own cells. This is achieved by so-called pattern recognition receptors, which display specificity for distinct molecular entities exclusively present in microbes.

With regard to function, the acquired immune response is composed of only two basic mechanisms, namely, direct destruction of infected target cells and activation or inhibition of effector cells. In the first mechanism, the immune system accepted damage to the host as the price to be paid for destroying the pathogen. The second mechanism is essential for regulating both the acquired and innate immune responses. In doing so, distinct functions such as antibody secretion by B cells, target cell killing by cytolytic T lymphocytes, and activation of macrophages and granulocytes must all be achieved. Moreover, this mechanism is also responsible for the downregulation of an immune response once the pathogen has been eradicated. It can be easily guessed that such a wide spectrum of effects cannot be achieved via a single route and that segregation into different routes is required. The appropriate route is selected by the innate immune system rapidly after the pathogen enters the host. Thus, acquired immunity and innate immune response regulate each other reciprocally. As we understand it now, the innate and acquired immune responses are interwoven in a mutual discourse at many stages.

It is the goal of this book to show how the dialogue between different types of pathogen and the host immune system, as well as the cross talk between the different components of the immune response, works. Although pathogen eradication is the major task of the immune response, protection is not always achieved without a price. Therefore, pathologic sequelae of infection, microbial evasion mechanisms, and the genetics of host susceptibility are all discussed in equal depth. Finally, we have turned our attention to novel ways of applying this knowledge to improve "our" side of the scale. Strategies of immune intervention will be discussed paradigmatically with two major microbial killers of humans.

I. THE PATHOGENS

Chapter 1

Overview of the Bacterial Pathogens

MICHAEL KUHN, WERNER GOEBEL, DANA J. PHILPOTT, AND PHILIPPE J. SANSONETTI

Pathogenic bacteria cause many different infectious diseases like diarrhea, typhoid fever, tuberculosis, leprosy, gastroenteritis, whooping cough, pneumonia, and meningitis. Despite the availability of therapeutic measures like antibiotics, these and other infectious diseases are still the main cause of human mortality, at least in developing countries. The increase in the resistance of many pathogenic bacteria to the currently available antibiotics observed in recent years will further complicate the problem of infectious diseases in the future (Liu, 1999).

Only detailed knowledge of the mechanisms of bacterial pathogenicity will allow us to find new ways of protection against and treatment of infectious diseases and hence will contribute to our assault on this major health problem of mankind. The last two decades have seen a tremendous increase in our understanding of the genetic, biochemical, and cellular mechanisms underlying many infectious diseases (Finlay and Falkow, 1997). The combination of molecular and cellular methods and the development of in vitro (cell culture) and in vivo (animal) models, together with the recent burst of genomic sequence data (see http://www.tigr.org/tdb/mdb/mdb.html for a summary of ongoing and finished bacterial genomic sequencing projects), have particularly improved our understanding of the mechanisms of bacterial pathogenicity.

The present chapter will not introduce all human bacterial pathogens. Instead, the most important findings on bacterial virulence factors and mechanisms of infection are summarized in Table 1 (gram-negative pathogens), Table 2 (gram-positive pathogens), and Table 3 (spirochetal pathogens). Some selected and extensively studied model organisms are described in more detail below, with a focus on the bacterial virulence factors and their role in infection and disease.

EXTRACELLULAR BACTERIA

Helicobacter pylori

Gastric infection by the gram-negative bacterium *Helicobacter pylori* is associated with a number of clinical outcomes including gastritis, peptic ulcer disease, mucosa-associated lymphoid tissue lymphoma, and adenocarcinoma of the stomach (Parsonnet et al., 1997). In many cases, however, successful colonization of the gastric mucosa by *H. pylori* leads to lifelong persistence of the organism in the absence of clinical manifestations. How is it that this organism can be capable of producing such diverse disease outcomes? It is likely that the genetics of both the host and the infecting strain of *H. pylori* play key roles in the manifestation and outcome of the disease. A number of different genetic approaches have shown a vast genetic diversity among strains of *H. pylori*. One striking example is the presence or absence of a large pathogenicity island (PAI) in the *H. pylori* chromosome (Tomb et al., 1997). PAIs are distinct stretches of DNA that are located within the bacterial chromosome and encode virulence factors associated with pathogenesis (Hacker et al., 1997). These discrete regions of DNA have a different G+C content from the rest of the bacterial chromosome and were probably inherited by horizontal transfer from an unknown microbial ancestor. In *H. pylori*, the cag pathogenicity island is found on a 40-kb stretch of DNA with approximately 40 open reading frames (Tomb et al., 1997). Strains of *H. pylori* with the cag PAI

Michael Kuhn and Werner Goebel • Lehrstuhl für Mikrobiologie, Biozentrum, Am Hubland, 97074 Würzburg, Germany. **Dana J. Philpott and Philippe J. Sansonetti** • Unité de Pathogénie Microbienne Moléculaire, INSERM U 389, Institut Pasteur, 25–28 Rue du Docteur Roux, 75724 Paris Cedex 15, France.

Table 1. Some characteristics of gram-negative human pathogens

Species	Disease(s)	Putative virulence factors	Activity	Function	Reference
Vibrio cholerae	Cholera	Cholera toxin	ADP-ribosylates host cell G proteins	Enterotoxin	Herrington et al. (1988)
		Toxin-coregulated pilus	Adhesin	Colonization of intestinal tract	
Campylobacter jejuni	Gastroenteritis; Guillain-Barré syndrome (autoimmune disease)	Flagella	Adhesin?	Motility; adhesion to intestinal cells?	Wooldridge and Ketley (1997)
		Heat-labile enterotoxin (LT-like)	ADP-ribosylates host cell G proteins	Enterotoxin	
		Endotoxin (LPS)	Molecular mimicry with host gangliosides	Anti-LPS antibody cross-reaction with neural tissue	
Pseudomonas aeruginosa	Opportunistic lung infection associated with cystic fibrosis; wound and burn infections	PilA	Adhesin	Colonization	Tan and Ausubel (2000)
		Exoenzyme S (Exos)	ADP-ribosylates host cell G proteins; GTPase-activating factor for Rho GTPases	Antiphagocytic activity	
		Exotoxin A (ExoA)	ADP-ribosylates EF-2	Tissue damage; anti-phagocytic activity	
		Alginate	Adhesin	Adhesion; antiphagocytic activity	
		LasA, LasB	Elastolytic activity	Tissue damage; immune complex deposition	
Legionella pneumophilia	Pneumonia, mainly in compromised hosts	Cap	Type IV pili	Adhesion to macrophages and epithelial cells	Vogel and Isberg (1999)
		Dot/Icm	Type IV secretion system and effector proteins?	Required for intracellular replication; cytotoxicity	
		Msp	Protease		
Neisseria spp.	Meningitis (N. meningitidis); gonorrhea (N. gonorrhoeae)	PilC	Pili	Adhesion to CD46 on host cells	Nassif et al. (1999)
		Opa proteins (OpaA–OpaK); Opc proteins	Outer membrane proteins	Adhesion; invasion and transcytosis (Opa proteins recognize heparan sulphate, vitronectin, fibronectin, and CD66)	
		PorA, PorB	Porins	Calcium influx and apoptosis of target cells (PorB)	
Bordetella pertussis	Whooping cough	Pertussis toxin	ADP-ribosylates host cell G proteins	Adhesion; increased respiratory secretions?	Ladant and Ullmann (1999)
		Adenylate cyclase toxin (CyaA)	Calmodulin-activated adenylate cyclase	Cytotoxicity; apoptosis	
		Filamentous hemagglutinin (Fha)	Hemagglutination	Colonization	
Rickettsia rickettsii	Rocky Mountain spotted fever	Phospholipase A	Phospholipase activity	Cell invasion	Silverman et al. (1992)

Table 2. Some characteristics of gram-positive human pathogens

Species	Disease(s)	Putative virulence factors	Activity	Function	Reference(s)
Staphylococcus aureus	Skin and mucosal infections, septicemia, endocarditis, toxic shock syndrome	Alpha-hemolysin (alpha-toxin)	Pore formation; hemolysis		Dinges et al. (2000), Krakauer (1999)
		Beta-hemolysin	Sphingomyelinase; hemolysis		
		Gamma-hemolysin (leucocidin)	Leukotoxin; hemolysis	Inhibition of phagocytosis	
		Delta-hemolysin	Cytolysis		
		Exfoliative toxins A and B	Serine proteases	Dermonecrosis; superantigens	
		Erythrogenic toxins A, B, and C		Superantigens	
		Enterotoxin		Superantigen	
		TSST-1[a]		Superantigen	
		ClfA (clumping factor)	Fibrinogen binding	Adhesion	
		Protein A (SpA)	Immunoglobulin binding, opsonization	Inhibition of phagocytosis	
Streptococcus pyogenes (group A streptococci)	Skin infections, scarlet fever, glomerulonephritis	M-protein	Antiphagocytic activity; complement inactivation	Inhibition of phagocytosis	Stevens (1997), Cleary and Retnoningrum (1994)
		Streptolysin O	Pore formation; hemolysis	Inhibition of phagocytosis	
		Streptolysin S	Cytolysis		
		Pyrogenic toxins A and C		Superantigens	
		Pyrogenic toxin B	Cysteine protease	Tissue destruction	
		C5a peptidase	C5a cleavage[b]	Complement inactivation	
		Streptokinase	Fibronectin binding	Adhesion	
Streptococcus pneumoniae	Pneumonia, bronchitis, sepsis, meningitis, otitis media, sinusitis	Polysaccharide capsule	Antiphagocytic activity	Inhibition of phagocytosis	Paton et al. (1993)
		Pneumolysin	Pore formation, cytotoxic activity, complement activation		
		Autolysin	Cell lysis	Release of pneumolysin	
		PspA	Adhesion		
		IgA protease	IgA cleavage		
Corynebacterium diphtheriae	Diphtheria	Diphtheria toxin AB	ADP-ribosylation of elongation factor EF-2	Inhibition of protein biosynthesis	Passador and Iglewski (1994)
Clostridium botulinum	Botulism	Botulinal neurotoxin	Proteolytic cleavage of synaptobrevin, syntaxin, and SNAP-25[c]	Inhibition of neurotransmitter release	Johnson (1999), Aktories (1997)
		C2 toxin	ADP-ribosylation of actin	Disruption of cytoskeleton	
		C3 toxin	ADP-ribosylation of Rho and Rac	Disruption of cytoskeleton	
Clostridium tetani	Tetanus	Tetanus neurotoxin	Proteolytic cleavage of synaptobrevin, syntaxin, and SNAP-25	Inhibition of neurotransmitter release	Johnson (1999)

[a] TSST-1, toxic shock syndrome toxin 1.
[b] Complement component C5a.
[c] SNAP-25, synaptosome-associated 25-kDa protein.

Table 3. Some characteristics of spirochetal human pathogens

Species	Disease(s)	Putative virulence factors	Activity	Function	References
Borrelia burgdorferi	Lyme disease	OspA, OspC	Lipoproteins	? (OspA is vaccine candidate)	Nordstrand et al. (2000)
		DbpA, DbpB	Lipoproteins, adhesins	Mediation of attachment to extracellular matrix	
		Other lipoproteins	Binding of toll-like receptor 2 (TLR2)	Stimulation of innate immune responses	
Treponema pallidum	Syphilis	Tpr proteins	Major surface proteins	Adhesion?	Weinstock et al. (1998)
		Hly proteins	Putative hemolysins[a]		
		Gcp	Putative metalloprotease[a]		

[a] Based on sequence data.

are referred to as type I, whereas strains without the PAI are termed type II. Although both types of *H. pylori* strains are associated with human disease, it is generally thought that strains possessing the cag PAI are more virulent (Censini et al., 1996).

Investigation of the interaction of *H. pylori* with epithelial cells in vitro has led to the description of a number of phenotypic changes that *H. pylori* induces in host cells. During infection, *H. pylori* closely apposes the host cell membrane, forming a modified cup-like structure that partially surrounds the organism. Accompanying this event is modification of host cytoskeletal elements resulting in the accumulation of actin beneath the sites of bacterial attachment (Segal et al., 1996). Additionally, a protein of 145 kDa phosphorylated on tyrosine residues was identified in extracts of cells that had been infected with *H. pylori* (Segal et al., 1997). Although this protein was originally thought to be a host cell protein, several studies have recently identified it as an *H. pylori* protein called CagA (Asahi et al., 2000; Odenbreit et al., 2000; Segal et al., 1999; Stein et al., 2000). CagA is an immunodominant protein of *H. pylori* encoded by the cag PAI. Upon translocation of CagA into the host cytosol, it becomes phosphorylated on tyrosine by a host tyrosine kinase that has yet to be identified (Fig. 1). Although its specific role in *H. pylori* pathogenesis is unknown, CagA may be involved in phenotypic changes induced in infected cells. Infection of cells with *H. pylori* strains possessing the cag PAI induces a growth factor-like phenotype in which infected cells spread out and become grossly elongated. An isogenic mutant strain of *H. pylori* lacking CagA is unable to stimulate this phenotype in infected cells (Segal et al., 1999).

A number of gram-negative pathogenic bacteria have evolved specialized systems for the delivery of virulence factors directly into the host cytosol. One such system is the type III secretion system, in which bacterial proteins lacking a typical signal sequence are secreted directly from the bacteria into the cytosol of infected cells. Structurally, the type III secretion apparatus resembles the flagellum, with components of the type III machine having homology to the basal-body proteins of flagella (Hueck, 1998). A system that was recently shown to be functionally equivalent to type III is the type IV secretion system, originally described as a DNA conjugal system for the delivery of DNA from *Agrobacterium tumefaciens* into plant cells (Burns, 1999). The cag PAI of *H. pylori* encodes a type IV secretion apparatus, and recent studies have shown for the first time that this secretion system is capable of translocating a bacterial protein into host cells. Strains possessing the cag PAI translocate CagA into infected cells, where

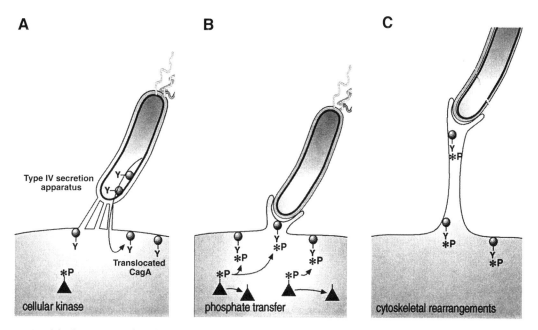

Figure 1. Model of type IV-mediated secretion of the virulence protein, CagA, into the eukaryotic cytosol by *H. pylori*. (A and B) CagA is translocated into the host cytosol by the type IV secretion system (A), where it becomes phosphorylated on tyrosine residues by a host tyrosine kinase (B). (C) Phosphorylated CagA triggers cytoskeletal rearrangements, leading to pedestal formation. Reproduced from Stein et al. (2000) with permission of the National Academy of Sciences.

it is phosphorylated on tyrosine, whereas strains that have nonpolar mutations in key components of the type IV system can no longer translocate CagA (Asahi et al., 2000; Stein et al., 2000). It will be interesting to see whether other *H. pylori* proteins are translocated into the host by this system and what role these proteins play in the pathogenesis of *H. pylori*.

Infection with *H. pylori* strains possessing the cag PAI is also associated with a number of signal transduction events within host cells. Activation of these pathways culminates in the induction of the eukaryotic transcription factors NF-κB and AP-1 (Naumann et al., 1999). These transcription factors are both key players in the regulation of inflammatory responses because a number of proinflammatory genes are under their transcriptional control. One gene that is regulated by both of these transcription factors encodes the chemokine interleukin-8 (IL-8), a potent chemoattractant for neutrophils (Harada et al., 1994). It is thought that the local production of IL-8 in the gastric mucosa in response to *H. pylori* infection of gastric epithelial cells recruits neutrophils to the infected site, resulting in inflammation. Although the bacterial product(s) responsible for NF-κB and AP-1 activation are not known, it appears that a functional type IV system is required, since mutations in components of the type IV machinery block activation of these inflammatory regulators (Covacci and Rappuoli, 2000).

Other virulence factors of *H. pylori* that have been associated with pathogenesis include urease, vacuolating toxin (VacA), and neutrophil-activating protein (HP-NAP). Urease is thought to be required to neutralize acid in the gastric mucosa, enabling *H. pylori* to colonize the harsh environment of the stomach. Its expression by *H. pylori* strains is required for virulence in animal models (Eaton et al., 1991). VacA induces the formation of large vacuoles within the cytosol of the infected cell. Recently, a yeast two-hybrid approach was used to identify eukaryotic binding partners of VacA. A novel protein, termed VIP54, which is an intermediate filament-interacting protein, was shown to specifically interact with VacA. It is speculated that this protein is involved in vacuole biogenesis during *H. pylori* infection (de Bernard et al., 2000). HP-NAP is an immunodominant protein of *H. pylori* and is capable of recruiting and activating neutrophils (Satin et al., 2000). However, the precise roles of these proteins in *H. pylori* disease pathogenesis are unknown. Future studies that apply such techniques as signature-tagged mutagenesis (Hensel et al., 1995) may be useful in identifying specific virulence factors necessary for pathogenesis in vivo.

Enteropathogenic *Escherichia coli*

A number of diarrheagenic enteropathogens including enteropathogenic *Escherichia coli* (EPEC), enterohemorrhagic *E. coli, Citrobacter rodentium,* and *Hafnia alvei* induce a characteristic adherence phenotype following infection of epithelial cells. This histopathological alteration of target cells is referred to as the attaching and effacing (A/E) lesion, and the inducing organisms are known as A/E pathogens. The A/E lesion results from the loss of apical microvilli on intestinal epithelial cells, which occurs through the reorganization of the underlying cytoskeleton (Moon et al., 1983). At the site of bacterial attachment, cytoskeletal rearrangements lead to the formation of an actin-rich pedestal on which A/E pathogens adhere (Color Plate 1A). Since the molecular mechanisms underlying the pathogenesis of EPEC have been the most extensively studied, the focus will be on this particular A/E pathogen.

The genes required for A/E lesion formation are present within a 35-kb PAI on the EPEC chromosome called the locus for enterocyte effacement (LEE). Transfer of this region into *E. coli* K-12 strains is sufficient to induce A/E lesion formation by this normally nonpathogenic *E. coli* strain (McDaniel and Kaper, 1997). Sequencing of the LEE PAI, in conjunction with a number of genetic studies, has identified genes encoding a type III secretion system, several secreted proteins, the outer membrane protein intimin, and its translocated receptor Tir. Mutations in any of these bacterial factors except for a secreted protein called EspF prevents A/E lesion formation in cultured epithelial cell models (Celli et al., 2000).

Recent studies of the role of the LEE-encoded secreted proteins in EPEC pathogenesis have demonstrated the potential involvement of EspA, EspB, and EspD as structural components of the secretion apparatus (Frankel et al., 1998). EspA is secreted by the type III secretion system and forms filamentous structures on the bacterial surface (Knutton et al., 1998). EspA filaments are thought to form a channel through which other secreted proteins are delivered into the host cytosol. EspB and EspD are inserted into the host plasma membrane (Wachter et al., 1999), and, because of their structural similarity to YopB and YopD of *Yersinia,* it is hypothesized that these two proteins may form a pore in the host cell membrane through which the other EPEC effector proteins are delivered (Celli et al., 2000) (Color Plate 1B).

Another EPEC protein that is secreted by the type III secretion system is the translocated intimin receptor, Tir. Although Tir was previously identified as a host cell protein (Rosenshine et al., 1992), it is now clear that it is an EPEC protein that is inserted into the host plasma membrane concurrent with host-induced modifications including phosphoryla-

tion on tyrosine residues (Kenny et al., 1997). Tir is predicted to form a hairpin structure; it has two transmembrane domains that span the host cell membrane, the N- and C-terminal regions are located within the host cytosol, and the region between the TMDs forms an extracellular loop (DeVinney et al., 1999). A number of studies have shown that the EPEC outer membrane protein intimin binds to the extracellular loop of Tir that extends from the surface of the host cell (Color Plate 1B). Tir binding to intimin appears to be essential for pedestal formation and actin condensation beneath the adherent bacteria since strains with mutations in *tir* can no longer form A/E lesions in tissue culture cells (Kenny et al., 1997).

The location of Tir at the tip of the EPEC pedestal and the orientation of its N- and C-terminal regions within the host cytosol suggest that it is a likely candidate to link EPEC with regulators of the host cytoskeleton in order to initiate the actin changes required for A/E lesion formation (Celli et al., 2000). Key regulators of actin dynamics are the family of small GTPases, comprising RhoA, Rac1, and Cdc42 (Hall, 1998). Although these GTPases play key roles in changes in the host actin dynamics induced by *Shigella,* they are not required for actin polymerization processes leading to EPEC pedestal formation (Ebel et al., 1998). Recently, however, the Wiskott-Aldrich syndrome protein (WASP) was demonstrated to be central to the A/E process induced by EPEC. WASP is an adapter protein that interacts with Cdc42 and the Arp2/3 complex, a complex of proteins that nucleates actin. Transfection of epithelial cells with mutant WASP that no longer interacts with Arp2/3 prevents the recruitment of the Arp2/3 complex to sites of bacterial attachment and also prevents actin polymerization leading to pedestal formation by EPEC (D. Kalman et al., 1999). What are the regulatory proteins that link Tir with WASP? Tir has no obvious similarities to eukaryotic proteins involved in cytoskeletal dynamics, suggesting the existence of an intermediary protein between Tir and WASP. However, the proline-rich N-terminal region of Tir and its C-terminal cytosolic tail that is phosphorylated on tyrosine residues may be key docking or recruitment sites for signaling molecules that link EPEC to regulators of the host cytoskeleton (Celli et al., 2000). Future studies will elucidate how this extracellular organism can trigger these complex cytoskeletal responses at the cell surface, leading to the morphologically distinct A/E phenotype.

Yersinia spp.

Three species of *Yersinia* are pathogenic to humans: *Yersinia pestis,* an arthropod-borne infection responsible for bubonic and pneumonic plague, and *Y. enterocolitica* and *Y. pseudotuberculosis* which are both enteropathogens that cause self-limiting infections of the gastrointestinal tract. All three species appear to have a tropism for lymphoid tissue and a common capacity to escape the nonspecific immune response. Histopathological examination of tissue from experimentally infected animals shows bacteria in extracellular microcolonies. In accordance with these in vivo findings, *Yersinia* spp. resist phagocytosis by macrophages and polymorphonuclear cells in vitro. Taken together, these findings indicate that yersiniae lead an extracellular life-style within their host. All three species possess a 70-kb plasmid encoding the Yop virulon, which is required for virulence (Cornelis and Wolf-Watz, 1997; Cornelis et al., 1998).

The Yop virulon encodes a number of secreted proteins called Yops and a type III secretion apparatus that is required for their delivery into the host cytosol. Yop delivery, however, requires adhesion of the bacteria to their target cells. In *Y. pseudotuberculosis,* Inv is the main adhesin promoting Yop translocation (Persson et al., 1995), whereas in *Y. enterocolitica,* the YadA adhesin appears to be more important, although either adhesin will suffice to allow contact with epithelial cells and subsequent Yop translocation (Sory and Cornelis, 1994). Once contact has been established, the type III secretion system is deployed. The Ysc secretion machinery in yersiniae is encoded by four contiguous loci, and a total of 29 genes have been identified (Cornelis et al., 1998). It is hypothesized that these proteins form a biological syringe, much like that identified for *Shigella* and *Salmonella* (see below), that directs the delivery of effector proteins from the bacterial cytoplasm into the host. YopB and YopD are secreted by this system and are inserted into the host plasma membrane, where they probably form a pore through which the other Yops are translocated.

Six Yop effector proteins are translocated into the cytosol of target cells by extracellular yersiniae: YopE, YopH, YopO/YpkA, YopP/YopJ, YopM, and YopT. Of these, YopE, YopH, and YopT have dramatic effects on the host cytoskeleton and appear to mediate the antiphagocytic effects of yersiniae (Cornelis et al., 1998; Bliska, 2000). YopE is a 23-kDa cytotoxin that, when targeted into epithelial cells, leads to cell rounding and detachment from the extracellular matrix. Although the mechanism by which YopE affects the host cytoskeleton is not known, recent studies suggest that the Rho family of small GTPases are potential targets; YopE accelerates GTP hydrolysis of all three Rho family members (Bliska, 2000). YopT is unique in that it appears to be the only effector protein that is not produced by all three pathogenic *Yersinia* spp. since virulent strains of *Y. pseudotuberculosis* lack this Yop. YopT appears to have cytotoxic effects in eukaryotic cells much like that of YopE. Studies have indicated that YopT leads to a modification and redistribution of RhoA in treated cells (Zumbihl et al., 1999). YopH is a powerful protein tyrosine phosphatase. It is thought to contribute to the inhibition of yersinia uptake by interfering with signaling from integrins. This protein dephosphorylates p130^{Cas} and focal adhesion kinase, and this leads to a disruption of focal adhesion complexes and stress fibers. In contrast, the role played by YopO/YpkA and YopM in yersinia pathogenesis is much less clear. YopO/YpkA is a serine/threonine protein kinase; however, its intracellular target is not known (Cornelis et al., 1998). The target of YopM is also not known, although studies indicate that this protein is trafficked to the cell nucleus (Skrzypek et al., 1998).

YopP/YopJ (YopP in *Y. enterocolitica* and YopJ in *Y. pseudotuberculosis* and *Y. pestis*) is a potent anti-inflammatory protein. This virulence factor perturbs many signaling pathways in eukaryotic cells, including inhibition of the extracellular signal-regulated kinase (ERK), c-Jun NH$_2$-terminal kinase (JNK), and p38-mitogen-activated protein kinase (p38-MAPK) pathways as well as the signaling pathway leading to NF-κB activation (Schesser et al., 1998; Palmer et al., 1998). Interruption of these pathways suppresses the production of proinflammatory cytokines, including tumor necrosis factor-alpha (TNF-α) and IL-8, that would normally be induced in infected cells by lipopolysaccharide (LPS) shed from the infecting organism (Ruckdeschel et al., 1997, 1998). These cytokines play an essential role in the inflammatory response to bacterial infection and are crucial in limiting the severity of yersinia infections. YopP/YopJ also induces apoptosis in infected macrophages (Mills et al., 1997; Monack et al., 1997) by a process dependent on the ability of this virulence factor to block NF-κB induction (Ruckdeschel et al., 1998). In addition to its role in cytokine gene expression, NF-κB regulates the production of antiapoptotic factors that are critical to balance proapoptotic signals in order to inhibit cell death.

A yeast two-hybrid screen was recently used to identify mammalian binding partners of YopJ of *Y. pseudotuberculosis*. Three MAPK kinases (MKKs) were shown to specifically interact with YopJ, and these interactions lead to the inability of MKKs to become phosphorylated and thus activated in a number of signal transduction pathways (Orth et al., 1999). Additionally, it was demonstrated that YopJ inhibits the NF-κB activation pathway, possibly by interfering with an unidentified MKK upstream of the IκB kinase complex. Thus, YopJ simultaneously blocks ERK, JNK, p38-MAPK, and NF-κB pathways by targeting an upstream activator common to all of these pathways. In this way, it inhibits proinflammatory cytokine production, as well as tipping the cellular balance to the accumulation of proapoptotic factors, leading to programmed cell death of macrophages.

FACULTATIVE INTRACELLULAR BACTERIA

Shigella spp.

Shigella spp. are gram-negative facultatively intracellular pathogens that invade the colonic and rectal mucosae of humans, causing bacillary dysentery. Four species of *Shigella* cause these infections, with *Shigella flexneri* accounting for most of the endemic disease. The pathogenesis of infection centers on the ability of *S. flexneri* to invade epithelial cells and initiate an intense inflammatory reaction.

All bacterial factors required for epithelial cell invasion reside in a 30-kb entry region on a 200-kb virulence plasmid of wild-*type S. flexneri* (Sansonetti, 1991). The invasion plasmid antigens (Ipa proteins) orchestrate the cytoskeletal rearrangements necessary for bacterial entry. These proteins also direct many of the other virulence properties of *S. flexneri*, including escape from the phagocytic vacuole and induction of apoptosis of macrophages and resulting inflammation. Also within the entry region are the *mxi/spa* genes, which encode proteins comprising a type III secretion system necessary for the translocation of Ipa proteins directly into host cells. The gene *icsA*, also present on the virulence plasmid, is necessary and sufficient to induce actin-based motility of *S. flexneri* within infected cells (Bernardini et al., 1989).

The type III secretion apparatus of *S. flexneri* was recently examined by electron microscopy and shown to be made up of three distinct components: an external needle, a neck domain, and a large proximal bulb (Blocker et al., 1999) (Fig. 2). These findings are similar to those published by Kubori et al. (1998) on the supramolecular structure of the *Salmonella* secretion apparatus and confirm the flagellum-like appearance of the secretion machine, which is extended by a rod-like structure protruding from the bacterial surface. Future studies will aim to identify the protein components of this apparatus and the molecular mechanisms of apparatus assembly and protein translocation.

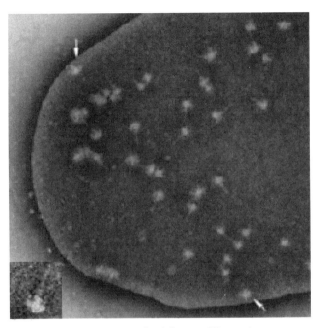

Figure 2. Electron micrograph of the type III secretion apparatus from *S. flexneri*. A negative stain of osmotically shocked *S. flexneri* is shown. Arrows point to type III secretons on the surface of the bacteria. The inset shows an individual secreton at higher magnification, revealing the tripartite nature of the apparatus: needle, neck, and bulb domains are clearly visible. Adapted from Blocker et al. (1999) with permission of The Rockefeller University Press.

In total, approximately 20 proteins that are secreted through the type III secretion system by *S. flexneri* in vitro (Sansonetti et al., 1999; P. J. Sansonetti et al., unpublished data). So far, only IpaA, IpaB, IpaC, and IpaD appear to play a role in entry into epithelial cells. IpaD and IpaB appear to be the plug in the type III secretion apparatus, preventing nonproductive secretion, and may thereby regulate the translocation of effector proteins into the host cytosol (Ménard et al., 1994). IpaB and IpaC form a translocation pore in the host cell membrane through which other effector molecules are secreted (Blocker et al., 1999; Ménard et al., 1994). IpaC is not only a component of the pore but also a key regulator of the cytoskeletal dynamics that are required for *Shigella* entry. Introduction of IpaC into the host cytosol induces actin polymerization and the formation of filopodial and lamellipodial structures on the cell surface in a Cdc42- and Rac1-dependent manner (Tran Van Nhieu et al., 1999) (Color Plate 2). IpaC leads to the activation of these small GTPases, which are required for *S. flexneri* entry. While IpaA is not strictly required for *S. flexneri* invasion, it modifies the entry focus of *S. flexneri* to allow for more efficient entry (Tran Van Nhieu et al., 1997). IpaA interacts with vinculin, a component of adhesion structures, and recent studies have shown that this interaction induces a conformational change in vinculin that allows it to then interact with F-actin (Bourdet-Sicard et al., 1999) (Color Plate 2). In this way, IpaA is implicated in the early entry process of *S. flexneri*. Another *S. flexneri* protein secreted by the type III secretion system is IpgD. Recent studies suggest that this protein is also implicated in *S. flexneri* entry since strains with mutations in *ipgD* display an altered phenotype during epithelial-cell infection. Both immunofluorescence and electron microscopy of epithelial cells infected with strains deficient in *ipgD* demonstrate an altered entry focus in which the *S. flexneri*-induced membrane ruffles are severely diminished compared to those induced by the wild-type strain (Niebuhr et al., 2000). Continued studies will clarify the role of this secreted protein in *S. flexneri* pathogenesis.

In contrast to entry into epithelial cells, uptake of *S. flexneri* by macrophages does not require the virulence plasmid and presumably occurs by normal phagocytic mechanisms. The fate of *S. flexneri* following phagocytosis was first studied in the late 1980s using a murine macrophage cell line (Clerc et al., 1987). Uptake of *S. flexneri* results in lysis of the phagocytic vacuole and rapid killing of the infected cell. It was not until 5 years later, however, that macrophage cell death was shown to occur by apoptosis (Zychlinsky et al., 1992). Apoptosis is not seen with the plasmid-cured strain, leading to the identification of the plasmid-encoded protein IpaB as the mediator of cell death (Zychlinsky et al., 1994). IpaB gains access to the cytosol, where it binds and activates caspase-1, also known as IL-1 converting enzyme (ICE), which leads to programmed cell death (Chen et al., 1996). Activation of caspase-1 is absolutely required for *S. flexneri*-induced apoptosis since cell death is not observed in *S. flexneri*-infected macrophages from caspase-1 knockout mice (Hilbi et al., 1998). The subsequent events that promote apoptosis during *S. flexneri* infection of macrophages are unknown.

Apoptosis is normally viewed as an immunologically silent cell death process unaccompanied by inflammation. However, this is clearly not the case for the caspase-1-dependent apoptosis induced by *S. flexneri*. Caspase-1 is a cysteine protease that cleaves the proinflammatory cytokine IL-1β and IL-18, a gamma-interferon-inducing cytokine (Ghayur et al., 1997). Murine macrophages release large amounts of mature IL-1β during the *Shigella*-induced apoptotic process (Zychlinsky et al., 1994). More recently, the roles played by caspase-1, IL-1β, and IL-18 in the pathogenesis of *S. flexneri* infection was tested directly by using knockout mice deficient in one of these proteins. Using the murine lung infection

model, it was shown that caspase-1 knockout mice exhibit less inflammation than do wild-type mice yet are unable to control the infection, since the bacterial load in the infected lungs continues to increase with time. The administration of recombinant IL-1β or IL-18 to caspase-1-deficient mice or the infection of mice deficient in these cytokines has demonstrated two points. IL-1β appears to be important for the acute inflammation observed during shigellosis, whereas IL-18 is required to elicit an effective antibacterial response in order to clear the bacteria from the infected tissue (Sansonetti et al., 2000). These studies indicate that caspase-1 activation by *S. flexneri* and the resulting cleavage and release of IL-1β and IL-18 from apoptotic macrophages are part of an innate program of host defense committed to clearing the infecting pathogen from the tissues. Therefore, it appears that although *S. flexneri*-induced inflammation is damaging to the host and probably accounts for the symptoms of the disease, this severe inflammatory reaction is necessary to rid the host of the infecting pathogen.

Salmonella spp.

Salmonella spp. have developed sophisticated mechanisms to modulate host cell functions in order to allow bacterial entry as well as to promote survival within membrane-bound vacuoles of both macrophages and epithelial cells. *Salmonella* possesses two PAIs, SPI-1 and SPI-2, each encoding a type III secretion system with structural similarity, however, they appear to be required at different stages of the infectious process. The SPI-1 system, encoded at centisome 63, functions early in the infection cycle since it is necessary for invasion of epithelial cells (Galan and Curtis, 1989; Galán, 1996). In contrast, SPI-2, which is encoded at centisome 30, plays a crucial role in the systemic growth of the organism and appears to be required for survival and proliferation within macrophages (Shea et al., 1996; Ochman et al., 1996).

The SPI-1 system is required for a number of effects in epithelial cells, including the induction of cytoskeletal changes required for entry and the activation of transcription factors that then regulate the production of inflammatory cytokines by infected cells. The majority of effector molecules of the SPI-1 system are encoded within the PAI, except for SopB, which is encoded by a small PAI called SPI-5, and SopE, which is encoded by a temperate bacteriophage (Galán, 1996; Wood et al., 1998; Hardt et al., 1998). Effector molecules of SPI-1 can be classified into four different categories: (i) proteins that are required for the secretion process (InvJ and

SpaO), (ii) regulators of the secretion process (SipD), (iii) proteins that promote translocation (i.e., components of the pore SipB, SipC, and SipD), and (iv) secreted effector proteins that are delivered into the host cytosol (SipA, SptP, SopB, SopE, and AvrA) (Galán, 1999).

Upon contact with epithelial cells, *Salmonella* induces pronounced rearrangements of the host actin cytoskeleton, leading to membrane ruffling and subsequent bacterial uptake (Galán, 1999). Induction of membrane ruffling has been shown previously to involve the small GTPases (Hardt et al., 1998); therefore, it was hypothesized that *Salmonella*-triggered cytoskeletal changes occurred via the activation of this group of regulators of actin dynamics. Subsequently, SopE, an effector of the SPI-1 system, was shown to have guanine nucleotide exchange factor activity, resulting in the activation of both Cdc42 and Rac1 and thereby suggesting a role for SopE in *Salmonella* uptake (Hardt et al., 1998). Another SPI-1 effector protein, SptP, acts as a GTPase-activating protein by inactivating Cdc42 and Rac1 (Fu and Galán, 1999). Thus, SopE and SptP appear to play opposing roles: SopE stimulates the cytoskeletal changes required for efficient entry of *Salmonella* into the host cell, while SptP restores the normal cytoskeletal architecture following entry. However, effector proteins other than SopE must be required for *Salmonella* entry into epithelial cells since deletion of *sopE* does not eliminate membrane ruffles altogether and since *Salmonella* invasion is only subtly affected early in infection (Lesser et al., 2000). Other candidates are SipA, a protein that binds actin, and SipC, a potential component of the translocation apparatus that may nucleate and bundle actin filaments on insertion into the host membrane (Zhou et al., 1999; Hayward and Koronakis, 1999). Both of these effector molecules are implicated in the initial entry process.

The presence of SPI-1 also correlates with the ability of *Salmonella* to stimulate the production of proinflammatory cytokines from infected epithelial cells. *Salmonella* infection results in the activation of the eukaryotic transcription factor NF-κB and, through the stimulation of the MAPK cascades, AP-1 (Hobbie et al., 1997). As mentioned above, both of these transcription factors play key roles in the regulation of genes involved in inflammation. *Salmonella* mutants defective in SPI-1-mediated secretion are unable to stimulate cytokine production in infected epithelial cells.

SPI-2 is required for the survival and replication of *Salmonella* in macrophages (Hensel et al., 1995; Shea et al., 1996). Following entry of the bacterium into macrophages, the *Salmonella*-containing vacuole becomes acidified, and it appears that this is the trigger for SPI-2-mediated secretion; induction of SPI-2 can also occur in vitro under acidic conditions (Beuzón et al., 1999). SpiC was demonstrated to be the first effector protein of the SPI-2 type III secretion system (Uchiya et al., 1999). *Salmonella* strains harboring a mutation in *spiC* no longer survive within macrophages and are attenuated in the mouse model. SpiC inhibits the fusion of *Salmonella*-containing vacuoles with lysosomes and endosomes as well as interfering with trafficking of vesicles devoid of microorganisms (Uchiya et al., 1999). Another protein recently shown to be an effector of SPI-2 is SifA (Beuzón et al., 2000). The *sifA* gene was originally shown to be required for the formation of tubular structures rich in lysosomal membrane glycoproteins in epithelial cells infected with *Salmonella* (Garcia-del Portillo et al., 1993; Stein et al., 1996). Although these structures are not observed in infected macrophages, SifA was shown to be important in intracellular growth within macrophages. SifA appears to be required for the maintenance of the vacuolar membrane surrounding infecting bacteria since *sifA* mutants lose their vacuoles and are found free in the host cell cytosol. These mutants appear to be unable to replicate in such an environment (Beuzón et al., 2000). These interesting results indicate that in contrast to other intracellular pathogens including *Listeria* and *Shigella,* which can replicate within the cytosol of macrophages, *Salmonella* is unable to exploit this environment for growth.

Listeria monocytogenes

The gram-positive bacterium *Listeria monocytogenes* is the only human pathogen of the genus *Listeria*. The bacteria, which are widespread in nature, are taken up orally through the ingestion of contaminated food. They penetrate the intestinal epithelium, grow intracellularly in hepatocytes of the liver and macrophages of the spleen, and finally cause a systemic infection resulting in sepsis, menigitis, and encephalitis. A number of crucial virulence factors which allow the bacteria to invade and multiply in the cytosol of different mammalian host cells were identified and characterized. A cluster of virulence genes necessary for the intracellular life cycle was identified; it consisted of six genes, coding for a cholesterol-dependent cytolysin called listeriolysin O (LLO), two phospholipases (PlcA and PlcB), a metalloprotease (Mpl), a protein inducing actin polymerization (ActA), and a positive regulatory factor (PrfA) necessary for the efficient transcription of the virulence genes of the cluster during infection (Kuhn and Goebel, 1999) (Fig. 3). Not closely linked to the vir-

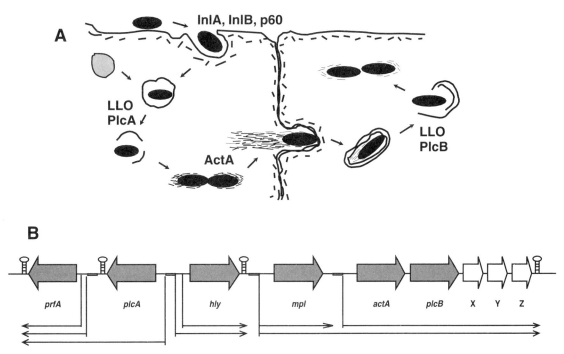

Figure 3. The intracellular life cycle (A) and virulence gene cluster (B) of *L. monocytogenes*. (A) *L. monocytogenes* enters mammalian cells through interaction of the surface proteins InlA, InlB, and p60 with mammalian cell receptors. The phagosome is lysed by the action of the pore-forming cytolysin LLO and a phosphatidylinositol-specific phospholipase C (PlcA), and the cytosolic bacteria induce the polymerization of host cell actin filaments by their surface protein ActA. Moving bacteria induce the formation of protrusions, which invade neighboring cells. The secondary vacuole is lysed by the action of LLO and a lecithinase (PlcB). (B) Virulence gene cluster, containing the genes *prfA* (encoding the positive regulatory factor A), *plcA* (PlcA), *hly* (LLO), *mpl* (encoding a metalloprotease involved in PlcB maturation), *actA* (ActA), and *plcB* (PlcB). Reproduced from Kuhn and Goebel (2000) with permission of Plenum Press.

ulence gene cluster are the genes encoding the members of the internalin family. Two (InlA and InlB) of the known eight internalins from *L. monocytogenes* mediate invasion into normally nonprofessional phagocytic cells. The roles of the other internalin family members are currently unknown. The internalins are surface proteins characterized by a central leucine-rich repeat region which is essential for their function in invasion (at least true for InlA and InlB) (Cossart and Lecuit, 1998). InlA mediates the invasion of human epithelial cells, and human E-cadherin was identified as its mammalian receptor (Mengaud et al., 1996). Surprisingly, mutation of a single amino acid in E-cadherin, rendering the molecule "mouse-like," results in a complete lack of InlA binding (Lecuit et al., 1999). This finding helped to explain earlier data on the lack of a phenotype of Δ*inlA* mutants in mouse virulence assays. InlB mediates invasion into epithelial cells, hepatocytes, and endothelial cells. It binds to the gC1q receptor found on many mammalian cells (Braun et al., 2000). InlB binding to mammalian cells results in activation of the cellular phosphatidylinositol 3-kinase, whose products, phosphatidylinositol-bisphosphate (PIP_2) and phosphatidylinositol-trisphosphate (PIP_3), may lead to

cytoskeletal rearrangements necessary for the uptake of the bacteria (Ireton et al., 1996). Shortly after phagocytosis by nonprofessional phagocytic cells or by macrophages, *L. monocytogenes* is found in a vacuole, which rapidly acidifies and is then lysed by the combined action of LLO and the two phospholipases (Fig. 3). LLO is the preeminent player in phagosomal lysis, since LLO-negative strains stay entrapped within the phagosome in almost all cells tested and such strains are drastically impaired in virulence. Lysis of the phagosomal membrane allows bacteria to escape into the cytosol, where extensive multiplication takes place. Efficient intracellular multiplication is also dependent on the presence of the transcriptional regulator PrfA. This seems to be due to PrfA-dependent expression of glucose-1-phosphate utilization in *L. monocytogenes*, indicating that the bacteria use this carbon source during replication in the host cell cytosol (Ripio et al., 1997; Goebel and Kuhn, 2000).

The surface molecule ActA then recruits the cellular actin assembly machinery, comprising the Arp2/3 complex, profilin, and vasodilator-stimulated phosphoprotein (VASP), to the bacterial surface in order to induce F-actin polymerization which results in the formation of actin tails behind the bacterium, pushing it through the cytosol. The role, if any, of the recruitment of the newly identified cellular proteins LaXp180 and stathmin for the intracellular movement is currently unknown (Pfeuffer et al., 2000). Reaching the cellular membrane, moving bacteria induce the formation of finger-like protrusions with a bacterium at the tip and the actin tail behind. These protrusions invaginate adjacent cells. They are then phagocytosed, resulting in bacteria surrounded by a double membrane vacuole. This secondary phagosome is again lysed by the action of LLO and the lecithinase PlcB. Once in the cytosol of the new host cell, the bacteria again start to replicate and to move intracellularly (Cossart and Lecuit, 1998; Kuhn and Goebel, 1999). Besides the well-characterized virulence factors of *L. monocytogenes* mentioned above, a number of virulence-associated genes and proteins were identified. The protein p60, encoded by the *iap* gene, was originally identified as an invasion-associated protein and later found to have murein hydrolase activity. p60 obviously plays a role in fibroblast and macrophage adhesion and invasion, but the exact role in host cell interaction is still unknown, in part due to the lack of well-defined in-frame deletion mutants (Kuhn and Goebel, 2000). The role of catalase and superoxide dismutase in the virulence of *L. monocytogenes* was investigated using mutants with in-frame deletions of the respective genes. Whereas single deletions (i.e., deletions of either gene) did not result in significant virulence reduction, a double deletion resulted in a strong decrease in virulence, pointing to a role for both enzymes in listerial pathogenesis, most probably in the survival of the oxidative attack by macrophages shortly after phagocytosis (Kuhn and Goebel, 1999). The recent identification of a gene, *clpC*, required for stress tolerance and intracellular survival (Rouquette et al., 1996, 1998) showed that proteins shared by many pathogenic and nonpathogenic bacteria may also contribute to virulence. The ClpC ATPase is required for virulence due to its role in supporting the early escape of *L. monocytogenes* from phagosomes. Deletion of *clpC* results in enhanced killing of intracellular *L. monocytogenes* in macrophages and leads to a significant reduction in virulence. It may thus act together with catalase and superoxide dismutase to allow prolonged survival inside phagosomes, permitting the bacteria to express phospholipases and LLO and allowing them to escape into the safe environment of the host cell cytosol.

Mycobacterium tuberculosis

Mycobacterium tuberculosis is still one of the most important human pathogens, infecting around one-third of the total population worldwide and killing about 3 million people each year. The disease is spread directly from person to person via aerosols, which, upon inhalation, bring *M. tuberculosis* immediately to the site of entry and growth in the lung tissue. *M. tuberculosis* is a gram-positive facultative intracellular bacterium that survives and grows in phagosomes of mononuclear phagocytes. The difficulties in growing *M. tuberculosis* in vitro and its highly hydrophobic cell wall have greatly limited the development of molecular biological tools required for the study of the virulence mechanisms of this important pathogen. However, the cell biology of the most striking ability of *M. tuberculosis,* its ability to survive inside phagosomes, is now well understood (see below). The recent completion of the genome sequence (Cole et al., 1998) represents a great leap forward and will certainly lead to further studies, which will result in an increasing understanding of *M. tuberculosis.* The invasion of mononuclear phagocytes is the key feature of *M. tuberculosis* pathogenesis, but the unequivocal identification of an invasion-mediating factor is still lacking. Arruda et al. (1993) identified an open reading frame (*mce*), which, on being cloned in *E. coli,* induced the uptake of the recombinant bacteria into HeLa cells. Disruption of the *mce* gene in *Mycobacterium bovis* BCG rendered this organism less invasive for HeLa cells. However, the role of *mce* in *M. tuberculosis* invasion is still unknown. Much more is known about the contribution of *M. tuberculosis* cell wall polymers to the uptake of the bacterium by phagocytes and its interaction with phagocyte receptors (Ehlers and Daffe, 1998). In vitro infection studies with mammalian phagocytes have established that *M. tuberculosis* adheres both directly and after opsonization to a set of receptors found on the surface of phagocytic cells, including complement receptor types 1, 3, and 4 (CR1, CR3, and CR4); the mannose receptor (MR); and the surfactant protein A receptor (SPA-R). Fc receptors are not used. CR3 is a principal phagocytic receptor on monocytes and neutrophils and forms elaborate connections with the actin cytoskeleton and intracellular signaling pathways. It has broad ligand specificity and appears to be the preferred receptor for diverse pathogens. The best ligand for CR3 is the complement factor C3bi, and CR3 is regarded as the dominant receptor for complement-opsonized particles. However, the availability of complement factors in the quiescent lung is still under debate, and it was proposed that nonopsonic *M. tuberculosis* might directly bind CR3 via *M. tuberculosis* surface polysaccharides, like D-glucan. MR is strongly expressed in resident macrophages and binds virulent but not avirulent nonopsonic *M. tu-*

berculosis strains, hence being ideally placed to promote entry. SPA-R may contribute to binding on opsonization of *M. tuberculosis* with mannose binding protein or SPA.

Once inside the host cell phagosome, virulent strains of *M. tuberculosis* are able to convert the hostile environment of the phagosome into a replication-supporting niche by inhibition of acidification and interference with phagosomal maturation, resulting in the inhibition of phagosome-lysosome fusion (Deretic and Fratti, 1999). In a first step, *M. tuberculosis* blocks the acquisition of the vacuolar proton-pumping ATPase complex and hence blocks the normal acidification of the phagosome (Sturgill-Koszycki et al., 1994). The *M. tuberculosis* phagosome maturation is arrested at an early stage; this step is characterized by the persistence of early endosomal markers (like the transferrin receptor) and limited acquisition of late endosomal markers (like the mannose-6-phosphate receptor and the glycoproteins Lamp-1 and Lamp-2) (Fig. 4). The persistent staining of *M. tuberculosis* phagosomes for transferrin receptor indicates that the phagosome is in an early state of continuous communication with the transferrin receptor-recycling compartment (Deretic and Fratti, 1999). The normal sequential interaction of phagosomes with early and late endosomes, culminating in maturation into a phagolysosome, requires the multicomponent vesicle docking and fusion machinery and is regulated by small GTPases of the Rab family. Rab5, which is implicated in the interaction between phagosomes and the endocytic pathway in macro-

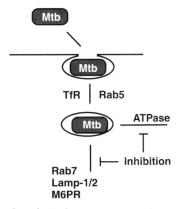

Figure 4. *M. tuberculosis* phagosome maturation arrest. Accumulation of Rab5 and TfR demonstrates the early endosomal characteristic of the vacuole. The late endosomal markers Rab7, Lamp-1, Lamp-2, and M6PR are largely absent from the *M. tuberculosis* vacuole. Delivery of the proton pumping ATPase to the vacuole is also inhibited. Rab proteins control membrane trafficking within endosomal compartments. Rab5, endocytosis and fusion between early endosomes; Rab7, late endosome and mature phagosomes; Mtb, *M. tuberculosis*; TfR, transferrin receptor; Lamp-1/2, glycoproteins; M6PR, mannose-6-phosphate receptor.

phages, accumulates on *M. bovis* BCG phagosomes. Rab7, which regulates late endosomal membrane trafficking, is not present on mycobacterial phagosomes, in contrast to the situation for normal phagosomes, which go through sequential acquisition of Rab5 and Rab7. Hence, the accumulation of Rab5 and the exclusion of Rab7 define precisely the checkpoint that has been compromised in the maturation of mycobacterial phagosomes (Via et al., 1997).

Mycobacterium leprae

Mycobacterium leprae, the causative agent of the ancient and dreaded disease leprosy, has never been grown on artificial media, which has hampered the study of its virulence mechanisms. Although the route of entry of *M. leprae* into the body and the method of its migration to the peripheral nervous system are unknown, it is known that *M. leprae* preferentially invades Schwann cells and that this represents the early crucial step that leads to sensorimotor loss. Infection of Schwann cells by *M. leprae* is followed by nerve damage, irrespective of the immunological status of the patient. The molecular mechanisms of the *M. leprae* tropism for peripheral nerves were, until recently, totally obscure. The recent progress described here was reviewed in detail recently (Rambukkana, 2000).

Nonmyelinated and myelinated Schwann cell axon units are found in peripheral nerves, but in both cases the system is completely surrounded by the basal lamina. As such, it is reasonable that the tropism for Schwann cells might involve components of the Schwann cell basal lamina, which is composed mainly of laminin-2, collagen IV, heparin sulfate proteoglycan, and entactin/nidogen. By in vitro analysis of purified native components of the basal lamina, it was found that *M. leprae* preferentially binds to laminin-2 (Rambukkana et al., 1997). Laminin-2 is a large glycoprotein composed of three polypeptide chains, $\alpha 2$, β, and γ, which are assembled into a cruciform structure. It was further demonstrated that *M. leprae* specifically interacts with the globular G domain at the carboxy-terminal end of the $\alpha 2$ chain of laminin-2. Since laminin-2 is specific for Schwann cells, the *M. leprae* specificity for this molecule elegantly explains the tropism of *M. leprae* for this cell type.

Laminin-2 is a component of the extracellular matrix and hence, by itself, is unlikely to trigger cell invasion by *M. leprae*. Laminin-2 is anchored to the Schwann cell surface via highly glycosylated dystroglycan receptors, composed of the transmembrane protein β-dystroglycan and the extracellular protein α-dystroglycan. It was demonstrated that *M. leprae* binds to α-dystroglycan only in the presence of laminin-2, which obviously forms a bridge between *M. leprae* and the α/β-dystroglycan receptor complex (Rambukkana et al., 1998) (Fig. 5). As a bacterial ligand of laminin-2, a major 21-kDa protein of the *M. leprae* cell wall was recently identified and designated the 21-kDa laminin-2 binding protein of *M. leprae* (ML-LBP21) (Shimoji et al., 1999). Since ML-LBP21-coated beads are engulfed by Schwann cells, this *M. leprae* protein is a very likely candiate for the adhesion- and invasion-promoting factor of the *M. leprae* surface involved in Schwann cell invasion. The identification of laminin-2, its receptor α/β-dystroglycan, and ML-LBP21 from *M. leprae* represents a major step forward in our understanding of *M. leprae* pathogenesis, especially its tropism for peripheral nerves, the key feature of its pathogenicity.

OBLIGATE INTRACELLULAR BACTERIA

Obligate intracellular bacterial pathogens like *Chlamydia*, *Rickettsia*, and *Coxiella* species are less well characterized than facultative intracellular pathogens. This is mainly due to difficulties in growing these bacteria and the lack of genetic tools to manipulate them. We therefore discuss recent progress in our understanding of the cell biology only of *Chlamydia* infections.

Members of the genus *Chlamydia* are obligate intracellular bacterial pathogens which are characterized by small genomes, limited biosynthetic capabilities, and a biphasic intracellular life cycle. *Chlamydia* species are the causative agents of a number of different and medically important infectious diseases. *C. trachomatis* causes trachoma, associated with infective blindness, and a number of sexually transmitted diseases. *C. pneumoniae* is a major pneumonia-causing pathogen and was recently also suspected to be the cause of systemic infections resulting in artherosclerosis.

The intracellular life cycle of all *Chlamydia* species is characterized by the transition of the infective but metabolically inactive elementary bodies into replicative but noninfective reticulate bodies and vice versa (Fig. 6) (Moulder, 1991). *Chlamydia* elementary bodies attach to and enter eukaryotic epithelial cells of mucosal surfaces. Entry of chlamydiae into host cells does not require metabolic activity by the microbe and is thought to occur by receptor-mediated endocytosis. Since the interaction of chlamydiae with their host cells can be inhibited by the addition of heparin or heparan sulfate, it was speculated that glycosaminoglycans found on the bacterial surface could be ligands for cellular receptors. A series of elegant studies showed that the heparan sulfate-like molecules on the bacterial surface are not derived from host cells and that the bacteria synthesize the heparan sulfate-like ligand that mediates in-

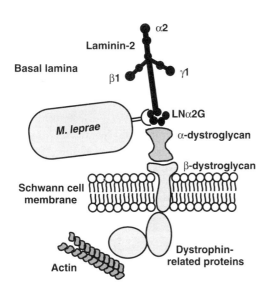

Figure 5. Model for the molecular basis of *M. leprae* interaction with Schwann cells. *M. leprae* binds to the LNα2G domain of laminin-2. α-Dystroglycan forms a bridge between laminin-2 and the membrane protein β-dystroglycan, which could act as a signaling receptor by its connections to the actin cytoskeleton. Reproduced from Rambukkana (2000) with permission of Elsevier Science.

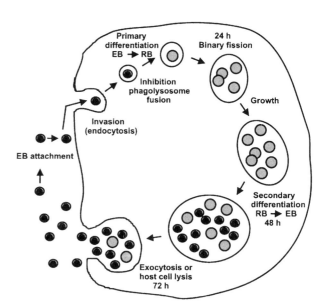

Figure 6. Diagram of the developmental cycle of *C. trachomatis*. The small, dark structures represent infectious elementary bodies (EBs). The larger, grey structures represent replicative reticulate bodies (RBs). Reproduced from Beatty et al. (1994) with permission of Elsevier Science.

fectivity (Zhang and Stephens, 1992; Stephens, 1994). Whereas some bacteria use host cell heparan sulfate proteoglycans as receptors for their invasion-triggering surface proteins, *Chlamydia* species produce the glycosaminoglycans to stimulate adhesion and invasion. The glycosaminoglycan binding protein of the chlamydiae is not known, but a 58-kDa outer membrane protein shows characteristics which make it a likely candidate for this activity (Stephens, 1994).

Once taken up by their host cell, the chlamydiae stay in a membrane-bound vacuole called the chlamydial inclusion, which is the only known environment to support chlamydial replication (Hackstadt et al., 1997). The inclusion is a specific cellular compartment since it lacks markers of early and late endosomes as well as lysosomal markers. In contrast, the membrane of the inclusion is supplied with sphingomyelin derived from the Golgi network, and this sphingomyelin is later also found in the chlamydiae themselves. The delivery of sphingomyelin from the Golgi network to the chlamydial inclusion and the complete lack of endosomal and lysosomal markers suggest that the inclusion represents a *trans*-Golgi compartment completely separate from the normal cellular endocytic trafficking. The inclusion therefore more closely resembles an exocytic vesicle in which transport to and fusion with the plasma membrane are inhibited or severely delayed. By appearing as a secretory vesicle, the chlamydial inclusion is not perceived by the host cell as a vesicle destined to fuse with lysosomes. Consistent with this interpretation is the observation that some serovars of *Chlamydia* do not lyse the cell at the completion of replication but are released by a process in which the inclusion membrane fuses with the plasma membrane to release its contents to the environment (Todd and Caldwell, 1985).

Since chlamydiae are membrane bound during their entire intracellular life cycle, all metabolites required for growth must cross this barrier. The bacteria must therefore have specialized mechanisms for acquiring nutrients from the host cytosol. The chlamydial inclusion does not allow the diffusion of even small molecules, and it is not known whether the sphingomyelin delivered to the inclusion is metabolized by the chlamydiae. Whether chlamydiae insert specific transporters into the inclusion membrane and whether the large number of chlamydial outer membrane proteins (see below) serve as importers for metabolites from the host cell cytosol is also still hypothetical (Hackstadt et al., 1997).

The absence of synthetic media for the growth of *Chlamydia* in vitro and the lack of any molecular genetic methods for working with *Chlamydia* have resulted in a severe restriction of our knowledge of chlamydial virulence factors. The recent sequencing of several chlamydial genomes revealed the presence of a number of genes which are likely to encode virulence factors (S. Kalman et al., 1999). A large multigene family of putative outer membrane transport proteins were identified which are chlamydia specific. They are thought to be necessary for the uptake of nutrients and cofactors from the host cell. Genes encoding complete type III secretion systems were detected in all *Chlamydia* strains sequenced, but the effector molecules transported by the systems are yet to be identified. The type III systems might be critical for the delivery into the host cell of bacterial proteins required for the interference with cellular vacuole trafficking that is necessary for development of the chlamydial inclusion. Spike-like protein complexes spanning the bacterial membranes and the inclusion membrane, which most probably represent type III secretion machineries, were found in early electron microscopic studies (Matsumoto, 1982). All chlamydiae produce and release a collection of proteins, termed Inc proteins, which are localized to the inclusion membrane. The Inc proteins are the only known bacterial proteins that reside in a parasitophorous vacuole. The function of the proteins is unknown, but it was speculated that they might be involved in different aspects of the intracellular life cycle of the chlamydiae and might hence represent important virulence factors of the bacteria (Bannantine et al., 2000).

Acknowledgments. D.J.P. and P.J.S. are grateful to Maria Mavris and Richard Ferrero for critical review of the manuscript. We also thank our colleagues for many discussions and for allowing us to cite unpublished data. D.J.P. is supported by a Marie Curie Fellowship from the European Community. Research in the Sansonetti laboratory is supported by grants from the Ministère de l'Education Nationale de la Recherche et de la Technologie (Programme BIOTECH and Programme de Recherche Fondamentale en Microbiologie). Research in the Goebel laboratory is supported by the Deutsche Forschungsgemeinschaft through SFB 479.

REFERENCES

Aktories, K. 1997. Bacterial toxins that target Rho proteins. *J. Clin. Investig.* 99:827–829.

Arruda, S., G. Bomfim, R. Knights, T. Huima-Byron, and L. W. Riley. 1993. Cloning of an *M. tuberculosis* DNA fragment associated with entry and survival inside cells. *Science* 261:1454–1457.

Asahi, M., T. Azuma, S. Ito, Y. Ito, H. Suto, Y. Nagai, M. Tsubokawa, Y. Tohyama, S. Maeda, M. Omata, T. Suzuki, and C. Sasakawa. 2000. *Helicobacter pylori* CagA protein can be tyrosine phosphorylated in gastric epithelial cells. *J. Exp. Med.* 191:593–602.

Bannantine, J. P., R. S. Griffiths, W. Viratyosin, W. J. Brown, and D. D. Rockey. 2000. A secondary structure motif predictive of protein localization to the chlamydial inclusion membrane. *Cell. Microbiol.* 2:35–47.

Beatty, W. L., G. I. Byrne, and R. P. Morrison. 1994. Repeated and persistent infection with *Chlamydia* and the development of chronic inflammation and disease. *Trends Microbiol.* 2:94–98.

Bernardini, M. L., J. Mounier, H. d'Hauteville, M. Coquis-Rondon, and P. J. Sansonetti. 1989. Identification of icsA, a plasmid locus of *Shigella flexneri* that governs bacterial intra- and intercellular spread through interaction with F-actin. *Proc. Natl. Acad. Sci. USA* 86:3867–3871.

Beuzón, C. R., G. Banks, J. Deiwick, M. Hensel, and D. W. Holden. 1999. pH-dependent secretion of SseB, a product of the SPI-2 type III secretion system of *Salmonella typhimurium*. *Mol. Microbiol.* 33:806–816.

Beuzón, C. R., S. Méresse, K. E. Unsworth, J. Ruiz-Albert, S. Garvis, S. Waterman, T. A. Ryder, E. Boucrot, and D. W. Holden. 2000. *Salmonella* maintains the integrity of its intracellular vacuole through the action of SifA. *EMBO J.* 19:3235–3249.

Bliska, J. B. 2000. Yop effectors of *Yersinia* spp. and actin rearrangements. *Trends Microbiol.* 8:205–208.

Blocker, A., P. Gounon, E. Larquet, K. Niebuhr, V. Cabiaux, C. Parsot, and P. J. Sansonetti. 1999. The tripartite type III secreton of *Shigella flexneri* inserts IpaB and IpaC into host membranes. *J. Cell Biol.* 147:683–693.

Bourdet-Sicard, R., M. Rudiger, B. M. Jockusch, P. Gounon, P. J. Sansonetti, and G. T. Nhieu. 1999. Binding of the *Shigella* protein IpaA to vinculin induces F-actin depolymerization. *EMBO J.* 18:5853–5862.

Braun, L., B. Ghebrehiwet, and P. Cossart. 2000. gC1q-R/p32, a C1q-binding protein, is a novel receptor for *Listeria monocytogenes*. *EMBO J.* 19:1458–1466.

Burns, D. L. 1999. Biochemistry of type IV secretion. *Curr. Opin. Microbiol.* 2:25–29.

Celli, J., W. Deng, and B. B. Finlay. 2000. Enteropathogenic *Escherichia coli* (EPEC) attachment to epithelial cells: exploiting the host cell cytoskeleton from the outside. *Cell. Microbiol.* 2:1–9.

Censini, S., C. Lange, Z. Xiang, J. E. Crabtree, P. Ghiara, M. Borodovsky, R. Rappuoli, and A. Covacci. 1996. cag, a pathogenicity island of *Helicobacter pylori*, encodes type I-specific and disease-associated virulence factors. *Proc. Natl. Acad. Sci. USA* 93:14648–14653.

Chen, Y., M. R. Smith, K. Thirumalai, and A. Zychlinsky. 1996. A bacterial invasin induces macrophage apoptosis by binding directly to ICE. *EMBO J.* 15:3853–3860.

Cleary, P., and D. Retnoningrum. 1994. Group A streptococcal immunoglobulin-binding proteins: adhesins, molecular mimicry or sensory proteins? *Trends Microbiol.* 2:131–136.

Clerc, P., A. Ryter, J. Mounier, and P. J. Sansonetti. 1987. Plasmid-mediated early killing of eucaryotic cells by *Shigella flexneri* as studied by infection of J774 macrophages. *Infect. Immun.* 55:521–527.

Cole, S. T., R. Brosch, J. Parkhill, et al. 1998. Deciphering the biology of *Mycobacterium tuberculosis* from the complete genome sequence. *Nature* 393:537–544.

Cornelis, G. R., A. Boland, A. P. Boyd, C. Geuijen, M. Iriarte, C. Neyt, M. P. Sory, and I. Stainier. 1998 The virulence plasmid of *Yersinia*, an antihost genome. *Microbiol. Mol. Biol. Rev.* 62:1315–1352.

Cornelis, G. R., and H. Wolf-Watz. 1997. The *Yersinia* Yop virulon: a bacterial system for subverting eukaryotic cells. *Mol. Microbiol.* 23:861–867.

Cossart, P., and M. Lecuit. 1998. Interactions of *Listeria monocytogenes* with mammalian cells during entry and actin-based movement: bacterial factors, cellular ligands and signaling. *EMBO J.* 17:3797–3806.

Covacci, A., and R. Rappuoli. 2000. Tyrosine-phosphorylated bacterial proteins: Trojan horses for the host cell. *J. Exp. Med.* 191:587–592.

de Bernard, M., M. Moschioni, G. Napolitani, R. Rappuoli, and C. Montecucco. 2000. The VacA toxin of *Helicobacter pylori* identifies a new intermediate filament-interacting protein. *EMBO J.* 19:48–56.

Deretic, V., and R. A. Fratti. 1999. *Mycobacterium tuberculosis* phagosome. *Mol. Microbiol.* 31:1603–1609.

DeVinney, R., A. Gauthier, A. Abe, and B. B. Finlay. 1999. Enteropathogenic *Escherichia coli*: a pathogen that inserts its own receptor into host cells. *Cell. Mol. Life Sci.* 55:961–976.

Dinges, M. M., P. M. Orwin, and P. M. Schlievert. 2000. Exotoxins of *Staphylococcus aureus*. *Clin. Microbiol. Rev.* 13:16–34.

Eaton, K. A., C. L. Brooks, D. R. Morgan, and S. Krakowka. 1991. Essential role of urease in pathogenesis of gastritis induced by *Helicobacter pylori* in gnotobiotic piglets. *Infect. Immun.* 59:2470–2475.

Ebel, F., C. von Eichel-Streiber, M. Rohde, and T. Chakraborty. 1998. Small GTP-binding proteins of the Rho- and Ras-subfamilies are not involved in the actin rearrangements induced by attaching and effacing *Escherichia coli*. *FEMS Microbiol. Lett.* 163:107–112.

Ehlers, M. R., and M. Daffe. 1998. Interactions between *Mycobacterium tuberculosis* and host cells: are mycobacterial sugars the key? *Trends Microbiol.* 6:328–335.

Finlay, B. B., and S. Falkow. 1997. Common themes in microbial pathogenicity revisited. *Microbiol. Mol. Biol. Rev.* 61:136–169.

Frankel, G., A. D. Phillips, I. Rosenshine, G. Dougan, J. B. Kaper, and S. Knutton. 1998. Enteropathogenic and enterohaemorrhagic *Escherichia coli*: more subversive elements. *Mol. Microbiol.* 30:911–921.

Fu, Y., and J. E. Galán. 1999. A *Salmonella* protein antagonizes Rac-1 and Cdc42 to mediate host-cell recovery after bacterial invasion. *Nature* 401:293–297.

Galán, J. E. 1996. Molecular genetic bases of *Salmonella* entry into host cells. *Mol. Microbiol.* 20:263–271.

Galán, J. E. 1999. Interaction of *Salmonella* with host cells through the centisome 63 type III secretion system. *Curr. Opin. Microbiol.* 2:46–50.

Galán, J. E., and R. D. Curtiss. 1989. Cloning and molecular characterization of genes whose products allow *Salmonella typhimurium* to penetrate tissue culture cells. *Proc. Natl. Acad. Sci. USA* 86:6383–6387.

Garcia-del Portillo, F., M. B. Zwick, K. Y. Leung, and B. B. Finlay. 1993. *Salmonella* induces the formation of filamentous structures containing lysosomal membrane glycoproteins in epithelial cells. *Proc. Natl. Acad. Sci. USA* 90:10544–10548.

Ghayur, T., S. Banerjee, M. Hugunin, D. Butler, L. Herzog, A. Carter, L. Quintal, L. Sekut, R. Talanian, M. Paskind, W. Wong, R. Kamen, D. Tracey, and H. Allen. 1997. Caspase-1 processes IFN-γ-inducing factor and regulates LPS-induced IFN-γ production. *Nature* 386:619–623.

Goebel, W., and M. Kuhn. 2000. Bacterial replication in the host cell cytosol. *Curr. Opin. Microbiol.* 3:49–53.

Hacker, J., G. Blum-Oehler, I. Mühldorfer, and H. Tschäpe. 1997. Pathogenicity islands of virulent bacteria: structure, function and impact on microbial evolution. *Mol. Microbiol.* 23:1089–1097.

Hackstadt, T., E. R. Fischer, M. A. Scidmore, D. D. Rockey, and R. A. Heinzen. 1997. Origins and functions of the chlamydial inclusion. *Trends Microbiol.* 5:288–293.

Hall, A. 1998. Rho GTPases and the actin cytoskeleton. *Science* 279:509–514.

Harada, A., N. Sekido, T. Akahoshi, Y. Wada, N. Mukaida, and K. Matsushima. 1994. Essential involvement of interleukin-8 (IL-8) in acute inflammation. *J. Leukoc. Biol.* **56:**559–564.

Hardt, W. D., L. M. Chen, K. E. Schuebel, X. R. Bustelo, and J. E. Galán. 1998. *S. typhimurium* encodes an activator of Rho GTPases that induces membrane ruffling and nuclear responses in host cells. *Cell* **93:**815–826.

Hardt, W. D., H. Urlaub, and J. E. Galán. 1998. A substrate of the centisome 63 type III protein secretion system of *Salmonella typhimurium* is encoded by a cryptic bacteriophage. *Proc. Natl. Acad. Sci. USA* **95:**2574–2579.

Hayward, R. D., and V. Koronakis. 1999. Direct nucleation and bundling of actin by the SipC protein of invasive *Salmonella*. *EMBO J.* **18:**4926–4934.

Hensel, M., J. E. Shea, C. Gleeson, M. D. Jones, E. Dalton, and D. W. Holden. 1995. Simultaneous identification of bacterial virulence genes by negative selection. *Science* **269:**400–403.

Herrington, D. A., R. H. Hall, G. Losonsky, J. J. Mekalanos, R. K. Taylor, and M. M. Levine. 1988. Toxin, toxin-coregulated pili, and the toxR regulon are essential *for Vibrio cholerae* pathogenesis in humans. *J. Exp. Med.* **168:**1487–1492.

Hilbi, H., J. E. Moss, D. Hersh, Y. Chen, J. Arondel, S. Banerjee, R. A. Flavell, J. Yuan, P. J. Sansonetti, and A. Zychlinsky. 1998. *Shigella*-induced apoptosis is dependent on caspase-1 which binds to IpaB. *J. Biol. Chem.* **273:**32895–32900.

Hobbie, S., L. M. Chen, R. J. Davis, and J. E. Galan. 1997. Involvement of mitogen-activated protein kinase pathways in the nuclear responses and cytokine production induced by *Salmonella typhimurium* in cultured intestinal epithelial cells. *J. Immunol.* **159:**5550–5559.

Hueck, C. J. 1998. Type III protein secretion systems in bacterial pathogens of animals and plants. *Microbiol. Mol. Biol. Rev.* **62:** 379–433.

Ireton, K., B. Payrastre, H. Chap, W. Ogawa, H. Sakaue, M. Kasuga, and P. Cossart. 1996. A role for phosphoinositide 3-kinase in bacterial invasion. *Science* **274:**780–782.

Johnson, E. A. 1999. Clostridial toxins as therapeutic agents: benefits of nature's most toxic proteins. *Annu. Rev. Microbiol.* **53:** 551–575.

Kalman, D., O. D. Weiner, D. L. Goosney, J. W. Sedat, B. B. Finlay, A. Abo, and J. M. Bishop. 1999. Enteropathogenic *E. coli* acts through WASP and Arp2/3 complex to form actin pedestals. *Nat. Cell. Biol.* **1:**389–391.

Kalman, S., W. Mitchell, R. Marathe, C. Lammel, J. Fan, R. W. Hyman, L. Olinger, J. Grimwood, R. W. Davis, and R. S. Stephens. 1999. Comparative genomes of *Chlamydia pneumoniae* and *C. trachomatis. Nat. Genet.* **21:**385–389.

Kenny, B., R. DeVinney, M. Stein, D. J. Reinscheid, E. A. Frey, and B. B. Finlay. 1997. Enteropathogenic *E. coli* (EPEC) transfers its receptor for intimate adherence into mammalian cells. *Cell* **91:**511–520.

Knutton, S., I. Rosenshine, M. J. Pallen, I. Nisan, B. C. Neves, C. Bain, C. Wolff, G. Dougan, and G. Frankel. 1998. A novel EspA-associated surface organelle of enteropathogenic *Escherichia coli* involved in protein translocation into epithelial cells. *EMBO J.* **17:**2166–2176.

Krakauer, T. 1999. Immune response to staphylococcal superantigens. *Immunol. Res.* **20:**163–173.

Kubori, T., Y. Matsushima, D. Nakamura, J. Uralil, M. Lara-Tejero, A. Sukhan, J. E. Galan, and S. I. Aizawa. 1998. Supramolecular structure of the *Salmonella typhimurium* type III protein secretion system. *Science* **280:**602–605.

Kuhn, M., and W. Goebel. 1999. Pathogenesis of *Listeria monocytogenes,* p. 97–130. *In* E. T. Ryser and E. H. Marth (ed.), *Listeria, Listeriosis, and Food Safety,* 2nd ed. Marcel Dekker, Inc., New York, N.Y.

Kuhn, M., and W. Goebel. 2000. Internalization of *Listeria monocytogenes* by nonprofessional and professional phagocytes. *Subcell. Biochem.* **33:**411–436.

Ladant, D., and A. Ullmann. 1999. *Bordetella pertussis* adenylate cyclase: a toxin with multiple talents. *Trends Microbiol.* **7:**172–176.

Lecuit, M., S. Dramsi, C. Gottardi, M. Fedor-Chaiken, B. Gumbiner, and P. Cossart. 1999. A single amino acid in E-cadherin responsible for host specificity towards the human pathogen *Listeria monocytogenes. EMBO J.* **18:**3956–3963.

Lesser, C. F., C. A. Scherer, and S. I. Miller. 2000. Rac, ruffle and Rho: orchestration of *Salmonella* invasion. *Trends Microbiol.* **8:** 151–152.

Liu, H. H. 1999. Antibiotic resistance in bacteria. A current and future problem. *Adv. Exp. Med. Biol.* **455:**387–396.

Matsumoto, A. 1982. Electron microscopic observations of surface projections on *Chlamydia psittaci* reticulate bodies. *J. Bacteriol.* **150:**358–364.

McDaniel, T. K., and J. B. Kaper. 1997. A cloned pathogenicity island from enteropathogenic *Escherichia coli* confers the attaching and effacing phenotype on E. coli K-12. *Mol. Microbiol.* **23:**399–407.

Ménard, R., P. J. Sansonetti, and C. Parsot. 1994. The secretion of the *Shigella flexneri* Ipa invasins is induced by epithelial cells and controlled by IpaB and IpaD. *EMBO J.* **13:**5293–5302.

Ménard, R., P. J. Sansonetti, C. Parsot, and T. Vasselon. 1994. Extracellular association and cytoplasmic partitioning of the IpaB and ipaC invasins of *Shigella flexneri. Cell* **79:**515–525.

Mengaud, J., H. Ohayon, P. Gounon, R.-M. Mege, and P. Cossart. 1996. E-cadherin is the receptor for internalin, a surface protein required for entry *of L. monocytogenes* into epithelial cells. *Cell* **84:**923–932.

Mills, S. D., A. Boland, M. P. Sory, P. van der Smissen, C. Kerbourch, B. B. Finlay, and G. R. Cornelis. 1997. *Yersinia enterocolitica* induces apoptosis in macrophages by a process requiring functional type III secretion and translocation mechanisms and involving YopP, presumably acting as an effector protein. *Proc. Natl. Acad. Sci. USA* **94:**12638–12643.

Monack, D. M., J. Mecsas, N. Ghori, and S. Falkow. 1997. *Yersinia* signals macrophages to undergo apoptosis and YopJ is necessary for this cell death. *Proc. Natl. Acad. Sci. USA* **94:**10385–10390.

Moon, H. W., S. C. Whipp, R. A. Argenzio, M. M. Levine, and R. A. Giannella. 1983. Attaching and effacing activities of rabbit and human enteropathogenic *Escherichia coli* in pig and rabbit intestines. *Infect. Immun.* **41:**1340–1351.

Moulder, J. W. 1991. Interaction of chlamydiae and host cells in vitro. *Microbiol. Rev.* **55:**143–190.

Nassif, X., C. Pujol, P. Morand, and E. Eugene. 1999. Interactions of pathogenic *Neisseria* with host cells. Is it possible to assemble the puzzle? *Mol. Microbiol.* **32:**1124–1132.

Naumann, M., S. Wessler, C. Bartsch, B. Wieland, A. Covacci, R. Haas, and T. F. Meyer. 1999. Activation of activator protein 1 and stress response kinases in epithelial cells colonized by *Helicobacter pylori* encoding the cag pathogenicity island. *J. Biol. Chem.* **274:**31655–31662.

Niebuhr, K., N. Jouihri, A. Allaoui, P. Guonon, P. J. Sansonetti, and C. Parsot. 2000. IpgD, a protein secreted by the type III secretion machinery of *Shigella flexneri,* is chaperoned by IpgE and implicated in entry focus formation. *Mol. Microbiol.* **38:**8–19.

Nordstrand, A., A. G. Barbour, and S. Bergström. 2000. *Borrelia* pathogenesis research in the post-genomic and post-vaccine era. *Curr. Opin. Microbiol.* **3:**86–92.

Ochman, H., F. C. Soncini, F. Solomon, and E. A. Groisman. 1996. Identification of a pathogenicity island required for *Sal*-

monella survival in host cells. *Proc. Natl. Acad. Sci. USA* 93: 7800–7804.

Odenbreit, S., J. Puls, B. Sedlmaier, E. Gerland, W. Fischer, and R. Haas. 2000. Translocation of *Helicobacter pylori* CagA into gastric epithelial cells by type IV secretion. *Science* 287:1497–1500.

Orth, K., L. E. Palmer, Z. Q. Bao, S. Stewart, A. E. Rudolph, J. B. Bliska, and J. E. Dixon. 1999. Inhibition of the mitogen-activated protein kinase kinase superfamily by a *Yersinia* effector. *Science* 285:1920–1923.

Palmer, L. E., S. Hobbie, J. E. Galan, and J. B. Bliska. 1998. YopJ of *Yersinia pseudotuberculosis* is required for the inhibition of macrophage TNF-α production and downregulation of the MAP kinases p38 and JNK. *Mol. Microbiol.* 27:953–965.

Parsonnet, J., G. D. Friedman, N. Orentreich, and H. Vogelman. 1997. Risk for gastric cancer in people with CagA positive or CagA negative *Helicobacter pylori* infection. *Gut* 40:297–301.

Passador, L., and W. Iglewski. 1994. ADP-ribosylating toxins. *Methods Enzymol.* 235:617–631.

Paton, J. C., P. W. Andrew, G. J. Boulnois, and T. J. Mitchell. 1993. Molecular analysis of the pathogenicity of *Streptococcus pneumoniae:* the role of pneumococcal proteins. *Annu. Rev. Microbiol.* 47:89–115.

Persson, C., R. Nordfelth, A. Holmstrom, S. Hakansson, R. Rosqvist, and H. Wolf-Watz. 1995. Cell-surface-bound *Yersinia* translocate the protein tyrosine phosphatase YopH by a polarized mechanism into the target cell. *Mol. Microbiol.* 18:135–150.

Pfeuffer, T., W. Goebel, J. Laubinger, M. Bachmann, and M. Kuhn. 2000. LaXp180, a mammalian ActA-binding protein, identified with the yeast two-hybrid system colocalizes with intracellular *Listeria monocytogenes*. *Cell. Microbiol.* 2:101–114.

Rambukkana, A. 2000. How does *Mycobacterium leprae* target the peripheral nervous system? *Trends Microbiol.* 8:23–28.

Rambukkana, A., J. L. Salzer, P. D. Yurchenco, and E. I. Tuomanen. 1997. Neural targeting of *Mycobacterium leprae* mediated by the G domain of the laminin-α2 chain. *Cell* 88:811–821.

Rambukkana, A., H. Yamada, G. Zanazzi, T. Mathus, J. L. Salzer, P. D. Yurchenco, K. P. Campbell, and V. A. Fischetti. 1998. Role of α-dystroglycan as a Schwann cell receptor for *Mycobacterium leprae*. *Science* 282:2076–2079.

Ripio, M. T., K. Brehm, M. Lara, M. Suarez, and J. A. Vazquez-Boland. 1997. Glucose-1-phosphate utilization by *Listeria monocytogenes* is PrfA dependent and coordinately expressed with virulence factors. *J. Bacteriol.* 179:7174–7180.

Rosenshine, I., M. S. Donnenberg, J. B. Kaper, and B. B. Finlay. 1992. Signal transduction between enteropathogenic *Escherichia coli* (EPEC) and epithelial cells: EPEC induces tyrosine phosphorylation of host cell proteins to initiate cytoskeletal rearrangement and bacterial uptake. *EMBO J.* 11:3551–3560.

Rouquette, C., C. de Chastellier, S. Nair, and P. Berche. 1998. The ClpC ATPase of *Listeria monocytogenes* is a general stress protein required for virulence and promoting early bacterial escape from the phagosome of macrophages. *Mol. Microbiol.* 27:1235–1245.

Rouquette, C., M. T. Ripio, E. Pellegrini, J. M. Bolla, R. I. Tascon, J.-A. Vazquez-Boland, and P. Berche. 1996. Identification of a ClpC ATPase required for stress tolerance and in vivo survival of *Listeria monocytogenes*. *Mol. Microbiol.* 21:977–987.

Ruckdeschel, K., S. Harb, A. Roggenkamp, M. Hornef, R. Zumbihl, S. Köhler, J. Heesemann, and B. Rouot. 1998. *Yersinia enterocolitica* impairs activation of transcription factor NF-κB: involvement in the induction of programmed cell death and in the suppression of the macrophage tumor necrosis factor alpha production. *J. Exp. Med.* 187:1069–1079.

Ruckdeschel, K., J. Machold, A. Roggenkamp, S. Schubert, J. Pierre, R. Zumbihl, J. P. Liautard, J. Heesemann, and B. Rouot. 1997. *Yersinia enterocolitica* promotes deactivation of macrophage mitogen-activated protein kinases extracellular signal-regulated kinase-1/2, p38, and c-Jun NH$_2$-terminal kinase. Correlation with its inhibitory effect on tumor necrosis factor-alpha production. *J. Biol. Chem.* 272:15920–15927.

Sansonetti, P. J. 1991. Genetic and molecular basis of epithelial cell invasion by *Shigella* species. *Rev. Infect. Dis.* 13:S285–S292.

Sansonetti, P. J., A. Phalipon, J. Arondel, K. Thirumalai, S. Banerjee, K. Takeda, and A. Zychlinsky. 2000. Caspase-1 activation of IL-1β and IL-18 are essential for *Shigella flexneri* induced inflammation. *Immunity* 12:581–590.

Sansonetti, P. J., G. Tran Van Nhieu, and E. Egile. 1999. Rupture of the intestinal epithelial barrier and mucosal invasion by *Shigella flexneri*. *Clin. Infect. Dis.* 28:466–475.

Satin, B., G. Del Giudice, V. Della Bianca, S. Dusi, C. Laudanna, F. Tonello, D. Kelleher, R. Rappuoli, C. Montecucco, and F. Rossi. 2000. The neutrophil-activating protein (HP-NAP) of *Helicobacter pylori* is a protective antigen and a major virulence factor. *J. Exp. Med.* 191:1467–1476.

Schesser, K., A. K. Spiik, J. M. Dukuzumuremyi, M. F. Neurath, S. Pettersson, and H. Wolf-Watz. 1998. The *yopJ* locus is required for *Yersinia*-mediated inhibition of NF-κB activation and cytokine expression: YopJ contains a eukaryotic SH2-like domain that is essential for its repressive activity. *Mol. Microbiol.* 28:1067–1079.

Segal, E. D., J. Cha, J. Lo, S. Falkow, and L. S. Tompkins. 1999. Altered states: involvement of phosphorylated CagA in the induction of host cellular growth changes by *Helicobacter pylori*. *Proc. Natl. Acad. Sci. USA* 96:14559–14564.

Segal, E. D., S. Falkow, and L. S. Tompkins. 1996. *Helicobacter pylori* attachment to gastric cells induces cytoskeletal rearrangements and tyrosine phosphorylation of host cell proteins. *Proc. Natl. Acad. Sci. USA* 93:1259–1264.

Segal, E. D., C. Lange, A. Covacci, L. S. Tompkins, and S. Falkow. 1997. Induction of host signal transduction pathways by *Helicobacter pylori*. *Proc. Natl. Acad. Sci. USA* 94:7595–7599.

Shea, J. E., M. Hensel, C. Gleeson, and D. W. Holden. 1996. Identification of a virulence locus encoding a second type III secretion system in *Salmonella typhimurium*. *Proc. Natl. Acad. Sci. USA* 93:2593–2597.

Shimoji, Y., V. Ng, K. Matsumura, V. A. Fischetti, and A. Rambukkana. 1999. A 21-kDa surface protein of *Mycobacterium leprae* binds peripheral nerve laminin-2 and mediates Schwann cell invasion. *Proc. Natl. Acad. Sci. USA* 96:9857–9862.

Silverman, D. J., L. A. Santucci, N. Meyers, and Z. Sekeyova. 1992. Penetration of host cells by *Rickettsia rickettsii* appears to be mediated by a phospholipase of rickettsial origin. *Infect. Immun.* 60:2733–2740.

Skrzypek, E., C. Cowan, and S. C. Straley. 1998. Targeting of the *Yersinia pestis* YopM protein into HeLa cells and intracellular trafficking to the nucleus. *Mol. Microbiol.* 30:1051–1065.

Sory, M. P., and G. R. Cornelis. 1994. Translocation of a hybrid YopE-adenylate cyclase from *Yersinia enterocolitica* into HeLa cells. *Mol. Microbiol.* 14:583–594.

Stein, M. A., K. Y. Leung, M. Zwick, F. Garcia-del Portillo, and B. B. Finlay. 1996. Identification of a *Salmonella* virulence gene required for formation of filamentous structures containing lysosomal membrane glycoproteins within epithelial cells. *Mol. Microbiol.* 20:151–164.

Stein, M., R. Rappuoli, and A. Covacci. 2000. Tyrosine phosphorylation of the *Helicobacter pylori* CagA antigen after cag-driven host cell translocation. *Proc. Natl. Acad. Sci. USA* 97:1263–1268.

Stephens, R. S. 1994. Molecular mimicry and *Chlamydia trachomatis* infection of eukaryotic cells. *Trends Microbiol.* 2:99–101.

Stevens, D. L. 1997. The toxins of group A streptococcus, the flesh eating bacteria. *Immunol. Invest.* 26:129–150.

Sturgill-Koszycki, S., P. H. Schlesinger, P. Chakraborty, P. L. Haddix, H. L. Collins, A. K. Fok, R. D. Allen, S. L. Gluck, J. Heuser, and D. G. Russell. 1994. Lack of acidification in *Mycobacterium* phagosomes produced by exclusion of the vesicular proton-ATPase. *Science* 263:678–681.

Tan, M. W., and F. M. Ausubel. 2000. *Caenorhabditis elegans*: a model genetic host to study *Pseudomonas aeruginosa* pathogenesis. *Curr. Opin. Microbiol.* 3:29–34.

Todd, W. J., and H. D. Caldwell. 1985. The interaction of *Chlamydia trachomatis* with host cells: ultrastructural studies of the mechanism of release of a biovar II strain from HeLa 229 cells. *J. Infect. Dis.* 151:1037–1044.

Tomb, J. F., O. White, A. R. Kerlavage, R. A. Clayton, G. G. Sutton, R. D. Fleischmann, K. A. Ketchum, H. P. Klenk, S. Gill, B. A. Dougherty, K. Nelson, J. Quackenbush, L. Zhou, E. F. Kirkness, S. Peterson, B. Loftus, D. Richardson, R. Dodson, H. G. Khalak, A. Glodek, K. McKenney, L. M. Fitzegerald, N. Lee, M. D. Adams, J. C. Venter, et al. 1997. The complete genome sequence of the gastric pathogen *Helicobacter pylori*. *Nature* 388:539–547.

Tran Van Nhieu, G., A. Ben-Ze'ev, and P. J. Sansonetti. 1997. Modulation of bacterial entry into epithelial cells by association between vinculin and the *Shigella* IpaA invasin. *EMBO J.* 16:2717–2729.

Tran Van Nhieu, G., E. Caron, A. Hall, and P. J. Sansonetti. 1999. IpaC induces actin polymerization and filopodia formation during *Shigella* entry into epithelial cells. *EMBO J.* 18:3249–3262.

Uchiya, K., M. A. Barbieri, K. Funato, A. H. Shah, P. D. Stahl, and E. A. Groisman. 1999. A *Salmonella* virulence protein that inhibits cellular trafficking. *EMBO J.* 18:3924–3933.

Via, L. E., D. Deretic, R. J. Ulmer, N. S. Hibler, L. A. Huber, and V. Deretic. 1997. Arrest of mycobacterial phagosome maturation is caused by a block in vesicle fusion between stages controlled by rab5 and rab7. *J. Biol. Chem.* 272:13326–13331.

Vogel, J. P., and R. R. Isberg. 1999. Cell biology of *Legionella pneumophilia*. *Curr. Opin. Microbiol.* 2:30–34.

Wachter, C., C. Beinke, M. Mattes, and M. A. Schmidt. 1999. Insertion of EspD into epithelial target cell membranes by infecting enteropathogenic *Escherichia coli*. *Mol. Microbiol.* 31:1695–1707.

Weinstock, G. M., J. M. Hardham, M. P. McLeod, E. J. Sodergren, and S. J. Norris. 1998. The genome of *Treponema pallidum*: new light on the agent of syphilis. *FEMS Micriobiol. Rev.* 22:323–332.

Wood, M. W., M. A. Jones, P. R. Watson, S. Hedges, T. S. Wallis, and E. E. Galyov. 1998. Identification of a pathogenicity island required for *Salmonella* enteropathogenicity. *Mol. Microbiol.* 29:883–891.

Wooldridge, K. G., and J. M. Ketley. 1997. *Campylobacter*-host cell interactions. *Trends Microbiol.* 5:96–102.

Zhang, J. P., and R. S. Stephens. 1992. Mechanism of *C. trachomatis* attachment to eukaryotic host cell. *Cell* 69:861–869.

Zhou, D., M. S. Mooseker, and J. E. Galan. 1999. Role of the *S. typhimurium* actin-binding protein SipA in bacterial internalization. *Science* 283:2092–2095.

Zumbihl, R., M. Aepfelbacher, A. Andor, C. A. Jacobi, K. Ruckdeschel, B. Rouot, and J. Heesemann. 1999. The cytotoxin YopT of *Yersinia enterocolitica* induces modification and cellular redistribution of the small GTP-binding protein RhoA. *J. Biol. Chem.* 274:29289–29293.

Zychlinsky, A., C. Fitting, J. N. Cavaillon, and P. J. Sansonetti. 1994. Interleukin 1 is released by macrophages during apoptosis induced by *Shigella flexneri*. *J. Clin. Investig.* 94:1328–1332.

Zychlinsky, A., B. Kenny, R. Ménard, M. C. Prevost, I. B. Holland, and P. J. Sansonetti. 1994. IpaB mediates macrophage apoptosis induced by *Shigella flexneri*. *Mol. Microbiol.* 11:619–627.

Zychlinsky, A., M.-C. Prévost, and P. J. Sansonetti. 1992. *Shigella flexneri* induces apoptosis in infected macrophages. *Nature* 358:167–169.

Immunology of Infectious Diseases
Edited by S. H. E. Kaufmann, A. Sher, and R. Ahmed
© 2002 ASM Press, Washington, D.C.

Chapter 2

Overview of the Fungal Pathogens

Luigina Romani

Fungi (*L. fungus,* mushroom) are eukaryotic microorganisms. The systematic study of these organisms is approximately 150 years old, yet the practical manifestations of these organisms have been known since antiquity. Mycologists estimate that there are approximately 1.5 million species of fungi, of which approximately 400 species have proved to be agents of disease in humans and animals.

Fungi form a diverse group of organisms that occupy many niches in the environment. In general they are abundant in nature and are free living as saprobes or symbionts, with only a few living as commensals of the normal microbiota of humans. Many are plant parasites of great importance. With few exceptions, most fungal infections are accidental and originate from an exogenous source, either by inhalation or by traumatic implantation. In addition to their disease-producing potential in humans, fungi are directly or indirectly harmful in many other ways. Negative or damaging effects produced by substances derived from fungi or mushrooms may be due to toxic, teratogenous, carcinogenic or hallucinogenic effects. Human history has been affected by fungi; notable examples include the potato famine, which caused mass migration from Ireland to the New World, and the discovery of a fungal waste product, penicillin, which ushered in the new age of chemotherapy and antibiotics.

Like saprobes, fungi share with bacteria a role in the decay of complex plant and animal remains in soil and can also be specifically beneficial to humans. Numerous fungal species, mostly belonging to the class Basidiomycetes, with large fructification bodies, are edible. Fungi have been the basis of biotechnology over the last 4,500 years. As a "cell factory," they are used for the preparation (fermentation) of food and beverages (bread, cakes, cheese, wine, and beer) and for the production of antibiotics, enzymes, steroids, and other substances required in biotechnology and industry. Finally, fungi serve as scientific models in studies of genetics, biochemical processes, and relationships involving parasites and hosts.

This chapter provides readers with the basic knowledge of fungal biology that is necessary for proper comprehension of the intimate mechanisms and strategies that fungi have adopted in causing infections and diseases.

OUTLINE OF FUNGAL BIOLOGY

Most 19th century biologists considered fungi to be primitive plants and grouped them in the Kingdom Plantae. Serious challenges to the prevailing ideas began in the 1950s, when Copeland envisioned four kingdoms: plants, animals, protists, and bacteria. Finally, in 1969, Whittaker published his five-kingdom modifications of Copeland's Schema in *Science* (Whittaker, 1969). Whittaker's five kingdoms are as follows:

I. Monera: Prokaryotes (bacteria, actinomycetes, and blue-green algae)
II. Protista: Eukaryotes (protozoan and other unicellular organisms)
III. Fungi: Eukaryotes
IV. Plantae: Eukaryotes
V. Animalia: Eukaryotes

The classification of fungi is based primarily on reproductive structures, although the basis of fungal taxonomy has begun to reflect data from molecular genetics. For example, the taxonomic position of *Pneumocystis carinii* has long been a matter of controversy because it shares morphologic and structural

Luigina Romani • Microbiology Section, Department of Experimental Medicine and Biochemical Sciences, School of Medicine, University of Perugia, Via del Giochetto, 06122 Perugia, Italy.

features with both fungi and protozoa (Mandell, 2000). However, *P. carinii* is different from true fungi in that it lacks ergosterol in the membrane and responds better to antiprotozoal agents. Studies of the small-subunit rRNA have revealed that the 16S-like rRNA of *P. carinii* has substantial sequence homology to various species of ascomycetous fungi (Edman et al., 1988).

Pathogenic fungi belong to four of the six phyla included in the kingdom Fungi (Table 1). The deuteromycetes (also known as Fungi Imperfecti) include the vast majority of fungal human pathogens. They are often referred to as imperfect fungi because no sexual phase has yet been observed. Within the Fungi Imperfecti, three classes are recognized; of these, the Blastomycetes (yeasts) and Hyphomycetes (molds) accommodate almost all the medically important species. Fungi can also be classified according to the site of infection, route of acquisition, and virulence, as discussed further below.

The scientific botanic name of a fungus is written in Latin, the first letter of the genus but not that of the species is capitalized, and both terms are italicized. However, the fungal nomenclature is subject to continuous changes that arise from increasing knowledge of fungal taxonomy. Readers interested in obtaining in-depth information on fungal taxonomy are advised to refer to the classification systems presented by Guarro et al. (1999).

Morphology and Morphogenesis

Fungi can be divided into different morphologic forms (Fig. 1). The two basic morphologic forms, yeasts and molds, are not always mutually exclusive; a fungus may assume one or both of these forms under different growth conditions. Yeasts are unicellular oval or spherical cells, usually about 3 to 5 μm in diameter, and reproduce asexually by a process termed blastoconidia formation (budding) or by fis-

sion. Yeast cells of *Cryptococcus neoformans* are surrounded by a mucoid capsule. The multiple budding yeast or "steering wheel" is characteristic and diagnostic of *Paracoccidioides brasiliensis*. In molds, spores germinate to produce branching filaments called hyphae, about 2 to 10 μm in diameter, which may be divided (septate hyphae) or not (coenocytic or nonseptate hyphae) into cells by septa. Filaments elongate by apical growth and by producing side branches. As a colony, or thallus, grows, its hyphae form a mass of intertwining strands called mycelium (Gr. *mykes*, mushroom), which is delineated into two types that differ in function: the vegetative mycelium, responsible for nutrition, and the aerial or reproductive mycelium. Aerial hyphae often produce specialized structures called conidia (i.e., asexual reproductive elements also called propagules) that are easily airborne and disseminated into the environment. The shape and size, together with certain developmental features of conidia, are useful to the mycologist in identifying the specific species (Kwon-Chung and Bennett, 1992; Sutton et al., 1998).

Some fungi (e.g., *Histoplasma capsulatum*, *Blastomyces dermatitidis*, *Coccidioides immitis*, *P. brasiliensis*, *Penicillium marneffei*, and *Sporothrix schenckii*) can exist in a mycelial or yeast morphology depending on the environmental conditions of growth (Vanden Bossche et al., 1993, Mandell et al., 2000). This capacity is known as dimorphism and is clinically important because most of the more pathogenic fungi are dimorphic: they usually appear in infected tissues as yeastlike cells but in cultures as saprobes or as typical molds. *Coccidioides* also has a parasitic stage, which is not a budding yeast but a spherule with internal spore formation. In these cases, the organisms are stimulated primarily by temperature and tissue environment and thus are thermal dimorphic organisms. However, dimorphism is regulated by many other factors (CO_2 concentration,

Table 1. Taxonomy of medically important fungi

Phylum	Sexual characteristics	Genus
Zygomycota	Sexual reproduction through zygospores; asexual reproduction through sporangiospores	*Mucor, Rhizopus, Absidia*
Ascomycota	Sexual reproduction through ascospores within sacs or asci; asexual reproduction through blastoconidia or conidia on conidiophores	*Microsporum, Piedraia Trichophyton, Aspergillus, Histoplasma, Blastomyces*
Basidiomycota	Sexual reproduction through basidiospores on the surface of basidium; asexual reproduction through conidiogenesis	*Cryptococcus*
Deuteromycota	Sexual stage is absent; asexual reproduction through conidiogenesis	*Candida, Malassezia, Trichosporon, Coccidioides, Paracoccidioides, Penicillium, Epidermophyton*

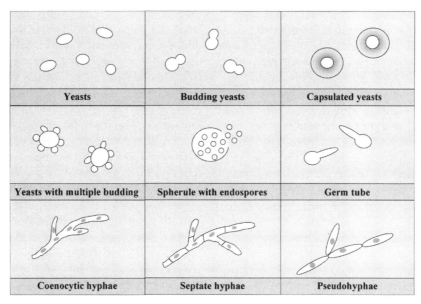

Figure 1. The different yeast and hyphal morphologies.

pH, and level of cysteine or other sulfhydryl-containing compounds). Induced yeastlike growth may be concomitant with increased pathogenic potential in some species. The morphology of *Candida albicans,* part of the microbiota of the mouth, gastrointestinal tract, and membranes lining the mucosa of other cavities and tissues, is unique. In addition to being yeastlike or filamentous, this organism can assume a yeastlike, filamentous, germ tube (the small hypha originating from yeast germination) and pseudohyphal morphology, wherein the cells are elongated and linked like sausages. Pseudohyphal development is an exaggerated form of budding; the newly formed cells do not take on an oval shape and separate from the parent but, rather, remain attached and continue to elongate. The coincident occurrence of yeastlike cells and hyphae in the species of *Candida* when found in tissues is also referred to as dimorphism (Odds, 1988).

Fungal morphogenesis, dimorphism, and phenotypic switching are now beginning to be explored at the molecular and genetic levels. Filamentation-regulatory gene products include several transcription factors and signal-transducing pathway components, including the mitogen-activated protein kinase cascade (Mitchell, 1998; Banuett, 1998; Brown and Gow, 1999; Wang and Heitman, 1999). They work in coordination to regulate responses to external signals (such as osmotic stress, pheromones and hormones, perturbations of cell wall integrity, pH, and interaction with host cells), perceived by a variety of types of receptors (Maresca et al., 1994; Staib et al., 1999). Filamentation (Kobayashi and

Cutler, 1998; Gale et al., 1998), conidial morphology (Tsai et al., 1998), dimorphism (Maresca et al., 1994; Mitchell, 1998), and phenotypic variation (Slutsky et al., 1985; Goldman et al., 1998) are all recognized major virulence factors of fungi (Hogan et al., 1996). Therefore, the identification of regulatory mechanisms and genes involved in all these processes represents one of the most advanced attempts to oppose fungal infectivity and prevent fungal infections (Kwon-Chung, 1998).

Cell Structure

Fungi have structures typical of eukaryotic cells. They possess a complex cytosol that contains microvesicles, microtubules, ribosomes, mitochondria, Golgi apparatus, nuclei, a double-membraned endoplasmic reticulum, and other structures. Fungal nuclei are variable in size, shape, and number. Enclosing the complex cytosol is another membrane called the plasmalemma. Fungal plasma membranes are similar to mammalian plasma membranes in that they contain lipids and proteins along with small quantities of carbohydrates, but they differ in that they contain the nonpolar sterol ergosterol rather than cholesterol as the principal sterol. The plasma membrane regulates the permeability of cells, and sterols provide structure and regulate membrane fluidity. Most current antifungal strategies interfere with ergosterol synthesis.

Unlike mammalian cells, fungi possess a multilayered rigid cell wall immediately exterior to the plasmalemma. It consists of chitinous microfibrils embedded in a matrix of small polysaccharides, proteins, lipids, inorganic salts, and pigments that provides skeletal support and shape. The outer cell wall of dermatophytes contains glycopeptides, which may evoke both immediate and delayed cutaneous hypersensitivity. The proportion of these components varies greatly among fungi. Chitin is a β-1,4-linked polymer of N-acetyl-D-glucosamine and is produced in the cytosol by chitin synthetase, located in chitosomes. The major polysaccharides of the cell wall matrix consist of glucans, made up of β-1,6-linked D-glucose residues with β-1,3-linked branches at frequent intervals; mannan, an α-1,6-linked polymer of D-mannose with α-1,2 and α-1,3 branches; chitosans (polymers of glucosamine); and galactans (polymers of galactose). Mannans, galactomannans, and, less frequently, rhamnomannans are responsible for the immunologic response to medically important fungi. *Cryptococcus neoformans* produces a capsular polysaccharide composed of at least three distinct polymers: glucoronoxylomannan, galactoxylomannan, and mannoprotein. On the basis of the proportion of these components, isolates of *C. neoformans* can be separated into four antigenic groups designated A, B, C, and D.

Metabolism and Nutritional Requirements

Most fungi are obligate aerobes that grow at the optimal temperature of 25 to 35°C and preferably at an acidic pH. They are heterotrophs, requiring a carbon and nitrogen source for the synthesis of amino acids for proteins, purines and pyrimidines for nucleic acids, glucosamine for chitin, and various vitamins. None can fix atmospheric nitrogen. Glucose is the best source of carbon, and organic nitrogen and ammonium compounds are the best sources of nitrogen for the majority of fungi.

Reproduction

Fungi reproduce by two general types of reproduction: sexual and asexual. The inherent pathogenicity of fungi is not related to their sexual or asexual states. Asexual reproduction in the majority of yeasts is achieved primarily by budding of somatic cells. Fission rarely occurs. In molds, reproductive units are of several types. Asexual propagules are represented by spores or conidia, depending on the mode of reproduction, and arise following mitosis of the parent nucleus. Asexual spores are commonly formed by consecutive cleavages within specialized saclike swellings called sporangia, common among the Zygomycota. Conidia are produced free, either by fragmentation of hyphae (arthroconidia) or by budding of a conidiogenous hypha (conidiophores), or from the thickened wall of hyphae (chlamydioconidia). Among dermatophytes, in which different sizes of conidia are produced, the terms "microconidia" (usually unicellular) and "macroconidia" (often multicellular) are used. Asexual structures of fungi are referred to as anamorphs; sexual structures are known as teleomorphs; and the whole fungus is known as the holomorph. Conidia are produced either exclusively as the anamorphs of Deuteromycota or in addition to sexual or asexual spores (in Zygomycota, Ascomicota, and Basidiomycota). The characteristics of the conidia (usually simple and unicellular but also multicellular and of various shapes, size, colors, morphologies, and architectures), as well as their mode formation, the locus of conidiogenesis, and the sequence of conidiogenesis, are used to distinguish the three major classes of anamorphs. In medical mycology, these attributes are particularly important, since the teleomorph state is seldom found. Asexual forms of reproduction represent the major method for the maintenance and dissemination of the species among many groups of fungi, including most of the medically important species. On rare occasions only, many perfect fungi reproduce sexually. Sexual methods of reproduction involve plasmogamy, karyogamy, genetic recombination, and meiosis. The resulting haploid spore is said to be a sexual spore. There are three morphological types: zygospores (large, thick-walled spores), ascospores (generally four to eight spores within a saclike structure called an ascus), and basidiospores (spores formed on the surface of a specialized club-shaped cell, the basidium). The morphology of sexual spores is an important attribute in the classification of fungi (Cole and Hoch, 1991; Sutton et al., 1998).

Despite the absence of meiosis during the life cycle of imperfect fungi, recombination of hereditary properties and genetic variation still occur by a mechanism called parasexuality, a process resulting from many events, including segregation and crossing over during mitosis and haploidization of the diploid nuclei.

FUNGAL DISEASES

In 1835, the monk Agostino Bassi published his classic research paper entitled "Del mal del segno, calcinaccio o moscardino," in which he reported his experimental work demonstrating for the first time that the fungus *Beauvaria bassiana* could cause disease in animals (silkworms). Two years later, Robert Remak observed the presence of hyphae in the crusts associated with tinea favosa. His observation was important because he was the first to incriminate a microorganism as the cause of human infection. Following these two important contributions, David Grub reported in 1841 that he had isolated a fungus from a patient with ringworm and then experimentally showed that the fungus causes ringworm when inoculated onto normal skin.

Fungi are capable of causing a wide spectrum of diseases and infections (Odds et al., 1992; Murphy et al., 1993; Mandell et al., 2000). Micetism and mycotoxicosis cause intoxication through ingestion of poisonous mushrooms or preformed toxic metabolites. Allergic diseases typically consist of hypersensitivity to the inhalation of fungal spores, conidia, or fungal fragments (Romani, 1997). Hypersensitive pneumonitis with cough, fever, lethargy, and pulmonary infiltrates may result following the patient's exposure to conidia of *Alternaria alternata*. *Aspergillus fumigatus* can cause allergic aspergillosis that may occur as extrinsic asthma, extrinsic allergic alveolitis, or allergic bronchopulmonary aspergillosis. Hypersensitivity may occur in association with the state of colonization observed with a fungus ball that forms in an ectatic bronchus, and even in the nasal sinuses. However, growth of the fungus in tissues is not required for hypersensitivity to occur (Latgè, 1999).

Infections caused by fungi are called mycoses, a term coined by the pathologist R. Virchow in 1856. Because human mycoses are poorly communicable from person to person, they are often endemic but rarely epidemic. Morbidity and exact mortality rates of fungal infections are not well known, since mycoses do not belong to the group of diseases which are strictly controlled and have to be reported. However, opportunistic and nosocomial mycoses have greatly increased over the past decades (Fridkin and Jarvis, 1996). Quite a few mycoses (histoplasmosis, coccidioidomycosis, paracoccidioidomycosis, and blastomycosis) occur in regions of endemic infection and are geographically limited to certain areas. In these regions, the mycoses are generally considered to be primary mycoses but may also occur as opportunistic mycoses. By contrast, the opportunistic fungi (such as *Aspergillus* spp. and zygomycetes) are ubiquitously distributed with the frequency of infection being dependent upon a population of immunocompromised hosts. *Penicillium marneffei,* an opportunistic pathogen, appears to be geographically restricted to East Asia, particularly Thailand and China.

Fungal infections are classified according to the primary site of infection, route of acquisition, and type of virulence (Table 2). According to the site of infection, mycoses are designated superficial, cutaneous, subcutaneous, and systemic or deep. These clinical classifications blend into each other; for ex-

Table 2. Classification of fungal infections

Site of infection	Route of acquisition	Virulence
Superficial	Exogenous	Primary
Cutaneous	Endogenous	Opportunistic
Subcutaneous		
Deep or systemic		

ample, a deep mycosis, such as coccidioidomycosis, may begin with cutaneous lesions, and a subcutaneous mycosis, such as sporotrichosis, may disseminate to become a systemic disease. Superficial mycoses are limited to the stratum corneum and essentially elicit no inflammation. Cutaneous infections involve the integument and its appendages, including hair and nails. Infection may involve the stratum corneum or deeper layers of the epidermis. Inflammation of the skin is elicited by the organism or its products. Subcutaneous mycoses include a range of different infections characterized by infection of the subcutaneous tissues, usually at the point of traumatic inoculation. An inflammatory response develops in the subcutaneous tissue, frequently with extension into the epidermis. Deep mycoses involve the lungs, abdominal viscera, bones, and central nervous system. The most common portals of entry are the respiratory tract, gastrointestinal tract, and blood vessels.

When classified according to the route of acquisition, a fungal infection may be designated exogenous (transmitted by airborne, cutaneous, or percutaneous routes) or endogenous (acquired from colonization or reactivation of a fungus from a latent infection) origin. When classified according to virulence, fungi may act as primary, inherently virulent, or opportunistic low-virulence pathogens, depending on whether they establish infection in an immunologically intact or compromised host.

Superficial and Cutaneous Mycoses

Superficial mycoses are usually cosmetic problems that are easily diagnosed and treated. These include infections of the outermost layers of skin (pityriasis versicolor and tinea nigra) and hair (black piedra and white piedra). Cutaneous mycoses are caused by a group of keratinophilic dermatophytes (of the genera *Epidermophyton, Microsporum,* and *Trichophyton*) and by nonkeratinophilic (e.g., *Candida* spp.) fungi. The clinical manifestations of these infections are referred to as tinea (L. *tinea,* worm) or ringworm, already described by Sabouraud in his famous monograph "Les Teignes" in the early 1900s.

Subcutaneous Mycoses

Subcutaneous mycoses include chromoblastomycosis, mycetoma, and sporothricosis. All appear to be caused by traumatic inoculation of the etiological fungi into the subcutaneous tissue, from where local and distal spread along cutaneous lymphatics may occur.

Deep Mycoses

Deep mycoses are caused by primary pathogenic (*Histoplasma capsulatum, Coccidioides immitis, Paracoccidioides brasiliensis,* and *Blastomyces dermatitidis*) and opportunistic (*Candida* spp., *Aspergillus* spp., the zygomycetes, *Cryptococcus neoformans, Pneumocystis carinii, Penicillium marneffei,* and *Fusarium* spp.) fungal pathogens. The primary pathogenic fungi establish infection usually via the respiratory tract, whereas the opportunistic fungi invade via the respiratory and alimentary tracts or intravascular devices.

Primary mycoses

The inherent virulence of the primary pathogenic fungi relies mostly on their dimorphism. They grow as filamentous molds as saprobes and in culture at 25°C; however, when they infect humans or are cultured at 37°C, they undergo transition to the yeastlike morphology seen in infected tissues. Each of these fungi exhibits biochemical and morphological features that enable it to evade host defenses (see below). Primary pulmonary infection occurs as a result of inhalation of conidia from the mycelial phase, which convert to the parasitic phase. In otherwise healthy people living or traveling in areas of endemic infection, the respiratory infections are asymptomatic or of very short duration, resolve rapidly without therapy, and are accompanied by the development of resistance to reinfection. However, patients exposed to a high inoculum of organisms or those with altered host defenses may suffer life-threatening progression or reactivation of latent foci of infection. In such cases, spread outside the lungs may occur, with each organism exhibiting a characterictic pattern of dissemination to secondary organs, such as brain, bone, bone marrow, liver, spleen, and skin.

Opportunistic mycoses

As emphasized above, humans are constantly exposed to viable fungal elements, yet pathological sequelae rarely develop, except for allergic reactions. At least two reasons may account for this. First, healthy immunocompetent humans have a high level of innate resistance to fungal colonization (Murphy et al., 1993). Intact skin serves as a primary barrier to any infection caused by fungi that primarily colonize the superficial, cutaneous, and subcutaneous layers of skin. Fatty acid content, pH, epithelial turnover, local humoral factors, and microbial antagonism appear to contribute to antifungal host resistance (Weitzman and Summerbell, 1995). Iron restriction, by limiting fungal growth, also contributes to natural resistance (Howard, 1998; Ramana and Wang, 2000). Second, the majority of fungi have a low inherent virulence (Murphy et al., 1993). However, their virulence can be greatly increased in patients with specific immunological defects. It is said that no fungus can be classified as nonpathogenic in the clinical setting of nosocomial fungal infections. This reflects a sophisticated degree of adaptation that the opportunistic fungi have evolved through exploitation of their own strategies and by flaws in host defense mechanisms. *C. albicans* is an example of the perfect fungal parasite, since it is capable of colonizing, infecting, immunizing, and persisting on mucosal surfaces of humans. The clinical spectrum of *Candida* infections ranges from mucocutaneous to systemic life-threatening infections. The principal risk factors predisposing to severe candidal infections are congenital or acquired defects of host cell-mediated immune mechanisms, including quantitative and qualitative defects in polymorphonuclear neutrophils and aberrant T-helper (Th) reactivity (Puccetti et al., 1995; Romani, 1999). Likewise, neutropenia due to cytotoxic chemotherapy and systemic corticosteroids is a common predisposing factor for invasive aspergillosis. The infection comes about through inhalation of small airborne *A. fumigatus* conidia (2 to 3 μm in diameter) and involves the lungs and the paranasal sinuses, from where germinated conidia may disseminate to the brain, kidneys, liver, heart, and bones. Septate branching hyphae are a common finding in tissues. The clinical entity zygomycosis, also termed mucormycosis or phycormycosis, encompasses a spectrum of infections similar to aspergillosis. Like candidiasis or aspergillosis, several underlying factors lead to increased susceptibility to fungi belonging to the zygomycetes. Most notable are metabolic acidosis, diabetes mellitus, leukopenia, and hyperglycemia. The monomorphic yeast *C. neoformans* typically causes primary pulmonary infections, from where hematogenous spread to the meninges frequently occurs. Pneumonia and meningitis are classical manifestations of the infection caused by inhalation of small basidiospores (1.8 to 2 μm in diameter). The fungus grows in infected tissues as a budding yeast. The most distinctive feature of this fungus is the presence of an acidic mucopolysaccharide capsule, which is required for virulence and is important diagnostically. Defective cellular immunity, especially that associated with AIDS, is the most common risk factor for developing cryptococcosis. *P. carinii,* a commensal of many wild and domestic animals, can be a major pulmonary opportunistic pathogen in immunodeficient individuals and in patients receiving immunosuppressive therapy. Airborne transmission has been established, but the actual source is still uncertain. After inhalation, the fungus, presumably in its yeast form, attaches to type 1 pneumocytes, a process which seems to be a critical step in the subsequent alveolar infection and acute respiratory insufficiency. Finally, hyalohyphomycosis, caused by any of a variety of normally saprophytic fungi with hyaline hyphal elements (for example *Fusarium* spp.), is an opportunistic infection of neutropenic patients that manifests itself as pneumonia, fungemia, and cutaneous lesions. Readers interested in in-depth information on mycoses are advised to refer to Kwon-Chung and Bennett (1992) and Mandell et al. (2000).

Pathogenicity and Virulence

It is often argued that fungi have evolved for a saprophytic existence and that mammalian infection is not necessary for the survival of any fungal species. However, in this context, it would make little teleological sense that fungi have a low inherent virulence. Instead, the observation that most fungi are opportunists and show infectivity only in patients with a variety of immunologic defects indicates that a high degree of coexistence has evolved between fungi and their mammalian hosts, which deviates into overt disease only under certain circumstances.

Although not unique among infectious agents, fungi possess complex and unusual relationships with the vertebrate immune system, partly due to some prominent features. These include their ability to exist in different forms and to reversibly switch from one to the other in infection. This implicates the existence of a multitude of host recognition and effector mechanisms to oppose fungal infectivity at different body sites. For commensals, two prominent features are also important, the highly effective strategies of immune evasion they must have evolved to survive in the host environment and the prolonged antigenic stimulation of the host, which can have profound immunoregulatory consequences. Thus, in the context of the antagonistic relationships that characterize the host-pathogen interactions, the strategies used by the host to limit fungal infectivity are necessarily disparate (Romani and Howard, 1995)

and, in retaliation, fungi have developed their own elaborate tactics to evade or overcome these defenses (Vartivarian, 1992; Calderone, 1994; Hogan et al., 1996; Kurokawa et al., 1998). This makes it extremely difficult to determine the importance of various microbial virulence factors and to evaluate the relative contributions of individual aspects of host defenses in limiting microbial replication. As a result, a variety of new strategies have been developed to investigate this interplay. Recent advances in fungal molecular biology, by cloning the genes responsible for producing putative virulent factors, have begun to clarify the nature of virulence determinants that are important in host-parasite interactions.

Unlike the potent toxins produced by many bacterial pathogens, pathogenic fungi do not seem to produce overtly toxic products that contribute directly to signs and symptoms of infection. The pathogenesis of fungal infections involves several virulence factors that allow fungal survival and persistence in the host, eventually leading to tissue damage. Some virulence factors are of obvious importance, such as compatibility of size with alveolar spaces, allowing deposition of fungi acquired by inhalation of airborne spores, and thermotolerance. Indeed, the ability of fungi to grow at 37°C is a prerequisite for dissemination to visceral organs. Therefore, thermotolerance can influence the pathogenic potential of fungi and correlates with the ability to produce heat shock proteins and the presence of fatty saturated acid in the fungal membranes (Maresca et al., 1994). However, the role of stress proteins in fungal diseases goes beyond their role in response to a variety of stressful stimuli, to encompass a function in morphogenesis and immunity (Matthews et al., 1998). It is worth mentioning that for commensals, such as *C. albicans,* the abilities to survive and persist in the host are not virulence factors per se, provided that a defense system efficiently opposes fungal infectivity. This highlights the concept that the pathogenesis of fungal infections is multifactorial and undoubtedly a function of both virulence factors and immunological status of the host, the relative importance of which may vary depending on the fungus. Virulence factors that allow fungi to elude host immune resistance are the most relevant in the medically important fungi.

For fungi to cause disease, they need to (i) adhere to and invade host tissues, (ii) multiply, (iii) evade or subvert the host immune system, and (iv) damage the host. The success of each process will depend on virulence factors of fungi.

Adherence

Adherence to host tissues is considered the pivotal first step in the pathogenesis of fungal infections.

Through mimicry of host antigens (see below) and antigenic variation, fungi may evade recognition by host cells. For instance, *P. carinii* expresses several different major surface proteins at any one time and is involved in lung attachment, through binding the mannose receptors (MRs), fibronectin, and surfactant proteins (Mandell et al., 2000). Under some circumstances, *C. albicans* is able to switch at a high frequency (10^{-5} to 10^{-2} switches per generation) among several phenotyes (Slutsky et al., 1985). These switches are extremely pleiotropic and affect colony morphology and cell shape and size, as well as virulence and antigenicity. Differences in the expression of these phenotypes may also determine the relative susceptibility to neutrophil fungicidal mechanisms. Phenotypic switching in *C. neoformans* results in qualitative changes of the capsule polysaccharide, one major virulence factor of the fungus (Goldman et al., 1998). The capsule is a prominent virulence factor because it is antiphagocytic (mainly by increasing the negative cellular charge and by impeding opsonization) and tolerogenic. Given the low level of encapsulation of yeast cells recovered from the environment, it appears that the capsule has evolved as a virulence factor to resist mammalian phagocytosis. The high levels of CO_2 in the lungs favor capsule formation by the fungus. Acapsular strains are avirulent in experimental models of cryptococcal infection. Additional important activities of capsular polysaccharides include blocking the recruitment of inflammatory cells and the induction of costimulatory molecules, inhibition of *Cryptococcus*-specific T-cell and antibody reactivity, and impairment of macrophage antifungal effector and secretory functions (Rodrigues et al., 1999).

Fungi possess a variety of complementary structures by which they adhere to cell surfaces and the extracellular matrix. This is best exemplified by the colonization of various human tissues by *Candida* spp. and the subsequent development of invasive candidiasis. The fungus possesses many structurally and functionally different adhesion molecules (Calderone and Fonzi, 2001; Hostetter, 1996). Various adherence mechanisms have been reported, and factors determining adherence may differ between organs. Adherence is influenced by fungal cell morphology and hydrophobicity, enviromental factors, pH, temperature, and the presence of other colonizing microorganisms. Adhesins may mediate additional fungal functions, such as morphogenesis and signaling. However, strains with reduced adherence in vitro are also avirulent in experimental models of infection, a finding that points to a direct link between adherence and virulence. The use of genes encoding proteins with adherent properties (Gale et al.,

1998; Sundstrom, 1999) has provided insight into the topology of protein adhesins. HWP1, a developmentally regulated adhesin of germ tubes and hyphae, attaches to buccal epithelial cells by an unconventional, transglutaminase-mediated mechanism of adhesion. By behaving like mammalian transglutaminase substrates, HWP1 enables yeast cells to form stable attachment to epithelial cells. Cells lacking the HWP1 gene lose adherence and virulence (Staab et al., 1999).

Common among fungi is the observation that adhesins are differentially expressed in the different forms of a fungus, a finding suggesting that adhesins mediate virulence associated with morphogenesis (Hostetter, 1999). Thus, adhesins are differentially expressed in *C. albicans* blastoconidia and hyphae, as well as in inhaled or swallowed conidia of *A. fumigatus*. Indeed, when conidia of *A. fumigatus* or spores of *Rhizopus* are inhaled and deposited in lung tissues, they are in a relatively quiescent metabolic state. They are coated with a thick, hydrophobic outer wall containing carbohydrate and protein molecules that mediate binding to host proteins, such as extracellular matrix proteins (Latgè, 1999). If conditions in the lungs are appropriate, the outer coat of the conidia of spores is shed and they swell and become more metabolically active. The differences in adherence and in host responses elicited by resting or swollen conidia are profound. Fungal adhesins also bind to many recognition molecules on host cells, including lectin, complement receptor 3 (CR3), and the CD14 receptor for lypolysaccharide. For instance, adhesins of *H. capsulatum* bind to CR3 (Marth and Kelsall, 1997), while the WI-1 adhesin of *B. dermatitidis* yeasts binds specifically to CD14 on macrophages (Klein and Newman, 1996). The WI-1 level of expression is altered in hypovirulent mutants, and targeted gene disruption revealed that this adhesin is indispensable for pathogenicity (Brandhorst et al., 1999). The binding to extracellular matrix protein, such as laminin, collagen, or fibronectin, is clearly an obvious important step in the dissemination of fungi.

Invasion

Fungi secrete a variety of enzymes, such as proteases, elastases, and phospholipases, which are considered to be major virulence factors, because they cause host cell damage and lysis and impair antifungal host defenses (Hube, 1996; Latgè, 1999, Ghannoum, 2000). For instance, they may cleave immunoglobulins G and A and may cause the release of proinflammatory cytokines. However, most of the evidence linking the production of lytic enzymes with the ability to cause disease is circumstantial. These enzymes are probably involved in the successful survival of the fungus as saprobes, with no obvious implications for survival as saprophytes. However, the recent findings that mutant cells lacking phospholipases and proteases are avirulent have confirmed the presence of a direct correlation between enzyme production and fungal virulence. More recent studies corroborate these findings, by showing that the expression of protease genes occurs differently during different types of infection (De Bernardis et al., 1998) and depends on the progress of the infection (Staib et al., 2000). Enzyme activity also contributes to tissue damage in infection (Schaller et al., 1999).

Evasion and Subversion of Host Immune Defenses

To escape elimination by host immune defense mechanisms, fungi have adopted a number of strategies. These strategies are particularly sophisticated for fungi living as commensals and for those to which humans are constantly exposed. In vertebrates, cellular and humoral components of the innate and adaptive immune system are major effector mechanisms of host resistance to fungi. Professional phagocytes, such as polymorphonuclear neutrophils and mononuclear leukocytes, engulf opsonized and unopsonized fungi through various receptors, including the CRs, Fc receptors, CD14, and the MRs (Romani, 2001). MRs are known to work as Toll-like receptors (TLRs), recognizing invariant structures on pathogens (Kopp and Medzhitov, 1999; McKnight and Gordon, 2000). They govern the ability of phagocytes to discriminate not only among fungi but also between the different forms of fungi and to originate discriminative response to them (Romani, 2000). The engagement of each receptor may result in profoundly different downstream intracellular events, which have important consequences in the expression of the overall antifungal immune defense.

Receptors for the C3 component of complement are also expressed on the surface of many fungi and may act as fungal adhesins (Kozel, 1996). All fungi studied to date have the ability to activate the alternative pathway leading to deposition of opsonic C3 on cell surfaces. C3 deposition is greatly accelerated through activation of the classical pathway by antibodies specific for antigen on the cell surface. It is interesting that C3 activation depends on the morphologic and structural characteristics of fungi. Encapsulated cryptococci are powerful activators of the complement system, while nonencapsulated cryptococci initiate the classical pathway (Kozel, 1996). The capsular size and serotype are, among others, the major variables that influence activation of the complement system. Likewise, resting conidia, swollen conidia, and hyphae of *Aspergillus* differ in the mode of initiation of the complement cascade (Kozel, 1996; Latgè, 1999).

CR3 engagement is most efficient in the uptake of opsonized yeasts. However, for effective killing and cytokine release to occur, the concomitant engagement of the Fc receptors is required (Romani, 2001). Indeed, CR3 activation leads to suppression of the oxidative burst and production of interleukin-12 in response to fungi (Marth and Kelsall, 1997; Romani, 2000). Failure to induce interleukin-12 may account for the lack of development of protective response to fungi (Romani et al., 1997). This means that the use of the different receptors, either alone or simultaneously, may result in coupling or uncoupling phagocytosis with inflammatory and immunological responses, including cytokine production, to fungi. Therefore, subversion of host phagocyte receptors by fungal pathogens represents a most successful strategy to escape elimination by the host immune system (Mosser and Karp, 1999).

One important observation is that cytokines may greatly influence the functioning of the recognition receptors (Romani, 2001). In addition, cytokines with activating or deactivating signals for effector phagocytes and Th cells are differentially produced on engagement of TLRs and other receptors. Thus, in addition to what is already known about cytokines (Stevens et al., 1998; Murphy et al., 1998), they may contribute to fungal virulence by interfering with receptor-mediated activation of phagocytic cells in response to fungi.

Upon attachment to phagocytic cells, fungi are destroyed either through a phagocytic process that provides an immediate innate cellular immune response to fungi residing intracellularly or through the secretion of microbicidal compounds against fungi residing extracellularly or against uningestible fungal elements. Fungal infectivity, however, can also be efficiently opposed by interfering with dimorphism and phenotypic variability (Romani, 2001).

The restriction of fungal growth occurs by both oxygen-dependent and independent mechanisms, intracellular or extracellular release of effector molecules, and other mechanisms. The oxidative killing occurs through production of toxic reactive oxygen intermediate, whose nature varies depending on the nature of the pathogens and the type of phagocytic cells. In retaliation, fungi have evolved strategies to selectively inhibit the respiratory burst, and fungal antioxidants have attracted considerable interest as virulence determinants (Hamilton and Holden, 1999). Melanin and mannitol are potent free radical scavengers produced by *Cryptococcus neoformans* and, probably, by *Aspergillus fumigatus*. Superoxide dismutases are important housekeeping antioxidants that may also play a role in fungal virulence, as catalases produced by *Candida albicans* and *A. fumigatus*. Therefore, antioxidant secretion may account for fungal intracellular survival and parasitism. However, intracellular survival may also depend on additional virulence factors, such as the ability to modulate phagolysosomal pH and to overcome iron restriction by phagocytes (Vartivarian, 1992; Calderone, 1994; Kurokawa et al., 1998).

An interesting recent observation is that fungal virulence genes are differentially activated during infection (Staib et al., 2000). The finding that the expression of virulence genes is affected by interaction with phagocytic cells (Colonna-Romano et al., 1998) indicates that the antifungal effector activity of the phagocytic system goes beyond the previously recognized functions, to include an activity on fungal gene expression.

Dimorphism

Dimorphism plays an essential role in the pathogenesis of infections caused by the dimorphic fungi.

This phenotypic change is associated with differences in the interaction between the organisms and cells of the host immune system, such as the ability to evade fungicidal mechanisms, the synthesis of the $\alpha 1-3$ glucan cell wall polysaccharide (which protects the fungus from digestive enzymes of host phagocytes), and the expression of specific genes (Maresca et al., 1994; Hogan et al., 1996; Colonna-Romano et al., 1998).

C. albicans can switch from a unicellular yeast form to various filamentous forms, all of which can be found in infected tissues (Odds, 1988). The ability to reversibly switch between these forms is thought to be important for *Candida* virulence (Kobayashi and Cutler, 1998). Although recent studies have clearly shown that the ability to switch from yeast to filamentous forms is required for virulence (Lo et al., 1997; Gale et al., 1998), it is not known whether the yeast or the hyphal form is responsible for pathogenicity. Other pathogenic fungi appear to proliferate in the host exclusively as yeast form cells. One possibility is that the filamentous form is required to evade the cells of the immune system whereas the yeast form is used for proliferation in infected tissues. Recent studies indicate that the innate immune sys-

Table 3. Fungal virulence and evasion mechanisms from host immune defenses

Virulence factors	Evasion mechanisms	Reference
Dimorphism	Hiding inside the cells as yeast (e.g., dimorphic fungi)	Medoff et al. (1987), Kurokawa et al. (1998)
	Filamentation (e.g., *Candida albicans*)	Gale et al. (1998)
Phenotypic switching	Evasion of inflammatory response	Goldman et al. (1998)
Cell wall structures	Masking of antigens and protection from lytic enzymes (e.g., α-glucan in dimorphic fungi)	Kurokawa et al. (1998)
	Production of inhibitory Th2 cytokines	Wang et al. (1998)
Capsule	Inhibition of phagocytosis, inflammatory reaction, antifungal effector activities, and T cell and antibody reactivity (e.g., *Cryptococcus neoformans*)	Rodrigues et al. (1999)
Complement binding	Iron uptake (e.g., *Candida albicans*)	Moors et al. (1992)
	CR3-dependent inhibition of antifungal responses and IL-12 (e.g., *Histoplasma capsulatum*)	Marth and Kelsall (1997)
Adhesins	Host mimicry	Calderone (1994)
	Receptor-mediated subversion of phagocyte responses	Romani (2001)
Antigens, allergens	Diversion from protective Th1 responses	Romani (1999)
Enzymes	Degradation of humoral immune reactivity	Hube (1996)
Fungal metabolites	Immunosuppression (e.g., NF-κB inhibition by gliotoxin)	Pahl et al. (1996)
pH and iron regulation	Survival and multiplication inside the cell (e.g., *Histoplasma* parasitism)	Kurokawa et al. (1998)
Antioxidants	Resistance to oxidative killing (e.g., production of melanin, mannitol, catalase, and superoxide dismutase)	Hamilton and Holden (1999)
Intracellular trafficking	Escape from the phagosome into the cytosol (e.g., *Candida albicans*)	Fè d'Ostiani et al. (2000)

tem fulfills the requirement of a discriminative system capable of sensing the two forms of *C. albicans* in terms of the type of immune response elicited. Ingestion of yeasts activates dendritic cells for antifungal effector functions and the ability to prime Th1 cells, while ingestion of hyphae inhibits those functions. Yeasts and hyphae appear to enter through distinct phagocytic morphologies and receptors. Moreover, once inside the cells, hyphae, but not yeasts, escape the phagosome and are found lying free within the cytoplasm. Strikingly, the different response of dendritic cells to the two forms of the fungus is dependent on cytokine environment (Fè d'Ostiani et al., 2000). Therefore, these findings suggest that virulence is associated with, but not directly related to, the hyphal forms, and that escape from the phagosome into the cytosol and the cytokine environment may act as important cofactors of virulence. It appears that virulence results from the ability to discriminate among the different forms of fungi at the single cell level. That virulence cannot be dogmatically assigned to the hyphal forms of fungi also comes from the observation that none of the monomorphic molds, which depend on hyphal growth in the host (e.g., *Aspergillus* and *Mucorales* species), or *C. albicans,* that may grow as hyphae in tissues, usually affect normal people.

Interestingly, fungal dimorphism and morphogenesis are affected by steroid hormones. High-affinity binding proteins for steroid hormones have been identified in many fungi (Loose et al., 1983; Hernandez-Hernandez et al., 1998). This finding may explain gender-based differences in susceptibility to fungal infections and the occurrence and recurrence of fungal infection in the setting of hormonal dysfunctions. Evasion and virulence mechanisms of pathogenic fungi are summarized in Table 3.

CONCLUSIONS

Progress toward understanding the epidemiology and pathogenesis of fungal infections has been slow, as has the progress in the area of diagnosis and treatment. There is a need for additional strategies of prevention and treatment of fungal infections. This demands the continuation of studies aimed at the molecular typing of fungi, fungal virulence genes, and host-specific immune reactivity that limit fungal infectivity. The final identification of candidate fungal vaccine will rely on a combined effort of fungal molecular biology and immunology.

Acknowledgments. Many thanks are due to Jo-Anne Rowe for invaluable secretarial support. This work was supported by a grant from the AIDS 50B.33 project.

REFERENCES

Banuett, F. 1998. Signalling in the yeasts: an informational cascade with links to the filamentous fungi. *Microbiol. Mol. Biol. Rev.* **62:**249–274.

Brandhorst, T. T., M. Wuthrich, T. Warner, and B. Klein. 1999. Targeted gene disruption reveals an adhesin indispensable for pathogenicity of *Blastomyces dermatitidis. J. Exp. Med.* **189:**1207–1216.

Brown, A. J. P., and N. A. R. Gow. 1999. Regulatory networks controlling *Candida albicans* morphogenesis. *Trends Microbiol.* **7:**333–338.

Calderone, R. A. 1994. Molecular pathogenesis of fungal infections. *Trends Microbiol.* **2:**461–463.

Calderone, R. A., and W. A. Fonzi. 2001. Virulence factors of *Candida albicans. Trends Microbiol.* **9:**327–335.

Cole, G. T., and H. C. Hoch. (ed.). 1991. *The Fungal Spore and Disease Initiation in Plants and Animals.* Plenum Press, New York, N.Y.

Colonna-Romano, S., A. Porta, A. Franco, G. S. Kobayashi, and B. Maresca. 1998. Identification and isolation by DDRT-PCR of genes differentially expressed by *Histoplasma capsulatum* during macrophage infection. *Microb. Pathog.* **25:**55–66.

De Bernardis, F., F. A. Mühlschlegel, A. Cassone, and W. A. Fonzi. 1998. The pH of the host niche controls gene expression in and virulence of *Candida albicans. Infect. Immun.* **66:**3317–3325.

Edman, J. C., J. A. Kovacs, H. Masur, D. V. Santi, H. J. Elwood, and M. L. Sogin. 1988. Ribosomal RNA sequence shows *Pneumocystis carinii* to be a member of the fungi. *Nature* **334:**519–522.

Fè d'Ostiani, C., G. del Sero, A. Bacci, C. Montagnoli, P. Ricciardi-Castagnoli, A. Spreca, and L. Romani. 2000. Dendritic cells discriminate between yeasts and hyphae of the fungus Candida albicans: implications for initiation of Th immunity in vivo and in vitro. *J. Exp. Med.* **191:**1661–1673.

Fridkin, S. K., and W. R. Jarvis. 1996. Epidemiology of nosocomial fungal infections. *Clin. Microbiol. Rev.* **9:**499–511.

Gale, C. A., C. M. Bendel, M. McClellan, M. Hauser, J. M. Becker, J. Berman, and M. K. Hostetter. 1998. Linkage of adhesion, filamentous growth, and virulence in *Candida albicans* to a single gene, INT1. *Science* **279:**1355–1358.

Ghannoum, M. A. 2000. Potential role of phospholipases in virulence and fungal pathogenesis. *Clin Microbiol. Rev.* **13:**122–143.

Goldman, D. L., B. C. Fries, S. P. Franzot, L. Montella, and A. Casadevall. 1998. Phenotypic switching in the human pathogenic fungus *Cryptococcus neoformans* is associated with changes in virulence and pulmonary inflammatory response in rodents. *Proc. Natl. Acad. Sci. USA* **8:**14967–14972.

Guarro, J., J. Gené, and A. M. Stchigel. 1999. Developments in fungal taxonomy. *Clin. Microbiol. Rev.* **12:**454–500.

Hamilton, A. J., and M. D. Holden. 1999. Antioxidant systems in the pathogenic fungi of man and their role in virulence. *Med. Mycol.* **37:**375–389.

Hernandez-Hernandez, F., R. Lopez-Martinez, I. Camacho-Arroyo, and C. A. Mendoza-Rodriguez. 1998–1999. Detection and expression of corticosteroid binding protein gene in human pathogenic fungi. *Mycopathologia* **143:**127–130.

Hogan, L. H., B. S. Klein, and S. M. Levitz. 1996. Virulence factors of medically important fungi. *Clin. Microbiol. Rev.* **9:**469–488.

Hostetter, M. K. 1996. An integrin-like protein in *Candida albicans:* implications for pathogenesis. *Trends Microbiol.* **4:**242–245.

Hostetter, M. K. 1999. Integrin-like proteins in *Candida* spp. and other microorganisms. *Fungal Genet. Biol.* **28:**135–145.

Howard, D. H. 1999. Acquisition, transport and storage of iron by pathogenic fungi. *Clin. Microbiol. Rev.* **12:**394–404.

Hube, B. 1996. *Candida albicans* secreted aspartyl proteinases. *Curr. Top. Med. Mycol.* **7:**55–69.

Klein, B. S., and S. L. Newman. 1996. Role of cell-surface molecules of *Blastomyces dermatitidis* in host-pathogen interaction. *Trends Microbiol.* **4:**246–251.

Kobayashi, S. D., and J. E. Cutler. 1998. *Candida albicans* hyphal formation and virulence: is there a clearly defined role? *Trends Microbiol.* **6:**92–94.

Kopp, E. B., and R. Medzhitov. 1999. The Toll-receptor family and control of innate immunity. *Curr. Opin. Immunol.* **11:**13–18.

Kozel, T. R. 1996. Activation of the complement system by pathogenic fungi. *Clin. Microbiol. Rev.* **9:**34–46.

Kurokawa, C. S., M. F. Sugizaki, and M. T. S. Peraçoli. 1998. Virulence factors in fungi of systemic mycoses. *Rev. Inst. Med. Trop. Sao Paulo* **40:**125–135.

Kwon-Chung, K. J. 1998. Gene disruption to evaluate the role of fungal candidate virulence genes. *Curr. Opin. Microbiol.* **1:**381–389.

Kwon-Chung, K. J., and J. E. Bennett. 1992. *Medical Mycology.* Lea & Febiger, Philadelphia, Pa.

Latgè, J.-P. 1999. *Aspergillus fumigatus* and aspergillosis. *Clin. Microbiol. Rev.* **12:**310–350.

Lo, H.-J., J. R. Kohler, B. DiDomenico, D. Loebenberg, A. Cacciapuoti, and G. R. Fink. 1997. Nonfilamentous *C. albicans* mutants are avirulent. *Cell* **90:**939–949.

Loose, D. S., E. P. Stover, A. Restrepo, D. A. Stevens, and D. Feldman. 1983. Estradiol binds to a receptor-like cytosol binding protein and initiates a biological response in *Paracoccidioides brasiliensis. Proc. Natl. Acad. Sci. USA* **80:**7659–7663.

Mandell, G. L., R. G. Douglas, and J. E. Bennett. 2000. Mycoses, p. 2655–2795. *In* G. L. Mandell, J. E. Bennett, and R. Dolin (ed.), *Principles and Practice of Infectious Diseases,* 5th ed. Churchill Livingstone, Inc., Philadelphia, Pa.

Maresca, B., L. Carratu, and G. S. Kobayashi. 1994. Morphological transition in the human fungal pathogen *Histoplasma capsulatum. Trends Microbiol.* **2:**110–114.

Marth, T., and B. L. Kelsall. 1997. Regulation of interleukin–12 by complement receptor 3 signalling. *J. Exp. Med.* **185:**1987–1995.

Matthews, R. C., B. Maresca, J. P. Burnie, A. Cardona, L. Carratu, S. Conti, G. S. Deepe, A. M. Florez, S. Franceschelli, E. Garcia, L. S. Gragano, G. S. Kobayashi, J. G. McEwen, B. L. Ortiz, A. M. Oviedo, L. Polonelli, L. Ponton, A. Restrepo, and A. Storlazzi. 1998. Stress proteins in fungal infections. *Med. Mycol.* **36**(Suppl. 1):45–51.

McKnight, A., and S. Gordon. 2000. Forum in Immunology: innate recognition systems. *Microbes Infect.* **2:**239–336.

Medoff, G., A. Painter, and G. S. Kobayashi. 1987. Mycelial- to yeast-phase transitions of the dimorphic fungi *Blastomyces dermatitidis* and *Paracoccidioides brasiliensis. J. Bacteriol.* **169:**4055–4060.

Mitchell, A. P. 1998. Dimorphism and virulence in *Candida albicans. Curr. Opin. Microbiol.* **1:**687–692.

Moors, M. A., T. L. Stull, K. J. Blank, H. R. Buckley, and D. M. Moser. 1992. A role for complement-like molecules in iron acquisition by *Candida albicans. J. Exp. Med.* **175:**1643–1651.

Mosser, D. M., and C. L. Karp. 1999. Receptor mediated subversion of macrophage cytokine production by intracellular pathogens. *Curr. Opin. Immunol.* **11:**406–411.

Murphy, J. W., F. Bistoni, G. S. Deepe, Jr., R. A. Blackstock, K. Buchanan, R. B. Ashman, L. Romani, A. Mencacci, E. Cenci, C. Fè d'Ostiani, G. Del Sero, V. L. Calich, and S. S. Kashino. 1998. Type 1 and type 2 cytokines: from basic science to fungal infections. *Med. Mycol.* **36:**109–118.

Murphy, J. W., H. Friedman, and M. Bendinelli (ed.). 1993. *Fungal Infections and Immune Responses.* Plenum Press, New York, N.Y.

Odds, F. C. 1988. *Candida and Candidosis.* 2nd ed. Baillière-Tindall, London, United Kingdom.

Odds, F. C., T. Arai, A. F. Disalvo, E. G. Evans, R. J. Hay, H. S. Randhawa, M. G. Rinaldi, and T. J. Walsh. 1992. Nomenclature of fungal diseases: a report and recommendations from a Sub-Committee of the International Society for Human and Animal Mycology (ISHAM). *J. Med. Vet. Mycol.* **30:**1–10.

Pahl, H. L., B. Krauß, K. Schulze-Osthoff, T. Decker, E. B. Traenckner, M. Vogt, C. Myers, T. Parks, P. Warring, A. Mühlbacher, A. Czernilofsky, and P. A. Baeuerle. 1996. The immunosuppressive fungal metabolite gliotoxin specifically inhibits transcription factor NF-κB. *J. Exp. Med.* **183:**1829–1840.

Puccetti, P., L. Romani, and F. Bistoni. 1995. A T_H1-T_H2-like switch in candidiasis: new perspectives for therapy. *Trends Microbiol.* **3:**237–240.

Ramana, N., and Y. Wang. 2000. A high-affinity iron permease essential for *Candida albicans* virulence. *Science* **288:**1062–1064.

Rodrigues, M. L., C. S. Alviano, and L. R. Travassos. 1999. Pathogenicity of *Cryptococcus neoformans:* virulence factors and immunological mechanisms. *Microbes Infect.* **1:**293–301.

Romani, L. 1997. The T cell response to fungal infections. *Curr. Opin. Immunol.* **9:**484–490.

Romani, L. 1999. Immunity to *Candida albicans:* Th1, Th2 and beyond. *Curr. Opin. Microbiol.* **2:**363–367.

Romani, L. 2001. Innate immunity against fungal pathogens, p. 401–432. *In* R. Chilar and R. Calderone (ed.), *Fungal Pathogenesis: Principles and Clinical Applications.* Marcel-Dekker, Inc., New York, N.Y.

Romani, L., and D. H. Howard. 1995. Mechanisms of resistance to fungal infections. *Curr. Opin. Immunol.* **7:**517–523.

Romani, L., P. Puccetti, and F. Bistoni. 1997. Interleukin-12 in infectious diseases. *Clin. Microbiol. Rev.* **10:**611–636.

Schaller, M., H. C. Korting, W. Schafer, J. Bastert, W. Chen, and B. Hube. 1999. Secreted aspartic proteinase (Sap) activity contributes to tissue damage in a model of human oral candidosis. *Mol. Microbiol.* **34:**169–180.

Slutsky, B., J. Buffo, and D. R. Soll. 1985. High-frequency switching of colony morphology in *Candida albicans. Science* **230:**666–669.

Staab, J. F., S. D. Bradway, P. L. Fidel, and P. Sundstrom. 1999. Adhesive and mammalian transglutaminase substrate properties of *Candida albicans* Hwp1. **283:**1535–1538.

Staib, P., M. Kretschmar, T. Nichterlein, H. Hof, and J. Morschhauser. 2000. Differential activation of a *Candida albicans* virulence gene family during infection. *Proc. Natl. Acad. Sci. USA* **97:**6102–6107.

Staib, P., M. Kretschmar, T. Nichterlein, G. Kohler, S. Michel, H. Hof, J. Hacker, and J. Morschhauser. 1999. Host-induced, stage-specific virulence gene activation in *Candida albicans* during infection. *Mol. Microbiol.* **32:**533–546.

Stevens, D. A., T. J. Walsh, F. Bistoni, E. Cenci, K. V. Clemons, G. Del Sero, C. Fè d'Ostiani, B. J. Kulberg, A. Mencacci, and L. Romani. 1998. Cytokines and mycoses. *Med. Mycol.* **36:**174–182.

Sundstrom, P. 1999. Adhesins in *Candida albicans*. *Curr. Opin. Microbiol.* **2:**353–357.

Sutton, D. A., A. W. Fothergill, and M. G. Rinaldi. 1998. *Guide to Clinically Significant Fungi*. Williams & Wilkins Co., Baltimore, Md.

Tsai, H. F., Y. C. Chang, R. G. Washburn, M. H. Wheeler, and K. J. Kwon-Chang. 1998. The developmentally regulated *alb1* gene of *Aspergillus fumigatus:* its role in modulation of conidial morphology and virulence. *J. Bacteriol.* **180:**3031–3038.

Vanden Bossche, H., F. C. Odds, and D. Kerridge (ed). 1993. *Dimorphic Fungi in Biology and Medicine*. Plenum Press, New York, N.Y.

Vartivarian, S. E. 1992. Virulence properties and nonimmune pathogenic mechanisms of fungi. *Clin. Infect. Dis.* **14:**S30–S36.

Wang, P., and J. Heitman. 1999. Signal transduction cascades regulating mating, filamentation, and virulence in *Cryptococcus neoformans. Curr. Opin. Microbiol.* **2:**358–362.

Wang, Y., S. P. Li, S. A. Moser, K. L. Bost, and J. E. Domer. 1998. Cytokine involvement in immunomodulatory activity affected by *Candida albicans* mannan. *Infect. Immun.* **66:**1384–1391.

Weitzman, I., and R. C. Summerbell. 1995. The dermatophytes. *Clin. Microbiol. Rev.* **8:**240–259.

Whittaker, R. H. 1969. New concepts of kingdoms of organisms. *Science* **163:**150–160.

Immunology of Infectious Diseases
Edited by S. H. E. Kaufmann, A. Sher, and R. Ahmed
© 2002 ASM Press, Washington, D.C.

Chapter 3

Overview of the Parasitic Pathogens

Edward J. Pearce and Rick L. Tarleton

The term "parasite" encompasses an enormous variety of protozoan and metazoan organisms. Acknowledging that parasites are an extremely important cause of disease in animals, this chapter will nevertheless focus primarily on endoparasites (parasites that live within rather than on their hosts) that represent a significantly prevalent and severe risk to human health (Murray et al., 2000); many of these parasites cause zoonotic diseases. Genetic and biological complexity clearly distinguishes the protozoan and metazoan parasites from viruses and bacteria. In contrast to the smaller genomes of viruses and bacteria, these eukaryotic parasites have on the order of 7,000 to 20,000 predicted protein-encoding genes. While this increased level of genetic complexity may be a requirement for being a eukaryote, multicellularity in the metazoans and the presence of multiple stages adapted to survival in intermediate and definitive hosts and under different environmental conditions in both protozoan and metazoan parasites are also likely to contribute to the need for larger genomes.

Although some infections, notably malaria, can cause significant acute mortality, almost all of the major parasitic diseases are chronic. Chronicity is a clear indication that the immune system is unable to eradicate the pathogen, and this in turn indicates that parasites possess the ability to subvert or evade the immune response in some way. It appears likely that parasites have made a considerable investment in the generation and retention of genes involved primarily in evading the host immune effector mechanism. For some organisms, such as African trypanosomes and, to a lesser though growing extent, *Plasmodium* (the causative agent of malaria), the molecular basis of immune evasion is quite well understood while for others, e.g., schistosomes, the evidence for immune evasion is striking but the mechanisms are unclear.

The genetic and morphologic complexity of parasites makes them challenging targets for immunological studies. Nevertheless, considerable strides have been made in recent years in understanding immune control of protozoans and metazoans, and indeed some of these organisms and the infections that they cause have become mainline models for the study of basic immunological principles. These studies have helped reveal some of the many complexities of immune induction and control, particularly with respect to cytokines and their roles in determining the course and intensity of immune responses.

MAJOR PARASITES AND THE DISEASES THEY CAUSE

Protozoa

Among the parasitic protozoa, there are two major pathogenic groups, the apicomplexans, which include *Plasmodium* spp., *Toxoplasma gondii,* and *Cryptosporidium parvum,* and the kinetoplastids, which include *Trypanosoma* and *Leishmania* spp. Other medically important although phylogenetically distinct protozoa include the intestinal parasites *Entamoeba histolytica* and, to a lesser extent, *Giardia lamblia* (which is not discussed further). Apicomplexan parasites have evolved to live intracellularly and are named for their anterior complex of distinct organelles that play a central role in the host cell invasion process; there are no free-living apicomplexans. Life cycle complexity is marked in these parasites, with various cell types being favored for infection depending on the stage of development. Kinetoplastids live either extracellularly within the blood or central nervous system (*Trypanosoma brucei*) or intracellularly in any cell type (*T. cruzi*) or

Edward J. Pearce • Department of Microbiology and Immunology, College of Veterinary Medicine, Cornell University, Ithaca, NY 14853. **Rick L. Tarleton** • Department of Cellular Biology, University of Georgia, Athens, GA 30602.

specifically within macrophages or cells that have features in common with macrophages, such as dendritic cells (*Leishmania* spp.).

Toxoplasma gondii

Toxoplasma infection in humans arises from the consumption of undercooked infected meat or through contact with the feces of an infected cat. In immunocompetent populations, this parasite causes a prevalent but relatively unimportant infection. Its prominence in immunology and parasitology has emerged due to its significance as an opportunistic infection in AIDS patients who do not have access to appropriate anti-*Toxoplasma* chemotherapy (Seitz and Trammer, 1998), from its great usefulness as a tool for understanding cell-mediated immunity (Yap and Sher, 1999), and as a result of its accessibility for cell biological studies (Roos et al., 2000). Most recently, it has been seen to have use as a model for studying *Plasmodium* biology; the malaria parasite is less amenable to experimentation (Crawford et al., 1999). The cat is the definitive host for *T. gondii,* and the parasite's sexual stage occurs intracellularly within the epithelial cells of the cat intestine. The product of sexual reproduction is an oocyst, which is shed with the feces and which upon digestion (by any mammal or bird or even some cold-blooded vertebrates) releases the tachyzoite stage of the parasite, which is able to invade any cell type within the body. Invasion is analogous to the process by which *Plasmodium* parasites enter their host cell, although due to its experimentally accessible biology, the process is better understood in *Toxoplasma*. Host cell recognition is in part via glycosaminoglycans, which are expressed on most (or all) vertebrate cells, helping to explain the broad host cell range (Carruthers et al., 2000a). Adhesion to the host cell occurs via secreted proteins MIC1 and MIC2, and invasion utilizes an actin-myosin-based process with which the parasite glides into a vacuole that it creates mostly from material secreted by its apical organelles (discussed by Carruthers et al., 2000b). As the vacuolar membrane forms, it excludes host surface transmembrane proteins and appears to fail to initiate host cell signaling (Mordue et al., 1999). Inside the host cell, the parasite remains within the parasitophorous vacuole, significantly altering it as it matures by inserting proteins through the membrane and preventing the cell from fusing with the vesicular system of the host cell and therefore from acidifying or fusing with lysosomes (discussed by Carruthers et al. [2000a]). The parasite divides, and daughter organisms leave the cell to find additional host cells. Within skeletal muscles and brain tissue especially, the tachyzoites trans-form into bradyzoites and encyst (Weiss and Kim, 2000). This stage can reactivate when eaten by another mammal, and the tachyzoites can continue the asexual life cycle in all mammals and initiate the sexual cycle if eaten by a cat. Continued encystment in infected organisms is dependent on an ongoing type 1-mediated immune response to the parasite in which gamma interferon (IFN-γ), CD4 and CD8 cells play central protective roles (Sher and Yap, 1999).

Plasmodium spp.

The species of *Plasmodium* that cause disease in humans are, in decreasing order of importance, *P. falciparum, P. vivax, P. malariae,* and *P. ovale*. Malaria parasites enter the bloodstream of the host when an infected mosquito takes a blood meal. The infectious sporozoite stage of the parasite remains in the bloodstream for only a few hours before invading a hepatocyte. A dominant surface protein called the circumsporozoite protein, in combination with a second protein, thrombospondin-related adhesive protein, allows recognition of glycosoaminoglycans in the liver and provides at least part of the targeting mechanism that allows the parasite to reach the correct cell for invasion (Frevert, 1994; Bujard et al., 1993). Inside the hepatocyte, the parasite divides to produce merozoites that are released from the liver cell and invade erythrocytes. Merozoite surface proteins EBA 175 and MSP-1 play roles in recognition of and adhesion to the erythrocyte, binding to glycophorin A in a process that is host sialic acid dependent (Klotz et al., 1992; Perkins and Rocco, 1998). Inside the erythrocyte, the parasite begins to digest hemoglobin, utilizing released amino acids for its own protein synthesis, and then divides to produce more merozoites, which emerge from the ruptured cell to infect new erythrocytes. A subset of parasites differentiate to produce male or female gametes that, if taken up by a blood-feeding mosquito, will fuse to form a zygote, and this zygote will proceed to infect the mosquito and divide to produce sporozoites capable of infecting additional humans. Fertilization is dependent on the Pfs48/45 proteins, which are expressed on the gamete surfaces (Carter et al., 2000).

Disease resulting from malaria infection can be due to anemia associated with excessive erythrocyte loss following high parasitemia or, more seriously and usually in children, to cerebral disease (coma) and metabolic acidosis (Chen et al., 2000). Adults may suffer from acute renal failure, jaundice, and pulmonary edema (Chen et al., 2000). Major-organ disease associated with infection results from changes in microcirculatory flow associated with adherence of the infected erythrocytes and from a tendency of infected cells to rosette or clump with noninfected erythrocytes, plus a poorly understood change in the deformability of uninfected cells that contributes to reduced flow (Dondorp et al., 2000). Impaired microcirculatory flow, combined with inflammation initiated by the interaction of the infected cells with the endothelium and the release of parasites following rupture of the infected erythrocytes, can lead to death. In pregnant women a similar process can occur within the placenta, especially in individuals carrying a first baby; this is also life-threatening. Parasitized erythrocytes adhere to endothelial cells primarily via proteins called PfEMP1, which are expressed in modified areas of the erythrocyte membrane called knobs. PfEMP1 binds to a variety of receptors on the endothelium including CD36, intercellular cell adhesion molecule (ICAM), thrombospondin, PECAM-1, and, especially in the placenta, hyaluronic acid and chondroitin sulfate A. PfEMP1 is also implicated in rosetting.

Immunity to *Plasmodium* appears to be complex and stage specific, with IFN-γ made by CD8 and CD4 cells playing a role in the response to liver stages and antibody being the primary protective mediator against blood stages.

Trypanosoma brucei

T. brucei is endemic in sub-Saharan Africa, where it is transmitted between humans by blood-feeding tsetse flies. The parasites live extracellularly within the plasma and can enter the central nervous system. The way in which they cause disease is unclear, although it appears likely that it is due to their existing in large numbers and stimulating the production of inflammatory mediators, such as NO, that cause the characteristic coma state that precedes death in this disease (discussed by MacLean et al. [1999]). The success of the infection is linked directly to the parasite's ability to select for expression between hundreds of genes that encode the major surface antigen, the variant surface glycoprotein (VSG) (Donelson et al., 1998; Rudenko, 1999). As the immune response leads to the production of high levels of antibodies against one variant and consequently to the demise of that line, parasites expressing a different VSG gene begin to proliferate to fill the niche, and they persist until the immune response leads to their demise; the pattern is then repeated. The extracellular existence of these parasites within the bloodstream makes antibody a crucial immune effector mechanism (reviewed by Hertz and Mansfield [1999]).

Trypanosoma cruzi

T. cruzi is endemic in several Central and South American countries, where it is the leading cause of a heart and gut disease known as Chagas' disease. Infection with *T. cruzi* is generally initiated by the deposition on the skin of metacyclic trypomastigotes by the blood-feeding reduviid bug intermediate host. Parasites then enter mammalian hosts via a break in the skin or mucosa. Metacyclic and bloodstream form trypomastigotes are nonreplicating forms; entry into host cells and conversion into replicating amastigote forms is required for expansion of the parasite population. A wide range of host cell types can support parasite entry and replication, but the receptor-ligand pairs involved in parasite entry are not well defined. Interaction between trypomastigotes and host cells leads to the recruitment of host cell lysosomes to the plasma membrane, where they coalesce and fuse, thereby creating a compartment which the parasite is able to enter (Burleigh, 2000). The signaling event necessary for this process is initiated by a parasite oligopeptidase B, which triggers transient elevations in the intracellular free calcium concentration ($[Ca^{2+}]_i$) in the host cells (Burleigh, 2000). Following the enforced and highly unusual phagocytosis, the parasite leaves the membrane-bound compartment by releasing molecules which dissolve the parasitophorous vacuole membrane, allowing the parasite to enter the cytoplasm. Disease due to *T. cruzi* is the result of continuing infection of crucially important muscle cells in the heart and/or alimentary tract, although autoimmunity has also been suggested to play a role in disease development. CD4 Th1 cells, CD8 cells, and antibody play important roles as effectors against this parasite, which inhabits a mixture of intracellular and extracellular locations (Tarleton, 1996).

Leishmania spp.

Leishmania spp. cause human disease in many countries in Africa and Asia, Central and South America, and Mediterranean Europe. Some species cause cutaneous disease, whereas others visceralize and are thus much more serious. The stage of the parasite infectious for humans, the promastigote, is introduced by the bite of the sandfly vector and targets macrophages for infection. Promastigotes are coated with a lipophosphoglycan (LPG). The phosphoglycan portion of this virulence factor (LPG mutants are minimally infective) extends from the surface of the parasite to form a glycocalyx that both activates host complement, becoming the target for C3 deposition, and at the same time sterically prevents membrane attack complex from being inserted into the membrane of the parasite (Sacks, 1992). Acquired C3 acts as an opsonin that, in concert with other molecules on the surface of the parasite, such as gp63, targets the parasite for phagocytosis by the desired host cell, the macrophage. Once inside the macrophage, the parasites are trafficked to the lysosomal compartment, where they transform into amastigotes, cease to express LPG, and persist and replicate (Alexander et al., 1999). Upon uptake by blood-feeding sandfly vectors, the amastigotes transform into promastigotes and reexpress LPG. Developmentally linked changes in LPG composition and expression allow what is basically the same molecule to play important roles in parasite biology within the insect vector, where it allows parasite adherence to the midgut wall until the blood meal has passed and eventually allows deadherence and movement toward the head, ready for transfer into the mammalian host at the time of biting (Sacks, 1992; Beverley and Turco, 1998).

Within the macrophage, *Leishmania* parasites act through mechanisms that are poorly understood (but see below) to inhibit the completion of signaling events that normally would lead to macrophage activation and parasite killing (McDowell and Sacks, 1999). However, IFN-γ is able to activate macrophages to overcome this parasite-induced block and, by inducing inducible NO synthase (iNOS) expression and NO production, is able to promote parasite killing (Bogdan et al., 2000). Importantly, one of the major signaling pathways targeted by the parasite is that which leads to interleukin-12 (IL-12) production, thereby minimizing the potential for immediate local activation by IL-12 of T cells or NK cells to make IFN-γ (McDowell and Sacks, 1999). The *L. major*-mouse model of human cutaneous leishmaniasis provides a valuable model for examining the roles of Th1 and Th2 cells in vivo; in this setting, Th1 cells are host protective whereas Th2 responses exacerbate disease and allow uncontrolled infection (Reiner and Locksley, 1995). In humans, disease develops as a result of poorly controlled parasite replication leading to the development of skin or mucosal lesions (*L. major, L. amazonensis, L. braziliensis*, and *L. chagasi*), visceralization and major-organ involvement (*L. donovani*, and *L. braziliensis*) or excessive and damaging immune responses to the parasite (mucocutaneous leishmaniasis due to *L. amazonensis*).

Entamoeba histolytica

Transmission of *Entamoeba histolytica* is via the fecal-oral route, in which infectious cysts excreted from infected individuals contaminate drinking water. Within the gut, the parasite excysts and colonizes the intestinal mucosal epithelium but has the potential to invade across the epithelium, causing severe gastrointestinal distress (Espinosa-Cantellano and Martinez-Palomo, 2000). Following invasion, colonization of the liver and other organs may occur. In these cases, amebic abscesses can develop and prove fatal. Recently, *E. histolytica* has definitively been shown to be a distinct species from a nonpathogenic parasite, *E. dispar*, which had been thought to be a nonpathogenic variant of the species *E. histolytica*. *E. histolytica* utilizes a series of virulence factors during infection, including a surface membrane Gal-GalNAc lectin that allows adherence and plays a role in the invasion process by inducing cytolysis plus a cysteine proteinase (CP5) that can participate in the induction of apoptosis in cells that the amoeba contacts (Gilchrist and Petri, 1999). The latter process is considered to be a protective mechanism against host effector cells such as neutrophils. Systemic and mucosal cellular and humoral immunity both appear to play a role in protection against this parasite (Gilchrist and Petri, 1999), but the details are unclear. A mouse model of intestinal amebiasis would greatly facilitate advances in this area.

Helminths

When considering metazoan helminth parasites, there are three major pathogenic groups: the cestodes, trematodes, and nematodes. Defining the parasitic niche of these parasites is not straightforward since most of them exist in numerous developmental life stages that are migratory or live within specific tissues that may differ from those inhabited by the adult parasites. As adults, nematode parasites, which are related to the free-living *Caenorhabditis elegans* worm, parasitize many niches within the human host, including the gut, lymphatics, and subcutis. Although nematode parasite development within the human host follows a predictable pattern through two defined larval stages followed by adulthood, this group of organisms exhibits a bewildering array of life cycle patterns, employing infection strategies as diverse as direct skin penetration, being eaten, and being delivered by the bite of a blood-feeding insect. Cestodes and trematodes, although related to each other, are phylogenetically quite distinct from nematodes. In humans, trematodes live either within the bloodstream or within the lungs or intestine. Cestodes are more commonly known as tapeworms and live as adults within the intestine but are pathogenic as larval stages which grow as cysts within tissues.

Cestodes

The most important cestodes that infect humans are *Taenia saginata, T. solium,* and *Echinococcus* spp. The first two parasites live as tapeworms within the human intestine and are transmitted through intermediate bovine or porcine hosts, respectively. Eggs produced by the adult parasites enter the environment and are eaten by the intermediate hosts, in which they hatch, and the emergent invasive larval stages penetrate the intestinal mucosa and migrate to muscles and other organs and encyst. Transmission occurs when undercooked meat is eaten by the human host and the cyst stage is activated and develops into the tapeworm within the gut. Human disease is caused when eggs are accidentally autoingested and cyst development proceeds. Disease is usually apparent as neurological symptoms associated with cysts within the brain. *Echinococcus* spp. are tapeworms in canines, sheep, or related animals acting as intermediate hosts in which cyst forms are found. Humans are affected when they inadvertently ingest eggs from contaminated canine feces. Cyst formation ensues, usually within the abdomen. These cysts are metastatic if ruptured and require surgical intervention for removal. Relatively little is known about virulence factors with these parasites or about the phenotype of protective immune responses in humans (but see Laclette et al. [1992] and White et al. [1997]).

Trematodes

The most important trematode parasites of humans are the *Schistosoma* spp., which cause disease by inducing a classic granulomatous immunopathology (Cheever and Yap, 1997; Dunne and Pearce, 1999). The infectious stage, the cercaria, released from an infected snail intermediate host, penetrates through the skin of the definitive host by secreting a broad-spectrum proteinase (elastase); following a period of days within the skin, it enters the vasculature and migrates via the lungs to the portal venous system (in the case of *S. mansoni* and *S. japonicum*). At these sites, the parasites mature and mate and female parasites first begin to produce eggs at approximately 4 to 6 weeks postinfection. Egg passage through the intestinal wall allows release to the exterior, where the life cycle can continue via infection of the snail intermediate host. Because the eggs are deposited intravascularly, there is the potential for them to be carried in the direction of the blood flow towards the liver, where they become trapped in the sinusoids. Once trapped, the eggs induce a strong Th2 immune response that orchestrates the formation of a granu-

lomatous lesion around them, essentially sequestering them from the host tissue and limiting what can otherwise be lethal inflammation associated with this massive antigen burden. The granulomatous lesions resolve once the encapsulated eggs die, but they leave behind fibrotic scars, the severity of which is controlled by qualitative facets of the immune response. In total, these pathologic changes can give rise to a potentially lethal increase in portal blood pressure. *S. hematobium* adult parasites live in the blood vessels around the bladder, and egg passage across the bladder wall leads to damage to this organ that can significantly increase the risk of cancer.

Immunological assessment of individuals living in areas where schistosomiasis is endemic has revealed that children are highly susceptible to superinfection or reinfection following treatment whereas adults are significantly immune and that resistance correlates with levels of parasite-specific immunoglobulin E, suggesting a role for this antibody in protective immunity (Butterworth et al., 1996).

Nematodes

Intestinal nematodes are the most prevalent parasites on Earth. Species such as *Ascaris lumbricoides,* the various hookworms (*Ancylostoma* and *Necator*) and whipworms (*Trichuris*), and, to a lesser extent, other parasites such as *Strongyloides* and *Trichinella* infect billions of people. While hookworms, which feed on blood ingested from the intestinal mucosal surface, can cause anemia, these parasites, which as a whole live largely within the intestinal lumen, are less obviously pathogenic than those which are more invasive. Nevertheless, subtle, chronic disease symptoms associated with malnutrition and delayed onset of puberty are very important manifestations of infections of this type (Chan et al., 1994). Experimental work with murine intestinal nematodes (*Heligmosomoides polygyrus* and *Trichuris muris,* as well as *Nippostrongylus brasiliensis* and the promiscuous parasite *Trichinella spiralis*) has been instrumental in defining a protective role for Th2 responses to this class of organisms and in demonstrating that Th1 responses can lead to chronicity of infection (Bancroft and Grencis, 1998). In addition to their importance in establishing effector roles for Th2 cells and in providing an underlying explanation of chronicity, these studies provide a highly relevant counterpoint to the "Th1 is protective, Th2 is exacerbative" model established with the *Leishmania* system.

More severe and obvious pathological changes are caused by filarial nematodes (Ong and Doyle, 1998; de Almeida and Freedman, 1999). *Wuchereria bancrofti* and *Brugia malayi* are transmitted by mosquito intermediate hosts. Larval stages mature into adults that live within the lymphatics, where females release microfilarial larvae that circulate within the bloodstream waiting for transmission to the intermediate insect host. Impaired lymphatic drainage associated with the adult parasites living within the lymph vessels can lead to elephantiasis, a self-explanatory condition in which there is severe swelling of the limb extremities, genitalia, and breasts. The other pathogenic filarial worm is *Onchocerca volvulus.* Transmitted by the bite of a blackfly, these parasites live as adults within subcutaneous nodules and release microfilariae that migrate through the skin, from which they can be transmitted to the intermediate host. The microfilariae cause severe itching and, by migrating through the conjunctiva, can precipitate the changes that lead to river blindness, a profound loss of sight associated with ongoing chronic inflammation in the eyes, in which Th2 responses appear to play a central role (Hall and Pearlman, 1999). In the absence of amenable model systems, experimental immunological studies of these infections have been limited (a problem perhaps soon to be solved by the reemergence of *Litomosoides sigmodontis,* a filarial infection of mice, as a model for human filariases) and the focus has been on studies of immune responses in humans living in areas of endemic infection. These have revealed correlations between the production of IFN-γ by blood leukocytes and severe pathological manifestations (King et al., 1993).

EXPANSION OF THE PARASITE POPULATION WITHIN THE HOST

An additional component of life cycle complexity is whether an individual parasite has the potential to proliferate within its host. A conventional view of infection based on bacterial or viral diseases is that an infectious organism enters the host and then, via rapid replication usually accompanied by host tissue damage, proliferates and initiates a race between itself and the host immune system. This scenario is appropriate for most parasitic protozoa, although the situation is complex in that following an initial period of proliferation, many parasites become relatively quiescent and persist chronically within the host. An alternative strategy of immune evasion by antigenic variation predisposes to population contraction and expansion as the host immune response limits the growth of one clonotype but is outmaneuvered by a newly emergent antigenically variant clone. As a result of parasite replication within the

host, parasitemia during protozoal infections is a reflection of the replicative rate of the parasite balanced against the efficacy of the host immune response. Parasite division can lead to an increase in the size of the population of a particular life cycle stage or may be linked to differentiation into a distinct life cycle stage that is destined to be transmitted to an intermediate host. For intracellular protozoans, unregulated parasite division leads to host cell death and ensuing tissue damage that can precipitate disease. Another consequence of population expansion within the host is that for extremely virulent parasites, one organism can constitute a lethal inoculum.

In contrast to the protozoa, with helminths it is the size of the infectious inoculum that directly dictates the size of the infectious burden. For example, one infectious schistosome larva can give rise to only one adult parasite, which, if it is able to mate with a parasite of the opposite sex, will reproduce sexually, resulting in the production of parasite eggs that leave the body to continue the life cycle. For schistosomiasis, infection intensity is maximally equivalent to the number of exposures the host has received. This is true for most helminths, where production of stages intended to transmit the infection, such as eggs or L1 larvae, leads to an increased burden of parasite antigen within the host. Indeed, it is the continued production and accumulation of stages intended for transmission that is most often the cause of disease during helminth infection. Eggs or larvae trapped or migrating through tissue initiate inflammatory responses that usually underlie the pathological manifestations of infection.

IMMUNITY TO PARASITES: GENERAL PRINCIPLES

A number of tools, in particular neutralizing antibodies, recombinant cytokines, and genetically manipulated mouse strains, have provided considerable new insights into the immune effector mechanisms involved in parasite control. The specifics of some of these mechanisms are dealt with more fully in chapters 9 and 17. Here we consider a few general characteristics of immunity to parasites that deserve special attention.

Parasite Biology Determines What Constitutes an Effective Immune Response

The diversity of lifestyles seen in parasites brings with it the requirement that an effective immune response be tailored to the individual parasite: one size does not fit all. The site of infection and persistence, whether the parasite lives intracellularly or extracellularly and (if the former) whether in a vacuole or not, whether the potential for replication exists, or whether antigenically distinct progeny are produced (e.g., production of eggs or larvae in the helminths) are all determining factors in what constitutes an effective immune response.

The clarity with which the mouse leishmaniasis model supported the in vitro studies that first described the Th1/Th2 paradigm (see chapter 12), led to the adoption of this model as the prototype of how protective immunity works against parasites. This system is characterized by the fact that the majority of mouse strains control *L. major* infection while one strain is highly susceptible and succumbs following exposure. Resistance is tightly coupled to the expression of a Th1 response, while susceptibility is coupled to the development of a Th2 response (Reiner and Locksley, 1995). After these early findings, there was an expectation that protective immune responses would invariably be Th1 in nature while Th2 responses would invariably be associated with a failure to resist infection. Work on immunity to intestinal helminths has clearly shown this view to be incorrect. For these parasites, it appears clear that exactly the opposite of the *Leishmania* system is operating, where Th2-like responses allow the resolution of infection and expulsion of parasites whereas Th1 responses promote chronicity (Bancroft and Grencis, 1998). Thus, as might be considered logical, the various components of the immune system do appear to play important roles in protective immunity against the spectrum of different parasites, and the real issue becomes whether the appropriate response is mounted following infection. Superficially, this might be thought of as providing parasites with the opportunity to evolve to become capable of preferentially inducing the type of immune response that cannot kill them. The outcome of such a strategy has been examined indirectly by using murine hosts that, through gene deletions, have been rendered incapable of mounting the type of immune response normally exhibited by wild-type mice. In these animals, infection usually has one of two consequences. For mice infected by parasites that replicate in the host, the forced induction of the opposite immune response usually leads to uncontrolled proliferation, excessive parasitemia, and death (see, e.g., Tarleton et al. [2000]). Alternatively, the opposite immune response turns out to be highly immunopathological and the host dies not from an increased parasite burden but as a result of the inappropriate immune response that the infection promotes (see, e.g. Gazzinelli et al. [1996]). In either case, the result is similar in the sense that host fitness is extremely compromised and thus the likelihood of transmission is reduced.

Infection studies in gene knockout mice, although sometimes highly artificial, may represent extreme examples of what happens more subtly in natural, immunocompetent hosts. The failure of the immune system to develop an appropriate response (defined as the requisite array of responses, the required diversity in the antigens recognized, and/or a sufficiently vigorous response) results in either an inability to tightly control the infection and/or a pathological response. The relationship between immune responses and disease development in parasitic infections is explored more fully below and in detail in chapter 21.

Although the Th1/Th2 paradigm has been an important guide for understanding and manipulating immune responses to parasites, this paradigm, like most, cannot fully explain such complex phenomena as the immune responses to parasites. Certainly, the views that a Th1 response alone is sufficient for immune control of intracellular pathogens while a Th2 response is a prerequisite for control of extracellular pathogens, that Th1 responses are solely involved in cellular immune responses and Th2 cells are the primary inducers of antibody production, and that Th2 responses are necessary to regulate a potentially overactive Th1 response are all too simplistic. Even in *Leishmania* infections, where the Th1/Th2 paradigm was largely validated, Th1 and Th2 responses alone cannot explain all. For example in models of *Leishmania* infection, the production of immunoregulatory cytokines such as transforming growth factor β (Wilson et al., 1998) or the responsiveness to cytokines such as IL-12 (Jones et al., 2000) and not the Th1/Th2 balance per se may be a better predictor of susceptibility and/or resistance.

Immune Control of Parasitic Infections Is Complex

Many parasite go through a series of developmental changes as they establish and grow or proliferate within the host. The net result of this is that although infected with only one species, a host may in fact be exposed to numerous sets of novel antigens as a result of the infectious organism proceeding through its developmental pathway. A perhaps extreme example of this is provided by the malaria organism. Infection with *Plasmodium* exposes the host to at least four distinct extracellular life cycle stages, the sporozoite, the merozoite, and the male and female gametocytes, plus additional forms that live within either hepatocytes or erythrocytes. While these life cycle stages share the expression of a basic set of genes, they each also express genes that encode proteins which serve stage-specific functions. Thus, primary exposure to malaria involves an immune response to what could be considered a series of related but distinct and therefore antigenically different organisms. This point of view can be extended to helminth parasites, where infection is invariably established following exposure to a larval worm that undergoes a complex developmental process to become an adult. Mature helminth parasites produce eggs or larvae which are morphologically and antigenically distinct from the adult forms and thus stimulate a series of new immune responses. For example, in schistosomiasis, adult schistosomes produce eggs that stimulate a very strong Th2 response, which is not apparent in mice infected with either male or female parasites alone or during prepatent infections (Grzych et al., 1991).

Hosts deal with the life cycle and antigenic complexity of parasites by invoking a similarly complex set of immune responses, complex both in terms of the effector mechanisms activated and in terms of the variety of antigens that are the targets of these effectors. The relative contribution of the various immune mechanisms to the overall control of the infection is not clear in many cases and may change throughout the course of the infection. For example, the early CD8 T-cell response is important in the control of infected hepatocytes in *Plasmodium* infections but is largely irrelevant once the parasites move from the liver into the erythrocytes (Good and Doolan, 1999). In contrast, maintenance of multiple immune effector responses, including potent antibody responses, Th1 cells, and CD8 T cells, is required for control of *T. cruzi* infection both in the acute stage and throughout the chronic infection (Tarleton, 1996). The need on the part of the host to generate multiple effector responses creates potential problems of compatibility among these different immune effector mechanisms (e.g., is it possible to generate effective Th1 and Th2 responses simultaneously, or do these responses counterregulate each other, resulting in an overall suboptimal response?).

In sharp contrast to the apparent situation in viral and in some bacterial infections, the immunodominance of a single antigen appears to be the exception rather than the rule in parasitic infections. Although the immune response to the full complement of antigens for any parasite has yet to be studied (not surprising, since there are 10,000 or more potential antigens), studies to date suggest that in most parasitic infections the immune system sees and responds to a wide variety of antigens. Exceptions include the VSGs of *T. brucei*, each of which is also quantitatively dominant in the parasite population but only for a brief period, and the LACK antigen in

L. major, which appears to be immunodominant only in the BALB/c mouse strain (Fowell and Locksley, 1999).

Complexity in the immune mechanisms and in the antigens which are the targets of these responses presents special challenges to vaccine development. Yet to be determined is whether vaccine strategies can be developed that will elicit multiple immune effector responses to a potentially large set of parasite antigens. It is also not trivial to determine which of the many antigens that are the target of these complex responses are necessary for immune control, and thus should be a part of a vaccine cocktail, and which are dispensable.

Persistence, Chronicity, and Evasion

Although often studied as agents of acute infections, most parasites have evolved to persist within the majority of hosts for prolonged periods, causing chronic rather than short-lived diseases. This clearly provides an advantage to the parasite in terms of increasing its ability to disseminate. However, chronicity brings with it problems for both the parasite and the host, requiring of the pathogen that it in some way evade the immune response and of the host that it regulate prolonged immune responsiveness to minimize pathologic effects. Failure of the parasite to evade the immune response leads to parasite death, and failure on the part of the host to make the correct immune response decision or to appropriately regulate the immune response in the face of ongoing infection usually leads to disease. In practice, chronicity of infection implies success for the parasite and host since both are able to survive over the relatively long term.

For several important protozoal parasites, chronicity is attained by evading the host immune response through antigenic variation. In African trypanosomes, which live extracellularly within the bloodstream in an environment that contains very high concentrations of antibodies, immune evasion is accomplished by selecting for expression one gene from a repertoire of hundreds of variant genes encoding the major surface glycoprotein (the VSG [see above]). While the immune response is appropriate and successful in recognizing and killing trypanosomes through an antibody-mediated attack directed against the dominant surface antigen, the switch in antigen phenotype by a parasite(s) allows escape and expansion of a temporarily invisible population. In this way, the host is relegated to playing catch-up while the parasite persists in numbers sufficient to allow transmission. In this disease situation, in the absence of drug intervention, the host eventually succumbs following a period during which immune responsiveness is generally diminished.

Antigenic variation is also utilized by malaria parasites to avoid immune system-based destruction (Newbold, 1999). In this situation, the parasites are living within erythrocytes and modify the surface of the infected cells with a series of proteins, one of which, PfEMP1, serves to allow interaction with the endothelium (see above). This is considered to be an important adaptation since it prevents the parasitized erythrocytes from being swept to the spleen, where they risk being removed due to the aberrant shape that they assume when parasitized. By inserting its own proteins in the surface of its host cell, the parasite of course runs the risk of being identified by the immune response, and the data indicate that this is in fact what occurs. Antibodies specific for PfEMP1 are thought to be able to block interaction of the parasitized cells with endothelium, thereby preventing sequestration and promoting transit of these cells to the spleen. In response to this, the parasite is able to select for expression any one of hundreds of PfEMP1-encoding VAR genes. Genome sequencing and other approaches have revealed the presence in *Plasmodium* of other families of clonally variant antigens (rifins, stevors) that are likely to also be involved in immune evasion.

Although it was initially believed that intracellular protozoans such as *Trypanosoma cruzi, Toxoplasma gondii,* and *Leishmania* might use the intracellular environment as a refuge from immune detection, it is clear that parasite proteins released within the host cell are processed and presented to the immune system and thus trigger cell-mediated immune responses. The location of *T. cruzi* in the cytoplasm of host cells makes class I major histocompatibility complex (MHC)-dependent activation of CD8 T cells particularly important in the control of this infection (Tarleton et al., 1996). CD8 T-cell recognition of *T. gondii-* and *Leishmania*-infected cells has also been reported, but the vacuolar location and the preference for infection of class II MHC-expressing macrophages in the case of *Leishmania* make CD4$^+$ T cells more critical direct mediators of intracellular parasite control in this infection (Overath and Aebischer, 1999).

The mechanisms of evasion of cellular immune responses elicited by these intracellular protozoans are not well understood. In contrast to viruses, which have mechanisms to restrict antigen processing and presentation in host cells, the evidence that protozoans can prevent class I or class II presentation of parasite-derived peptides is more limited. Metacyclic forms of *Leishmania* activate and bind C3b and C3bi, ligands which allow preferential entry into the phag-

ocyte host cells via CR1 and CR3 receptors (Alexander et al., 1999). This mode of entry avoids triggering the macrophage respiratory burst or nitric oxide production and suppresses IL-12 production, thus promoting the survival of *Leishmania* in an otherwise potentially hostile host cell (Mosser and Karp, 1999; McDowell and Sacks, 1999). There are also alternative receptors for host cell entry by the infective metacylic forms and an additional set of entry ligands used by amastigotes of *Leishmania* to avoid activation of macrophages by the entering parasite. Once within a macrophage vacuole, *Leishmania* may limit antigen presentation via the class II MHC pathway, although this remains controversial (Overath and Aebischer, 1999; Alexander et al., 1999).

Rather than restricting protein release into the antigen-processing pathways in host cells, parasites like *T. cruzi* may use an alternative strategy and actually release many different or related proteins (e.g., members of the large *trans*-sialidase family [Frasch, 2000]) into the MHC class I processing pathway. Peptides derived from these proteins could elicit suboptimal immune responses either by competing with each other for binding to MHC for presentation on the host cell surface or by acting as inhibitory altered peptide ligands for each other (Vidal and Allen, 1996). Such altered peptide ligand effects on immunity to *Plasmodium* have been documented (Plebanski et al., 1997). Chronicity also brings with it a restriction in the cell types and tissues in which some intracellular pathogens can survive. For example, both *T. cruzi* and *T. gondii* appear to become largely restricted to muscles and the nervous system (especially the brain) during the chronic infection. This restriction could be due to one or more factors, including anatomical barriers to immune detection, the relatively poor antigen-presenting capacity of the host cells, and an anti-inflammatory environment in these tissues (Alexander and Hunter, 1998).

There is no evidence to date that parasitic helminths use antigenic variation to evade the immune response and persist as chronic infections. Nevertheless, many helminths do avoid damage even though they are living within animals that are mounting intense immune responses to them. The detailed mechanism by which this happens is currently unclear. However, recent data from the filarial nematode field indicate that these organisms may produce molecules that are profoundly anti-inflammatory, thereby effectively silencing the effector arms of any immune responses that may be directed toward them (Pastrana et al., 1998). Given the wealth of evidence that infection with tissue helminths is accompanied by strong immune responsiveness, coupled with the inexplicable observation that the response seems incapable of focusing on the parasites, this seems like a very attractive possibility.

RELATIONSHIP BETWEEN IMMUNITY AND DISEASE

In many parasitic infections, the host appears to be faced with a seemingly impossible task: to control a persistent infection for decades without destroying substantial amounts of self tissue. For most infections, the mechanisms of the pathological changes are still not well understood. Furthermore, the association between the antiparasite response and the pathogenic response is not clear. In nearly all parasitic infections, there are a substantial percentage of hosts—generally the majority of infected hosts—that control an infection without experiencing a resulting development of clinical disease. There may even be hosts who actually cure these infections without developing disease (although this has been extremely difficult to document in most infections). These cases reinforce the point that clinical pathology is not a necessary consequence of infection, even when that infection is a chronic one. The determinants of the outcome of the host-parasite interaction in terms of immune control and disease development include host and parasite genetics, the immunological status of the host at the time of initial infection and afterwards, including prior and concurrent infections, and other physiological experiences (e.g., age, pregnancy, and hormonal and nutritional status). However, the consensus view is that control of the infection without overwhelming tissue destruction requires a delicate balance between the induction and maintenance of effective antiparasite immune responses and the regulation of that response.

The best-studied models of immune responses to infection—primarily in viral and bacterial systems—suggest that the immune system responds vigorously to infection, committing resources to the rapid expansion of pathogen-specific lymphocytes. As the pathogen is cleared, the pathogen-specific T and B cells decrease in frequency due to cell death (Welsh and McNally, 1999). The decrease in the number of pathogen-induced lymphocytes presumably rids the host of lymphocytes which are no longer required to contain an infection (while at the same time retaining a memory population) and also provides "space" in the lymphocyte pool for the expansion of clones specific for other antigens or pathogens that the host may encounter. This cell death may also provide a means for the deletion of potentially autoreactive lymphocytes induced during the course of an infection.

Less well studied is what happens to the pathogen-specific lymphocytes in cases where the inducing pathogen is not cleared but instead persists for years or decades in the host, which occurs from most parasitic infections. Is the immune system capable of maintaining for years a high frequency of activated parasite-specific lymphocytes? Does a memory population ever form? What are the consequences for both the control of the pathogen and the immunopathology of constant activation due to pathogen persistence? In cases of persistent viral infections, these pathogen-specific lymphocytes persist but become at least partially anergic. Is this also the case in persistent parasitic infections?

In addition to direct destruction of host tissues by parasites or parasite-derived molecules, there are a number of ways in which pathological effects might occur during the course of parasitic infections: (i) failure of the host to sufficiently regulate an otherwise protective antiparasite response, (ii) generation of a vigorous but ineffective (and thus potentially host-destructive) antiparasite response, and (iii) development of anti-self or autoimmune responses. The immune response to pathogens can be viewed as a continuum: too little of a response results in failure to control the infection, an overwhelming parasite load, and death of the host, while too much of the same response may control the parasite load better but at the cost of increased immunopathology. The "optimal" response is judged to be somewhere in between—sufficient to control the infection while minimizing damage to self. Studies with mice lacking the ability to produce immunoregulatory cytokines clearly demonstrate the pathological consequences of the failure to regulate an otherwise protective antiparasite immune response (Neyer et al., 1997; Hunter et al., 1997; Rosa Brunet et al., 1997). However, one aspect lacking in such a simple model is the fact that the immune system is not a single response set at high, medium, or low but instead is multidimensional. The generation of a protective immune response involves not only making a quantitatively strong response but also making the appropriate set of immune responses. During the evolution of the response to a pathogen, the immunodominance (or not) of particular antigens is established and T cells are selected for development of particular cytokine response patterns. An equally vigorous immune response dominated by either type 1 cytokines (IFN-γ, IL-12, and IL-18) or type 2 cytokines (IL-4, IL 5, and IL-13) or focused on one subset of antigens rather than another can have very different consequences in terms of pathogen control and disease development. Immunopathology in many infections is more likely to be the result of a potent but poorly focused immune response (the result of making the "wrong choice") rather than too much of an otherwise protective response.

Prime examples of making the wrong choices include the generation of predominantly Th2 responses to intracellular pathogens (e.g., the course of *Leishmania* major infection in the BALB/c mouse) and of Th1 responses to intestinal helminths (e.g., *T. muris* infection in the Akr mouse). Qualitative differences in immune responses which may appear to have only subtle effects on the pathogen in the acute phase of an infection can nonetheless have dramatic effects on the course of disease when compounded over many months or years. For example, mice with and without the ability to generate substantial type 2 cytokine responses are equally able to control acute infection with *T. cruzi* but Th2-deficient mice do a better job of controlling the chronic infection and consequently of limiting the severity of chronic disease (Tarleton et al., 2000). The reduction in parasite load that an efficient and effective immune response can bring about may be overlooked as a determinant of disease severity. The relative ability of immune responses to reduce pathogen load by limiting host cell invasion or parasite replication in protozoal infections or by reducing the numbers of adults or their fecundity in helminth infections determines the level of continued antigenic stimulation and hence, in some respect, the chances for development of immunopathology.

The view that the pathological effects during parasitic infection are the result of induction of anti-self immune responses has been particularly well developed for *T. cruzi* infection and Chagas' disease (Kierszenbaum, 1999). *T. cruzi* may produce proteins which mimic self proteins, or, alternatively, the continued antigenic stimulation inherent in such a persistent infection could disrupt regulatory controls in the immune system, resulting in anti-self immune responses and subsequent clinical disease. However, such regulatory defects have not been promoted as the cause of disease in other persistent parasitic infections, and the characteristics of *T. cruzi* or the infection that it causes that would uniquely predispose the host toward an anti-self response are not clear. Thus, it has been argued that Chagas' disease is much like other persistent parasitic infections, where disease is more likely to be a consequence of pathogen persistence and a continuous anti-parasite immune response of variable efficiency (Tarleton and Zhang, 1999).

The site of parasitism can have a profound effect on pathogenicity. Generally, the least pathogenic organisms live within the intestinal lumen while, as might be expected, severely pathogenic parasites live within the bloodstream or one of the major organ systems. This oversimplified categorization is of course affected by the genetics of the individual host and of the parasite. Perhaps most importantly, some organs are less tolerant of infection than are others. For example, the brain can accept *Toxoplasma gondii* infection as long as the immune response is sufficient and appropriate to control parasite replication and ensure continued encystment. In patients with deficiencies in their ability to make IFN-γ, cysts can activate and the brain damage that results from waves of infection and cell lysis that ensues can be lethal. For *Taenia solium,* another parasite that has a propensity to establish infection within the brain, damage can develop when the extracellular cyst grows and compresses surrounding tissue. Both *Taenia* and *Toxoplasma* can parasitize additional organs, including muscle, but the threat they pose to life is less severe in these cases.

Since much of the pathology of parasitic infections is associated with the production of mediators by the immune system, there is the potential for different organs to mount certain types of responses to affect the outcome of parasitic infection on an organ-by-organ basis. This is apparent in *L. donovani* infection, where liver damage is light in experimental mice and is controlled within months of infection whereas splenic damage is severe and chronic. These different effects are associated with the relative inability during this infection of splenic marginal-zone macrophages versus hepatic macrophages to become activated to make mediators, such as NO, that are cytotoxic for the parasite.

EMERGING AREAS

Despite success in controlling ulcerative disease caused by the nematode *Dracunculus* and the projection by the World Health Organization and related organizations that additional helminth (lymphatic filaria) and protozoan (*T. cruzi*) infections can be controlled, the threat to human health from parasitic infections remains greater today than at any other time. Following the development, at a startling pace, of drug resistance, malaria has reemerged as one of the world's most prevalent and dangerous infectious diseases. In the wake of civil war and the breakdown of community health care and monitoring programs, sleeping sickness, a disease for which there is no safe chemotherapy, is again epidemic in several countries in central and northeastern Africa. Despite the availability for decades of excellent drugs, the number of cases of schistosomiasis is not in decline. In addition to these continuing problems and the reemergence of infections once thought to be under control, parasites previously unrecognized as major human pathogens have emerged as significant risks to human health. This is exemplified by the recent outbreaks of *Cryptosporidium parvum* infection in various communities in the United States; this apicomplexan parasite is spread by ingestion of encysted forms in water contaminated with fecal material from infected individuals (Griffiths and Tzipori, 1998) and is thus an example of a failure in a developed country of sewage treatment plants or of water purification processes to protect the general populace against parasitic diseases. With global warming, there is also an expectation that parasites previously considered to be largely tropical pathogens will move north and south of their traditional areas of endemicity to cause disease in formerly temperate zones. The ready spread of parasitic pathogens is also enhanced by the greater ease of global travel and by the global transportation of food (a factor in outbreaks of foodborne *Cyclospora* infection in the United States).

The effect on the immune system of infection with parasitic organisms is an area of increasing interest. In many areas of the world, individuals proceed through life carrying one or more chronic parasitic infections. Each infection stimulates an immune response that may render the host more or less susceptible to infection with another organism or to the development of diseases caused by the immune system such as autoimmunities and chronic inflammatory conditions of unknown etiology. A recent report in the popular press (*New York Times,* 7 September 1999) of the cessation of the symptoms of chronic inflammatory bowel disease in patients treated by infection with a nematode that normally is parasitic in the intestines of pigs (and which causes a self-limiting infection in humans) illustrates this point. Moreover, it has become clear that chronic helminth infections can influence the nature of the immune response induced by certain vaccines (Sabin et al., 1996; Cooper et al., 1999) and, in experimental settings, the responses to other pathogens (see, e.g., Curry et al. [1995]). The full impact of these kinds of interactions has yet to be defined.

The lack of effective vaccines for any human parasitic infection is a reflection of the complexity of defining protective immune responses in many cases and the perceived difficulty of improving on the normal course of infection, where the best outcome one can expect is survival with minimal pathological effects; as highlighted above, there are relatively few examples of sterile immunity against parasites. Vaccine development requires a firm understanding of immune mechanisms and ways to elicit these responses (which are lacking in a number of these pathogens) and good models in which to test vaccines. With major international financial and political support, malaria remains the focus of much immunoparasitology vaccine research. Recent completion of the sequence of the genome of a *P. falciparum* isolate has provided the library of sequences from which selection of vaccine antigens will be made and has increased our expectations for success in this arena. Work with experimental vaccines in mice and in humans has shown that partial protection can be achieved with a variety of inocula inducing a spectrum of effector mechanisms including antibody and CD4 and CD8 cells (as both cytolytic cells and cytokine producers), and roles for NK cells in amplifying the protective response and for NO as an effector mediator have been proposed. Nevertheless, definition of the appropriate immune response to target for induction and identification of the best antigens to utilize in a vaccine continue to be major hurdles that are unlikely to be overcome in the immediate future.

The situation may be brighter in some cases, and the emergence of new technologies and approaches holds great promise for advances in the future. For some infections (e.g., with *T. cruzi, Leishmania,* and intestinal helminths), there are excellent models and at least a reasonable if not full understanding of immune effector mechanisms and how to simulate these responses. Projects to sequence the genomes of many of these pathogens will soon reveal the entire genetic composition of many parasites, providing the raw material for vaccine discovery and perhaps additional insights into immune evasion mechanisms. This information provides an unprecedented opportunity for the discovery of vaccine candidates to proceed genomewide rather than one gene or protein at a time. New technologies such as genetic immunization, expression library immunization, prime-boost regimens, and recombinant viruses will aid in the discovery and/or delivery of vaccines. Additional means are being developed and used to help sift through these genomes, including DNA microarrays to identify parasite genes that are expressed at particular points in the life cycle or under certain environmental conditions and host genes that are activated by the infection process (Hayward et al., 2000; Manger and Relman, 2000). Functional assays for tagging or blocking the expression of potentially each and every protein and bioinformatic approaches to predict the localization of gene products and thus their potential to be recognized by an effective immune response are emerging. The ability to assimilate this coming flood of information and to apply it to enhance immune control of parasites may be our next challenge.

REFERENCES

Alexander, J., and C. A. Hunter. 1998. Immunoregulation during toxoplasmosis. *Chem. Immunol.* 70:81–102.

Alexander, J., A. R. Satoskar, and D. G. Russell. 1999. *Leishmania* species: models of intracellular parasitism. *J. Cell Sci.* 112:2993–3002.

Araujo, M. I., E. M. Carvalho, E. J. Pearce, and E. A. Sabin. 1996. Impairment of tetanus toxoid-specific Th1-like immune responses in humans infected with *Schistosoma mansoni. J. Infect. Dis.* 173:269–272.

Bancroft, A., A. J. Curry, D. W. Dunne, K. J. Else, R. K. Grencis, and J. Jones. 1995. Evidence that cytokine-mediated immune interactions induced by *Schistosoma mansoni* alter disease outcome in mice concurrently infected with *Trichuris muris. J. Exp. Med.* 181:769–774.

Bancroft, A. J., and R. K. Grencis. 1998. Th1 and Th2 cells and immunity to intestinal helminths. *Chem. Immunol.* 71:192–208.

Beverley, S. M., and S. J. Turco. 1998. Lipophosphoglycan (LPG) and the identification of virulence genes in the protozoan parasite *Leishmania. Trends Microbiol.* 6:35–40.

Bogdan, C., A. Diefenbach, and M. A. Rollinghoff. 2000. The role of nitric oxide in innate immunity. *Immunol. Rev.* 173:17–26.

Bujard, H., A. Crisanti, M. R. Hollingdale, H. M. Muller, I. Reckmann, and K. J. Robson. 1993. Thrombospondin related anonymous protein (TRAP) of *Plasmodium falciparum* binds specifically to sulfated glycoconjugates and to HepG2 hepatoma cells suggesting a role for this molecule in sporozoite invasion of hepatocytes. *EMBO J.* 12:2881–2889.

Burleigh, B. A. 2000. Lysosome exocytosis and invasion of non-phagocytic host cells by *Trypanosom cruzi*, p. 195–212. *In* C. Tschudi and E. J. Pearce (ed.), *Biology of Parasitism.* Kluwer Academic Publishers, Boston, Mass.

Butterworth, A. E., D. W. Dunne, A. J. Fulford, J. H. Ouma, and R. F. Sturrock. 1996. Immunity and morbidity in *Schistosoma mansoni* infection: quantitative aspects. *Am. J. Trop. Med. Hyg.* 55(Suppl.):109–115.

Carruthers, V. B., O. K. Giddings, S. Hakansson, and L. D. Sibley. 2000a. *Toxoplasma gondii* uses sulfated proteoglycans for substrate and host cell attachment. *Infect. Immun.* 68:4005–4011.

Carruthers, V. B., G. D. Sherman, and L. D. Sibley. 2000b. The *Toxoplasma* adhesive protein MIC2 is proteolytically processed at multiple sites by two parasite-derived proteases. *J. Biol. Chem.* 275:14346–14353.

Carter, R., K. N. Mendis, L. H. Miller, L. Molineaux, and A. Saul. 2000. Malaria transmission-blocking vaccines—how can their development be supported? *Nat. Med.* 6:241–244.

Chan, M. S., G. F. Medley, P. Jaimison, and D. A. P. Bundy. 1994. The evaluation of potential global morbidity attributable to intestinal nematode infections. *Parasitology* 109:373–387.

Cheever, A. W., and G. S. Yap. 1997. Immunologic basis of disease and disease regulation in schistosomiasis. *Chem. Immunol.* 66:159–176.

Chen, Q., M. Wahlgren, and M. Schlichtherle. 2000. Molecular aspects of severe malaria. *Clin. Microbiol. Rev.* 13:439–450.

Cooper, P. J., I. Espinel, M. Espinel, R. H. Guderian, T. B. Nutman, W. Paredes, and M. Wieseman. 1999. Human onchocerciasis and tetanus vaccination: impact on the postvaccination antitetanus antibody response. *Infect. Immun.* 67:5951–5957.

Crawford, M. J., R. G. Donald, L. M. Fohl, K. M. Hager, J. C. Kissinger, M. G. Reynolds, D. S. Roos, B. Striepen, and W. J. Sullivan, Jr. 1999. Transport and trafficking: *Toxoplasma* as a model for *Plasmodium. Novartis Found. Symp.* 226:176–195, discussion 195–198.

de Almeida, A. B., and D. O. Freedman. 1999. Epidemiology and immunopathology of bancroftian filariasis. *Microbes Infect.* 1:1015–1022.

Dondorp, A. M., P. A. Kager J. Vreeken, and N. J. White. 2000. Abnormal blood flow and red blood cell deformability in severe malaria. *Parasitol. Today* 16:228–232.

Donelson, J. E., N. M. El-Sayed, and K. L. Hill. 1998. Multiple mechanisms of immune evasion by African trypanosomes. *Mol. Biochem. Parasitol.* 91:51–66.

Dunne, D. W., and E. J. Pearce. 1999. Immunology of hepato-splenic schistosomiasis mansoni: a human perspective. *Microbes Infect.* 17:553–560.

Engwerda, C. R., and P. M. Kaye. 2000. Organ-specific immune responses associated with infectious disease. *Immunol. Today* 21:73–78.

Espinosa-Cantellano, M., and A. Martinez-Palomo. 2000. Pathogenesis of intestinal amebiasis: from molecules to disease. *Clin. Microbiol. Rev.* 13:318–331.

Fowell, D. J., and R. M. Locksley. 1999. *Leishmania* major infection of inbred mice: unmasking genetic determinants of infectious diseases. *Bioessays* 21:510–518.

Frasch, A. C. 2000. Functional diversity in the trans-sialidase and mucin families in *Trypanosoma cruzi. Parasitol. Today* 16:282–286.

Frevert, U. 1994. Malaria sporozoite-hepatocyte interactions. *Exp. Parasitol.* 79:206–210.

Gazzinelli, R. T., M. Wysocka, S. Hieny, T. Scharton-Kersten, A. Cheever, R. Kuhn, W. Muller, G. Trinchieri, and A. Sher. 1996. In the absence of endogenous IL-10, mice acutely infected with *Toxoplasma gondii* succumb to a lethal immune response dependent on CD4[+] T cells and accompanied by overproduction of IL-12, IFN-gamma and TNF-alpha. *J. Immunol.* 157:798–805.

Gilchrist, C. A., and W. A. Petri. 1999. Virulence factors of *Entamoeba histolytica Curr. Opin. Microbiol.* 2:433–437.

Good, M. F., and D. L. Doolan. 1999. Immune effector mechanisms in malaria. *Curr. Opin. Immunol.* 11:412–419.

Griffiths, J. K., and S. Tzipori. 1998. Natural history and biology of *Cryptosporidium parvum. Adv. Parasitol.* 40:5–36.

Grzych, J. M., E. Pearce, A. Cheever, Z. A. Caulada, P. Caspar, S. Heiny, F. Lewis, and A. Sher. 1991. Egg deposition is the major stimulus for the production of Th2 cytokines in murine schistosomiasis mansoni. *J. Immunol.* 146:1322–1327.

Hall, L. R., and E. Pearlman. 1999. Pathogenesis of onchocercal keratitis (River blindness). *Clin. Microbiol. Rev.* 12:445–453.

Hayward, R. E., J. L. Derisi, S. Alfadhli, D. C. Kaslow, P. O. Brown, and P. K. Rathod. 2000. Shotgun DNA microarrays and stage-specific gene expression in *Plasmodium falciparum* malaria. *Mol. Microbiol.* 35:6–14.

Hertz, C. J., and J. M. Mansfield. 1999. IFN-gamma-dependent nitric oxide production is not linked to resistance in experimental African trypanosomiasis. *Cell Immunol.* 192:24–32.

Hoffman, S. L., A. A. Mahmoud, H. W. Murray, T. B. Nutman, and J. Pepin. 2000. Tropical medicine. *Br. Med. J.* 320:490–494.

Hunter, C. A., L. A. Ellis-Neyes, T. Slifer, S. Kanaly, G. Grunig, M. Fort, D. Rennick, and F. G. Araujo. 1997. IL-10 is required to prevent immune hyperactivity during infection with *Trypanosoma cruzi. J. Immunol.* 158:3311–3316.

Huston, C., and W. A. Petri, Jr. 1998. Host-pathogen interaction in amebiasis and progress in development. *Eur. J. Clin. Microbiol. Infect. Dis.* 17:601–614.

Jones, D. E., L. U. Buxbaum, and P. Scott. 2000. IL-4-independent inhibition of IL-12 responsiveness during *Leishmania amazonensis* infection. *J. Immunol.* 165:364–372.

Kierszenbaum, F. 1999. Chagas' disease and the autoimmunity hypothesis. *Clin. Microbiol. Rev.* **12:**210–223.

King, C. L., S. Mahanty, V. Kumaraswami, J. S. Abrams, J. Regunathan, K. Jayaraman, E. A. Ottesen, and T. B. Nutman. 1993. Cytokine control of parasite-specific anergy in human lymphatic filariasis. Preferential induction of a regulatory T helper type 2 lymphocyte subset. *J. Clin. Investig.* **92:**1667–1673.

Klotz, F. W., J. D. Haynes, and P. A. Orlandi. 1992. A malaria invasion receptor, the 175-kilodalton erythrocyte binding antigen of *Plasmodium falciparum,* recognizes the terminal Neu5Ac(alpha 2-3)Gal- sequences of glycophorin A. *J. Cell Biol.* **116:**901–909.

Laclette, J. P., C. B. Shoemaker, D. Richter, D. L. Arcos, N. Pante, C. Cohen, D. Bing, and A. Nicholson-Weller. 1992. Paramyosin inhibits complement C1. *J. Immunol.* **148:**124–128.

MacLean, L., M. Odiit, D. Okitoi, and J. M. Sternberg. 1999. Plasma nitrate and interferon gamma in Trypanosoma brucei rhodesiense infections: evidence that nitric oxide production is induced during both early blood-stage and late meningoencephalitic-stage infections. *Trans. R. Soc. Trop. Med. Hyg.* **93:**169–170.

Manger, I. D., and D. A. Relman. 2000. How the host 'sees' pathogens: global gene expression responses to infection. *Curr. Opin. Immunol.* **12:**215–221.

McDowell, M. A., and D. L. Sacks. 1999. Inhibition of host cell signal transduction by *Leishmania:* observations relevant to the selective impairment of IL-12 responses. *Curr. Opin. Microbiol.* **2:**438–443.

Mordue, D. G., N. Desai, M. Dustin, and L. D. Sibley. 1999. Invasion by *Toxoplasma gondii* establishes a moving junction that selectively excludes host cell plasma membrane proteins on the basis of their membrane anchoring. *J. Exp. Med.* **190:**1783–1792.

Mosser, D. M., and C. L. Karp. 1999. Receptor mediated subversion of macrophage cytokine production by intracellular pathogens. *Curr. Opin. Immunol.* **11:**406–411.

Murray, H. W., J. Pepin, T. B. Nutman, S. L. Hoffman, and A. A. Nahmoud. 2000. Tropical medicine. *Br. Med. J.* **320:**490–494.

Newbold, C. I. 1999. Antigenic variation in *Plasmodium falciparum:* mechanisms and consequences. *Curr. Opin. Microbiol.* **2:**420–425.

Neyer, L. E., G. Grunig, M. Fort, J. S. Remington, D. Rennick, and C. A. Hunter. 1997. Role of interleukin-10 in regulation of T-cell-dependent and T-cell-independent mechanisms of resistance to *Toxoplasma gondii. Infect. Immun.* **65:**1675–1682.

Ong, R. K., and R. L. Doyle. 1998. Tropical pulmonary eosinophilia. *Chest* **113:**1673–1679.

Overath, P., and T. Aebischer. 1999. Antigen presentation by macrophages harboring intravesicular pathogens. *Parasitol. Today* **15:**325–332.

Pastrana, D., V. N. Raghavan, P. FitzGerald, S. W. Eisinger, C. Metz, R. Bucala, R. P. Schleimer, C. Bickel, and A. L. Scott. 1998. Filarial nematode parasites secrete a homologue of the human cytokine macrophage migration inhibitory factor. *Infect. Immun.* **66:**5955–5963.

Perkins, M. E., and L. J. Rocco. 1988. Sialic acid-dependent binding of *Plasmodium falciparum* merozoite surface antigen, Pf200, to human erythrocytes. *J. Immunol.* **141:**3190–3196.

Plebanski, M., E. A. Lee, and A. V. Hill. 1997. Immune evasion in malaria: altered peptide ligands of the circumsporozoite protein. *Parasitology* **115**(Suppl.):S55–S66.

Reiner, S. L., and R. M. Locksley. 1995. The regulation of immunity to *Leishmania major. Annu. Rev. Immunol.* **13:**151–177.

Roos, D., J. A., Darling, K. M. Hager, J. Kissinger, M. G. Reynold, and B. Striepen. 2000. *Toxoplasma* as a model apicomplexan parasite: biochemistry, cell biology, molecular genetics, genomics and beyond, p. 143–168. *In* C. Tschudi and E. J. Pearce (ed.), *Biology of Parasitism.* Kluwer Academic Publishers, Boston, Mass.

Rosa Brunet, L., F. D. Finkelman, A. W. Cheever, M. A. Kopf, and E. J. Pearce. 1997. IL-4 protects against TNF-alpha-mediated cachexia and death during acute schistosomiasis. *J. Immunol.* **159:**777–785.

Rudenko, G. 1999. Genes involved in phenotypic and antigenic variation in African trypanosomes and malaria. *Curr. Opin. Microbiol.* **2:**651–656.

Sacks, D. L. 1992. The structure and function of the surface lipophosphoglycan on different developmental stages of *Leishmania* promastigotes. *Infect. Agents Dis.* **14:**200–206.

Seitz, H. M., and T. Trammer. 1998. Opportunistic infections caused by protozoan parasites. *Tokai J. Exp. Clin. Med.* **23:**249–257.

Tarleton, R. L. 1996. Immunity to *Trypanosoma cruzi,* p. 227–247. *In* S. H. E. Kaufmann (ed.), *Host Response to Intracellular Pathogens.* R. G. Landes Co., Austin, Tex.

Tarleton, R. L., M. J. Grusby, M. Postan, and L. H. Glimcher. 1996. *Trypanosoma cruzi* infection in MHC-deficient mice: further evidence for the role of both class I- and class II-restricted T cells in immune resistance and disease. *Int. Immunol.* **8:**13–22.

Tarleton, R. L., and L. Zhang. 1999. Chagas disease etiology: autoimmunity or parasite persistence? *Parasitol. Today* **15:**94–99.

Tarleton R. L., M. J. Grusby, and L. Zhang. 2000. Increased susceptibility of Stat4-deficient and enhanced resistance in Stat6-deficient mice to infection with *Trypanosoma cruzi. J. Immunol.* **165:**1520–1525.

Vidal, K., and P. M. Allen. 1996. The effect of endogenous altered peptide ligands on peripheral T-cell responses. *Semin. Immunol.* **8:**117–122.

Weiss, L. M., and K. Kim. 2000. The development and biology of bradyzoites of *Toxoplasma gondii. Front. Biosci.* **5:**D391–D405.

Welsh, R. M., and J. M. McNally. 1999. Immune deficiency, immune silencing, and clonal exhaustion of T cell responses during viral infections. *Curr. Opin. Microbiol.* **2:**382–387.

White, A. C., Jr., P. Robinson, and R. Kuhn. 1997. *Taenia solium* cysticercosis: host-parasite interactions and the immune response. *Chem. Immunol.* **66:**209–230.

Wilson, M. E., B. M. Young, B. L. Davidson, K. A. Mente, and S. E. McGowan. 1998. The importance of TGF-beta in murine visceral leishmaniasis. *J. Immunol.* **161:**6148–6155.

Yap, G. S., and A. Sher. 1999. Cell-mediated immunity to *Toxoplasma gondii:* initiation, regulation and effector function. *Immunobiology* **201:**240–247.

Immunology of Infectious Diseases
Edited by S. H. E. Kaufmann, A. Sher, and R. Ahmed
© 2002 ASM Press, Washington, D.C.

Chapter 4

Overview of the Viral Pathogens

JONATHAN W. YEWDELL AND JACK R. BENNINK

Viruses are small segments of nucleic acid wrapped in a protein or lipoprotein shell. They have the ability to penetrate host cells and use the host machinery to reproduce. At their simplest, viruses consist of a few genes that encode a nucleic acid polymerase and several proteins that comprise the virion. At their most complex, viruses contain several hundred genes encoding numerous viral structural proteins, proteins that alter cellular metabolism to favor virus replication (or enable virus to persist in a latent state), and proteins that modify the host immune response to favor virus transmission. Viruses are always completely dependent on cells for the production of energy, the provision of raw materials (amino acids, lipids, and sugars), and protein synthesis.

Viruses are an inescapable product of evolution, and every living species is accompanied by a unique set of viruses capable of infecting species members. Virus sets overlap considerably and even dynamically, since viruses exhibit an extremely high mutation rate relative to their hosts and are constantly changing genetically, with the consequence that their host range is in constant flux. Many hundreds of viruses are known to be capable of infecting humans, and there are probably thousands more that remain to be discovered.

Viruses, like all life forms, are selected simply to replicate and do not particularly care to harm their hosts. Indeed, killing all of their hosts is a suicidal mechanism, and over time evolution selects for a balance between viruses and their hosts. On the other hand, the genetic variability of viruses means that mutants with enhanced potential for causing mayhem are constantly generated. Moreover, encounters between species enable the introduction of new viruses, with the possibility of tremendous lethality for the new host until a new equilibrium is reached. Con-

sequently, all species, from *Escherichia coli* to redwoods to blue whales, evolve strategies for controlling virus replication. How this is achieved by simple organisms is an interesting question that is beyond the scope of this chapter (but well worth pondering). Vertebrates have gone to great lengths to protect themselves from viruses (and other pathogens, of course) by evolving intricate systems of innate and adaptive immunity.

There are at least four practical reasons for immunologists to have a good working knowledge of virology. The first is that viruses remain a major cause of human morbidity and mortality and pose a constant potential for causing devastating plagues (Table 1). Second, viruses are important vectors for vaccines against viral and nonviral pathogens. Third, viruses are evolution's gift to gene therapists. Finally, viruses are extremely useful experimental tools and probes for understanding the biology of cells and organisms. Given the brevity of this chapter, we have set only the modest goal of providing a simple introduction to viruses, with the hope of piquing the reader's interest to study the subject in more depth. We encourage readers to explore in detail *Principles of Virology* (Flint et al., 2000), a marvelous textbook with superb diagrams and figures that provides profound insights into the biology and evolution of viruses. There are a number of other excellent texts that cover more specialized aspects of virology or virus-host interactions (Coffin et al., 1997; Ewald, 1994; Fields et al., 1996; Granoff and Webster, 1999; McCance, 1998; Plotkin and Orenstein, 1999; Richman et al., 1997; Scheld et al., 1998, 1999). In addition, throughout this chapter we refer to textbooks and reviews as jumping-off points for those who would like to further explore a given topic.

Jonathan W. Yewdell and Jack R. Bennink • Laboratory of Viral Diseases, National Institute of Allergy and Infectious Diseases, Bethesda, MD 20892-0440.

Table 1. Leading virus-associated diseases[a]

Cause of disease	No. of deaths	DALYs[b]	No. of carriers
Respiratory viruses (pneumonia and influenza)[c]	3,500,000	83,000,000	
Gastrointestinal viruses (all causes)[c]	2,200,000	73,000,000	
HIV	2,285,000	71,000,000	33,600,000
Measles virus	888,000	30,000,000	
Hepatitis virus	92,000	1,700,000	
Chronic hepatitis B virus	700,000[d]		350,000,000
Chronic hepatitis C virus			170,000,000
Dengue virus	15,000	558,000	
Japanese encephalitis virus	3,000	503,000	
Poliovirus	2,000	213,000	

[a] World Health Organization (1999).
[b] DALY, disability-adjusted life year, defined as disability years lost in 1998 due to the disease.
[c] Includes nonviral infectious disease mortality.
[d] Chronic hepatitis B contributes to these deaths from liver cirrhosis and cancer.

STRUCTURAL PROPERTIES

Virions range in diameter from 18 nm (parvoviruses) to 450 nm (poxviruses) (amounting to a 25-fold difference in diameter and a 15,000-fold difference in volume). They may be composed of just a few different proteins or many tens of proteins, and their genomes range in size from 3.2 kb (hepadnaviruses) to 350 kb (iridoviruses) (Table 2) (Chiu et al., 1997).

For the purposes of the immune system, the most important structural distinction in viruses is their outer covering. Naked viruses possess a protein shell, while enveloped viruses possess an envelope derived from host cell membrane (usually the plasma membrane, but some viruses use membranes from the endoplasmic reticulum or Golgi complex). Viral envelopes are composed of cellular lipids and viral proteins. Most enveloped viruses contain minimal amounts of host proteins, but others are more pro-

Table 2. Virus classification

Virus family (abbreviation)	Genome[a]	Genome size (kb)	Coat
DNA viruses			
Adenoviridae (ADE)	DS DNA	36–38	Naked
Baculoviridae	DS DNA	100	Enveloped
Hepadnaviridae (HEP)	DS/NS DNA	3.2	Enveloped
Herpesviridae (HER)	DS DNA	120–200	Enveloped
Iridoviridae	DS DNA	150–350	Naked/enveloped
Papovaviridae (PAP)	DS DNA	45–55	Naked
Parvoviridae (PAR)	NS DNA	18–26	Naked
Poxviridae (POX)	DS DNA	170–200	Enveloped
RNA viruses			
Arenaviridae (ARE)	NS RNA	10–14	Enveloped
Astroviridae (AST)	PS RNA	7.2–7.9	Naked
Birnaviridae	DS RNA	7	Naked
Bunyaviridae (BUN)	NS RNA	13.5–21	Enveloped
Caliciviridae (CAL)	PS RNA	8	Naked
Coronaviridae (COR)	PS RNA	16–21	Enveloped
Filoviridae (FIL)	NS RNA	12.7	Enveloped
Flaviviridae (FLA)	PS RNA	10	Enveloped
Orthomyxoviridae (ORTH)	NS RNA	13.6	Enveloped
Paramyxoviridae (PARA)	NS RNA	16–20	Enveloped
Picornaviridae (PIC)	PS RNA	7.2–8.4	Naked
Reoviridae (REO)	DS RNA	22–27	Naked
Retroviridae (RET)	PS RNA	3.5–9	Enveloped
Rhabdoviridae (RHA)	NS RNA	13–16	Enveloped
Togaviridae (TOG)	PS RNA	12	Enveloped

[a] DS, double stranded; NS, minus strand; PS, plus strand.

miscuous and may contain relatively large amounts of host proteins, including class I or II molecules of the major histocompatibility complex (MHC). The presence of such polymorphic host molecules provides potential additional targets for immune recognition.

The structures of both naked and enveloped viruses are highly repetitive, providing the immune system an opportunity for a high-avidity interaction on the basis of multivalent recognition by low-affinity receptors. Enveloped viruses usually require membrane integrity for infection, making them vulnerable to the complement system or membrane-disrupting peptides. Enveloped viruses also tend to be more fragile than nonenveloped (naked) viruses, making their transmission more dependent on intimate contact between hosts. Some of these viruses can be transferred only by exchange of body fluids. The surface proteins of both naked and enveloped viruses are highly resistant to proteases present in extracellular fluids and, when required, even to the harsh conditions of the upper gastrointestinal tract.

The outer virion shell protects the viral nucleic acid, which is complexed to viral structural proteins that enable its packaging into the virion during virus biogenesis. Viruses are grouped into six categories based on the nucleic acid present in infectious virions and the immediate nucleic acid product produced in infected cells: minus-strand RNA (noncoding) transcribed into plus-strand RNA, plus-strand RNA transcribed into minus-strand RNA, plus-strand RNA transcribed into minus-strand DNA, double-stranded RNA, single-stranded DNA, and double-stranded DNA. Many viruses carry their own nucleic acid polymerases to initiate the infectious cycle, which can occur either in the cytosol or the nucleus.

A common feature of animal viruses is their high particle-to-infectivity ratio, i.e., the number of particles required to initiate an infection. With very few exceptions, this is greater than 10, commonly greater than 100, and occasionally even greater than 1,000. It is difficult to determine the extent to which this reflects structural defects in a high percentage of viruses or a relatively low probability of even a perfect virion for initiating infection. Since this is invariably determined in vitro, it is unclear whether the ratio is higher in vivo, as seems likely. If structural defects are common, they are relatively minor, at least as far as the humoral immune system is concerned, since there is little evidence to suggest that distinct antibody responses are elicited by infectious versus noninfectious virions. Indeed, the induction of antibody responses by purposely inactivated viruses is a principal strategy of antiviral vaccination.

The prodigious reproductive potential of viruses gives them extreme latitude in producing mutants—given hundreds of offspring each with a generation of time of less than 12 h, it is advantageous to possess a high mutation rate, many orders of magnitude higher than multicellular organisms such as ourselves. The high mutation rate, in conjunction with selection pressure for packaging efficiency, makes multiple copies of genes in a virion a liability, and only retroviruses are known to deliberately incorporate more than a single copy of their genomes into virions.

STRATEGIES OF VIRUS ENTRY

Organism

Virus survival requires transmission between hosts. The route of transmission is a critical aspect of viral biology since it dictates (or vice versa) in what cells the infection of host is initiated and what cells must produce the virus for transmission to occur. The transmission of a given virus is usually restricted to a single anatomical location, which provides an opportunity to focus immunity to a given pathogen to a limited number of sites in an organism (Table 3). For example, influenza virus and other respiratory viruses which replicate in the columnar epithelium of the upper airway are transmitted strictly through this portal, and a local immune response in the upper airway is sufficient to block infection. By contrast, enteric viruses like rotavirus infect only via the gastrointestinal tract. Vaccines to these agents should therefore focus on generating effective immune responses in the respiratory and gastrointestinal systems, respectively. Similarly, virus dissemination can be prevented by local immunity at the site of transmission. Thus, human immunodeficiency virus (HIV)-infected individuals could be potentially removed from the virus transmission cycle, without requiring global eradication of virus replication, by immune removal of virus from the organs of dissemination (Flint et al., 2000; Mims et al., 2001).

As the largest single organ in humans and the most external, the skin is an obvious target for initiation of viral infections, sufficiently obvious, in fact, that the cornified epithelium is an extremely effective barrier against virus transmission and only a few viruses have managed the trick of penetrating this barrier on their own. Transmission through the skin can be achieved by physical introduction past the keratinocytes by either natural (insect or animal bites) or artificial (hypodermic) means. In the former case,

Table 3. Sites of viral infection[a]

Skin
RNA viruses
Coxsackievirus (PIC)
Human immunodeficiency virus (RET)
Measles virus (PAR)
Rubella virus (TOG)

DNA viruses
B virus (HER)
Cytomegalovirus (HER)
Epstein-Barr virus (HER)
Herpes simplex virus (HER)
Human herpesvirus 6 (HER)
Human herpesvirus 8 (HER)
Orf virus (POX)
Papillomavirus (PAP)
Parvovirus B19 (PAR)
Molluscum contagiosum virus (POX)
Vaccinia virus (POX)
Varicella-zoster virus (HER)

Lymphoid system and macrophages
RNA viruses
Alphavirus (TOG)
Ebola virus (FIL)
Enterovirus (PIC)
Flavivirus (FLA)
Guanarito virus (ARE)
Human immunodeficiency virus (RET)
Junin virus (ARE)
Lassa virus (ARE)
Lymphocytic choriomeningitis virus (ARE)
Machupo virus (ARE)
Marburg virus (FIL)
Mumps virus (PAR)
Poxvirus (POX)
Rubella virus (TOG)
Sabia virus (ARE)

Respiratory system
RNA viruses
Coronavirus (COR)
Enteroviruses (PIC)
Influenza virus types A and B (ORTH)
Measles virus (PAR)
Parainfluenza virus types 1, 2, and 3 (PARA)
Polyomavirus (PAP)
Respiratory syncytial virus (PARA)
Rhinoviruses (PIC)

DNA viruses
Adenovirus (ADE)
B virus (HER)
Cytomegalovirus (HER)
Epstein-Barr virus (HER)
Herpes simplex virus (HER)
Varicella-zoster virus (HER)

Central nervous system
RNA viruses
California encephalitis virus (BUN)
Colorado tick fever virus (REO)
Coxsackievirus (PIC)
Eastern equine encephalitis virus (TOG)
Echovirus (PIC)
Influenza virus (ORTH)
Japanese encephalitis virus (FLA)
Human immunodeficiency virus type 1 (RET)
Lymphocytic choriomeningitis virus (ARE)
Measles virus (PAR)
Mumps virus (PAR)
Murray Valley fever virus (FLA)
Poliovirus (PIC)
Rabies virus (RHA)
St. Louis encephalitis virus (FLA)
Tick-borne encephalitis virus (FLA)
Venezuelan equine encephalitis virus (TOG)
Western equine encephalitis virus (TOG)
West Nile fever virus (FLA)

Heart and muscle
RNA viruses
Alphavirus (FLA)
Coxsackievirus (PIC)
Dengue virus (FLA)
Echovirus (PIC)
Hepatitis A virus (PIC)
Human immunodeficiency virus (RET)
Influenza virus (ORTH)
Lymphocytic choriomeningitis virus (ARE)
Measles virus (PAR)
Mumps virus (PAR)
Poliovirus (PIC)
Rabies virus (RHA)
Rubella virus (TOG)
Yellow fever virus (FLA)

DNA viruses
Adenovirus (ADE)
Cytomegalovirus (HER)
Epstein-Barr virus (HER)
Hepatitis B virus (HEP)
Herpes simplex virus (HER)
Varicella-zoster virus (HER)

Liver
RNA viruses
Ebola virus (FIL)
Echovirus (PIC)
Enterovirus (PIC)
Hepatitis A virus (PIC)
Hepatitis C virus (FLA)
Hepatitis D virus (DEL)
Hepatitis E virus
Hepatitis G virus
Junin virus (ARE)
Lassa virus (ARE)
Machupo virus (ARE)
Marburg virus (FIL)
Rubella virus (TOG)
Rift Valley fever virus (BUN)
Yellow fever virus (FLA)

DNA viruses
Epstein-Barr virus (HER)
Cytomegalovirus (HER)
Human herpesvirus 6 (HER)
Human herpesvirus 7 (HER)
Varicella-zoster virus (HER)

Hemorrhagic fever
RNA viruses
Congo-Crimean hemorrhagic fever (BUN)
Dengue virus (FLA)
Ebola virus (FIL)
Guanarito virus (ARE)
Hantaan virus (HAN)
Junin virus (ARE)
Kyasanur Forest virus (FLA)
Lassa virus (ARE)
Machupo virus (ARE)
Marbug virus (FIL)
Omsk virus (FLA)
Rift Valley fever virus (BUN)
Sabia virus (ARE)

Gonads
RNA viruses
Ebola virus (FIL)
Marburg virus (FIL)
Mumps virus (PAR)

DNA viruses
Adenovirus (ADE)
B virus (HER)
Cytomegalovirus (HER)
Epstein-Barr virus (HER)
Herpes simplex virus types 1 and 2 (HER)
Human herpesvirus 6 (HER)
Polyomavirus (PAP)
Vaccinia virus (POX)
Varicella-zoster virus (HER)

Kidneys
RNA viruses
Ebola virus (FIL)
Marburg virus (FIL)
Polyomavirus (PAP)

DNA viruses
Adenovirus (ADE)
Cytomegalovirus (HER)

Gastrointestinal tract
RNA viruses
Astrovirus (AST)
Calicivirus (CAL)
Rotavirus types A, B, and C (REO)

DNA viruses
Adenovirus (ADE)

Liver
DNA viruses
Adenovirus (ADE)
Epstein-Barr virus (HER)
Hepatitis B virus (HEP)
Herpes simplex virus (HER)
Varicella-zoster virus (HER)

Eye
RNA viruses
Coxsackievirus type A24 (PIC)
Enterovirus type 70 (PIC)
Influenza virus (ORTH)
Human immunodeficiency virus (RET)
Measles virus (PAR)
Mumps virus (PAR)
Newcastle disease virus (PAR)
Rubella virus (TOG)

DNA viruses
Adenovirus (ADE)
Cytomegalovirus (HER)
Epstein-Barr virus (HER)
Herpes simplex virus (HER)
Molluscum contagiosum virus (POX)
Papillomavirus (PAP)
Vaccinia virus (POX)
Varicella-zoster virus (HER)

[a] Abbreviations of families are defined in Table 2.

transmission may be a natural part of the virus life cycle or may be unrelated to virus evolution (but still detrimental to unlucky individuals infected with West Nile virus, for example). Mammalian (or avian) cells differ considerably from insect cells, and the ability to productively infect members of both phyla implies an importance in cross-species transmission to viral survival.

Cells

Viral replication requires delivery of the viral nucleic acid to the cytosol, where it can initiate the replication cycle immediately or after transport to the nucleus. Penetration can occur in two locales: either directly at the plasma membrane or after internalization into an endosome or other internal cellular membrane system (e.g., some viruses are thought to penetrate cells from the endoplasmic reticulum). Enveloped viruses penetrate by fusion of their membranes with cell membranes, while naked viruses penetrate by disrupting cell membranes. In either case, viruses must first adhere to the target cell by binding to a cellular receptor, which can be virtually any molecule on the cell surface (Fig. 1). The specificity of cellular receptors ranges from highly specific, e.g., a ligand expressed in a single cell type in a single tissue, to completely promiscuous, e.g., a molecule expressed by every cell, such as sialic acid, which is a receptor for many viruses. In the former case, the receptor is usually responsible for viral tropism, while in the latter case, viral tropism depends on other factors (such as the route of entry into the host and the ability to penetrate the cell or replicate once inside). Viral penetration is usually a complicated affair that entails conformational alterations in viral surface proteins and interactions with additional cell surface proteins. There are ample opportunities for the immune system to block penetration by preventing viral binding to host cells or by preventing downstream events in the penetration and uncoating process (Berger, 1997; Doms, 2000; Kasamatsu and Nakanishi, 1998; Klasse et al., 1998; McDermott and Murphy, 2000; Norkin, 1995; Sodeik, 2000; Whittaker et al., 2000).

The requirement of viral genomes to reach the cytosol provides an early opportunity for recognition by the adaptive immune system in the absence of viral gene expression. Antigenic peptides can be generated from viral proteins that accompany the viral genomes into the cytosol. Since peptide generation is often quite inefficient, this usually requires that thousands of copies of the source protein be delivered, which limits this pathway to highly abundant proteins from large viruses. There is evidence, however, that this skews adaptive responses in some systems.

OUTCOMES OF CELLULAR INFECTION

Viral penetration of cells has four potential outcomes (with all gradations in between). First, the cell may be completely inhospitable and the viral proteins and nucleic acids are disposed of with minimal perturbation of the host cells. Second, viral replication initiates but fails to produce infectious progeny, with consequences for the cell ranging from minimal transient perturbations to death. Third, viral replication results in the generation of infectious progeny and

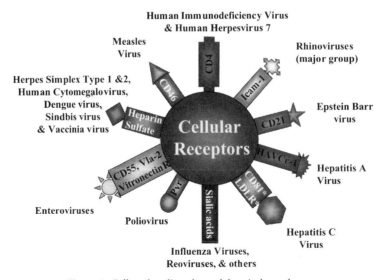

Figure 1. Cell surface ligands used for viral attachment.

cells either are killed immediately or remain persistently infected and continue to function as they produce progeny viruses. Fourth, the virus enters a latent state and essentially disappears until it is triggered to reactivate, with the production of infectious progeny.

These outcomes are not mutually exclusive, and even in a given individual harboring a virus, these processes can occur simultaneously depending on the nature of the cell infected and the exact conditions of infection (number of viruses infecting the cell [multiplicity of infection], exposure of the cell to cytokines, cell cycle status). As always, evolution selects only for the transmission of virus between hosts (the selection of viruses replicating within any given organism is only an intermediate in the ultimate process). In some circumstances, even a nonproductive infection in cells may be selected evolutionarily if it facilitates virus transmission. For example, a virus may nonproductively infect immune cells, disabling the cells and thereby enhancing viral growth in productively infected cells. On the other hand, most examples of nonproductive infection are not a result of evolutionary selection but simply an example of the law of biological entropy: there are many more ways for things to go wrong than to go right.

The mechanisms that viruses use to achieve these outcomes vary tremendously with the virus, but all viruses must fulfill several basic tasks: (i) produce mRNA to generate viral proteins on cellular ribosomes; (ii) replicate their genome; (iii) assemble their genomes with viral (and sometimes cellular) proteins, and release progeny from the cells (Doms et al., 1993; Garoff et al., 1998); and (iv) modify the host cellular metabolism to optimize viral replication.

A productive viral infection usually results in the generation of hundreds to thousands (or more) progeny. The shortest infectious cycles can be completed in 4 h. This capacity for replication provides a serious challenge to the immune system, since just three or four infectious cycles over the course of a single day can be sufficient to produce enough virus to infect every cell in a target organ. The host must therefore mount an immediate response to such rapid cytopathic viruses, and this is, no doubt, one of the major selective forces for the evolution of the innate immune system.

Coordinated Gene Expression

Following cellular penetration, viruses usually have a precise plan of attack that entails the temporally coordinated transcription and expression of subsets of their genes. Within any given segment of the infectious cycle, different viral gene products are often expressed in widely different quantities depending on the function of the gene product. This plan can vary from cell type to cell type, and abortive infections often result from failing to successfully negotiate the transition from one stage to another. Often the plan of expression is based on genome replication, and viral genes can be classified as early (before genome replication) and late (after genome replication). The times of genome replication can vary widely but generally are between 2 and 12 h after infection. At the great risk of oversimplification, the enzymes required for viral replication and modification of cellular functions are expressed immediately on penetration whereas many of the proteins that make up virions are produced late in the infectious cycle. For the adaptive immune system, the most important aspect of coordinated gene expression is that not all infected cells express the full range of viral gene products, and antigens presented by infected professional antigen-presenting cells may be limited to early-gene products.

GENETIC INSTABILITY OF VIRUSES

Genetic instability is the sine qua non of viruses. Indeed, the mutation rate of RNA viruses is sufficiently high that despite possessing a tiny genome relative to other life forms, virtually every individual in a population is still unique. DNA viruses are generally more stable, but they still exhibit mutation rates several orders of magnitude higher than those of host cells. It is therefore necessary to think of viruses as dynamic populations of related genomes and not as monolithic entities (Domingo and Holland, 1997; Koonin, 1992; Shadan and Villarreal, 1996).

Although virus recombination is probably a relatively infrequent occurrence, it still is probably very important for most viruses, which have a haploid genome and therefore can profit by a mechanism that enables them to escape from lethal mutations. Indeed, it is often observed that serial plaque purification of viruses ultimately results in the generation of poorly replicating viruses, suggesting that recombination is probably an important mechanism for maintaining functional genomes. A number of RNA viruses foster recombination by possessing segmented genomes. Recombination also occurs as a result of polymerases shifting from one genome to another (predominantly in RNA viruses) and of strand breakage and rejoining (predominantly in DNA viruses).

The genetic instability of RNA viruses in particular makes them elusive targets for the immune system. For many viruses, mutants that escape neutralization by monoclonal antibodies arise with a frequency of 10^{-5}. This can result in antigenic drift, in which the humoral immune system selects for neutralization-resistant mutants. This, of course, is a significant problem in influenza vaccination. Influenza virus, as a segmented virus, also undergoes antigenic shift, in which the viral surface proteins are exchanged in recombination events. This can result in the introduction of novel surface proteins from animal influenza viruses and hence in devastating epidemics. Hepatitis C virus, an increasingly important human pathogen, is so highly variable that multiple serotypes are often isolated from the same individual.

For genetic instability to be of any use to the virus, the resulting gene products must be sufficiently plastic to utilize the mutations to produce a novel (and useful) phenotype. This is not uniform among viral proteins, and it is commonly found that mutation rates among viral proteins vary hugely. At the risk of oversimplification, the extracellular domains of membrane proteins of envelope viruses demonstrate the greatest flexibility for accepting mutations while proteins involved in protein-protein interactions, for example the coat proteins of naked viruses or viral replication proteins, are less tolerant of mutations.

Capturing Host Genes

Another potential source of genetic variability is the capture of host genes. This happens most often with retroviruses due to their unique life cycle, which entails integration into the host genome (the retroviral capture and mutation of host cell genes involved in cellular proliferation led to the identification of oncogenes as altered cellular genes). Small viruses are under heavy selection pressure to minimize genome size, which makes host genes difficult to swallow.

For the large DNA viruses such as *Herpesviridae* and *Poxviridae* family members, however, insertion of even large amounts of foreign genes has no discernible effect on virus function, so there is the potential for capturing host genes. These viruses often possess sophisticated programs for manipulating host immunity, and clearly these genes are often derived from the host. Such genes are, however, usually distantly related to host genes, so that these events are probably extremely infrequent. Thus, for all viruses but retroviruses, capture of host genes was probably important in their early evolution but is less important over a human time frame (Alcami and Koszinowski, 2000; Becker, 1996; McFadden et al., 1998; Tortorella et al., 2000; Weinberg, 1997).

TISSUE TROPISM

A critical aspect of viral infections is that replication is usually limited to anatomical locations and cell types (Table 3). There are a number of contributing factors. The first is physical isolation of viruses due to anatomical barriers. For example, enteric viruses may never have the opportunity to escape the gastrointestinal system, even though they would be capable of infecting other cell types. The second is the specificity of viral receptors and the limited distribution of cellular factors required for viral penetration. HIV, for example, requires the cellular expression of CD4, which is limited to a small subset of cells, and also requires host cells to express certain chemokine receptors to enable fusion of viral and cellular membranes. The third factor is that even given entry to the cytosol, viruses can be rather finicky about replicating, and very few (if any) have the ability to productively replicate in every cell type in the body. This implies a requirement for nonhousekeeping cellular genes for productive infection, but identifying cellular gene products that positively (or negatively) influence virus infection is extremely difficult in practice.

One aspect of viral tropism is particularly important to the immune system. If viruses are unable to infect professional antigen-presenting cells, an alternative mechanism must be used for presenting viral antigens to naïve CD8 T cells. It is thought that under these circumstances presentation occurs via cross-priming, a process in which professional antigen-presenting cells acquire viral proteins produced by infected cells and process them for presentation to T cells.

Kinetic Aspects of Infection

Many viruses replicate in a host by a program that requires the dissemination of virus from one organ to another. Virus dissemination can occur via either the blood or the lymph. Since lymphatics are more accessible to extracellular particles than are capillaries, this is a more likely route of dissemination (the lymphatics function to collect foreign material from the periphery to the lymph nodes). Viruses also have an opportunity to reach the blood via the lymphatics, if they manage to avoid sequestration in the lymph nodes on the way to the venous system.

Virions probably have a difficult time spreading in this direct manner, and in many cases virus spread is mediated by infected white blood cells (red blood cells cannot be infected since they lack essential biosynthetic functions). Since these cells have the intrinsic ability to leave the blood or lymph and infiltrate tissues (diapedesis), they can provide a direct route for virus entry into organs. Lacking a cellular carrier, viruses must rely on other ways to breach the barriers that guard the tissues. Some viruses are capable of being transcytosed by endothelial cells into the underlying tissues. In tissues with sinusoids (adrenals, bone marrow, liver, and spleen), viruses may be transcytosed by resident macrophages that line the sinusoids. In other organs (kidneys, pancreas, and gut), many of the capillaries are fenestrated, providing a direct route for viral penetration. Finally, some connective tissues, muscles, and the central nervous system (CNS) are highly resistant to direct penetration, since the endothelial cells of the capillaries are backed by a formidable basement membrane. In this case, virus penetration from the blood probably occurs by diapedesis.

The pattern of virus spread can be dependent on the mechanism of virus maturation. Enveloped viruses can dictate whether they mature from the apical or luminal surface of polarized epithelial cells by taking advantage of the signals used by the cells to maintain polarization. Respiratory viruses often mature from the apical surface of epithelial cells, limiting their spread to the surface of the airway. Presumably this is a way of increasing their chance of transmission by maximizing their concentration in respiratory fluids. Other viruses with less restricted tissue tropism mature from the basolateral surface. This increases their chances of hematogenous spread.

Viruses capable of infecting neurons (neurotropic viruses) take advantage of the transport capacity of neurons to travel from the periphery to the ganglia or the CNS. Such traffic can be bidirectional. Herpesviruses, the geniuses of latency, persist in a latent state in the ganglia or spine and upon reactivation are transported to the periphery, where they bud from sensory nerve termini to be transmitted to new hosts via intimate contact. Rabies virus travels to the CNS from sensory neurons in the vicinity of an animal bite, multiplies in the CNS, and then leaves via efferent neurons to the salivary glands, where virus is manufactured for saliva-borne transmission. Incredibly, the viral replication in the CNS is sufficiently specific to induce the rabid behavior essential to transmission. All of this is accomplished by using the information encoded by just 12,000 nucleotides (Scheld et al., 1991).

Another mode of virus spread is from mother to fetus. For noncytopathogenic viruses, this can ensure virus maintenance in a species. For retroviruses, which integrate into the genome, the line between virus and host becomes blurred, as viral genes are transmitted in the genome. For cytopathic viruses, this mode of transmission may have catastrophic medical consequences to the host but little evolutionary benefit to the virus, since a dead fetus or infant has little potential for transmitting the virus to another host.

SPECIES SPECIFICITY

The fact that receptor-independent tissue tropism of viruses is common indicates that virus replication in cells is often a complicated business that in many circumstances requires very specific factors in differentiated cells. It should come as no surprise, then, that most viruses have a very limited capacity to infect other species. Even in situations where this can occur, the features of infection in different hosts may differ enormously. The practical consequence for biomedical research is that it is extremely difficult to find accurate animal models for human viral diseases. For immunologists it is crucial to recognize that different elements of the immune system may be used for combating infections with the same virus in different species. Moreover, molecules that evolve to interfere with host responses may be highly species specific and can even interact with different target molecules in other species.

An important element in virus evolution becomes apparent when viruses cross species barriers, particularly when the species are closely related. Very few viral infections of natural hosts have high mortality rates—this is a consequence of maximizing transmission, where it rarely benefits a virus to kill the host. Just how easy it is for a virus to increase its lethality becomes apparent when the virus jumps to a species related sufficiently closely to the natural host to support virus replication. In this case, the brakes on virus replication imposed by natural selection may be inoperative and the virus can be highly lethal. Indeed, the most virulent viruses for humans result from such species jumping. These include herpes B virus (African green monkeys), filoviruses such as Lassa fever and Marburg viruses (natural host unknown), HIV (chimpanzee or other primates), and hantaviruses (mice). Most of these viruses do not pose much of a public health risk, since their transmission between humans is limited. On the other hand, the potential danger of a newly introduced virus is illustrated by HIV, which in the course of adapting to a new host will kill tens of millions. Tragically, the high rate of transmission of HIV in sub-Saharan Africa is providing a real-time lesson in the coevolution of virus and host. This horror is not without precedent in human history: the arrival of the Europeans in the Americas introduced a number of viral diseases (smallpox and influenza) that the native peoples had not experienced in many generations (if ever). The devastating consequences of these diseases were a major factor in the rapid ascendancy of the Europeans.

The balance between host and virus is most vividly illustrated by the introduction of the rabbitpox virus myxoma virus into the rabbit population of Australia. European rabbits were established in Australia from a few individuals and consequently exhibited very little genetic polymorphism. Myxoma virus evolved in a different species of rabbit, where it causes skin lesions, but was remarkably lethal for the Australian rabbits, with a 99.8% mortality rate. A single year, however, was sufficient for the selection both of rabbits resistant to lethal infection and of less virulent virus stains, with net results that the virus was more efficiently transmitted in the population and rabbits continue their assault on Australian ecosystems.

PATHOGENICITY

Viruses need not be pathogenic, since, as discussed above, evolution selects viruses for maximal transmissibility between hosts. Pathogenicity can be a positive factor in transmissibility, e.g., for respiratory viruses, which are most efficiently spread by coughing, sneezing, and the outpouring of mucus in response to destruction of the respiratory epithelium. A special case is when virus infection of immune cells causes a generalized immunosuppression, resulting in infection with other organisms that favor the transmission of the original infecting virus (Fauci, 1996; Levy, 1998; Mims et al., 2001; Nathanson, 1997; Oldstone, 1996; Wright, 1996).

Pathogenicity can be caused by direct destruction of cells by the virus, secretion or release of toxic substances by virus-infected cells, or the host immune response to the virus. In the last example, the process of inflammation itself may cause tissue destruction or direct immune recognition of virus-infected cells. Inasmuch as this is a normal protective response, it is not truly immunopathological. A relatively uncommon outcome of viral infections is transformation of infected cells into benign or malignant tumor cells. This can be a direct effect of viral proteins, as occurs for human papillomavirus, or an indirect effect of cellular proliferation induced by chronic virus infections, as occurs for hepatitis B virus.

Hepatitis B virus infection is one example where the immune system steps over the line of protection into the realm of immunopathology. Viral replication in hepatocytes appears to be innocuous, with the damage coming over many years from virus-specific CD8 T cells that infiltrate the liver and destroy infected cells. Hepatitis B virus infections (which feature the release of enormous amounts of virus into the plasma) also provide another example of immunopathology in the deposition of immune complexes composed of viral antigens and antibodies. This can

destroy the kidneys. Surprisingly, this is not known to occur for other virus infections in humans. Less well established are cases of immune mimicry, when viral antigens induce responses that cross-react with cellular antigens, breaking down the normally operative tolerance mechanisms. Tolerance to self antigens may also be subverted by the process of inflammation induced by viral infections.

VULNERABILITY TO IMMUNE ATTACK

Whether by choice or necessity, viruses offer numerous opportunities for attack by the vertebrate immune system. The earliest is to prevent infection at the site of entry. This can occur by either non-antibody- or antibody-mediated mechanisms. Protection against membrane viruses can be mediated by defensins (small proteins that are secreted by neutrophils, monocytes, and Paneth cells and that compromise membrane integrity), complement components, and possibly other serum proteins. Natural antibodies, i.e., antibodies induced without exposure to the pathogen or closely related viruses, can also play a protective role against infection. Humans produce large amounts of antibodies specific for terminal galactose residues linked to a penultimate galactose by a 1-3α bond. This oligosaccharide is absent in human and other primates but is present in gut bacteria, which induce the antibody response. Interestingly, other mammals and insects can also generate this oligosaccharide linkage, and membrane viruses produced by these species may express surface glycoproteins with the oligosaccharide. It appears that humans are protected by infection from a number of viruses by such antibodies. Antibodies induced by prior exposure to a virus (or viral vaccine) are often the most efficient means of protection against viral infection and can play an important role in clearing an infection.

A number of features of virus replication in host cells result in detection of the virus and counterattack by the immune system. First, the replication of RNA viruses (and even DNA viruses) results in the presence of unusually large amounts of double-stranded RNA in the cytoplasm. This rapidly triggers the production of interferons by infected cells. Interferon induction is perhaps the most critical early warning signal in virus infections, since it produces an antiviral state in both the infected cell and surrounding uninfected cells and also provides perhaps the initial warning signal to the immune system. The presence of strange nucleic acids in the cytosol can also activate a cellular system that degrades double-stranded RNA, compromising viral replication. Second, the requirement for viral protein synthesis on ribosomes enables the cell to sample cellular ribosomes and display peptides from viral gene products on the cell surface in association with MHC class I molecules. Third, viruses with "hit-and-run" strategies usually try to maximize virus production by monopolizing the cellular biosynthetic metabolism and as a result shutting down host cell protein synthesis. This results in decreases in MHC class I expression, which can be detected by NK cells; these cells can kill infected cells or release cytokines with antiviral activities. Cytokines released by NK cells augment the cytokines released by infected cells, and this process serves as an important accelerant in the immune response. Fourth, the changes in cellular metabolism induced by virus infection can trigger cellular apoptosis in an attempt to prevent the release of viral progeny— the Cartonian nobility of this gesture ("It is a far, far better thing that I do, than I have ever done before . . .") is somewhat compromised by the likelihood of cell death from the later stages of viral infection (Miller and White, 1998; O'Brien, 1998; Teodoro and Branton, 1997).

The innate immune system has nearly complete responsibility for controlling infections for the first 3 to 5 days after infection with an infectious agent that the host has not previously experienced (or any antigenically cross-reactive viruses). Perhaps this is sufficient to completely contain low-level infections with some viruses, but for the more serious threats the adaptive immune system must be mobilized to contain and clear the infection. The adaptive immune system has a variety of effector mechanisms for this purpose, all based on the specificity of antibodies and T-cell receptors for viral antigens. The genes encoding these remarkable molecules are the only genes in vertebrates that are routinely subject to somatic mutation and rearrangement. This enables the immune system to keep pace with genetic variability of viruses (and other pathogens), maintaining the capacity to respond specifically to virtually any virus-encoded protein.

Our level of knowledge about how the innate and adaptive immune systems are used to control viral infection is described in chapters 11, 18, 24, and 28.

REFERENCES

Alcami, A., and U. H. Koszinowski. 2000. Viral mechanisms of immune evasion. *Immunol. Today* **21**:447–455.

Becker, Y. 1996. A short introduction to the origin and molecular evolution of viruses. *Virus Genes* **11**:73–77.

Berger, E. A. 1997. HIV entry and tropism: the chemokine receptor connection. *AIDS* **11**:S3–S16.

Chiu, W., R. M. Burnett, and R. L. Garcea. 1997. *Structural Biology of Viruses*. Oxford University Press, New York, N.Y.

Coffin, J. M., S. H. Hughes, and H. E. Varmus (ed.). 1997. *Retroviruses*. Cold Spring Harbor Laboratory Press, Cold Spring Harbor, N.Y.

Domingo, E., and J. J. Holland. 1997. RNA virus mutations and fitness for survival. *Annu. Rev. Microbiol.* **51**:151–178.

Doms R. W. 2000. Beyond receptor expression: The influence of receptor conformation, density and affinity in HIV-1 infection. *Virology* **276**:229–237.

Doms, R. W., R. A. Lamb, J. K. Rose, and A. Helenius. 1993. Folding and assembly of viral membrane proteins. *Virology* **193**:545–562.

Ewald, P. W. 1994. *Evolution of Infectious Disease*. Oxford University Press, Oxford, United Kingdom.

Fauci, A. S. 1996. Host factors and the pathogenesis of HIV-induced disease. *Nature* **384**:529–533.

Fields, B. N., D. M. Knipe, and P. M. Howley. 1996. *Fields Fundamental Virology*, 3rd ed. Lippincott-Raven, Philadelphia, Pa.

Flint, S. J., L. W. Enquist, R. M. Krug, V. R. Racaniello, and A. M. Skalka. 2000. *Principles of Virology: Molecular Biology, Pathogenesis, and Control*. ASM Press, Washington, D.C.

Garoff, H., R. Hewson, and D.-J. E. Opstelten. 1998. Virus maturation by budding. *Microbiol. Mol. Biol. Rev.* **62**:1170–1190.

Granoff, A., and R. G. Webster. 1999. *Encyclopedia of Virology*, 2nd ed. Academic Press, Ltd., London, United Kingdom.

Kasamatsu, H., and A. Nakanishi. 1998. How do animal DNA viruses get to the nucleus? *Annu. Rev. Microbiol.* **52**:627–686.

Klasse P. J., R. Bron, and M. Marsh. 1998. Mechanisms of enveloped virus entry into animal cells. *Adv. Drug Delivery Rev.* **34**:65–91.

Koonin, E. V. 1992. Evolution of viral genomes. *Semin. Virol.* **3**:311–417.

Levy, J. A. 1998. *HIV and the Pathogenesis of AIDS*, 2nd ed. ASM Press, Washington, D.C.

McCance, D. J. (ed.). 1998. *Human Tumor Viruses*. ASM Press, Washington, D.C.

McDermott, D. H., and P. M. Murphy. 2000. Chemokines and their receptors in infectious disease. *Springer Semin. Immunol.* **22**:393–416.

McFadden, G., A. Lalani, H. Everett, P. Nash, and X. Xu. 1998. Virus-encoded receptors for cytokines and chemokines. *Semin. Cell Dev. Biol.* **9**:359–368.

Miller, L. K., and E. White (ed.). 1998. Apoptosis in virus infection. *Semin. Virol.* **8**:443–523.

Mims, C., A. Nash, and J. Stephen. 2001. *Mims' Pathogenesis of Infectious Disease*, 5th ed. Academic Press, Inc., San Diego, Calif.

Nathanson, N. (ed.). 1997. *Viral Pathogenesis*. Lippincott-Raven Publishers, Philadelphia, Pa.

Norkin, L. C. 1995. Virus receptors: implications for pathogenesis and the design of antiviral agents. *Clin. Microbiol. Rev.* **8**:293–315.

O'Brien, V. 1998. Viruses and apoptosis. *J. Gen. Virol.* **79**:1833–1845.

Oldstone, M. B. A. 1996. Principles of viral pathogenesis. *Cell* **87**:799–801.

Plotkin, S. A., and W. A. Orenstein. 1999. *Vaccines*, 3rd ed. Harcourt-Brace, Philadelphia, Pa.

Richman, D. D., R. J. Whitley, and F. G. Hayden (ed.). 1997. *Clinical Virology*. Churchill Livingstone, Inc., New York, N.Y.

Scheld, W. M., D. Armstrong, and J. M. Hughes (ed.). 1998. *Emerging Infections 1*. ASM Press, Washington, D.C.

Scheld, W. M., W. A. Craig, and J. M. Hughes (ed.). 1999. *Emerging Infections 2.* ASM Press, Washington, D.C.

Scheld, W. M., R. J. Whitley, and D. T. Durack (ed.). 1991. *Infections of the Central Nervous System.* Raven Press, New York, N.Y.

Shadan, F. F., and L. P. Villarreal. 1996. The evolution of small DNA viruses of eukaryotes: past and present considerations. *Virus Genes* **11:**239–257.

Sodeik, B. 2000. Mechanisms of viral transport in the cytoplasm. *Trends Microbiol.* **8:**465–472.

Teodoro, J. G., and P. E. Branton. 1997. Regulation of apoptosis by viral gene products. *J. Virol.* **71:**1739–1746.

Tortorella, D., B. E. Gewurz, M. H. Furman, D. J. Schust, and H. L. Ploegh. 2000. Viral subversion of the immune system. *Annu. Rev. Immunol.* **18:**861–926.

Weinberg, R. A. 1997. The cat and mouse games that genes, viruses and cells play. *Cell* **88:**573–575.

Whittaker, G. R., M. Kann, and A. Helenius. 2000. Viral entry into the nucleus. *Ann. Rev. Cell Dev. Biol.* **16:**627–651.

World Health Organization. 1999. *World Health Organization Infectious Disease Report.* WHO/CDS/99.1. World Health Organization, Geneva, Switzerland.

Wright, P. F. 1996. *Seminars in Virology,* vol. 7. *Viral Pathogenesis.* The W. B. Saunders Co., Philadelphia, Pa.

II. THE ANTI-INFECTIVE IMMUNE RESPONSE

Immunology of Infectious Diseases
Edited by S. H. E. Kaufmann, A. Sher, and R. Ahmed
© 2002 ASM Press, Washington, D.C.

Chapter 5

Evolution of the Host Defense System

AUSTIN L. HUGHES

The vertebrate immune system includes the suite of cellular and molecular mechanisms which vertebrates use to recognize and eliminate parasites. (Here "parasite" is used in the evolutionary sense to refer to any organism that lives at the expense of and inside the body of another, including viruses, bacteria, fungi, protists, and metazoan parasites.) Invertebrate animals, plants, and even bacteria possess mechanisms that may be characterized as "immune," but the vertebrate immune system includes a number of aspects not shared with any other immune system. Traditionally, mechanisms of the vertebrate immune system have been classified under two main headings: (i) innate or nonspecific immunity and (ii) specific immunity. Specific immunity involves mechanisms for somatically generating receptor proteins that are highly specific for particular molecules of parasite origin (antigens). Specific immunity is sometimes referred to as adaptive immunity because it has the capacity to adapt (somatically) to new antigens. However, this terminology is somewhat unfortunate, since in evolutionary biology the term "adaptive" refers to any trait that confers a selective advantage on its bearer; in this sense, the mechanisms of innate immunity are just as adaptive as those of specific immunity.

The specific immune system includes several unique molecules found only in vertebrates: the immunoglobulins (Ig), the T-cell receptors (TCR), and the class I and class II molecules of the major histocompatibility complex (MHC). None of these has been found outside the jawed vertebrates (Gnathostomata), and repeated attempts to locate homologues in the jawless vertebrates (Agnatha) have so far failed. On the other hand, all jawed vertebrates possess Ig, TCR, and MHC in fully functional form. From an evolutionary point of view, the appearance of this complex suite of adaptations within only one lineage of life represents an intriguing unsolved problem.

In contrast to the specific immune system, vertebrate innate immunity shows some functional similarities to the immune systems of invertebrate animals, insofar as these are known. Some immunologists have even argued that there is an evolutionary continuity between invertebrate immune mechanisms and the vertebrate immune system. On this view, vertebrates inherited a basic immune system from their invertebrate ancestors, and the specific immune system was added on top of the preexisting system. Until recently, many biologists believed that the modern animal phyla all originated in a relatively short time span in the Cambrian period (the so-called Cambrian explosion). Recent molecular data have argued against this scenario (Fig. 1), but it still has many adherents. Given the widespread belief in a very narrow time span for the origin of vertebrates, the appearance of a full-blown innate immune system in the vertebrates appeared particularly remarkable and difficult to explain.

Many of the molecules involved in immunity are characterized by an extraordinary diversity. Particularly in the specific immune system, diversity stored in the germ line serves as a basis for the somatic generation of a wide variety of specific receptors. Such diversity indeed seems a prerequisite for any system adapted for recognizing each of the wide and unpredictable array of potential antigens an individual may encounter in its lifetime. In this chapter, I review recent evidence from molecular evolutionary studies regarding (i) the origin of the vertebrate immune system and (ii) the molecular mechanisms by which families of immune system genes have been diversified. These two questions involve rather different time frames. The basic molecules of specific immunity

---

Austin L. Hughes • Department of Biological Sciences, University of South Carolina, Columbia, SC 29208.

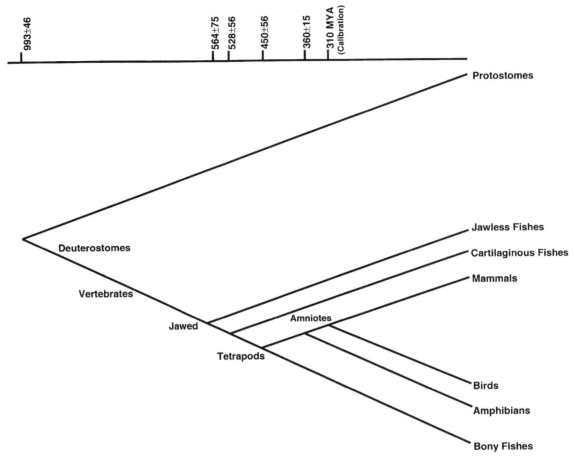

Figure 1. Phylogeny and estimated divergence times of major vertebrate clades. Divergence times are based on data of Kumar and Hedges (1998) and Wang et al. (1999).

were present in the vertebrate lineage before the divergence of cartilaginous and bony fishes, which is estimated to have occurred about 528 million years ago (Kumar and Hedges, 1998). By contrast, the diversification of immune system molecules is an ongoing process and is as evident in very recent vertebrate evolution as it was in the beginning. Nonetheless, similar evolutionary mechanisms—particularly gene duplication, mutation in its various forms, and natural selection—can be seen at work in both cases.

ORIGIN OF VERTEBRATE IMMUNITY: WAS THERE A "BIG BANG"?

The Cambrian period lasted from roughly 590 million to 505 million years ago, and until recently it was generally accepted that the major animal phyla diverged within this period. However, recent analyses of molecular data have suggested that the divergence of major lineages of animals occurred well

prior to the Cambrian. This revised timescale suggests the need for corresponding modifications in our views of the origins of both innate and specific immunity in vertebrates.

Innate Immune Mechanisms

As mentioned above, many researchers studying innate immunity have proposed that innate immune mechanisms of vertebrates share an evolutionary ancestry with those of invertebrates. For example, Habicht wrote, "It is gratifying to find that defenses that are considered to be primitive in vertebrate species are indeed phylogenetically ancient. . . . Invertebrates possess a variety of host defense-related molecules that have been conserved in vertebrates" (G. S. Habicht, Editorial, *Ann. N. Y. Acad. Sci.* 712: ix–xi, 1994). Hughes (1998a) tested this hypothesis of evolutionary continuity by reconstructing phylogenetic relationships of nine protein families including members having immune system functions in both vertebrates and arthropods. In most cases, the phylogenies showed evidence that immune system functions have evolved independently in arthropods and vertebrates.

One recently identified aspect of vertebrate innate immunity that suggests evolutionary continuity is the expression of a homologue of the *Drosophila* Toll protein in macrophages and other cells involved in regulating innate immune responses (Medzhitov et al., 1997; Underhill et al., 1999). In *Drosophila,* the Toll protein controls both dorsoventral patterning in embryos and the antifungal immune response of adults. Recent sequencing has revealed Toll to be a member of an extensive multigene family of cell surface receptors in both insects and vertebrates that is characterized by an extracellular domain involving leucine-rich repeats and an intracellular domain involved in signal transduction by the NF-kB pathway (Rock et al., 1998).

Insect Toll-related receptors include several (such as 18w and Tollo) which are not known to be involved in the immune response. In mammals, of a number of Toll-like receptor proteins (TLRs) so far discovered, only TLR2 is now known to have an immune system involvement (Medzhitov et al., 1997; Underhill et al., 1999). A phylogenetic analysis of vertebrate and *Drosophila* Toll-related proteins is shown in Fig. 2; the phylogenetic tree is rooted with *Drosophila* Slit and its vertebrate homologues, which are involved in nervous-system development (Fig. 2). Even if mammalian TLR1 to TLR6 all turn out to play immune system roles, the phylogeny in Fig. 2 is most consistent with independent evolution of an immune system function in vertebrate and invertebrate members of this family, since both the outgroup and certain insect Toll-related proteins lack an immune system function. The Toll phylogeny thus does not support the hypothesis of an evolutionary continuity of vertebrate and invertebrate immune responses, as noted previously by Hughes (1998a) and Luo and Zheng (2000).

The available evidence thus suggests that even innate immune mechanisms of vertebrates have evolved independently of those in protostomes such as insects. A recent analysis of molecular data has estimated the divergence time of deuterostome and protostome lineages at 993 million ± 46 million years ago (Fig. 1) (Wang et al., 1999). If this is true, there was no Cambrian explosion and the vertebrate lineage has been evolving independently for twice as long a time as was previously supposed. Given this long period of separation, it is not surprising that immune mechanisms have evolved independently in the deuterostome and protostome lineages.

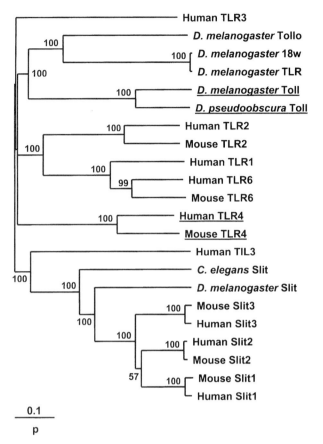

Figure 2. Phylogeny of Toll-related proteins, reconstructed by the neighbor-joining method of Saitou and Nei (1987) on the basis of the proportion of amino acid difference (p). Numbers on the branches are bootstrap percentages (i.e., the percentage of 1,000 pseudosamples constructed from the data by sampling sites from the data with replacement) which support the branch (Felsenstein, 1985). Only values of ≥50% are shown. Names of molecules with known immune system expression are underlined.

Specific Immunity

Probably because it was assumed that the unique adaptations constituting the vertebrate-specific immune system must have evolved very rapidly, a number of authors have invoked extraordinary mechanisms to explain the origin of these adaptations. However, the arguments advanced for these extraordinary mechanisms are problematic. In general, it seems preferable to assume that the evolutionary mechanisms that operated early in vertebrate history were akin to those we have observed in more recent vertebrate history rather than to invoke special mechanisms of which we have no evidence in recent populations. The two mechanisms most commonly invoked to explain specific immunity—whole-genome duplication by polyploidization and horizontal gene transfer—are not documented as giving rise to any major adaptive advance in recent vertebrate populations. I have termed the invocation of such mechanisms "genomic catastrophism," by analogy to catastrophism in geology (Hughes, 1999a). As in geology, it seems preferable in studying the history of genomes to adopt a position of genomic uniformitarianism unless there is compelling evidence for some spectacular mechanism. In early vertebrate evolution, there is no compelling evidence for either genome duplication or horizontal gene transfer.

Ohno (1970) was the first to suggest that polyploidization played an important role in early vertebrate evolution. In retrospect, we can see that Ohno emphasized polyploidization because an incorrect theory regarding the mechanism of gene expression in eukaryotes led him to doubt that tandem gene duplication could ever lead to new adaptations. Actually, all gene duplications which we know to have led to new protein functions have occurred by tandem duplication and none have occurred by polyploidization (Hughes, 1999b). In any event, a version of Ohno's hypothesis which postulated two rounds of genome duplication early in vertebrate history (the 2R hypothesis) has recently been very popular among developmental biologists (see, e.g., Sidow, 1996).

However, there is no good evidence that even one round of genome duplication occurred early in vertebrate history (Skrabanek and Wolfe, 1998). Advocates of the 2R hypothesis have adduced as evidence for this hypothesis the existence of gene families having four members in vertebrates (Sidow, 1996). In fact, this is true only if the family in question duplicated within the vertebrate lineage and shows a topology of a particular form, namely, a topology consisting of two clusters of two members, a form designated (AB) (CD) (Skrabanek and Wolfe, 1998; Hughes, 1999b, 1999c). Hughes (1999c) tested these predictions by a phylogenetic analysis of 13 gene families that had previously been adduced as supporting the 2R hypothesis. In only one of these was a topology of the (AB) (CD) form observed, and statistical support for that topology was very weak. In all other cases, the phylogenetic analyses indicated either that the genes duplicated before the origin of vertebrates or that the topology was of a form not predicted by the 2R hypothesis (Hughes, 1999c). Thus, the 2R hypothesis resoundingly failed the one rigorous test to which it has so far been subjected.

Some authors (see, e.g., Kasahara et al., 1997) have tried to implicate polyploidization in the origin of vertebrate-specific immunity. Aside from the fact that there is no evidence that polyploidization occurred early in vertebrate history, there are other problems with this view. For one thing, polyploidization can lead to duplication only of what is already present; it cannot explain the origin of gene families

unique to vertebrates, such as Ig, TCR, and MHC. Thus, for example, the 2R hypothesis, if it were true, might explain why vertebrates have α, β, γ, and δ TCR, but it cannot explain how TCR arose in the first place. However, the latter is the crucial question for explaining the origin of specific immunity.

One popular form of evidence for polyploidization consists of lists of paralogous genes located on different chromosomes. For example, Kasahara et al. (1997) provided a list of gene families including paralogues located in particular regions of human chromosomes 1, 6, 9, and 19 (Table 1). They claimed that these paralogues were duplicated by the alleged two rounds of polyploidization early in vertebrate history. The relevance to the origin of specific immunity lies in the fact that the chromosome 6 region involved is the region where the MHC genes are located. However, phylogenetic analyses have provided strong evidence that these duplications occurred at widely different times over the history of life on Earth (Table 1).

In most vertebrate species, the production of antibodies involves a process of somatic rearrangement of gene segments; among the proteins required for this process are the recombination activators RAG1 and RAG2. Bernstein et al. (1996) observed some amino acid sequence similarity between RAG1 and RAG2 and certain bacterial integrases involved in site-specific recombination. On the basis of this similarity, they proposed that the ancestors of RAG1 and RAG2 were acquired by vertebrate ancestors by horizontal gene transfer from bacteria. However, RAG1 and RAG2 actually show substantial sequence similarity to certain DNA-binding proteins of fungi. For example, there are striking similarities between RAG1 and a yeast protein called RAD18 (Hughes, 1999a). Thus, it seems most likely that the ancestors of RAG1 and RAG2 have been in eukaryotes at least since the common ancestor of animals and fungi.

A similar argument was made by Agrawal et al. (1998), who showed that RAG1 and RAG2 together can act as a transposase in vitro. They argued on the basis of this observation that these genes originated as a transposon that was "captured" and "tamed" by ancient vertebrates to serve as a basis for specific immunity. It is possible that this theory is correct, but the results of Agrawal et al. (1998) certainly do not prove it. Functional similarities between RAG1-RAG2 and transposases may be fortuitous. Alternatively, transposons themselves may originate from recombination-promoting genes of cellular organisms that have "escaped" rather than the other way around. At present, we know nothing of the evolutionary origin of transposable elements in general. Given our ignorance about the origin of transposons,

Table 1. Duplication times of some genes on human chromosomes 1, 6, 9, and 19 alleged to be involved in polyploidization events early in vertebrate history

Gene duplication (human chromosomal location)	Divergence time	Reference
TAP transporters (6)–ABC2 (9)	Before eukaryote-eubacterium divergence	Hughes (1998b)
LMP2, LMP7 (6)–PSMB7 (9)	Before animal-fungus divergence	Hughes (1998b)
HSP70 (6)–GRP78 (9)	Before animal-fungus divergence	Hughes (1998b)
Notch4 (6)–Notch1, Notch2, and Notch3 (1, 9, 19)	Before deuterostome-protostome divergence	Hughes (1999c)
CYP21 (6)–CYP2 (19)	Before deuterostome-protostome divergence	Yeager and Hughes (1999)
CD1 (1)–MHC class I (6)	After tetrapod origin	Hughes (1991a)

[a] Divergence times were all based on phylogenetic analyses using a method (Saitou and Nei, 1987) that does not assume a molecular clock.

it would be presumptuous to invoke transposons as the origin of any adaptive feature of eukaryotes.

GENERATION AND MAINTENANCE OF DIVERSITY

Balancing Selection: the MHC

The MHC molecules are cell surface glycoproteins that function to present peptides to T cells (Klein, 1986). There are two major families: class I molecules, which have a near-universal expression pattern and present peptides to cytotoxic T cells, and class II molecules, which are expressed on antigen-presenting cells of the immune system and present peptides to helper T cells. It has long been known that in humans, mice, and several other vertebrate species, certain MHC loci are highly polymorphic; indeed, the polymorphism of these loci was discovered before their function was known (Klein, 1986). For example, the database of named human MHC alleles as of this writing contains sequences for the following number of alleles at the three polymorphic class I loci: 168 alleles at HLA-A, 342 alleles at HLA-B, and 90 alleles at HLA-C. Such extensive polymorphism is known at no other human locus.

There are four separate lines of evidence favoring the hypothesis that MHC polymorphism is maintained by a form of balancing selection; thus, unlike the vast majority of genetic polymorphisms of which we are aware (Nei, 1987), it is not a selectively neutral polymorphism. Briefly, the lines of evidence are as follows.

1. The frequency distribution of MHC alleles differs significantly from the neutral expectation (Hedrick and Thompson, 1983). In neutral polymorphism, we expect generally to see one common allele and one or a few rarer alleles. In the MHC, however, there is a large number of alleles of intermediate frequency.

2. MHC polymorphisms are long-lasting evolutionarily, much more so than neutral polymorphisms are expected to be (Mayer et al., 1988). As a result, MHC polymorphisms can often pre-date speciation events, a phenomenon that has been referred to as transspecies polymorphism (Mayer et al., 1988). For example, Fig. 3 shows a phylogenetic tree of class II MHC DQ β-chain genes of sheep and cattle. The fact that certain genes of sheep cluster closer to certain genes of cattle than they do to other genes

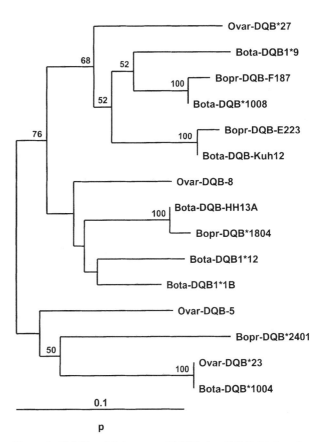

Figure 3. Neighbor-joining tree of MHC class II DQ β1 domains from *Bos taurus* (Bota-), *Bos primigenius indicus* (Bopr-), and *Ovis aries* (Ovar-) based on the proportion of amino acid difference (p). Numbers on the branches are as in Fig. 2.

of sheep is evidence that allelic lineages pre-date the divergence of these two species, which is estimated to have occurred about 20 million years ago.

3. MHC genes typically show a highly unusual pattern of nucleotide substitution, which is expected only for positive Darwinian selection favoring diversity at the amino acid level. In most protein-coding genes, the number of synonymous nucleotide substitutions per synonymous site (d_S) exceeds the number of nonsynonymous (amino acid-altering) nucleotide substitutions per nonsynonymous site (d_N) (Nei, 1987). This occurs because a majority of nonsynonymous mutations are deleterious to protein structure and thus are eliminated by so-called purifying selection (Kimura, 1977). On the other hand, if natural selection actually favors amino acid diversity, d_N can exceed d_S (Hughes, 1999b). For both polymorphic class I and class II loci, it has been shown that d_N significantly exceeds d_S in the codons encoding the peptide-binding region (PBR) of the molecule whereas in the rest of the gene d_S exceeds d_N (Hughes and Nei, 1988, 1989; Hughes et al., 1994). Figure 4 illustrates this pattern for human class I alleles.

4. Polymorphic MHC loci show a pattern whereby the introns of these genes are homogenized relative to exons by recombination and subsequent genetic drift (Cereb et al., 1997). As a result, the introns of MHC genes are not as old as the exons and do not show a "transspecies" pattern of evolution. This is precisely what is expected theoretically for a gene region not under balancing selection (such as introns in MHC genes) linked to another region under balancing selection (such as the exons containing the PBR codons) (Nei and Li, 1980; Strobeck, 1983). The evidence for this phenomenon is illustrated in Fig. 5. In pairwise comparisons among alleles within human class I loci, d_S in exons 2 and 3 (which encode the PBR) is almost always greater than the number of nucleotide substitutions per site (d) in intron 3 (the longest intron in the gene) (Fig. 5A). This is an unusual pattern because in most genes d in introns and d_S in exons are virtually identical (Hughes, 1999c). One hypothesis that might seem to explain this pattern is that the intron sequence is conserved because of some as yet unknown functional constraint. However, the results of comparisons between loci argue strongly against this hypothesis, since in these comparisons d_S in exons is no greater than d in introns (Fig. 5B). The only interpretation consistent with the results of both within- and between-locus comparisons is that the introns are homogenized relative to the exons by recombination and subsequent genetic drift (Cereb et al., 1997). This would be evidence of balancing selection acting on MHC exons, even if we knew nothing else about MHC polymorphism.

A

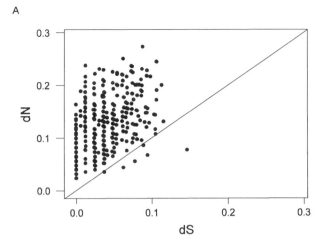

B

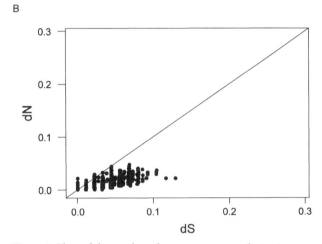

Figure 4. Plots of the number of nonsynonymous substitutions per nonsynonymous site (d_N) versus the number of synonymous substitutions per synonymous site (d_S) (Nei and Gojobori, 1986) for pairwise comparisons among alleles at the human MHC class I *HLA-A, HLA-B,* and *HLA-C* loci. Separate plots were constructed for the codons encoding PCR (A) and the remainder of exons 2 and 3 (encoding the $\alpha 1$ and $\alpha 2$ domains) (B). Only within-locus comparisons are included in this figure, but the relationships are essentially the same for between-locus comparisons (data not shown). In each case, a 45° line is drawn for reference.

The MHC thus provides a textbook example of the effects of balancing selection at the DNA level. With respect to host-parasite coevolution, the most revealing aspect of MHC polymorphism is the fact that this selection is focused on the PBR. This implies that selection is favoring diversity in the PBR. Since different forms of the PBR are known to confer different peptide-binding specificities, this implies that the ability to bind a diverse array of peptides confers an advantage on the individual (Hughes and Nei, 1988). Presumably, this advantage arises from the fact that an individual able to bind a diverse array of peptides has broader parasite defense than one able to bind only a limited peptide repertoire. Essentially

A

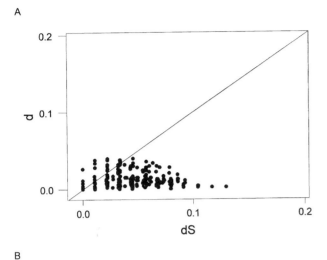

B

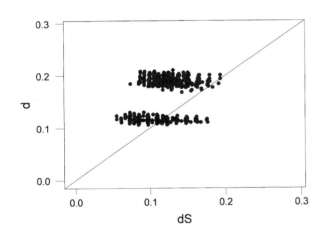

Figure 5. Plots of the number of nucleotide substitutions per site (*d*) in intron 3 versus the number of synonymous substitutions per synonymous site (*d*$_S$) in exons 2 and 3 in within-locus comparisons (A) and between-locus comparisons (B) of human genes from the *HLA-A, HLA-B,* and *HLA-C* loci. In each case, a 45° line is drawn for reference.

this argument was made by Doherty and Zinkernagel (1975) shortly after the first evidence of the peptide-binding function of MHC molecules. Subsequent results have strongly supported this hypothesis (Hughes and Yeager, 1998).

One prediction of this hypothesis is that peptide binding by vertebrate host MHC will exert selection on the regions of parasite genes which encode MHC-bound peptides. This selection will favor escape mutants, which the host MHC cannot recognize or recognizes poorly. Perhaps the most convincing experimental examples of natural selection favoring escape mutants have involved the simian immunodeficiency virus in rhesus macaques. In a study by Evans et al. (1999), monkeys of known class I MHC genotype were infected with simian immunodeficiency virus and sequences were obtained throughout

the course of infection. A significantly higher d_N than d_S was seen in portions of viral proteins bound by the host MHC but not in those bound by other rhesus MHC types. This indicates that natural selection favored amino acid changes specifically in peptides bound by the host MHC.

In altered peptide ligand (APL) antagonism, a small alteration in a peptide bound by class I MHC will downregulate the cytotoxic T-cell response to the original peptide by an unknown mechanism (Gilbert et al., 1998). Thus, APL antagonism is expected to favor genetic diversity in the parasite population. One interesting example of apparent APL antagonism involves the circumsporozoite protein (CSP) of the most virulent human malaria parasite, *Plasmodium falciparum*. The CSP is abundantly expressed on the surface of the sporozoite, the infective stage of the parasite, and there is evidence of positive selection ($d_N > d_S$) on regions of the CSP gene encoding known MHC-bound peptides (Hughes, 1991b; Hughes and Hughes, 1995).

Diversification of Multigene Families

According to Ohno's widely cited model for the origin of new protein function, gene duplication is typically followed by a period during which the two duplicate genes are redundant (Ohno, 1973). This theory holds that a redundant gene copy can by chance accumulate mutations that fortuitously adapt it to some new function. However, recent molecular evidence has contradicted Ohno's model in several respects, and it seems very unlikely that Ohno's mechanism is typical of the way in which genes with new functions evolve (Hughes, 1994, 1999b). An important line of evidence against this model is that, as shown by analysis of patterns of nucleotide substitution, in many cases amino acid changes that adapt duplicate genes to specific functions are fixed by positive Darwinian selection rather than being the result of mutations fixed by chance in a period of redundancy.

The immune system has provided several examples of positive selection after gene duplication in multigene families. One of the first examples involved variable region genes of Ig heavy chains (V$_H$ genes). The production of Ig heavy chains involves somatic rearrangement of V$_H$, D$_H$, J$_H$, and C$_H$ segments. There are three complementarity-determining regions (CDR1 to CDR3), which determine the specificity of the antibody; CDR1 and CDR2 are encoded in the V$_H$ segment, while CDR3 is contributed by D$_H$ and J$_H$ (Kabat et al., 1991). In some mammals, antibodies involved in the primary antibody response result solely from this process of rearrangement; humans and mice are examples.

In humans and mice, V_H genes belong to distinct families, some of which are quite ancient, pre-dating the origin of mammals (Ota and Nei, 1994). However, more recent duplications of V_H gene segments have often occurred. When Tanaka and Nei (1989) examined rates of nucleotide substitution in comparisons among recently duplicated human and mouse V_H regions, they found evidence, in the form of an enhanced rate of nonsynonymous substitution in the codons encoding the CDR, that natural selection has acted to diversify the CDR among these genes. This pattern is seen only in comparisons among closely related V_H genes. Thus, it seems that once an advantageous new form of the CDR is obtained, purifying selection takes over, as with most genes. A similar pattern was observed in the gene segments encoding the V regions of TCR β chains (Allen et al., 1996).

Interestingly, natural selection favoring diversity at the amino acid level is a characteristic not only of the specific immune system but also of some innate immune system genes. Defensins are antimicrobial peptides found in mammals; apparently related genes are found in insects, suggesting that the presence of defensins may be one aspect of innate immunity that shows evolutionary continuity between invertebrates and vertebrates (Hughes, 1999d). In mammals, there are two families of defensins, designated α and β. The α defensins, in particular, show signs of having recently duplicated independently in several mammalian lineages, and β defensins have duplicated within the ruminants. Natural selection has acted to diversify these gene families, apparently as an adaptation to newly encountered bacterial pathogenes (Hughes, 1999d). Thus, although ancient and relatively unsophisticated, these innate defenses of mammals are still actively engaged in an arms race with parasites.

REFERENCES

Agrawal, A., Q. E. Eastmann, and D. G. Schatz. 1998. Transposition mediated by RAG1 and RAG2 and its implications for the evolution of the immune system. *Nature* 394:744–751.

Allen, T. M., J. S. Lanchbury, A. L. Hughes, and D. I. Watkins. 1996. The T cell receptor b chain-encoding gene repertoire of a New World primate species, the cottontop tamarin. *Immunogenetics* 45:151–160.

Bernstein, R. M., S. F. Schluter, H. Bernstein, and J. J. Marchalonis. 1996. Primordial emergence of the recombination activating gene 1 (RAG1): sequence of the complete shark gene indicates homology to microbial integrases. *Proc. Natl. Acad. Sci. USA* 93:9454–9459.

Cereb, N., A. L. Hughes, and S. Y. Yang. 1997. Locus-specific conservation of the HLA class I introns by intra-locus homogenization. *Immunogenetics* 47:30–36.

Doherty, P. C., and R. M. Zinkernagel. 1975. Enhanced immunologic surveillance in mice heterozygous at the *H-2* gene complex. *Nature* 256:50–52.

Evans, D. T., D. H. O'Connor, P. Jing, J. L. Dzuris, J. Sidney, J. da Silva, T. M. Allen, H. Horton, J. E. Venham, R. A. Rudersdorf, T. Vogel, C. D. Pauza, R. E. Bontrop, R. DeMars, A. Sette, A. L. Hughes, and D. I. Watkins. 1999. Virus-specific cytotoxic T-lymphocyte responses select for amino-acid variation in simian immunodeficiency virus Env and Nef. *Nat. Med.* 5:1270–1276.

Felsenstein, J. 1985. Confidence limits on phylogenies: an approach using the bootstrap. *Evolution* 39:783–791.

Gilbert, S. C., M. Plebanski, S. Gupta, J. Morris, M. Cox, M. Aidoo, D. Kwiatkowski, B. M. Greenwood, H.C. Whittle, and A. V. S. Hill. 1998. Association of malaria parasite population structure, HLA, and immunological antagonism. *Science* 279:1173–1177.

Hedrick, P. W., and G. Thompson. 1983. Evidence for balancing selection at HLA. *Genetics* 104:449–456.

Hughes, A. L. 1991a. Evolutionary origin and diversification of the mammalian CD1 antigen genes. *Mol. Biol. Evol.* 8:185–201.

Hughes, A. L. 1991b. Circumsporozoite genes of malaria parasites (*Plasmodium* spp.): evidence for positive selection on immunogenic regions. *Genetics* 127:345–353.

Hughes, A. L. 1994. The evolution of functionally novel proteins after gene duplication. *Proc. R. Soc. London Ser. B* 256:119–124.

Hughes, A. L. 1998a. Protein phylogenies provide evidence of a radical discontinuity between arthropod and vertebrate immune systems. *Immunogenetics* 47:283–296.

Hughes, A. L. 1998b. Phylogenetic tests of the hypothesis of block duplication of homologous genes on human chromosomes 6, 9, and 1. *Mol. Biol. Evol.* 15:854–870.

Hughes, A. L. 1999a. Genomic catastrophism and the origin of vertebrate immunity. *Arch. Immun. Ther. Exp.* 47:347–353.

Hughes, A. L. 1999b. *Adaptive Evolution of Genes and Genomes.* Oxford University Press, New York, N.Y.

Hughes, A. L. 1999c. Phylogenies of developmentally important proteins do not support the hypothesis of two rounds of genome duplication early in vertebrate history. *J. Mol. Evol.* 48:565–576.

Hughes, A. L. 1999d. Evolutionary diversification of the mammalian defensins. *Cell. Mol. Life Sci.* 56:94–103.

Hughes, A. L., and M. Nei. 1988. Pattern of nucleotide substitution at major histocompatibility complex class I genes reveals overdominant selection. *Nature* 335:167–170.

Hughes, A. L., and M. Nei. 1989. Nucleotide substitution at major histocompatibility complex class II loci: evidence for overdominant selection. *Proc. Natl. Acad. Sci. USA* 86:958–962.

Hughes, A. L., and M. Yeager. 1998. Natural selection at major histocompatibility complex loci of vertebrates. *Annu. Rev. Genet.* 32:415–435.

Hughes, A. L., M. K. Hughes, C. Y. Howell, and M. Nei. 1994. Natural selection at the class II major histocompatibility complex loci of mammals. *Philos. Trans. R. Soc. London Ser. B* 345:359–367.

Hughes, M. K., and A. L. Hughes. 1995. Natural selection on *Plasmodium* surface proteins. *Mol. Biochem. Parasitol.* 71:99–113.

Kabat, E. A., T. T. Wu, H. M. Perry, K. S. Gottesman, and C. Foller. 1991. *Sequences of Proteins of Immunological Interest.* U.S. Department of Health and Human Services, Washington, D.C.

Kasahara, M., J. Nakaya, Y. Satta, and N. Takahata. 1997. Chromosomal duplication and the emergence of the adaptive immune system. *Trends Genet.* 13:90–92.

Kimura, M. 1977. Preponderance of synonymous changes as evidence for the neutral theory of molecular evolution. *Nature* 267:275–276.

Klein, J. 1986. *Natural History of the Major Histocompatibility Complex.* John Wiley & Sons, Inc., New York, N.Y.

Kumar, S., and S. B. Hedges. 1998. A molecular timescale for vertebrate evolution. *Nature* 392:917–920.

Luo, C., and L. Zheng. 2000. Independent evolution of Toll and related genes in insects and mammals. *Immunogenetics* 51:92–98.

Mayer, W. E., D. Jonker, D. Klein, P. Ivanyi, G. van Seventer, and J. Klein. 1988. Nucleotide sequence of chimpanzee MHC class I alleles: evidence for transspecies mode of evolution. *EMBO J.* 7:2765–2774.

Medzhitov, R., P. Preston-Hurlburt, and C. A. Janeway, Jr. 1997. A human homologue of the *Drosophila* Toll protein signals activation of adaptive immunity. *Nature* 388:394–397.

Nei, M. 1987. *Molecular Evolutionary Genetics.* Columbia University Press, New York, N.Y.

Nei, M., and T. Gojobori. 1986. Simple methods for estimating the numbers of synonymous and nonsynonymous nucleotide substitutions. *Mol. Biol. Evol.* 3:418–426.

Nei, M., and W.-H. Li. 1980. Non-random association between electromorphs and inversion chromosomes in finite populations. *Genet. Res.* 35:65–83.

Ohno, S. 1970. *Evolution by Gene Duplication.* Springer-Verlag, New York, N.Y.

Ohno, S. 1973. Ancient linkage groups and frozen accidents. *Nature* 244:259–262.

Ota, T., and M. Nei. 1994. Divergent evolution and evolution by the birth-and-death process in the immunoglobulin V_H gene family. *Mol. Biol. Evol.* 11:469–482.

Rock, F. L., G. Hardiman, J. C. Timans, R. A. Kastelein, and F. Bazan. 1998. A family of human receptors structurally related to *Drosophila* Toll. *Proc. Natl. Acad. Sci. USA* 95:588–593.

Saitou, N., and M. Nei. 1987. The neighbor-joining method: a new method for reconstructing phylogenetic trees. *Mol. Biol. Evol.* 4:406–425.

Sidow, A. 1996. Gen(om)e duplications in the evolution of early vertebrates. *Curr. Opin. Genet. Dev.* 6:715–722.

Skrabanek, L., and K. H. Wolfe. 1998. Eukaryote genome duplication—where's the evidence? *Curr. Opin. Genet. Dev.* 8:694–700.

Strobeck, C. 1983. Expected linkage disequlibrium for a neutral locus linked to a chromosomal rearrangement. *Genetics* 103:545–555.

Tanaka, T., and M. Nei. 1989. Positive Darwinian selection observed at the variable-region genes of immunoglobulin. *Mol. Biol. Evol.* 6:447–459.

Underhill, D. M., A. Ozinsky, A. M. Hajjar, A. Stevens, C. B. Wilson, M. Bassetti, and A. Aderem. 1999. The Toll-like receptor 2 is recruited to macrophage phagosomes and discriminates between pathogens. *Nature* 401:811–815.

Wang, D. Y., S. Kumar, and S. B. Hedges. 1999. Divergence time estimates for the early history of animal phyla and the origin of plants, animals, and fungi. *Proc. R. Soc. London Ser. B* 266:163–171.

Yeager, M., and A. L. Hughes. 1999. Evolution of the mammalian MHC: natural selection, recombination, and concerted evolution. *Immunol. Rev.* 167:45–58.

III. INNATE IMMUNITY

Immunology of Infectious Diseases
Edited by S. H. E. Kaufmann, A. Sher, and R. Ahmed
© 2002 ASM Press, Washington, D.C.

Chapter 6

Phagocytes and Anti-Infective Immunity

GORDON D. BROWN AND SIAMON GORDON

In the body, human cells are outnumbered 10 to 1 by microbes, almost all of which are capable of utilizing the abundant carbon, nitrogen, phosphorus, and other essential nutrients present in these cells. The ability of these microbes to proliferate in immunocompromised individuals demonstrates the need for an immune system to prevent inundation by a multitude of invaders. Even in the presence of such a system, the niche provided by human and animal tissues has given rise to pathogenic organisms that are able to overcome these defense mechanisms.

In healthy individuals, the immune system is composed of two interrelated parts, the innate and adaptive systems, whose response depends on the type of microbial invader. The innate response is composed principally of phagocytic cells and is capable of immediately recognizing and responding to microbial invasion. Phagocytes are also critical for the appropriate initiation of the adaptive response and the generation of specific immunity. The adaptive response, in turn, may utilize the phagocytes as effector cells to help resolve the infection. The actions of phagocytes are therefore central in the response to microbial invaders.

In this chapter, we present an overview of the role played by phagocytes in anti-infective immunity. We describe the various types and functions of phagocytic cells, the mechanisms they utilize for microbial recognition, uptake, and killing; and their involvement with the adaptive immune system. Where appropriate, we also demonstrate how pathogens have overcome the various anti-infective phagocyte functions and indicate where these microbial mechanisms have aided the understanding of phagocyte cell biology.

TYPES AND FUNCTIONS OF PHAGOCYTES

Metchnikoff first proposed a role for phagocytes in anti-infective immunity in the late 19th century, when he demonstrated that phagocytosis was important in wound healing, inflammation, and host defense. The main phagocytic cells in mammals are polymorphonuclear leukocytes (neutrophils), monocytes, and macrophages (Mϕ) (Gordon, 1999c; Rabinovitch, 1995). These cells have been termed "professional" phagocytes by virtue of their ability to ingest a variety of particles, and they are largely responsible for the recognition and control of invading microbes. "Paraprofessional" phagocytes include dendritic cells (DC), which display selective phagocytic ability and which, along with macrophages, are important in inducing the adaptive response by presenting antigen. Other cells, such as fibroblasts and epithelial cells, are also capable of phagocytosis but do not respond to particle uptake in the same fashion as the professional phagocytes. The ability to induce phagocytosis in these "nonprofessional" phagocytes is exploited by a variety of intracellular pathogens to escape the microbicidal responses of the professional phagocytes.

DC originate from both myeloid and lymphoid precursors, the former are involved in the induction of the adaptive immune response, while the latter may function in peripheral tolerance (Banchereau and Steinman, 1998; Bell et al., 1999; Reis e Sousa et al., 1999; Rescigno et al., 1999a, 1999b). DCs of the myeloid lineage derive from blood mononuclear cells and have two distinct functional stages, the immature and mature stages. The immature cells are found in most tissues and are able to take up and process antigen, whereas the mature cells lose this ability but acquire the unique ability to present an-

Gordon D. Brown and Siamon Gordon • Sir William Dunn School of Pathology, University of Oxford, South Parks Road, Oxford, OX1 3RE, United Kingdom.

tigen to naïve T cells after migration to lymphoid organs. After presentation and activation of lymphocytes, DCs undergo apoptosis. The migratory ability of DCs is an important attribute, stemming in part from changes in chemokine receptor expression patterns during maturation. During the transitional phases of maturation, stimulated by microbes, microbial products, and inflammatory cytokines, these cells also produce a number of chemokines to attract other immune cells including Mφ, neutrophils, natural killer (NK) cells, and immature DCs. DCs are paraprofessional phagocytes in that they are capable of phagocytosing microbes only during their immature antigen-processing stage; maturation results in the down regulation of this activity. DCs are also capable of engulfing apoptotic bodies and presenting the antigens they contain, a phenomenon known as cross-priming. Thus, the major role of DCs in anti-infective immunity is as an accessory cell in inducing the immune response, capturing and presenting antigen to prime the adaptive immune response, and attracting other immune cells to sites of infection.

Neutrophils are short-lived but essential effector cells involved in the control of extracellular bacterial and fungal infections; they have also been implicated in the control of some intracellular bacterial infections (Cossart et al., 2000; Hampton et al., 1998). The importance of neutrophils is exemplified in neutropenia, which results in an increased susceptibility to bacterial and fungal infections. Neutrophils are among the first cells to arrive at the site of infection, attracted from the blood by a variety of chemoattractants including CXC chemokines released by macrophages and other cells, microbial products, and the products of complement activation. Neutrophils can restrict microbial spread through phagocytosis of the pathogens, especially after opsonization (see below), and destruction of the pathogens via a variety of microbicidal mechanisms. They also release a number of cytokines and chemokines to attract other cells of both the innate and adaptive immune systems. In contrast to DCs and Mφ, neutrophils lack the accessory molecules required to present antigen to lymphocytes. Neutrophils therefore contribute to the resolution of infection by directly destroying microbial invaders and targeting the specific immune response to the site of infection.

Mφ originate from blood monocytes, are distributed widely in all tissues, and represent a first line of defense against invading microbes (Gordon, 1999a). Mφ are key cells in anti-infective immunity, since they are important in both the innate and adaptive responses. The functions of Mφ, listed with mechanisms and examples in Table 1, include the ability to detect microbial invasion, respond to and

Table 1. Mechanisms and examples of Mφ functions

Detection of microbial invasion
    Opsonic and nonopsonic receptors for microbes and their
    products (Fig. 1)

Restriction of microbial spread
    Phagocytosis
    Granuloma formation
    Intracellular killing

Recruitment of immune cells
    Release of cytokines and other inflammatory mediators

Accessory cells in lymphocyte activation
    Antigen processing and presentation
    Costimulatory molecules
    Cytokines

Effector cells in cell-mediated immunity
    Increased phagocytosis
    Increased intracellular killing
    Clearance of apoptotic cells

Participation in humoral immunity
    Receptors for antibody and complement

restrict microbial spread, recruit other immune cells to the site of infection, act as accessory cells in secondary lymphocyte activation and as effector cells in cell-mediated immunity, and participate in humoral immunity by eliminating foreign antigens. Mφ are also important in the clearance of apoptotic cells. Since the functions of Mφ are enhanced when these cells are activated by interactions with T cells, cytokines such as gamma interferon (IFN-γ), or bacterial products such as lipopolysaccharide (LPS), Mφ activation represents a crucial step in anti-infective immunity, and defects in this activation result in an increased susceptibility to pathogens. Mφ can also produce a number of anti-inflammatory molecules, such as transforming growth factor β (TGF-β) and interleukin 10 (IL-10), which contribute to the resolution of inflammatory responses. With such an important role in anti-infective immunity, the Mφ also provides an ideal niche for many pathogens able to modify Mφ functions and/or overcome the antimicrobial host defenses. This is discussed in more detail below and in later chapters.

The actions of phagocytes are, however, not always protective and can lead to tissue injury and disease, an important cause of morbidity and mortality in humans (Gallin et al., 1999). The extracellular release of toxic oxidants and hydrolytic enzymes (see below) can lead to tissue damage, while inflammatory mediators, such as tumor necrosis factor alpha (TNF-α) and IL-1, can lead to fever, wasting, and septic shock. Persistent infections may lead to chronic inflammation, mediated in part by phagocytes and resulting in fever, secondary infections, cachexia, or even death. Phagocytes can contribute to the generation of autoimmune diseases by presenting microbial epitopes to lymphocytes which are cross-reactive to self molecules. Phagocytes may also act as "Trojan horses," aiding in the dissemination of pathogens throughout the host. These and other aspects of infectious pathologic responses are discussed in detail in later chapters.

MICROBIAL RECOGNITION

Since most microbes can proliferate far more quickly than the host can mount a specific antimicrobial response, the innate immune system must be able to recognize quickly and control an invader while the adaptive immune response is initiated. This has been achieved by the evolution of a set of germ line-encoded proteins, termed pattern recognition receptors (PRRs), which are either free in the plasma or membrane bound and are capable of recognizing conserved microbial molecules, termed pathogen-associated microbial patterns (Medzhitov and Janeway, 1997). These microbial molecules include lipoteichoic acid of gram-positive bacteria and LPS of gram-negative bacteria. By recognizing the pathogen-associated microbial patterns, the PRRs enable the host to recognize a wide variety of microbes with a limited set of molecules. The PRRs determine the mechanism of uptake (phagocytosis) and influence the maturation pathway of the resultant phagosome and the inflammatory responses mediated by the phagocyte. PRRs also provide a means of entry for intracellular pathogens.

The plasma-derived PRRs include the collectins, pentraxins, and complement, which coat the microbe (opsonization), allowing recognition and binding by opsonic receptors on host phagocytes (Medzhitov and Janeway, 1997). After the induction of acquired immunity, opsonic recognition is enhanced by the production of specific antimicrobe antibodies. The best-characterized opsonic receptors on phagocytes are the complement and antibody receptors. The direct or nonopsonic recognition and binding of microbes is mediated by a variety of membrane-bound PRRs on phagocytes, including C-type lectins, leucine-rich proteins, scavenger receptors, and integrins (Aderem and Underhill, 1999; Gordon, 1999c; Ofek et al., 1995). The structure and properties of a member of each of the membrane-bound PRR families and some of their endogenous and microbial ligands are presented in Fig. 1.

PRRs act as receptors for the binding and entry of many intracellular pathogens. *Mycobacterium tuberculosis,* for example, utilizes complement receptors (CRs), the mannose receptor, CD14, and the surfactant protein A (collectin) receptor to bind to host macrophages (Ehlers and Daffe, 1998). Since the various receptors can generate different host cell responses (see below), the intracellular survival of pathogens may depend on which receptor they utilize to gain entry into the host cell. *Toxoplasma gondii,* for example, is killed by the antimicrobial respiratory burst after entry through the Fc receptor but survives after entry through CR3, which does not lead to a respiratory burst (Gordon, 1999b). Although less well characterized, receptors other than the PRRs are also used by pathogens to bind to and/or enter host cells; an example is provided by Dr-fimbriated *Escherichia coli,* which binds to epithelial cells via decay-accelerating factor (CD55) (Selvarangan et al., 2000). Extracellular pathogens, on the other hand, have evolved a number of mechanisms to avoid recognition, such as the capsules of staphylococcal and streptococcal pathogens, which prevent complement deposition on the bacterial surface and contact with host phagocytes (Peterson et al., 1978; Whitnack et al., 1981).

MICROBIAL UPTAKE

The receptor-mediated binding of microbes to the phagocyte surface initiates transmembrane activation signals, which lead to microbial engulfment and internalization. This process, termed phagocytosis, is complex, heterogeneous, and not fully understood, but depends on actin polymerization and is used by cells to take up large particles (>0.5 μm in diameter). There are a variety of phagocytic receptors, including the PRRs, each dictating the mechanism of phagocytosis. Many of these receptors also serve as adhesion molecules and may interact with other surface receptors, either stimulating or inhibiting phagocytosis. The likelihood that microbes are recognized by more than one receptor adds another layer of complexity. While extracellular pathogens have developed mechanisms to inhibit or avoid uptake, phagocytosis can be exploited by intracellular pathogens to gain access to host cells.

Our understanding of phagocytosis has evolved from studies of single receptor-ligand interactions, especially those involving the Fcγ receptor (FcγR) and CRs. Early work on the FcγR led to the development of the zipper model, proposed in the 1970s (Griffin et al., 1975, 1976). In this model, actin-rich pseudopodia extend circumferentially over the par-

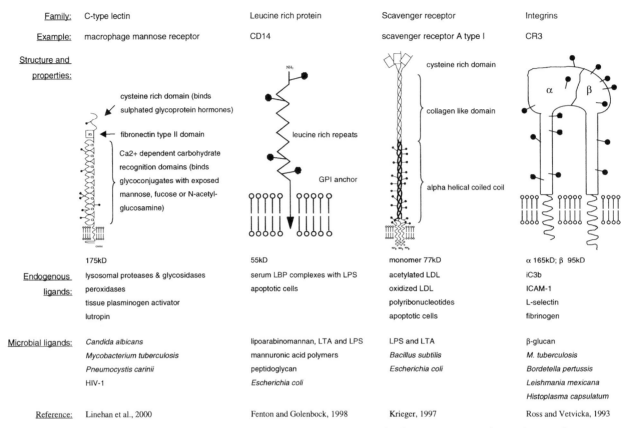

Family:	C-type lectin	Leucine rich protein	Scavenger receptor	Integrins
Example:	macrophage mannose receptor	CD14	scavenger receptor A type I	CR3
Structure and properties:	175kD	55kD	monomer 77kD	α 165kD; β 95kD
Endogenous ligands:	lysosomal proteases & glycosidases peroxidases tissue plasminogen activator lutropin	serum LBP complexes with LPS apoptotic cells	acetylated LDL oxidized LDL polyribonucleotides apoptotic cells	iC3b ICAM-1 L-selectin fibrinogen
Microbial ligands:	Candida albicans Mycobacterium tuberculosis Pneumocystis carinii HIV-1	lipoarabinomannan, LTA and LPS mannuronic acid polymers peptidoglycan Escherichia coli	LPS and LTA Bacillus subtilis Escherichia coli	β-glucan M. tuberculosis Bordetella pertussis Leishmania mexicana Histoplasma capsulatum
Reference:	Linehan et al., 2000	Fenton and Golenbock, 1998	Krieger, 1997	Ross and Vetvicka, 1993

In the structure diagram: cysteine rich domain (binds sulphated glycoprotein hormones); fibronectin type II domain; Ca2+ dependent carbohydrate recognition domains (binds glycoconjugates with exposed mannose, fucose or N-acetyl-glucosamine); leucine rich repeats; GPI anchor; cysteine rich domain; collagen like domain; alpha helical coiled coil; α; β

Figure 1. Properties and ligands of selected PRRs. Abbreviations: LBP, LPS-binding protein; LTA, lipoteichoic acid; LDL, low-density lipoprotein; ICAM-1, intercellular cell adhesion molecule 1. The structures of the various receptors are reprinted, with permission, from *The Leukocyte Antigen FactsBook,* 2nd edition (Barclay et al., 1997).

ticle surface through the sequential binding of cell surface receptors to ligands on the microbial surface. The host plasma membrane ultimately engulfs the entire particle, forming a particle-shaped phagosome surrounded by F-actin, the actin cup. More recent studies have shown that phagocytosis is initiated by receptor clustering occurring from receptor-ligand interactions (Aderem and Underhill, 1999). The clustering results in cytoplasmic ITAMs (immunoglobulin gene family tyrosine activation motif) becoming tyrosine phosphorylated. These ITAMs are either part of the FcγR (FcγRIIA) or located on dimerized γ chains which associate with the receptors (FcγRI and FcγRIIIA) (shown schematically in Fig. 2), and their initial phosphorylation may be due to src family kinases. A second tyrosine kinase, Syk, then binds to the phosphorylated ITAMs and initiates a number of signaling cascades, which are thought to occur through the participation of Cdc42, phosphatidylinositol 3-kinase (PI3-kinase), Rac1, and ARF6, resulting in actin assembly, membrane protrusion, pseudopod extension, and, finally, closure of the phagocytic cup. Fcγ-mediated phagocytosis is also negatively regulated by another src kinase, Fgr,

which associates with an immunoreceptor tyrosine-based inhibition motif (ITIM)-containing receptor, signal regulatory protein α (Aderem and Underhill, 1999; Gordon, 1999c; Gresham et al., 2000; Swanson and Baer, 1995; Turner et al., 2000). The exact mechanism of FcγR-induced actin polymerization and phagosome formation, however, is still unclear.

Phagocytosis mediated by CRs is less well understood and is different from that mediated by the FcγRs (Aderem and Underhill, 1999; Gordon, 1999c). Unlike FcγR, the internalization of bound particles by CRs is not blocked by inhibitors of tyrosine kinases and requires an additional stimulus such as TNF-α or attachment to extracellular matrix proteins. Furthermore, internalization requires intact microtubules and occurs with the particle appearing to sink into the cell and not being engulfed by pseudopodia, as occurs with FcγR. The phagosomal membrane is also less adherent, held by point-like contacts to the particle that are enriched with cytoskeletal proteins including F-actin, vinculin, α-actinin, and paxillin. In contrast to FcγR, phagocytosis mediated by CRs does not elicit the production of proinflammatory mediators, such as

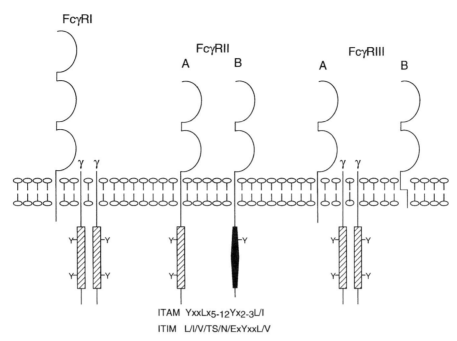

Figure 2. FcγR and their isoforms. Shown are the tyrosine residues present in the ITAM (striped box) or ITIM (shaded box), which become phosphorylated after receptor cross-linking. The ITAM and ITIM sequences are also indicated.

arachidonic acid metabolites, or induce the respiratory burst (see below). Consequently, CRs are commonly utilized by intracellular pathogens to gain access to host cells.

Intracellular pathogens make use of similar and unique mechanisms to gain entry into professional and nonprofessional phagocytes (Finlay and Falkow, 1997; Wright and Silverstein, 1983). To gain entry into epithelial cells, for example, *Listeria monocytogenes* utilizes a host adhesion molecule, E-cadherin, in a PI3-kinase-dependent zipper mechanism (Cossart and Lecuit, 1998). *Salmonella* species gain entry into macrophages and epithelial cells by using type III secretion systems to deliver proteins into the host cytosol and stimulating macropinocytosis, an actin-based trigger mechanism of uptake (Goosney et al., 1999). *Legionella pneumophila* binds to macrophages via CR3 and enters the cell by inducing an extended pseudopod, which coils around the bacterium, a mechanism termed coiling phagocytosis (Horwitz, 1984). These specialized entry mechanisms are used to avoid the normal maturation of the phagosome and the associated antimicrobial events which occur after phagocytosis (see below). This can also be achieved by an extracellular lifestyle, exemplified by pathogens such as *Yersinia,* which use a type III secretion system to actively prevent phagocytosis by blocking the signaling mechanisms controlling cytoskeletal rearrangements (Cornelis, 1998).

PHAGOSOMAL MATURATION

After internalization, the phagosome matures through a number of sequential steps involving extensive vesicle budding and fusion, generating an increasingly antimicrobial environment in which the ingested microbe is ultimately killed and digested (Aderem and Underhill, 1999; Berón et al., 1995; Cox et al., 2000; Desjardins et al., 1994; Gordon, 1999c; Sinai and Joiner, 1997). The first step after internalization is depolymerization of F-actin from the phagosome and fusion with early endosomes. This fusion requires the small GTPase Rab5, generating a dynamic compartment which continually undergoes vesicle fusion and fission and which may access the recycling endosomal network. Over time, selective protein sorting results in the maturation of the phagosome, which loses its early endosomal markers, such as Rab5, and acquires markers of late endocytic vesicles. These markers include Rab7, which mediates the progression from early to late endosome, hydrolytic enzymes such as cathepsin D, and the proton pump ATPase, which contributes to the lowering of the phagosome pH. The final stage of maturation is fusion with lysosomes, generating a low-pH phagolysosomal compartment containing a variety of degradative hydrolases. During maturation, microtubules facilitate movement of the phagosome from the periphery to a perinuclear location.

The current understanding of these maturation pathways has been greatly aided by the subversive abilities of intracellular pathogens, which have evolved mechanisms to interfere with these processes. A schematic overview of phagocytosis and phagosomal maturation, along with some examples of where pathogens interfere with this process, is shown in Fig. 3. Intracellular pathogens display a range of life-styles from those that have adapted to life within the low pH of degradative phagolysosomes, such as *Leishmania* and *Coxiella*, to those which avoid this environment completely by disrupting the phagosomal membrane and escaping into the host cytosol, such as *Shigella* and *Listeria*. Some pathogens, such as *Mycobacterium*, arrest maturation of the phagosome, while others, such as *Legionella*, convert the phagosome to a unique vacuole which has limited intersection with the host endosomal network. Although the general pathway of phagosomal maturation is outlined here, most of the mechanisms regulating this maturation process are still unknown.

MICROBIAL KILLING

The microbicidal environment of the maturing phagosome is generated by a number of interrelated mechanisms which often work synergistically (Cossart et al., 2000; Gordon, 1999c). Microbial killing is accomplished by the low pH of the phagosome, the fusion with lysosomes, the limitation of nutrients, and the generation of reactive oxygen and nitrogen intermediates. The lysosomal contents which are released into the phagosomal vacuole include a number of antimicrobial peptides, proteins, and acid hydrolases such as the membrane-permeabilizing peptide defensins, which have a broad spectrum of microbial targets (discussed in more detail in chapter 8), and lysozyme, which attacks the peptidoglycan layer of bacterial cell walls.

The limitation of nutrients, especially iron, that are essential for microbial growth is also an effective antimicrobial mechanism. Although the containment of the microbe within the phagosome itself limits nutrient availability, delivery of iron via the endosomal recycling pathway is further limited through the down regulation of transferrin receptors (Sunder-Plassmann et al., 1999). Another molecule, natural resistance-associated macrophage protein 1 (Nramp-1) localizes to the phagosome after microbial uptake and is thought to play a role in the removal of iron and other divalent cations from the phagosome (Blackwell and Searle, 1999; Canonne-Hergaux et al., 1999; Gruenheid et al., 1997). Polymorphisms in Nramp-1 have been linked to susceptibility to tuber-

culosis and leprosy in humans, and mutations in Nramp-1 in inbred mice result in susceptibility to a number of intracellular parasites such as *Salmonella*, *Leishmania*, and *Mycobacterium*.

The respiratory burst of phagocytes that culminates in the production of reactive oxygen intermediates is one of the best characterized antimicrobial defenses (Clark, 1999; Hampton et al., 1998). When activated, the phagocyte NADPH oxidase (phox), a membrane-associated protein complex, generates superoxide (O_2^-) by transferring electrons from NAPDH to O_2. The superoxide then reacts within the phagosomal lumen to produce toxic oxidants including hydroxyl radicals and hydrogen peroxide. The hydrogen peroxide is then converted by myeloperoxidase to hypochlorous acid, one of the most effective bactericidal oxidants produced by the cell. Activation of the oxidase complex is incompletely understood but involves numerous proteins, including PI3-kinase, phospholipase C, protein kinase C, and GTP-binding proteins such as Rac in signal transduction pathways leading from the cellular receptor involved in the recognition of the microbe to phosphorylation of one the cytosolic phox proteins (p47[phox]). Mutations in the phox proteins result in chronic granulomatous disease, a disease characterized by recurrent infections with a number of bacteria and fungi and an inability of these phagocytes to kill in vitro.

The other key enzyme involved in intracellular killing of microbes is the inducible nitric oxide synthase (iNOS) of phagocytes (Burgner et al., 1999; Shiloh et al., 1999). The induction of iNOS leads to the production of large amounts of nitric oxide (NO) through the oxidative deamination of L-arginine. NO then reacts with superoxide, generated by the respiratory burst, or thiol groups to produce antimicrobial compounds such as peroxynitrite and nitrosothiols. iNOS can be induced either individually or synergistically by bacterial products such as LPS and proinflammatory cytokines including TNF-α, IFN-γ, and IL-1β (discussed below). The role of iNOS in the control of many murine infections such as leishmaniasis, tuberculosis, and malaria has been well established through inhibitor studies and with the use of knockout animals. Mice doubly deficient in both iNOS and phox proteins displayed enhanced susceptibility even to normal commensal organisms, although Mϕ from these mice still had a limited capacity to kill microbes, demonstrating the limited effectiveness of the other antimicrobial mechanisms. In contrast, the role of iNOS in host defense in humans has been controversial since the induction of high levels of NO by human blood-derived leuko-

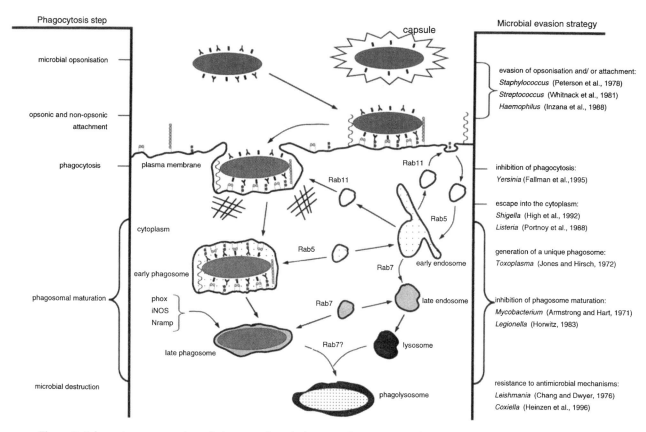

Phagocytosis step

microbial opsonisation

opsonic and non-opsonic
attachment

phagocytosis — plasma membrane

cytoplasm

early phagosome

phagosomal maturation — phox
iNOS
Nramp

late phagosome

microbial destruction

capsule

Rab11
Rab11
Rab5
Rab5
Rab7
Rab7
Rab7?

early endosome
late endosome
lysosome
phagolysosome

Microbial evasion strategy

evasion of opsonisation and/ or attachment:
Staphylococcus (Peterson et al., 1978)
Streptococcus (Whitnack et al., 1981)
Haemophilus (Inzana et al., 1988)

inhibition of phagocytosis:
Yersinia (Fallman et al.,1995)

escape into the cytoplasm:
Shigella (High et al., 1992)
Listeria (Portnoy et al., 1988)

generation of a unique phagosome:
Toxoplasma (Jones and Hirsch, 1972)

inhibition of phagosome maturation:
Mycobacterium (Armstrong and Hart, 1971)
Legionella (Horwitz, 1983)

resistance to antimicrobial mechanisms:
Leishmania (Chang and Dwyer, 1976)
Coxiella (Heinzen et al., 1996)

Figure 3. Schematic representation of phagocytosis and phagosomal maturation. Also shown are the strategies used by microbes to evade or modulate these processes.

cytes has not been clearly demonstrated. It is thought, however, that the regulation of this enzyme is more complex than in mice and that there is sufficient circumstantial evidence to substantiate the role of this enzyme in host defense.

The development of these antimicrobial mechanisms has in turn led to the evolution of a number of resistance mechanisms in pathogens. *Mycobacterium*, for example, blocks acidification of its phagosomes by exclusion of the vesicular proton ATPase (Sturgill-Koszycki et al., 1994). Acidification also triggers membrane lysis by pathogens, such as *Listeria*, which escape into the cytoplasm (Beauregard et al., 1997). *Leishmania* cells are covered in lipophosphoglycan, which helps them resist the degradative environment within the phagolysosome (Descoteaux and Turco, 1999). Pathogens acquire essential nutrients such as iron by binding transferrin or lactoferrin, as occurs with *Neisseria*, or secreting siderophores, such as the mycobactins and exochelins of *Mycobacterium*, which bind iron with a higher affinity than the host molecules do (De Voss et al., 1999; Schryvers and Stojiljkovic, 1999). However, the mechanisms by which microbes acquire nutrients within the phagosome are mostly unknown. The res-

piratory burst can be avoided by entry through specific receptors (see above) or by suppression of the initiating signaling cascade, as occurs with *Yersinia* (Cornelis, 1998). Microbes such as *Salmonella* produce enzymes such as catalase, glutathione reductase, and superoxide dismutase, which break down toxic oxidants (Storz et al., 1990). Resistance to reactive nitrogen intermediates is mediated by the same enzymes as well as by alkyl hydroperoxide reductase, an enzyme found in most organisms and shown to contribute to the intracellular survival of *Salmonella* and *Mycobacteria* (Manca et al., 1999; Storz et al., 1990).

Finally, programmed cell death, or apoptosis, is also an important component of anti-infective immunity, although its role is unclear. In some cases apoptosis appears to favor the pathogen, while in other cases it appears to favor the host (Fratazzi et al., 1999; Weinrauch and Zychlinsky, 1999). Many pathogens with different cellular niches, such as *Yersinia, Shigella,* and *Salmonella,* actively induce apoptosis in phagocytes by a variety of mechanisms, possibly to take advantage of the suppressive effects of apoptosis on the inflammatory response. Others, such as *Leishmania, Chlamydia,* and a number of viruses, inhibit apoptosis to prolong their intracellular growth. In contrast, apoptosis is beneficial to the host during mycobacterial infections, resulting in intracellular killing and prevention of mycobacterial spread. Thus, apoptosis may be an important defense mechanism, limiting the spread and growth of intracellular organisms.

PRODUCTION OF SOLUBLE MEDIATORS

In conjunction with their ability to recognize, take up, and kill microbes, phagocytes must rapidly signal and recruit other cells to the sites of infection. Furthermore, the adaptive immune system must be primed and a specific immune response must be initiated to remove the invader. The signaling and recruitment of cells are achieved through the release of soluble mediators, such as cytokines and chemokines, which are generated after recognition and/or uptake of the microbial invader. These mediators, along with antigen presentation to lymphocytes, help direct the generation of the adaptive immune response (see "Antigen Presentation" below). The development of the final immune response is complex and depends greatly on the types of soluble mediators produced and the interplay of these factors among the various immune cells.

The binding of microbes or their products to PRRs results, in most cases, in the production and/or release of proinflammatory mediators, such as reactive oxygen intermediates and arachidonic acid metabolites, as well as a number of proinflammatory cytokines. Although not all the signaling pathways leading to the NFκB-dependent expression of these cytokines are completely understood, the recently identified Toll-like receptors (TLR) are important components (Underhill et al., 1999; Wright, 1999). The TLRs, originally identified in *Drosophila*, are a family of receptors with homology to the IL-1 receptor. They are recruited to the phagosome and can distinguish between various pathogens; TLR2 recognizes fungi and gram-positive bacteria, while TLR4 recognizes LPS and gram-negative bacteria. Similar to the IL-1 receptor, signaling through the TLRs occurs via MyD88 and IRAK to activate NFκB. A number of other TLRs have been identified and, although not yet characterized, may also be involved in microbial discrimination and cytokine release.

Cytokines are central molecules of the immune response, forming a complex network that mediates and regulates both innate and adaptive immunity (Billiau et al., 1998; Biron, 1998; Paludan, 1998; Pretolani, 1999; Thomson, 1998). Cytokines bind

to their cognate cell surface receptors and signal through a variety of pathways, although many signal through the Janus family kinases (Jaks) and signal transducer and activator of transcription (Stat) proteins. Table 2 lists the properties and characteristics of various selected pro- and anti-inflammatory cytokines involved in these responses. IL-12, IL-18, and IFN-γ are central in macrophage activation and the generation of a Th1-type response (see below). IL-12 released by Mφ stimulates NK cells and T cells to produce IFN-γ, which in turn augments IL-12 secretion, generating a positive feedback loop. Activation by IFN-γ stimulates phagocytosis and induces phagosome-lysosome fusion, the respiratory burst, and the production of NO intermediates. Mφ can also be activated by IFN-α/β, stimulating antiviral and antimicrobial mechanisms. IL-4 and IL-13, on the other hand, stimulate an alternative form of Mφ activation, while IL-10 leads to Mφ deactivation. The formation of granulomas, organized lesions of T cells and Mφ at the site of infection and often critical in restricting microbial dissemination, depends on cytokines such as TNF-α and IFN-γ and various chemotactic cytokines (chemokines). Cytokines such as TGF-β are also critical in the suppression and resolution of the immune response.

Chemokines signal cells through seven transmembrane G-protein-coupled receptors, and they function to recruit neutrophils, monocytes, immature DC, and activated T cells to the sites of infection (Thomson, 1998). Chemokines are divided into four families based on the number and position of conserved cysteines: C, CC, CXC, and the CX_3C chemokines. In general, CXC chemokines, such as IL-8, attract neutrophils, while CC and C chemokines, such as monocyte chemotactic protein 1 (MCP-1) and lymphotactin, attract monocytes and lymphocytes. Chemokines can also induce the release of proinflammatory mediators and stimulate the respiratory burst.

Pathogens modulate cytokine networks to favor their survival, either by inhibiting the production of proinflammatory cytokines or by stimulating the production of anti-inflammatory cytokines. Examples include the poxviruses and herpesviruses, which produce virokines, mimics of anti-inflammatory cytokines, and viroceptors, soluble mimics of proinflammatory cytokine receptors (Mosser and Karp, 1999). Other examples include mycobacterial deactivation of Mφ, making these phagocytes refractory to activating cytokines and stimulating them to produce TGF-β, and the ability of *Yersinia* to inhibit NFκB activation, thereby preventing the expression

Table 2. Selected cytokines important in anti-infective immunity

Cytokine	Effect	Primary role
IL-4/IL-13	CD4$^+$ Th2 differentiation T-cell proliferation B-cell isotype switching (IgE) Alternative Mϕ activation ↑ MHC class II, B7-1, B7-2 ↑ giant-cell formation ↓ IL-1, TNF-α, IL-6, IL-12	Th2-mediated immunity
IL-6	B- and T-cell growth ↑ acute-phase protein levels	Lymphocyte stimulator
IL-10	Mϕ deactivation ↓ IL-1, TNF-α, IL-6, IL-12 ↓ MHC class II, B7-1, B7-2 ↓ T-cell proliferation	Anti-inflammatory effect
IL-12	T-cell proliferation CD4$^+$ Th1 differentiation ↑ IFN-γ ↑ CTL^a activity	Th1-mediated immunity
IL-18	T-cell proliferation CD4$^+$ Th1 differentiation ↑ IFN-γ ↓ IL-10	Th1-mediated immunity
IFN-γ	Mϕ and neutrophil activation CD4$^+$ Th1 differentiation B-cell isotype switching (IgG2a, IgG3)^a ↑ NK-cell cytolytic activity ↑ vascular adhesion molecule levels ↑ MHC classes I and II ↑ TNF-α, IL-1, IL-12, IFN-β ↓ IL-10	Th1-mediated immunity
IFN-α/β	Mϕ and NK-cell activation ↑ CTL activity ↑ MHC class I	Antiviral and antimicrobial immunity
TNF-α	Mϕ and neutrophil activation Inflammatory-cell recruitment ↑ vascular adhesion molecules ↑ MHC class I ↑ acute-phase protein levels ↑ T-cell apoptosis	Proinflammatory effect

^{a} CTL, cytotoxic T lymphocyte; IgG, immunoglobulin G.

of proinflammatory cytokines (Fitzpatrick and Bielefeldt-Ohmann, 1999; Wilson et al., 1998).

ANTIGEN PRESENTATION

A central role of phagocytes, particularly DC, in the generation of adaptive immunity is that of antigen presentation (Banchereau and Steinman, 1998; Fearon and Locksley, 1996; Romagnani, 1996). These interactions with T cells are critical in the control and resolution of infections; CD8$^+$ T cells lyse cells infected with cytosolic pathogens, aiding in or directly killing these pathogens and also activating macrophages, while CD4$^+$ Th1 cells are critical in the resolution of intracellular infections, activating Mϕ to increase their ability to phagocytose and kill pathogens. CD4$^+$ Th2 cells mediate Mϕ-independent responses to extracellular parasites, such as helminths. CD4$^+$ T cells also provide help to antigen-stimulated B cells to generate antimicrobial antibodies. The role of T and B cells is detailed briefly below, but is discussed in greater detail in later chapters. The pathways of antigen processing and presentation are detailed schematically in Fig. 4.

The presentation of peptide antigens to receptor-specific T cells requires the noncovalent association of the peptides with major histocompatibility complex (MHC) molecules, of which there are two main classes with different structures, class I and class II. Almost all nucleated cells express MHC class I molecules, which present antigenic peptides to cytotoxic CD8$^+$ T cells (Pamer and Cresswell, 1998). These peptides come from either host cell-derived or microbe-derived proteins originating from the cytosol and are produced by a cytoplasmic proteolytic complex, the proteasome, some of whose components can be induced by IFN-γ. These peptides are translocated into the endoplasmic reticulum by TAP (transporter associated with antigen processing) proteins, where they associate with the MHC class I molecules and β_2-microglobulin (β_2m) and are subsequently transported to the cell surface. Since the presented peptides originate from the cytosol, MHC class I presentation is important in the control of cytosolic pathogens, such as viruses. MHC class I molecules can also present antigenic peptides originating from the phagosome, normally presented by MHC class II molecules (see below), although the mechanisms involved are unknown (Wick and Ljunggren, 1999).

MHC class II molecules are mainly restricted to Mϕ, DC, and B cells. MHC class II expression is increased after activation of Mϕ and upon maturation in DC, as described previously (Cresswell, 1994). These cells are capable of taking up exogenous antigens and generating the peptides required through the actions of peptidases in acidified late endosomal and/or phagosomal compartments. The peptides are thought to be loaded onto MHC class II molecules in a specialized compartment, the MIIC compartment, for subsequent presentation to CD4$^+$ Th cells. To prevent association with endogenous peptides during synthesis, MHC class II molecules are associated with an invariant chain (Ii), which directs the transport out of the endoplasmic reticulum and Golgi. Ii is removed by proteolysis and by the actions of an auxiliary molecule, HLA-DM, in the MIIC compartment, allowing the binding of foreign peptide and transport to the cell surface. Since peptides derived from the endosomal/phagosomal pathway are presented through MHC class II, this presentation pathway is critical for the control of intracellular pathogens.

Two other classes of molecules, MHC class Ib and CD1, also present antigen to T cells (Lindahl et al., 1997; Park et al., 1998; Porcelli et al., 1998; Schaible et al., 1999). MHC class Ib molecules present short N-formylmethionine-containing peptides of bacterial and/or mitochondrial origin to CD8$^+$ T cells. Although MHC class Ib is structurally similar to MHC class I and noncovalently linked to β_2m, the processing and peptide loading mechanisms are un-

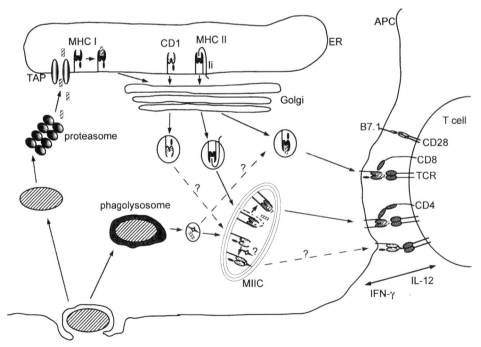

Figure 4. Schematic representation of the antigen-processing and antigen presentation pathways for MHC class I, MHC class II, and CD1 molecules. Dashed arrows indicate putative and/or unknown pathways.

clear and may be TAP independent. CD1 is structurally related to MHC class I, associates with β_2m, and is expressed mainly by activated Mϕ, DC, and B cells. The five identified CD1 genes fall into two classes; CD1d is found in many mammals, including rats and mice, and CD1a, CD1b, CD1c, and CD1e are found only in humans. The latter class of molecules are capable of presenting glycolipid and microbial lipid antigens, such as mycolic acids from mycobacteria, to cytotoxic CD4$^-$ CD8$^-$ T cells and possibly CD8$^+$ T cells. The site and mechanisms of antigen loading and processing are unknown but are TAP independent and may occur in the MIIC compartment.

The generation of an appropriate T-cell response depends on costimulatory molecules and cytokines (Fearon and Locksley, 1996). Activation of T cells requires not only the T-cell receptor (TCR) but also a second signal mediated by costimulatory molecules such as CD40L, CD28, and CTLA4, which interact with CD40, B7-1, and B7-2 on antigen-presenting cells (APCs). These interactions not only activate the APCs but also modulate T-cell activation and proliferation and mediate the type of CD4$^+$ Th cell (Th1 or Th2) produced. Cytokines generated by the APCs have a major influence on the differentiation of CD4$^+$ T cells into Th1- or Th2-type cells. Peripheral activation of APCs by microbes and cross-linking of CD40 during antigen presentation bias the development of naïve T cells to the Th1 type through the actions of IL-12 (see above), whereas the generation of Th2 T cells requires IL-4. The role and generation of Th1 and Th2 T cells in infection are discussed in greater detail in chapter 12.

Intracellular pathogens, such as *Listeria,* have greatly aided the elucidation of many of these antigen presentation pathways (Busch et al., 1999). However, the critical role of antigen presentation in the control of intracellular infections has been exploited by a number of intracellular pathogens to avoid immune recognition. For example, viruses have evolved a number of ways of preventing MHC class I presentation, including inhibition of protein processing (Epstein-Barr virus), inhibition of MHC class I assembly (cytomegalovirus), and inhibition of TAP transport (herpes simplex virus) (Yewdell and Bennink, 1999). Intracellular pathogens such as *Mycobacterium* down regulate the surface expression of MHC class II and CD1, although the mechanisms controlling this are unclear (Schaible et al., 1999). Some bacteria and viruses produce superantigens which bind to MHC class II molecules outside the peptide binding groove and cause extensive nonspecific T-cell activation (Herman et al., 1991).

CONCLUDING REMARKS

Phagocytes play a central role in anti-infective immunity, which is important in all aspects of the immune response. As we have shown, phagocytes recognize and destroy microbial invaders, release cytokines and chemokines to attract and activate other immune cells, and play an important part in the generation of adaptive immunity. Pathogens have evolved numerous strategies to overcome these defenses, which has been useful in the elucidation of the various anti-infective mechanisms. An understanding of these mechanisms is important for the control of infection as well as disease, and although these mechanisms are becoming more defined, many aspects remain unclear. Among these are the following.

1. How do intracellular pathogens obtain nutrients? Is there any way of stimulating the cell to prevent pathogens from acquiring these nutrients, or, conversely, can the mechanisms used by microbes to access intracellular nutrients be targeted by novel drugs?

2. What are the factors governing the presentation of antigens to T cells which result in the generation of a Th1 and a Th2 response? What factors skew this response to favor the microbe?

3. What are the relative roles of infected Mϕ and DC in the induction of cellular immunity to intracellular pathogens?

4. What factors are involved in maturation of the phagosome, what are the mechanisms used by pathogens to control this process, and can we overcome these mechanisms?

5. What are the mechanisms of exogenous antigen presentation on MHC class I molecules?

Acknowledgments. We acknowledge the Wellcome Trust and the Medical Research Council, UK, for financial support. We thank Philip Taylor, Leanne Peiser, and Janet Willment for critically reading the manuscript. In memory of Albert D. Beyers.

REFERENCES

Aderem, A., and D. M. Underhill. 1999. Mechanisms of phagocytosis in macrophages. *Annu. Rev. Immunol.* **17**:593–623.

Armstrong, J., and P. Hart. 1971. Response of cultured macrophages to *Mycobacterium tuberculosis* with observations on fusion of lysosomes with phagosomes. *J. Exp. Med.* **134**:713–740.

Banchereau, J., and R. M. Steinman. 1998. Dendritic cells and the control of immunity. *Nature* **392**:245–252.

Barclay, A. N., M. H. Brown, S. K. A. Law, A. J. McKnight, M. G. Tomlinson, and P. A. van der Merwe. 1997. *The Leucocyte Antigen FactsBook,* 2nd ed. Academic Press, Inc., San Diego, Calif.

Beauregard, K. E., K. D. Lee, R. J. Collier, and J. A. Swanson. 1997. pH-dependent perforation of macrophage phagosomes by listeriolysin O from *Listeria monocytogenes*. *J. Exp. Med.* **186:** 1159–1163.

Bell, D., J. W. Young, and J. Banchereau. 1999. Dendritic cells. *Adv. Immunol.* **72:**255–324.

Berón, W., C. Alvarez-Dominguez, L. Mayorga, and P. D. Stahl. 1995. Membrane trafficking along the phagocytic pathway. *Trends Cell Biol.* **5:**100–104.

Billiau, A., H. Heremans, K. Vermeire, and P. Matthys. 1998. Immunomodulatory properties of interferon-gamma. An update. *Ann. N. Y. Acad. Sci.* **856:**22–32.

Biron, C. A. 1998. Role of early cytokines, including alpha and beta interferons (IFN-alpha/beta), in innate and adaptive immune responses to viral infections. *Semin. Immunol.* **10:**383–390.

Blackwell, J. M., and S. Searle. 1999. Genetic regulation of macrophage activation: understanding the function of Nramp1 (=Ity/Lsh/Bcg). *Immunol. Lett.* **65:**73–80.

Burgner, D., K. Rockett, and D. Kwiatkowski. 1999. Nitric oxide and infectious diseases. *Arch. Dis. Child.* **81:**185–188.

Busch, D. H., K. Kerksiek, and E. G. Pamer. 1999. Processing of *Listeria monocytogenes* antigens and the in vivo T-cell response to bacterial infection. *Immunol. Rev.* **172:**163–169.

Canonne-Hergaux, F., S. Gruenheid, G. Govoni, and P. Gros. 1999. The Nramp1 protein and its role in resistance to infection and macrophage function. *Proc. Assoc. Am. Physicians* **111:**283–289.

Chang, K. P., and D. M. Dwyer. 1976. Multiplication of a human parasite (Leishmania donovani) in phagolysosomes of hamster macrophages in vitro. *Science* **193:**678–680.

Clark, R. A. 1999. Activation of the neutrophil respiratory burst oxidase. *J. Infect. Dis.* **179**(Suppl. 2):S309–S317.

Cornelis, G. R. 1998. The *Yersinia* deadly kiss. *J. Bacteriol.* **180:** 5495–5504.

Cossart, P., P. Boquet, S. Normark, and R. Rappuoli (ed.). 2000. *Cellular Microbiology*. ASM Press, Washington, D.C.

Cossart, P., and M. Lecuit. 1998. Interactions of Listeria monocytogenes with mammalian cells during entry and actin-based movement: bacterial factors, cellular ligands and signaling. *EMBO J.* **17:**3797–3806.

Cox, D., D. J. Lee, B. M. Dale, J. Calafat, and S. Greenberg. 2000. A Rab11-containing rapidly recycling compartment in macrophages that promotes phagocytosis. *Proc. Natl. Acad. Sci. USA* **97:**680–685.

Cresswell, P. 1994. Assembly, transport, and function of MHC class II molecules. *Annu. Rev. Immunol.* **12:**259–293.

Descoteaux, A., and S. J. Turco. 1999. Glycoconjugates in *Leishmania* infectivity. *Biochim. Biophys. Acta* **1455:**341–352.

Desjardins, M., L. A. Huber, R. G. Parton, and G. Griffiths. 1994. Biogenesis of phagolysosomes proceeds through a sequential series of interactions with the endocytic apparatus. *J. Cell Biol.* **124:**677–688.

De Voss, J. J., K. Rutter, B. G. Schroeder, and C. E. Barry III. 1999. Iron acquisition and metabolism by mycobacteria. *J. Bacteriol.* **181:**4443–4451.

Ehlers, M. R., and M. Daffe. 1998. Interactions between *Mycobacterium tuberculosis* and host cells: are mycobacterial sugars the key? *Trends Microbiol.* **6:**328–335.

Fallman, M., K. Andersson, S. Hakansson, K. E. Magnusson, O. Stendahl, and H. Wolf-Watz. 1995. Yersinia pseudotuberculosis inhibits Fc receptor-mediated phagocytosis in J774 cells. *Infect. Immun.* **63:**3117–3124.

Fearon, D. T., and R. M. Locksley. 1996. The instructive role of innate immunity in the acquired immune response. *Science* **272:** 50–53.

Fenton, M. J., and D. T. Golenbock. 1998. LPS-binding proteins and receptors. *J. Leukoc. Biol.* **64:**25–32.

Finlay, B. B., and S. Falkow. 1997. Common themes in microbial pathogenicity revisited. *Microbiol. Mol. Biol. Rev.* **61:**136–169.

Fitzpatrick, D. R., and H. Bielefeldt-Ohmann. 1999. Transforming growth factor beta in infectious disease: always there for the host and the pathogen. *Trends Microbiol.* **7:**232–236.

Fratazzi, C., R. D. Arbeit, C. Carini, M. K. Balcewicz-Sablinska, J. Keane, H. Kornfeld, and H. G. Remold. 1999. Macrophage apoptosis in mycobacterial infections. *J. Leukoc. Biol.* **66:**763–764.

Gallin, J. I., R. Snyderman, D. T. Fearon, B. F. Haynes, and C. Nathan (ed.). 1999. *Inflammation: Basic Principles and Clinical Correlates,* 3rd ed. Lippincott Williams & Wilkins, Philadelphia, Pa.

Goosney, D. L., D. G. Knoechel, and B. B. Finlay. 1999. Enteropathogenic *E. coli, Salmonella,* and *Shigella:* masters of host cell cytoskeletal exploitation. *Emerg. Infect. Dis.* **5:**216–223.

Gordon, S. 1999a. Macrophages and the immune response, p. 533–545. *In* W. E. Paul (ed.), *Fundamental Immunology*, 4th ed. Lippincott-Raven Publishers, Philadelphia, Pa.

Gordon, S. (ed.). 1999b. *Phagocytosis: Microbial Invasion*, vol. 6. JAI Press Inc., Stamford, Conn.

Gordon, S. (ed.). 1999c. *Phagocytosis: the Host*, vol. 5. JAI Press Inc., Stamford, Conn.

Gresham, B. H., B. M. Dale, J. W. Potter, P. W. Chang, C. M. Vines, C. A. Lowell, C. F. Lagenaur, and C. L. Willman. 2000. Negative regulation of phagocytosis in murine macrophages by the Src kinase family member, Fgr. *J. Exp. Med.* **191:**515–528.

Griffin, F. M., Jr., J. A. Griffin, J. E. Leider, and S. C. Silverstein. 1975. Studies on the mechanism of phagocytosis. I. Requirements for circumferential attachment of particle-bound ligands to specific receptors on the macrophage plasma membrane. *J. Exp. Med.* **142:**1263–1282.

Griffin, F. M., Jr., J. A. Griffin, and S. C. Silverstein. 1976. Studies on the mechanism of phagocytosis. II. The interaction of macrophages with anti-immunoglobulin IgG-coated bone marrow-derived lymphocytes. *J. Exp. Med.* **144:**788–809.

Gruenheid, S., E. Pinner, M. Desjardins, and P. Gros. 1997. Natural resistance to infection with intracellular pathogens: the Nramp1 protein is recruited to the membrane of the phagosome. *J. Exp. Med.* **185:**717–730.

Hampton, M. B., A. J. Kettle, and C. C. Winterbourn. 1998. Inside the neutrophil phagosome: oxidants, myeloperoxidase, and bacterial killing. *Blood* **92:**3007–3017.

Heinzen, R. A., M. A. Scidmore, D. D. Rockey, and T. Hackstadt. 1996. Differential interaction with endocytic and exocytic pathways distinguish parasitophorous vacuoles of *Coxiella burnetii* and *Chlamydia trachomatis*. *Infect. Immun.* **64:**796–809.

Herman, A., J. W. Kappler, P. Marrack, and A. M. Pullen. 1991. Superantigens: mechanism of T-cell stimulation and role in immune responses. *Annu. Rev. Immunol.* **9:**745–772.

High, N., J. Mounier, M. C. Prevost, and P. J. Sansonetti. 1992. IpaB of *Shigella flexneri* causes entry into epithelial cells and escape from the phagocytic vacuole. *EMBO J.* **11:**1991–1999.

Horwitz, M. A. 1983. Formation of a novel phagosome by the Legionnaires' disease bacterium (*Legionella pneumophila*) in human monocytes. *J. Exp. Med.* **158:**1319–1331.

Horwitz, M. A. 1984. Phagocytosis of the Legionnaires' disease bacterium (*Legionella pneumophila*) occurs by a novel mechanism: engulfment within a pseudopod coil. *Cell* **36:**27–33.

Inzana, T. J., J. Ma, T. Workman, R. P. Gogolewski, and P. Anderson. 1988. Virulence properties and protective efficacy of the capsular polymer of *Haemophilus* (*Actinobacillus*) pleuropneumoniae serotype 5. *Infect. Immun.* **56:**1880–1889.

Jones, T. C., and J. G. Hirsch. 1972. The interaction between *Toxoplasma gondii* and mammalian cells. II. The absence of lysosomal fusion with phagocytic vacuoles containing living parasites. *J. Exp. Med.* **136**:1173–1194.

Krieger, M. 1997. The other side of scavenger receptors: pattern recognition for host defense. *Curr. Opin. Lipidol.* **8**:275–280.

Lindahl, K. F., D. E. Byers, V. M. Dabhi, R. Hovik, E. P. Jones, G. P. Smith, C. R. Wang, H. Xiao, and M. Yoshino. 1997. H2-M3, a full-service class Ib histocompatibility antigen. *Annu. Rev. Immunol.* **15**:851–879.

Linehan, S. A., L. Martinez-Pomares, and S. Gordon. 2000. Macrophage lectins in host defence. *Microbes Infect.* **2**:279–288.

Mahoney, J. A., and S. Gordon. 1998. Macrophage receptors and innate immunity. *Biochemistry* **20**:12–16.

Manca, C., S. Paul, C. E. Barry III, V. H. Freedman, and G. Kaplan. 1999. Mycobacterium tuberculosis catalase and peroxidase activities and resistance to oxidative killing in human monocytes in vitro. *Infect. Immun.* **67**:74–79.

Medzhitov, R., and C. A. Janeway, Jr. 1997. Innate immunity: impact on the adaptive immune response. *Curr. Opin. Immunol.* **9**:4–9.

Mosser, D. M., and C. L. Karp. 1999. Receptor mediated subversion of macrophage cytokine production by intracellular pathogens. *Curr. Opin. Immunol.* **11**:406–411.

Ofek, I., J. Goldhar, Y. Keisari, and N. Sharon. 1995. Nonopsonic phagocytosis of microorganisms. *Annu. Rev. Microbiol.* **49**:239–276.

Paludan, S. R. 1998. Interleukin-4 and interferon-gamma: the quintessence of a mutual antagonistic relationship. *Scand. J. Immunol.* **48**:459–468.

Pamer, E., and P. Cresswell. 1998. Mechanisms of MHC class I—restricted antigen processing. *Annu. Rev. Immunol.* **16**:323–358.

Park, S. H., Y. H. Chiu, J. Jayawardena, J. Roark, U. Kavita, and A. Bendelac. 1998. Innate and adaptive functions of the CD1 pathway of antigen presentation. *Semin. Immunol.* **10**:391–398.

Peterson, P. K., B. J. Wilkinson, Y. Kim, D. Schmeling, and P. G. Quie. 1978. Influence of encapsulation on staphylococcal opsonization and phagocytosis by human polymorphonuclear leukocytes. *Infect. Immun.* **19**:943–949.

Porcelli, S. A., B. W. Segelke, M. Sugita, I. A. Wilson, and M. B. Brenner. 1998. The CD1 family of lipid antigen-presenting molecules. *Immunol. Today* **19**:362–368.

Portnoy, D. A., P. S. Jacks, and D. J. Hinrichs. 1988. Role of hemolysin for the intracellular growth of *Listeria monocytogenes*. *J. Exp. Med.* **167**:1459–1471.

Pretolani, M. 1999. Interleukin-10: an anti-inflammatory cytokine with therapeutic potential. *Clin. Exp. Allergy.* **29**:1164–1171.

Rabinovitch, M. 1995. Professional and non-professional phagocytes: an introduction. *Trends Cell Biol.* **5**:85–87.

Reis e Sousa, C., A. Sher, and P. Kaye. 1999. The role of dendritic cells in the induction and regulation of immunity to microbial infection. *Curr. Opin. Immunol.* **11**:392–399.

Rescigno, M., F. Granucci, S. Citterio, M. Foti, and P. Ricciardi-Castagnoli. 1999a. Coordinated events during bacteria-induced DC maturation. *Immunol. Today* **20**:200–203.

Rescigno, M., F. Granucci, and P. Ricciardi-Castagnoli. 1999b. Dendritic cells at the end of the millennium. *Immunol. Cell Biol.* **77**:404–410.

Romagnani, S. 1996. Understanding the role of Th1/Th2 cells in infection. *Trends Microbiol.* **4**:470–473.

Ross, G. D., and V. Vetvicka. 1993. CR3 (CD11b, CD18): a phagocyte and NK cell membrane receptor with multiple ligand specificities and functions. *Clin. Exp. Immunol.* **92**:181–184.

Schaible, U. E., H. L. Collins, and S. H. Kaufmann. 1999. Confrontation between intracellular bacteria and the immune system. *Adv. Immunol.* **71**:267–377.

Schryvers, A. B., and I. Stojiljkovic. 1999. Iron acquisition systems in the pathogenic *Neisseria*. *Mol. Microbiol.* **32**:1117–1123.

Selvarangan, R., P. Goluszko, V. Popov, J. Singhal, T. Pham, D. M. Lublin, S. Nowicki, and B. Nowicki. 2000. Role of decay-accelerating factor domains and anchorage in internalization of Dr-fimbriated *Escherichia coli*. *Infect. Immun.* **68**:1391–1399.

Shiloh, M. U., J. D. MacMicking, S. Nicholson, J. E. Brause, S. Potter, M. Marino, F. Fang, M. Dinauer, and C. Nathan. 1999. Phenotype of mice and macrophages deficient in both phagocyte oxidase and inducible nitric oxide synthase. *Immunity* **10**:29–38.

Sinai, A. P., and K. A. Joiner. 1997. Safe haven: the cell biology of nonfusogenic pathogen vacuoles. *Annu. Rev. Microbiol.* **51**:415–462.

Storz, G., L. A. Tartaglia, and B. N. Ames. 1990. The OxyR regulon. *Antonie Leeuwenhoek* **58**:157–161.

Sturgill-Koszycki, S., P. H. Schlesinger, P. Chakraborty, P. L. Haddix, H. L. Collins, A. K. Fok, R. D. Allen, S. L. Gluck, J. Heuser, and D. G. Russell. 1994. Lack of acidification in *Mycobacterium* phagosomes produced by exclusion of the vesicular proton-ATPase. *Science* **263**:678–681. (Erratum, **263**:1359.)

Sunder-Plassmann, G., S. I. Patruta, and W. H. Horl. 1999. Pathobiology of the role of iron in infection. *Am. J. Kidney Dis.* **34**:S25–S29.

Swanson, J. A., and S. C. Baer. 1995. Phagocytosis by zippers and triggers. *Trends Cell Biol.* **5**:89–93.

Thomson, A. (ed.). 1998. *The Cytokine Handbook*, 3rd ed. Academic Press, Inc., San Diego, Calif.

Turner, M., E. Schweighoffer, F. Colucci, J. P. Di Santo, and V. L. Tybulewicz. 2000. Tyrosine kinase SYK: essential functions for immunoreceptor signaling. *Immunol. Today* **21**:148–154.

Underhill, D. M., A. Ozinsky, A. M. Hajjar, A. Stevens, C. B. Wilson, M. Bassetti, and A. Aderem. 1999. The Toll-like receptor 2 is recruited to macrophage phagosomes and discriminates between pathogens. *Nature* **401**:811–815.

Weinrauch, Y., and A. Zychlinsky. 1999. The induction of apoptosis by bacterial pathogens. *Annu. Rev. Microbiol.* **53**:155–187.

Weis, W. I., M. E. Taylor, and K. Drickamer. 1998. The C-type lectin superfamily in the immune system. *Immunol. Rev.* **163**:19–34.

Whitnack, E., A. L. Bisno, and E. H. Beachey. 1981. Hyaluronate capsule prevents attachment of group A streptococci to mouse peritoneal macrophages. *Infect. Immun.* **31**:985–991.

Wick, M. J., and H. G. Ljunggren. 1999. Processing of bacterial antigens for peptide presentation on MHC class I molecules. *Immunol. Rev.* **172**:153–162.

Wilson, M., R. Seymour, and B. Henderson. 1998. Bacterial perturbation of cytokine networks. *Infect. Immun.* **66**:2401–2409.

Wright, S. D. 1999. Toll, a new piece in the puzzle of innate immunity. *J. Exp. Med.* **189**:605–609.

Wright, S. D., and S. C. Silverstein. 1983. Receptors for C3b and C3bi promote phagocytosis but not the release of toxic oxygen from human phagocytes. *J. Exp. Med.* **158**:2016–2023.

Yewdell, J. W., and J. R. Bennink. 1999. Mechanisms of viral interference with MHC class I antigen processing and presentation. *Annu. Rev. Cell Dev. Biol.* **15**:579–606.

Immunology of Infectious Diseases
Edited by S. H. E. Kaufmann, A. Sher, and R. Ahmed
© 2002 ASM Press, Washington, D.C.

Chapter 7

Innate Immunity in Bacterial Infections

EMIL R. UNANUE

The host response to pathogens is extraordinarily diverse. Much of the host response centers on the pathogen and the route and extent of the infection. This chapter analyzes some general features of host-pathogen interaction and discusses general principles of them. The chapter is based on a recent one that also dealt with general aspects of innate immunity and considered aspects of innate immunity studied mainly in mice (Unanue, 2000).

Two interactions take place between the host and pathogen, distinguished by the extent of involvement of the lymphocyte. Responses independent of lymphocytes have been termed natural immunity, innate immunity, or T-independent responses (Bancroft et al., 1991; Fearon and Locksley, 1996; Medzhitov and Janeway, 1998). Responses involving lymphocytes are the adaptive responses. The innate response includes the response of various leukocytes, in particular the cells of the mononuclear phagocyte system (the macrophages), the cells of the dendritic cell lineage, the granulocytes, and the natural killer (NK) cells. All of them are mobilized and activated on challenge with infectious organisms, without the need for direct participation by the T cell. Their response to pathogens is fast and immediate, which has led to the concept that the innate cellular response is the initial step in the host response. The cells of the innate response also cooperate with the lymphocytes through two distinct processes. One is by presenting antigens in the form of peptide fragments. The T-cell system recognizes peptide fragments only when they are bound to molecules of the major histocompatibility complex (MHC) system. The second process is by releasing modulatory molecules, which are made up predominantly of cytokines. The cells of the innate system regulate and poise the adaptive response when it comes into operation (Unanue, 1997).

INNATE RESPONSE

Mutant mice that are congenitally without lymphocytes constitute the best experimental system for the analysis of the innate system of defense (reviewed by Bancroft et al. [1991] and Unanue [1997]). These mice survive only because of the function of their innate system. These strains include the SCID mice, a strain found by Bosma that lacks all lymphocytes, but has normal hematopoiesis and normal macrophages, granulocytes, and NK cells. SCID mice have a defect in one of the enzymes, DNA-PK, involved in the recombination of the V gene segments required to form the mature antigen receptor of T and B cells. Other mice have been produced, by gene ablation techniques, that lack other enzymes in this recombination process, like Rag and Kμ proteins, and that also exhibit a selective absence of lymphocytes.

SCID mice develop normally and can live without many problems in relatively clean environments. (Table 1). These mice have a strong line of defense toward many pathogens and can restrict or delay the course of infection. Inflammatory responses are normal, and all leukocytes can be mobilized. Their extent of resistance depends strongly on the pathogen. While many bacterial infections can be controlled, SCID mice do not do well in combating viruses. Infections with common murine pathogens, including viruses, and other pathogens, like *Pneumocystis carinii*, occasionally develop.

The three central cells of the innate response that operate in the SCID mice are the macrophages, neutrophils, and NK cells. In particular, macrophages and NK cells release early cytokines that are involved in inflammation and participate in a cascade of cell-to-cell interactions that result in the activation of macrophages and neutrophils. There are two major

Emil R. Unanue • Department of Pathology and Immunology, Washington University School of Medicine, St. Louis, MO 63110.

Table 1. Properties of SCID mice

1. Complete absence of B and T lymphocytes
2. A cellular thymus with only stromal cells; very atrophic lymph nodes and spleen with about 1/10 the number of cells
3. Normal number of granulocytes, macrophages, and NK cells
4. Leukocyte mobilization in response to sterile or infectious inflammation
5. Normal antigen-presenting function: class I and II expression normal, allogeneic or syngeneic T-cell responses stimulated by APC
6. No cytokine release by spleen cells on addition of mitogens (like concanavalin A); IL-1, IL-12, and TNF released by addition of some microbes
7. Induction of IFN-γ release from NK cells by macrophage-NK cell interaction
8. Partially resistant to microbial infections: reduced microbial growth, development of a carrier state of resistance, but no sterilizing immunity
9. Production of number of cytokines from macrophages and NK cells; these cytokines include IL-1α, IL-1β, TNF-α, TNF-β, IL-6, IL-10, and IL-12 (all from macrophages) and IFN-γ (from NK cells); no production of IL-2, IL-4, or IL-5.
10. Immune function reconstituted to normal by addition of T cells (or bone marrow stem cells)

differences in the response of SCID mice to pathogens from that of normal mice. First, SCID mice show no sterilizing immunity; thus, the growth of the pathogens can only be partially controlled but not eliminated. Second, SCID mice do not develop a memory or secondary response following a primary infection. The state of cellular activation is limited and cannot be perpetuated unless lymphocytes are present. The response of SCID mice to the pathogen *Listeria monocytogenes* is discussed later in this chapter.

RECOGNITION OF THE PATHOGEN BY THE INNATE SYSTEM: COMPARISON WITH THE ADAPTIVE SYSTEM

The manner in which the innate system recognizes a foreign element is quite distinct from that used by the adaptive system. The first difference lies in the nature of the molecules involved in the recognition. The surface structures on macrophages, neutrophils, and other cells involved in recognition of pathogens are expressed in all cells and do not involve recombination of the DNA segments encoding their combining site. In contrast, the hallmarks of the lymphocyte receptors that recognize foreign elements are that they form a cellular system involving receptors expressed in a clonal fashion and resulting from the recombination of gene segments that encode a different portion of the combining site.

Another major difference between the innate and the lymphocyte systems lies in the nature of the molecules that are recognized. The innate system recognizes the display of complex carbohydrates or lipoproteins that form the walls of the microbes. These structures may be shared among microbes. Many of these molecules are presented as repeating units that permit the extensive association with the cellular recognition molecules, a circumstance that favors interactions of higher avidity, which result in signaling and uptake by phagocytosis. To quote Hoffman et al. (1999) (Medzhitov and Janeway, 1998), who have long studied the innate system, "the repetitive structure permits all the prongs to engage." In contrast, lymphocytes recognize small segments of proteins or glycoproteins, either directly as in the B cells or following intracellular protein processing as in T cells (see "Symbiosis between the innate cellular system and the T-cell response" below).

The innate system recognizes pathogens by way of surface receptors as well as by using circulating blood proteins. A variety of surface molecules, found mostly in macrophages and neutrophils but also in epithelial cells, are involved: some primarily recognize and bind to the pathogen, and others are primarily involved in signaling or in promoting phagocytosis. The blood protein system is involved in recognition of the pathogen, leading to the deposition on their surface of proteins that either kill the pathogen or allow leukocytes to phagocytize it.

Among the cell surface receptors identified in phagocytes are the family of scavenger receptors (Freeman et al., 1991), the Toll-like receptors (TLR), and a number of diverse receptors for polysaccharides (including macrosialin [CD68] and the mannose receptor), microbial lipoproteins (CD14), and immunoglobulin G (IgG) and complement (C) proteins (reviewed by Franc et al. [1999]).

Several members of the scavenger receptors have been cloned (receptors A, type I and II, and type B, CD36, and others). These surface proteins have broad specificity and interact with gram-positive and -negative bacteria, participating in their clearance from the circulation. Scavenger receptors also bind to negatively charged molecules, low-density lipoproteins, polynucleotides, and anionic polysaccharides, and phospholipids. Scavenger receptors have homologies to structures found in hemocytes of insects, presumably the early evolutionary counterparts of phagocytes.

In analogy to invertebrates, the Toll system of surface molecules is centrally involved in the processes that lead to recognition of the pathogen and activation of the effector cell. The Toll molecules were identified in the fruit fly *Drosophila melanogas-*

ter as developmental molecules involved in the dorsoventral organization. They were also found to be required in the antifungal response of the fly. Interaction with Toll resulted in the activation of several genes that encode peptides that kill the fungi. Other molecules in *Drosophila,* like 18-wheeler, are involved in responses to bacteria (Color Plate 3).

In vertebrates, several TLR have been identified (Medzhitov et al., 1997). The TLR are transmembrane proteins with extracellular leucine-rich repeats, a transmembrane segment, and a cytoplasmic domain with homology to the interleukin-1 (IL-1) receptor. Up to nine different TLR have now been identified, and each may serve to primarily interact with a given pathogen. TLR-2, for example is involved in interactions with gram-positive bacteria and yeasts, while TLR-4 is involved in interaction with the lipopolysaccharides (LPS) of gram-negative organisms. The importance of TLR-4 was first noted in a strain of mice that was unresponsive to the endotoxin and which had a mutation.

The mechanism by which TLR interact with the microbial surface is the subject of much analysis at present. Recognition of the microbe may well involve more than one receptor with which TLR associate or form part of the recognition unit. For the recognition of LPS, the surface molecule CD14 is involved by binding to it, yet it does not signal the cell unless it acts in concert with TLR-4. All the TLR molecules signal through NF-κB and a series of adapter molecules, resulting in the transcription of genes that encode cytokines and costimulator molecules. Signaling takes place by way of the IL-1 receptor family of cytoplasmic domains, which include the IL-1 and IL-18 receptors.

The Fc and C receptors are of major importance since they promote, by several thousand-fold, the uptake of microbes containing bound antibody and/or C proteins (Ravetch and Clynes, 1998). Various Fc receptors for IgG (FcγRI, FcγRII, FcγRIII) have been identified and cloned.

The C system is involved both in recognizing pathogens and in inducing inflammation (Fig. 1) (reviewed by Abbas et al. [2000]). C includes a number of blood proteins as well as molecules on the surface of leukocytes. Once the system is initiated or activated, a series of protein-to-protein interactions take place, some involving enzymatic reactions that result in partial proteolysis of key C proteins, with the release of biologically active peptides and the deposition of fragments on target cells. The surface molecules include receptors for some of the C proteins and also molecules that regulate the interactions of the C proteins when deposited on the cell membrane. Through the cascade of interactions de-

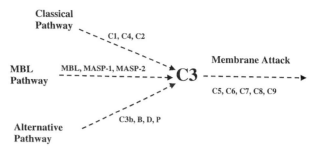

Figure 1. The various pathways that result in activation of the C3 protein. Once C3 is cleaved, the C system proceeds in protein-protein interactions involving the indicated C proteins. Figure courtesy of John P. Atkinson.

picted in Color Plate 3, three important biological effects are generated. First is the deposition on the target cell surface of C proteins, most prominently C3, a central protein in the cascade. When C3 is specifically activated, the partially cleaved fragments are deposited on the cell. The C receptors CR1, CR2, and CR3 show specificity for cleaved C3 fragments. These receptors are expressed in monocytes, macrophages, neutrophils, and B cells to various degrees (Fearon and Locksley, 1996). The target cell is now "opsonized" and can interact with specific C receptors on leukocytes. Since the original description of its phenomenon, opsonization has become recognized as a major step in the clearance and elimination from the blood and extracellular fluids of many microbes and proteins. Following adhesion of the target cell to the leukocyte, phagocytosis takes place, resulting in the internalization of the target cell and, depending on its nature, on its killing by the leukocyte.

Other important biological activities of C result from the release of small peptides derived from the cleavage of the C proteins. These peptides cause inflammation: some, like the fragment C3a, lead mast cells to degranulate and to release vasoactive amines that result in blood vessel dilatation and increase blood flow; others, like the C5a fragment, are potent chemoattractants for neutrophils. Finally, the deposition of the terminal C proteins, i.e., the last series of proteins that join the cascade, causes the formation of a pore on the surface with changes in water and electrolyte flow and eventual osmotic death of the cell. Thus, target cells can be eliminated by either phagocytosis or direct membrane alterations, while at the same time inflammation takes place with changes in blood vessels and the arrival of neutrophils.

The key point with this important protein system is the mode of initiation that leads to the one central step of partial cleavage of C3 (to C3b). The

C system can be activated through three distinct pathways, two of which are part of the innate system. The classical pathway is mediated by the antibody molecule binding to its target cell and activating the first protein in the cascade, C1q. The other two pathways are phylogenetically distant, appearing in the invertebrates, and include the alternative pathway and the lectin pathway. In the alternative pathway, a small amount of C3b is spontaneously deposited on the surface of the target cells, most probably because of a low level of C3 degradation from serum enzymes. In mammalian cells this deposition is limited and regulated by a number of surface proteins that control such activation. The normal surface glycoproteins containing terminal sialic acid are important in fostering the interaction for one critical regulatory protein, factor H, which inhibits interactions of C3b with other C proteins. In contrast, no such regulation occurs when C3b is deposited on microbial surfaces, and activation proceeds. This alternative pathway of complement activation is thought to be vital in the clearance of many encapsulated organisms. Indeed, a genetic defect in C3, the key opsonic protein that deposits on microbe surfaces, is incompatible with life, resulting in pronounced infections with diverse microorganisms, particularly extracellular bacteria (reviewed by Carrol [1998]).

The third pathway of C activation involves proteins that directly interact with carbohydrates and lead to C3 cleavage. Included in this group is a serum protein made in the liver, termed mannose binding protein (MBP) (Turner, 1996). MBP has structural similarities to C1q, having 18 binding subunits with a C-terminal lectin domain and a collagen-like amino terminus. MBP forms part of a group of proteins, the collectins, which are considered a first line of defense through their interactions with polysaccharides and glycoproteins (Epstein et al., 1996). Collectins have general structural features; they are polymers made of subunits, each with a carbohydrate recognition unit and a collagen-like stalk. Other collectins are the serum bovine protein conglutinin and the lung surfactant proteins A and D. (The lung surfactants are thought to be involved in the rapid clearance of inhaled bacteria at the level of lung alveoli, most probably through a mechanism of opsonization involving the uptake and elimination of the bacteria by the alveolar macrophages [Turner, 1996].) MBP interacts with mannose and n-acetylglucosamine residues on bacterial surfaces. It does not interact with mammalian surface glycoproteins. MBP circulates complexed with inactive enzymes (MASP-1 and MASP-2), but following binding to carbohydrates, the two serine proteases are activated, leading to the cleavage of C3 and initiation of the cascade. MBP is believed to be the most primitive of the proteins associated with the C system and was perhaps the first to develop. Some mutations in MBP are believed to influence susceptibility to microbial infection (Turner, 1996). Other circulating proteins, with a general structural similarity to collectins, are the ficolins, which interact with n-acetylglucosamine of bacteria. Ficolins also associate with MASP and cleave C3 (Matsushita et al., 2000).

CELLULAR RESPONSE

Activated Macrophages

The mononuclear phagocyte system includes the circulating monocytes and their products of differentiation, the various tissue macrophages, and the dendritic cell lineage (Gordon et al., 1995). Macrophages are found in all tissues, usually near epithelial surfaces and blood vessels. Macrophages constitute a first barrier to the dissemination of exogenous material. Mononuclear phagocytes are also involved in the reorganization of tissue during inflammation and in wound healing and are involved in the removal of tissue debris and apoptotic cells. Macrophages function in part by the release of mediators that affect the surrounding cells. The early release of cytokines by macrophages is an important response to microbes. Macrophages also express histocompatibility molecules and participate in interactions with CD4 and CD8 T cells (Tables 2 and 3).

The production and differentiation of macrophages are under the control of colony-stimulating factors (CSF), of which CSF-1 is the major member. CSF-1 is a protein elaborated by many cells including mesenchymal cells. Its absence translates into a deficit of mature macrophages in some organs, resulting in the pathologic manifestations exhibited by the osteopetrotic mouse. These mice show an increase in bone formation because of the normal formation of bone matrix by osteoblasts, which is not balanced by its removal by osteoclasts, the multinucleated giant cells derived from blood monocytes.

Macrophages are activated in response to foreign stimuli. An activated macrophage is a large cell, with an increase in the number of vacuoles and more active pinocytic activity (Mackaness, 1964). In culture, activated macrophages spread avidly on the culture dish, in contrast to resting macrophages, which are loosely attached. Notably, activated macrophages express a number of cytocidal molecules that enable them to control the growth of intracellular pathogens. Among these are reactive oxygen and nitrogen metabolites (Klebanoff, 1998; Nathan, 1997). Highly

Table 2. Properties of macrophages

1. Membrane receptors for diverse chemical structures
   Scavenger receptor
   C receptors
   Fcγ receptors
   Sialoadhesin
   Mannose receptors
   Macrosialin
   Cytokine receptors (IFN-γ, TNF)
   CD14-LPS receptor

2. Production of cytokines
   IL-1α, IL-1β
   TNF-α
   IL-12
   IL-10
   IL-6
   Fibroblast growth factor

3. Antigen presentation

4. Production of enzymes involved in antimicrobial responses
   and/or acting on connective tissue proteins and cells
   Collagenase
   Elastase
   Lysozyme
   Lysosomal enzymes

5. Production of bioactive lipid and small radicals
   Prostaglandins
   Platelet-activating factor
   Reactive oxygen intermediates
   Reactive nitrogen intermediates

Table 3. Generation of activated macrophages

Pathway I (T-cell independent)
1. Microbe → macrophage receptors (TLR and others)
2. Release of early cytokines by macrophages (IL-12, TNF-α, IL-1β, IL-6)
3. IL-12 + TNF → NK cell
4. NK cells produce IFN-γ

Pathway II (T-cell dependent)
1. Microbe → macrophages
2. Release of early cytokines by macrophages as in step above
3. Presentation of microbial peptides to T cells by macrophages
4. Upregulation of B7-1 and B7-2 by macrophages
5. T-cell activation
   TCR engaged by peptide-MHC complex of the macrophage
   T-cell–APC interaction fostered by adhesion/costimulatory molecules/CD40-CD40L molecules
6. Differentiation of T cells to Th1 pattern of differentiation through IL-12 release

reactive oxygen derivatives are formed during the consumption of oxygen by the macrophages. The reactions involve the assembly of a phagocyte oxidase (phos) that utilizes NADPH. The oxidase contains three cytosolic proteins and a unique membrane cytochrome b, which uses NADPH to transfer oxygen. The oxidant species that are made include the superoxide anion (O_2^-), the perhydroxyl radical ($HO_2\cdot$), and the hydroxyl radical ($OH\cdot$). Reactive oxygen intermediates are important cytocidal molecules that kill a variety of bacteria, particularly the extracellular pyogenic species (like staphylococci, streptococci, pneumococci, and *Haemophilus*). A striking clinical observation that indicates the importance of this pathway is the congenital disease chronic granulomatous disease, in which the patients are highly sensitive to infections with pyogenic organisms (reviewed by Rosen [1993]). Several defects have been found to be responsible for chronic granulomatous disease, each being associated with mutations in the components of the oxidase, particularly of the *phos* gene.

The production of NO· by activated macrophages results from the expression of an inducible enzyme, inducible nitric oxide synthase. (There are two constitutive isoforms of the enzyme, the endothelial and neuronal forms.) Nitric oxide is produced from the metabolism of arginine to citrulline. Nitration of a number of enzymes, including ribonucleoside reductase, results in the impaired growth of cells. Activated macrophages that are infected with pathogens restrict their growth, and part, or all, of this restriction can be attributed to nitric oxide production. For example, inhibition of nitric oxide production in mice infected with a number of intracellular facultative bacteria or with a variety of viruses resulted in uncontrolled infection. The same effects were found in mice lacking the gene for the inducible nitric oxide synthase. Under these situations, mice resist infections with pyogenic bacteria. In contrast, mice defective in the oxidase are susceptible to extracellular bacteria. While defects in one or the other cytocidal pathway can usually be compensated for, combined defects of both results in severe infections with opportunistic organisms (Shiloh et al., 1999).

The activated macrophage, first described in tuberculosis infection, is the cellular hallmark of the response to intracellular pathogens, as is most evident in the formation of the tuberculous granuloma (Lurie, 1964; Mackaness, 1964). The granuloma consists of activated macrophages, some of which contain the bacilli, while others form multinucleated giant cells. (This capacity of macrophages to organize in infective foci and restrict the spread of microbes is a primitive evolutionary behavior. A similar behavior is noted in invertebrates as a response to exogenous stimuli, e.g., an accumulation of hemocytes that restrict the dissemination of the phlogogenic material.)

The relationship between activated macrophages and the control of the infection with intracellular pathogens was highly emphasized in the classical studies of Lurie and collaborators (Lurie, 1964) in experimental tuberculosis. Their studies made the important point that it was the activated macrophages that curbed the growth of the tubercule bacilli, while serum antibodies were ineffective. This relationship was subsequently established in murine infections with *Listeria monocytogenes,* particularly by the Mackaness group (Mackaness, 1964). Their observations led to the concept that defense against some intracellular pathogens was dependent not on antibody molecules but on the activated macrophage. In striking contrast, defense against extracellular toxins, against infections with many extracellular pyogenic bacteria, and against the blood and extracellular stages of some viral infections included a strong involvement by serum antibodies that either neutralized the phlogogen or opsonized it for phagocytosis or for attack by C activation.

The activation of macrophages is mainly the result of the interaction of macrophages with the cytokine gamma interferon (IFN-γ) (Bach et al., 1997), which binds to specific receptors found in many different cells, including those of the mononuclear phagocyte lineage. Neutralizing IFN-γ in mice by injection of monoclonal antibodies or infecting mice that do not produce IFN-γ or do not respond to it because of lack of the IFN-γ receptor or the IFN signaling molecules like STAT-1 (i.e., by gene ablation techniques) results in overwhelming infection with intracellular pathogens and the absence of activated macrophages. In humans, genetic defects in the receptor or in STAT-1 result in high susceptibility to infections with mycobacteria and salmonellae (Newport et al., 1996). IFN-γ is the most important of the cytokines produced during the early stages of an infection, since it regulates a number of cellular effector pathways by activating a number of important genes (including LMP2 and LMP7, involved in proteasome activation and NO synthase gene involved in NO production).

There are two important issues to note. The first is that the effect of IFN-γ on macrophages is markedly potentiated by second stimuli, which include interaction with bacteria or their products (LPS are the most notable) or with cytokines, particularly tumor necrosis factor (TNF). The second is that macrophage activation can be inhibited, in particular by cytokines like IL-4, IL-10, and transforming growth factor β, which are anti-inflammatory. The way in which the balance of IFN-γ versus these anti-inflammatory cytokines occurs during an infectious process can be critical and needs to be evaluated, particularly in chronic situations (Moore et al., 1993).

Because both NK cells and T cells produce IFN-γ, the activated macrophage is found as a result of activation of either the innate system or the T-cell system (Table 3). The innate system becomes activated when macrophages interact with microbes, leading to the release of early cytokines that then interact with other cells, particularly NK cells (Unanue, 1997). The adaptive T-cell system is activated in a clonal manner when the antigen-reactive cloned T cells recognize the specific peptides from pathogens presented by histocompatibility molecules.

Neutrophils

Neutrophils are the major cells controlling the growth of extracellular bacteria as well as some intracellular facultative pathogens. Neutrophils are the main phagocytic cells in human blood but are less represented in the mouse. They are terminal cells that do not divide, and they have a short life span (6 to 8 h). In humans, neutrophils are produced in large numbers (about 10^{11} per day) under normal circumstances, under the influence of G-CSF. Neutrophils die by apoptosis and are then eliminated by macrophages through phagocytosis. Neutropenic individuals are highly sensitive to infections with extracellular bacteria, which usually are eliminated by the neutrophil microbicidal mechanisms.

The neutrophil utilizes both oxidative and nonoxidative mechanisms to kill bacteria. The oxidative burst, as described above for activated macrophages, involves the activation of the NADPH oxidase with the generation of superoxide anion. In the neutrophil much of the O_2^- is converted to hydrogen peroxide, which in turn reacts with Cl^- ions to generate hypochlorous acid (HOCl); this reaction is catalyzed by the enzyme myeloperoxidase. This is a short-lived compound that can also react with amines to form the more stable microbicidal N-chloramines. The importance of the NADPH oxidase became evident in studies of chronic granulomatous disease, where defects in the elimination of gram-positive organisms are evident. The nonoxidative mechanisms of neutrophils involve cationic peptides of the neutrophil granule. The defensins comprise a family of antimicrobial peptides, some located in their primary granules (Ganz and Lehrer, 1997; Boman, 1998). (Defensins and related molecules are also produced in epithelial cells and serve as major microbicidal molecules in infections of respiratory and gastrointestinal epithelia. Similar molecules have been identified in invertebrates and could represent the most primitive line of defense.)

The migration of neutrophils to sites of inflammation is critical. Directed migration or chemotaxis takes place when the neutrophil recognizes a gradient of the chemoattractant. Among the chemoattractants are products derived from C activation (e.g., C5a), small lipids (e.g., leukotriene B$_4$, from the leukotriene cascade of mediators), microbial products, and a large family of small polypeptides, the chemokine family. Chemokines comprise about a dozen or more small proteins, now classified into three groups, CXC, CC, and C chemokines, depending on the presence of terminal cysteine residues (reviewed by Rollins [1997] and Mantovani [1999]). The CXC chemokines (i.e., those with two terminal cysteines with a residue in between) are powerful neutrophil chemoattractants, while the CC and C chemokines attract monocytes and lymphocytes. More than one chemokine can interact with each receptor: promiscuity in binding is extensive. Chemokines are induced strongly by interaction with a range of bacteria. Particularly prominent is the release of CXC family members as a consequence of infection with streptococci and staphylococci. The interplay between host and microbes in the context of chemokines is critical. This issue will become clearly understood now that the major chemical moieties (and their receptors) have been identified.

The neutrophil is activated by interactions with microbes, particularly if these are opsonized, as described in the previous section. Cytokines also contribute to the activation. At present, some discussion has developed concerning the participation of neutrophils in infections with intracellular pathogens. Clearly, neutrophils are found in tuberculous granulomas, but their role is not clear. With some intracellular pathogens, neutrophils do have an effect in reducing the microbial load (Unanue, 1997).

In summary, the above discussions about activated macrophages and neutrophils point to two effector systems that restrict the growth of microbes. In the innate immune reactions, extracellular, pyogenic bacteria interact directly with membrane receptors of phagocytes or indirectly by way of the C system activated through either the alternative pathway or the lectin pathway. In adaptive immunity, antibody molecules opsonize extracellular pyogenic bacteria, together with the complement protein C3. In either circumstances, the opsonized bacteria taken up, particularly by neutrophils, are killed in a process involving the respiratory burst with the generation of oxygen intermediates. In contrast, the many facultative and obligate intracellular pathogens are not entirely or partially eliminated by neutrophils, even if opsonized. They are eliminated by macrophages only when activated by IFN-γ. IFN-γ is released by NK cells during innate stages of infections and/or by CD4 CD8 T cells during the adaptive phase. Under normal circumstances, the innate and adaptive systems act in synchrony.

The NK Cell Response

NK cells, which represent about 10% of circulating blood cells, constitute an early line of defense against viruses and intracellular pathogenic bacteria. NK cells derive from stem cells of the bone marrow, and they mature in the absence of lymphocytes. Athymic (SCID) mice have a normal number of NK cells while being devoid of T cells (Table 1) (Trinchieri, 1989). NK cells were first identified by their capacity to kill target cells without the need for prior sensitization or priming. NK cells participate in the early stages of the response to many viruses like vaccinia virus, mousepox virus, and cytomegalovirus. Their deletion results in widespread viral dissemination. Inbred strains of mice vary in their susceptibility to viral growth through variations in genes that affect NK cell function. NK cells have also been implicated in the control of infection with intracellular bacteria (e.g., *Listeria*, and the control of some parasitic infections (e.g., with *Toxoplasma gondii*). Tumor growth and tumor metastasis can be influenced by NK cells (Trinchieri, 1989).

When NK cells establish contact with the target cell, the NK cells degranulate and release granule-associated proteins. Two key proteins of the granule are the granzymes and perforin, which cooperate in bringing about the death of the target cell: perforin released from the granule forms a pore on the membrane of target cells, and the granzymes then enter the target cell through the pore made by perforin and kill the cell, via apoptosis.

NK cells are also involved in the response to intracellular pathogens, by virtue of their strong production of cytokines, particularly IFN-γ, as described above in the discussion of activated macrophages (Unanue, 1997). The production of IFN-γ can be extensive, placing the NK cell as a central component of the regulation of the early stages of an infectious process, particularly by intracellular pathogens. Indeed, IFN-γ plays an essential role in cellular activation besides having an antiviral effect.

Although NK cells can produce cytokines after their interaction with target cells, the main stimuli for their cytokine production derives from macrophages. A pathway of stimulation from macrophages to NK cells has been identified in which the macrophage interacts with pathogenic organisms and this interaction results in the release of the cytokines IL-12 and TNF (reviewed by Unanue [1997]). The production of cytokines by the macrophage first involves its activation with the TLR induced by interaction with the organism. Both IL-12 and TNF bind to specific receptors on the NK cells, activating them and inducing them to produce IFN-γ. Other cytokines are also released from the macrophages, like IL-1α, IL-1β, IL-18, and IL-6, and each has a predominant target of action. This pathway of cytokine cascade, i.e., pathogen → macrophages → IL-12 + TNF → NK cells = IFN-γ, operates in a variety of infections, particularly with intracellular pathogenic bacteria, parasites, and some viruses. Upon production of IFN-γ, the macrophage system is activated and primed to become a highly cytocidal cell. NK cells are also regulated by a number of cytokines that promote their growth and activation. Among these are IL-2 and IL-15 molecules, as well as IFN-α/β.

Recently, there has been much interest in the mechanism used by NK cells to recognize their target cells and the factors that regulate their activities (Lanier, 1997) The evidence points to two sets of surface receptors: the activation receptors, which permit recognition and killing of target cells, and, importantly, the inhibitory receptors, which, if engaged, inhibit the activation of the NK cell. The nature of all the activating receptors is not entirely known. Another activating receptor is the FcγRIII (CD16), which allows the interaction of NK cells with target cells bound to antibody molecules. There are examples of receptors (see below) that can be inhibitory or activating depending on the presence or absence of inhibitory signals in their cytosolic domains. The inhibitory receptors interact with various forms of class I MHC molecules. An NK cell that interacts with a target cell bearing class I MHC molecules may be inhibited from killing the target cell. As a proof of the involvement of class I MHC molecules, this inhibition can be released by blocking and/or removing the class I MHC molecules (this is the missing-self hypothesis proposed by Karre) (Karre et al., 1986). Thus, the NK cells may favor recognition of target cells bearing low levels or abnormal forms of class I MHC molecules, as can occur with some virally infected or tumor cells. The inhibitory receptors are diverse and are represented by two sets of molecules, C-type lectin receptors and Ig-like receptors. The former are disulfide-linked type 2 integral membrane dimers (e.g., human CD94 and mouse Ly49A). The Ig-like receptors, which have been termed KIR, are diverse membrane proteins that vary in their expression of Ig domains. NK cells appear to vary in the extent and diversity of NK-cell-inhibiting

receptors. Different allelic forms of receptors exist. All these express cytoplasmic tyrosine inhibitory products (ITIM), which associate upon their phosphorylation with tyrosine phosphatases, antagonizing the activation of tyrosine protein kinases. It is noteworthy that some viruses express a class I-like MHC molecule which can have biological consequence by engaging and neutralizing the NK cell receptors. This has been documented for murine cytomegalovirus.

CELLULAR INTERACTION IN INNATE RESPONSES TO MICROBES: LESSONS FROM *LISTERIOSIS*

L. monocytogenes infection in the SCID mouse has served as a basic experimental model to examine the interactions of microbes with the innate immune system, in the complete absence of lymphocytes (Fig. 2; Table 3). Similar results have now been found in infections by other intracellular pathogens, so some general principles can be deduced on how these infections are partially controlled. In the *Listeria* infection in SCID mice, exponential growth of *Listeria* takes place after systemic infection. The rate of growth is about the same as in normal mice. After a

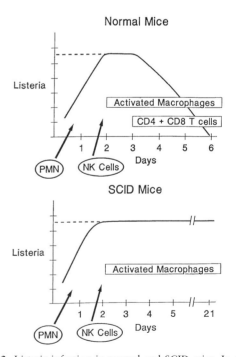

Figure 2. *Listeria* infection in normal and SCID mice. In normal mice there is exponential growth of bacteria followed by control of the infection. The cells involved at different stages are indicated. In SCID mice the absence of lymphocytes results in persistence of the infection. The early components of the infection involve neutrophils and NK cells, while lymphocytes are essential for clearance of the infection.

few days, the growth of *Listeria* stops but the numbers of bacteria are maintained at about a steady state for prolonged periods. During the growth phase, *Listeria* cells are contained in small granulomas. In normal mice, at about the same time, the number of *Listeria* cells progressively decreases, leading to their complete elimination. *Listeria* cells can reach the cytosol as a consequence of their production of the pore-forming protein listeriolysin O (reviewed by Unanue [1997]). This cytosolic stage allows *Listeria* cells to pass among cells in tissues apparently without an extracellular phase (Tilney and Portnoy, 1989). The vacuolar and cytosolic stages of *Listeria* generate peptides for either class II or I MHC molecules, which will trigger T-cell activation. Sterilizing immunity in *Listeria* infection results from CD4 and/or CD8 T cells that are generated during presentation of *Listeria* antigens by the macrophages or dendritic cells (Kaufmann, 1993; North et al., 1997; Pamer et al., 1997).

Listeria infection proceeds through a number of stages, each of which involves the action of particular cells and cytokines. The early exponential growth of *Listeria* is controlled by neutrophils within a few hours of the infection (Unanue, 1997). The activated macrophages do not become apparent until 2 or 3 days later. Involved in the early neutrophil phase is the cytokine IL-1, most probably by modulating the appearance of chemokines. Among the chemokines involved in the recruitment of monocytes is MCP-1. Indeed, mice lacking expression of CCR2, the receptor for MCP-1, as a result of gene ablation do not recruit macrophages and are highly sensitive to *Listeria* infection. The role of neutrophils is not only to curb the dissemination of the microbe but also to control the liver infection. *Listeria* infects hepatocytes, where it grows exuberantly unless restricted by neutrophils. Ablation of neutrophils results in dissemination of the microbe throughout the parenchyma, with widespread death of liver cells by apoptosis: mice die of acute liver failure. (The importance of the neutrophils is also apparent in normal mice and in the secondary challenge of normal previously infected mice.) The complete dependency on neutrophils for control of the early growth of *Listeria* indicates clearly how different cells and effector mechanisms cooperate in bringing about control of the infection.

Following the early growth phase, NK cells come into action through the release of IFN-γ, which leads to macrophage activation. Interestingly, both normal and SCID mice produce the same number of activated macrophages. In SCID mice, the induction of IFN-γ by NK cells results from cytokines released by macrophages, IL-12, and TNF. (In normal mice,

the clonal *Listeria* T cells also respond after recognizing immunogenic peptides from the *Listeria* presented by antigen-presenting cells [APC].) In normal mice, the NK- and T-cell stages rapidly blend with each other.

Examination of the macrophages discloses a heightened expression of MHC class II molecules and of their antigen-presenting capabilities. The macrophages show enhanced microbicidal activity and all the properties of activated macrophages, including the production of nitric oxide and oxygen radicals. The activated macrophages restrict the growth of *Listeria* in the granulomas in a process that involves the release of nitric oxide.

Despite this extensive macrophage activation noted in both SCID and normal mice, the difference in the infections by the two strains is marked: it was mentioned above that the normal strain develops sterilizing immunity; the SCID strain, on the other hand, becomes a chronic carrier of the infection. The conclusion is that activated macrophages by themselves are not capable of entirely eliminating an infection by intracellular pathogens and that lymphocytes must play a role in complete microbial elimination beyond that of activating macrophages by IFN.

Listeria organisms are powerful agonists for macrophage release of cytokines. The elements in *Listeria* that induce this response probably involve more than one chemical entity. Not all microbes induce this powerful macrophage response, and thus the extent to which SCID mice mobilize the innate system will vary. The SCID mouse responds to *Listeria* uptake by the release of IL-12 and TNF by macrophages that have taken up the microbe. Both these cytokines play seminal roles in the regulation of the innate system, along with the lymphocytes. IL-12 and TNF both bind to specific receptors and drive NK cells for the expression of IFN-γ. As with IFN-γ, neutralization of these cytokines by specific antibodies, or by gene ablation, results in uncontrolled infection. The role of TNF is, however, much broader than that of IL-12. TNF acts not only on various leukocytes but also in the vascular endothelium. TNF-activated endothelia express adhesion molecules (E-selectin, intercellular cell adhesion molecule [ICAM]) that promotes the adhesion of leukocytes and their migration to the extracellular milieu.

SYMBIOSIS BETWEEN THE INNATE CELLULAR SYSTEM AND THE T-CELL RESPONSE: THE MHC SYSTEM

T-cell responses depend on their recognition of peptides derived from the intracellular processing of protein antigens, an event carried out by the macrophages or DC, major cells of the innate system. Peptides derived from antigen processing bind to the MHC molecules. MHC molecules are peptide-binding molecules that save peptides from intracellular digestion and transport them to the cell surface (Babbitt et al., 1985). The peptide-MHC molecular complex is the molecular substrate that engages the T-cell receptor for antigen.

The composition of the peptide-MHC complex reflects the intracellular milieu of the APC. Class I MHC molecules sample peptides from proteins localized to the cytosol. In contrast, the peptides bound to class II molecules derive mainly from proteins taken by the vesicular system of the APC. The class I MHC molecules are central to the presentation of peptides derived from viruses or bacteria that reach the cytosol. CD8 T cells have cytolytic properties and will lyse infected cells and also release cytokines with antiviral effects, like IFN-α/β and IFN-γ. An important point is that class I MHC molecules are expressed in most cells. Thus, most infected cells can signal their infection through class I MHC molecules. The class II MHC system samples proteins found in the vesicular system, i.e., proteins that are internalized from the extracellular milieu by either receptor-mediated or fluid-phase endocytosis. Thus, the MHC class II molecules are essential for presentation of many of the microbes that have entered the APC through phagocytosis. CD4 T cells recognize the MHC class II-peptide complex and are the central cells in the response to intracellular pathogens. Thus, it is via the two major sets of MHC molecules—the class I and class II MHC proteins—that the T-cell system is informed whether an abnormal or previously unrecognized molecule has entered the APC. The MHC molecules thus connect the innate cellular response with the T-cell response (Babbitt et al., 1985; Bjorkman et al., 1987; reviewed by Latek and Unanue [1999]).

The presentation of a peptide-MHC complex by the APC initiates the activation of the T cells; on T-cell activation, a series of cellular events profoundly changes the cellular environment. Following the presentation of the peptide-MHC complex, APC express adhesion and stimulatory molecules that serve to foster close cell adhesion as well as activation of the T cells. Activated T cells will proliferate and release cytokines like IL-2, IL-4, IL-6, lymphotoxin, and IFNs, which alter the environment; they also direct cellular interactions that can activate or kill cells. Prominent among these interactions are those of CD4 T cells with B cells, which result in antibody formation, those of CD4 or CD8 T cells with APC, releasing IFN-γ and activating the macrophage system, and those of CD8 T cells with APC or other MHC-bearing cells, causing their death.

REFERENCES

Abbas, A. K., A. H. Lichtman, and J. S. Pober. 2000. *The Complement System in Cellular and Molecular Immunology*, 4th ed., p. 316. The W. B. Saunders Co., Philadelphia, Pa.

Babbitt, B. P., P. M. Allen, G. Matsueda, E. Haber, and E. R. Unanue. 1985. Binding of immunogenic peptides to Ia histocompatibility molecules. *Nature* 317:359–363.

Bach, E. A., M. Aguet, and R. D. Schreiber. 1997. The IFN-γ receptor: a paradigm for cytokine receptor signalling. *Annu. Rev. Immunol.* 15:563–591.

Bancroft, G. J., R. D. Schreiber, and E. R. Unanue. 1991. Natural immunity: a T-cell-independent pathway of macrophage activation, defined in the SCID mouse. *Immunol. Rev.* 124:5–24.

Bjorkman, P. J., B. Saper, B. Samraoui, W. S. Bennett, J. L. Strominger, and D. C. Wiley. 1987. The foreign antigen binding site and T cell recognition regions of class I histocompatibility regions. *Nature* 329:512–515.

Boman, H. G. 1998. Gene-encoded peptide antibiotics and the concept of innate immunity: an update review. *Scand. J. Immunol.* 48:15–25.

Carrol, M. C. 1998. The role of complement and complement receptors in the induction and regulation of immunity. *Annu. Rev. Immunol.* 16:545–568.

Eggleton, P., and K. B. M. Reid. 1999. Lung surfactant proteins involved in innate immunity. *Curr. Opin. Immunol.* 11:28–33.

Epstein, J., Q. Eichbaum, S. Sheriff, and A. B. Ezekowitz. 1996. The collectins in innate immunity. *Curr. Opin. Immunol.* 8:29–35.

Fearon, D. T., and R. M. Locksley. 1996. The instructive role of innate immunity in the acquired immune response. *Science* 272:50–54.

Franc, N. C., K. White, and R. A. B. Ezekowitz. 1999. Phagocytosis and development: back to the future. *Curr. Opin. Immunol.* 11:47–52.

Freeman, M., J. Ashkenas, D. J. Rees, D. M. Kingsley, N. G. Copeland, N. A. Jenkins, and M. Krieger. 1991. An ancient, highly conserved family of cysteine-rich protein domains revealed by cloning type I and II murine macrophage scavenger receptors. *Proc. Natl. Acad. Sci. USA* 88:4931–4935.

Ganz, T., and R. I. Lehrer. 1997. Antimicrobial peptides of leukocytes. *Curr. Opin. Hematol.* 4:53–58.

Gordon, S., S. Clark, D. Greaves, and A. Doyle. 1995. Molecular immunobiology of macrophages: recent progress. *Curr. Opin. Immunol.* 7:24–33.

Hoffman, J. A., F. C. Kafatos, C. A. Janeway, Jr., and R. A. B. Ezekowitz. 1999. Phylogenetic perspectives in innate immunity. *Science* 284:1313–1318.

Karre, K., H.-G. Ljunggren, G. Piontek, and R. Kiessling. 1986. Selective rejection of H-2 deficient lymphoma variants suggest alternate immune defense strategy. *Nature* 319:675–678.

Kaufmann, S. H. E. 1993. Immunity to intracellular bacteria. *Annu. Rev. Immunol.* 11:129–163.

Klebanoff, S. J. 1998. Microbicidal mechanisms, oxygen dependent, 1713–1728. *In* P. J. Delves (ed), *Encyclopedia of Immunology*, 2nd ed., Academic Press, Inc., New York, N.Y.

Lanier, L. L. 1997. Natural killer cells—from no receptor to too many. *Immunity* 6:371–378.

Latek R. R., and E. R. Unanue. 1999. Mechanisms of consequences of peptide selection by the I-A^k class II molecule. *Immunol. Rev.* **172**:209–228.

Lemaitre, B., E. Nicolas, L. Michant, J. M. Reichhart, and J. A. Hoffman. 1996. The dorsoventral regulatory gene cassette spatzle/Toll/cactus controls the potent anti fungal response in *Drosophila* adults. *Cell* **86**:973–983.

Lurie, M. B. 1964. *Resistance to Tuberculosis: Experimental Studies in Native and Acquired Defensive Mechanisms.* Harvard University Press, Cambridge, Mass.

Mackaness, G. B. 1964. The immunological basis of acquired cellular resistance. *J. Exp. Med.* **120**:105–113.

Mantovani, A. 1999. The chemokine system: redundancy for robust outputs. *Immunol. Today* **20**:254–256.

Matsushita, M., Y. Endo, and T. Fujita. 2000. Cutting edge: complement-activating complex of ticolin and mannose-binding lectin-associated serine protease. *J. Immunol.* **164**:2281–2284.

Medzhitov, R., and C.A. Janeway, Jr. 1998. An ancient system of host defense. *Curr. Opin. Immunol.* **10**:12–15.

Medzhitov, R., P. Preston-Huribut, and C. A. Janeway. 1997. A human homologue of the *Drosophila* Toll protein signals activation of adaptive immunity. *Nature* **388**:394–397.

Moore, K. V., A. O'Garra, R. de Waal Malefyt, P. Vieira, and T. R. Mosman. 1993. Interleukin 10. *Annu. Rev. Immunol.* **11**:165–184.

Nathan, C. 1997. Perspective series. Nitric oxide and nitric oxide synthases. Inducible nitric oxide synthase: what difference does it make? *J. Clin. Investig.* **100**:2417–2423.

Newport, M. J., C. M. Huxley, S. Lamhamedi, P. Revy, J. F. Emile, M. Newport, M. Levin, S. Blanche, E. Seboun, A. Fischer, and J. L. Casonova. 1996. Interferon-gamma receptor deficiency in an infant with fatal bacille Calmette-Guerin infection. *N. Engl. J. Med.* **335**:1956–1961.

North, R. J., P. L. Dunn, and J. W. Conlan. 1997. Murine listeriosis as a model of anti-microbial defense. *Immunol. Rev.* **158**:27–36.

Pamer, E. G., A. J. A. M. Sijts, M. S. Villanueva, D. H. Busch, and S. Vijh. 1997. MHC class I antigen processing of *Listeria monocytogenes* proteins: implications for dominant and subdominant CTL responses. *Immunol. Rev.* **158**:129–136.

Ravetch, J. V., and R. A. Clynes. 1998. Divergent roles for Fc receptors and complement in vivo. *Annu. Rev. Immunol.* **16**:421–432.

Rollins, B. J. 1997. Chemokines. *Blood* **90**:909–928.

Rosen, F. S. 1993. The primary specific immunodeficiencies, p. 1271–1291. *In* P. J. Lachman (ed), *Clinical Aspects of Immunology*, 3rd ed., Blackwell Publishing Co., Boston.

Shiloh, M. W., J. D. MacMicking, S. Nicholson, J. E. Brause, S. Potter, M. Marino, F. Fang, M. Dinauer, and C. Nathan. 1999. Phenotype of mice and macrophages deficient in both phagocytic oxidase and inducible nitric oxide synthase. *Immunity* **10**:29–38.

Tilney, L. G., and D. A. Portnoy. 1989. Actin filaments and the growth, movement and spread of the intracellular parasite *Listeria monocytogenes*. *J. Cell Biol.* **109**:1597–1608.

Trinchieri, G. 1989. Biology of natural killer cells. *Adv. Immunol.* **47**:187–376.

Turner, M.W. 1996. Mannose binding lectin: the pluripotent molecule of the innate immune system. *Immunol. Today* **17**:532–536.

Unanue, E. R. 1997. Studies in Listeriosis show the strong symbiosis between the innate cellular system and the T cell response. *Immunol. Rev.* **158**:11–25.

Unanue, E. R. 2000. Interaction of pathogens with the innate and adaptive immune system, p. 291–311. *In* P. Cossart, P. Boquet, S. Normark, and R. Rappuoli (ed.), *Cellular Microbiology.* ASM Press, Washington, D.C.

Immunology of Infectious Diseases
Edited by S. H. E. Kaufmann, A. Sher, and R. Ahmed
© 2002 ASM Press, Washington, D.C.

Chapter 8

Defensins and Cathelicidins: Antimicrobial Peptide Effectors of Mammalian Innate Immunity

TOMAS GANZ AND ROBERT I. LEHRER

Initial contacts between microbes and their animal hosts typically occur on surfaces that interface with the environment. The skin's horny layer forms a physical barrier whose surface and foundations are impregnated with antimicrobial substances. Moist membranes are surmounted by a mucus blanket that entraps microbes, facilitates their mechanical disposal, and exposes them to various antimicrobial substances, including endogenous antimicrobial peptides and proteins. If the microbes persist and gain attachment, the underlying epithelial cells can respond by releasing antimicrobial molecules and chemokines that attract phagocytes from the blood and surrounding tissues. Phagocytes can sequester microbes to deprive them of essential nutrients and expose them to multiple antimicrobial substances, including an array of defensive peptides, proteins, and enzymes. Moreover, some of the molecules generated or released by phagocytes can attract dendritic cells and lymphocytes and may help in other ways to initiate and augment adaptive immune responses.

Whatever the initial circumstances, most encounters between microbes and hosts end successfully from the host's point of view. This review will center on antimicrobial peptides, effector molecules that generally act by disrupting microbial membranes.

DEFENSINS

Human defensins (Ganz and Lehrer, 1995; Lehrer et al., 1993) belong to a widely distributed family of microbicidal peptides with a conserved six-cysteine, three-disulfide motif. Defensin peptides are present in various host defense settings, including the cytoplasmic granules of phagocytic and secretory cells and on epithelial surfaces that are routinely exposed to microbes. Three closely related defensins, human neutrophil peptides HNP-1, HNP-2, and HNP-3, are major components of the neutrophil's dense azurophil granules. A fourth defensin, HNP-4, shares this location but is about 100-fold less abundant. When human neutrophils ingest *Salmonella enterica* serovar Typhimurium in the presence of radioactive iodide, defensins are the most abundant radioiodinated polypeptides in phagocytic vacuoles (Joiner et al., 1989). Since iodination is produced by the neutrophil's myeloperoxidase-hydrogen peroxide system, iodinated defensins provide evidence that the neutrophil's oxidative and nonoxidative systems operate concurrently within the phagosome. Two human defensins, HD-5 and HD-6, are located in the granules of Paneth cells (Porter et al., 1997a, 1997b; Jones and Bevins, 1993). These specialized, long-lived epithelial cells are positioned at the bottom of small intestinal crypts and are involved in local host defense. When stimulated by bacteria or cholinergic stimuli, murine Paneth cells release antimicrobial activity that is largely due to their highly abundant defensins (Ayabe et al., 2000). The granules of Paneth cells also contain lysozyme and phospholipase A2, both of which have antimicrobial properties. Two more recently characterized defensins (Bensch et al., 1995; Zhao et al., 1996; Harder et al., 1997), human beta-defensins HBD-1 and HBD-2, differ from the classical "alpha"-defensins in the spacing and connectivity of their cysteine residues. Their mRNAs are expressed in epithelial organs, with HBD-1 being most abundant in the kidneys and HBD-2 being most abundant in inflamed skin. HBD-2 synthesis is induced by inflammation, most probably by an NF-

Tomas Ganz • Departments of Medicine and Pathology, UCLA School of Medicine, Los Angeles, CA 90095-1690. **Robert I. Lehrer** • Department of Medicine, UCLA School of Medicine, Los Angeles, CA 90095-1690.

κB-dependent transcriptional control mechanism analogous to that described for bovine lingual and tracheal epithelial defensins (Diamond et al., 1991, 1996; Schonwetter et al., 1995). Although defensins have been found in the granulocytes and epithelial cells of many vertebrate species, their production by mononuclear phagocytes appears to be more restricted, having been shown for alpha-defensins only in rabbit alveolar macrophages (Ganz et al., 1989) and for beta-defensins only in bovine alveolar macrophages (Ryan et al., 1998).

Under low-salt conditions (e.g., 10 mM sodium phosphate), defensins are microbicidal at micromolar (low-microgram-per-milliliter) concentrations against many gram-positive and gram-negative bacteria, yeast, and fungi and certain enveloped viruses (Ogata et al., 1992; Miyasaki et al., 1990; Lehrer et al., 1989; Daher et al., 1986; Ganz et al., 1985). Increasing salt concentrations competitively inhibit defensin activity (Lehrer et al., 1985, 1988a), but the inhibitory effect is modulated by the properties of the target microbe. For example, at electrolyte concentrations that prevail in extracellular fluids, HD-5 (100 μg/ml) killed more than 90% of an inoculum of *Listeria monocytogenes* in 3 h but showed little activity against *S. enterica* serovar Typhimurium (Porter et al., 1997b). Estimates of defensin concentrations in the phagocytic vacuoles of neutrophils are in the high-milligram-per-milliliter range, a concentration that may be sufficient to overcome inhibition by extracellular ion concentrations. Similar considerations also apply to the activity of intestinal defensins ("cryptdins") in the narrow (diameter, 5 to 10 μm) intestinal crypt lumens into which Paneth cells secrete their defensin-containing granules. Some defensins display additional in vitro activities relevant to inflammation and repair, including inhibition of adrenocorticotropin-stimulated cortisol production, inhibition of fibrinolysis, and a mitogenic effect on fibroblasts (Higazi et al., 1995; Murphy et al., 1993; Singh et al., 1988; Zhu et al., 1987). Defensins may also function as early chemotactic signals to cells that initiate adaptive immune responses, dendritic cells, and memory T cells (Yang et al., 1999). This activity is mediated by the interaction of specific defensins (HBD-1 and HBD-2) with the chemokine receptor CCR6. Although the crystal structure of one of these defensins, HBD-2, was recently solved (Hoover, 2000), the structural basis for its interaction with the chemokine receptor CCR6 has not yet been elucidated.

The microbicidal and cytotoxic activity of defensins is thought to involve several steps (Lehrer et al., 1985, 1988b, 1989; Lichtenstein et al., 1986, 1988). Initially, defensins bind to target cell membranes and make them permeable to small molecules such as trypan blue (molecular weight, 960) and smaller molecules, such as o-nitrophenyl-β-D-galactopyranoside (ONPG) (a disaccharide-like molecule) and various β-lactam antibiotics. Both electrostatic interaction and transmembrane electromotive force play a role in defensin-mediated permeabilization of biological membranes (White et al., 1995; Wimley et al., 1994; Fujii et al., 1993; Kagan et al., 1990; Lehrer et al., 1988a, 1989; Lichtenstein et al., 1988). Studies with planar lipid bilayer model systems showed that formation of defensin pores required the application of a *trans*-negative electromotive force to pull the cationic defensin molecules into the membrane. In anionic phospholipid liposomes (but not zwitterionic or mixed liposomes), human defensin HNP-2 induced leakage of vesicle contents through stable pores, whose diameter approximated 25 Å, based on the passage of size-specified dextran markers. Based on this estimated pore size and other considerations, a model pore structure—essentially a ring of six defensin homodimers—has been proposed. However, rabbit defensins permeabilize phospholipid vesicles in a graded rather than an all-or-none fashion, suggesting that the formation of well-defined, stable pores may not be the only mechanism whereby defensins mediate membrane disruption.

Human defensins are encoded by at least nine different genes (Liu et al., 1997, 1998; Linzmeier et al., 1993; Sparkes et al., 1989; Jones and Bevins, 1992, 1993) that cluster in the *def* locus on chromosome band 8p23. This locus includes all the known defensin genes, irrespective of their site(s) of expression in neutrophils, Paneth cells, or other epithelial cells. The adjacent genomic location of the alpha- and beta-defensins and their similar fold (Zimmermann et al., 1995) supports the notion that these genes diverged from a common precursor. Each mature alpha-defensin is produced by posttranslational processing from a preprodefensin, which typically contains a signal sequence, an anionic propiece, and the C-terminally located mature defensin (Ganz et al., 1993). The anionic charge of the propiece often balances the cationic charge of the mature peptide and may assist its folding and posttranslational processing. Beta-defensins frequently lack anionic propieces and contain an α-helical N-terminal extension (Hoover et al., 2000). An interesting and unusual circular (θ) defensin was recently found in the neutrophils of rhesus monkeys (Tang et al., 1999) that also contain several more conventional alpha-defensins. The defensin is produced by circular splicing from two truncated alpha-defensin-like precursors, each of which donates three cysteines. With the exception of murine Paneth cell defensins (cryptdins), where the metalloprotease matrilysin plays an important role as a processing enzyme that generates mature defensins (Wilson et al., 1999), little is known about the enzymes that generate active defensins.

That defensins are of ancient origin is suggested by their occurrence in the phagocytes, secretory glands, and epithelia of mammals, the duck-billed platypus (a monotreme), chickens, and turkeys and in rattlesnake venom (crotoxins). The similarly named but less obviously homologous peptides called insect and plant defensins occur in various invertebrates and plants, where their synthesis can be induced by microbial invasion. There is impressive interspecies variation in the expression of defensins as well as of other antimicrobial polypeptides. Neutrophil alpha-defensins have been found in humans and other primates, rabbits, guinea pigs, hamsters, and rats, and beta-defensins have been found in the cattle and fowl (chickens and turkeys) and in venom from the male platypus. In contrast, defensins are absent from the leukocytes of mice, pigs, horses, sheep, and goats. Presumably, adverse consequences from the lack of neutrophil defensins in these species are mitigated by the presence of other antimicrobial effector mechanisms, such as NADPH oxidase, inducible nitric oxide synthase, cathelicidins, serprocidins, and other antimicrobial polypeptides.

CATHELICIDINS

Cathelicidins (Zanetti et al., 1995) are a large family of microbicidal peptide precursors that contain a conserved N-terminal cathelin domain with about 100 amino acid residues and a C-terminal peptide with 12 to 80 amino acid residues. The C-terminal peptide structure is highly variable, and peptides ranging from α-helical to β-sheet and other more complex structures are all found associated with the cathelin domain. The cathelin domain bears an intriguing resemblance to the cystatin domain found in the precursor of the inflammatory peptide bradykinin and in precursors of other bioactive polypeptides. Many cathelicidins undergo extracellular processing (proteolytic cleavage) that frees the antimicrobial C-terminal peptide from the precursor (Panyutich et al., 1997; Zanetti et al., 1991, 1995; Scocchi et al., 1992), while others may be active (e.g., in binding lipopolysaccharide) in the uncleaved form (Levy et al., 1993; Zarember et al., 1997). The only known human cathelicidin has been designated hCAP18 or FALL39/LL-37 by the three groups (Agerberth et al., 1995; Cowland et al., 1995; Larrick et al., 1995) that described its cDNA, gene and

peptide forms. Unlike defensins, which are stored in their mature form in the granules of neutrophils, hCAP18/LL-37 is stored as a 16-kDa (140-amino-acid) proform. Defensins are stored within the primary (azurophil) granules of neutrophils, organelles whose contents are translocated to phagocytic vacuoles. In contrast, hCAP18/LL-37 is present in the secondary (specific) granules, whose contents are largely secreted. During or after secretion, hCAP18 undergoes proteolytic processing (Gudmundsson et al., 1996) to the 4.5-kDa, 37-amino-acid peptide called LL-37. The analogous processing of bovine cathelicidins, probactenecins proBac5 and proBac7, and porcine cathelicidins, proprotegrins proPG1-3, is mediated by trace amounts of neutrophil elastase (Panyutich et al., 1997; Scocchi et al., 1992), but processing of the human peptide has not yet been analyzed. mRNA for the human cathelicidin was also found in the testis (Agerberth et al., 1995) and/or epididymis, and it occurs at high concentration (40 to 140 μg/ml) in normal semen, mostly attached to spermatozoa, perhaps as a deterrent to microbial hitchhikers (Malm et al., 2000). hCAP18/LL-37 expression is prominently induced by inflammation in human keratinocytes (Frohm et al., 1997; Agerberth et al., 1995). Unlike defensins, which are rich in β-sheet type structure, LL-37 is expected to assume an amphipathic α-helical conformation. In vitro, the human peptide LL-37 displayed both lipopolysaccharide-binding (Hirata et al., 1995) and microbicidal activities (Agerberth et al., 1995) against *Escherichia coli*. Human neutrophils have about one-third as much cathelicidin in their specific granules as they have either lactoferrin or lysozyme (Borregaard et al., 1995). High levels of hCAP18/LL-37 RNA were also found in surface airway epithelial cells and in submucosal gland cells of the human lungs (Bals et al., 1998).

Cathelicidins have also been found in neutrophils of cows, pigs, rabbits, and mice (Gennaro et al., 1989; Marzari et al., 1988; Romeo et al., 1988; Kokryakov et al., 1993; Mirgorodskaya et al., 1993; Levy et al., 1993; Larrick et al., 1994; Zanetti et al., 1995; Moscinski and Hill, 1995). They are especially abundant in the neutrophils of pigs and cattle, species with multiple cathelicidin genes that generate a large variety of peptide forms. For example, bovine bactenecins Bac5 and Bac7 (Frank et al., 1990) and porcine PR-39 (Agerberth et al., 1991) are proline- and arginine-rich peptides with repetitive segments. Porcine prophenins (Harwig et al., 1995) have repetitive proline- and phenylalanine-rich segments. Bovine indolicidin (Del Sal et al., 1992; Selsted et al., 1992) is an unusually tryptophan-rich tridecapeptide.

We have been especially intrigued by the porcine protegrin family cathelicidin peptides, whose mature domains have 16 to 18 amino acid residues, among which are multiple arginine residues and four conserved cysteines (Kokryakov et al., 1993; Aumelas et al., 1996; Fahrner et al., 1996). Mature protegrins have a general resemblance to tachyplesins, small β-sheet peptides found in the hemocytes of horseshoe crabs (Nakamura et al., 1988), and a closer resemblance to RTD-1, an 18-residue circular defensin recently found in *Macaca mulatta*, the rhesus monkey (Tang et al., 1999).

Some cathelicidins, including the polypeptides p15A and p15B found in rabbit granulocytes, are not cleaved after secretion from neutrophils (Levy et al., 1993; Weinrauch et al., 1995; Zarember et al., 1997). When released from secondary granules, p15 peptides synergize with bactericidal permeability-inducing protein (an azurophil granule protein) to inhibit the growth of *E. coli* in rabbit peritoneal exudates. Because rabbit defensins also synergize with BPI (Levy et al., 1995) and because similar effects were described for other polypeptide combinations (Odeberg and Olsson, 1976; Miyasaki and Bodeau, 1992), in vivo effectiveness of antimicrobial peptides may also benefit from neutrophil-administered polypharmacy.

CONCLUSION

Defensins and cathelicidins are antimicrobial peptides that are found early and in abundance in host defense contexts. Baseline expression of these peptides at sites vulnerable to infection is augmented by specific mechanisms that enhance the delivery of these peptides to infected or inflamed tissues. These include transcriptional induction of defensin and cathelicidin synthesis, stimulated degranulation of cells that store the peptides or their precursors, and recruitment of additional cells that release stored peptides. Individual peptides differ in their antimicrobial spectrum, and early evidence suggests that they sometimes act synergistically with each other or with larger antimicrobial polypeptides. At sites that are more distant from the infected or inflamed locus, lower concentrations of defensins may act as signaling molecules, similarly to chemokines. Recent progress in the definition of the specific role of individual defensins and cathelicidins has been all the more impressive when we consider their multiplicity and potentially overlapping activity, the marked interspecies variability of primary structures and patterns of tissue expression, and the very high

biological concentrations which have hindered the experimental use of neutralizing antibodies.

REFERENCES

Agerberth, B., H. Gunne, J. Odeberg, P. Kogner, H. G. Boman, and G. H. Gudmundsson. 1995. FALL-39, a putative human peptide antibiotic, is cysteine-free and expressed in bone marrow and testis. *Proc. Natl. Acad. Sci. USA* 92:195–199.

Agerberth, B., J. Y. Lee, T. Bergman, M. Carlquist, H. G. Boman, V. Mutt, and H. Jornvall. 1991. Amino acid sequence of PR-39. Isolation from pig intestine of a new member of the family of proline-arginine-rich antibacterial peptides. *Eur. J. Biochem.* 202:849–854.

Aumelas, A., M. Mangoni, C. Roumestand, L. Chiche, E. Despaux, G. Grassy, B. Calas, and A. Chavanieu. 1996. Synthesis and solution structure of the antimicrobial peptide protegrin-1. *Eur. J. Biochem.* 237:575–583.

Ayabe, T., D. P. Satchell, C. L. Wilson, W. C. Parks, M. E. Selsted, and A. J. Ouellette. 2000. Secretion of microbicidal a-defensins by intestinal Paneth cells in response to bacteria. *Nat. Immunol.* 1:113–118.

Bals, R., X. Wang, M. Zasloff, and J. M. Wilson. 1998. The peptide antibiotic LL-37/hCAP-18 is expressed in epithelia of the human lung where it has broad antimicrobial activity at the airway surface. *Proc. Natl. Acad. Sci. USA* 95:9541–9546.

Bensch, K. W., M. Raida, H. J. Magert, P. Schulz-Knappe, and W. G. Forssmann. 1995. hBD-1: a novel beta-defensin from human plasma. *FEBS Lett.* 368:331–335.

Borregaard, N., M. Sehested, B. S. Nielsen, H. Sengelov, and L. Kjeldsen. 1995. Biosynthesis of granule proteins in normal human bone marrow cells. Gelatinase is a marker of terminal neutrophil differentiation. *Blood* 85:812–817.

Cowland, J. B., A. H. Johnsen, and N. Borregaard. 1995. hCAP-18, a cathelin/pro-bactenecin-like protein of human neutrophil specific granules. *FEBS Lett.* 368:173–176.

Daher, K. A., M. E. Selsted, and R. I. Lehrer. 1986. Direct inactivation of viruses by human granulocyte defensins. *J. Virol.* 60:1068–1074.

Del Sal, G., P. Storici, C. Schneider, D. Romeo, and M. Zanetti. 1992. cDNA cloning of the neutrophil bactericidal peptide indolicidin. *Biochem. Biophys. Res. Commun.* 187:467–472.

Diamond, G., J. P. Russell, and C. L. Bevins. 1996. Inducible expression of an antibiotic peptide gene in lipopolysaccharide-challenged tracheal epithelial cells. *Proc. Natl. Acad. Sci. USA* 93:5156–5160.

Diamond, G., M. Zasloff, H. Eck, M. Brasseur, W. L. Maloy, and C. L. Bevins. 1991. Tracheal antimicrobial peptide, a cysteine-rich peptide from mammalian tracheal mucosa: peptide isolation and cloning of a cDNA. *Proc. Natl. Acad. Sci. USA* 88:3952–3956.

Fahrner, R. l., T. Dieckmann, S. S. Harwig, R. I. Lehrer, D. Eisenberg, and J. Feigon. 1996. Solution structure of protegrin-1, a broad-spectrum antimicrobial peptide from porcine leukocytes. *Chem. Biol.* 3:543–550.

Frank, R. W., R. Gennaro, K. Schneider, M. Przybylski, and D. Romeo. 1990. Amino acid sequences of two proline-rich bactenecins. Antimicrobial peptides of bovine neutrophils. *J. Biol. Chem.* 265:18871–18874.

Frohm, M., B. Agerberth, G. Ahangari, M. Stahle-Backdahl, S. Liden, H. Wigzell, and G. H. Gudmundsson. 1997. The expression of the gene coding for the antibacterial peptide LL-37 is induced in human keratinocytes during inflammatory disorders. *J. Biol. Chem.* 272:15258–15263.

Fujii, G., M. E. Selsted, and D. Eisenberg. 1993. Defensins promote fusion and lysis of negatively charged membranes. *Protein Sci.* 2:1301–1312.

Ganz, T., and R. I. Lehrer. 1995. Defensins. *Pharmacol.Ther.* 66:191–205.

Ganz, T., L. Liu, E. V. Valore, and A. Oren. 1993. Posttranslational processing and targeting of transgenic human defensin in murine granulocyte, macrophage, fibroblast, and pituitary adenoma cell lines. *Blood* 82:641–650.

Ganz, T., J. R. Rayner, E. V. Valore, A. Tumolo, K. Talmadge, and F. Fuller. 1989. The structure of the rabbit macrophage defensin genes and their organ-specific expression. *J. Immunol.* 143:1358–1365.

Ganz, T., M. E. Selsted, D. Szklarek, S. S. Harwig, K. Daher, D. F. Bainton, and R. I. Lehrer. 1985. Defensins. Natural peptide antibiotics of human neutrophils. *J. Clin. Investig.* 76:1427–1435.

Gennaro, R., B. Skerlavaj, and D. Romeo. 1989. Purification, composition, and activity of two bactenecins, antibacterial peptides of bovine neutrophils. *Infect. Immun.* 57:3142–3146.

Gudmundsson, G. H., B. Agerberth, J. Odeberg, T. Bergman, B. Olsson, and R. Salcedo. 1996. The human gene FALL39 and processing of the cathelin precursor to the antibacterial peptide LL-37 in granulocytes. *Eur. J. Biochem.* 238:325–332.

Harder, J., J. Bartels, E. Christophers, and J.-M. Schroeder. 1997. A peptide antibiotic from human skin. *Nature* 387:861–862.

Harwig, S. S., V. N. Kokryakov, K. M. Swiderek, G. M. Aleshina, C. Zhao, and R. I. Lehrer. 1995. Prophenin-1, an exceptionally proline-rich antimicrobial peptide from porcine leukocytes. *FEBS Lett.* 362:65–69.

Higazi, A. A., I. I. Barghouti, and R. Abu-Much. 1995. Identification of an inhibitor of tissue-type plasminogen activator-mediated fibrinolysis in human neutrophils. A role for defensin. *J. Biol. Chem.* 270:9472–9477.

Hirata, M., J. Zhong, S. C. Wright, and J. W. Larrick. 1995. Structure and functions of endotoxin-binding peptides derived from CAP18. *Prog. Clin. Biol. Res.* 392:317–326.

Hoover, D. M., K. R. Rajashankar, R. Blumenthal, A. Puri, J. J. Oppenheim, O. Chertov, and J. Lubkowski. 2000. The structure of human beta-defensin-2 shows evidence of higher-order oligomerization. *J. Biol. Chem.* 275:32911–32918.

Joiner, K. A., T. Ganz, J. Albert, and D. Rotrosen. 1989. The opsonizing ligand on Salmonella typhimurium influences incorporation of specific, but not azurophil, granule constituents into neutrophil phagosomes. *J. Cell Biol.* 109:2771–2782.

Jones, D. E., and C. L. Bevins. 1992. Paneth cells of the human small intestine express an antimicrobial peptide gene. *J. Biol. Chem.* 267:23216–23225.

Jones, D. E., and C. L. Bevins. 1993. Defensin-6 mRNA in human Paneth cells: implications for antimicrobial peptides in host defense of the human bowel. *FEBS Lett.* 315:187–192.

Kagan, B. L., M. E. Selsted, T. Ganz, and R. I. Lehrer. 1990. Antimicrobial defensin peptides form voltage-dependent ion-permeable channels in planar lipid bilayer membranes. *Proc. Natl. Acad. Sci. USA* 87:210–214.

Kokryakov, V. N., S. S. Harwig, E. A. Panyutich, A. A. Shevchenko, G. M. Aleshina, O. V. Shamova, H. A. Korneva, and R. I. Lehrer. 1993. Protegrins: leukocyte antimicrobial peptides that combine features of corticostatic defensins and tachyplesins. *FEBS Lett.* 327:231–236.

Larrick, J. W., M. Hirata, R. F. Balint, J. Lee, J. Zhong, and S. C. Wright. 1995. Human CAP18: a novel antimicrobial lipopolysaccharide-binding protein. *Infect. Immun.* 63:1291–1297.

Larrick, J. W., M. Hirata, H. Zheng, J. Zhong, D. Bolin, J. M. Cavaillon, H. S. Warren, and S. C. Wright. 1994. A novel granulocyte-derived peptide with lipopolysaccharide-neutralizing activity. *J. Immunol.* 152:231–240.

Lehrer, R. I., A. Barton, K. A. Daher, S. S. Harwig, T. Ganz, and M. E. Selsted. 1989. Interaction of human defensins with *Escherichia coli*. Mechanism of bactericidal activity. *J. Clin. Investig.* 84:553–561.

Lehrer, R. I., A. Barton, and T. Ganz. 1988a. Concurrent assessment of inner and outer membrane permeabilization and bacteriolysis in *E. coli* by multiple-wavelength spectrophotometry. *J. Immunol. Methods* 108:153–158.

Lehrer, R. I., T. Ganz, D. Szklarek, and M. E. Selsted. 1988b. Modulation of the in vitro candidacidal activity of human neutrophil defensins by target cell metabolism and divalent cations. *J. Clin. Investig.* 81:1829–1835.

Lehrer, R. I., A. K. Lichtenstein, and T. Ganz. 1993. Defensins: antimicrobial and cytotoxic peptides of mammalian cells. *Annu. Rev. Immunol.* 11:105–128.

Lehrer, R. I., D. Szklarek, T. Ganz, and M. E. Selsted. 1985. Correlation of binding of rabbit granulocyte peptides to *Candida albicans* with candidacidal activity. *Infect. Immun.* 49:207–211.

Levy, O., C. E. Ooi, P. Elsbach, M. E. Doerfler, R. I. Lehrer, and J. Weiss. 1995. Antibacterial proteins of granulocytes differ in interaction with endotoxin. Comparison of bactericidal/permeability-increasing protein, p15s, and defensins. *J. Immunol.* 154:5403–5410.

Levy, O., J. Weiss, K. Zarember, C. E. Ooi, and P. Elsbach. 1993. Antibacterial 15-kDa protein isoforms (p15s) are members of a novel family of leukocyte proteins. *J. Biol. Chem.* 268:6058–6063.

Lichtenstein, A., T. Ganz, M. E. Selsted, and R. I. Lehrer. 1986. In vitro tumor cell cytolysis mediated by peptide defensins of human and rabbit granulocytes. *Blood* 68:1407–1410.

Lichtenstein, A. K., T. Ganz, T. M. Nguyen, M. E. Selsted, and R. I. Lehrer. 1988. Mechanism of target cytolysis by peptide defensins. Target cell metabolic activities, possibly involving endocytosis, are crucial for expression of cytotoxicity. *J. Immunol.* 140:2686–2694.

Linzmeier, R., D. Michaelson, L. Liu, and T. Ganz. 1993. The structure of neutrophil defensin genes. *FEBS Lett.* 321:267–273.

Liu, L., L. Wang, H. P. Jia, C. Zhao, H. H. Q. Heng, B. C. Schutte, P. B. J. McCray, and T. Ganz. 1998. Structure and mapping of the human β-defensin HBD-2 gene and its expression at sites of inflammation. *Gene* 222:237–244.

Liu, L., C. Zhao, H. H. Q. Heng, and T. Ganz. 1997. The human β-defensin-1 and α-defensins are encoded by adjacent genes: two peptide families with differing disulfide topology share a common ancestry. *Genomics* 43:316–320.

Malm, J., O. Sorensen, T. Persson, M. Frohm-Nilsson, B. Johansson, A. Bjartell, H. Lilja, M. Stahle-Backdahl, N. Borregaard, and A. Egesten. 2000. The human cationic antimicrobial protein (hCAP-18) is expressed in the epithelium of human epididymis, is present in seminal plasma at high concentrations, and is attached to spermatozoa. *Infect. Immun.* 68:4297–4302.

Marzari, R., B. Scaggiante, B. Skerlavaj, M. Bittolo, R. Gennaro, and D. Romeo. 1988. Small, antibacterial and large, inactive peptides of neutrophil granules share immunoreactivity to a monoclonal antibody. *Infect. Immun.* 56:2193–2197.

Mirgorodskaya, O. A., A. A. Shevchenko, K. O. Abdalla, I. V. Chernushevich, T. A. Egorov, A. X. Musoliamov, V. N. Kokryakov, and O. V. Shamova. 1993. Primary structure of three cationic peptides from porcine neutrophils. Sequence determination by the combined usage of electrospray ionization mass spectrometry and Edman degradation. *FEBS Lett.* 330:339–342.

Miyasaki, K. T., and A. L. Bodeau. 1992. Human neutrophil azurocidin synergizes with leukocyte elastase and cathepsin G in the killing of *Capnocytophaga sputigena*. *Infect. Immun.* **60**:4973–4975.

Miyasaki, K. T., A. L. Bodeau, T. Ganz, M. E. Selsted, and R. I. Lehrer. 1990. In vitro sensitivity of oral, gram-negative, facultative bacteria to the bactericidal activity of human neutrophil defensins. *Infect. Immun.* **58**:3934–3940.

Moscinski, L. C., and B. Hill. 1995. Molecular cloning of a novel myeloid granule protein. *J. Cell. Biochem.* **59**:431–442.

Murphy, C. J., B. A. Foster, M. J. Mannis, M. E. Selsted, and T. W. Reid. 1993. Defensins are mitogenic for epithelial cells and fibroblasts. *J. Cell. Physiol.* **155**:408–413.

Nakamura, T., H. Furunaka, T. Miyata, F. Tokunaga, T. Muta, S. Iwanaga, M. Niwa, T. Takao, and Y. Shimonishi. 1988. Tachyplesin, a class of antimicrobial peptide from the hemocytes of the horseshoe crab (*Tachypleus tridentatus*). Isolation and chemical structure. *J. Biol. Chem.* **263**:16709–16713.

Odeberg, H., and I. Olsson. 1976. Microbicidal mechanisms of human granulocytes: synergistic effects of granulocyte elastase and myeloperoxidase or chymotrypsin-like cationic protein. *Infect. Immun.* **14**:1276–1283.

Ogata, K., B. A. Linzer, R. I. Zuberi, T. Ganz, R. I. Lehrer, and A. Catanzaro. 1992. Activity of defensins from human neutrophilic granulocytes against *Mycobacterium avium-Mycobacterium intracellulare*. *Infect. Immun.* **60**:4720–4725.

Panyutich, A., J. Shi, P. L. Boutz, C. Zhao, and T. Ganz. 1997. Porcine polymorphonuclear leukocytes generate extracellular microbicidal activity by elastase-mediated activation of secreted proprotegrins. *Infect. Immun.* **65**:978–985.

Porter, E. M., L. Liu, A. Oren, P. A. Anton, and T. Ganz . 1997a. Localization of human intestinal defensin 5 in Paneth cell granules. *Infect. Immun.* **65**:2389–2395.

Porter, E. M., E. van Dam, E. V. Valore, and T. Ganz. 1997b. Broad-spectrum antimicrobial activity of human intestinal defensin 5. *Infect. Immun.* **65**:2396–2401.

Romeo, D., B. Skerlavaj, M. Bolognesi, and R. Gennaro. 1988. Structure and bactericidal activity of an antibiotic dodecapeptide purified from bovine neutrophils. *J. Biol. Chem.* **263**:9573–9575.

Ryan, L. K., J. Rhodes, M. Bhat, and G. Diamond. 1998. Expression of beta-defensin genes in bovine alveolar macrophages. *Infect. Immun.* **66**:878–881.

Schonwetter, B. S., E. D. Stolzenberg, and M. A. Zasloff. 1995. Epithelial antibiotics induced at sites of inflammation. *Science* **267**:1645–1648.

Scocchi, M., B. Skerlavaj, D. Romeo, and R. Gennaro. 1992. Proteolytic cleavage by neutrophil elastase converts inactive storage proforms to antibacterial bactenecins. *Eur. J. Biochem.* **209**:589–595.

Selsted, M. E., M. J. Novotny, W. L. Morris, Y. Q. Tang, W. Smith, and J. S. Cullor. 1992. Indolicidin, a novel bactericidal tridecapeptide amide from neutrophils. *J. Biol. Chem.* **267**:4292–4295.

Singh, A., A. Bateman, Q. Z. Zhu, S. Shimasaki, F. Esch, and S. Solomon. 1988. Structure of a novel human granulocyte peptide with anti-ACTH activity. *Biochem. Biophys. Res. Commun.* **155**:524–529.

Sparkes, R. S., M. Kronenberg, C. Heinzmann, K. A. Daher, I. Klisak, T. Ganz, and T. Mohandas. 1989. Assignment of defensin gene(s) to human chromosome 8p23. *Genomics* **5**:240–244.

Tang, Y. Q., J. Yuan, G. Osapay, K. Osapay, D. Tran, C. J. Miller, A. J. Ouellette, and M. E. Selsted. 1999. A cyclic antimicrobial peptide produced in primate leukocytes by the ligation of two truncated alpha-defensins. *Science* **286**:498–502.

Weinrauch, Y., A. Foreman, C. Shu, K. Zarember, O. Levy, P. Elsbach, and J. Weiss. 1995. Extracellular accumulation of potently microbicidal bactericidal/permeability-increasing protein and p15s in an evolving sterile rabbit peritoneal inflammatory exudate. *J. Clin. Investig.* **95**:1916–1924.

White, S. H., W. C. Wimley, and M. E. Selsted. 1995. Structure, function, and membrane integration of defensins. *Curr. Opin. Struct. Biol.* **5**:521–527.

Wilson, C. L., A. J. Ouellette, D. P. Satchell, T. Ayabe, Y. S. Lopez-Boado, J. L. Stratman, S. J. Hultgren, L. M. Matrisian, and W. C. Parks. 1999. Regulation of intestinal alpha-defensin activation by the metalloproteinase matrilysin in innate host defense. *Science* **286**:113–117.

Wimley, W. C., M. E. Selsted, and S. H. White. 1994. Interactions between human defensins and lipid bilayers: evidence for formation of multimeric pores. *Protein Sci.* **3**:1362–1373.

Yang, D., O. Chertov, S. N. Bykovskaia, Q. Chen, M. J. Buffo, J. Shogan, M. Anderson, J. M. Schroder, J. M. Wang, O. M. Howard, and J. J. Oppenheim. 1999. Beta-defensins: linking innate and adaptive immunity through dendritic and T cell CCR6. *Science* **286**:525–528.

Zanetti, M., R. Gennaro, and D. Romeo. 1995. Cathelicidins: a novel protein family with a common proregion and a variable C-terminal antimicrobial domain. *FEBS Lett.* **374**:1–5.

Zanetti, M., L. Litteri, G. Griffiths, R. Gennaro, and D. Romeo. 1991. Stimulus-induced maturation of probactenecins, precursors of neutrophil antimicrobial polypeptides. *J. Immunol.* **146**:4295–4300.

Zarember, K., P. Elsbach, K. Shin-Kim, and J. Weiss. 1997. p15s (15-kD antimicrobial proteins) are stored in the secondary granules of rabbit granulocytes: implications for antibacterial synergy with the bactericidal/permeability-increasing protein in inflammatory fluids. *Blood* **89**:672–679.

Zhao, C. Q., I. Wang, and R. I. Lehrer. 1996. Widespread expression of beta-defensin HBD-1 in human secretory glands and epithelial cells. *FEBS Lett.* **396**:319–322.

Zhu, Q. Z., A. V. Singh, A. Bateman, F. Esch, and S. Solomon. 1987. The corticostatic (anti-ACTH) and cytotoxic activity of peptides isolated from fetal, adult and tumor-bearing lung. *J. Steroid. Biochem.* **27**:1017–1022.

Zimmermann, G. R., P. Legault, M. E. Selsted, and A. Pardi. 1995. Solution structure of bovine neutrophil beta-defensin-12: the peptide fold of the beta-defensins is identical to that of the classical defensins. *Biochemistry* **34**:13663–13671.

Immunology of Infectious Diseases
Edited by S. H. E. Kaufmann, A. Sher, and R. Ahmed
© 2002 ASM Press, Washington, D.C.

Chapter 9

Innate Immunity to Parasitic Infections

CHRISTOPHER A. HUNTER AND ALAN SHER

Although parasitism implies coexistence of the host and infectious agent, the immune response plays a critical role in the establishment and maintenance of this balance. Traditionally, the control of parasitic infections was thought to be the exclusive domain of the acquired immune system. However, during the past decade it has been recognized that innate immunity can shape the outcome of the host-parasite encounter. The abilities of phagocytes to engulf and destroy cells and of complement components to kill extracellular parasites appear as simple effector mechanisms. However, the innate events that underlie these functions are complex and suggest the existence of receptors that recognize parasites specifically or a surveillance system that simply distinguishes self from nonself. The new information emerging from this rapidly expanding research area is the focus of this chapter.

As noted previously in this volume, parasitic organisms are diverse in their biology, host habitats, and the type of immune responses they elicit. Helminths are unique among infectious agents in that they are multicellular and, with few exceptions, fail to replicate in their definitive hosts. Moreover, resistance to these infections is dependent on a highly polarized Th2-type cytokine response pattern that is reminiscent of the patterns seen in allergy. Protozoa, on the other hand, are unicellular and occupy intracellular and/or extracellular host niches. They typically elicit strong cell-mediated responses associated with protective immunity, with Th1 cytokines playing a dominant role. The highly divergent lifestyles and patterns of associated adaptive immune responses to helminth and protozoan parasites are also reflected in the distinct innate responses they trigger and in their consequences for the pathogen. For protozoa, innate immunity is thought to play an important role in limiting early parasite replication until cognitive T- and B-lymphocyte responses can take over. On the other hand, the innate recognition of helminths may function to limit the number of invading infective larvae and perhaps slow their development prior to the onset of adaptive immunity.

Although the innate immune system is the first to be triggered during the response to invading pathogens, it is now appreciated that vertebrate innate immune recognition can determine the class of the subsequent adaptive immune response. Thus, the highly polarized Th1 and Th2 responses elicited by different parasites or the same parasite (e.g., *Leishmania major* in different genetic settings) are thought to be determined, at least in part, by innate recognition events. An important question now under intensive investigation is how the innate immune system distinguishes "Th1" from "Th2" parasites and communicates this decision to differentiating T cells.

To be successful, parasites have to survive the innate response, and as a consequence the innate immune system represents a powerful selective pressure. This is evident from the numerous mechanisms employed by protozoa and helminths for evading innate immunity and underscores the importance of studying innate immunity to understand the host-parasite adaptation, as well as to define strategies to control these pathogens. Since by definition the protective mechanisms in question do not depend on conventional T- and B-cell recognition, they may be of particular use for limiting infection in immunocompromised individuals. Finally, by defining the pathways through which these pathogens polarize adaptive immune effector function, studies of the innate immune response to parasites may lead to the discovery of new approaches for improving the effi-

Christopher A. Hunter • Department of Pathobiology, School of Veterinary Medicine, University of Pennsylvania, 3800 Spruce St., Philadelphia, PA 19104. **Alan Sher** • Laboratory of Parasitic Diseases, NIAID, NIH, Building 4, Room 126, Bethesda, MD 20892-0425.

cacy of vaccination and directing the development of appropriate adaptive responses.

HUMORAL MECHANISMS OF INNATE IMMUNITY

Activation of Complement and Its Evasion by Vertebrate Life Cycle Stages

Perhaps the simplest forms of innate immunity are represented by the presence of preexisting, soluble factors that can recognize and destroy invading parasites. The alternative pathway of complement activation represents one of the oldest defense mechanisms and is a first line of defense against extracellular parasites. This system of innate recognition is based on the continuous turnover of C3b on all surfaces, but this molecule is normally inactivated by different complement regulatory factors such as factors H and I. However, the surfaces of most parasites lack these regulatory proteins and can actually repel factor H and so will not degrade C3b, resulting in the initiation of a series of events that lead to the activation of the complement cascade and formation of the membrane attack complex (MAC). There is also a lectin-mediated pathway, in which mannose residues on parasite surfaces are recognized by a mannan-binding protein which initiates complement activation. Irrespective of how the complement system becomes activated, the formation of the MAC can lead to direct parasite lysis while the deposition of complement components will opsonize parasites for phagocytosis. In addition, complement activation components are chemotactic and attract immune cells to the site of infection (Fig. 1).

Because the complement system represents such an important first line of defense in resistance to pathogens, successful parasites have developed a variety of developmentally regulated strategies to subvert complement-mediated attack. For example, while many of the parasitic stages found in insect vectors are susceptible to lysis via the alternative pathway of complement activation, infective forms have developed mechanisms of resistance. Thus, different stages of the African trypanosome, such as procyclics and epimastigotes found in the tsetse fly, are highly susceptible to the alternative pathway of complement activation (Ferrante and Allison, 1983). However, as these forms develop into the infective metacyclic stage, they develop a thick surface coat that is a physical barrier protecting against the MAC. While it is likely that this coat first developed as a means of evading complement-mediated lysis, the ability to express antigenically distinct forms of the variable surface glycoprotein, the major component of this coat, forms the basis for antigenic variation, which allows this parasite to persist in the face of an adaptive immune response.

Similar to the African trypanosomes, the epimastigote stage of *Trypanosoma cruzi*, found in the insect vector, is susceptible to the alternative pathway of complement, whereas the infective extracelluar trypomastigote of *T. cruzi* is resistant. This resistance to complement is multifactorial, and trypomastigotes have several mechanisms that either prevent efficient complement activation or lead to its shedding from the surface. Initial studies suggested that trypomastigotes have a developmentally regulated factor that permits them to evade the lytic action of complement (Joiner et al., 1988; Rimoldi et al., 1988). The identification of the trypomastigote gp160 antigen as a

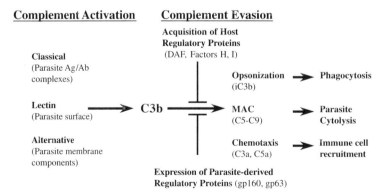

Figure 1. Complement system. The activation of the complement system through either the classical, lectin, or alternative pathways converges on the deposition of C3b on the parasite surface. In the absence of host (or parasite) regulatory proteins, this cascade proceeds to the assembly of the MAC, the opsonization of parasites, and the release of chemotactic peptides. Developmental stages of protozoan parasites found in insects are highly susceptible to lysis via the alternative pathway of complement activation, whereas the stages specific for the mammalian hosts have developed a variety of strategies to evade this mechanism of host resistance. Ag, antigen; Ab antibody.

homologue of the host complement regulatory protein decay-accelerating factor (Norris et al., 1991) was an important step in understanding how these parasites evade complement. Like decay-accelerating factor, gp160 can bind to C3b and C4b (Norris and Schrimpf, 1994) and inhibit the uptake of subsequent members of this complement cascade, thus preventing convertase formation and lysis of the parasite. In addition, the binding of C3b to gp160 allows a parasite protease to cleave this complex, which may represent a mechanism to avoid lysis as well as complement-mediated opsonization. Importantly, whereas complement-sensitive epimastigotes fail to express gp160, epimastigotes transfected with gp160 are resistant to complement-mediated lysis (Norris, 1998).

The extracellular promastigote stage of *Leishmania* spp. is found in the sandfly vector and can activate the alternative and lectin-mediated pathways of complement (Green et al., 1994, Mosser and Edelson, 1984). However, as promastigotes develop into the infective metacyclic stage, their membrane is altered to prevent the insertion of the lytic C5b–C9 complex (Puentes et al., 1990). This correlates with their ability to express a modified form of a surface lipophosphoglycan (LPG) which is approximately twice as long as the form on promastigotes and which may inhibit the insertion of the MAC into the surface membrane of the parasite (Saraiva et al., 1995). However, the importance of LPG in the virulence of different *Leishmania* species appears to differ, since studies which used gene targeting to generate LPG mutants indicate that promastigotes of *L. mexicana* which lack LPG are still infective (Ilg, 2000) whereas promastigotes of *L. major* which lack LPG are highly attenuated (Spath et al., 2000). Another developmental change that occurs during the generation of metacyclics is increased expression of the surface proteinase gp63 (Kweider et al., 1989), which can cleave C3b to the inactive iC3b form and so prevent deposition of the C5b–C9 complex (Mosser and Brittingham, 1997). However, iC3b will opsonize the parasites for phagocytosis through complement receptors such as Mac-1 (Blackwell et al., 1985; Mosser and Edelson, 1985). This process of complement-mediated phagocytosis is important because it targets the parasites to the macrophage, their host cell of choice and is also important for the intracellular survival of the parasite (Mosser and Edelson, 1987). A similar mechanism is used by *Babesia rodhani,* which, by activating complement, allows it to bind CR1 and penetrate erythrocytes (Jack and Ward, 1980). The finding that two unrelated intracellular parasites have used a similar strategy to target their host cells illustrates how parasites can subvert a normally protective innate immune response to promote their own survival.

The protozoan *Entamoeba histolytica* normally produces a nonpathogenic infection in the gut. However, under certain circumstances it will invade mucosal surfaces and in severe cases it can also invade tissues of the host and result in the development of liver abscesses. The events that result in the invasion of tissues are uncertain, with contradictory reports on the ability of pathogenic versus nonpathogenic forms to activate the alternative complement pathway and their susceptibility to lysis. However, there are several studies indicating that these amoebae have developed mechanisms to prevent complement-mediated lysis. The identification of a galactose-specific adhesin that confers resistance to complement-sensitive amoebae (Braga et al., 1992) suggests that this may be a virulence factor, but how this lectin varies between strains of *E. histolytica* that differ in their relative susceptibility to complement is not known. In addition, the ability of these parasites to incorporate host complement-regulatory proteins into their membranes can help to prevent the insertion of the MAC (Gutierrez-Kobeh et al., 1997). Moreover, the extracellular cysteine proteinase of *E. histolytica* can specifically cleave C3, and while this leads to activation of the alternative pathway, it may also inactivate C3a and C5a and so prevent their immunoregulatory and chemotactic effects (Reed et al., 1995).

Although helminths have evolved a sophisticated set of molecular inhibitors of complement activation (Fishelson, 1995) they also exploit host complement-regulatory proteins by acquiring them on their surfaces. The hydatid cyst of *Echinococcus granulosus* contains the host complement regulatory protein factor H (Diaz et al., 1997), while larvae and adults of *Schistosoma mansoni* express host decay-accelerating factor on their tegumental surfaces (Pearce et al., 1990). These examples demonstrate that the ability of parasites to mimic complement-regulatory molecules or to acquire them from the host represents a central strategy for evading complement-mediated damage by the innate immune system.

Alternative Mediators of Innate Immunity to *Trypanosoma brucei*

Besides complement, there are other soluble factors that mediate innate immunity to parasitic infections. In particular, the resistance of humans to *T. brucei* is determined in part by a primate-specific, innate cytolytic defense mechanism that restricts the host range of African trypanosomes (Tomlinson and Raper, 1998). Biochemical analysis revealed that high-density lipoproteins were part of a complex that mediates this cytolytic effect (Rifkin, 1978), and subsequent studies demonstrated that this complex, trypanosome lysis factor 1 (TLF1), is composed of several common apoplipoproteins, as well as a haptoglobin-related protein (Hpr) (Hajduk et al., 1989; Smith et al., 1995). A second cytolytic complex, TLF2, has also been identified which shares many of the components of TLF1 but contains a unique immunoglobulin M (IgM) component and has a lower lipid content (Raper et al., 1999). To mediate cytotoxicity, TLF has to undergo receptor-mediated uptake and enter an intracellular acidic compartment (Hager and Hajduk, 1997), and the peroxidase activity associated with TLF suggests that lysis of trypanosomes may be due to oxidative damage (Smith et al., 1995). Figure 2 outlines a proposed mechanism of action for TLF. Recent findings suggest that there is a similar role for TLF in killing of *Plasmodium* spp., an observation that may explain the long-standing difficulty associated with adapting malaria parasites to in vitro culture in media containing human serum (K. P. Day and S. L. Hajduk, personal communication).

Whereas TLF is capable of killing *T. brucei*, the subspecies that infect humans, *T. b. gambiense* and

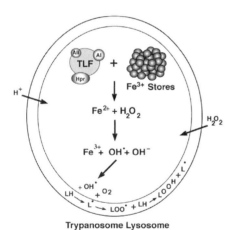

Figure 2. Mechanism of TLF killing of *T. b. brucei*. TLF binds to high-affinity receptors on the surface of *T. b. brucei* and is endocytosed and targeted to the lysosome. At low lysosomal pH and in the presence of high intracellular concentrations of hydrogen peroxide, TLF facilitates the release of Fe^{2+} from iron stores. Fe^{2+} ions react with H_2O_2 via the Fenton reaction to form hydroxyl radicals. Hydroxyl radicals produced in this reaction attack polyunsaturated fatty acids (LH), causing lipid free-radical formation (L·). The lipid free radical forms a lipid peroxyl radical (LOO·) in the presence of O_2, which peroxidates adjacent lipids, creating a chain reaction. The lipid hydroperoxides (LOOH) formed are unstable, resulting in a wide variety of products that can cause membrane breakdown and release of lysosomal contents. This model was supplied by Joseph Bishop and Steve Hajduk from the University of Alabama at Birmingham.

T. b. rhodesiense, are resistant to TLF-mediated cytolysis. Possible mechanisms that underlie resistance to TLF include the inability of these parasites to internalize TLF (Hager and Hajduk, 1997) and the expression of higher levels of antioxidants that protect them from TLF-mediated peroxidase activity (Tomlinson and Raper, 1998). A molecular basis for the resistance to TLF is provided by studies which have correlated resistance to TLF with the expression of a serum resistance-associated (SRA) gene, whose product is homologous to the variant surface glycoprotein (De Greef and Hamers, 1994). The expression of SRA is associated with resistance to TLF, and transfection of SRA into *T. brucei* confers resistance to human serum, identifying this gene as critical for the adaptation of *T. b. rhodesiense* to survive in humans (Xong et al., 1998).

Although cytokines are normally associated with regulation and activation of cells of the immune system, there is evidence that tumor necrosis factor alpha (TNF-α) is directly involved in innate imunity to *T. brucei*. The ability of TNF-α to bind to and be internalized by *T. brucei* results in cytolysis of this protozoan (Magez et al., 1997). The susceptibility of parasites to this mechanism of killing is specific because insect stages are resistant to lysis and only parasites isolated during the peak of parasitemia are lysed by TNF-α. Support for this mechanism in vivo is provided by studies in which neutralization of TNF-α in mice infected with *T. brucei* results in an increase in parasitemia (Magez et al., 1997). Nevertheless, it is not clear whether these findings are due to a lack of TNF-α-mediated cytolysis of parasites or to an immunoregulatory effect of TNF-α depletion.

CELLULAR MECHANISMS OF INNATE IMMUNITY

Innate Defenses Mediated by Phagocytes

The most basic cellular mechanisms of resistance to infection are associated with the ability of phagocytes to engulf invading microorganisms. Phagocytosis by macrophages exposes parasites to a respiratory burst and a hostile lysosomal compartment which in many cases is lethal to microorganisms. Neutrophils and macrophages represent an innate first line of defense that alone, or in combination with complement, can result in killing of many parasites. Thus, mononuclear phagocytes can kill schistosomula (Peck et al., 1983) and tachyzoites of *Toxoplasma gondii* (Catterall et al., 1987). At the same time, many pathogens have developed strategies to evade these responses and survive inside host cells. Moreover, the ability of many parasites to survive inside macrophages when phagocytosed or to actively invade cells provides a mechanism for evading humoral effector molecules. The ability of *Leishmania* spp. to gain access to the macrophage via the CR1 and CR3 receptors, which fail to trigger the respiratory burst, is probably an important factor in allowing them to survive within these cells. The intracellular survival of *Trypanosoma cruzi* is dependent on the ability of the parasite to escape from the phagolysosome. This process may be facilitated by the expression by *T. cruzi* of a homologue of C9 that can disrupt the phagosome membrane, allowing escape of the parasite into the cytoplasm (Andrews et al., 1990). The ability of *Toxoplasma gondii* to actively invade cells enables it to form a parasitophorous vacuole, which fails to undergo acidification (Sibley et al., 1985). If, instead, the parasite is forced to enter the cell by a phagocytic pathway, it is exposed to the normal phagolysosomal system and is killed (Joiner et al., 1990).

Cytokine-Dependent Innate Resistance to Intracellular Parasites

The ability of certain parasites to invade and replicate within host cells allows them to evade the humoral immune response. Therefore, a recognition process is required to alert the immune system to the presence of infected cells, along with a series of effector mechanisms to control parasite replication. One of the most important cytokines in the initiation of cell-mediated immunity is interleukin-12 (IL-12). The production of IL-12 in response to infection plays a critical role in the activation of NK cells to produce gamma interferon (IFN-γ), which in turn is responsible for the activation of effector mechanisms required to control replication of intracellular pathogens (Fig. 3). There are several cellular sources of IL-12 that can be triggered to initiate this innate mechanism of resistance during infection. Inflammatory macrophages can respond to *Toxoplasma gondii* and *Trypanosoma cruzi* to produce IL-12 (Aliberti et al., 1996; Gazzinelli et al., 1993). In addition, purified mouse and human neutrophils will make IL-12 when stimulated with extracts of *T. gondii* (Bliss et al., 1999), and this may explain previous studies which indicated a protective role for neutrophils in resistance to *T. gondii* (Sayles and Johnson, 1996). The ability of CD8α^+ dendritic cells to produce IL-12 in response to soluble antigens of *T. gondii* (Reis e Sousa et al., 1997) indicates that they may be an important source of IL-12, especially during the initial stages of *Toxoplasma* infection (Fig. 4). Although IL-12 is important for the development of

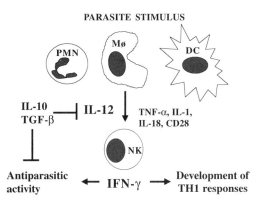

Figure 3. Regulation of innate cell-mediated immunity to parasites. Infection with various parasites can stimulate the production of proinflammatory cytokines from several sources including neutrophils (PMN), macrophages (Mø), and dendritic cells (DC). IL-12, in combination with other cofactors, plays an important role in stimulating NK-cell production of IFN-γ, which mediates antiparasitic activity and may contribute to the development of Th1-type responses. IL-10 and TGF-β are inhibitors of this innate mechanism of immunity, either acting directly on accessory cell populations or NK cells to inhibit the production of proinflammatory cytokines or antagonizing the effector mechanisms required to control parasite replication.

protective immunity to leishmaniasis, early studies indicated that promastigotes of *Leishmania major* do not activate macrophages to produce IL-12 (Carrera et al., 1996; Reiner et al., 1994) and that infected macrophages have an impaired ability to produce this cytokine (Belkaid et al., 1998). It is now recognized that murine dendritic cells have the capacity to make IL-12 in response to *Leishmania* amastigotes and promastigotes (Gorak et al., 1998; von Stebut et al., 1998) and thus may provide the initial source of the cytokine during *Leishmania* infection.

The ability of macrophages, neutrophils, mast cells, and dendritic cells to respond in an innate manner to parasite antigens implies the presence of specific receptors, pattern recognition molecules, or unusual signaling mechanisms that initiate this response. The glycosylphosphatidylinositol (GPI) lipid anchors of many parasite surface proteins are capable of activating protein kinases and stimulating the production of proinflammatory cytokines. Thus, GPIs of *T. brucei*, *L. mexicana*, and *Plasmodium falciparum* can stimulate macrophages to upregulate inducible nitric oxide synthase and produce TNF-α and IL-1 (Magez et al., 1998; Schofield and Hackett, 1993). Similarly, the GPI anchor fraction of mucin-like molecules from *T. cruzi* trypomastigotes stimulates macrophage production of IL-12 and TNF-α (Camargo et al., 1997). Interestingly, the GPI from epimastigotes of *T. cruzi* are unable to stimulate cytokine production. This difference in the ability of GPI from trypomastigotes and epimastigotes to stimulate the

CD11c   IL-12p40

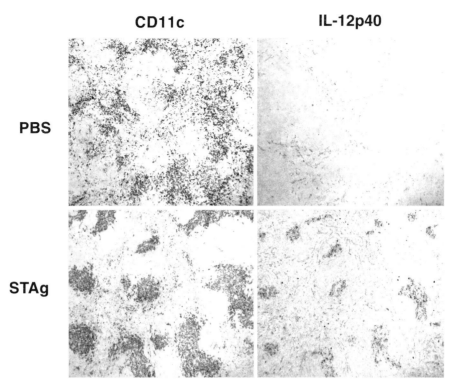

Figure 4. Activation of splenic dendritic cells by *Toxoplasma* products. The mobilization and activation of dendritic cells are likely to be key steps in the initiation of cell-mediated responses to intracellular pathogens. This figure demonstrates the response of splenic dendritic cells to a soluble extract of *Toxoplasma* tachyzoites (STAg) 6 h after intravenous injection. In the left-hand panels, spleen cells were stained with the DC cell surface marker CD11c, while the right-hand panels show serial sections from the same spleens stained with an anti-IL-12 p40 monoclonal antibody. As can be seen, the *Toxoplasma* products induce a massive mobilization of dendritic cells into the T-cell areas of the spleen, and many of these dendritic cells produce IL-12, a cytokine crucial for the induction of IFN-γ dependent resistance to the parasite.

production of cytokines is associated with additional galactose residues and unsaturated fatty acids present in the GPI anchors isolated from trypomastigotes (Almeida et al., 2000).

In contrast to the activating effects of many parasite GPIs, the LPG and GIPLS of *Leishmania* have a number of downmodulatory effects on macrophage function, including inhibition of IL-12 production as well as reduced expression of inducible nitric oxide synthese and TNF-R (Carrera et al., 1996; Proudfoot et al., 1995). An insight into the molecular basis for these events is provided by studies in which it was shown that LPG can interfere with signaling in infected cells and is unable to activate protein kinase C (Descoteaux et al., 1991; Feng et al., 1999). Thus, it appears that variation in structure of parasite GPIs imparts different properties of signal transduction to this class of glycolipid (Tachado et al., 1999). Nevertheless, it is not clear if these events depend on some as yet unidentified host receptors or if GPIs can directly signal cells through their nonspecific interaction with different membrane components.

Regulation of NK Cell Responses to Parasites

The recognition that cytokines are involved in the regulation of cellular immunity provided a framework to understand how different cell populations could interact to provide a sophisticated form of innate immunity. This is best illustrated by the complex mechanisms used to regulate the ability of natural killer (NK) cells to mediate innate resistance to many parasites (Fig. 3). NK cells are large granular lymphocytes which have many functions in common with T cells. For example, they can recognize class I molecules, have cytotoxic functions, and, like T cells, produce IFN-γ, TNF-α, IL-5, IL-10, and IL-13. These common features suggest that T and NK cells have a common developmental pathway but that unlike T cells, NK-cell development and function are independent of gene rearrangement and NK cells lack a T-cell receptor and cannot directly recognize foreign antigens. Historically, it was recognized that infection of mice with different parasitic organisms or challenge with parasite antigens resulted in a transient increase in NK-cell activity (as measured by

NK-cell cytolytic activity) (see, e.g., Hauser et al. [1983]). Similarly, stimulation of human peripheral blood mononuclear cells with subcellular components of *T. gondii* will activate human NK cells to produce IFN-γ (Sharma et al., 1986). Subsequent studies established that NK cells produce IFN-γ in response to monokines produced by adherent cells stimulated with protozoan antigens (Sher et al., 1993). Although long-term control of these infections is clearly dependent on T cells, the early production of IFN-γ by NK cells may be an important mechanism which prevents parasites from overwhelming the host prior to the development of adaptive responses. This NK-cell-dependent mechanism of resistance is relevant to many other intracellular pathogens in addition to *Leishmania* and *Toxoplasma*. These include *Trypanosoma cruzi* (Cardillo et al., 1996), *E. histolytica* (Seydel et al., 2000), *Cryptosporidium parvum* (McDonald et al., 1992), and *Plasmodium chabaudi* (Mohan et al., 1997).

Although IL-12 is a critical cytokine required to stimulate NK-cell production during parasitic infections, its ability to stimulate NK cells to produce high levels of IFN-γ is dependent on other soluble and cell-bound ligands. Several studies have identified TNF-α and IL-1 as being important cofactors for IL-12-induced NK-cell production of IFN-γ during toxoplasmosis (Hunter et al., 1995b; Sher et al., 1993). Costimulation also plays a role in the NK-cell-mediated response to intracellular parasites, and cells infected with *T. gondii* or *T. cruzi* have been shown to upregulate the expression of B7, the ligand for the costimulatory molecule CD28 (see, e.g., Frosch et al. [1997]). Interestingly, activated NK cells express CD28, the ligand for B7, and stimulation through this interaction enhances IL-12-induced NK-cell production of IFN-γ and innate resistance to *T. gondii* (Hunter et al., 1997). Thus, the ability of *L. donovani* to prevent infected macrophages from upregulating the expression of costimulatory molecules may allow the parasite to subvert optimal innate and adaptive responses (Kaye et al., 1994). These findings correlate with the ability of *L. donovani* to bypass NK-cell production of IFN-γ (Kaye and Bancroft, 1992).

During many parasitic infections, there is an initial peak of NK cell activity which is followed by a sharp fall in NK cell activity, which indicates that there is a mechanism(s) to switch off NK-cell responses. At least two cytokines (IL-10 and transforming growth factor β [TGF-β]) play a role in the inhibition of NK cell responses during parasitic infections. IL-10 can inhibit macrophage expression of B7 molecules and their production of TNF-α, IL-1, and IL-12 (Moore et al., 1993). Similarly, TGF-β (a product of many cell types, including macrophages

and NK cells) inhibits NK-cell production of IFN-γ and resistance to *T. gondii* (Hunter et al., 1995a). In addition, the production of IL-10 and TGF-β during parasitic infection can antagonize macrophage effector functions and so enhance the survival of intracellular parasites (Gazzinelli et al., 1992). However, it is unclear whether the production of these inhibitory cytokines represents a parasite strategy to inhibit protective host responses or simply reflects a balanced host response required to prevent the development of immunopathology.

Mast Cells and Eosinophils as Effectors of Innate Immunity

Although humoral mechanisms are normally associated with resistance to helminths, there are several innate interactions of these parasites with cell types associated with Th2-type responses. Mast cells are important in resistance to nematodes, but many of their effects are essentially T-cell dependent (Else and Finkelman, 1998). However, cercariae of *Schistosoma mansoni* are capable of activating the release of histamine from mast cells in vitro independently of adherence or complement. These events could be important in attracting inflammatory cells into areas where these parasites are migrating (Catto et al., 1980). The role of mast cells in innate immunity to other helminths remains unclear, with reductions in mast cell numbers not affecting the expulsion of *Trichuris muris* or *Nippostrongylus brasiliensis*, although they are important for resistance to *Trichinella spiralis* (Alizadeh and Murrell, 1984). Mast cells may also play a role in directing resistance to protozoans, and although they are weakly phagocytic, they can be activated by direct contact with promastigotes of *Leishmania* spp. to release preformed TNF-α (Bidri et al., 1997).

There is little evidence for a role of eosinophils in resistance to protozoa, although, when activated, these cells can kill virulent *E. histolytica* without the help of opsonins (Lopez-Osuna et al., 1992). Eosinophils appear to be more important in resistance to helminth infections, and eosinophilia is a characteristic feature of these infections. The observation that eosinophils kill opsonized schistosomula of *S. mansoni* in vitro and the histological association of these cells with dead or dying larval stages of various helminths suggested an important role for this cell population in resistance to the tissue-migratory, larval stages of various helminths (Butterworth, 1984). However, many of these events were dependent on the opsonic effects of antibody, and eosinophilia is thought to be largely dependent on the production of IL-5 by T cells. Nevertheless, there is also a T-cell-independent eosinophilia in mice infected with *Tox-ocara canis,* which is dependent on IL-5 (Takamoto et al., 1995). Since NK cells can produce IL-5 (Warren et al., 1995) and regulate eosinophila during an allergic reaction (Walker et al., 1998), this may be a mechanism whereby NK cells can influence the development of effector mechanisms required for resistance to worms. For example, the production of IL-5 by NK cells appears to be important in the regulation of eosinophilia in response to *Heligmosomoides polygyrus* (Svetic et al., 1993). In direct contrast, it has been reported that the growth of the filarial worm *Brugia malayi* is dependent on host NK-cell function. Thus, comparisons of worm survival and development in different strains of mice with different levels of NK-cell activity reveal that mice with reduced NK-cell activity were nonpermissive to growth of *B. malayi* whereas SCID mice with normal NK-cell activity are permissive and depletion of NK cells in SCID mice prevented growth of *B. malayi* (Babu et al., 1998).

Effector Cells Which Bridge Innate and Adaptive Immunity

The hallmark of the adaptive response is the selection of T and B cells which have undergone somatic gene rearrangement and which are selectively expanded following antigenic stimulation. However, there are B- and T-cell populations which undergo limited gene rearrangements and which may represent a population of cells primed to respond in an innate manner to microrganisms. This section deals with three cell types that appear to represent a bridge between innate and adaptive immunity.

B1 cells

CD5$^+$ B1 cells produce low-affinity polyreactive antibodies that can recognize polysaccharides and are a source of IL-10. These unique cells arise early in ontogeny before conventional B cells, are present in large numbers in the body cavity, and utilize a limited set of V genes for their B-cell receptors. In addition, these B cells do not undergo somatic hypermutation and as a consequence have a limited diversity of VDJ junctions compared to conventional B cells. The role of B1 cells in the immune response to parasites remains understudied, but these cells will proliferate and produce IL-10 in response to a polylactosamine antigen present on eggs of *S. mansoni* (Velupillai and Harn, 1994) which may drive the development of egg-specific Th2-type responses. Resistance to the filarial parasite *B. malayi* is associated with the presence of B1 lymphocytes, and it has been proposed

that an early B1 response is responsible for the attrition of infective larvae whereas clearance of surviving parasites is dependent on cellular immunity (Paciorkowski et al., 2000).

γδ and NK T cells

Since γδ and NK T cells express T-cell receptor chains which are invariant or possess a highly limited genetic diversity, it has been proposed that these cells may recognize a narrow range of antigens. Although γδ T cells represent a small percentage of lymphocytes in the periphery, they are abundant in epithelial and mucosal tissues, the sites of initial infection by many parasites. A role for γδ T cells in resistance to infection is indicated by studies in which stimulation of human peripheral blood mononuclear cells from naive individuals with *T. gondii* or *P. falciparum* results in an expansion of γδ T cells (Goerlich et al., 1991; Subauste et al., 1995). Moreover, these in vitro results are mirrored during the acute stage of these infections in humans (Roussilhon et al., 1990; Scalise et al., 1992). The activity of γδ T cells is not restricted to protozoan infections, since there is also an expansion of γδ T cells in response to *N. brasiliensis* (Rosat et al., 1995) and these cells represent a source of IL-4 during this infection that may be important for the development of Th2 responses (Ferrick et al., 1995). The events that lead to activation and expansion of γδ T cells following infection have not been well defined. However, γδ T cells can respond to heat shock proteins (HSP) and since invasion and intracellular replication by different parasites result in increased expression of HSP, this may provide a mechanism that allows γδ T cells to recognize infected cells. Thus, the ability of *T. gondii* to induce HSP by host cells is associated with a protective role for γδ T cells in murine models (Hisaeda et al., 1997) and is probably due to the ability of γδ T cells to lyse infected cells and produce IFN-γ in response to this infection (Hisaeda et al., 1995; Kasper et al., 1996; Subauste et al., 1995). The function of γδ T cells in resistance to malaria is less clear, with data indicating that γδ T cells can recognize parasite HSPs (Kopacz and Kumar, 1999) and that γδ T cells play a role in resistance to liver stages (Tsuji et al., 1994) as well as in the control of parasitemia (Elloso et al., 1994). Recent studies suggest that HSP may also play an immunomodulatory role, and the ability of HSP to stimulate the production of proinflammatory cytokines (Asea et al., 2000) and be involved in the generation of cytotoxic T cells (Cho et al., 2000) provides an alternative explanation for the role of HSP in resistance to these parasites.

NK T cells form a lymphocyte subset with a distinct surface phenotype and reactivity to CD1. NK T cells express several markers that are typically associated with NK cells, but which express an invariant T-cell receptor. Members of the CD1 family of proteins are involved in the presentation of foreign lipids and glycolipids. Although CD1 is structurally similar to other major histocompatibility complex (MHC) molecules, it has a more open configuration in the antigen binding sites that is likely to account for its ability to present many different lipid antigens. NK T cells can produce high levels of IL-4 when they are stimulated through their T-cell receptor and it was proposed that this response is important in directing Th2 development during parasitic infections. However, NK T cells are not required for development of Th2 cytokine responses in BALB/c mice infected with *L. major* or in mice injected with schistosome eggs (Brown et al., 1996). An alternative role for NK T cells may be in the generation of antibody responses unrestricted by classical MHC genes. Thus, evidence has been presented arguing that the CD1d-restricted recognition of the GPI-anchored surface antigens of *Plasmodium* and *Trypanosoma* by NK T cells regulates the development of IgG antibodies against these molecules (Schofield et al., 1999). However, recent studies indicate that IgG responses to the GPI-anchored circumsporozoite protein is independent of CD1 and is dependent on the more classical MHC class II pathway (Molano et al., 2000).

ROLE OF THE INNATE RESPONSE TO PARASITES IN DETERMINING THE NATURE OF ADAPTIVE IMMUNITY

Although innate immunity plays an important role in resistance to acute parasitic infections, the adaptive response is required to provide long-term protective immunity. The development of adaptive T- and B-cell responses following infection is dependent on the innate ability of accessory cells to present antigen, provide costimulation, and produce cytokines that affect the onset, duration, magnitude, and character of the adaptive immune response. There is now recognition that cross talk between the innate and adaptive arms of the immune system is required for an integrated and efficient effector response with the correct functional phenotype.

Initiation of Th1 Responses

While innate production of IL-12 is important for NK-cell activation, this cytokine is also critical for the development of protective T-cell responses re-

quired for long-term control of many intracellular parasites (Gazzinelli et al., 1994; Sypek et al., 1993). In contrast, the production of IL-12 antagonizes the development of protective Th2-type responses during helminth infection and results in increased susceptibility to these parasites (Else and Finkelman, 1998). Thus, although innate production of IL-12 is associated with resistance to protozoa, it can contribute to susceptibility to various helminths.

The ability of IL-12 to drive the development of Th1-type responses is due to both direct and indirect activities of the cytokines. IL-12 has direct effects on the development of Th1 responses, but its ability to stimulate the production of IFN-γ by NK cells early in the course of infection can also influence the development of subsequent antigen-specific Th1 CD4$^+$ T cells required for resistance to *L. major* (Scharton and Scott, 1993). The mechanism whereby IFN-γ affects the development of Th1 responses is not clear but may be due to its ability to directly inhibit the development of Th2 responses (Pernis et al., 1995). However, while NK cells may help in this process, they are not essential for the development of the protective Th1 responses required for ultimate control of *L. major* (Scharton and Scott, 1993; Wakil et al., 1998).

Other cytokines, such as TNF-α and IL-1, are also involved in the development of T-cell responses, and IL-18, a novel cytokine which shares many properties with IL-1 and IL-12, is a potent inducer of NK- and T-cell production of IFN-γ (Okamura et al., 1995). Since IL-18 exists as a preformed cytokine which can be released rapidly, it is an ideal candidate for the regulation of innate immunity to parasites. Our understanding of the role of IL-18 in innate immunity to parasitic infections is far less comprehensive than our understanding of IL-12. Mice deficient in IL-18 mount less efficient Th1-type responses following infection with *L. major,* associated with increased susceptibility to this infection (Wei et al., 1999), although these mice appear to ultimately control this infection (Ohkusu et al., 2000). Whether this behavior is a consequence of an altered innate response or can be attributed solely to a defect in T-cell differentiation or the responses of differentiated T cells is not yet clear. Nevertheless, exogenous IL-18 can be used to augment NK-cell-mediated resistance to *T. gondii*, although this effect is largely dependent on endogenous IL-12 (Cai et al., 2000a).

Initiation of Th2 Responses

IL-4 plays an important role in the development of Th2-type responses, which are generally associated with resistance to helminths and susceptibility to protozoan parasites. Thus, the early burst of IL-4 produced in BALB/c mice infected with *L. major* downregulates IL-12 receptor β2-chain expression on CD4$^+$ T cells and so inhibits the development of protective Th1 responses (Himmelrich et al., 1998; Jones et al., 1998). Since increasing evidence indicates a stochastic component to the development of Th1 and Th2 responses (Reiner and Seder, 1999), the exact role played by IL-4 (or other factors produced by the innate immune system) in directing Th2 development remains an important unanswered question. Several cell types are associated with the production of IL-4, including mast cells (Plaut et al., 1989), basophils (Seder et al., 1991), NK T cells (Yoshimoto and Paul, 1994), and eosinophils (Sabin et al., 1996). The involvement of the innate system as the early source of IL-4 in BALB/c mice infected with *L. major* remains unclear, although there is a restricted population of CD4$^+$ T cells specific for the parasite LACK antigen, which produces high levels of IL-4 during early infection (Launois et al., 1997). The cytokine IL-13 (which shares elements of the IL-4 signaling pathway) is also important in susceptibility to *L. major* (Matthews et al., 2000; Noben-Trauth et al., 1999) and resistance to *N. brasiliensis* (Urban et al., 1998). Many cell types, including mast cells and basophils (Marone et al., 1997) as well as NK cells (Hoshino et al., 1999), can make this cytokine, and whether innate production of IL-13 is involved in directing the development of Th2 responses or in regulating effector cell functions in parasitic infection is an important area for future research.

SUMMARY AND CONCLUSIONS

Historically, the concept that innate immunity is important in resistance to parasites was based on the identification of cells with nonspecific effector functions against these pathogens. The field has now advanced to provide an understanding of the cytokines and costimulatory molecules which regulate these innate effector functions and is beginning to address the molecular signaling pathways involved. For example, recent studies with parasitic systems have identified distinct roles for various transcription factors in innate resistance to infection. Thus, the IFN consensus binding protein is required for innate IL-12 responses to *T. gondii* (Scharton-Kersten et al., 1997), while RelB and STAT4 are important in regulating the innate production of IFN-γ (Caamaño et al., 1999; Cai et al., 2000b). However, many questions remain concerning the interactions between the innate immune system and parasites. In particular,

the initial mechanisms that allow a host to recognize parasites are poorly defined. Parasite-specific receptors, similar to the Toll receptors which are triggered by bacterial products (Medzhitov et al., 1997), may exist which can recognize parasite GPIs or other moieties. Alternatively, other mechanisms may alert the immune system to the presence of invading parasites, and there may be a unique system that allows mammalian cells to distinguish among parasitic eukaryotes. In particular, many parasites are cytolytic or cause tissue destruction during migration, and this may provide a nonspecific "danger" signal (Matzinger, 1998). However, if the initiation of the innate response is due to a nonspecific signal, it is still not clear that such a signal can influence the development of appropriate polarized adaptive responses. Interestingly, two recent studies indicate important roles for chemokine-mediated signaling in the initiation of protective immunity to *T. gondii*. In one study, IP-10 was shown to be essential for the recruitment of T cells and the development of protective immunity (Khan et al., 2000), and the other study provides evidence that signaling through CCR5 stimulates CD8α$^+$ dendritic cells to produce IL-12, which is essential for resistance to *T. gondii* (Aliberti et al., 2000).

Understanding the cellular and molecular basis of the mechanisms that underlie innate immunity to parasitic diseases may also provide important information for the rational design of immunotherapies or vaccines. At present there is a paucity of vaccines which protect against parasitic diseases, and understanding how innate immunity initiates the development of long-lived, protective responses to these parasites may provide new approaches to vaccination. Perhaps the best example of how understanding the mechanisms of innate immunity to infection can influence the development of new approaches to deal with parasitic infections is provided by IL-12. The identification of a key role for IL-12 in the activation of NK cells and the development of Th1-type responses has led to its use in models of parasitic diseases to enhance host resistance to many parasitic infections (Gazzinelli et al., 1993; Sedegah et al., 1994; Sypek et al., 1993; Urban et al., 1996). In addition, IL-12 has been used to modulate vaccination responses to enhance immunity to intracellular parasites and in the development of an antipathology vaccine (Afonso et al., 1994; Gurunathan et al., 1998; Wynn et al., 1995). An important challenge now is to determine if other elements of the innate immune response can be utilized in the design of more efficient vaccines and/or immunotherapies.

Acknowledgments. We thank George Yap, David Mosser, Steve Hajduk, Steve Beverly, and Phillip Scott for their helpful discussions and criticism during the preparation of this chapter.

REFERENCES

Afonso, L. C. C., T. M. Scharton, L. Q. Vieira, M. Wysocka, G. Trinchieri, and P. Scott. 1994. The adjuvant effect of interleukin-12 in a vaccine against *Leishmania major*. *Science* 263:235–237.

Aliberti, J., C. Reis e Sousa, M. Schito, S. Hieny, T. Wells, G. B. Huffnagle, and A. Sher. 2000. CCR5 provides a signal for microbial induced production of IL-12 by CD8α+ dendritic cells. *Nat. Immunol.* 1:83–87.

Aliberti, J. C., M. A. G. Cardoso, G. A. Martins, R. T. Gazzinelli, L. Q. Vieira, and J. S. Silva. 1996. Interleukin-12 mediates resistance to *Trypanosoma cruzi* in mice and is produced by murine macrophages in response to live trypomastigotes. *Infect. Immun.* 64:1961–1967.

Alizadeh, H., and K. D. Murrell. 1984. The intestinal mast cell response to *Trichinella spiralis* infection in mast cell-deficient w/wv mice. *J. Parasitol.* 70:767–773.

Almeida, I. C., M. M. Camargo, D. O. Procopio, L. S. Silva, A. Mehlert, L. R. Travassos, R. T. Gazzinelli, and M. A. J. Ferguson. 2000. Highly purified glycosylphosphatidylinositols from *Trypanosoma cruzi* are potent proinflammatory agents. *EMBO J.* 19:101–110.

Andrews, N. W., C. K. Abrams, S. L. Slatin, and G. Griffiths. 1990. A *T. cruzi*-secreted protein immunologically related to the complement component C9: evidence for membrane pore-forming activity at low pH. *Cell* 61:1277–1287.

Asea, A., S. K. Kraeft, E. A. Kurt-Jones, M. A. Stevenson, L. B. Chen, R. W. Finberg, G. C. Koo, and S. K. Calderwood. 2000. HSP70 stimulates cytokine production through a CD14-dependent pathway, demonstrating its dual role as a chaperone and cytokine. *Nat. Med.* 6:435–442.

Babu, S., P. Porte, T. R. Klei, L. D. Shultz, and T. V. Rajan. 1998. Host NK cells are required for the growth of the human filarial parasite *Brugia malayi* in mice. *J. Immunol.* 161:1428–1432.

Belkaid, Y., B. Butcher, and D. L. Sacks. 1998. Analysis of cytokine production by inflammatory mouse macrophages at the single cell level: selective impairment of IL-12 induction in *Leishmania*-infected cells. *Eur. J. Immunol.* 28:1389–1400.

Bidri, M., I. Vouldoukis, M. D. Mossalayi, P. Debre, J. J. Guillosson, D. Mazier, and M. Arock. 1997. Evidence for direct interaction between mast cells and *Leishmania* parasites. *Parasite Immunol.* 19:475–483.

Blackwell, J. M., R. A. Ezekowitz, M. B. Roberts, J. Y. Channon, R. B. Sim, and S. Gordon. 1985. Macrophage complement and lectin-like receptors bind *Leishmania* in the absence of serum. *J. Exp. Med.* 162:324–331.

Bliss, S. K., A. J. Marshall, Y. Zhang, and E. Y. Denkers. 1999. Human polymorphonuclear leukocytes produce IL-12, TNF-α, and the chemokines macrophage-inflammatory protein-1α and -1β in response to *Toxoplasma gondii* antigens. *J. Immunol.* 162:7369–7375.

Braga, L. L., H. Ninomiya, J. J. McCoy, S. Eacker, T. Wiedmer, C. Pham, S. Wood, P. J. Sims, and W. A. Petri, Jr. 1992. Inhibition of the complement membrane attack complex by the galactose-specific adhesion of *Entamoeba histolytica*. *J. Clin. Investig.* 90:1131–1137.

Brown, D. R., D. J. Fowell, D. B. Corry, T. A. Wynn, N. H. Moskowitz, A. W. Cheever, R. M. Locksley, and S. L. Reiner. 1996. β2-Microglobulin-dependent NK1.1+ T cells are not essential for T helper cell 2 immune responses. *J. Exp. Med.* 184:1295–1304.

Butterworth, A. E. 1984. Cell-mediated damage to helminths. *Adv. Parasitol.* 23:143–235.

Caamaño, J., J. Alexander, L. Craig, R. Bravo, and C. A. Hunter. 1999. The NF-κB family member RelB is required for innate and adaptive immunity to *Toxoplasma gondii*. *J. Immunol.* 163:4453–4461.

Cai, G., R. Kastelein, and C. A. Hunter. 2000a. Interleukin-18 (IL-18) enhances innate IL-12-mediated resistance to *Toxoplasma gondii*. *Infect. Immun.* 68:6932–6938.

Cai, G., T. Radzanowski, E. Villegas, R. Kastelein, and C. A. Hunter. 2000b. Identification of STAT4-dependent and independent mechanisms of resistance to *Toxoplasma gondii*. *J. Immunol.* 165:2619–2627.

Camargo, M. M., I. C. Almeida, M. E. S. Pereira, M. A. J. Ferguson, L. R. Travassos, and R. T. Gazzinelli. 1997. Glycosylphosphatidylinositol-anchored mucin-like glycoproteins isolated from *Trypanosoma cruzi* trypomastigotes initiate the synthesis of proinflammatory cytokines in macrophages. *J. Immunol.* 158:5890–5901.

Cardillo, F., J. C. Voltarelli, S. G. Reed, and J. S. Silva. 1996. Regulation of *Trypanosoma cruzi* infection in mice by gamma interferon and interleukin 10: role of NK cells. *Infect. Immun.* 64:128–134.

Carrera, L., R. T. Gazzinelli, R. Badolato, S. Hieny, W. Muller, R. Kuhn, and D. Sacks. 1996. Leishmania promastigotes selectively inhibit interleukin 12 induction in bone marrow-derived macrophages from susceptible and resistant mice. *J. Exp. Med.* 183:515–526.

Catterall, J. R., C. M. Black, J. P. Leventhal, N. W. Rizk, J. S. Wachtel, and J. S. Remington. 1987. Nonoxidative microbicidal activity in normal human alveolar and peritoneal macrophages. *Infect. Immun.* 55:1635–1640.

Catto, B. A., F. A. Lewis, and E. A. Ottesen. 1980. Cercaria-induced histamine release: a factor in the pathogenesis of schistosome dermatitis? *Am. J. Trop. Med. Hyg.* 29:886–889.

Cho, B. K., D. Palliser, E. Guillen, J. Wisniewski, R. A. Young, J. Chen, and H. N. Eisen. 2000. A proposed mechanism for the induction of cytotoxic T lymphocyte production by heat shock fusion proteins. *Immunity* 12:263–272.

De Greef, C., and R. Hamers. 1994. The serum resistance-associated (SRA) gene of *Trypanosoma brucei rhodesiense* encodes a variant surface glycoprotein-like protein. *Mol. Biochem. Parasitol.* 68:277–284.

Descoteaux, A., S. J. Turco, D. L. Sacks, and G. Matlashewski. 1991. *Leishmania donovani* lipophosphoglycan selectively inhibits signal transduction in macrophages. *J. Immunol.* 146:2747–2753.

Diaz, A., A. Ferreira, and R. B. Sim. 1997. Complement evasion by *Echinococcus granulosus*: sequestration of host factor H in the hydatid cyst wall. *J. Immunol.* 158:3779–3786.

Elloso, M. M., H. C. van der Heyde, J. A. vande Waa, D. D. Manning, and W. P. Weidanz. 1994. Inhibition of *Plasmodium falciparum* in vitro by human γδ T cells. *J. Immunol.* 153:1187–1194.

Else, K. J., and F. D. Finkelman. 1998. Intestinal nematode parasites, cytokines and effector mechanisms. *Int. J. Parasitol.* 28:1145–1158.

Feng, G. J., H. S. Goodridge, M. M. Harnett, X. Q. Wei, A. V. Nikolaev, A. P. Higson, and F. Y. Liew. 1999. Extracellular signal-related kinase (ERK) and p38 mitogen-activated protein (MAP) kinases differentially regulate the lipopolysaccharide-mediated induction of inducible nitric oxide synthase and IL-12 in macrophages: *Leishmania* phosphoglycans subvert macrophage IL-12 production by targeting ERK MAP kinase. *J. Immunol.* 163:6403–6412.

Ferrante, A., and A. C. Allison. 1983. Alternative pathway activation of complement by African trypanosomes lacking a glycoprotein coat. *Parasite Immunol.* 5:491–498.

Ferrick, D. A., M. D. Schrenzel, T. Mulvania, B. Hsieh, W. G. Ferlin, and H. Lepper. 1995. Differential production of interferon-g and interleukin-4 in response to Th1- and Th2-stimulating pathogens by γδ T cells in vivo. *Nature* 373:255–257.

Fishelson, Z. 1995. Novel mechanisms of immune evasion by *Schistosoma mansoni*. *Mem. Inst. Oswaldo Cruz* 90:289–292.

Frosch, S., D. Kuntzlin, and B. Fleischer. 1997. Infection with *Trypanosoma cruzi* selectively upregulates B7-2 molecules on macrophages and enhances their costimulatory activity. *Infect. Immun.* 65:971–977.

Gazzinelli, R. T., S. Hieny, T. A. Wynn, S. Wolf, and A. Sher. 1993. Interleukin 12 is required for the T-lymphocyte-independent induction of interferon γ by an intracellular parasite and induces resistance in T-cell deficient hosts. *Proc. Natl. Acad. Sci. USA* 90:6115–6119.

Gazzinelli, R. T., I. P. Oswald, S. Hieny, S. L. James, and A. Sher. 1992. The microbicidal activity of interferon-γ-treated macrophages against *Trypanosoma cruzi* involves an L-arginine-dependent, nitrogen oxide-mediated mechanism inhibitable by interleukin-10 and transforming growth factor-β. *Eur. J. Immunol.* 22:2501–2506.

Gazzinelli, R. T., M. Wysocka, S. Hayashi, E. Y. Denkers, S. Hieny, P. Caspar, G. Trinchieri, and A. Sher. 1994. Parasite-induced IL-12 stimulates early IFN-γ synthesis and resistance during acute infection with *Toxoplasma gondii*. *J. Immunol.* 153:2533–2543.

Goerlich, R., G. Hacker, K. Pfeffer, K. Heeg, and H. Wagner. 1991. *Plasmodium falciparum* merozoites primarily stimulate the Vγ9 subset of human γ/δ T cells. *Eur. J. Immunol.* 21:2613–2616.

Gorak, P. M. A., C. R. Engwerda, and P. M. Kaye. 1998. Dendritic cells, but not macrophages, produce IL-12 immediately following *Leishmania donovani* infection. *Eur. J. Immunol.* 28:687–695.

Green, P. J., T. Feizi, M. S. Stoll, S. Thiel, A. Prescott, and M. J. McConville. 1994. Recognition of the major cell surface glycoconjugates of *Leishmania* parasites by the human serum mannan-binding protein. *Mol. Biochem. Parasitol.* 66:319–328.

Gurunathan, S., C. Prussin, D. L. Sacks, and R. A. Seder. 1998. Vaccine requirements for sustained cellular immunity to an intracellular parasitic infection. *Nat. Med.* 4:1409–1415.

Gutierrez-Kobeh, L., N. Cabrera, and R. Perez-Montfort. 1997. A mechanism of acquired resistance to complement-mediated lysis by *Entamoeba histolytica*. *J. Parasitol.* 83:234–241.

Hager, K. M., and S. L. Hajduk. 1997. Mechanism of resistance of African trypanosomes to cytotoxic human HDL. *Nature* 385:823–826.

Hajduk, S. L., D. R. Moore, J. Vasudevacharya, H. Siqueira, A. F. Torri, E. M. Tytler, and J. D. Esko. 1989. Lysis of *Trypanosoma brucei* by a toxic subspecies of human high density lipoprotein. *J. Biol. Chem.* 264:5210–5217.

Hauser, W. E., S. D. Sharma, and J. S. Remington. 1983. Augmentation of NK cell activity by soluble and particulate fractions of *Toxoplasma gondii*. *J. Immunol.* 131:458–463.

Himmelrich, H., C. Parra-Lopez, F. Tacchini-Cottier, J. A. Louis, and P. Launois. 1998. The IL-4 rapidly produced in BALB/c mice after infection with *Leishmania major* down-regulates IL-12 receptor β2-chain expression on CD4+ T cells resulting in a state of unresponsiveness to IL-12. *J. Immunol.* 161:6156–6163.

Hisaeda, H., H. Nagasawa, K. Maeda, Y. Maekawa, H. Ishikawa, Y. Ito, R. A. Good, and K. Himeno. 1995. γδ T cells play an important role in hsp65 expression and in acquiring protective immune responses against infection with *Toxoplasma gondii*. *J. Immunol.* 154:244–251.

Hisaeda, H., T. Sakai, H. Ishikaw, Y. Maekawa, K. Yasutomo, R. A. Good, and K. Himeno. 1997. Heat shock protein 65 induced by γδ T cells prevents apoptosis of macrophages and contributes to host defense in mice infected with *Toxoplasma gondii*. *J. Immunol.* 159:2375–2381.

Hoshino, T., R. H. Wiltrout, and H. A. Young. 1999. IL-18 is a potent coinducer of IL-13 in NK and T cells: a new potential role for IL-18 in modulating the immune response. *J. Immunol.* 162:5070–5077.

Hunter, C. A., L. Bermudez, H. Beernink, W. Waegell, and J. S. Remington. 1995a. Transforming growth factor–β inhibits interleukin-12-induced production of interferon-γ by natural killer cells: a role for transforming growth factor-β in the regulation of T-cell independent resistance to *Toxoplasma gondii*. *Eur. J. Immunol.* 25:994–1000.

Hunter, C. A., R. Chizzonite, and J. S. Remington. 1995b. Interleukin 1β is required for the ability of IL-12 to induce production of IFN-γ by NK cells: a role for IL-1β in the T cell independent mechanism of resistance against intracellular pathogens. *J. Immunol.* 155:4347–4354.

Hunter, C. A., L. Ellis-Neyer, K. Gabriel, M. Kennedy, P. Linsley, and J. S. Remington. 1997. The role of the CD28/B7 interaction in the regulation of NK cell responses during infection with *Toxoplasma gondii*. *J. Immunol.* 158:2285–2293.

Ilg, T. 2000. Lipophosphoglycan is not required for infection of macrophages or mice by *Leishmania mexicana*. *EMBO J.* 19:1953–1962.

Jack, R. M., and P. A. Ward. 1980. *Babesia rodhaini* interactions with complement: relationship to parasitic entry into red cells. *J. Immunol.* 124:1566–1573.

Joiner, K. A., W. D. daSilva, M. T. Rimoldi, C. H. Hammer, A. Sher, and T. L. Kipnis. 1988. Biochemical characterization of a factor produced by trypomastigotes of *Trypanosoma cruzi* that accelerates the decay of complement C3 convertases. *J. Biol. Chem.* 263:11327–11335.

Joiner, K. A., S. A. Fuhrman, H. M. Miettinen, L. H. Kasper, and I. Mellman. 1990. *Toxoplasma gondii*: fusion competence of parasitophorous vacuoles in Fc receptor-transfected fibroblasts. *Science* 249:641–646.

Jones, D., M. M. Elloso, L. Showe, D. Williams, G. Trinchieri, and P. Scott. 1998. Differential regulation of the interleukin-12 receptor during the innate immune response to *Leishmania major*. *Infect. Immun.* 66:3818–3824.

Kasper, L. H., T. Matsuura, S. Fonseka, J. Arruda, J. Y. Channon, and I. A. Khan. 1996. Induction of γδ T cells during acute murine infection with *Toxoplasma gondii*. *J. Immunol.* 157:5521–5527.

Kaye, P. M., and G. J. Bancroft. 1992. *Leishmania donovani* infection in scid mice: lack of tissue response and in vivo macrophage activation correlates with failure to trigger natural killer cell-derived gamma interferon production in vitro. *Infect. Immun.* 60:4335–4342.

Kaye, P. M., N. J. Rogers, A. J. Curry, and J. C. Scott. 1994. Deficient expression of co-stimulatory molecules on *Leishmania*-infected macrophages. *Eur. J. Immunol.* 24:2850–2854.

Khan, I. A., J. A. MacLean, F. S. Lee, L. Casciotti, E. DeHaan, J. D. Schwartzman, and A. D. Luster. 2000. IP-10 is critical for effector T cell trafficking and host survival in *Toxoplasma gondii* infection. *Immunity* 12:483–494.

Kopacz, J., and N. Kumar. 1999. Murine gd T lymphocytes elicited during *Plasmodium yoelii* infection respond to *Plasmodium* heat shock proteins. *Infect. Immun.* 67:57–63.

Kweider, M., J. L. Lemesre, F. Santoro, J. P. Kusnierz, M. Sadigursky, and A. Capron. 1989. Development of metacyclic *Leishmania* promastigotes is associated with the increasing expression of GP65, the major surface antigen. *Parasite Immunol.* **11:**197–209.

Launois, P., I. Maillard, S. Pingel, K. G. Swihart, I. Xenarios, H. Acha-Orbea, H. Diggelmann, R. M. Locksley, H. R. MacDonald, and J. A. Louis. 1997. IL-4 rapidly produced by Vβ4 Vα8 CD4⁺ T cells instructs Th2 development and susceptibility to *Leishmania major* in BALB/c mice. *Immunity* **6:**541–549.

Lopez-Osuna, M., J. Arellano, and R. R. Kretschmer. 1992. The destruction of virulent *Entamoeba histolytica* by activated human eosinophils. *Parasite Immunol.* **14:**579–586.

Magez, S., M. Geuskens, A. Beschin, H. del Favero, H. Verschueren, R. Lucas, E. Pays, and P. de Baetselier. 1997. Specific uptake of tumor necrosis factor-alpha is involved in growth control of *Trypanosoma brucei*. *J. Cell Biol.* **137:**715–727.

Magez, S., B. Stijlemans, M. Radwanska, E. Pays, M. A. Ferguson, and P. De Baetselier. 1998. The glycosyl-inositol-phosphate and dimyristoylglycerol moieties of the glycosylphosphatidylinositol anchor of the trypanosome variant-specific surface glycoprotein are distinct macrophage-activating factors. *J. Immunol.* **160:**1949–1956.

Marone, G., V. Casolaro, V. Patella, G. Florio, and M. Triggiani. 1997. Molecular and cellular biology of mast cells and basophils. *Int. Arch. Allergy Immunol.* **114:**207–217.

Matthews, D. J., C. L. Emson, G. J. McKenzie, H. E. Jolin, J. M. Blackwell, and A. N. McKenzie. 2000. IL-13 is a susceptibility factor for *Leishmania major* infection. *J. Immunol.* **164:**1458–1462.

Matzinger, P. 1998. An innate sense of danger. *Semin. Immunol.* **10:**399–415.

McDonald, V., R. Deer, S. Uni, M. Iseki, and G. J. Bancroft. 1992. Immune responses to *Cryptosporidium muris* and *Cryposporidium parvum* in adult immunocompromised (nude and SCID) mice. *Infect. Immun.* **60:**3325–3331.

Medzhitov, R., P. Preston-Hurlburt, and C. A. Janeway. 1997. A human homologue of the *Drosophila* Toll protein signals activation of adaptive immunity. *Nature* **388:**394–397.

Mohan, K., P. Moulin, and M. M. Stevenson. 1997. Natural killer cell cytokine production, not cytotoxicity, contributes to resistance against blood-stage *Plasmodium chabaudi* AS infection. *J. Immunol.* **159:**4990–4998.

Molano, A., S. H. Park, Y. H. Chiu, S. Nosseir, A. Bendelac, and M. Tsuji. 2000. The IgG response to the circumsporozoite protein is MHC class II-dependent and CD1d-independent: exploring the role of GPIs in NK T cell activation and antimalarial responses. *J. Immunol.* **164:**5005–5009.

Moore, K. W., A. O'Garra, R. de Waal Malefyt, P. Vieira, and T. R. Mossman. 1993. Interleukin 10. *Annu. Rev. Immunol.* **11:**165–190.

Mosser, D. M., and A. Brittingham. 1997. Leishmania, macrophages and complement: a tale of subversion and exploitation. *Parasitology* **115:**S9–S23.

Mosser, D. M., and P. J. Edelson. 1984. Activation of the alternative complement pathway by *Leishmania* promastigotes: parasite lysis and attachment to macrophages. *J. Immunol.* **132:**1501–1505.

Mosser, D. M., and P. J. Edelson. 1985. The mouse macrophage receptor for C3bi (CR3) is a major mechanism in the phagocytosis of *Leishmania* promastigotes. *J. Immunol.* **135:**2785–2789.

Mosser, D. M., and P. J. Edelson. 1987. The third component of complement (C3) is responsible for the intracellular survival of *Leishmania major*. *Nature* **327:**329–331.

Noben-Trauth, N., W. E. Paul, and D. L. Sacks. 1999. IL-4- and IL-4 receptor-deficient BALB/c mice reveal differences in susceptibility to *Leishmania major* parasite substrains. *J. Immunol.* **162:**6132–6140.

Norris, K. A. 1998. Stable transfection of *Trypanosoma cruzi* epimastigotes with the trypomastigote-specific complement regulatory protein cDNA confers complement resistance. *Infect. Immun.* **66:**2460–2465.

Norris, K. A., B. Bradt, N. R. Cooper, and M. So. 1991. Characterization of a *Trypanosoma cruzi* C3 binding protein with functional and genetic similarities to the human complement regulatory protein, decay-accelerating factor. *J. Immunol.* **147:**2240–2247.

Norris, K. A., and J. E. Schrimpf. 1994. Biochemical analysis of the membrane and soluble forms of the complement regulatory protein of *Trypanosoma cruzi*. *Infect. Immun.* **62:**236–243.

Ohkusu, K., T. Yoshimoto, K. Takeda, T. Ogura, S. Kashiwamura, Y. Iwakura, S. Akira, H. Okamura, and K. Nakanishi. 2000. Potentiality of interleukin-18 as a useful reagent for treatment and prevention of *Leishmania major* infection. *Infect. Immun.* **68:**2449–2456.

Okamura, H., H. Tsutsui, T. Komatsu, M. Yutsudo, A. Hakura, T. Tanimoto, K. Torigoe, T. Okura, Y. Nukada, K. Hattori, K. Akita, M. Namba, F. Tanabe, K. Konishi, S. Fukuda, and M. Kurimoto. 1995. Cloning of a new cytokine that induces IFN-γ production by T cells. *Nature* **378:**88–91.

Paciorkowski, N., P. Porte, L. D. Shultz, and T. V. Rajan. 2000. B1 B lymphocytes play a critical role in host protection against lymphatic filarial parasites. *J. Exp. Med.* **191:**731–736.

Pearce, E. J., B. F. Hall, and A. Sher. 1990. Host-specific evasion of the alternative complement pathway by schistosomes correlates with the presence of a phospholipase C-sensitive surface molecule resembling human decay accelerating factor. *J. Immunol.* **144:**2751–2756.

Peck, C. A., M. D. Carpenter, and A. A. Mahmoud. 1983. Species-related innate resistance to *Schistosoma mansoni*. Role of mononuclear phagocytes in schistosomula killing in vitro. *J. Clin. Investig.* **71:**66–72.

Pernis, A., S. Gupta, K. J. Gollob, E. Garfein, R. L. Coffman, C. Schindler, and P. Rothman. 1995. Lack of interferon γ receptor β chain and the prevention of interferon γ signalling in TH1 cells. *Science* **269:**245–247.

Plaut, M., J. H. Pierce, C. J. Watson, J. Hanley-Hyde, R. P. Nordan, and W. E. Paul. 1989. Mast cell lines produce lymphokines in response to cross-linkage of FcεRI or to calcium ionophores. *Nature* **339:**64–67.

Proudfoot, L., C. A. O'Donnell, and F. Y. Liew. 1995. Glyco-inositolphospholipids of *Leishmania major* inhibit nitric oxide synthesis and reduce leishmanicidal activity in murine macrophages. *Eur. J. Immunol.* **25:**745–750.

Puentes, S. M., R. P. Da Silva, D. L. Sacks, C. H. Hammer, and K. A. Joiner. 1990. Serum resistance of metacyclic stage *Leishmania major* promastigotes is due to release of C5b-9. *J. Immunol.* **145:**4311–4316.

Raper, J., R. Fung, J. Ghiso, V. Nussenzweig, and S. Tomlinson. 1999. Characterization of a novel trypanosome lytic factor from human serum. *Infect. Immun.* **67:**1910–1916.

Reed, S. L., J. A. Ember, D. S. Herdman, R. G. DiScipio, T. E. Hugli, and I. Gigli. 1995. The extracellular neutral cysteine proteinase of *Entamoeba histolytica* degrades anaphylatoxins C3a and C5a. *J. Immunol.* **155:**266–274.

Reiner, S. L., and R. A. Seder. 1999. Dealing from the evolutionary pawnshop: how lymphocytes make decisions. *Immunity* **11:**1–10.

Reiner, S. L., S. Zheng, Z. E. Wang, L. Stowring, and R. M. Locksley. 1994. Leishmania promastigotes evade interleukin 12 induction by macrophages and stimulate a broad range of cytokines from CD4⁺ T cells during initiation of infection. *J. Exp. Med.* **179:**447–456.

Reis e Sousa, B. C., S. Hieny, T. Scharton-Kersten, D. Jankovic, H. Charset, R. N. Germain, and A. Sher. 1997. In vivo microbial stimulation induces rapid CD40 ligand-independent production of interleukin 12 by dendritic cells and their redistribution to T cell areas. *J. Exp. Med.* 186:1819–1829.

Rifkin, M. R. 1978. Identification of the trypanocidal factor in normal human serum: high density lipoprotein. *Proc. Natl. Acad. Sci. USA* 75:3450–3454.

Rimoldi, M. T., A. Sher, S. Heiny, A. Lituchy, C. H. Hammer, and K. Joiner. 1988. Developmentally regulated expression by *Trypanosoma cruzi* of molecules that accelerate the decay of complement C3 convertases. *Proc. Natl. Acad. Sci. USA* 85:193–197.

Rosat, J.-P., F. Conceicao-Silva, G. A. Waanders, F. Beermann, A. Wilson, M. J. Owen, A. C. Hayday, S. Huang, M. Aguet, H. R. MacDonald, and J. A. Louis. 1995. Expansion of $\gamma\delta^+$ T cells in BALB/c mice infected with *Leishmania major* is dependent upon Th2-type CD4$^+$ T cells. *Infect. Immun.* 63:3000–3004.

Roussilhon, C., M. Agrapart, J. J. Ballet, and A. Bensussan. 1990. T lymphocytes bearing the $\gamma\delta$ T cell receptor in patients with acute *Plasmodium falciparum* malaria. *J. Infect. Dis.* 162:283–285.

Sabin, E. A., M. A. Kopf, and E. J. Pearce. 1996. *Schistosoma mansoni* egg-induced early IL-4 production is dependent upon IL-5 and eosinophils. *J. Exp. Med.* 184:1871–1878.

Saraiva, E. M., P. F. Pimenta, T. N. Brodin, E. Rowton, G. B. Modi, and D. L. Sacks. 1995. Changes in lipophosphoglycan and gene expression associated with the development of *Leishmania major* in *Phlebotomus papatasi*. *Parasitology* 111:275–287.

Sayles, P. C., and L. L. Johnson. 1996. Exacerbation of toxoplasmosis in neutrophil-depleted mice. *Nat. Immun.* 15:249–258.

Scalise, F., R. Gerli, G. Castellucci, F. Spinozzi, G. M. Fabietti, S. Crupi, L. Sensi, R. Britta, R. Vaccaro, and A. Bertotto. 1992. Lymphocytes bearing the $\gamma\delta$ T-cell receptor in acute toxoplasmosis. *Immunology* 76:668–670.

Scharton, T. M., and P. Scott. 1993. Natural killer cells are a source of interferon γ that drives differentiation of CD4$^+$ T cell subsets and induces early resistance to *Leishmania major* in mice. *J. Exp. Med.* 178:567–577.

Scharton-Kersten, T., C. Contursi, A. Masumi, A. Sher, and K. Ozato. 1997. Interferon consensus sequence binding protein-deficient mice display impaired resistance to intracellular infection due to a primary defect in interleukin 12 p40 induction. *J. Exp. Med.* 186:1523–1534.

Schofield, L., and F. Hackett. 1993. Signal transduction in host cells by a glycosylphosphatidylinositol toxin of malaria parasites. *J. Exp. Med.* 177:145–153.

Schofield, L., M. J. McConville, D. Hansen, A. S. Campbell, B. Fraser-Reid, M. J. Grusby, and S. D. Tachado. 1999. CD1d-restricted immunoglobulin G formation to GPI-anchored antigens mediated by NKT cells. *Science* 283:225–229.

Sedegah, M., F. Finkelman, and S. L. Hoffman. 1994. Interleukin 12 induction of interferon γ-dependent protection against malaria. *Proc. Natl. Acad. Sci. USA* 91:10700–10702.

Seder, R. A., W. E. Paul, A. M. Dvorak, S. J. Sharkis, A. Kagey-Sobotka, Y. Niv, F. D. Finkelman, S. A. Barbieri, S. J. Galli, and M. Plaut. 1991. Mouse splenic and bone marrow cell populations that express high-affinity Fce receptors and produce interleukin 4 are highly enriched in basophils. *Proc. Natl. Acad. Sci. USA* 88:2835–2839.

Seydel, K. B., S. J. Smith, and S. L. Stanley, Jr. 2000. Innate immunity to amebic liver abscess is dependent on gamma interferon and nitric oxide in a murine model of disease. *Infect. Immun.* 68:400–402.

Sharma, S. D., J. Verhoef, and J. S. Remington. 1986. Enhancement of human natural killer cell activity by subcellular components of *Toxoplasma gondii*. *Cell. Immunol.* 86:317–326.

Sher, A., I. P. Oswald, S. Hieny, and R. Gazzinelli. 1993. *Toxoplasma gondii* induces a T-independent IFN-γ response in natural killer cells that requires both adherent accessory cells and tumor necrosis factor-α. *J. Immunol.* 150:3982–3989.

Sibley, L. D., E. Weidner, and J. L. Krahenbuhl. 1985. Phagosome acidification blocked by intracellular *Toxoplasma gondii*. *Nature* 315:416–419.

Smith, A. B., J. D. Esko, and S. L. Hajduk. 1995. Killing of trypanosomes by the human haptoglobin-related protein. *Science* 268:284–286.

Spath, G. F., L. Epstein, B. Leader, S. M. Singer, H. A. Avila, S. J. Turco, and S. M. Beverley. 2000. Lipophosphoglycan is a virulence factor distinct from related glycoconjugates in the protozoan parasite *Leishmania major*. *Proc. Natl. Acad. Sci. USA* 97:9258–9263.

Subauste, C. S., J. Y. Chung, D. Do, A. H. Koniaris, C. A. Hunter, J. G. Montoya, S. Porcelli, and J. S. Remington. 1995. Preferential activation and expansion of human peripheral blood $\gamma\delta$ T cells in response to *Toxoplasma gondii* in vitro and their cytokine production and cytotoxic activity against *T. gondii*-infected cells. *J. Clin. Investig.* 96:610–619.

Svetic, A., K. B. Madden, X. D. Zhou, P. Lu, I. M. Katona, F. D. Finkelman, J. F. Urban, Jr., and W. C. Gause. 1993. A primary intestinal helminthic infection rapidly induces a gut-associated elevation of Th2-associated cytokines and IL-3. *J. Immunol.* 150:3434–3441.

Sypek, J. P., C. L. Chung, S. E. H. Mayor, J. M. Subramanyam, S. J. Goldman, D. S. Sieburth, S. F. Wolf, and R. G. Schaub. 1993. Resolution of cutaneous leishmaniasis: Interleukin 12 initiates a protective T helper type I immune response. *J. Exp. Med.* 177:1797–1802.

Tachado, S. D., R. Mazhari-Tabrizi, and L. Schofield. 1999. Specificity in signal transduction among glycosylphosphatidylinositols of *Plasmodium falciparum*, *Trypanosoma brucei*, *Trypanosoma cruzi* and *Leishmania* spp. *Parasite Immunol.* 21:609–617.

Takamoto, M., Y. Kusama, K. Takatsu, H. Nariuchi, and K. Sugane. 1995. Occurrence of interleukin-5 production by CD4$^-$ CD8$^-$ (double-negative) T cells in lungs of both normal and congenitally athymic nude mice infected with *Toxocara canis*. *Immunology* 85:285–291.

Tomlinson, S., and J. Raper. 1998. Natural immunity to trypanosomes. *Parasitol. Today* 14:354–359.

Tsuji, M., P. Mombaerts, L. Lefrancois, R. S. Nussenzweig, F. Zavala, and S. Tonegawa. 1994. $\gamma\delta$ T cells contribute to immunity against the liver stages of malaria in $\alpha\beta$ T cell deficient mice. *Proc. Natl. Acad. Sci. USA* 91:345–349.

Urban, J. F., R. Fayer, S.-J. Chen, W. C. Gause, M. K. Gately, and F. D. Finkelman. 1996. IL-12 protects immunocompetent and immunodeficient neonatal mice against infection with *Cryptosporidium parvum*. *J. Immunol.* 156:263–268.

Urban, J. F., N. Noben-Trauth, D. D. Donaldson, K. B. Madden, S. C. Morris, M. Collins, and F. D. Finkelman. 1998. IL-13, IL-4Rα, and STAT6 are required for the expulsion of the gastrointestinal nematode parasite *Nippostrongylus brasiliensis*. *Immunity* 8:255–264.

Velupillai, P., and D. A. Harn. 1994. Oligosaccharide-specific induction of interleukin 10 production by B220$^+$ cells from schistosome-infected mice: a mechanism for regulation of CD4$^+$ T-cell subsets. *Proc. Natl. Acad. Sci. USA* 91:18–22.

von Stebut, E., Y. Belkaid, T. Jakob, D. L. Sacks, and M. C. Udey. 1998. Uptake of *Leishmania major* amastigotes results in activation and interleukin 12 release from murine skin-derived dendritic cells: implications for the initiation of anti-*Leishmania* immunity. *J. Exp. Med.* **188:**1547–1552.

Wakil, A. E., Z. E. Wang, J. C. Ryan, D. J. Fowell, and R. M. Locksley. 1998. Interferon γ derived from CD4$^+$ T cells is sufficient to mediate T helper cell type 1 development. *J. Exp. Med.* **188:**1651–1656.

Walker, C., J. Checkel, S. Cammisuli, P. J. Leibson, and G. J. Gleich. 1998. IL-5 production by NK cells contributes to eosinophil infiltration in a mouse model of allergic inflammation. *J. Immunol.* **161:**1962–1969.

Warren, H. S., B. F. Kinnear, J. H. Phillips, and L. Lanier. 1995. Production of IL-5 by human NK cells and regulation of IL-5 secretion by IL-4, IL-10, and IL-12. *J. Immunol.* **154:**5144–5152.

Wei, X. Q., B. P. Leung, W. Niedbala, D. Piedrafita, G. F. Feng, M. Sweet, L. Dobbie, A. J. Smith, and F. Y. Liew. 1999. Altered immune responses and susceptibility to *Leishmania major* and *Staphylococcus aureus* infection in IL-18-deficient mice. *J. Immunol.* **163:**2821–2828.

Wynn, T. A., A. W. Cheever, D. Jankovic, R. W. Poindexter, P. Caspar, F. A. Lewis, and A. Sher. 1995. An IL-12 based vaccination method for preventing fibrosis induced by schistosome infection. *Nature* **376:**594–596.

Xong, H. V., L. Vanhamme, M. Chamekh, C. E. Chimfwembe, J. Van Den Abbeele, A. Pays, N. Van Meirvenne, R. Hamers, P. De Baetselier, and E. Pays. 1998. A VSG expression site-associated gene confers resistance to human serum in *Trypanosoma rhodesiense*. *Cell* **95:**839–846.

Yoshimoto, T., and W. E. Paul. 1994. CD4$^+$, NK1.1$^+$ T cells promptly produce interleukin 4 in response to in vivo challenge with anti-CD3. *J. Exp. Med.* **179:**1285–1295.

Immunology of Infectious Diseases
Edited by S. H. E. Kaufmann, A. Sher, and R. Ahmed
© 2002 ASM Press, Washington, D.C.

Chapter 10

Innate Immunity and Fungal Infections

AMY C. HERRING AND GARY B. HUFFNAGLE

Innate immunity is central to host defense against fungi. For many types of fungal infections, innate immunity is solely responsible for host defense. However, even for fungal infections that require an adaptive immune response for clearance, innate immunity plays a key role in the effective development of adaptive immunity.

The innate immune system employs broad, non-specific mechanisms to either completely destroy a microbial pathogen or contain the infection until an adaptive immune response is generated. Macrophages, neutrophils, and monocytes (i.e., phagocytic cells) are essential for resistance to fungal infections (Table 1). NK cells, mast cells, and $\gamma\delta$ T cells are also important; however, their relative contribution is determined largely by the type of fungal insult. Nonhematopoietic cells such as epithelial and endothelial cells also participate in innate immune surveillance against fungal infection. Many of the classic mechanisms of an innate response are utilized against fungi; these include (i) opsonization and phagocytosis by complement and pattern recognition receptors, (ii) induction of oxygen-dependent and -independent fungicidal activity, and (iii) production of proinflammatory mediators. The production of early cytokines by innate cells is a key aspect of the host response to fungal infection. These mediators play a critical role in activating phagocytes and orchestrating the development of adaptive immunity to fungi (Fig. 1). Thus, innate immunity is an integral part of host defense against all fungal infections.

INNATE IMMUNITY AS THE FIRST LINE OF DEFENSE

Several broad effector mechanisms are induced early to combat a fungal infection. Complement, mannose binding protein (MBP), and surfactant proteins promote initial recognition (opsonization) of fungi. Subsequent binding and phagocytosis of fungi are mediated by both complement receptors and pattern recognition receptors (PRRs) expressed on the surface of phagocytes and nonphagocytic cells. The binding of fungi is accompanied by the activation of oxygen-dependent and -independent killing mechanisms in addition to proinflammatory signal generation.

The complement pathways are an essential part of the innate response to fungi. Several experimental models have shown that mice deficient in C3 or C5 components exhibit decreased resistance to *Cryptococcus neoformans*, *Candida albicans*, *Aspergillus fumigatus*, and *Paracoccidioides brasiliensis* (reviewed by Kozel [1998]). The presence of fungi rapidly triggers the activation of the alternate complement pathway, resulting in deposition of large amounts of C3b on the pathogen surface. *C. neoformans* is a potent activator of the alternate pathway, and C3 binds extensively to the capsule of *Cryptococcus* (reviewed by Kozel [1998]). *C. albicans* also activates complement, leading to the rapid deposition of C3b on the surface of this yeast (reviewed by Kozel [1998]). This process serves to opsonize fungi for recognition by phagocytic cells.

Opsonization can also be mediated by MBP via recognition and binding to complex carbohydrates (e.g., D-mannose and N-acetylglucosamine) on fungal surfaces. Several studies suggest the participation of MBP in the innate response to fungi. For example, levels of MBP in serum are significantly decreased 1 h following intravenous infection with *C. albicans* (Tabona et al., 1995). MBP binds only to acapsular strains of *C. neoformans* (Schelenz et al., 1995) and was recently shown to bind strongly to several *Can-*

Amy C. Herring and Gary B. Huffnagle • Pulmonary Division, Department of Internal Medicine, University of Michigan Medical Center, Ann Arbor, MI 48109.

Table 1. Cells of the innate and adaptive immune response that are sources of signal molecules

Primary innate cells[a]	Other innate cells[b]	Adaptive cells[c]
Monocytes/macrophages	Epithelial cells	$\alpha\beta$ T cells
Neutrophils	Fibroblasts	$\gamma\delta$ T cells
Eosinophils	Endothelial cells	B cells
Mast cells	Muscle cells	
NK cells	Neural cells	
$\gamma\delta$ T cells		

[a] Cells that cannot modify their antigen receptors.
[b] Cells that possess few or no antigen receptors.
[c] Cells that can modify their antigen receptors.

dida species and *A. fumigatus* (Neth et al., 2000). These findings suggest a role for MBP during fungal infection, and it is likely that MBP is involved in the early recognition of other fungal pathogens. In addition to functioning as an opsonin, MBP activates components of the complement cascade (Kawasaki, 1999) and presumably amplifies the opsonization and recognition of fungi.

During pulmonary infections, surfactant proteins may also opsonize fungi and participate in host defense. Surfactant proteins A (SP-A) and D (SP-D) interact with a variety of respiratory pathogens including *C. neoformans, A. fumigatus,* and *Pneumocystis carinii.* SP-A and SP-D bind to *Aspergillus* and *Pneumocystis* and increase their phagocytosis by macrophages (Madan et al., 1997; O'Riordan et al., 1995a). Similarly, SP-D can bind to acapsular forms of *C. neoformans* (Schelenz et al., 1995). These observations suggest that surfactant proteins contribute to pulmonary defense mechanisms by opsonizing and enhancing clearance of respiratory fungal pathogens.

The phagocytosis of fungi is mediated by both complement receptors and PRRs expressed on the surface of phagocytes. Complement receptors 1, 3, and 4 (CR1, CR3, and CR4) can mediate the uptake of opsonized *Cryptococcus* (Casadevall and Perfect, 1998). The presence of CR3 is important for resistance to cryptococcal infection. Administration of anti-CR3 antibody during infection resulted in significant mortality (Cross et al., 1997). Phagocytosis can also occur in the absence of opsonization and is mediated primarily by PRRs that recognize invariant

microbial constituents. The mannose and β-glucan receptors are two PRRs that are potentially involved in the phagocytosis of fungi by recognizing mannan/mannoproteins and glucan, respectively, on the fungal surface. Mannan and glucan are major components of the *Candida* cell wall, and mannose receptors are important for phagocytosis of several *Candida* species (Vazquez-Torres and Balish, 1997). The involvement of mannose and β-glucan receptors in the phagocytosis of acapsular *C. neoformans* in vitro has been described (Cross and Bancroft, 1995). The mannose receptor also interacts with glycoprotein A of *Pneumocystis,* facilitating uptake by macrophages (O'Riordan et al., 1995b). The contribution of glucan receptors in the phagocytosis of *C. albicans* and other fungi is not well characterized. Toll receptors are also members of the PRR family and play an essential role in the innate recognition of microorganisms. The specific involvement of mammalian Toll-like receptors (TLRs) in host defense against fungi has yet to be established; however, recent evidence demonstrates a preference of TLR2 for phagosomes containing yeast (Underhill et al., 1999). Future studies will continue to elucidate the role of specific TLRs in innate responses to fungi.

The activation of oxygen-dependent (i.e., NO, reactive oxygen intermediates, reactive nitrogen intermediates, and peroxynitrite) and oxygen-independent (i.e., cationic proteins, lysozyme, defensins, arachidonic acid metabolites, and myeloperoxidase) killing mechanisms has been detected during fungal infections. Both effector mechanisms can be utilized by macrophages and neutrophils; however, the importance of these cells is dependent on the nature of the infection. Neutrophils are essential for resistance to *Aspergillus* infection, while macrophages play a supporting role. In contrast, macrophages are key in *Cryptococcus, Coccidioides, Histoplasma,* and *Blastomyces* infections whereas neutrophils play a secondary role. Neutrophils and macrophages are both essential for host defense against *Candida* and *Paracoccidioides.* The

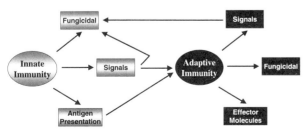

Figure 1. Functions and interplay of innate and adaptive immunity.

involvement of reactive oxygen and nitrogen intermediates has been described for several fungal infection models including *C. neoformans* and *C. albicans*. NO and reactive nitrogen intermediates are toxic to *Cryptococcus* (Casadevall and Perfect, 1998). Alveolar macrophages produce NO in response to *C. neoformans* or *A. fumigatus* (Gross et al., 1999). Peroxynitrite is also an important molecule involved in killing fungal pathogens. Small antimicrobial proteins such as defensins, lactoferrin, and calprotectin are released from phagocytic cells to aid in the killing of fungi. Mice deficient in myeloperoxidase showed increased susceptibility following infection with *C. albicans* (Aratani et al., 1999). Productive destruction of fungal pathogens involves the cooperation of both oxygen-dependent and oxygen-independent fungicidal mechanisms. In addition to reactive intermediates and reactive proteins, activated macrophages and neutrophils release several proinflammatory mediators. The role of these early signals during fungal infections will be discussed in detail below.

Although phagocytes are central to the elimination of fungi, other cells of the innate immune system can contribute to this process. NK cells serve two main functions: (i) the direct killing or growth inhibition of a pathogen and (ii) the production of cytokines (e.g., gamma interferon [IFN-γ], and tumor necrosis factor alpha [TNF-α]) to activate phagocytic responses. In general, NK cells play a supporting role during the course of a fungal infection. NK cells can exert direct effects on *C. neoformans* by inhibiting its growth; therefore, NK cells may be involved in host protection from *Cryptococcus* (Casadevall and Perfect, 1998). Depletion of NK cells during *C. neoformans* infection in the intravenous model enhances early counts of fungi in the lungs (Salkowski and Balish, 1991). With respect to *C. albicans*, NK cells do not appear to be essential for controlling infection. Studies performed with SCID mice report no difference in survival, and NK-cell depletion fails to increase the susceptibility to *Candida* (Greenfield et al., 1993; Romani et al., 1993). NK-cell activity is increased during *Coccidioides* but not *Aspergillus* infection (Petkus, 1987; Roilides et al., 1998b).

The spectrum of participation of γδ T cells in host defense against fungal infections is not well defined. However, γδ T cells play a role in resistance to mucosal *Candida* infection. Specifically, depletion of γδ T cells results in increased susceptibility to *C. albicans* infection. An expansion of γδ T cells occurred at 72 h postinfection, and these cells produce IFN-γ which enhances the anticandidal activity of macrophages (Jones-Carson et al., 1995). These findings suggest a role for γδ T cells in the early phase of immunity to *C. albicans*. Future studies are needed to elucidate the specific involvement of γδ T cells during other fungal infections.

THE LINK BETWEEN INNATE IMMUNITY AND ADAPTIVE IMMUNITY

The cells of the innate immune system possess many immunoregulatory functions, along with potent antifungal effector mechanisms that can be activated by adaptive immunity. There are a number of points in host defense at which there is a link between innate and adaptive immunity: (i) early signal generation, (ii) antigen presentation, and (iii) effector cell activity. These are discussed in detail below. Thus, even for fungal infections that require an adaptive immune response for clearance, innate immunity plays a key role in the effective development of adaptive immunity.

Early Signal Generation

The cells of the innate immune system rapidly release cytokines in response to fungal products and binding of opsonized fungi. The phagocytic cells are important sources of TNF-α, interleukin-12 (IL-12), macrophage inflammatory protein 1α (MIP-1α), and IL-1 whereas NK cells and γδ T cells can synthesize IFN-γ. Epithelial cells and other structural cells are major sources of monocyte chemotactic protein 1 (MCP-1). These early signals from innate immunity (i) result in cellular activation and maturation, (ii) result in cellular migration and recruitment, and (iii) upregulate adhesion molecule expression. Together, these signals focus the innate and adaptive responses to the site of infection and enhance the fungicidal activity of the recruited leukocytes (Table 2, Fig. 2).

TNF-α, IL-12, IL-18, and IFN-γ

TNF-α, IL-12, IL-18, and IFN-γ strongly promote the development of Th1-type antifungal re-

Table 2. Effect of signals from innate immunity on the development of adaptive immunity

Th1 response	Th2 response
IL-18	IL-4
IL-12	IL-10
IFN-γ	IL-6
TNF-α	PGE$_2$[a]
IL-1	IL-1
MCP-1	MCP-1
MIP-1α	

[a] PGE$_2$, prostaglandin E$_2$.

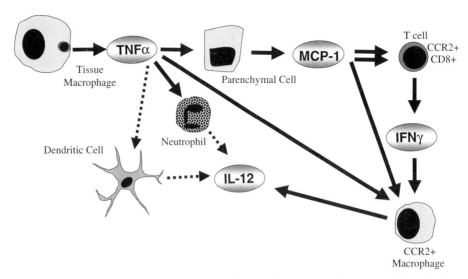

Figure 2. Cytokine networks in the innate response to *C. neoformans* that promote adaptive T1-cell-mediated immunity. This is a working model of early signal generation in response to pulmonary *C. neoformans* infection. The solid arrows represent information proven experimentally, whereas the dashed arrows represent hypothesized interactions. IL-18, IL-1, and MIP-1α, which also drive Th1 responses to *Cryptococcus,* are not included here.

sponses and are therefore essential for resistance to a variety of fungi including *C. neoformans* and *C. albicans.*

TNF-α is an early-response cytokine, and several lines of evidence demonstrate a critical role for TNF-α during fungal infections. The production of TNF-α during pulmonary cryptococcosis is essential for resistance to *C. neoformans*. TNF-α is induced early in the course of a *C. neoformans* infection and precedes the inflammatory response in infected mice (Huffnagle et al., 1996). Intraperitoneal administration of TNF-α also increased the survival rate of animals infected with a highly virulent strain of *Cryptococcus* (Kawakami et al., 1996a). In contrast, neutralization of TNF-α at the time of *C. neoformans* infection permanently skews the immune response and alters the production of subsequent innate signals. Administration of anti-TNF-α monoclonal antibody on day 0 results in significant reduction of IL-12, IFN-γ, and MCP-1 production at week 1 postinfection (A. C. Herring, unpublished observation). TNF-α neutralization on day 0 also causes a shift from a Th1-type immune response to a Th2-like response in the lungs of infected mice. Anti-TNF-α-treated mice fail to generate a delayed-type hypersensitivity response to *C. neoformans* antigen and exhibit elevated IL-5 production and pulmonary eosinophilia (J. L. Lee, G. B. Toews, R. McDonald, A. C. Herring, and G. B. Huffnagle, submitted for publication).

A similar role for TNF-α has been described in other fungal infection models. Mice deficient in both TNF-α and lymphotoxin develop a Th2 response to

C. albicans infection and have high levels of IL-4 and IL-10 (Mencacci et al., 1998a). The survival of these TNF/LT$^{-/-}$ animals was also significantly decreased and correlated with elevated fungal counts in organs (Netea et al., 1999). In addition, neutralization of TNF-α impairs resistance to *A. fumigatus* (Mehrad et al., 1999b), *Histoplasma capsulatum* (Allendoerfer and Deepe, 1998), and *P. carinii* (Chen et al., 1992). TNF-α can also be induced from cultured macrophages in the presence of *A. fumigatus* (Taramelli et al., 1996). Taken together, these findings strongly suggest that TNF-α is a critical proximal mediator and is important for establishing host resistance to a variety of fungal pathogens.

The importance of IL-12 in the early phase of fungal infections has been well characterized using *C. albicans*. In a murine model of systemic candidiasis, induction of IL-12 RNA expression was detected in resistant mice but was undetectable in susceptible mice (Romani et al., 1994b). Furthermore, neutralization of IL-12 in the resistant animals resulted in a progressive, nonhealing infection and a shift to a Th2-type response (Romani et al., 1994a). These findings suggested that the early production of IL-12 plays a critical role in the development of protective Th1 immunity to *Candida*. Interestingly, neutrophils are an essential source of early IL-12 during an infection with *C. albicans*. Neutrophil depletion at the time of infection renders mice susceptible to *C. albicans* and induces a Th2 cytokine profile (Romani et al., 1997). Several studies have also described an essential role for IL-12 in establishing resistance to *C. neoformans* infection. *C. neoformans* can induce significant IL-12 production (Herring, unpublished; Pitzurra et al., 2000). Administration of IL-12 during the first week of a cryptococcal infection increased long-term survival and prevented dissemination to the brain (Kawakami et al., 1996c). Conversely, anti-IL-12 treatment inhibited pulmonary clearance and caused a switch from Th1 to Th2 immunity (Hoag et al., 1997). IL-12 p35 or p40 knockout mice also exhibited Th2 polarization in response to *Cryptococcus* (Decken et al., 1998). The induction of IL-12 appears to be important during *H. capsulatum* infection because IL-12 RNA is detected on day 3 post-infection (Cain and Deepe, 1998) and IL-12 neutralization increased the mortality due to *Histoplasma* infection (Zhou et al., 1995). Thus, early production of IL-12 is critical for the initiation of protective Th1 immunity to fungi.

The production of IFN-γ is essential for protection against fungi. IFN-γ is a potent activator of fungicidal activity for cells of the innate immune system. However, IFN-γ also drives Th1 responses to fungal infections. In experimental models of IFN-γ deficiency, diminished IFN-γ levels result in a switch from protective Th1 to nonprotective Th2 responses. For example, neutralization of IL-12 in a variety of fungal infection models results in significant reduction of IFN-γ production (Cenci et al., 1998; Decken et al., 1998; Kawakami et al., 1996b; Zhou et al., 1995). TNF-α neutralization also inhibits early IFN-γ production in the lungs of *C. neoformans*-infected mice (Herring, unpublished). The importance of IFN-γ in resistance to fungal infection has been strengthened further by studies performed in knockout animals. Mice deficient in IFN-γ display increased organ burden and enhanced susceptibility to both *C. albicans* and *H. capsulatum* (Allendoerfer and Deepe, 1997; Balish et al., 1998; Kaposzta et al., 1998; Lavigne et al., 1998). A similar increase in mortality due to *Cryptococcus* and *Aspergillus* infection has been demonstrated using anti-IFN-γ antibody (Kawakami et al., 1996b; Nagai et al., 1995). IFN-γ receptor knockout mice develop a Th2 bias and fail to generate protective Th1 immunity to *C. albicans* (Cenci et al., 1998). The presence of IFN-γ also appears to be important for the induction of chemokines in response to *C. neoformans* (Kawakami et al., 1999b). Therefore, the early production of TNF-α and IL-12 induces IFN-γ and a protective Th1 response is generated. Any perturbation of these early signals abrogates IFN-γ production and shifts the response to a Th2 phenotype demonstrating that IFN-γ is required for host resistance to fungi.

To date, the involvement of IL-18 in innate responses to fungi has not been extensively analyzed. The role of IL-18 in host resistance to *C. neoformans* was examined recently in IL-18 deficient mice. The levels of IL-12 and IFN-γ were significantly reduced in the IL-18$^{-/-}$ animals and correlated with reduced clearance of *C. neoformans* from the lungs (Kawakami et al., 2000a). Similar results have been reported following neutralization of IL-18 during pulmonary cryptococcal infection (Kawakami et al., 2000b). In addition, administration of murine recombinant IL-18 enhanced fungal clearance from the lungs and prevented brain dissemination of a highly virulent strain of *Cryptococcus* (Kawakami et al., 1997a). These findings suggest that IL-18 plays a supporting role in host defense against *C. neoformans*. Based on this model of infection, it is likely that IL-18 will prove to be an important mediator in host responses to a variety of other fungal pathogens.

IL-4 and IL-10

IL-4 and IL-10 can also be produced by cells of the innate immune system and have profound adverse consequences on the subsequent development of adaptive immunity to fungi. Although T helper cells are major sources of IL-4, mast cells can also synthesize IL-4. Interestingly, while IL-10 is produced by Th2 cells, large amounts of IL-10 are made by macrophages and neutrophils. Neutralization of IL-4 facilitates clearance and prolongs survival following *C. neoformans* or *C. albicans* infection (Kawakami et al., 1999a; Tonnetti et al., 1995). Similarly, treatment with soluble IL-4 receptor protects animals from either *Candida* or *Aspergillus* (Cenci et al., 1995, 1997). IL-4 knockout mice are also more resistant to *A. fumigatus* and shift from a Th2-type response to a Th1-type response (Cenci et al., 1999; Kurup et al., 1999). The absence of IL-10 produces similar results. IL-10-deficient mice exhibit upregulated Th1 cytokine responses and increased resistance to *C. albicans* and *A. fumigatus* (Del Sero et al., 1999; Vazquez-Torres et al., 1999). Neutralization of IL-10 also increased innate fungal resistance to *Candida* and facilitated the development of Th1 protective immunity (Mencacci et al., 1998b; Tonnetti et al., 1995). Therefore, IL-4 and IL-10 drive nonprotective Th2 immune responses to fungi and suppress protective Th1 immunity, thereby enhancing susceptibility to fungal infection.

Chemokines

Fungal infections induce the production of both C-C and C-X-C chemokines (for a more comprehensive review of chemokines in fungal infections, please see reference (Traynor and Huffnagle, 2001). Both C-C and C-X-C chemokines are important in granulocyte and mononuclear cell recruitment to the site of infection. Chemokine production in concert with upregulation of adhesion molecule expression (reviewed by Huffnagle and Toews [1997]) mediate leukocyte extravasation and migration into sites of fungal infection. However, recent evidence also indicates that chemokine production by the innate immune system is also important in cell activation and promoting adaptive immunity.

As an example of the roles of chemokines in leukocyte recruitment, the C-C chemokines, MCP-1, MIP-1α, and T-cell activator gene 3 all play important roles in leukocyte recruitment during fungal infection. MCP-1 is induced in response to pulmonary *C. neoformans* infection and is correlated with inflammatory cell recruitment and subsequent clearance of *Cryptococcus* from the lungs (Huffnagle et al., 1995b). Mice deficient in CCR2, the primary receptor for MCP-1, have defects in monocyte and CD8 T-cell recruitment in response to a pulmonary *C. neoformans* infection (Traynor et al., 2000) MIP-1α is also induced in the lungs of *C. neoformans*-infected mice (Huffnagle et al., 1997). Neutralization of MIP-1α or TCA-3 inhibits leukocyte recruitment to the site of *C. neoformans* infection or antigen challenge (Doyle and Murphy, 1997, 1999; Huffnagle et al., 1997). C-C chemokines are probably also important in leukocyte recruitment during other fungal infections. As an example, stimulation of peripheral blood mononuclear cells with *C. albicans* induces significant production of MCP-1 (Jiang et al., 1996), and MCP-1 and MIP-1α are also induced in the lung following pulmonary challenge with *A. fumigatus* (Schelenz et al., 1999; Shahan et al., 1998). Finally, the role of C-X-C chemokines in fungal infections has not received as much attention as that of C-C chemokines, but C-X-C chemokines are clearly important for neutrophil recruitment (Mehrad et al., 1999a).

In terms of innate immunity, it is becoming increasingly clear that C-C chemokines also modulate the development of antifungal adaptive immunity. MCP-1 is produced by almost all cell types. Mice deficient in CCR2, the primary receptor for MCP-1, develop a Th2 response to *C. neoformans* characterized by pulmonary eosinophilia and the production of IL-4 and IL-5 (Traynor et al., 2000). Elevated MCP-1 levels are detected during vaginal *C. albicans* infection, and neutralization of MCP-1 results in increased fungal burden, suggesting that MCP-1 serves a protective role during this mucosal infection (Saavedra et al., 1999); however, leukocyte recruitment is unaffected, suggesting an immunoregulatory role. MCP-1 drives Th2-type responses to *Leishmania*, *Schistosoma*, and autoimmune encephalitis and in

OVA TcR transgenic mice (Gu et al., 2000; Karpus and Kennedy, 1997; Karpus et al., 1997; Warmington et al., 1999). However, data from fungal infections clearly indicate that MCP-1 is important for establishing Th1 immunity to fungal pathogens. Thus, the specific role of MCP-1 in modulating the Th1 or Th2 immune response is determined by the nature of the microbial infection. MIP-1α-deficient mice develop a nonprotective Th2 response to highly virulent strains of *C. neoformans* characterized by pulmonary eosinophilia and elevated immunoglobulin E (IgE) and IL-4 production (Olszewski et al., 2000). Based on preliminary data with a number of *C. neoformans* isolates, it appears that MIP-1α actually prevents Th2 immune responses during a pulmonary cryptococcal infection rather than promoting Th1 responses (M. A. Olszewski, unpublished observation). Future studies will continue to elucidate the specific involvement of these and other chemokines during the course of a variety of fungal infections. However, it appears that production of C-C chemokines by the innate immune system is critical for the development of protective Th1 adaptive immunity.

Antigen Presentation

Antigen presentation is a specialized function of cells of the innate immune system that links innate and adaptive immunity. Effective presentation of fungal antigens is required for the development of protective immunity. Here we provide only a conceptual overview since antigen presentation is covered in more detail in other chapters in this book. The major antigen-presenting cells (APC) include dendritic cells, B cells, and macrophages. Other resident cells such as epithelial cells and fibroblasts can also be activated to express major histocompatibility complex class II antigens and thus present fungal antigens to recently activated T cells during an inflammatory response. B cells express major histocompatibility complex class II antigens, and activated B cells in the lymph nodes probably also play an important role in driving early immune responses. Dendritic cells are particularly numerous in the epithelium of mucosal surfaces and take up antigen and carry it to the lymph nodes to initiate primary immune responses. Dendritic cells are the most effective APC for stimulating naive T cells and are probably key APC in initiating Th1-type cell-mediated immunity against fungi. Macrophages have a key regulatory function in regulating APC activity, either enhancing or suppressing types of immune responses depending on the stimulus (and production of fungal virulence factors [described below]).

Effector Cell Activity

Following the development of Th1 or Th2 responses, the signals from adaptive immunity can influence fungal killing by innate immunity (phagocytes). It is well established that IFN-γ and granulocyte-macrophage colony-stimulating factor (GM-CSF) induce the fungicidal activity of macrophages. For example, the activation of rat alveolar macrophages with IFN-γ or GM-CSF induced the ingestion and killing of *C. neoformans* (Chen et al., 1994; Mody et al., 1991). Similar studies with human peripheral blood mononuclear cells revealed that GM-CSF and IL-2 induced anticryptococcal activity in these cells (Levitz, 1991). The IFN-γ-mediated activation of NO is clearly an important antifungal mechanism; however, the specific details are beyond the scope of this chapter. In contrast, IL-4 and IL-10 increase the susceptibility to fungal infections by inhibiting the antifungal activity of macrophages. NO secretion and fungal killing of *C. albicans* are suppressed in the presence of IL-4 and IL-10 (Cenci et al., 1993; Roilides et al., 1998a). IL-4 can also inhibit the uptake of *Candida* by mononuclear phagocytes (Roilides et al., 1997). Therefore, adaptive immunity modulates fungicidal mechanisms of phagocytes by enhancing fungal killing through Th1 cytokines and dampening antifungal activity through Th2 cytokines.

MODULATION OF INNATE IMMUNITY BY FUNGAL VIRULENCE FACTORS

Pathogenic fungi produce a number of virulence factors (Table 3). In this chapter, we are defining a virulence factor as a microbial product that allows the microbe to avoid being eliminated by the host. There are a number of points in host defense at which fungal virulence factors and secreted/shed fungal products can facilitate evasion:

1. Modulate afferent-phase cytokine signals by (i) downregulating proinflammatory cytokines, (ii) upregulating anti-inflammatory cytokines, and (iii) promoting switching of the immune response
2. Alter antigen processing

Table 3. Fungal virulence factors

Adhesins	Catalase
Proteases	Toxins
Superoxide dismutase	Mannitol
Phospholipase	Capsule
Pigments	Eicosanoids
Urease	

3. Block leukocyte recruitment to the site of infection
4. Inhibit effector phase mechanisms

Most of the work in this area has concentrated on *C. neoformans,* but it is likely that many of the virulence mechanisms utilized by *C. neoformans* are also used by other fungi. In the broader context of microbiology, it should be kept in mind that pathogenic fungi are predominantly environmental microbes (with the possible exceptions of *Pneumocystis* and *C. albicans*). Thus, the primary role of fungal virulence factors is to enhance survival of the fungus outside the host (in the environment). However, the difference between pathogenic and nonpathogenic species of fungi is the production of factors that enhance fungal survival in a host, i.e., virulence factors.

Inhibition of early signal molecule generation is a target for fungal virulence factors. The increased virulence of some strains of *C. neoformans* is largely due to inhibition of TNF-α, IL-12, IL-18, and IFN-γ production during the first week of infection (Huffnagle et al., 1995, 1996; Kawakami et al., 1996a, 1996b, 1996c, 1997a, 1997b). Intraperitoneal administration of TNF-α, IL-12, or IL-18 can increase survival and decrease dissemination of these cryptococcal strains (Kawakami et al., 1996a, 1996c, 1997a). Addition of polysaccharide capsule from *C. neoformans* decreases TNF-α and IL-1β production by macrophages in vitro (Vecchiarelli et al., 1995). The capsule also induces IL-10 production, thereby providing a mechanism by which the capsule may downregulate macrophage activation and protective Th1 responses (Levitz et al., 1996; Monari et al., 1997; Vecchiarelli et al., 1996). Melanin can also reduce TNF-α production by alveolar macrophages (Huffnagle et al., 1995a). NK-cell production of TNF-α is also inhibited by coculture with cryptococci (Murphy et al., 1997). The polysaccharide capsule and melanin also interfere with effector phase killing mechanisms such as phagocytosis and oxidant-mediated killing (Jacobson and Tinnell, 1993; Kozel and Mastroianni, 1976; Wang and Casadevall, 1994).

Cryptococcal virulence factors can also interfere with antigen presentation and leukocyte recruitment. Cryptococcal polysaccharide and melanin both interfere with antigen presentation and subsequent cytokine signaling by macrophages for *Cryptococcus*-specific lymphocyte proliferation (Collins and Bancroft, 1991; Huffnagle et al., 1995a; Vecchiarelli et al., 1994). In addition, cryptococcal antigen and polysaccharide induce immunologic unresponsiveness to subsequent challenge with *C. neoformans* (Murphy, 1989). Another mechanism of evasion is by blocking adhesion molecule-leukocyte interactions on the endothelium, thereby interfering with leukocyte recruitment to the site of infection (Dong and Murphy, 1996)

SUMMARY

Innate immunity is central to host defense against fungi even for fungal infections that require an adaptive immune response for clearance. Several broad effector mechanisms are induced early to combat the fungal infection and to promote subsequent signal generation. The cells of the innate immune system possess many immunoregulatory functions (providing a link between innate and adaptive immunity), along with potent antifungal effector mechanisms that can be activated by adaptive immunity. Fungal virulence factors and secreted or shed fungal products can interfere with a number of innate mechanisms, resulting in a dynamic interaction between microbe and host. This interplay between innate immunity and fungal virulence factors determines how the infection is initially handled and how adaptive immunity ultimately develops.

REFERENCES

Allendoerfer, R., and G. S. J. Deepe. 1997. Intrapulmonary response to *Histoplasma capsulatum* in gamma interferon knockout mice. *Infect. Immun.* 65:2564–2569.

Allendoerfer, R., and G. S. J. Deepe. 1998. Blockade of endogenous TNF-alpha exacerbates primary and secondary pulmonary histoplasmosis by differential mechanisms. *J. Immunol.* 160:6072–6082.

Aratani, Y., H. Koyama, S. Nyui, K. Suzuki, F. Kura, and N. Maeda. 1999. Severe impairment in early host defense against *Candida albicans* in mice deficient in myeloperoxidase. *Infect. Immun.* 67:1828–1836.

Balish, E., R. D. Wagner, A. Vazquez-Torres, C. Pierson, and T. Warner. 1998. Candidiasis in interferon-gamma knockout (IFN-gamma$^{-/-}$) mice. *J. Infect. Dis.* 178:478–487.

Cain, J. A., and G. S. J. Deepe. 1998. Evolution of the primary immune response to *Histoplasma capsulatum* in murine lung. *Infect. Immun.* 66:1473–1481.

Casadevall, A., and J. R. Perfect. 1998. *Cryptococcus neoformans*, p. 177–222. American Society for Microbiology, Washington, D.C.

Cenci, E., A. Mencacci, G. Del Sero, A. Bacci, C. Montagnoli, C. F. d'Ostiani, P. Mosci, M. Bachmann, F. Bistoni, M. Kopf, and L. Romani. 1999. Interleukin-4 causes susceptibility to invasive pulmonary aspergillosis through suppression of protective type 1 responses. *J. Infect. Dis.* 180:1957–1968.

Cenci, E., A. Mencacci, G. Del Sero, C. F. d'Ostiani, P. Mosci, A. Bacci, C. Montagnoli, M. Kopf, and L. Romani. 1998. IFN-gamma is required for IL-12 responsiveness in mice with *Candida albicans* infection. *J. Immunol.* 161:3543–3550.

Cenci, E., A. Mencacci, R. Spaccapelo, L. Tonnetti, P. Mosci, K. H. Enssle, P. Puccetti, L. Romani, and F. Bistoni. 1995. T helper cell type 1 (Th1) and Th2-like responses are present in mice with gastric candidiasis but protective immunity is associated with Th1 development. *J. Infect. Dis.* 171:1279–1288.

Cenci, E., S. Perito, K. H. Enssle, P. Mosci, J. P. Latge, L. Romani, and F. Bistoni. 1997. Th1 and Th2 cytokines in mice with invasive aspergillosis. *Infect. Immun.* 65:564–570.

Cenci, E., L. Romani, A. Mencacci, R. Spaccapelo, E. Schiaffella, P. Puccetti, and F. Bistoni. 1993. Interleukin-4 and interleukin-10 inhibit nitric oxide-dependent macrophage killing of *Candida albicans*. *Eur. J. Immunol.* 23:1034–1038.

Chen, G. H., J. L. Curtis, C. H. Mody, P. J. Christensen, L. R. Armstrong, and G. B. Toews. 1994. Effect of granulocyte-macrophage colony-stimulating factor on rat alveolar macrophage anticryptococcal activity in vitro. *J. Immunol.* 152:724–734.

Chen, W., E. A. Havell, and A. G. Harmsen. 1992. Importance of endogenous tumor necrosis factor alpha and gamma interferon in host resistance against *Pneumocystis carinii* infection. *Infect. Immun.* 60:1279–1284.

Collins, H. L., and G. J. Bancroft. 1991. Encapsulation of *Cryptococcus neoformans* impairs antigen-specific T-cell responses. *Infect. Immun.* 59:3883–3888.

Cross, C. E., and G. J. Bancroft. 1995. Ingestion of acapsular *Cryptococcus neoformans* occurs via mannose and β-glucan receptors, resulting in cytokine production and enhanced phagocytosis of the encapsulated form. *Infect. Immun.* 63:2604–2611.

Cross, C. E., H. L. Collins, and G. J. Bancroft. 1997. CR3-dependent phagocytosis by murine macrophages: different cytokines regulate ingestion of a defined CR3 ligand and complement-opsonized *Cryptococcus neoformans*. *Immunology* 91:289–296.

Decken, K., G. Kohler, K. Palmer-Lehmann, A. Wunderlin, F. Mattner, J. Magram, M. K. Gately, and G. Alber. 1998. Interleukin-12 is essential for a protective Th1 response in mice infected with *Cryptococcus neoformans*. *Infect. Immun.* 66:4994–5000.

Del Sero, G., A. Mencacci, E. Cenci, C. F. d'Ostiani, C. Montagnoli, A. Bacci, P. Mosci, M. Kopf, and L. Romani. 1999. Antifungal type 1 responses are upregulated in IL-10-deficient mice. *Microbes Infect.* 1:1169–1180.

Dong, Z. M., and J. W. Murphy. 1996. Cryptococcal polysaccharides induce ʟ-selectin shedding and tumor necrosis factor receptor loss from the surface of human neutrophils. *J. Clin. Investig.* 97:689–698.

Doyle, H. A., and J. W. Murphy. 1997. MIP-1 alpha contributes to the anticryptococcal delayed-type hypersensitivity reaction and protection against *Cryptococcus neoformans*. *J. Leukoc. Biol.* 61:147–155.

Doyle, H. A., and J. W. Murphy. 1999. Role of the C-C chemokine, TCA3, in the protective anticryptococcal cell-mediated immune response. *J. Immunol.* 162:4824–4833.

Greenfield, R. A., V. L. Abrams, D. L. Crawford, and T. L. Kuhls. 1993. Effect of abrogation of natural killer cell activity on the course of candidiasis induced by intraperitoneal administration and gastrointestinal candidiasis in mice with severe combined immunodeficiency. *Infect. Immun.* 61:2520–2525.

Gross, N. T., K. Nessa, P. Camner, and C. Jarstrand. 1999. Production of nitric oxide by rat alveolar macrophages stimulated by *Cryptococcus neoformans* or *Aspergillus fumigatus*. *Med. Mycol.* 37:151–157.

Gu, L., S. Tseng, R. M. Hornoer, C. Tam, M. Loda, and B. J. Rollins. 2000. Control of TH2 polarization by the chemokine monocyte chemoattractant protein-1. *Nature* 404:407–411.

Hoag, K. A., M. F. Lipscomb, A. A. Izzo, and N. E. Street. 1997. IL-12 and IFN-gamma are required for initiating the protective Th1 response to pulmonary cryptococcosis in resistant CB-17 mice. *Am. J. Respir. Cell Mol. Biol.* 17:733–739.

Huffnagle, G. B., G. H. Chen, J. L. Curtis, R. A. McDonald, R. M. Strieter, and G. B. Toews. 1995a. Down-regulation of the afferent phase of T cell-mediated pulmonary inflammation and immunity by a high melanin-producing strain of *Cryptococcus neoformans*. *J. Immunol.* **155:**3507–3516.

Huffnagle, G. B., R. M. Strieter, L. K. McNeil, R. A. McDonald, M. D. Burdick, S. L. Kunkel, and G. B. Toews. 1997. Macrophage inflammatory protein-1α (MIP-1α) is required for the efferent phase of pulmonary cell-mediated immunity to a *Cryptococcus neoformans* infection. *J. Immunol.* **159:**318–327.

Huffnagle, G. B., R. M. Strieter, T. J. Standiford, R. A. McDonald, M. D. Burdick, S. L. Kunkel, and G. B. Toews. 1995b. The role of monocyte chemotactic protein-1 (MCP-1) in the recruitment of monocytes and CD4+ T cells during a pulmonary *Cryptococcus neoformans* infection. *J. Immunol.* **155:**4790–4797.

Huffnagle, G. B., and G. B. Toews. 1997. Mechanisms of macrophage recruitment into infected lungs, p. 373–407. *In* M. F. Lipscomb and S. W. Russell (ed.), *Lung Macrophages and Dendritic Cells in Health and Disease.* Marcel Dekker, Inc., New York, N.Y.

Huffnagle, G. B., G. B. Toews, M. D. Burdick, M. B. Boyd, K. S. McAllister, R. A. McDonald, S. L. Kunkel, and R. M. Strieter. 1996. Afferent phase production of TNF-α is required for the development of protective T cell immunity to *Cryptococcus neoformans*. *J. Immunol.* **157:**4529–4536.

Jacobson, E. S., and S. B. Tinnell. 1993. Antioxidant function of fungal melanin. *J. Bacteriol.* **175:**7102–7104.

Jiang, Y., T. R. Russell, D. T. Graves, H. Cheng, S. H. Nong, and S. M. Levitz. 1996. Monocyte chemoattractant protein 1 and interleukin-8 production in mononuclear cell stimulated by oral microorganisms. *Infect. Immun.* **64:**4450–4455.

Jones-Carson, J., A. Vazques-Torres, H. C. van der Heyde, T. Warner, R. D. Wagner, and E. Balish. 1995. γδ T cell-induced nitric oxide production enhances resistance to mucosal candidiasis. *Nat. Med.* **1:**552–557.

Kaposzta, R., P. Tree, L. Marodi, and S. Gordon. 1998. Characteristics of invasive candidiasis in gamma interferon- and interleukin-4 deficient mice: role of macrophages in host defense against *Candida albicans*. *Infect. Immun.* **66:**1708–1717.

Karpus, W. J., and K. J. Kennedy. 1997. MIP-1 alpha and MCP-1 differentially regulate acute and relapsing autoimmune encephalomyelitis as well as Th1/Th2 lymphocyte differentiation. *J. Leukoc. Biol.* **62:**681–687.

Karpus, W. J., N. W. Lukacs, K. J. Kennedy, W. S. Smith, S. D. Hurst, and T. A. Barrett. 1997. Differential CC chemokine-induced enhancement of T helper cell cytokine production. *J. Immunol.* **158:**4129–4136.

Kawakami, K., M. Hossain Qureshi, T. Zhang, Y. Koguchi, Q. Xie, M. Kurimoto, and A. Saito. 1999a. Interleukin-4 weakens host resistance to pulmonary and disseminated cryptococcal infection caused by combined treatment with interferon-gamma-inducing cytokines. *Cell. Immunol.* **197:**55–61.

Kawakami, K., Y. Koguchi, M. H. Qureshi, Y. Kinjo, S. Yara, A. Miyazato, M. Kurimoto, K. Takeda, S. Akira, and A. Saito. 2000a. Reduced host resistance and Th1 response to *Cryptococcus neoformans* in interleukin-18 deficient mice. *FEMS Microbiol. Lett.* **186:**121–126.

Kawakami, K., X. Qifeng, M. Tohyama, M. H. Qureshi, and A. Saito. 1996a. Contribution of tumor necrosis factor-alpha (TNF-alpha) in host defense mechanism against *Cryptococcus neoformans*. *Clin. Exp. Immunol.* **106:**468–474.

Kawakami, K., M. H. Qureshi, T. Zhang, Y. Koguchi, K. Shibuya, S. Naoe, and A. Saito. 1999b. Interferon-gamma (IFN-gamma)-dependent protection and synthesis of chemoattractants for mononuclear leukocytes caused by IL-12 in the lungs of mice infected with *Cryptococcus neoformans*. *Clin. Exp. Immunol.* **117:**113–122.

Kawakami, K., M. H. Qureshi, T. Zhang, Y. Koguchi, S. Yara, K. Takeda, S. Akira, M. Kurimoto, and A. Saito. 2000b. Involvement of endogenously synthesized interleukin-18 in the protective effects of IL-12 against pulmonary infection with *Cryptococcus neoformans* in mice. *FEMS Immunol. Med. Microbiol.* **27:**191–200.

Kawakami, K., M. H. Qureshi, T. Zhang, H. Okamura, M. Kurimoto, and A. Saito. 1997a. IL-18 protects mice against pulmonary and disseminated infection with *Cryptococcus neoformans* by inducing IFN-γ production. *J Immunol.* **159:**5528–5534.

Kawakami, K., M. Tohyama, X. Qifeng, and A. Saito. 1997b. Expression of cytokines and inducible nitric oxide synthase mRNA in the lungs of mice infected with *Cryptococcus neoformans*: effects of interleukin-12. *Infect. Immun.* **65:**1307–1312.

Kawakami, K., M. Tohyama, K. Teruya, N. Kudeken, Q. Xie, and A. Saito. 1996b. Contribution of interferon-gamma in protecting mice during pulmonary and disseminated infection with *Cryptococcus neoformans*. *FEMS Immunol. Med. Microbiol.* **13:**123–130.

Kawakami, K., M. Tohyama, Q. Xie, and A. Saito. 1996c. IL-12 protects mice against pulmonary and disseminated infection caused by *Cryptococcus neoformans*. *Clin. Exp. Immunol.* **104:**208–214.

Kawasaki, T. 1999. Structure and biology of mannan-binding protein, MBP, an important component of innate immunity. *Biochim. Biophys. Acta* **1473:**186–195.

Kozel, T. R. 1998. Complement activation by pathogenic fungi. *Res. Immunol.* **149:**309–320.

Kozel, T. R., and R. P. Mastroianni. 1976. Inhibition of phagocytosis by cryptococcal polysaccharide: dissociation of the attachment and ingestion phases of phagocytosis. *Infect. Immun.* **14:**62–67.

Kurup, V. P., H. Y. Choi, P. S. Murali, J. Q. Xia, R. L. Coffman, and J. N. Fink. 1999. Immune responses to *Aspergillus* antigen in IL-4−/− mice and the effect of eosinophil ablation. *Allergy* **54:**420–427.

Lavigne, L. M., L. R. Schopf, C. L. Chung, R. Maylor, and J. P. Sypeck. 1998. The role of recombinant muring IL-12 and IFN-gamma in the pathogenesis of a murine systemic *Candida albicans* infection. *J. Immunol.* **160:**284–292.

Levitz, S. M. 1991. Activation of human peripheral blood mononuclear cells by interleukin-2 and granulocyte-macrophage colony-stimulation factor to inhibit *Cryptococcus neoformans*. *Infect. Immun.* **59:**3393–3397.

Levitz, S. M., A. Tabuni, S. H. Nong, and D. T. Golenbock. 1996. Effects of interleukin-10 on human peripheral blood mononuclear cell responses to *Cryptococcus neoformans, Candida albicans,* and lipopolysaccharide. *Infect. Immun.* **64:**945–951.

Madan, T., K. B. Reid, P. U. Sarma, S. S. Aggrawal, P. Strong, U. Kishore, and P. Eggleton. 1997. Binding of pulmonary surfactant proteins A and D to *Aspergillus fumigatus* conidia enhances phagocytosis and killing by human neutrophils and alveolar macrophages. *Infect. Immun.* **65:**3171–3179.

Mehrad, B., R. M. Strieter, T. A. Moore, W. C. Tsai, S. A. Lira, and T. J. Standiford. 1999a. CXC chemokine receptor-2 ligands are necessary components of neutrophil-mediated host defense in invasive pulmonary aspergillosis. *J. Immunol.* **163:**6086–6094.

Mehrad, B., R. M. Strieter, and T. J. Standiford. 1999b. Role of TNF-alpha in pulmonary host defense in murine invasive aspergillosis. *J. Immunol.* **162:**1633–1640.

Mencacci, A., E. Cenci, G. Del Sero, C. F. d'Ostiani, P. Mosci, C. Montagnoli, A. Bacci, F. Bistoni, V. F. J. Quesniaux, B. Ryffel, and L. Romani. 1998a. Defective co-stimulation and impaired Th1 development in tumor necrosis factor/lymphotoxin-α double-deficient mice infected with *Candida albicans*. *Int. Immunol.* 10:37–48.

Mencacci, A., E. Cenci, G. Del Sero, C. F. d'Ostiani, P. Mosci, G. Trinchieri, L. Adorini, and L. Romani. 1998b. IL-10 is required for development of protective Th1 responses in IL-12-deficient mice upon *Candida albicans* infection. *J. Immunol.* 161:6228–6237.

Mody, C. H., C. L. Tyler, R. G. Sitrin, C. Jackson, and G. B. Toews. 1991. Interferon-gamma activates rat alveolar macrophages for anticryptococcal activity. *Am. J. Respir. Cell Mol. Biol.* 5:19–26.

Monari, C., C. Retini, B. Palazzetti, F. Bistoni, and A. Vecchiarelli. 1997. Regulatory role of exogenous IL-10 in the development of immune response versus *Cryptococcus neoformans*. *Clin. Exp. Immunol.* 109:242–247.

Murphy, J. W. 1989. Clearance of *Cryptococcus neoformans* from immunologically suppressed mice. *Infect. Immun.* 57:1946–1952.

Murphy, J. W., A. Zhou, and S. C. Wong. 1997. Direct interactions of human natural killer cells with *Cryptococcus neoformans* inhibit granulocyte-macrophage colony-stimulating factor and tumor necrosis factor alpha production. *Infect. Immun.* 65:4564–4571.

Nagai, H., J. Guo, H. Choi, and V. P. Kurup. 1995. Interferon-gamma and tumor necrosis factor-alpha protect mice from invasive aspergillosis. *J. Infect. Dis.* 172:1554–1560.

Netea, M. G., L. J. van Tits, J. H. Curfs, F. Amiot, J. F. Meis, J. W. van der Meer, and B. J. Kullberg. 1999. Increased susceptibility of TNF-alpha lymphotoxin-alpha double knockout mice to systemic candidiasis through impaired recruitment of neutrophils and phagocytosis of *Candida albicans*. *J. Immunol.* 163:1498–1505.

Neth, O., D. L. Jack, A. W. Dodds, H. Holzel, N. J. Klein, and M. W. Turner. 2000. Mannose-binding lectin binds to a range of clinically relevant microorganisms and promotes complement deposition. *Infect. Immun.* 68:688–693.

Olszewski, M. A., G. B. Huffnagle, R. A. McDonald, D. M. Lindell, B. B. Moore, D. N. Cook, and G. B. Toews. 2000. The role of macrophage inflammatory protein 1α/CCL3 in regulation of T cell-mediated immunity to *Cryptococcus neoformans* infection. *J. Immunol.* 165:6429–6436.

O'Riordan, D. M., J. E. Standing, K.-Y. Kwon, D. Chang, E. C. Crouch, and A. H. Limper. 1995a. Surfactant protein D interacts with *Pneumocystis carinii* and mediates organism adherence to alveolar macrophages. *J. Clin. Investig.* 95:2699–2710.

O'Riordan, D. M., J. E. Standing, and A. H. Limper. 1995b. *Pneumocystis carinii* glycoprotein A binds macrophage mannose receptors. *Infect. Immun.* 63:779–784.

Petkus, A. F. 1987. Natural killer cell inhibition of young spherules and endospores of *Coccidioides immitis*. *J. Immunol.* 139:3107–3111.

Pitzurra, L., R. Cherniak, M. Giammarioli, S. Perito, F. Bistoni, and A. Vecchiarelli. 2000. Early induction of IL-12 by human monocytes exposed to *Cryptococcus neoformans* mannoproteins. *Infect. Immun.* 68:558–563.

Roilides, E., A. Anastasiou-Katsiardani, A. Dimitiadou-Georgiadou, I. Kadiltsoglou, S. Tsaparidou, C. Panteliadis, and T. J. Walsh. 1998a. Suppressive effects of interleukin-10 on human mononuclear phagocyte function against *Candida albicans* and *Staphylococcus aureus*. *J. Infect. Dis.* 178:1734–1742.

Roilides, E., I. Kadiltsoglou, A. Dimitiadou, M. Hatzistilianou, A. Manitsa, J. Karpouzas, P. A. Pizzo, and T. J. Walsh. 1997. Interleukin-4 suppresses antifungal activity of human mononuclear phagocytes against *Candida albicans* in association with

decreased uptake of blastoconidia. *FEMS Immunol. Med. Microbiol.* 19:169–180.

Roilides, E., H. Katsifa, and T. J. Walsh. 1998b. Pulmonary host defences against *Aspergillus fumigatus*. *Res. Immunol.* 149:454–465.

Romani, L., A. Mencacci, E. Cenci, G. Del Sero, F. Bistoni, and P. Puccetti. 1997. An immunoregulatory role for neutrophils in CD4⁺ T helper subset selection in mice with candidiasis. *J. Immunol.* 158:2356–2362.

Romani, L., A. Mencacci, E. Cenci, R. Spaccapelo, E. Schiaffella, L. Tonnetti, P. Puccetti, and F. Bistoni. 1993. Natural killer cells do not play a dominant role in CD4⁺ subset differentiation in *Candida albicans*-infected mice. *Infect. Immun.* 61:3769–3774.

Romani, L., A. Mencacci, L. Tonnetti, R. Spaccapelo, E. Cenci, P. Puccetti, S. Wolf, and F. Bistoni. 1994a. IL-12 is both required and prognostic in vivo for T helper type 1 differentiation in murine candidiasis. *J. Immunol.* 153:5167–5175.

Romani, L., A. Mencacci, L. Tonnetti, R. Spaccapelo, E. Cenci, S. Wolf, P. Puccetti, and F. Bistoni. 1994b. Interleukin-12 but not interferon-gamma production correlates with induction of T helper type-1 phenotype in murine candidiasis. *Eur. J. Immunol.* 24:909–915.

Saavedra, M., B. Taylor, N. Lukacs, and P. L. J. Fidel. 1999. Local production of chemokines during experimental vaginal candidiasis. *Infect. Immun.* 67:5820–5826.

Salkowski, C. A., and E. Balish. 1991. Role of natural killer cells in resistance to systemic cryptococcosis. *J. Leukoc. Biol.* 50:151–159.

Schelenz, S., R. Malhotra, R. B. Sim, U. Holmskov, and G. J. Bancroft. 1995. Binding of host collectins to the pathogenic yeast *Cryptococcus neoformans*: human surfactant protein D acts as an agglutinin for acapsular yeast cells. *Infect. Immun.* 63:3360–3366.

Schelenz, S., D. A. Smith, and G. J. Bancroft. 1999. Cytokine and chemokine responses following pulmonary challenge with *Aspergillus fumigatus*: obligatory role of TNF-alpha and GM-CSF in neutrophil recruitment. *Med. Mycol.* 37:183–194.

Shahan, T. A., W. G. Sorenson, J. D. Paulauskis, R. Morey, and D. M. Lewis. 1998. Concentration- and time-dependent up-regulation and release of the cytokines MIP-2, KC, TNF, and MIP-1alpha in rat alveolar macrophages by fungal spores implicated in airway inflammation. *Am. J. Respir. Cell Mol. Biol.* 18:435–440.

Tabona, P., A. Mellor, and J. A. Summerfield. 1995. Mannose binding protein is involved in first-line host defence: evidence from transgenic mice. *Immunology* 85:153–159.

Taramelli, D., M. G. Malabarba, G. Sala, N. Basilico, and G. Cocuzza. 1996. Production of cytokines by alveolar and peritoneal macrophages stimulated by *Aspergillus fumigatus* conidia or hyphae. *J. Med. Vet. Mycol.* 34:49–56.

Tonnetti, L., R. Spaccapelo, E. Cenci, A. Mencacci, P. Puccetti, R. L. Coffman, F. Bistoni, and L. Romani. 1995. Interleukin-4 and -10 exacerbate candidiasis in mice. *Eur. J. Immunol.* 25:1559–1565.

Traynor, T. R., and G. B. Huffnagle. 2001. Role of chemokines in fungal infections. *Med. Mycol.* 39:41–50.

Traynor, T. R., W. A. Kuziel, G. B. Toews, and G. B. Huffnagle. 2000. CCR2 expression determines T1 versus T2 polarization during pulmonary *Cryptococcus neoformans* infection. *J. Immunol.* 164:2021–2027.

Underhill, D. M., A. Ozinsky, A. M. Hajjar, A. Stevens, C. B. Wilson, M. Bassetti, and A. Aderem. 1999. The Toll-like receptor 2 is recruited to macrophage phagosomes and discriminates between pathogens. *Nature* 401:811–815.

Vazquez-Torres, A., and E. Balish. 1997. Macrophages in resistance to candidiasis. *Microbiol. Mol. Biol. Rev.* 61:170–192.

Vazquez-Torres, A., J. Jones-Carson, R. D. Wagner, T. Warner, and E. Balish. 1999. Early resistance of interleukin-10 knockout mice to acute systemic candidiasis. *Infect. Immun.* 67:670–674.

Vecchiarelli, A., D. Pietrella, M. Dottorini, C. Monari, C. Retini, T. Todisco, and F. Bistoni. 1994. Encapsulation of *Cryptococcus neoformans* regulates fungicidal activity and the antigen presentation process in human alveolar macrophages. *Clin. Exp. Immunol.* 98:217–223.

Vecchiarelli, A., C. Retini, C. Monari, C. Tascini, F. Bistoni, and T. R. Kozel. 1996. Purified capsular polysaccharide of *Cryptococcus neoformans* induces interleukin-10 secretion by human monocytes. *Infect. Immun.* 64:2846–2849.

Vecchiarelli, A., C. Retini, D. Pietrella, C. Monari, C. Tascini, T. Beccari, and T. R. Kozel. 1995. Downregulation by cryptococcal polysaccharide of tumor necrosis factor alpha and interleu-kin-1 beta secretion from human monocytes. *Infect. Immun.* 63:2919–2923.

Wang, Y., and A. Casadevall. 1994. Susceptibility of melanized and nonmelanized *Cryptococcus neoformans* to nitrogen- and oxygen-derived oxidants. *Infect. Immun.* 62:3004–3007.

Warmington, K. S., L. Boring, J. H. Ruth, J. Sonstein, C. M. Hogaboam, J. L. Curtis, S. L. Kunkel, I. R. Charo, and S. W. Chensue. 1999. Effect of C-C chemokine receptor 2 (CCR2) knockout on type-2 (schistosomal antigen-elicited) pulmonary granuloma formation: analysis of cellular recruitment and cytokine responses. *Am. J. Pathol.* 154:1407–1416.

Zhou, P., M. C. Sieve, J. Bennett, K. J. Kwon-Chung, R. P. Tewari, R. T. Gazzinelli, A. Sher, and R. A. Seder. 1995. IL-12 prevents mortality in mice infected with *Histoplasma capsulatum* through induction of IFN-gamma. *J. Immunol.* 155:785–795.

Immunology of Infectious Diseases
Edited by S. H. E. Kaufmann, A. Sher, and R. Ahmed
© 2002 ASM Press, Washington, D.C.

Chapter 11

Innate Immunity and Viral Infections

CHRISTINE A. BIRON, MARC DALOD, AND THAIS P. SALAZAR-MATHER

The two major functions of innate immune responses are (i) to mediate antimicrobial effects while adaptive immune responses are being expanded and activated and (ii) to provide conditions promoting the subset of adaptive immune responses most effective in defense against the particular pathogen being encountered. The host has evolved receptors specific for chemical characteristics of different infectious agents, distinct from host determinants, and has linked the binding of these receptors to induction of the innate cytokine responses most effective under the conditions of challenge being encountered. Cytokines classified as innate are those made by nonimmune cells or cells of the innate immune system. Some of these can access antimicrobial defense pathways in virtually every different kind of nucleated cell. In addition, they can activate other downstream effector mechanisms by inducing responses in cells of the innate immune system such as monocytic cells, natural killer (NK) cells, polymorphonuclear leukocytes, and dendritic cells (DCs) and in T and B lymphocytes of the adaptive immune system.

A variety of overlapping innate cytokine responses are induced during particular viral infections and infections with nonviral agents including certain bacteria and intracellular protozoan, but not extracellular, parasites (Fig. 1). These include tumor necrosis factor alpha (TNF-α), interleukin-12 (IL-12), and gamma interferon (IFN-γ). A characteristic of viral infections, however, which might predispose them to readily induce and be sensitive to a different subset of innate and adaptive immune responses, is the nature of their protein production and replication through the cytoplasm of infected host cells. Initial responses to challenge with a variety of viruses include several direct intracellular pathways to induction of the innate IFNs, i.e., IFN-α/β (Biron and

Sen, in press; Pfeffer et al., 1998). There are indications that IFN-α/β may be induced and function in innate immunity during certain nonviral infections (Ballas et al., 1996; Diefenbach et al., 1998; Tokunaga et al., 1992), but prominent systemic early IFN-α/β responses appear to be a unique or uniquely dominant characteristic of conditions during many viral infections. Moreover, certain of the effects induced by IFN-α/β are particularly important for antiviral defense. Taken together with the role of IFN-α/β in promoting expression of the class I major histocompatibility (MHC) molecules, which are important for the presentation of cytoplasmic antigens to CD8 T cells, and the contribution of CD8 T lymphocyte responses to resistance, a potential cascade of innate to adaptive immune responses particular to and directed by initial IFN-α/β induction during viral infections is suggested.

This chapter reviews current understanding of the induction and function of innate immune responses to viral infections. The focus is on the characteristics unique to or best characterized in the context of viral rather than nonviral infections. The material has been organized into six sections. The first reviews the literature on induction of innate cytokine proteins during in vivo infections. The second presents the known molecular pathways to cytokine induction. The third is an overview of biochemical pathways activated by key innate cytokines. The last three sections integrate this information to examine functions of innate cytokines in regulating endogenous immune responses, the accessing of innate cytokines by adaptive immune responses, and the contributions of innate cytokines to viral pathogenesis. In considering these materials, the reader should keep in mind the limitations restricting the synthesis of information. It is sobering to realize the influences,

Christine A. Biron, Marc Dalod, and Thais P. Salazar-Mather • Department of Molecular Microbiology and Immunology, Division of Biology and Medicine, Brown University, Providence, RI 02912.

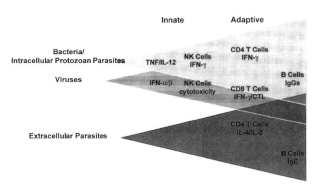

Figure 1. Distinguishing features of general pathways of innate to adaptive immune responses during infections with viruses, bacteria and intracellular protozoa, and parasites. Initial host cytokine responses to infectious agents are induced as a result of recognition, by specific receptors expressed in or on host cells, of unique microbial structures. Many viral infections induce innate cytokine responses overlapping with those seen during infections with bacteria or intracellular protozoa. These include IL-12 and NK-cell IFN-γ production, responses important for promoting downstream Th1-type responses with CD4 T-cell IFN-γ production. Responses to viruses can have dominant early IFN-α/β production induced by unique viral products. This response is associated with NK cell cytotoxicity but not IFN-γ production. There are prominent downstream CD8 T-cell responses including IFN-γ production and cytotoxic T-lymphocyte (CTL) function during many viral infections. Challenges with certain organisms of the viral, bacterial, or protozoan parasite classes also induce the proinflammatory cytokine cascade including TNF. Responses to extracellular parasites fail to elicit an early IL-12 production and are linked to Th2 responses with CD4 T-cell IL-4 and IL-5 production. The patterns are idealized, and there can be overlap. Ig, immunoglobulin. Adapted from Biron and Sen, 2001.

on the questions asked or not asked, resulting from the history of scientific research and the ease of approach for study. It is not always possible to directly compare responses and effects because the same studies simply have not been done. Moreover, innate immune responses to the pressures of assault by infectious agents are likely to be shaped by availability as well as efficacy of working components. It is unlikely that the pathways seeming most rational or functional to immunologists are always the ones selected during evolution of immune responses.

INNATE CYTOKINE RESPONSES TO VIRAL INFECTIONS

Studies of virus-induced innate cytokine expression and function in the context of a complete immune system generally have been done in the mouse. This is because it is difficult to detect the early phases of infections in humans. Indeed, most of the results on natural primary infections of humans are obtained at times after onset of illness when T cells are already

activated. T cells can produce certain cytokines identified as innate, i.e., IFN-γ and TNF-α, and their responses contribute at least in part to the expression of these factors at such times. There are a few reports of early responses during viral infections of nonhuman primates and during early phases after vaccination or challenge of humans with attenuated viruses. An overview, provided by the most informative reports, quantitating levels of protein production of innate cytokine responses during viral infections in mice, nonhuman primates, and humans is discussed below and presented in Table 1.

IFN-α/β Responses

The IFN-α/β gene family is composed of one IFN-β gene and multiple IFN-α genes (Biron and Sen, 2001; Pfeffer et al., 1998). If appropriately stimulated, any nucleated cell can make IFN-α/β. Viruses vary, however, both in their ability to induce IFN-α/β and in their sensitivity to the antiviral functions activated by these cytokines. Respiratory syncytial virus (RSV) is an example of a poor IFN inducer in culture (Chonmaitree et al., 1981; Roberts et al., 1992). In vivo, IFN-α/β are induced early after the onset of most of the mouse, nonhuman primate, and human viral infections studied to date. However, the more extensive studies of mouse infections indicate that the levels of induction vary widely depending on the agent used, the genetic background and age of the host, the dose and mode of inoculations, and the compartment examined. IFN-α/β and their functions are necessary for protection against replication of the virus, disease, and/or death during many viral infections in the mouse (Cousens et al., 1999; Muller et al., 1994; Ryman et al., 2000; van den Broek et al., 1995). The mechanisms for these effects, however, are incompletely understood. As discussed below, IFN-α/β can mediate a variety of functions and the protective effects could be delivered at the level of activation of antiviral mechanisms or of promotion of secondary immune defense pathways. Additionally or alternatively, they could result from limiting the spread of infection to different cell types. Extension of cell tropism and altered tissue distribution have been observed after blocking of endogenous IFN-α/β functions during infections of mice with lymphocytic choriomeningitis virus (LCMV) (Sandberg et al., 1994), influenza virus (Garcia-Sastre et al., 1998), herpes simplex virus (HSV) (Leib et al., 1999), and Sindbis virus (Ryman et al., 2000). In the last three infections, a change in tropism is observed as increases in the frequencies of infected macrophages and/or DCs. Such altered tropism might occur because increased viral replica-

Table 1. In vivo induction of innate cytokine protein expression early during viral infections

Species	Virus	Cytokine response		Remarks	References
		Detected	Not detected		
Mouse	MCMV	IFN-α/β, TNF-α, IL-1, IL-6, IL-12, IFN-γ, IL-18		This model of innate immune responses during virus infection is the best characterized one, with detailed studies of the kinetics of cytokine production early after infection in different compartments and analysis of their role in promoting local IFN-γ secretion by NK cells and protection from disease.	Grundy et al. (1982), Orange et al. (1995b, 1997), Orange and Biron (1996a, 1996b), Pien et al. (2000), Ruzek (1997, 1999), Salazar-Mather et al. (1996, 1998, 2000)
	LCMV	IFN-α/β	TNF-α,[a] IL-6,[a] IL-12, IFN-γ	IFN-α/β are inhibiting IL-12 expression and downstream IFN-γ production. Serum TNF-α and IFN-γ responses are low at very early times during infections with different strains, but there is variability between strains at later times.	Bukowski et al. (1983), Cousens et al. (1997), Muller et al. (1994), Orange and Biron (1996a), Salazar-Mather et al. (1996), Welsh (1978)
	Influenza virus	IFN-α/β, TNF-α, IL-1, IL-6, IL-12, IFN-γ		Cytokines are detectable between 1.5 and 4 days in bronchoalveolar lavage fluid but not in serum.	Conn et al. (1995), Hennet et al. (1992), Monteiro et al. (1998), Vackeron et al. (1990)
	Sindbis virus (neonatal)	IFN-α/β, TNF-α, IL-6, IFN-γ		Infection of neonatal immunocompetent mice leads to toxic shock with production of very high levels of cytokines in the serum and death before day 3.	Klimstra et al. (1999)
	Sindbis virus (adult)	IFN-α/β	TNF-α, IL-6, IL-12, IFN-γ	IFN-α/β are critical for protection against disease in adult mice. In the absence of their functions, high levels of TNF-α, IL-6, IL-12, and IFN-γ in serum are observed.	Ryman et al. (2000), Trgovcich et al. (1999), Viljeck (1964)
	HSV	IFN-α/β, IL-6, IL-12, IFN-γ		The major producers of IFN-α/β in the spleen of mice injected with UV-inactivated HSV are marginal metallophilic macrophages and marginal zone macrophages.	Eloranta and Alm (1999), He et al. (1999), Kanangat et al. (1996)
	RSV	IFN-γ		NK cells are the major producers of IFN-γ early after infection, and their accumulation in the lungs is correlated with the later recruitment of CD8 T cells in the absence of eosinophils	Hussell and Openshaw (1998)

Continued on following page

Table 1. In vivo induction of innate cytokine protein expression early during viral infections (*continued*)

Species	Virus	Cytokine response		Remarks	References
		Detected	Not detected		
Nonhuman primate macaque	SIV	IFN-α/β, TNF-α, IL-12, IFN-γ, IL-18		IFN-α/β is the first cytokine detectable in serum. The increase in IL-12 levels is only moderate and correlates inversely with IFN-α levels. IFN-γ and TNF-α are not always detected and are found only later on, when CD8 T cells are already activated.	Clayette et al. (1995), Giavedoni et al. (2000), Khatissian et al. (1996), Rosenberg et al. (1997)
baboon	Ebola virus	IFN-α/β, TNF-α		High levels of IFN-α and TNF-α in serum are detected and correlate with the severity of the pathological coagulation.	Ignatiev et al. (2000)
Human	Ebola virus	IFN-α/β, TNF-α, IL-1, IL-6, IL-12, IFN-γ, IL-18		Patients with fatal hemorrhagic fever versus asymptomatic infection have opposite patterns of cytokine levels in serum (IFN-γ high, TNF-α and IFN-α variable, no IL-6 versus IL-6, IL-1 and TNF-α high, no IFN-α, IL-12, and IFN-γ).	Leroy et al. (2000), Villinger et al. (1999)
	CMV	TNF-α, IL-6		Allogeneic bone marrow transplant patients with active CMV disease have significantly higher levels of serum IL-6 than patients who do not develop CMV disease.	Humar et al. (1999)
	Influenza virus	IFN-α/β, TNF-α, IL-6		Low levels of IFN-α/β, TNF-α, and IL-6 are detectable in nasal lavage fluid and in serum at early time after experimental influenza virus infection with a relatively mild virus. Levels of IFN-α/β measured in serum are lower than those reported earlier during natural infection.	Green et al. (1982), Hayden et al. (1998)
	HSV	IFN-α/β, TNF-α, IL-1, IL-6, IL-12, IFN-γ		These studies measure the early kinetics of cytokine production in vesicle fluid of recurrent herpetic lesions.	Mikloska et al. (1998), Torseth et al. (1987)
	RSV	IFN-α/β, TNF-α, IL-1, IL-6, IL-12		RSV has been reported to be a poor inducer of IFN-α/β in vitro. IFN-α/β are detected in the serum or nasal lavage fluid from infected infants in some but not all studies. IL-12 is reported to be induced during infection, but lower basal levels correlate with increased severity of disease.	Blanco-Quiros et al. (1999), Hall et al. (1978), Nakayama et al. (1993), Noah et al. (1995), Roberts et al. (1992)

Virus	Cytokines		Comments	References
EBV	IFN-α/β, TNF-α, IL-1, IFN-γ, IL-18	IL-6	In a case report, IFN-α/β is detected in serum very early after infection, before the onset of symptoms. No IFN-α/β is detected, but increased levels of IFN-γ, TNF-α, IL-1, and IL-18 are observed in other studies in patients enrolled later on, at the time of overt infectious mononucleosis, when CD8 T cells are already activated.	Biglino et al. (1996), Brewster et al. (1985), Linde et al. (1992), Setsuda et al. (1999), Svedmyr et al. (1984), Wright-Brown et al. (1998)
HIV	IFN-α/β, TNF-α, IL-1, IFN-γ	IL-6	Most of the studies have been performed in patients at or after the onset of symptoms, at a time when CD8 T cells are already activated. The levels of IFN-α/β and proinflammatory cytokines in serum are sustained or increase further with progression of the infection, and IL-6 becomes detectable in some patients, whereas defects in IL-12 and IFN-α/β production after in vitro restimulation have been described.	Biglino et al. (1996), Ferbas et al. (1995), Gaines et al. (1990), Gray et al. (1996), Marshall et al. (1999), Rizzardi et al. (1996), Sinicco et al. (1993)
Yellow fever virus	IFN-α/β, TNF-α	IFN-γ	These studies measure different immunological parameters at early times after vaccination. TNF-α is not detected in one study, and very low increases are observed in another.	Hacker et al. (1998), Reinhardt et al. (1998), Wheelock and Sibley (1965)
Dengue virus	IFN-α/β, TNF-α, IL-6, IL-12, IFN-γ, IL-18	IL-1	General increases are observed in proinflammatory cytokine levels except for IL-1 during early dengue virus infection. Patients with dengue hemorrhagic fever have higher levels of IFN-γ, TNF-α, and IL-18 in serum than do individuals with dengue fever, whereas the reverse is true for IL-12.	Chaturvedi et al. (2000), Green et al. (1999), Kurane et al. (1993)
Hantavirus	TNF-α, IL-1, IL-6, IFN-γ		These studies have been performed in patients at or after the onset of symptoms, at a time when T lymphocytes are already activated. The frequency of cells producing proinflammatory cytokines is especially elevated in the lungs and spleens of patients who died from hantavirus pulmonary syndrome.	Kanerva et al. (1998), Krakauer et al. (1995), Linderholm et al., (1996), Mori et al. (1999)

[a] C. A. Biron and M. C. Ruzek, unpublished data.

tion would be accompanied by generation of higher proportions of mutants with enhanced capabilities for replication in these different cell types. However, it has recently been shown that some DC lineage cells are major producers of IFN-α/β in humans. Therefore, an important mechanism in place to protect DCs from a natural vulnerability to viral infection would be lost if IFN-α/β functions are inhibited. In addition to interfering with antigen presentation for the development of protective adaptive immune responses, targeting of macrophages and DCs for infection might result in induction of other innate cytokines associated with more problematic consequences to the host. Thus, there are many mechanisms by which IFN-α/β can promote disease resistance during viral infections.

On the other hand, there are examples of correlations between IFN-α/β levels and disease severity. In nonhuman primates and in humans, high levels of IFN-α/β in serum are associated with a bad clinical outcome in acute Ebola virus (Ignatiev et al., 2000) and chronic human immunodeficiency virus (HIV) (Poli et al., 1994) infections. Based on such observation, IFN-α/β have been proposed to play a role in the immunopathogenesis of these infections, but no direct evidence has been obtained in this regard. Indeed, in mice infected with Sindbis virus, IFN-α/β are critical for protection against disease, even though there is a positive correlation between levels of IFN-α/β in serum and virus load (Ryman et al., 2000; Trgovcich et al., 1999). Moreover, in LCMV infections of mice, there are IFN-α/β effects in promoting lethal disease following intracranial infections. These have been suggested to result from an IFN-α/β-mediated inhibition of viral spread such that organism replication and T-cell responses are concentrated in the brain to result in a life-endangering T-cell-mediated immunopathology (Sandberg et al., 1994).

TNF-α, IL-1, and IL-6 Responses

Innate immune cells can make the proinflammatory cytokines TNF-α, IL-1, and IL-6. Certain nonimmune cells, such as vascular endothelial cells, can also produce them, but to different degrees. They can be detected early in most but not all viral infections. Their common kinetics of expression may be explained in part by shared regulatory pathways governing their induction and synthesis. Only LCMV in the mouse (C. Biron et al., unpublished data) and yellow fever virus in the human (Reinhardt et al., 1998) have been reported to be poor inducers of TNF-α. The mechanisms presiding over the different patterns of cytokine secretion in different host-virus

combinations are not well understood. They might be accounted for, in part, by different cell tropism of the viruses, especially by their respective abilities to infect macrophages and DCs, known major producers of proinflammatory cytokines. Because certain cytokines inhibit or enhance the expression of other cytokines, however, there also is likely to be significant cross-regulation shaping the composition of the overall cytokine responses to particular viruses. These two mechanisms may contribute to the very large amounts of proinflammatory cytokines observed during Sindbis virus infections of adult mice having had the IFN-α/β response neutralized (Ryman et al., 2000) because a consequence is a change in cell tropism and because IFN-α/β can inhibit expression of certain other innate cytokine responses (see below). In addition, in vitro studies have shown that particular viruses have specific molecular pathways to activate or inhibit the production of specific cytokines in infected cells. Finally, the genetics of the hosts must also be taken in account. Different strains of normal mice have different susceptibilities to the same virus infections, and this can be linked to qualitative or quantitative changes in the innate cytokine responses. Although several factors may contribute to the differences in cytokine expression, it has been reported that the allele for high production of TNF-α in humans may increase the susceptibility to developing severe nephropathia epidemica after infection with the hantavirus Puumala virus (Kanerva et al., 1998).

The very high levels of secretion of TNF-α, IL-1, and IL-6 observed in mouse Sindbis virus and human hantavirus or dengue virus infections have been implicated in the immunopathogenesis of the corresponding diseases. By contrast, a recent report suggests that early production of these cytokines, especially IL-6, may participate in the protection against hemorrhagic fever during Ebola virus infection in humans (Leroy et al., 2000). The ability of IL-6 to induce secretion of glucocorticoids (GCs) and therefore limit the extent of the pathologic inflammatory reactions, as demonstrated in mice infected with murine cytomegalovirus (MCMV) (Ruzek et al., 1997, 1999), may contribute to such a protective effect.

Other Innate Cytokine Responses

NK cells are a primary source of innate IFN-γ. IL-12 can be produced by a variety of innate immune cells including monocytic cells, polymorphonuclear leukocytes, and DCs. Early IFN-γ secretion has been found in many mouse and human viral infections. Where characterized, it depends on upstream IL-12 production (Biron et al., 1999). This pathway is inhibited by IFN-α/β during LCMV infection in the mouse (Cousens et al., 1997, 1999; Nguyen et al., 2000). Early IFN-γ production has also been reported to be lacking in one recent study of acute simian immunodeficiency virus infection even in the face of a weak induction of IL-12 (Giavedoni et al., 2000), but this observation remains controversial. Human volunteers vaccinated with yellow fever virus (Reinhardt et al., 1998) and individuals with asymptomatic Ebola virus infections (Leroy et al., 2000) do not have detectable levels of IFN-γ in serum. Most other studies of primary virus infections in humans have been performed at or after the onset of illness, at a time when the T lymphocytes are activated and contribute at least in part to the production of the IFN-γ observed. Therefore, additional studies of earlier time points during viral infections of monkeys or vaccination of volunteers with attenuated viruses will be necessary to better evaluate the innate cytokine responses in primates. It has been shown recently that the CD8 T-cell responses in HIV primary infection are weak, especially compared to those elicited during acute Epstein-Barr virus (EBV) infection (Dalod et al., 1999a). These different profiles of acquired immune responses in primary acute HIV and EBV infection may result from different innate cytokine responses. It is important, therefore, to analyze patterns of the very earliest innate immune responses to these agents after infections of monkeys identified as susceptible or resistant to SIV or HIV infection.

Little is known about the induction of two more recently described innate cytokines, i.e., IL-18 (Akira, 2000; Lebel-Binay et al., 2000) and IL-15 (Fehniger and Caligiuri, 2001; Waldmann and Tagaya, 1999). IL-18 is induced and functions to promote NK cell IFN-γ responses in some but not all compartments during MCMV infection (Pien et al., 2000). Monocytic cells are known to be able to produce these factors. IL-15, at least, is also made by other non-immune cell populations. Both cytokines are sometimes expressed at times overlapping with the proinflammatory cytokine responses to bacteria or bacterial products.

PATHWAYS INDUCING INNATE CYTOKINE RESPONSES

Much work has been done characterizing the virus-activated molecular pathways to induction of IFN-α/β. Less is known about the virus-induced mechanisms promoting other innate cytokine responses. The converse is true concerning responses to bacterial infections.

IFN-α/β

The large IFN-α/β gene family is likely to be in place to access or allow induction under a variety of conditions. Regulation of these genes is complex. The interaction of certain viruses with their cell surface receptors for infection may induce the production of IFN-α/β (Biron and Sen, 2001). There are, however, other intracellular receptors for viral products specifically linked to IFN-α/β induction. Certain viral infections induce the intracellular activation of a particular complex, called virus-activated factor, thought to be important for IFN-β expression because of its binding to the regulatory sequences of the gene (Wathelet et al., 1998). Double-stranded RNA (dsRNA), expressed as a result of viral replication in infected cells but not found in uninfected cells, is the oldest known and a potent inducer of IFN-α/β expression (Biron and Sen, 2001). Although a number of events may be in place to facilitate the process, protein kinase R (PKR) activation as a result of binding the dsRNA and effects on the IκB kinase complex have been demonstrated to promote activation of the NF-κB transcription factor. NF-κB is one of the factors required for inducing the IFN-β and certain IFN-α genes. Other activated factors needed constitute the family of interferon-regulatory factors (IRFs). One of these, IRF-3, is ubiquitous in uninfected cells and is used to directly promote IFN gene expression under conditions of challenge with particular viruses and/or viral products. Such pathways induce the expression of IFN-β and particular IFN-α genes. Remarkably, the first IFN protein products then act through the IFN-α/β receptor (IFN-α/βR) and its signaling pathways to promote the expression of another IRF molecule, IRF-7, and induce downstream activation of other IFN-α genes (Erlandsson et al., 1998; Juang et al., 1998; Marie et al., 1998). This mechanism appears to be important for in vivo magnitude of the overall IFN-α/β response, at least in the context of vaccinia virus (VV) infections of mice (Deonarain et al., 2000). Thus, there is an IFN-α/β–to–IFN-α/β cascade. This is presumably an amplification pathway for expression of these factors. Given that virtually all nucleated cells express IFN-α/βRs, such an amplification pathway is likely to be a major contributor to the magnitude of IFN-α/β responses elicited during viral infections directly inducing first IFN gene targets for expression. It is also likely to be very important for accessing antiviral defense mechanisms to protect the host.

DCs can produce IFN-α after exposure to a wide range of viruses. The response is not necessarily a result of infection, because mannose receptors, which play an important role in antigen capture by DCs, are required for the human DC responses to HSV, HIV, and influenza virus (Milone and Fitzgerald-Bocarsly, 1998). In contrast, Sendai virus induction of IFN-α expression occurs primarily through monocyte responses and does not appear to be mannose receptor dependent. DCs can also be directly stimulated through their CD40 molecules to express IFN-α (Cella et al., 1999). Thus, there are different cell surface receptors on DCs linked to IFN-α induction, and these receptors may function to induce this innate cytokine response under a variety of conditions in addition to viral infections. The DC IFN-α response contribution to overall IFN-α/β-mediated antiviral defense might be very small because all cells infected with viruses can produce the cytokines and many other cell types can be targets for infections. Given that DC IFN-α responses are very profound, however, they could specifically act to protect DCs and neighboring lymphocytes from infection while DCs are taking up viruses for antigen processing and presentation. The infection-independent pathways also have the potential to be important for inducing IFN-α during challenges not able to access other pathways of IFN-α/β induction, either viral or nonviral, and for activating DC IFN-α production to shape downstream adaptive immune responses (see below).

Other Cytokines

Much less is known about the molecular pathways accessed by viral products for induction of the other innate cytokines. Where characterized, an IL-12 response is required for innate IFN-γ induction. TNF-α, IL-6, and IL-1 can be induced as a cascade because TNF-α can promote IL-1 and IL-6 induction and IL-1 can enhance IL-6 production. Activated NF-κB can contribute to the transcription of a number of proinflammatory cytokines including TNF-α (Chandel et al., 2000). Thus, one of the aforementioned pathways, i.e., dsRNA working through PKR for NF-κB activation, has the potential to enhance the expression of many other innate cytokines. This may suggest a lack of specificity for IFN-α/β induction by the virus-induced signaling pathway. There are examples, however, of infections with high induction of an early systemic IFN-α/β without a significant TNF-α response (Table 1). The understanding of the many interactions with transcription factors and the positive or negative consequences of such interactions at different cytokine

gene regulatory regions is still limited. A number of different transcription factors are required for optimal gene expression, and the composite is likely to be different for different genes and/or in the context of exposure of different cell types or different mixtures of cytokines. NF-κB is just one piece of the puzzle. Nevertheless, it is interesting that EBV LMP1 acts to induce IL-12p40 and IL-12p35 gene expression and that there is evidence for NF-κB function in induction of at least the p40 chain (Yoshimoto et al., 1998). Furthermore, the IL-15 gene has an NF-κB motif in its regulatory region, and the human T-cell lymphotropic virus type 1 Tax protein accesses a direct pathway to the activation of IL-15 by working through this site (Azimi et al., 1998). The pathway does not appear to reflect an innate defense response but, rather, the usurpation of an innate response by the virus to promote its replication. The effect contributes to the lymphoproliferative aspects of human T-cell lymphotropic virus type 1 pathogenesis (Azimi et al., 1999). The HIV Nef protein also is reported to induce IL-15, along with TNF-α, IL-6, and IFN-γ (Quaranta et al., 1999), but the molecular intermediates contributing to the induction of these responses are not characterized.

DIRECT PATHWAYS USED BY INNATE CYTOKINE RESPONSES: MOLECULAR TARGETS FOR ANTIVIRAL FUNCTIONS, CYTOKINE/CHEMOKINE REGULATION, AND ANTIGEN PRESENTATION

The molecular pathways used by cytokines to mediate biological functions are being characterized at an extraordinary rate. Nevertheless, our understanding of the fast array of downstream effects and the complexities of their regulation in the context of the mixed cytokine responses elicited in vivo is only superficially understood. A few of the best-characterized mechanisms, with high known or potential relevance to viral infections, are reviewed below. In particular, pathways and effects activated by IFN-α/β and IFN-γ are discussed in some detail (Fig. 2). Remarkably, most cells express receptors for both types of IFNs. Thus, these factors affect a wide range of cell types. Moreover, they can modify the expression of large numbers of genes; gene array technology suggests that these might number in the hundreds (Der et al., 1998). Some of these are directly induced by activation of preexisting factors to facilitate the expression of gene targets with particular regulatory sequences. Others are induced in cascades initiated by the first direct products.

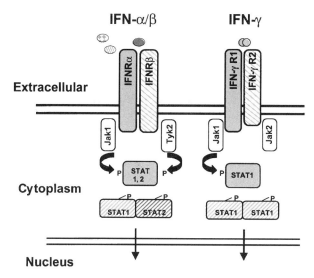

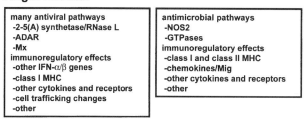

Figure 2. Simplified model of the pathways for signaling through the IFN-α/β and IFN-γ receptors to reach major target responses. There are specific heterodimeric receptors for these cytokines. These are linked to particular but overlapping kinases and STAT molecules to transmit the signal from cytokine exposure to the nucleus of the cell. IFN-α/β are particularly effective at activating a number of well-characterized biochemical pathways blocking viral replication. These include the 2-5(A) synthetase/RNase L system, ADAR, and Mx proteins. A variety of immunoregulatory effects also appear to be preferentially elicited in response to IFN-α/β compared to IFN-γ. These are up-regulation of other IFN-α/β genes. IFN-γ appears to be particularly effective at inducing NOS2 and a family of GTPases with antimicrobial functions. It also has unique function for promoting antigen-processing and presentation pathways to both class I and class II MHC molecules and inducing the expression of a variety of chemokines including Mig.

Signaling

IFN-α/β

The major effects induced by IFN-α/β result from binding to a specific heterodimeric receptor, with activation of the tyrosine kinases Tyk2 and Jak1 (Biron and Sen, 2001; Darnell et al., 1994; Ihle, 1995; Stark et al., 1998). These events precipitate activation, by phosphorylation, of signal-transducing proteins for gene induction. The most important mediators of IFN-α/β effects appear to be the signal

transducers and activators of transcription (STATs) STAT1 and STAT2. However, there are indications that a number of other pathways can be induced, including pathways through STAT4, particularly in the human (Cho et al., 1996; Farrar et al., 2000; Rogge et al., 1998), and the mitogen-activated protein kinase pathways. Phosphorylated STAT1-STAT2 heterodimers move from the cytoplasm to the nucleus. They form complexes with a specific member of the family of IRFs, identified as P48, to interact with the IFN-stimulated response elements (ISRE) in regulatory regions of IFN-α/β-inducible genes. The issue of STAT4 activation is important because STAT4 is a significant contributor to IFN-γ expression in response to IL-12 (Cho et al., 1996; Murphy et al., 2000). Thus, STAT4 activation may link IFN-α/β to IFN-γ expression and to downstream consequences activated by IFN-γ. The difference in ready activation of STAT4 by IFN-α/β in human compared to mouse cells is, at least in part, a result of difference in the STAT2 molecule produced by the two different species (Farrar et al., 2000).

IFN-γ

The IFN-γ receptor is a heterodimer with components specific for binding IFN-γ (Biron and Sen, 2001; Darnell et al., 1994; Ihle, 1995; Stark et al., 1998). These molecules use the Jak1 and Jak2 kinases to induce STAT1 phosphorylation. Phosphorylated STAT1 homodimers translocate to the nucleus to bind to gamma-activated sequences in regulatory regions of IFN-γ-inducible genes. Although this is the major pathway, IFN-γ can signal to the ISRE elements less effectively than IFN-α/β through undetermined *trans*-activating factors. Likewise, although ISRE is a major target for IFN-α/β-induced effects, STAT1 homodimers can be formed and bind to gamma-activated sequence elements during IFN-α/β signaling. These secondary pathways provide an explanation, in addition to possible induction of IFN-γ by IFN-α/β, of some of the redundancy of function observed with the two different types of IFNs.

Fine-tuning of responses

There are three requirements for any cytokine to mediate effects: (i) the protein has to be induced, (ii) specific cytokine receptors have to be present on the target cell(s), and (iii) appropriate intracellular signaling molecules must be present. Although there are a few well-described pathways for IFN signaling, our understanding of how these work in total during responses to infectious challenges is limited. This point has been recently highlighted by the demonstration of STAT1-dependent negative regulation of responses. A consequence of the phenomenon is that new IFN-α/β effects in the mouse, including induction of IFN-γ (Nguyen et al., 2000), and IFN-γ effects in human cells, including induction of the c-myc factor promoting cell proliferation (Ramana et al., 2000), have been revealed in the absence of STAT1. These results indicate that there must be STAT1-independent signaling pathways to IFN-α/β- and IFN-γ-mediated effects and that regulation of STAT1 levels or functions might change the consequences of exposure to these cytokines. In a broader view, they also suggest that the availability or ratio of particular signaling components in the cell might qualitatively regulate the downstream responses to any cytokine. Thus, much remains to be learned about the many effects induced by particular cytokines and how these might be regulated in the context of the complexities of endogenous immune responses to infections.

IFN-α/β Effects

Antiviral functions

A number of IFN-α/β-activated biochemical pathways to antiviral functions have been well characterized for some time, and others continue to be delineated (Biron and Sen, in press). Three of these pathways result in either inhibited or altered protein synthesis and use the binding of dsRNA as second regulators or substrates. The first pathway is initiated by IFN-α/β induction of 2-5(A) synthetases. Once activated by binding of dsRNA, these enzymes produce 2'-5' oligoadenylates to activate a latent RNase, identified as RNase L, which in turn cleaves viral and cellular RNAs to inhibit protein synthesis and viral replication. The second pathway is promoted by IFN-α/β-elicited enhancement of PKR expression. Upon binding of the dsRNA, this enzyme is activated to phosphorylate itself and then other proteins including the translation initiation factor eIF-2α. Phosphorylation of eIF-2α also inhibits protein synthesis and viral replication. The third is accessed by IFN-α/β induction of the dsRNA-specific adenosine deaminase ADAR. This enzyme uses dsRNA to catalyze the deamination of adenosine to iosine in viral and cellular RNAs. Such site-specific editing can result in the synthesis of proteins with altered functions. Other IFN-α/β-elicited pathways access members of a superfamily of GTPases involved in endocytosis and vesicle transport. These guanylate binding proteins, Mx and other related molecules, appear to be very effective at inhibiting the replication of a subset of RNA viruses. The mechanism of action is inhibition of viral nucleocapsid transport in the cell.

Cytokine regulation

IFN-α/β regulate the expression of a number of different cytokines and cytokine receptors. As stated above, after induction of IFN-β or particular IFN-α genes in response to challenge conditions, their products can access the IFN-α/β receptors to induce the expression of other members of the IFN-α/β family. The IL-15 gene also has been reported to be induced under conditions of exposure to IFN-α/β or chemical inducers of IFN-α/β (Durbin et al., 2000; Zhang et al., 1998). Constitutive IL-15 expression is dependent on IRF-1, and this molecule can be activated by stimulation with IFN-α/β or IFN-γ (Waldmann and Tagaya, 1999). Thus, there is the potential for IFNs to induce IL-15, but definitive demonstration of such a pathway requires characterization of IL-15 protein production.

The effects of IFNs on IL-12 expression and function as well as IFN-γ expression are complex. Extended expression of the heterodimeric high affinity receptor for IL-12 is promoted by IFN-α/β or IFN-γ in the human (Gollob et al., 1997; Rogge et al., 1997) and IFN-γ in the mouse (Szabo et al., 1997a). These effects may facilitate the induction of Th1-type responses by helping to maintain IL-12 responsiveness and downstream IL-12 induction of CD4 T cells expressing IFN-γ. Consistent with the changes in receptor expression, IFN-γ enhances the expression of the IL-12 p40 chain (Trinchieri, 1998). At high concentrations, however, the IFN-α/β cytokines inhibit the expression of IL-12 in both the mouse (Cousens, 1997) and the human (Karp et al., 2000; McRae et al., 1998). Moreover, the levels induced at early times during LCMV infections of mice also induce a state of NK cell refractoriness to IL-12 for IFN-γ stimulation despite the preservation of expression of the heterodimeric high-affinity IL-12 receptor (Nguyen et al., 2000; Pien and Biron, 2000). Thus, there appear to be pathways used by high conditions of IFN-α/β to limit IL-12 and its effects. On the other hand, the IFN-α/β cytokines promote IFN-γ expression by human T cells under a variety of culture conditions (Brinkmann et al., 1993; Manetti et al., 1995; Sareneva et al., 1998) and by mouse CD8 T cells activated in vivo during LCMV infections (Cousens et al., 1999). Thus, there are contrasting effects of IFN-α/β for IL-12 and IFN-γ responses, and these are in part a result of effects mediated by differences in concentrations and differences in states or phenotypes of target cells examined.

Antigen presentation

IFN-α/β have long been known to enhance the expression of the class I major histocompatibility (MHC) molecules (Boehm et al., 1997; Lindahl et al., 1976). Since antigen presentation by these molecules is important for activation of CD8 T cell responses, such a function might facilitate CD8 T-cell responses to viral infections.

IFN-γ Effects

Antiviral functions

IFN-γ is likely to access a variety of antiviral defense pathways, including those also accessed by IFN-α/β. Some, however, appear to be more readily activated by IFN-γ. Others have been studied only in the context of IFN-γ induction and await analysis following IFN-α/β exposure. The best-characterized pathways activated by IFN-γ are mediated as a result of induction of the enzyme nitric oxide synthase 2 (NOS2), also known as inducible nitric oxide synthase (MacMicking et al., 1997). IFN-γ is a potent inducer of this enzyme, but a number of different stimuli, including TNF-α alone or in synergy with IFN-α/β, also promote its expression. Once induced in activated macrophages, NOS2 facilitates a wide range of antimicrobial functions by catalyzing the production of nitric oxide (NO), which in turn can react with oxygen to yield other reactive molecules. These products mediate antiviral activity by chemically modifying proteins essential to viral functions. In addition to NOS2, there is a growing list of IFN-γ-inducible genes and molecules with homologies to GTPases and their genes (Carlow et al., 1998; Taylor et al., 1996, 2000). Certain of these are also induced by IFN-α/β (Carlow et al., 1998). To date, only two of these molecules have been characterized for antimicrobial function. One appears to be essential for defense against a protozoan parasitic infection but not for resistance to several different viral infections in vivo (Taylor et al., 2000). Another appears to confer resistance to vesicular stomatitis virus but not HSV in a culture system (Carlow et al., 1998). Given the number of these genes, the variety of viral pathogens, and the known antiviral functions of the Mx GTPases, many more antiviral functions are likely to be found for at least some of the products of these genes.

Cytokine regulation

As stated above, IFN-γ can promote the expression and function of IL-12. It also can enhance TNF responses by up-regulating TNF receptors. Interesting new information is available on the importance of IFN-γ for the induction of a subset of the low-molecular-weight chemotactic cytokines, i.e., chemokines. In particular, the monokine induced by IFN-γ (Mig), the IFN-induced protein of 10 kDa (IP-10), and interferon-inducible T-cell α chemoattractant (I-TAC) are induced by IFN-γ (Khan et al., 2000; Rossi and Zlotnik, 2000; Salazar-Mather et al., 2000). IP-10 and I-TAC can also be induced by cytokines other than IFN-γ, such as IFN-α/β and TNF-α, whereas the Mig gene has unique regulatory sequences with a stringent and specific requirement for IFN-γ induction (Farber, 1990; Wong et al., 1994; Wright and Farber, 1991). A common receptor is used by all of these chemokines and is expressed on activated lymphocytes. Thus, induction of the Mig, IP-10, and I-TAC chemokines in infected tissues may direct recruitment of activated cells to deliver antiviral effector mechanisms.

Antigen presentation

IFN-γ can induce the expression of class II as well as class I MHC molecules (Boehm et al., 1997; Fruh and Yang, 1999). The effects on class II expression would promote CD4 T-cell responses. IFN-γ does this by enhancing a number of accessory molecules involved in class II expression and function, including (i) the transcription factor CIITA required for expression of the class II complex genes, (ii) the invariant-chain protein and the two DM proteins promoting assembly and maturation of the class II complex, and (iii) the cathepsins thought to promote the processing of exogenous proteins into peptides for presentation. Interestingly, although both IFN-α/β and IFN-γ can induce the expression of class I molecules, IFN-γ appears to have unique or more extensive functions for induction of subunits of the proteasome-processing endogenous proteins into peptides for class I presentation, i.e., LMP-2 and LMP-7, and the proteasome regulator PA28 (Fruh and Yang, 1999). It has also been reported to induce the expression of molecules promoting the transport of peptides to the endoplasmic reticulum for loading onto class I molecules. Thus, IFN-γ mediates a number of functions, which could act to enhance or modify antigen presentation for stimulation of CD8 T-cell responses.

Others

A number of other innate cytokines are known to mediate important antiviral and immune regulatory effects. TNF-α deserves special consideration.

There are different receptors for TNF, types 1 (TNFR1) and 2 (TNFR2), found on a wide range of cell types. The cytoplasmic tails of the two receptors are distinct and can plug into different intracellular signaling pathways (Biron and Sen, 2001). Although TNF-α can mediate cytotoxic and necrotic effects, its major function may be to enhance inflammation. It can, however, also mediate a variety of other functions important in defense against viral infections, including enhancement of IFN-γ responses, upregulation of class I MHC expression, and activation of certain antiviral pathways including NOS2 induction. If induced at high systemic levels, TNF-α can promote life-threatening toxic shock conditions.

SHAPING OF ENDOGENOUS IMMUNE RESPONSES BY INNATE CYTOKINE RESPONSES: INDUCTION OF INNATE AND ADAPTIVE CELLULAR RESPONSES, AND DELIVERY OF EFFECTOR FUNCTIONS

Innate Responses

Responses elicited by IFN-α/β

A number of other cellular responses are elicited during viral infections through IFN-α/β-dependent mechanisms. The cytokines are potent inducers of NK-cell-mediated cytotoxicity (Biron et al., 1999). Although these cells can lyse certain virus-infected cells, the evidence for importance of this pathway in antiviral defense is still limited. In MCMV infections, NK cell cytotoxicity may help control infection in the spleen (Tay and Welsh, 1997) but it is not a critical mediator of defense in the liver (Orange et al., 1995b, Orange and Biron, 1996b; Tay and Welsh, 1997). The localized requirement may be a result of the fact that in the presence of IFN-α/β, NK-cell responsiveness to IL-12 for IFN-γ production is sustained for only short periods in the spleen compared to the liver (Nguyen et al., 2000; Pien and Biron, 2000). Nevertheless, since NK cell cytotoxity is always observed with IFN-α/β induction in vivo and is induced during LCMV infections of mice with no demonstrable role for NK cells in antiviral defense, the response must play a biologically important role. One intriguing possibility is that NK-cell cytotoxicity directs or limits adaptive responses. The contention is supported by importance of the perforin molecule, required for lytic function of both NK and T cells, in protection against a rare and devastating disease associated with immune disregulation, familial hemophagocytic lymphohistiocytosis (Stepp et al., 1999). Remarkably, characteristics of this disease are seen less severely or with a later onset in different groups of patients with hemophagocytic lymphohistocytosis and can be precipitated by viral infections. Moreover, dramatic modifications in immune cell distribution, characterized as leukopenia with decreases in thoracic duct drainages but increases in lymph node cellularity and redistribution of nucleated cells from splenic red to white pulp regions, are also induced by IFN-α/β exposure in vivo (Biron et al., 1999; Ishikawa and Biron, 1993). These effects may be in place to localize the repertoire of T and B cells and peripheral DCs to specialized sites of antigen processing and presentation and/or to promote the subclasses of adaptive immune responses needed for protection against viral infections. The conditions, however, are also accompanied by an NK-cell-dependent migration of bone marrow-derived cell populations to the marginal zone regions rich in monocyte/macrophage and DC lineage cells (Salazar-Mather et al., 1996). Thus, NK cell cytotoxicity may be activated by IFN-α/β to mediate important immunoregulatory functions.

IFN-α/β also induce the modest blastogenesis and proliferation of NK cells and memory CD8 T cells in vivo (Biron et al., 1999). Since they are not growth factors but, rather, can have antiproliferative functions at high concentrations, these effects are thought to be mediated by downstream intermediaries. If IL-15 is induced by IFN-α/β, it would be a candidate molecule for this function because the cytokine utilizes in its receptor the β and γ chains, common to the IL-2 receptor and expressed by NK and memory T-cell populations, along with a specific α chain (Fehniger and Caligiuri, 2001; Waldmann and Tagaya, 1999). However, there is no direct evidence demonstrating such a function for endogenous production of IL-15 in vivo.

Responses elicited by other cytokines

Although the overall contribution for NK-cell-mediated cytotoxicity to antiviral defense remains unclear, the importance of NK cells in early defense against a variety of viral infections has been definitively established (Biron et al., 1999). There is strong evidence for their significance in defense against herpesviruses in both the human and the mouse. The best-characterized pathways for NK-cell-mediated defense occur downstream of IFN-γ production. Production of this cytokine at early times after infection can promote access to the IFN-γ-activated biochemical pathways of antiviral defense described above. In particular, a variety of viruses are sensitive to effects accessed as a result of NOS2 functions, including the DNA viruses VV, EBV, HSV, and MCMV, and the RNA viruses vesicular stomatitis virus (VSV) and hepatitis B virus (Ahmed and Biron, 1998; Biron and Sen, 2001; Guidotti et al., 2000; Reiss and Komatsu, 1998). Moreover, as described below, NK-cell IFN-γ responses may have a number of functions that affect the antiviral state as a result of shaping or directing downstream adaptive immune responses. The NK-cell IFN-γ response during early infections of mice is clearly IL-12 dependent (Orange and Biron, 1996a). Surprisingly, there is a precise dichotomy of functions for the innate cytokine responses during MCMV infection, with activation of NK-cell cytotoxicity being IFN-α/β dependent but induction of NK-cell–IFN-γ production being IL-12 dependent (Orange and Biron, 1996b). Given that conditions of exposure to IL-12 also enhance NK-cell cytotoxicity, secondary effects elicited during or after viral infections may contribute to the separation of functions.

NK cells also have the potential to promote resistance to infection as a result of producing TNF-α. Many different cells of the innate immune system and even nonimmune cells, however, can produce this factor. In MCMV infections of mice, NK cells are not required for an innate TNF-α response (Orange et al., 1995b; Orange and Biron, 1996b). TNF-α can promote the migration of DCs from peripheral compartments to carry antigen to and present it in lymphoid organs (Roake et al., 1995; Wang et al., 1997).

Adaptive Responses

The importance of innate responses in directing adaptive responses has been underscored by the demonstration of the role for IL-12 in promoting Th1 CD4 T-cell responses producing IFN-γ (Trinchieri, 1998). A second component of this response is the early induction of NK-cell IFN-γ to help preserve the expression of the high-affinity IL-12 receptor on, and IL-12 responsiveness by, CD4 T cells (Szabo et al., 1997a). Signaling for this pathway is dependent on STAT4, and a transcription factor suggested to be a lineage commitment factor for Th1 CD4 T cells is T-bet (Murphy et al., 2000; Szabo et al., 2000). The absence of innate IL-12 and IFN-γ responses contributes to conditions promoting the Th2 CD4 T-cell responses associated with IL-4 and IL-5 production. Signaling for this pathway is thought to be dependent on another STAT molecule, STAT6 (Murphy et al., 2000), and the transcription factors suggested to be lineage commitment factors for Th1 CD4 T cells are GATA-3 and c-MAF (Murphy et al., 2000; Ouyang et al., 1998; Szabo et al., 1997b). These pathways have been thought to be in place to "hardwire" T-cell populations to particular lineages, but recent studies suggest that there is a long-term need for IL-

12 in maintaining Th1 responses (Park et al., 2000; Stobie et al., 2000; Yap et al., 2000). Idealized patterns (Fig. 1) suggest that Th1 responses are particularly important in defense against bacterial and intracellular protozoan infections because these agents are sensitive to some of the antimicrobial pathways activated by IFN-γ. In contrast, Th2 responses are associated with the appearance of eosinophils and immunoglobulin E antibody production, and these mediators are important in defense against extracellular parasitic infections. Since the major pathways have regulatory loops inhibiting the reciprocal response, induction of the "wrong" helper type response renders the host more susceptible to infection.

Innate response shaping of the quality or essence of T-cell immune responses to viral infections is less well understood. Certainly, IFN-γ is an important component of defense against many different kinds of viruses, and T-cell IFN-γ responses are induced at high levels during most of the viral infections characterized. By these criteria, protective responses might be characterized as Th1 type. CD4 T cells can be induced to express IFN-γ in response to viral infections. However, CD8 T cells are major contributors to the IFN-γ response during a number of viral infections including those due to LCMV (Butz and Bevan, 1998; Murali-Krishna et al., 1998; Su et al., 1998) and influenza virus (Flynn et al., 1998) infections in the mouse and HIV (Jassoy et al., 1993), EBV (Dalod, 1999b), and influenza virus (Lalvani et al., 1997) infections in the human. The CD8 T cells can also be induced to express TNF-α, and cytotoxic CD8 T-cell responses appear to be elicited during many viral infectons and are particularly high during some of them. Thus, there are numerous reasons to expect that T cells are regulated by unique mechanisms following challenges with viruses. Although the mechanisms remain poorly described, certain elements are beginning to be appreciated.

Regulation of IFN-γ expression

T-cell IFN-γ responses can be induced through IL-12-independent pathways during a number of different viral infections of mice, including LCMV (Cousens et al., 1999; Orange and Biron, 1996a; Oxenius et al., 1999), mouse hepatitis virus (Schijns et al., 1998), and influenza virus (Monteiro et al., 1998) infections. Moreover, the cytokine is not required for CD8 T-cell expansion during LCMV infections (Cousens et al., 1999). Likewise, IFN-α/β is not required for CD8 T-cell expansion or IFN-γ expression during LCMV infection (Cousens et al., 1999), even though these cytokines can promote IFN-γ under certain conditions. In the absence of IFN-α/β functions, however, an IL-12 response is revealed and contributes to the conditions promoting IFN-γ production during LCMV infections of mice (Cousens et al., 1999). Exogenous IL-12 is known to be a good inducer of activated T-cell IFN-γ production in culture (Trinchieri, 1998). Thus, there are "innate" cytokine pathways to IFN-γ production by T cells during viral infections. One of these is IFN-α/β dependent. Another is IL-12 dependent, is revealed in the absence of IFN-α/β functions, and overlaps with the pathway to NK-cell IFN-γ production at early times during viral and nonviral infections and with the well-characterized pathway to CD4 T-cell IFN-γ responses. It is interesting that RSV infections are not strong inducers of IFN-α/β. If the conditions of infection also elicit low levels of IL-12, the reported spectrum-like responses of sometimes Th1 type but sometimes Th2 type with the appearance of eosinophils, uncharacteristic of responses to most viral infections, might result from deficiencies in the availability of both of these innate cytokines.

Given the range of cells expressing the particular cytokines, the effects of IFN-α/β may be accessed as a result of production of IFN-α/β by virus-infected cells and/or appropriately stimulated DCs. The effects of IL-12, however, are more likely to be accessed as a result of cytokine production by DCs. It should be remembered, however, that stimulation of CD8 T cells through the T-cell receptor is a potent inducer of IFN-γ production. Endogenous IL-2 also enhances IFN-γ production by primed CD8 T cells (Cousens et al., 1995; Su et al., 1998). This is an example of an adaptive-response component facilitating T-cell cytokine responses, however, because IL-2 is largely a CD4 T-cell product acting on CD8 T cells. The importance of the contributions of each of the possible pathways to IFN-γ expression by T cells during viral infection may vary depending on how much of a particular cytokine is induced and/or how much antigen is present.

Regulation of TNF-α and perforin expression

Little is known about the factors promoting T-cell TNF-α and perforin responses during viral infections. IL-12 (Cousens et al., 1999; Orange and Biron, 1996a), IFN-γ (Graham et al., 1993), and IFN-α/β (van den Broek et al., 1995) are not absolutely essential by themselves for induction of cytotoxic T-cell function, although enhancing effects on CD8 T-cell responses have been demonstrated for each of the cytokines under particular conditions. An interesting question is how the T-cell IFN-γ, TNF-α, and perforin responses might be differentially regulated within individual cells. The system might have evolved unique pathways to specifically access or regulate these responses because certain effector mechanisms are more important in defense against a particular virus and/or are more prone to contribute to immunopathology under particular conditions. For example, although many viruses appear to be sensitive to antiviral defense mechanisms activated by IFN-γ, killing of infected cells through perforin-dependent mechanisms appears more important during infections with nonlytic than during infections with lytic viruses (Kagi and Hengartner, 1996). Moreover, cytotoxic CD8 T cells can be major contributors to immunopathology during viral infections, particular in the brain and liver. Thus, it might be important to be able to down-regulate such a response. Likewise, although TNF-α can access certain antiviral effects, it can promote cytokine-mediated disease if expressed at very high systemic levels, particularly in the context of IFN-γ induction. It has been recently shown that perforin but not IFN-γ responses are significantly reduced in CD8 T-cell populations isolated late during HIV infections (Appay et al., 2000). Although the issue of "fine-tuning" CD8 T-cell responses is an important one, little mechanistic information is available about how this might happen. Interestingly, however, there is a possibility that the development of cytotoxic T cell functions may require stronger T-cell receptor-initiated signal transduction than is required for induction of cytokine gene expression (She et al., 1999).

Directing Adaptive Responses to Infected Sites

Once appropriate defense mechanisms have been activated, cells with the ability to deliver these functions must be directed to sites of infections in solid tissues. One of the members of the family of β or CC chemokines, macrophage inflammatory protein 1α (MIP-1α), is important for inflammation during a number of viral infections of the mouse. Consistent with the chemotactic activity of MIP-1α for induced lymphocyte and macrophage populations in culture, mice genetically deficient in MIP-1α have profoundly reduced inflammation in response to a variety of viral challenges. The reduced responses include T-cell-associated inflammation in influenza virus-infected lungs on days 7 to 28 of infection (Cook, 1995), following cardiac coxsackievirus infection (Cook et al., 1995), and following corneal infections with HSV (Tumpey et al., 1998). The inflammatory responses under these conditions are accompanied by and contribute to marked immunopathology. In MCMV infections, MIP-1α is required for induction of an early NK-cell infiltration into livers (Salazar-

Mather et al., 1998). This trafficking of NK cells results in focal accumulations at sites of viral antigen expression in hepatic parenchyma at 2 to 3 days after initiation of infection. Peak defense against MCMV is dependent on MIP-1α. The specific requirement for this single cytokine in these systems is remarkable, given that chemokine responses are frequently induced in clusters and utilize overlapping receptors.

The mechanisms by which MIP-1α might be pivotal for inflammation and defense under these conditions are being elucidated. A chemokine-to-cytokine-to-chemokine cascade has been identified in infected livers (Fig. 3). NK cells are induced to express IFN-γ during MCMV infections. The NK-cell IFN-γ response is detected both systemically and in the splenic lymphoid organ for very brief periods but occurs for longer periods in infected livers. MIP-1α is required for the peak local liver NK-cell IFN-γ response but not the serum or spleen responses (Salazar-Mather et al., 2000). A downstream consequence of the MIP-1α-dependent NK-cell accumulation and NK-cell IFN-γ expression in the liver is induction of the α or CXC chemokine Mig, and Mig also is required for peak defense against MCMV infection (Salazar-Mather, 2000). As stated above, a number of chemokines including Mig, IP-10, and I-TAC can be induced by IFN-γ, but the Mig gene has a unique stringent requirement for IFN-γ induction. Mig is a potent chemoattractant for activated T lymphocytes.

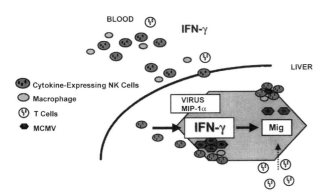

Figure 3. Chemokine-to-cytokine-to-chemokine cascade using innate NK-cell responses to direct localization of downstream adaptive responses. The model is based on studies of MCMV infections in livers. In the first step, NK cells are activated, in response to IL-12, to produce IFN-γ in a variety of host compartments. This production subsides rapidly in the periphery. In the second step, the expression of the chemokine MIP-1α is induced in response to viral challenge signals in the liver and promotes the recruitment of NK cells from the blood to the liver. In the third step, NK cells surround and sequester MCMV-infected cells, forming distinctive clusters of inflammatory foci. These events also serve to localize and sustain the production of IFN-γ. In the fourth step, there is induction of the γ-inducible chemokine Mig in response to localized production of IFN-γ. In the last step, Mig may be involved in the downstream recruitment of activated T cells into liver.

Thus, the conditions of MIP-1α-dependent accumulation of NK cells to deliver IFN-γ to infected livers set up for Mig induction, and Mig has the potential to promote the downstream accumulation of T lymphocytes and delivery of their antiviral functions to this site. The system is an example of how innate immune responses can regulate or direct adaptive immune responses by promoting the signals telling them where to go. The results might also explain how individual cytokines and chemokines might play key critical roles in antiviral defense.

ACCESSING INNATE RESPONSES BY ADAPTIVE IMMUNE RESPONSES

Activated T lymphocytes produce cytokines (IFN-γ, TNF-α, and the early T-lymphocyte activation-1 protein identified as Eta-1) and express TNF-related membrane molecules (CD40L and TRANCE). These factors and cell surface receptors can cooperate to provide the two signals required for differentiation and activation of innate cytokine production by DCs. CD40L is expressed transiently on CD4 T cells early after activation and can induce the differentiation of DCs into Th2-promoting DCs (DC2) in the absence of IFN-γ or into Th1-promoting, IL-12-secreting DCs (DC1) in the presence of IFN-γ (Hilkens et al., 1997; Ridge et al., 1998). Since they are very efficient producers of IFN-γ, activated CD8 T cells may cooperate with CD4 T cells to sustain IL-12 production by DCs and further amplify the Th1 responses in the course of infection. Eta-1 has also recently been shown to induce IL-12 secretion through ligation of the $\alpha_2\beta_3$ integrin on macrophages during corneal HSV infection in mice (Ashkar et al., 2000). TRANCE is expressed for several days after activation by both CD4 and CD8 T cells and shares with CD40L the ability to induce the transcription of various cytokine genes (IFN-α/β, TNF-α, IL-1, IL-6, IL-12, and IL-15) by DCs (Bachmann et al., 1999b). These two molecules can also cooperate with TNF-α to enhance the viability of DCs, in part by up-regulating the antiapoptotic molecule Bcl-XL. Activated T cells that express high levels of TRANCE could thus promote their own survival by interacting with DCs and inducing IL-15 production. Activated CD8 T cells may even modulate DC function independently of CD40L, i.e., independently of CD4 T cells. On the other hand, it has been shown that cytotoxic T cells may be implicated in the termination of immune responses on resolution of virus infection by killing virus antigen-expressing DCs. Clearly, much remains to be learned about how the positive and negative effects of CD8 and CD4 T cells are balanced to optimize these responses, but their interactions with DCs are likely to play an important role in accessing innate cytokines for protection of the host during acute viral infections.

Memory T lymphocytes express high levels of mRNA encoding IFN-γ, TNF-α, CD40L, and TRANCE, which can thus be synthesized very early after encounter of the specific antigen under conditions of secondary challenge. In particular, CD8 T cells are very fast and efficient producers of IFN-γ (Bachmann et al., 1999a; Lalvani et al., 1997; Zimmermann et al., 1999). Therefore, memory CD8 T cells are likely to be major contributors to the induction of innate cytokine production, especially IL-12, and to the downstream amplification of adaptive Th1 immune responses during secondary infections. They could interact very early with virus antigen-presenting macrophages and DCs. This hypothesis is supported by the observation that vaccination of mice with a recombinant VV encoding a strong CD8 epitope derived from RSV protects them from Th2 disease after challenge with the virus by promoting a protective Th1 response (Srikiatkhachorn and Braciale, 1997). Similar recent observations suggest a potential immunoregulatory role for memory CD8 T cells in promoting IL-12 secretion and Th1 immunity during protozoan parasitic infections of mice (Gurunathan et al., 2000). It is also interesting that memory T lymphocytes have been implicated in the overactivation of the inflammatory response and that dengue hemorrhagic fever occurs only after secondary infections with this virus (Chaturvedi et al., 2000).

CONTRIBUTIONS OF THE INNATE IMMUNE RESPONSE TO DISEASE

High levels of circulating proinflammatory cytokines have long been known to be detrimental to the host (Gutierrez-Ramos and Bluethmann, 1997). The conditions are associated with coagulation, necrosis, vascular collapse, and multiorgan failure. They have been best studied during gram-negative bacterial sepsis and/or experimentally after challenge with the endotoxin from these organisms, lipopolysaccharide (LPS). Under these conditions, IL-12 acts to induce IFN-γ and IFN-γ and TNF-α synergize to induce a variety of disease parameters and death. Thus, inhibiting either IFN-γ or TNF-α function alone protects the host. Until recently, however, little attention has been paid to the potential contribution of such responses to viral pathogenesis. It is now clear that systemic proinflammatory cytokines can be part of acute primary responses to some viruses and are likely to contribute to disease during adaptive responses to a number of viral infections.

Isolated Innate Responses

Cytokine-dependent disease can be observed during innate-phase immune responses to particular acute primary viral infections. The proinflammatory cytokine cascade induced during MCMV infections of immunocompetent mice, with significant levels of TNF-α, IL-6, IL-12, and IFN-γ in serum but low or undetectable IL-1 levels, is associated with a TNF-dependent liver necrosis (Orange et al., 1997). Although this cytokine-dependent disease is induced, it is quickly resolved. Remarkably, the cytokine cascade links IL-6 expression to the induction of an endogenous GC surge (Ruzek et al., 1997), and this response functions to limit the overall magnitude of cytokine expression and to protect against TNF-dependent death occurring acutely and with rapid onset, i.e., within 3 days of challenge (Ruzek et al., 1999). In contrast to LPS-induced death, the MCMV-induced death in the absence of GCs is IFN-γ independent. This might be because IFN-α/β also are induced and these cytokines can access some of the same functions as IFN-γ. Similar disease conditions are likely to be common to a number of viral infections. In particular, acute Sindbis virus infections of immunocompetent neonatal mice induce profound levels of IFN-α/β and TNF-α in serum, as well as IFN-γ production, and these infections can induce rapid death (within 3 days) (Klimstra et al., 1999). Moreover, the absence of IFN-α/β functions in adult mice renders them susceptible to virus-induced death associated with high levels of TNF-α (Ryman et al., 2000). Finally, IFN-α/β induced early during infections with vesicular stomatitis virus and LCMV sensitizes mice to LPS toxicity (Doughty et al., 2001; Nansen and Randrup-Thomsen, 2001).

Mixing of Adaptive and Innate Responses

A variety of pathways by which adaptive immune responses can act to access innate-immunity cytokines are reviewed above. Such pathways are likely to contribute to pathologic changes during infections with Dengue virus (Chaturvedi et al., 2000) and hantaviruses (Mori et al., 1999).

A threatening situation arises from the lack of general appreciation for how an ongoing viral infection might predispose individuals to toxicities resulting from secondary challenges with other infectious agents and/or cytokine administration. In both humans and mice, disease levels elicited by challenges with bacteria or bacterial products are increased during viral infections. The best-documented example in humans is that of influenza virus. After infection with this pathogen, infections with bacteria can lead to sudden and abrupt worsening of the condition. In mice, a number of viruses increase the susceptibility to death and disease after secondary challenges with such agents. For LPS challenge during adaptive immune responses to LCMV infections, the sensitivity is a consequence of priming for TNF-α, IL-12, and IFN-γ responses with both T and NK cells contributing to IFN-γ production (Nguyen and Biron, 1999). The conditions also predispose for sensitivity to the toxic effects of administered IL-12 (Orange et al., 1994, 1995a). Thus, the magnitudes of innate cytokine responses and sensitivities to innate cytokines are changed. Given that humans are constantly being bombarded with a variety of agents, virus-induced sensitization is likely to contribute to many different conditions of disease. In fact, the presence of an underlying subclinical viral infection may help explain how one individual experiences a critical condition whereas another tolerates a particular bacterial infection. Moreover, responding to exposure to enteric agents, as a result of procedural or disease-associated compromise of the bowel, may be significantly more difficult in the context of viral infections. As an example, virus-induced priming for sensitivity might contribute to the pathogenesis during Ebola virus infections, which are associated with both deterioration of the gut and extensive coagulation.

Acknowledgments. We thank Ganes Sen and Joan Durbin for sharing their expertise.

REFERENCES

Ahmed, R., and C. A. Biron. 1998. Immunity to viruses, p. 1295–1334. *In* W. E. Paul (ed.), *Fundamental Immunology,* 4th ed. Lippincott-Raven Publishers, Philadelphia, Pa.

Akira, S. 2000. The role of IL-18 in innate immunity. *Curr. Opin. Immunol.* **12**:59–63.

Appay, V., D. F. Nixon, S. M. Donahoe, G. M. Gillespie, T. Dong, A. King, G. S. Ogg, H. M. Spiegel, C. Conlon, C. A. Spina, D. V. Havlir, D. D. Richman, A. Waters, P. Easterbrook, A. J. McMichael, and S. L. Rowland-Jones. 2000. HIV-specific CD8(+) T cells produce antiviral cytokines but are impaired in cytolytic function. *J. Exp. Med.* **192**:63–76.

Ashkar, S., G. F. Weber, V. Panoutsakopoulou, M. E. Sanchirico, M. Jansson, S. Zawaideh, S. R. Rittling, D. T. Denhardt, M. J. Glimcher, and H. Cantor. 2000. Eta-1 (osteopontin): an early component of type-1 (cell-mediated) immunity. *Science* **287**:860–864.

Azimi, N., K. Brown, R. N. Bamford, Y. Tagaya, U. Siebenlist, and T. A. Waldmann. 1998. Human T cell lymphotropic virus type I Tax protein trans-activates interleukin 15 gene transcription through an NF-kappaB site. *Proc. Natl. Acad. Sci. USA* **95**:2452–2457.

Azimi, N., S. Jacobson, T. Leist, and T. A. Waldmann. 1999. Involvement of IL-15 in the pathogenesis of human T lymphotropic virus type I-associated myelopathy/tropical spastic paraparesis: implications for therapy with a monoclonal antibody directed to the IL-2/15R beta receptor. *J. Immunol.* **163**:4064–4072.

Bachmann, M. F., M. Barner, A. Viola, and M. Kopf. 1999a. Distinct kinetics of cytokine production and cytolysis in effector and memory T cells after viral infection. *Eur. J. Immunol.* **29**:291–299.

Bachmann, M. F., B. R. Wong, R. Josien, R. M. Steinman, A. Oxenius, and Y. Choi. 1999b. TRANCE, a tumor necrosis factor family member critical for CD40 ligand-independent T helper cell activation. *J. Exp. Med.* **189**:1025–1031.

Ballas, Z. K., W. L. Rasmussen, and A. M. Krieg. 1996. Induction of NK activity in murine and human cells by CpG motifs in oligodeoxynucleotides and bacterial DNA. *J. Immunol.* **157**:1840–1845.

Biglino, A., A. Sinicco, B. Forno, A. M. Pollono, M. Sciandra, C. Martini, P. Pich, and P. Gioannini. 1996. Serum cytokine profiles in acute primary HIV-1 infection and in infectious mononucleosis. *Clin. Immunol. Immunopathol.* **78**:61–69.

Biron, C. A., K. B. Nguyen, G. C. Pien, L. P. Cousens, and T. P. Salazar-Mather. 1999. Natural killer cells in antiviral defense: function and regulation by innate cytokines. *Annu. Rev. Immunol.* **17**:189–220.

Biron, C. A., and G. C. Sen. 2001. Interferons and other cytokines, p. 321–351. *In* D. Knipe, P. Howley, D. Griffin, R. Lamb, M. Martin, and S. Straus (ed.), *Fields Virology,* 4th ed. Lippincott, Williams & Wilkins, Philadelphia, Pa.

Blanco-Quiros, A., H. Gonzalez, E. Arranz, and S. Lapena. 1999. Decreased interleukin-12 levels in umbilical cord blood in children who developed acute bronchiolitis. *Pediatr. Pulmonol.* **28**:175–180.

Boehm, U., T. Klamp, M. Groot, and J. C. Howard. 1997. Cellular responses to interferon-gamma. *Annu. Rev. Immunol.* **15**:749–795.

Brewster, F. E., K. S. Byron, and J. L. Sullivan. 1985. Immunoregulation during acute infection with Epstein-Barr virus: dynamics of interferon and 2′,5′-oligoadenylate synthetase activity. *J. Infect. Dis.* **151**:1109–1115.

Brinkmann, V., T. Geiger, S. Alkan, and C. H. Heusser. 1993. Interferon alpha increases the frequency of interferon gamma-producing human CD4+ T cells. *J. Exp. Med.* **178**:1655–1663.

Bukowski, J. F., C. A. Biron, and R. M. Welsh. 1983. Elevated natural killer cell-mediated cytotoxicity, plasma interferon, and tumor cell rejection in mice persistently infected with lymphocytic choriomeningitis virus. *J. Immunol.* **131**:991–996.

Butz, E. A., and M. J. Bevan. 1998. Massive expansion of antigen-specific CD8+ T cells during an acute virus infection. *Immunity* **8**:167–175.

Carlow, D. A., S. J. Teh, and H. S. Teh. 1998. Specific antiviral activity demonstrated by TGTP, a member of a new family of interferon-induced GTPases. *J. Immunol.* **161**:2348–2355.

Cella, M., D. Jarrossay, F. Facchetti, O. Alebardi, H. Nakajima, A. Lanzavecchia, and M. Colonna. 1999. Plasmacytoid monocytes migrate to inflamed lymph nodes and produce large amounts of type I interferon. *Nat. Med.* **5**:919–923.

Chandel, N. S., W. C. Trzyna, D. S. McClintock, and P. T. Schumacker. 2000. Role of oxidants in NF-kappaB activation and TNF-alpha gene transcription induced by hypoxia and endotoxin. *J. Immunol.* **165**:1013–1021.

Chaturvedi, U. C., R. Agarwal, E. A. Elbishbishi, and A. S. Mustafa. 2000. Cytokine cascade in dengue hemorrhagic fever: implications for pathogenesis. *FEMS Immunol. Med. Microbiol.* **28**:183–188.

Cho, S. S., C. M. Bacon, C. Sudarshan, R. C. Rees, D. Finbloom, R. Pine, and J. J. O'Shea. 1996. Activation of STAT4 by IL-12 and IFN-alpha: evidence for the involvement of ligand-induced tyrosine and serine phosphorylation. *J. Immunol.* **157**:4781–4789.

Chonmaitree, T., N. J. Roberts, Jr., R. G. Douglas, Jr., C. B. Hall, and R. L. Simons. 1981. Interferon production by human mononuclear leukocytes: differences between respiratory syncytial virus and influenza viruses. *Infect. Immun.* **32**:300–303.

Clayette, P., R. Le Grand, O. Noack, B. Vaslin, R. Le Naour, O. Benveniste, F. Theodoro, P. Fretier, and D. Dormont. 1995. Tumor necrosis factor-alpha in serum of macaques during SIVmac251 acute infection. *J. Med. Primatol.* **24**:94–100.

Conn, C. A., J. L. McClellan, H. F. Maassab, C. W. Smitka, J. A. Majde, and M. J. Kluger. 1995. Cytokines and the acute phase response to influenza virus in mice. *Am. J. Physiol.* **268**:R78–R84.

Cook, D. N., M. A. Beck, T. M. Coffman, S. L. Kirby, J. F. Sheridan, I. B. Pragnell, and O. Smithies. 1995. Requirement of MIP-1 alpha for an inflammatory response to viral infection. *Science* **269**:1583–1585.

Cousens, L. P., J. S. Orange, and C. A. Biron. 1995. Endogenous IL-2 contributes to T cell expansion and IFN-gamma production during lymphocytic choriomeningitis virus infection. *J. Immunol.* **155**:5690–5699.

Cousens, L. P., J. S. Orange, H. C. Su, and C. A. Biron. 1997. Interferon-alpha/beta inhibition of interleukin 12 and interferon-gamma production in vitro and endogenously during viral infection. *Proc. Natl. Acad. Sci. USA* **94**:634–639.

Cousens, L. P., R. Peterson, S. Hsu, A. Dorner, J. D. Altman, R. Ahmed, and C. A. Biron. 1999. Two roads diverged: interferon alpha/beta- and interleukin 12-mediated pathways in promoting T cell interferon gamma responses during viral infection. *J. Exp. Med.* **189**:1315–1328.

Dalod, M., M. Dupuis, J. C. Deschemin, C. Goujard, C. Deveau, L. Meyer, N. Ngo, C. Rouzioux, J. G. Guillet, J. F. Delfraissy, M. Sinet, and A. Venet. 1999a. Weak anti-HIV CD8(+) T-cell effector activity in HIV primary infection. *J. Clin. Investig.* **104**:1431–1439.

Dalod, M., M. Sinet, J. C. Deschemin, S. Fiorentino, A. Venet, and J. G. Guillet. 1999b. Altered ex vivo balance between CD28+ and CD28− cells within HIV-specific CD8+ T cells of HIV-seropositive patients. *Eur. J. Immunol.* **29**:38–44.

Darnell, J. E., Jr., I. M. Kerr, and G. R. Stark. 1994. Jak-STAT pathways and transcriptional activation in response to IFNs and other extracellular signaling proteins. *Science* **264**:1415–1421.

Deonarain, R., A. Alcami, M. Alexiou, M. J. Dallman, D. R. Gewert, and A. C. Porter. 2000. Impaired antiviral response and alpha/beta interferon induction in mice lacking beta interferon. *J. Virol.* **74**:3404–3409.

Der, S. D., A. Zhou, B. R. Williams, and R. H. Silverman. 1998. Identification of genes differentially regulated by interferon alpha, beta, or gamma using oligonucleotide arrays. *Proc. Natl. Acad. Sci. USA* **95**:15623–15628.

Diefenbach, A., H. Schindler, N. Donhauser, E. Lorenz, T. Laskay, J. MacMicking, M. Rollinghoff, I. Gresser, and C. Bogdan. 1998. Type 1 interferon (IFNalpha/beta) and type 2 nitric oxide synthase regulate the innate immune response to a protozoan parasite. *Immunity* **8**:77–87.

Doughty, L. A., K. B. Nguyen, J. E. Durbin, and C. A. Biron. 2001. A role for IFN-α/β in virus infection-induced sensitization to endotoxin. *J. Immunol.* **166**:2658–2664.

Durbin, J. E., A. Fernandez-Sesma, C. K. Lee, T. D. Rao, A. B. Frey, T. M. Moran, S. Vukmanovic, A. Garcia-Sastre, and D. E. Levy. 2000. Type I IFN modulates innate and specific antiviral immunity. *J. Immunol.* **164**:4220–4228.

Eloranta, M. L., and G. V. Alm. 1999. Splenic marginal metallophilic macrophages and marginal zone macrophages are the major interferon-alpha/beta producers in mice upon intravenous challenge with herpes simplex virus. *Scand. J. Immunol.* **49**:391–394.

Erlandsson, L., R. Blumenthal, M. L. Eloranta, H. Engel, G. Alm, S. Weiss, and T. Leanderson. 1998. Interferon-beta is required for interferon-alpha production in mouse fibroblasts. *Curr. Biol.* **8**:223–226.

Farber, J. M. 1990. A macrophage mRNA selectively induced by gamma-interferon encodes a member of the platelet factor 4 family of cytokines. *Proc. Natl. Acad. Sci. USA* **87**:5238–5242.

Farrar, J. D., J. D. Smith, T. L. Murphy, S. Leung, G. R. Stark, and K. M. Murphy. 2000. Selective loss of type I interferon-induced STAT4 activation caused by a minisatellite insertion in mouse *Stat2*. *Nat. Immunol.* **1**:65–69.

Fehniger, T. A., and M. A. Caligiuri. 2001. Interleukin 15: biology and relevance to human disease. *Blood* **97**:14–32.

Ferbas, J., J. Navratil, A. Logar, and C. Rinaldo. 1995. Selective decrease in human immunodeficiency virus type 1 (HIV-1)-induced alpha interferon production by peripheral blood mononuclear cells during HIV-1 infection. *Clin. Diagn. Lab. Immunol.* **2**:138–142.

Flynn, K. J., G. T. Belz, J. D. Altman, R. Ahmed, D. L. Woodland, and P. C. Doherty. 1998. Virus-specific CD8+ T cells in primary and secondary influenza pneumonia. *Immunity* **8**:683–691.

Fruh, K., and Y. Yang. 1999. Antigen presentation by MHC class I and its regulation by interferon gamma. *Curr. Opin. Immunol.* **11**:76–81.

Gaines, H., M. A. von Sydow, L. V. von Stedingk, G. Biberfeld, B. Bottiger, L. O. Hansson, P. Lundbergh, A. B. Sonnerborg, J. Wasserman, and O. O. Strannegaard. 1990. Immunological changes in primary HIV-1 infection. *AIDS* **4**:995–999.

Garcia-Sastre, A., R. K. Durbin, H. Zheng, P. Palese, R. Gertner, D. E. Levy, and J. E. Durbin. 1998. The role of interferon in influenza virus tissue tropism. *J. Virol.* **72**:8550–8558.

Giavedoni, L. D., M. C. Velasquillo, L. M. Parodi, G. B. Hubbard, and V. L. Hodara. 2000. Cytokine expression, natural killer cell activation, and phenotypic changes in lymphoid cells from rhesus macaques during acute infection with pathogenic simian immunodeficiency virus. *J. Virol.* **74**:1648–1657.

Gollob, J. A., H. Kawasaki, and J. Ritz. 1997. Interferon-gamma and interleukin-4 regulate T cell interleukin-12 responsiveness through the differential modulation of high-affinity interleukin-12 receptor expression. *Eur. J. Immunol.* **27**:647–652.

Graham, M. B., D. K. Dalton, D. Giltinan, V. L. Braciale, T. A. Stewart, and T. J. Braciale. 1993. Response to influenza infection in mice with a targeted disruption in the interferon gamma gene. *J. Exp. Med.* **178**:1725–1732.

Gray, C. M., L. Morris, J. Murray, J. Keeton, S. Shalekoff, S. F. Lyons, P. Sonnenberg, and D. J. Martin. 1996. Identification of cell subsets expressing intracytoplasmic cytokines within HIV-1-infected lymph nodes. *AIDS* **10**:1467–1475.

Green, J. A., R. P. Charette, T. J. Yeh, and C. B. Smith. 1982. Presence of interferon in acute- and convalescent-phase sera of humans with influenza or influenza-like illness of undetermined etiology. *J. Infect. Dis.* **145**:837–841.

Green, S., D. W. Vaughn, S. Kalayanarooj, S. Nimmannitya, S. Suntayakorn, A. Nisalak, R. Lew, B. L. Innis, I. Kurane, A. L. Rothman, and F. A. Ennis. 1999. Early immune activation in acute dengue illness is related to development of plasma leakage and disease severity. *J. Infect. Dis.* **179**:755–762.

Grundy, J. E., J. Trapman, J. E. Allan, G. R. Shellam, and C. J. Melief. 1982. Evidence for a protective role of interferon in resistance to murine cytomegalovirus and its control by non-H-2-linked genes. *Infect. Immun.* **37**:143–150.

Guidotti, L. G., H. McClary, J. M. Loudis, and F. V. Chisari. 2000. Nitric oxide inhibits hepatitis B virus replication in the livers of transgenic mice. *J. Exp. Med.* **191**:1247–1252.

Gurunathan, S., L. Stobie, C. Prussin, D. L. Sacks, N. Glaichenhaus, D. J. Fowell, R. M. Locksley, J. T. Chang, C. Y. Wu, and R. A. Seder. 2000. Requirements for the maintenance of Th1 immunity in vivo following DNA vaccination: a potential immunoregulatory role for CD8+ T cells. *J. Immunol.* **165**:915–924.

Gutierrez-Ramos, J. C., and H. Bluethmann. 1997. Molecules and mechanisms operating in septic shock: lessons from knockout mice. *Immunol. Today* **18**:329–334.

Hacker, U. T., T. Jelinek, S. Erhardt, A. Eigler, G. Hartmann, H. D. Nothdurft, and S. Endres. 1998. In vivo synthesis of tumor necrosis factor-alpha in healthy humans after live yellow fever vaccination. *J. Infect. Dis.* **177**:774–778.

Hall, C. B., R. G. Douglas, Jr., R. L. Simons, and J. M. Geiman. 1978. Interferon production in children with respiratory syncytial, influenza, and parainfluenza virus infections. *J. Pediatr.* **93**:28–32.

Hayden, F. G., R. Fritz, M. C. Lobo, W. Alvord, W. Strober, and S. E. Straus. 1998. Local and systemic cytokine responses during experimental human influenza A virus infection. Relation to symptom formation and host defense. *J. Clin. Investig.* **101**:643–649.

He, J., H. Ichimura, T. Iida, M. Minami, K. Kobayashi, M. Kita, C. Sotozono, Y. I. Tagawa, Y. Iwakura, and J. Imanishi. 1999. Kinetics of cytokine production in the cornea and trigeminal ganglion of C57BL/6 mice after corneal HSV-1 infection. *J. Interferon Cytokine Res.* **19**:609–615.

Hennet, T., H. J. Ziltener, K. Frei, and E. Peterhans. 1992. A kinetic study of immune mediators in the lungs of mice infected with influenza A virus. *J. Immunol.* **149**:932–939.

Hilkens, C. M., P. Kalinski, M. de Boer, and M. L. Kapsenberg. 1997. Human dendritic cells require exogenous interleukin-12-inducing factors to direct the development of naive T-helper cells toward the Th1 phenotype. *Blood* **90**:1920–1926.

Humar, A., P. St Louis, T. Mazzulli, A. McGeer, J. Lipton, H. Messner, and K. S. MacDonald. 1999. Elevated serum cytokines are associated with cytomegalovirus infection and disease in bone marrow transplant recipients. *J. Infect. Dis.* **179**:484–488.

Hussell, T., and P. J. Openshaw. 1998. Intracellular IFN-gamma expression in natural killer cells precedes lung CD8+ T cell recruitment during respiratory syncytial virus infection. *J. Gen. Virol.* **79**:2593–2601.

Ignatiev, G. M., A. A. Dadaeva, S. V. Luchko, and A. A. Chepurnov. 2000. Immune and pathophysiological processes in baboons experimentally infected with Ebola virus adapted to guinea pigs. *Immunol. Lett.* **71**:131–140.

Ihle, J. N. 1995. Cytokine receptor signalling. *Nature* **377**:591–594.

Ishikawa, R., and C. A. Biron. 1993. IFN induction and associated changes in splenic leukocyte distribution. *J. Immunol.* **150**:3713–3727.

Jassoy, C., T. Harrer, T. Rosenthal, B. A. Navia, J. Worth, R. P. Johnson, and B. D. Walker. 1993. Human immunodeficiency virus type 1-specific cytotoxic T lymphocytes release gamma interferon, tumor necrosis factor alpha (TNF-α), and TNF-β when they encounter their target antigens. *J. Virol.* **67**:2844–2852.

Juang, Y., W. Lowther, M. Kellum, W. C. Au, R. Lin, J. Hiscott, and P. M. Pitha. 1998. Primary activation of interferon A and interferon B gene transcription by interferon regulatory factor 3. *Proc. Natl. Acad. Sci. USA* **95**:9837–9842.

Kagi, D., and H. Hengartner. 1996. Different roles for cytotoxic T cells in the control of infections with cytopathic versus noncytopathic viruses. *Curr. Opin. Immunol.* **8**:472–477.

Kanangat, S., J. Thomas, S. Gangappa, J. S. Babu, and B. T. Rouse. 1996. Herpes simplex virus type 1-mediated upregulation of IL-12 (p40) mRNA expression. Implications in immunopathogenesis and protection. *J. Immunol.* **156**:1110–1116.

Kanerva, M., A. Vaheri, J. Mustonen, and J. Partanen. 1998. High-producer allele of tumour necrosis factor-alpha is part of the susceptibility MHC haplotype in severe puumala virus-induced nephropathia epidemica. *Scand. J. Infect. Dis.* **30**:532–534.

Karp, C. L., C. A. Biron, and D. N. Irani. 2000. Interferon beta in multiple sclerosis: is IL-12 suppression the key? *Immunol. Today* **21**:24–28.

Khan, I. A., J. A. MacLean, F. S. Lee, L. Casciotti, E. DeHaan, J. D. Schwartzman, and A. D. Luster. 2000. IP-10 is critical for effector T cell trafficking and host survival in Toxoplasma gondii infection. *Immunity* **12**:483–494.

Khatissian, E., M. G. Tovey, M. C. Cumont, V. Monceaux, P. Lebon, L. Montagnier, B. Hurtrel, and L. Chakrabarti. 1996. The relationship between the interferon alpha response and viral burden in primary SIV infection. *AIDS Res. Hum. Retroviruses* **12**:1273–1278.

Klimstra, W. B., K. D. Ryman, K. A. Bernard, K. B. Nguyen, C. A. Biron, and R. E. Johnston. 1999. Infection of neonatal mice with Sindbis virus results in a systemic inflammatory response syndrome. *J. Virol.* **73**:10387–10398.

Krakauer, T., J. W. Leduc, and H. Krakauer. 1995. Serum levels of tumor necrosis factor-alpha, interleukin-1, and interleukin-6 in hemorrhagic fever with renal syndrome. *Viral Immunol.* **8**:75–79.

Kurane, I., B. L. Innis, S. Nimmannitya, A. Nisalak, A. Meager, and F. A. Ennis. 1993. High levels of interferon alpha in the sera of children with dengue virus infection. *Am. J. Trop. Med. Hyg.* **48**:222–229.

Lalvani, A., R. Brookes, S. Hambleton, W. J. Britton, A. V. Hill, and A. J. McMichael. 1997. Rapid effector function in CD8+ memory T cells. *J. Exp. Med.* **186**:859–865.

Lebel-Binay, S., A. Berger, F. Zinzindohoue, P. Cugnenc, N. Thiounn, W. H. Fridman, and F. Pages. 2000. Interleukin-18: biological properties and clinical implications. *Eur. Cytokine Netw.* **11**:15–26.

Leib, D. A., T. E. Harrison, K. M. Laslo, M. A. Machalek, N. J. Moorman, and H. W. Virgin. 1999. Interferons regulate the phenotype of wild-type and mutant herpes simplex viruses in vivo. *J. Exp. Med.* **189**:663–672.

Leroy, E. M., S. Baize, V. E. Volchkov, S. P. Fischer-Hoch, M. Georges-Courbot, J. Lansoud-Soukate, M. Capron, P. Debre, J. B. McCormick, and A. J. Georges. 2000. Human asymptomatic Ebola infection and strong inflammatory response. *Lancet* **355**:2210–2215.

Lindahl, P., I. Gresser, P. Leary, and M. Tovey. 1976. Interferon treatment of mice: enhanced expression of histocompatibility antigens on lymphoid cells. *Proc. Natl. Acad. Sci. USA* **73**:1284–1287.

Linde, A., B. Andersson, S. B. Svenson, H. Ahrne, M. Carlsson, P. Forsberg, H. Hugo, A. Karstorp, R. Lenkei, A. Lindwall, et al. 1992. Serum levels of lymphokines and soluble cellular receptors in primary Epstein-Barr virus infection and in patients with chronic fatigue syndrome. *J. Infect. Dis.* **165**:994–1000.

Linderholm, M., C. Ahlm, B. Settergren, A. Waage, and A. Tarnvik. 1996. Elevated plasma levels of tumor necrosis factor (TNF)-alpha, soluble TNF receptors, interleukin (IL)-6, and IL-

10 in patients with hemorrhagic fever with renal syndrome. *J. Infect. Dis.* **173**:38–43.

MacMicking, J., Q. W. Xie, and C. Nathan. 1997. Nitric oxide and macrophage function. *Annu. Rev. Immunol.* **15**:323–350.

Manetti, R., F. Annunziato, L. Tomasevic, V. Gianno, P. Parronchi, S. Romagnani, and E. Maggi. 1995. Polyinosinic acid: polycytidylic acid promotes T helper type 1-specific immune responses by stimulating macrophage production of interferon-alpha and interleukin-12. *Eur. J. Immunol.* **25**:2656–2660.

Marie, I., J. E. Durbin, and D. E. Levy. 1998. Differential viral induction of distinct interferon-alpha genes by positive feedback through interferon regulatory factor-7. *EMBO J.* **17**:6660–6669.

Marshall, J. D., J. Chehimi, G. Gri, J. R. Kostman, L. J. Montaner, and G. Trinchieri. 1999. The interleukin-12-mediated pathway of immune events is dysfunctional in human immunodeficiency virus-infected individuals. *Blood* **94**:1003–1011.

McRae, B. L., R. T. Semnani, M. P. Hayes, and G. A. van Seventer. 1998. Type I IFNs inhibit human dendritic cell IL-12 production and Th1 cell development. *J. Immunol* **160**:4298–4304.

Mikloska, Z., V. A. Danis, S. Adams, A. R. Lloyd, D. L. Adrian, and A. L. Cunningham. 1998. In vivo production of cytokines and beta (C-C) chemokines in human recurrent herpes simplex lesions—do herpes simplex virus-infected keratinocytes contribute to their production? *J. Infect. Dis.* **177**:827–838.

Milone, M. C., and P. Fitzgerald-Bocarsly. 1998. The mannose receptor mediates induction of IFN-alpha in peripheral blood dendritic cells by enveloped RNA and DNA viruses. *J. Immunol.* **161**:2391–2399.

Monteiro, J. M., C. Harvey, and G. Trinchieri. 1998. Role of interleukin-12 in primary influenza virus infection. *J. Virol.* **72**:4825–4831.

Mori, M., A. L. Rothman, I. Kurane, J. M. Montoya, K. B. Nolte, J. E. Norman, D. C. Waite, F. T. Koster, and F. A. Ennis. 1999. High levels of cytokine-producing cells in the lung tissues of patients with fatal hantavirus pulmonary syndrome. *J. Infect. Dis.* **179**:295–302.

Muller, U., U. Steinhoff, L. F. Reis, S. Hemmi, J. Pavlovic, R. M. Zinkernagel, and M. Aguet. 1994. Functional role of type I and type II interferons in antiviral defense. *Science* **264**:1918–1921.

Murali-Krishna, K., J. D. Altman, M. Suresh, D. J. Sourdive, A. J. Zajac, J. D. Miller, J. Slansky, and R. Ahmed. 1998. Counting antigen-specific CD8 T cells: a reevaluation of bystander activation during viral infection. *Immunity* **8**:177–187.

Murphy, K. M., W. Ouyang, J. D. Farrar, J. Yang, S. Ranganath, H. Asnagli, M. Afkarian, and T. L. Murphy. 2000. Signaling and transcription in T helper development. *Annu. Rev. Immunol.* **18**:451–494.

Nakayama, T., S. Sonoda, T. Urano, K. Sasaki, N. Maehara, and S. Makino. 1993. Detection of alpha-interferon in nasopharyngeal secretions and sera in children infected with respiratory syncytial virus. *Pediatr. Infect. Dis. J.* **12**:925–929.

Nansen, A., and A. Randrup-Thomsen. 2001. Viral infections cause rapid sensitization to lipopolysaccharide: central role of IFN-α/β. *J. Immunol.* **166**:982–988.

Nguyen, K. B., and C. A. Biron. 1999. Synergism for cytokine-mediated disease during concurrent endotoxin and viral challenges: roles for NK and T cell IFN-gamma production. *J. Immunol.* **162**:5238–5246.

Nguyen, K. B., L. P. Cousens, L. A. Doughty, G. C. Pien, J. E. Durbin, and C. A. Biron. 2000. Interferon α/β-mediated inhibition and promotion of interferon γ: STAT1 resolves a paradox. *Nat. Immunology* **1**:70–76.

Noah, T. L., F. W. Henderson, I. A. Wortman, R. B. Devlin, J. Handy, H. S. Koren, and S. Becker. 1995. Nasal cytokine pro-

duction in viral acute upper respiratory infection of childhood. *J. Infect. Dis.* **171**:584–592.

Orange, J. S., and C. A. Biron. 1996a. An absolute and restricted requirement for IL-12 in natural killer cell IFN-gamma production and antiviral defense. Studies of natural killer and T cell responses in contrasting viral infections. *J. Immunol.* **156**:1138–1142.

Orange, J. S., and C. A. Biron. 1996b. Characterization of early IL-12, IFN-alphabeta, and TNF effects on antiviral state and NK cell responses during murine cytomegalovirus infection. *J. Immunol.* **156**:4746–4756.

Orange, J. S., T. P. Salazar-Mather, S. M. Opal, and C. A. Biron. 1997. Mechanisms for virus-induced liver disease: tumor necrosis factor-mediated pathology independent of natural killer and T cells during murine cytomegalovirus infection. *J. Virol.* **71**:9248–9258.

Orange, J. S., T. P. Salazar-Mather, S. M. Opal, R. L. Spencer, A. H. Miller, B. S. McEwen, and C. A. Biron. 1995a. Mechanism of interleukin 12-mediated toxicities during experimental viral infections: role of tumor necrosis factor and glucocorticoids. *J. Exp. Med.* **181**:901–914.

Orange, J. S., B. Wang, C. Terhorst, and C. A. Biron. 1995b. Requirement for natural killer cell-produced interferon gamma in defense against murine cytomegalovirus infection and enhancement of this defense pathway by interleukin 12 administration. *J. Exp. Med.* **182**:1045–1056.

Orange, J. S., S. F. Wolf, and C. A. Biron. 1994. Effects of IL-12 on the response and susceptibility to experimental viral infections. *J. Immunol.* **152**:1253–1264.

Ouyang, W., S. H. Ranganath, K. Weindel, D. Bhattacharya, T. L. Murphy, W. C. Sha, and K. M. Murphy. 1998. Inhibition of Th1 development mediated by GATA-3 through an IL-4-independent mechanism. *Immunity* **9**:745–755.

Oxenius, A., U. Karrer, R. M. Zinkernagel, and H. Hengartner. 1999. IL-12 is not required for induction of type 1 cytokine responses in viral infections. *J. Immunol.* **162**:965–973.

Park, A. Y., B. D. Hondowicz, and P. Scott. 2000. IL-12 is required to maintain a Th1 response during *Leishmania major* infection. *J. Immunol.* **165**:896–902.

Pfeffer, L. M., C. A. Dinarello, R. B. Herberman, B. R. Williams, E. C. Borden, R. Bordens, M. R. Walter, T. L. Nagabhushan, P. P. Trotta, and S. Pestka. 1998. Biological properties of recombinant alpha-interferons: 40th anniversary of the discovery of interferons. *Cancer Res.* **58**:2489–2499.

Pien, G. C., and C. A. Biron. 2000. Compartmental differences in NK cell responsiveness to IL-12 during lymphocytic choriomeningitis virus infection. *J. Immunol.* **164**:994–1001.

Pien, G. C., A. R. Satoskar, K. Takeda, S. Akira, and C. A. Biron. 2000. Selective IL-18 requirements for induction of compartmental IFN-γ responses during viral infection. *J. Immunol.* **165**:4787–4791.

Poli, G., P. Biswas, and A. S. Fauci. 1994. Interferons in the pathogenesis and treatment of human immunodeficiency virus infection. *Antiviral Res.* **24**:221–233.

Quaranta, M. G., B. Camponeschi, E. Straface, W. Malorni, and M. Viora. 1999. Induction of interleukin-15 production by HIV-1 nef protein: a role in the proliferation of uninfected cells. *Exp. Cell Res.* **250**:112–121.

Ramana, C. V., N. Grammatikakis, M. Chernov, H. Nguyen, K. C. Goh, B. R. Williams, and G. R. Stark. 2000. Regulation of c-myc expression by IFN-gamma through Stat1-dependent and -independent pathways. *EMBO J.* **19**:263–272.

Reinhardt, B., R. Jaspert, M. Niedrig, C. Kostner, and J. L'Age-Stehr. 1998. Development of viremia and humoral and cellular parameters of immune activation after vaccination with yellow fever virus strain 17D: a model of human flavivirus infection. *J. Med. Virol.* **56:**159–167.

Reiss, C. S., and T. Komatsu. 1998. Does nitric oxide play a critical role in viral infections? *J. Virol.* **72:**4547–4551.

Ridge, J. P., F. Di Rosa, and P. Matzinger. 1998. A conditioned dendritic cell can be a temporal bridge between a CD4+ T-helper and a T-killer cell. *Nature* **393:**474–478.

Rizzardi, G. P., W. Barcellini, G. Tambussi, F. Lillo, M. Malnati, L. Perrin, and A. Lazzarin. 1996. Plasma levels of soluble CD30, tumour necrosis factor (TNF)-alpha and TNF receptors during primary HIV-1 infection: correlation with HIV-1 RNA and the clinical outcome. *AIDS* **10:**F45–F50.

Roake, J. A., A. S. Rao, P. J. Morris, C. P. Larsen, D. F. Hankins, and J. M. Austyn. 1995. Dendritic cell loss from nonlymphoid tissues after systemic administration of lipopolysaccharide, tumor necrosis factor, and interleukin 1. *J. Exp. Med.* **181:**2237–2247.

Roberts, N. J., Jr., J. Hiscott, and D. J. Signs. 1992. The limited role of the human interferon system response to respiratory syncytial virus challenge: analysis and comparison to influenza virus challenge. *Microb. Pathog.* **12:**409–414.

Rogge, L., L. Barberis-Maino, M. Biffi, N. Passini, D. H. Presky, U. Gubler, and F. Sinigaglia. 1997. Selective expression of an interleukin-12 receptor component by human T helper 1 cells. *J. Exp. Med.* **185:**825–831.

Rogge, L., D. D'Ambrosio, M. Biffi, G. Penna, L. J. Minetti, D. H. Presky, L. Adorini, and F. Sinigaglia. 1998. The role of Stat4 in species-specific regulation of Th cell development by type I IFNs. *J. Immunol.* **161:**6567–6574.

Rosenberg, Y. J., A. Cafaro, T. Brennan, J. G. Greenhouse, F. Villinger, A. A. Ansari, C. Brown, K. McKinnon, S. Bellah, J. Yalley-Ogunro, W. R. Elkins, S. Gartner, and M. G. Lewis. 1997. Virus-induced cytokines regulate circulating lymphocyte levels during primary SIV infections. *Int. Immunol.* **9:**703–712.

Rossi, D., and A. Zlotnik. 2000. The biology of chemokines and their receptors. *Annu. Rev. Immunol.* **18:**217–242.

Ruzek, M. C., A. H. Miller, S. M. Opal, B. D. Pearce, and C. A. Biron. 1997. Characterization of early cytokine responses and an interleukin (IL)-6-dependent pathway of endogenous glucocorticoid induction during murine cytomegalovirus infection. *J. Exp. Med.* **185:**1185–1192.

Ruzek, M. C., B. D. Pearce, A. H. Miller, and C. A. Biron. 1999. Endogenous glucocorticoids protect against cytokine-mediated lethality during viral infection. *J. Immunol.* **162:**3527–3533.

Ryman, K. D., W. B. Klimstra, K. B. Nguyen, C. A. Biron, and R. E. Johnston. 2000. Alpha/beta interferon protects adult mice from fatal Sindbis virus infection and is an important determinant of cell and tissue tropism. *J. Virol.* **74:**3366–3378.

Salazar-Mather, T. P., T. A. Hamilton, and C. A. Biron. 2000. A chemokine-to-cytokine-to-chemokine cascade critical in antiviral defense. *J. Clin. Investig.* **105:**985–993.

Salazar-Mather, T. P., R. Ishikawa, and C. A. Biron. 1996. NK cell trafficking and cytokine expression in splenic compartments after IFN induction and viral infection. *J. Immunol.* **157:**3054–3064.

Salazar-Mather, T. P., J. S. Orange, and C. A. Biron. 1998. Early murine cytomegalovirus (MCMV) infection induces liver natural killer (NK) cell inflammation and protection through macrophage inflammatory protein 1alpha (MIP-1alpha)-dependent pathways. *J. Exp. Med.* **187:**1–14.

Sandberg, K., P. Kemper, A. Stalder, J. Zhang, M. V. Hobbs, J. L. Whitton, and I. L. Campbell. 1994. Altered tissue distribution of viral replication and T cell spreading is pivotal in the protection against fatal lymphocytic choriomeningitis in mice after neutralization of IFN-alpha/beta. *J. Immunol.* **153:**220–231.

Sareneva, T., S. Matikainen, M. Kurimoto, and I. Julkunen. 1998. Influenza A virus-induced IFN-alpha/beta and IL-18 synergistically enhance IFN-gamma gene expression in human T cells. *J. Immunol.* **160:**6032–6038.

Schijns, V. E., B. L. Haagmans, C. M. Wierda, B. Kruithof, I. A. Heijnen, G. Alber, and M. C. Horzinek. 1998. Mice lacking IL-12 develop polarized Th1 cells during viral infection. *J. Immunol.* **160:**3958–3964.

Setsuda, J., J. Teruya-Feldstein, N. L. Harris, J. A. Ferry, L. Sorbara, G. Gupta, E. S. Jaffe, and G. Tosato. 1999. Interleukin-18, interferon-gamma, IP-10, and Mig expression in Epstein-Barr virus-induced infectious mononucleosis and post-transplant lymphoproliferative disease. *Am. J. Pathol.* **155:**257–265.

She, J., M. C. Ruzek, P. Velupillai, I. de Aos, B. Wang, D. A. Harn, J. Sancho, C. A. Biron, and C. Terhorst. 1999. Generation of antigen-specific cytotoxic T lymphocytes and regulation of cytokine production takes place in the absence of CD3zeta. *Int. Immunol.* **11:**845–857.

Sinicco, A., A. Biglino, M. Sciandra, B. Forno, A. M. Pollono, R. Raiteri, and P. Gioannini. 1993. Cytokine network and acute primary HIV-1 infection. *AIDS* **7:**1167–1172.

Srikiatkhachorn, A., and T. J. Braciale. 1997. Virus-specific CD8+ T lymphocytes downregulate T helper cell type 2 cytokine secretion and pulmonary eosinophilia during experimental murine respiratory syncytial virus infection. *J. Exp. Med.* **186:**421–432.

Stark, G. R., I. M. Kerr, B. R. Williams, R. H. Silverman, and R. D. Schreiber. 1998. How cells respond to interferons. *Annu. Rev. Biochem.* **67:**227–264.

Stepp, S. E., R. Dufourcq-Lagelouse, F. Le Deist, S. Bhawan, S. Certain, P. A. Mathew, J. I. Henter, M. Bennett, A. Fischer, G. de Saint Basile, and V. Kumar. 1999. Perforin gene defects in familial hemophagocytic lymphohistiocytosis. *Science* **286:**1957–1959.

Stobie, L., S. Gurunathan, C. Prussin, D. L. Sacks, N. Glaichenhaus, C. Y. Wu, and R. A. Seder. 2000. The role of antigen and IL-12 in sustaining Th1 memory cells in vivo: IL-12 is required to maintain memory/effector Th1 cells sufficient to mediate protection to an infectious parasite challenge. *Proc. Natl. Acad. Sci. USA* **11:**11.

Su, H. C., L. P. Cousens, L. D. Fast, M. K. Slifka, R. D. Bungiro, R. Ahmed, and C. A. Biron. 1998. CD4+ and CD8+ T cell interactions in IFN-gamma and IL-4 responses to viral infections: requirements for IL-2. *J. Immunol.* **160:**5007–5017.

Svedmyr, E., I. Ernberg, J. Seeley, O. Weiland, G. Masucci, K. Tsukuda, R. Szigeti, M. G. Masucci, H. Blomogren, and W. Berthold. 1984. Virologic, immunologic, and clinical observations on a patient during the incubation, acute, and convalescent phases of infectious mononucleosis. *Clin. Immunol. Immunopathol.* **30:**437–450.

Szabo, S. J., A. S. Dighe, U. Gubler, and K. M. Murphy. 1997a. Regulation of the interleukin (IL)-12R beta 2 subunit expression in developing T helper 1 (Th1) and Th2 cells. *J. Exp. Med.* **185:**817–824.

Szabo, S. J., L. H. Glimcher, and I. C. Ho. 1997b. Genes that regulate interleukin-4 expression in T cells. *Curr. Opin. Immunol.* **9:**776–781.

Szabo, S. J., S. T. Kim, G. L. Costa, X. Zhang, C. G. Fathman, and L. H. Glimcher. 2000. A novel transcription factor, T-bet, directs Th1 lineage commitment. *Cell* **100:**655–669.

Tay, C. H., and R. M. Welsh. 1997. Distinct organ-dependent mechanisms for the control of murine cytomegalovirus infection by natural killer cells. *J. Virol.* **71:**267–275.

Taylor, G. A., C. M. Collazo, G. S. Yap, K. Nguyen, T. A. Gregorio, L. S. Taylor, B. Eagleson, L. Secrest, E. A. Southon, S. W.

Reid, L. Tessarollo, M. Bray, D. W. McVicar, K. L. Komschlies, H. A. Young, C. A. Biron, A. Sher, and G. F. Vande Woude. 2000. Pathogen-specific loss of host resistance in mice lacking the IFN-gamma-inducible gene IGTP. *Proc. Natl. Acad. Sci. USA* 97:751–755.

Taylor, G. A., M. Jeffers, D. A. Largaespada, N. A. Jenkins, N. G. Copeland, and G. F. Vande Woude. 1996. Identification of a novel GTPase, the inducibly expressed GTPase, that accumulates in response to interferon gamma. *J. Biol. Chem.* 271: 20399–20405.

Tokunaga, T., O. Yano, E. Kuramoto, Y. Kimura, T. Yamamoto, T. Kataoka, and S. Yamamoto. 1992. Synthetic oligonucleotides with particular base sequences from the cDNA encoding proteins of *Mycobacterium bovis* BCG induce interferons and activate natural killer cells. *Microbiol. Immunol.* 36:55–66.

Torseth, J. W., B. J. Nickoloff, T. Y. Basham, and T. C. Merigan. 1987. Beta interferon produced by keratinocytes in human cutaneous infection with herpes simplex virus. *J. Infect. Dis.* 155: 641–648.

Trgovcich, J., J. F. Aronson, J. C. Eldridge, and R. E. Johnston. 1999. TNFalpha, interferon, and stress response induction as a function of age-related susceptibility to fatal Sindbis virus infection of mice. *Virology* 263:339–348.

Trinchieri, G. 1998. Interleukin-12: a cytokine at the interface of inflammation and immunity. *Adv. Immunol.* 70:83–243.

Tumpey, T. M., H. Cheng, D. N. Cook, O. Smithies, J. E. Oakes, and R. N. Lausch. 1998. Absence of macrophage inflammatory protein-1alpha prevents the development of blinding herpes stromal keratitis. *J. Virol.* 72:3705–3710.

Vacheron, F., A. Rudent, S. Perin, C. Labarre, A. M. Quero, and M. Guenounou. 1990. Production of interleukin 1 and tumour necrosis factor activities in bronchoalveolar washings following infection of mice by influenza virus. *J. Gen. Virol.* 71:477–479.

van den Broek, M. F., U. Muller, S. Huang, M. Aguet, and R. M. Zinkernagel. 1995. Antiviral defense in mice lacking both alpha/beta and gamma interferon receptors. *J. Virol.* 69:4792–4796.

Viljeck, J. 1964. Production of interferon by newborn and adult mice infected with Sindbis virus. *Virology* 22:651–652.

Villinger, F., P. E. Rollin, S. S. Brar, N. F. Chikkala, J. Winter, J. B. Sundstrom, S. R. Zaki, R. Swanepoel, A. A. Ansari, and C. J. Peters. 1999. Markedly elevated levels of interferon (IFN)-gamma, IFN-alpha, interleukin (IL)-2, IL-10, and tumor necrosis factor-alpha associated with fatal Ebola virus infection. *J. Infect. Dis.* 179:S188–S191.

Waldmann, T. A., and Y. Tagaya. 1999. The multifaceted regulation of interleukin-15 expression and the role of this cytokine in NK cell differentiation and host response to intracellular pathogens. *Annu. Rev. Immunol.* 17:19–49.

Wang, B., H. Fujisawa, L. Zhuang, S. Kondo, G. M. Shivji, C. S. Kim, T. W. Mak, and D. N. Sauder. 1997. Depressed Langerhans cell migration and reduced contact hypersensitivity response in mice lacking TNF receptor p75. *J. Immunol.* 159: 6148–6155.

Wathelet, M. G., C. H. Lin, B. S. Parekh, L. V. Ronco, P. M. Howley, and T. Maniatis. 1998. Virus infection induces the assembly of coordinately activated transcription factors on the IFN-beta enhancer in vivo. *Mol. Cell* 1:507–518.

Welsh, R. M., Jr. 1978. Cytotoxic cells induced during lymphocytic choriomeningitis virus infection of mice. I. Characterization of natural killer cell induction. *J. Exp. Med.* 148:163–181.

Wheelock, E. F., and W. A. Sibley. 1965. Circulating virus, interferon and antibody after vaccination with the 17-D strain of yellow-fever virus. *N. Engl. J. Med.* 273:194–198.

Wong, P., C. W. Severns, N. B. Guyer, and T. M. Wright. 1994. A unique palindromic element mediates gamma interferon induction of mig gene expression. *Mol. Cell. Biol.* 14:914–922.

Wright, T. M., and J. M. Farber. 1991. 5′ regulatory region of a novel cytokine gene mediates selective activation by interferon gamma. *J. Exp. Med.* 173:417–422.

Wright-Browne, V., A. M. Schnee, M. A. Jenkins, P. F. Thall, B. B. Aggarwal, M. Talpaz, and Z. Estrov. 1998. Serum cytokine levels in infectious mononucleosis at diagnosis and convalescence. *Leuk. Lymphoma* 30:583–589.

Yap, G., M. Pesin, and A. Sher. 2000. Cutting edge: IL-12 is required for the maintenance of IFN-gamma production in T cells mediating chronic resistance to the intracellular pathogen, *Toxoplasma gondii. J. Immunol.* 165:628–631.

Yoshimoto, T., H. Nagase, T. Yoneto, J. Inoue, and H. Nariuchi. 1998. Interleukin-12 expression in B cells by transformation with Epstein-Barr virus. *Biochem. Biophys. Res. Commun.* 252: 556–560.

Zhang, X., S. Sun, I. Hwang, D. F. Tough, and J. Sprent. 1998. Potent and selective stimulation of memory-phenotype CD8+ T cells in vivo by IL-15. *Immunity* 8:591–599.

Zimmermann, C., A. Prevost-Blondel, C. Blaser, and H. Pircher. 1999. Kinetics of the response of naive and memory CD8 T cells to antigen: similarities and differences. *Eur. J. Immunol.* 29:284–290.

IV. ACQUIRED IMMUNITY

Immunology of Infectious Diseases
Edited by S. H. E. Kaufmann, A. Sher, and R. Ahmed
© 2002 ASM Press, Washington, D.C.

Chapter 12

The Th1/Th2 Paradigm in Infections

TIM R. MOSMANN AND DEBORAH J. FOWELL

INTRODUCTION

Since the original identification of the Th1 and Th2 cytokine secretion phenotypes among long-term mouse T-cell clones, there has been an enormous amount of research aimed at defining the T-cell cytokine patterns that occur during different responses in mice and humans. As is usual in immunology, the real situation is much more complex than the starting model. The extent of the diversity of T-cell responses is much larger than the original Th1/Th2 dichotomy, raising questions about the significance of the original sharply defined Th1 and Th2 phenotypes, the extent of diversity of T-cell cytokine patterns, the information used by the immune system to decide which type of response to induce, the signals that induce differentiation into these and other phenotypes in vivo, and the extent to which differentiation and continued differentiation occur during normal responses.

Dichotomous Responses

The study of functional heterogeneity within the CD4$^+$ T-cell population with regard to infectious disease was prompted by studies in the early 1970s on the development of humoral and cell-mediated immunity to pathogens and experimental antigens. Two important observations from these early studies continue to drive investigations into immune regulation today; the first was that the two arms of the response (cell mediated versus humoral) were often unequally expressed, and the second was that the immune response type correlated with a healing or nonhealing phenotype in infected individuals. The Th1/Th2 dichotomy provided a cytokine-based framework for understanding CD4$^+$ T-cell heterogeneity during curative and pathogenic immune responses. An essential component of Th effector cell development is that the cytokines produced by Th1 and Th2 populations serve to augment the development of cells of the same subset while suppressing the expansion and functions of the other subset. This well-regulated mutual antagonism serves to focus, or polarize, the immune response toward an effector type most suited for the resolution of each microbial challenge.

Resistance to many intracellular pathogens, including bacteria, fungi, and protozoa, is characterized by the induction of a Th1 response. The production of gamma interferon (IFN-γ) and/or tumor necrosis factor alpha (TNF-α) by the Th1 population is essential for the activation of macrophages to a microbicidal state. In addition, IFN-γ stimulates the production of immunoglobulin G antibodies, which mediate opsonization and phagocytosis of particulate organisms. Th1 responses are also associated with viral infections; a direct role for CD4 cells in viral clearance has not been demonstrated for most viruses, but Th1 responses may support the expansion of CD8$^+$ antiviral effectors.

In contrast, extracellular pathogens, in particular parasitic helminths, are associated with the induction of Th2 responses. Unlike the clear activity of Th1-derived IFN-γ in activating macrophages for intracellular microbe killing, it is unclear how Th2 cytokines mediate protection from helminth infection. While the Th2-derived cytokines interleukin-4 (IL-4) and IL-5 mediate eosinophil and mast cell activation and IgE production, the use of mouse models where these effector populations can be experimentally ablated has failed to demonstrate an obligatory role in resistance to gut parasites. It is thought that IL-4 and IL-13 promote the expulsion of intestinal worms by directly mediating physiological changes that are detrimental to worm survival in the gut.

Tim R. Mosmann and Deborah J. Fowell • Center for Vaccine Biology and Immunology, University of Rochester Medical Center, 601 Elmwood Ave., Box 609, Rochester, NY 14642.

Dominance of the Th1/Th2 Model

Several features of this diversity have conspired to increase the emphasis on the Th1 and Th2 phenotypes. These represent extreme responses that have radically different effector functions, and the two responses cross-regulate each other (Mosmann and Coffman, 1989). For many of the experimental infectious-disease models studied in the mouse, infection drives the polarization to either a Th1 or Th2 response that is essential for successful control of infection (Abbas et al., 1996). Historically, however, our choice of pathogens may have overestimated the prevalence of the classical Th1/Th2 responses. Clear-cut conditions have been established for the in vitro differentiation of Th1 and Th2 cells, whereas the regulation of differentiation of other phenotypes is less well understood. Both Th1 and Th2 cells proliferate extensively in vitro, in contrast to Treg cells, which are more difficult to culture (Groux et al., 1997), because they have unusual growth requirements, have lower proliferative potential, or are not stable under in vitro conditions. Thus, there may be additional T-cell phenotypes that remain undiscovered because they have not yet been cultured and cloned in vitro—such cell types may include the legendary CD8 suppressor cell, which has been difficult to isolate and characterize in spite of abundant evidence for its presence in complex in vivo and in vitro responses.

WHAT IS THE ACTUAL DIVERSITY OF T-CELL CYTOKINE SECRETION PHENOTYPES IN VIVO?

Other Cytokine Secretion Phenotypes

Many mouse T-cell clones fit cleanly into the Th1 or Th2 definitions, namely, the secretion of IL-2, IFN-γ, and lymphotoxin by Th1 cells and the secretion of IL-4, IL-5, IL-9, IL-10, and IL-13 by Th2 cells. However, it was recognized almost immediately that many human T-cell clones (Maggi et al., 1988; Paliard et al., 1988) and some mouse clones (Firestein et al., 1989; Street et al., 1990) often synthesized the Th0 pattern, a mixture of these two sets of cytokines. Other patterns include mouse T-cell clones secreting IL-2, IL-4, and IL-5 but not IFN-γ (Street et al., 1990); T cells secreting IFN-γ and IL-10 but not IL-4 (Assenmacher et al., 1994); nonnaive T cells secreting only IL-2 (Sad and Mosmann, 1994; Sallusto et al., 1999); Th3 cells secreting transforming growth factor β (TGF-β) and IL-10 but not IL-4 (Chen et al., 1994); and Tr1 cells secreting IL-10 and/or TGF-β but not IL-4 (Groux et al., 1997).

Differentiation versus Temporary Modifications in Cytokine Secretion Patterns

The Th1 and Th2 patterns are relatively stable, and it is difficult to convert one cell type into the other or to induce either phenotype to revert to a naive cytokine pattern. Thus, these two phenotypes represent stable differentiation states. In contrast, cytokine secretion patterns can be temporarily altered, for example, IL-12 induces transient IFN-γ secretion by Th2 cells (Manetti et al., 1994; Yssel et al., 1994), and progesterone or prostaglandin E_2 induces a more Th2-like cytokine pattern in Th0 cells (Piccinni et al., 1995). These temporary changes should not be regarded as a change in phenotype but, rather, as a response by that phenotype to altered stimulation conditions. The physiological significance of these temporary changes in vivo remains to determined.

Do Th1, Th2 and Other Cytokine Secretion Patterns Represent Distinct Phenotypes?

Although the Th1 and Th2 phenotypes, as well as potentially other phenotypes, can be demonstrated to represent distinct differentiation states at the single-cell level, it has also been suggested that there is a continuum of individual cells secreting different patterns of cytokines and that Th1-biased or Th2-biased responses include more cells expressing Th1 or Th2 cytokines, respectively, even though each cell is not a prototypic Th1 or Th2. In some studies, the cytokine patterns appear to be random (Kelso, 1995), although in other studies with clones and freshly isolated cells, cytokine expression patterns are clearly nonrandom (Assenmacher et al., 1994; Street et al., 1990). It is difficult to reconcile the idea of a continuum of cytokine patterns expressed by single cells with the growing evidence for precise transcriptional control of cytokine gene expression in differentiated cell types. The Th1 and Th2 phenotypes clearly represent stable, terminally differentiated states with defined, regulated patterns of cytokine gene expression. However, the variety of cytokine patterns that have been described by different investigators raises the question of how many other discrete patterns of gene expression exist, and how they are regulated.

Monoallelic Expression of Cytokine Genes

Several cytokine genes, including those encoding IL-2, IL-3, IL-4, IL-5, IL-13, and possibly IFN-γ show an unusual pattern of expression—each gene is often expressed from only a single chromosome in differentiated T cells (Hollander et al., 1998; Bix and

Locksley, 1998; Hsieh et al., 2000). This partially monoallelic expression is not as complete as the exclusion seen for antibody and T-cell receptor (TCR) genes; nevertheless, this striking pattern of expression suggests that there may be a link to the mechanism(s) whereby a T cell switches on a particular set of cytokine genes.

Stochastic Model for Commitment of T cells to Different Cytokine Patterns

Based on cytokine patterns among T-cell clones and PCR analysis of early cells, it has been suggested that effector T-cell cytokine patterns are not fixed and dichotomous but are really random, with selection of the resulting patterns to give a population with Th1 or Th2 characteristics. The findings of monoallelic expression of cytokine genes are consistent with this idea that commitment to expression of each cytokine gene is random, since independent regulation of each cytokine allele would generate a diverse repertoire of combinatorially assorted cytokine gene expression patterns. An important component of this model is the requirement for a selection process to obtain the final cytokine patterns, such as Th1 or Th2, that are seen on long-term culture and cloning (Fig. 1A). This selection process would need to be specific for a small number of phenotypes out of the large number possible if initial cytokine gene expression is randomly assorted.

Model for Stochastic but Directed Differentiation

Instead of stochastic commitment to cytokine expression patterns followed by preferential death or proliferation to select the final phenotypes, T-cell differentiation might be due to a continued process of activation of different genes of a particular pattern, e.g., Th2, under the regulation of both TCR and cytokine signals (Fig. 1B). Thus, cytokine pressure could continue to induce the activation of additional genes until the full pattern was expressed. This is consistent with the derivation of mixed (Th0) patterns of cytokine synthesis by first culturing T cells under Th1 conditions and then switching them to Th2 conditions (Murphy et al., 1996). By this model, the choice of which group of genes to activate would be directed by TCR and/or cytokine signals whereas the sequence of activation of genes within that group would be stochastic. Monoallelic expression might occur by a feedback mechanism such that successful activation of, e.g., the IL-4 gene would result in termination of the activation process for that gene or group of genes. Activation of cytokine genes may proceed by a multistep process: although IL-4, IL-5,

and IL-13 are not always expressed together in early cultures, these closely linked cytokine genes are often expressed from the same chromosome in clones (Kelly and Locksley, 2000). This suggests that an initial step, such as long-range chromosomal activation and demethylation, could be monoallelic, and then the genes on that chromosomal segment could be activated randomly until the full Th2 pattern was achieved.

Early versus late cytokine gene expression may be regulated differently. Several lines of evidence suggest that there may be differences between newly differentiated and long-term effector T cells. In short-term cultures, monoallelic expression was unstable (Riviere et al., 1998), whereas long-term Th2 cells showed fidelity of expression from one allele (Riviere et al., 1998; Bix and Locksley, 1998). In CD8 T cells, the cytokine expression patterns are flexible for several generations after initial activation (Kelso and Groves, 1997) but the Tc1 and Tc2 patterns are stable after several days of proliferation in polarizing environments (Mosmann and Sad, 1996). Long-term clones of Th1 and Th2 cells have stable cytokine expression patterns, and subclones normally express the same patterns. Initial induction of phenotypes may be cytokine independent and modulated by the quality of T-cell–antigen-presenting cell (APC) interaction, for example the differentiation of limited numbers of cells into Th2 in IL-4 receptor (IL-4R) (Jankovic et al., 2000) knockout mice. Long-term cytokine gene expression may require cytokine signals for expansion or further stabilization of differentiation.

Do Differentiated T Cells Always Express All of Their Potential Cytokines?

An extra feature of T-cell cytokine gene expression makes "snapshot" data of cytokine synthesis very difficult to interpret. Even in fully differentiated T-cell clones, the individual cells within the clone do not always express all the cytokines that they are capable of expressing. For example, in Th1 clones, double labeling for cytokine mRNA (Bucy et al., 1994) or protein secretion (Karulin et al., 2000) shows that some cells produce only IL-2, some produce only IFN-γ, and some produce both. However, Th1 clones normally show good fidelity on subcloning, suggesting that each cell in the clonal population (or at least each clonable cell) has the potential to produce the full panoply of Th1 cytokines but that only a subset of the cytokines may be produced by a single cell on a single occasion.

This phenomenon introduces further difficulties in the measurement of differentiation of T cells into

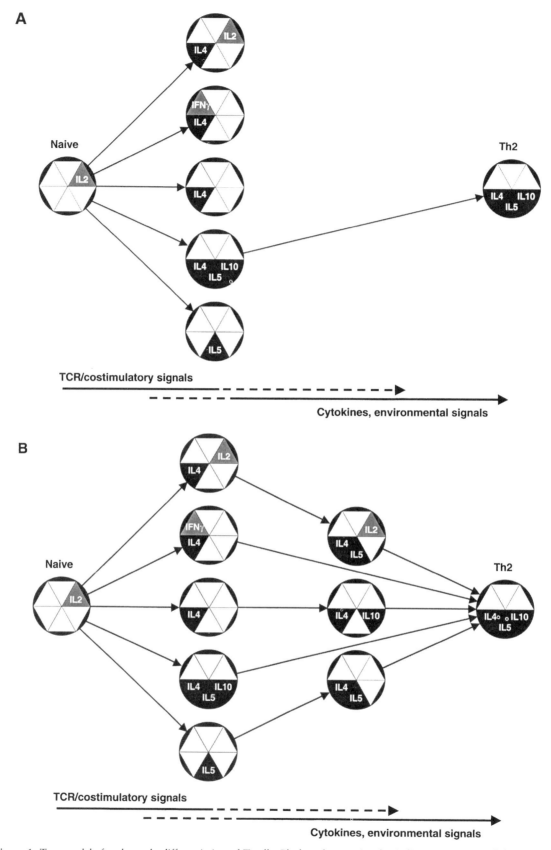

Figure 1. Two models for the early differentiation of T cells. Black and gray triangles indicate expression of the cytokine genes of the Th2 and Th1 patterns, respectively. (A) In the stochastic model, the initial differentiation event results in a variety of progeny cells expressing random cytokine patterns, and only those cells expressing the mature Th2 phenotype are selected for further proliferation. (B) In the stochastic but directed model, the initial differentiation event results in the same random mixture of patterns, but then each cell continues to differentiate, in response to environmental cues, towards the final Th2 pattern.

discrete cytokine patterns. For example, elegant single-cell PCR studies showed apparently random sets of cytokine expression in T cells during differentiation, rather than discrete phenotypes (Kelso et al., 1999). However, this method would not be able to measure the potential of each cell; instead, it measures the set of cytokines expressed on that particular occasion (subject to the possibility that cells expressing lower levels might not be detected). The expression by some cells of only a subset of their possible cytokines also introduces uncertainty into the assessment of cytokine patterns during in vivo responses—for example, the large numbers of cells secreting IL-2 but not IFN-γ, observed during in vivo responses (Karulin et al., 2000), could have been due either to Th1 cells that did not secrete IFN-γ on that particular occasion or to IL-2-producing precursor cells that do not secrete IFN-γ on any occasion (see below). It is not yet known whether the transient expression of limited sets of cytokines by individual committed cells is a random process or whether it is regulated by stimulation conditions such as the strength and duration of TCR signaling or the levels of costimulators on APC.

WHAT ARE THE CRITERIA USED TO DECIDE BETWEEN Th1 AND Th2 RESPONSES TO PARTICULAR INFECTIONS?

Coevolution of Host Immune Response and Microbial Pathogenesis

The outcome of infectious challenge is a tightly regulated balance between the survival of host and pathogen. For the infected host, the immune response has to be aggressive enough to eradicate the infection but sufficiently controlled to avoid immunopathology. In contrast, the pathogen needs to create an environment that allows its growth, development, and eventual transmission without necessarily destroying the host. For the most part, the coevolution of host and pathogen has generated highly effective pathogen-specific defense mechanisms. This tight relationship makes it difficult to assert accountability for a given response to host or pathogen. Similarly, a combination of host and parasite genetic variables generally conspires to create the disease state.

Initiation of the Immune Response Is Tightly Regulated by the Host

In the absence of infection, the immune system exists in a relatively quiescent state. The induction of

distinct Th subsets against individual pathogens is controlled in part by stringent activation criteria of the host immune system. Strict regulation of the selection and activation of the T-cell repertoire protects the mammalian host from inappropriate immune activation against tissue antigens and innocuous inhaled antigens and dietary proteins. For Th-cell activation to occur, the APC, namely, the dendritic cell (DC), must present pathogen-derived peptides in the context of major histocompatibility complex class II molecules and express costimulatory molecules such as B7.1/B7.2, CD40, intercellular cell adherence molecule 1 (ICAM-1), and/or OX40 ligand (Banchereau and Steinman, 1998). The acquisition of these immunostimulatory properties is carefully regulated. For the DC the capacity to activate T cells, in terms of both antigen-presenting capacity and expression of costimulatory molecules, is contingent on inflammatory stimuli such as bacterial lipopolysaccharide (Cella et al., 1997; Gallucci et al., 1999). Thus, the inception of the adaptive immune response is fine-tuned to occur only at the time of infectious challenge. How is the initial immune response further channeled toward a distinct effector program for specific pathogen clearance?

Factors Implicated in Driving Th1 and Th2 Responses

Studies using experimental protein antigens have reported numerous manipulations that can influence the Th1/Th2 decision (Abbas et al., 1996). Modulating factors at the time of T-cell priming include the cytokine milieu, dose of antigen, extent of TCR and costimulatory molecule ligation, and the type of APC. Apart from cytokine-mediated signals, most modulations center on the quality of the APC–T-cell interaction. The nature of the APC–T-cell interaction will presumably be translated within the T cell through the activation of as yet ill-defined kinase cascades that ultimately assemble the appropriate transcription complexes and ensure DNA accessibility for distinct cytokine gene expression (Glimcher and Murphy, 2000). The way in which the described experimental modulators of Th differentiation relate to situations of specific infectious challenge remains unclear.

Role of the Dendritic Cell

In the past year, there has been a wealth of reports suggesting that information pertinent to Th differentiation is carried by the DC from the tissue site of infection to the lymph node site of T-cell priming (Lanzavecchia and Sallusto, 2000; Kalinski et al.,

1999). Naive T cells do not enter non-lymphoid tissues and are therefore unlikely to receive direct pathogen signals for differential effector development on initial activation. In contrast, immature DCs reside in peripheral tissues and are activated by pathogens or pathogen-induced tissue damage. DC activation results in a transient increase in antigen uptake, assembly of peptide-major histocompatibility complex fusions, upregulation of costimulatory molecules, and migration to draining lymph nodes for priming of naive T cells. Recent reports suggest that DCs, in addition to T-cell activation signals, carry signals that bias effector differentiation appropriately for the specific microbe they encountered in the tissue (Reis e Sousa et al., 1999a). On encountering bacteria, intracellular protozoa, or viruses, DCs tend to upregulate IL-12 production. These IL-12-producing DCs efficiently promote Th1 development. In contrast, the lack of strong IL-12-inducing stimuli or the presence of prostaglandin E_2 has been demonstrated to drive DC maturation towards a Th2-inducing phenotype (Kalinski et al., 1999). Possibly the strongest evidence in support of DC discrimination on encountering a pathogen comes from studies on immune responses to the yeast and hyphae forms of the fungus *Candida albicans*. Ingestion of yeasts activated DCs for IL-12 production and priming for protective Th1 responses, whereas ingestion of hyphae inhibited IL-12 production and induced a nonprotective IL-4 response (d'Ostiani et al., 2000).

Little is known about the long-term stability of the cytokine profiles acquired by DCs during maturation. Some reports suggest that mature IL-12-producing DCs become resistant to modulating factors, while others report a change in DC polarizing potential over time (Langenkamp et al., 2000; Reis e Sousa, 1999b; Vieira et al., 2000). The stability question is an important one if DCs are to bear polarizing information that remains representative of the tissue environment from which they came. Future studies extending the observations to real infections will be required to validate the importance of the DC dichotomy in Th differentiation. Present studies have focused on cytokine-mediated signals from DCs for Th differentiation; however, it is likely that additional pathogen-derived information carried by DC, such as pathogen-related antigen dose and extent of costimulator upregulation, will also bias Th1/Th2 effector development.

Macrophage Involvement?

The macrophage is part of the front line of defense against invading microbes and is equipped with many antimicrobial responses. Phagocytosis of particles or organisms from the microenvironment triggers the induction of a number of proinflammatory mediators by the infected macrophage. Indeed, following uptake of intracellular pathogens such as mycobacteria, toxoplasmas, and listeriae, the macrophage upregulates the production of IL-12, TNF-α, and IL-1. T-cell priming within an IL-12-rich environment favors differentiation, growth, and survival of Th1 cells, accounting for the dominant Th1-like responses to these organisms (Hsieh et al., 1993). The extent to which macrophages influence the initiation of Th1 differentiation in vivo is unclear, since they would appear to be in the wrong anatomical site, i.e., the tissue rather than the lymph node. However, at the site of infection they may play an important role in sustaining the signals for Th1 expansion or may further promote Th1 differentiation in primed T cells that reach the infection site without prior adoption of a fixed effector program (see the section on uncommitted precursors, below).

Genetically Regulated Biases in Host Th1 and Th2 Responses

The genetic background of the infected host has a strong influence on Th differentiation. One of the classic examples of genetic control of Th1/Th2 development comes from the study of infection with the intracellular protozoan *Leishmania major* in inbred strains of mice (Fowell and Locksley, 1999). Resistance to *L. major* infection in most mouse strains, including the B10.D2 mouse, is dependent on the development of a robust Th1 response that activates the infected macrophage to a leishmaniacidal state. The BALB/c mouse strain is uniquely susceptible to *L. major* infection due to the development of a strong Th2 response, which fails to control parasite growth and eventually proves fatal. The genetic basis for the susceptibility of the BALB strain has not been fully characterized. At the T-cell level, a BALB-specific failure to retain expression of the IL-12R beta chain and a T-cell-intrinsic propensity for IL-4 production have been implicated in the aberrant Th2 response (Guler et al., 1996; Bix et al., 1998); the latter phenotype may drive susceptibility to *L. major* in vivo (Fowell et al., 1999).

The extent to which host genetic factors influence the effector choice will probably depend on the strength of polarizing cues from the infectious organism. For example, while BALB/c mice are highly susceptible to infection with *L. major* due to their failure to develop a Th1 response, their Th1-dependent control of intracellular organisms that induce a brisk IL-12 response is not impaired. Similarly, while C57BL/6 mice are susceptible to the nematode *Trichuris muris* due to their failure to develop a protective Th2 response, they mount strong protective Th2 responses on challenge with another nematode, *Nippostrongylus brasiliensis*. That inbred mouse strains appear exquisitely sensitive to infection in highly pathogen-specific ways demonstrates a high degree of redundancy within component parts of the differentiation pathways for Th1 and Th2 responses. Such a degree of redundancy was not anticipated from in vitro studies probably because the complexity of the immune response in vivo cannot be realized in the tissue culture dish. Indeed, human immunodeficiencies have provided the best examples of immune redundancy. Genetic deletions in IL-12, IL-12R, or IFN-γR genes cause highly restricted susceptibility to mycobacterial and salmonella infections (de Jong et al., 1998; Newport et al., 1996). Remarkably, these individuals were not susceptible to other viral, bacterial, or fungal infections, whose control was thought to be dependent on an IL-12- and/or IFN-γ-driven Th1 response.

The future challenge will be to relate the experimental data on criteria for Th1/Th2 differentiation to situations of microbial infection in vivo. Perhaps the strongest validation of the notion that experimental factors are biologically significant in Th differentiation comes from the exploitation of such components by pathogens for their survival.

Th1/Th2 Interference by the Pathogen

Pathogens that persist in infected hosts must evolve successful strategies to avoid a microbicidal immune response: these include the avoidance of immune recognition, suppression of a damaging immune response, and instruction of Th differentiation in favor of a beneficial immune response type. In general, pathogen immunomodulatory tactics are not designed to completely subvert the host immune response; instead, the best outcome is to generate an environment that supports their persistence without significant detriment to the host. Thus, pathogen-induced responses are often beneficial for pathogen and host alike. Subsequent chapters in this section of the book describe in detail the development of immune responses to individual pathogens. Here we give a general idea of the way in which pathogens have learned to manipulate Th1/Th2 differentiation.

Pathogen-Mediated Deviation of the Host Immune Response

Some microbes appear to produce products that actively bias the immune response in a Th1 or Th2 direction. On encountering the immune system, *Tox-*

oplasma gondii rapidly induces IL-12 production from DCs to promote a potent Th1 response (Sousa et al., 1997). The Th1 response is critical for host survival and pathogen latency, since *Toxoplasma* infection of IL-12- or IFN-γ-deficient mice is fatal as a result of high parasitemia. Surprisingly, *Toxoplasma*-derived proteins appear to further regulate host survival by limiting IL-12-mediated immunopathology. Soluble *T. gondii* antigens drive DCs to transiently produce IL-12 and then become refractory to further IL-12-inducing signals; this DC "paralysis" can last for up to a week (Reis e Sousa et al., 1999b). The specific factor from *Toxoplasma* extracts that drives IL-12 production remains elusive. Thus, the microbe both initiates a protective-Th1 response and limits the immunopathology by reducing prolonged exposure to IL-12. Similarly, mycobacterial infections are relatively nonpathogenic due to their active induction of a Th1 response. The Th1-driven inflammatory granulomatous response sequesters organisms in areas of liquefaction and tissue destruction (caseous necrosis), thus both containing the organism with minimal host tissue damage and enabling the organism to remain latent (Saunders and Cooper, 2000).

In contrast, helminth-secreted products have recently been shown to promote DCs to prime for Th2 responses (Whelan et al., 2000). The nematode *Ascaridia galli* expresses a prostaglandin H D-isomerase that mediates the synthesis of prostaglandin E$_2$, providing a mechanism for the generation of Th2-inducing DCs by nematodes (Meyer et al., 1996). It is unclear why the induction of a Th2 response is beneficial to the pathogen. It may be the lesser of two evils, since a proinflammatory Th1 response in the gut is unlikely to benefit host or pathogen. Indeed, the eggs of the parasitic worm *Schistosoma mansoni* induce the development of a potent Th2 response that appears to be necessary to downregulate the immunopathology that would arise if the production of nitric oxide were left unchecked (Brunet et al., 1999). In contrast, the blocking of IL-13 reduces the liver damage associated with the Th2-induced granuloma formation (Chiaramonte et al., 1999). The schistosomiasis infection model is a good example of how a careful Th1/Th2 balance is needed to prevent disease expression, involving an ultimate trade-off between containment of the pathogen and tissue damage.

Pathogen-Mediated Suppression of Th Differentiation

The production of proinflammatory cytokines including TNF-α, IL-1, and IL-12 by monocyte populations provides an early signal for protective Th1-

mediated immunity to intracellular pathogens. It is not surprising, therefore, that many prokaryotes and viruses have evolved ways to disrupt the production of these cytokines to aid pathogen survival. Infection of macrophages by the protozoan *Leishmania major* not only fails to induce inflammatory mediators such as IL-12 but also actively suppresses the induction of IL-12 expression by other inflammatory mediators (Reiner et al., 1994; Carrera et al., 1996). The evasion of macrophage inflammatory mediators presumably allows the infective promastigote form of *L. major* to survive within the macrophage long enough to transform into the more resistant amastigote forms. Measles virus infection also ablates infected monocyte production of IL-12 (Karp et al., 1996). Cross-linking of the monocyte complement-regulatory molecule CD46 downregulates IL-12 production, and measles virus appears to exploit this mechanism by expressing a hemagglutinin ligand for CD46 (Mosser and Karp, 1999). Other microbial strategies for manipulating macrophage activation and cytokine production include the activation of the cellular SHP-1 phosphatase (Knutson et al., 1998) and induction of the anti-inflammatory cytokine TGF-β by the mycobacterial lipoarabinomannan product (Dahl et al., 1996); the inhibition of NF-κB activation by preventing phosphorylation of its inhibitor, IκB, by the *Yersinia* YopJ molecule (Schesser et al., 1998); the production of TNF-α and TNF-β receptors by poxviruses (Spriggs, 1994); and the potential modulation of macrophage-migration inhibitory factor (MIF) by nematode-derived MIF orthologues (Pennock et al., 1998).

Pathogen-Mediated Suppression of Existing Effector Responses

Other pathogen schemes seek to modulate existing immune responses. Many persistent viruses have evolved to encode products that block or modulate Th1 responses, including the expression of proteins that bind IFNs by poxviruses (Alcami and Smith, 1996) and the production of an IL-10 homolog by Epstein-Barr virus (Moore et al., 1990). In addition, examples from both viruses and parasites suggest that immune responses can be modified by the generation of natural altered peptide ligands (Franco et al., 1995). Experimentally, the alteration of CD4$^+$ T-cell epitopes has been shown to influence Th1/Th2 differentiation in a number of model systems (Tao et al., 1997). While we do not understand the biochemical mechanism for the effect of altered peptide ligands, the phenomenon appears to have been exploited by pathogens to modulate immune responses in vivo. Naturally occurring polymor-

phisms in the *Plasmodium falciparum* protein that is the target of the early immune response were shown to induce a rapid change from IFN-γ production to production of the immunosuppressive cytokine IL-10 (Plebanski et al., 1999). It is thought that such polymorphisms may prevent the elimination of the parasite and contribute to the overall reduction in T-cell responses to malaria antigens in areas of endemic infection.

EXPANSION OF AN UNCOMMITTED PRECURSOR POPULATION DURING IMMUNE RESPONSES

Although differentiation into Th1, Th2, or other phenotypes secreting several potent cytokines is a common outcome of antigen stimulation of naive T cells, it is now clear that substantial numbers of T cells can be primed without differentiating into effector cells secreting one of these cytokine patterns. Stimulation of mouse naive CD4 T cells in vitro in the presence of TGF-β and anti-IFN-γ results in a proliferating precursor (Thpp) T-cell population that continues to express IL-2 and retains the ability to differentiate into either Th1 or Th2 cells (Sad and Mosmann, 1994). We have found similar proliferating, IL-2-secreting cells in vivo, which may constitute the majority of antigen-specific CD4 T cells during an immune response (X. Wang and T. R. Mosmann, unpublished data). A population of human memory CD4 T cells expressing the CCR7 chemokine receptor also displays the IL-2-only phenotype, suggesting that these "central memory" cells are a substantial population in humans (Sallusto et al., 1999; Lanzavecchia and Sallusto, 2000). Although the human IL-2-producing cells have not been shown directly to be uncommitted and multipotential, the CCR7$^+$ population includes precursors of IFN-γ- and IL-4-producing cells.

The requirements for these primed precursor cells to differentiate into Th1 or Th2 cells are similar or identical to the signals that induce naive T-cell differentiation: IL-4 and IFN-γ are required for differentiation into Th2 and Th1 cells, respectively. The addition of blocking monoclonal antibodies specific for these two cytokines is often sufficient to maintain the primed precursor cells in an uncommitted state, suggesting that one of the ways in which the primed precursor state is induced is simply antigen activation in the absence of strong differentiative signals. However, this is not a very satisfying explanation, because it would mean that the extent of differentiation was highly dependent on other responses in the vicinity. Since this would lead to unpredictable responses, we prefer a model in which at least part of the regulation of differentiation into primed precursor cells is active. The ability of TGF-β to prevent Th2 differentiation is an example of such active regulation, and we suggest that there will be an analogous signal that prevents differentiation into Th1 cells.

Do These Cells Differentiate More Rapidly than Naive Cells?

After stimulation with antigen or APC, naive T cells require about 3 to 5 days to differentiate into either Th1 or Th2 cells. Although the activated state of the in vitro-derived Thpp cells raised the possibility that they would differentiate more rapidly, the kinetics of differentiation of naive and Thpp cells were in fact very similar (Akai and Mosmann, 1999). In addition to testing the acquisition of the ability to secrete substantial amounts of IL-4 or IFN-γ, the kinetics of commitment were investigated; i.e., how long was required before naive or Thpp cells would express Th1 or Th2 cytokine patterns even if shifted back to nondifferentiative conditions? Again, naive and Thpp cells both required 3 to 5 days for this commitment. Thus, the kinetics of differentiation of Thpp cells do not appear to be more rapid, so that the advantage of the Thpp phenotype in future infections may be due only to the presence of an expanded pool of antigen-specific precursors rather than to a more rapid expression of effector phenotypes by individual cells.

Trafficking of Precursor Cells

Human IL-2-secreting "central memory" cells express cell surface markers that suggest that these cells may home preferentially to lymph nodes (Sallusto et al., 1999); they are defined by the expression of CCR7, which binds to the chemokines ELC and SLC and assists with entry into lymph nodes via high endothelial venules (HEV), and most but not all express CD62 ligand (CD62L), which binds to glycoproteins on HEV to mediate initial attachment. This is consistent with the possibility that these cells require "postgraduate education" to differentiate into the appropriate effector phenotype during a subsequent response and that this differentiation proceeds under the direction of the lymphoid microenvironment, including DCs that have acquired the ability to selectively stimulate one or other differentiation pathway (see above). However, it is also possible that the primed precursor cells may express a different phenotype when recently activated, as Thpp cells derived by antigen stimulation in vitro express low levels of CD62L (Sad and Mosmann, 1994), and the

antigen-specific IL-2-only CD4 T cells derived by immunization in vivo include similar numbers of both CD62Lhi and CD62Llo cells (Wang and Mosmann, unpublished). If these three populations of cells, producing IL-2 but not IFN-γ or IL-4, are all equivalent, this suggests that they can exist in different states expressing different cell surface markers and hence probably different homing properties. This raises the possibility that unlike naive T cells, the primed precursor cells may migrate into sites of inflammation or infection. The primed precursor cells may return to a CD62Lhi state as a long-term memory population but then may lose expression of CD62L during reactivation in lymph nodes, before circulating to nonlymphoid sites for further differentiation. Although naive T cells are thought to require priming by strong APC such as DCs, if the primed precursor cells can respond to other APC such as macrophages or B cells, this strengthens the possibility that such cells at a site of infection could control T-cell differentiation, not just as bystanders but as direct participants. This may provide more flexibility of input of differentiative signals. Also, previous studies showing effects of B cells on Th subset differentiation (Stockinger et al., 1996) may have analyzed the effects of B cells on the differentiation of activated Thpp cells rather than naive T cells. Thus, the primed but uncommitted T-cell phenotype may provide separation of the initial priming and activation event, in both time and location, from the induction of effector differentiation.

Bringing together the existence of IL-2-secreting precursor cells with the fact that differentiated Th1 cells sometimes secrete only a partial subset of their full cytokine pattern, it is clear that cells identified as secreting IL-2 but not IFN-γ might be either primed precursor cells or Th1 cells that are not synthesizing IFN-γ on that particular occasion. This introduces some uncertainty into single-cell measurements of cytokine production. If many cells in a population secrete IL-2 but very few secrete IFN-γ, this population probably includes mostly primed precursor or naive cells. On the other hand, if IL-2- and IFN-γ-secreting cells are present at similar frequencies, many of the IL-2-secreting cells may represent Th1 cells, even if two-color assays show that the cells are secreting only IL-2 but not IFN-γ. If the secretion of only some of the full complement of cytokines by a single effector T cell is due to variations in the stimulation conditions, it may be possible to identify conditions that will reliably induce each cell to produce its full potential set of cytokines, but if the expression of different cytokines on each occasion is a stochastic process, the true cytokine secretion potential of single cells could be determined only by repetitive stimulation or subcloning.

Biological Significance of Uncommitted Precursors

In both mouse and human immune responses, a substantial population of uncommitted CD4 antigen-specific cells may be useful for providing an expanded pool of antigen-specific cells without committing to a particular set of effector functions. These might then differentiate during the immune response to subsequent infections to provide the correct effector functions. This may serve two functions. First, the T cells induced by the first infection may cross-react with a similar but nonidentical pathogen in the second infection, and different effector functions may be required to combat the two pathogens. Second, T cells of the same specificity but different effector functions may be required to deal with different stages of the same pathogen, for example in malaria, in which Th1 and Th2 responses are required at different stages (Langhorne et al., 1989).

CONCLUSION

The importance of "classical" Th1 and Th2 responses in several well-characterized disease models is probably an example of the more general principle that diverse effector functions (often mediated by cytokines) are required for the eradication of different infections. We expect that T cells expressing non-Th1, non-Th2 patterns may be essential for other diseases and that the crucial differences between the immune responses may be subtle. The requirement for multiple effector phenotypes is almost certainly due to the intensive interplay between the host response and each pathogen, driving the evolution of complex host defense strategies and equally complex evasion and interference tactics by the pathogen. The induction of substantial numbers of antigen-specific but uncommitted T cells during an immune response may also provide the immune system with extra flexibility to adjust effector functions during ongoing or future infections.

REFERENCES

Abbas, A. K., K. M. Murphy, and A. Sher. 1996. Functional diversity of helper T lymphocytes. *Nature* **383:**787–793.

Akai, P. S., and T. R. Mosmann. 1999. Primed and replicating but uncommitted T helper precursor cells show kinetics of differentiation and commitment similar to those of naive T helper cells. *Microbes Infect.* **1:**51–68.

Alcami, A., and G. L. Smith. 1996. Receptors for gamma-interferon encoded by poxviruses: implications for the unknown origin of vaccinia virus. *Trends Microbiol.* **4:**321–326.

Assenmacher, M., J. Schmitz, and A. Radbruch. 1994. Flow cytometric determination of cytokines in activated murine T helper lymphocytes: expression of interleukin-10 in interferon-gamma and in interleukin-4-expressing cells. *Eur. J. Immunol.* **24:**1097–1101.

Bancereau, J., and R. M. Steinman. 1998. Dendritic cells and the control of immunity. *Nature* **392:**245–252.

Bix, M., and R. M. Locksley. 1998. Independent and epigenetic regulation of the interleukin-4 alleles in CD4+ T cells. *Science* **281:**1352–1354.

Bix, M., Z. E. Wang, B. Thiel, N. J. Schork, and R. M. Locksley. 1998. Genetic regulation of commitment to interleukin 4 production by a CD4(+) T cell-intrinsic mechanism. *J. Exp. Med.* **188:**2289–2299.

Brunet, L. R., M. Beall, D. W. Dunne, and E. J. Pearce. 1999. Nitric oxide and the Th2 response combine to prevent severe hepatic damage during *Schistosoma mansoni* infection. *J. Immunol.* **163:**4976–4984.

Bucy, R. P., A. Panoskaltsis-Mortari, G. Q. Huang, J. Li, L. Karr, M. Ross, J. H. Russell, K. M. Murphy, and C. T. Weaver. 1994. Heterogeneity of single cell cytokine gene expression in clonal T cell populations. *J. Exp. Med.* **180:**1251–1262.

Carrera, L., R. T. Gazzinelli, R. Badolato, S. Hieny, W. Muller, R. Kuhn, and D. L. Sacks. 1996. *Leishmania* promastigotes selectively inhibit interleukin 12 induction in bone marrow-derived macrophages from susceptible and resistant mice. *J. Exp. Med.* **183:**515–526.

Cella, M., A. Engering, V. Pinet, J. Pieters, and A. Lanzavecchia. 1997. Inflammatory stimuli induce accumulation of MHC class II complexes on dendritic cells. *Nature* **388:**782–787.

Chen, Y., V. K. Kuchroo, J. Inobe, D. A. Hafler, and H. L. Weiner. 1994. Regulatory T cell clones induced by oral tolerance: suppression of autoimmune encephalomyelitis. *Science* **265:**1237–1240.

Chiaramonte, M. G., D. D. Donaldson, A. W. Cheever, and T. A. Wynn. 1999. An IL-13 inhibitor blocks the development of hepatic fibrosis during a T-helper type 2-dominated inflammatory response. *J. Clin. Investig.* **104:**777–785.

Dahl, K. E., H. Shiratsuchi, B. D. Hamilton, J. J. Ellner, and Z. Toossi. 1996. Selective induction of transforming growth factor beta in human monocytes by lipoarabinomannan of *Mycobacterium tuberculosis*. *Infect. Immun.* **64:**399–405.

de Jong, R., F. Altare, I. A. Haagen, D. G. Elferink, T. Boer, P. J. van Breda Vriesman, P. J. Kabel, J. M. Draaisma, J. T. van Dissel, F. P. Kroon, J. L. Casanova, and T. H. Ottenhoff. 1998. Severe mycobacterial and *Salmonella* infections in interleukin-12 receptor-deficient patients. *Science* **280:**1435–1438.

d'Ostiani, C. F., G. Del Sero, A. Bacci, C. Montagnoli, A. Spreca, A. Mencacci, P. Ricciardi-Castagnoli, and L. Romani. 2000. Dendritic cells discriminate between yeasts and hyphae of the fungus *Candida albicans*. Implications for initiation of T helper cell immunity in vitro and in vivo. *J. Exp. Med.* **191:**1661–1674.

Firestein, G. S., W. D. Roeder, J. A. Laxer, K. S. Townsend, C. T. Weaver, J. T. Hom, J. Linton, B. E. Torbett, and A. L. Glasebrook. 1989. A new murine CD4+ T cell subset with an unrestricted cytokine profile. *J. Immunol.* **143:**518–525.

Fowell, D. J., and R. M. Locksley. 1999. *Leishmania major* infection of inbred mice: unmasking genetic determinants of infectious diseases. *Bioessays* **21:**510–518.

Fowell, D. J., K. Shinkai, X. C. Liao, A. M. Beebe, R. L. Coffman, D. R. Littman, and R. M. Locksley. 1999. Impaired NFATc translocation and failure of Th2 development in Itk-deficient CD4+ T cells. *Immunity* **11:**399–409.

Franco, A., C. Ferrari, A. Sette, and F. V. Chisari. 1995. Viral mutations, TCR antagonism and escape from the immune response. *Curr. Opin. Immunol.* 7:524–531.

Gallucci, S., M. Lolkema, and P. Matzinger. 1999. Natural adjuvants: endogenous activators of dendritic cells. *Nat. Med.* 5:1249–1255.

Glimcher, L. H., and K. M. Murphy. 2000. Lineage commitment in the immune system: the T helper lymphocyte grows up. *Genes Dev.* 14:1693–1711.

Groux, H., A. O'Garra, M. Bigler, M. Rouleau, S. Antonenko, J. E. de Vries, and M. G. Roncarolo. 1997. A CD4+ T cell subset inhibits antigen-specific T-cell responses and prevents colitis. *Nature* 389:737.

Guler, M. L., J. D. Gorham, C. S. Hsieh, A. J. Mackey, R. G. Steen, W. F. Dietrich, and K. M. Murphy. 1996. Genetic susceptibility to *Leishmania*: IL-12 responsiveness in TH1 cell development. *Science* 271:984–987.

Hollander, G. A., S. Zuklys, C. Morel, E. Mizoguchi, K. Mobisson, S. Simpson, C. Terhorst, W. Wishart, D. E. Golan, A. K. Bhan, and S. J. Burakoff. 1998. Monoallelic expression of the interleukin-2 locus. *Science* 279:2118–2121.

Hsieh, C. S., S. E. Macatonia, C. S. Tripp, S. F. Wolf, A. O'Garra, and K. M. Murphy. 1993. Development of TH1 CD4+ T cells through IL-12 produced by *Listeria*-induced macrophages. *Science* 260:547–549.

Hsieh, S., N. Chen, K. Tarbell, N. Liao, Y. Lai, K. Lee, K. Lee, S. Wu, H. Sytwu, S. Han, and H. McDevitt. 2000. Transgenic mice expressing surface markers for IFN-gamma and IL-4 producing cells. *Mol. Immunol.* 37:281–293.

Jankovic, D., M. C. Kullberg, N. Noben-Trauth, P. Caspar, W. E. Paul, and A. Sher. 2000. Single cell analysis reveals that IL-4 receptor/Stat6 signaling is not required for the in vivo or in vitro development of CD4+ lymphocytes with a Th2 cytokine profile. *J. Immunol.* 164:3047–3055.

Kalinski, P., C. M. Hilkens, E. A. Wierenga, and M. L. Kapsenberg. 1999. T-cell priming by type-1 and type-2 polarized dendritic cells: the concept of a third signal. *Immunol. Today* 20:561–567.

Karp, C. L., M. Wysocka, L. M. Wahl, J. M. Ahearn, P. J. Cuomo, B. Sherry, G. Trinchieri, and D. E. Griffin. 1996. Mechanism of suppression of cell-mediated immunity by measles virus. *Science* 273:228–231.

Karulin, A. Y., M. D. Hesse, M. Tary-Lehmann, and P. V. Lehmann. 2000. Single-cytokine-producing CD4 memory cells predominate in type 1 and type 2 immunity. *J. Immunol.* 164:1862–1872.

Kelly, B. L., and R. M. Locksley. 2000. Coordinate regulation of the IL-4, IL-13, and IL-5 cytokine cluster in Th2 clones revealed by allelic expression patterns. *J. Immunol.* 165:2982–2986.

Kelso, A. 1995. Th1 and Th2 subsets—paradigms lost. *Immunol. Today* 16:374–379.

Kelso, A., and P. Groves. 1997. A single peripheral Cd8(+) T cell can give rise to progeny expressing type 1 and/or type 2 cytokine genes and can retain its multipotentiality through many cell divisions. *Proc. Natl. Acad. Sci. USA* 94:8070–8075.

Kelso, A., P. Groves, L. Ramm, and A. G. Doyle. 1999. Single-cell analysis by RT-PCR reveals differential expression of multiple type 1 and 2 cytokine genes among cells within polarized CD4+ T cell populations. *Int. Immunol.* 11:617–621.

Knutson, K. L., Z. Hmama, P. Herrera-Velit, R. Rochford, and N. E. Reiner. 1998. Lipoarabinomannan of *Mycobacterium tuberculosis* promotes protein tyrosine dephosphorylation and inhibition of mitogen-activated protein kinase in human mononuclear phagocytes. Role of the Src homology 2 containing tyrosine phosphatase 1. *J. Biol. Chem.* 273:645–652.

Langenkamp, A., M. Messi, A. Lanzavecchia, and F. Sallusto. 2000. Kinetics of dendritic cell activation: impact on priming of Th1, Th2 and nonpolarized T cells. *Nat. Immunol.* 1:311–316.

Langhorne, J., S. J. Meding, K. Eichmann, and S. S. Gillard. 1989. The response of CD4+ T cells to *Plasmodium chabaudi* chabaudi. *Immunol. Rev.* 112:71–94.

Lanzavecchia, A., and F. Sallusto. 2000. Dynamics of T lymphocyte responses: intermediates, effectors, and memory cells. *Science* 290:92–97.

Maggi, E., G. Del Prete, D. Macchia, P. Parronchi, A. Tiri, I. Chretien, M. Ricci, and S. Romagnani. 1988. Profiles of lymphokine activities and helper function for IgE in human T cell clones. *Eur. J. Immunol.* 18:1045–1050.

Manetti, R., F. Gerosa, M. G. Giudizi, R. Biagiotti, P. Parronchi, M. P. Piccinni, S. Sampognaro, E. Maggi, S. Romagnani, and G. Trinchieri. 1994. Interleukin 12 induces stable priming for interferon gamma (IFN-gamma) production during differentiation of human T helper (Th) cells and transient IFN-gamma production in established Th2 cell clones. *J. Exp. Med.* 179:1273–1283.

Meyer, D. J., R. Muimo, M. Thomas, D. Coates, and R. E. Isaac. 1996. Purification and characterization of prostaglandin-H E-isomerase, a sigma-class glutathione S-transferase, from *Ascaridia galli*. *Biochem. J.* 313:223–227.

Moore, K. W., P. Vieira, D. F. Fiorentino, M. L. Trounstine, T. A. Khan, and T. R. Mosmann. 1990. Homology of cytokine synthesis inhibitory factor (IL-10) to the Epstein-Barr virus gene BCRFI. *Science* 248:1230–1234.

Mosmann, T. R., and R. L. Coffman. 1989. TH1 and TH2 cells: different patterns of lymphokine secretion lead to different functional properties. *Annu. Rev. Immunol.* 7:145–173.

Mosmann, T. R., and S. Sad. 1996. The expanding universe of T-cell subsets: Th1, Th2 and more. *Immunol. Today* 17:138–146.

Mosser, D. M., and C. L. Karp. 1999. Receptor mediated subversion of macrophage cytokine production by intracellular pathogens. *Curr. Opin. Immunol.* 11:406–411.

Murphy, E., K. Shibuya, N. Hosken, P. Openshaw, V. Maino, K. Davis, K. Murphy, and A. O'Garra. 1996. Reversibility of T helper 1 and 2 populations is lost after long-term stimulation. *J. Exp. Med.* 183:901–913.

Newport, M. J., C. M. Huxley, S. Huston, C. M. Hawrylowicz, B. A. Oostra, R. Williamson, and M. Levin. 1996. A mutation in the interferon-gamma-receptor gene and susceptibility to mycobacterial infection. *N. Engl. J. Med.* 335:1941–1949.

Paliard, X., R. de Waal Malefijt, H. Yssel, D. Blanchard, I. Chretien, J. Abrams, J. de Vries, and H. Spits. 1988. Simultaneous production of IL-2, IL-4, and IFN-gamma by activated human CD4+ and CD8+ T cell clones. *J. Immunol.* 141:849–855.

Pennock, J. L., J. M. Behnke, Q. D. Bickle, E. Devaney, R. K. Grencis, R. E. Isaac, G. W. Joshua, M. E. Selkirk, Y. Zhang, and D. J. Meyer. 1998. Rapid purification and characterization of L-dopachrome-methyl ester tautomerase (macrophage-migration-inhibitory factor) from *Trichinella spiralis*, *Trichuris muris* and *Brugia pahangi*. *Biochem. J.* 335:495–498.

Piccinni, M. P., M. G. Giudizi, R. Biagiotti, L. Beloni, L. Giannarini, S. Sampognaro, P. Parronchi, R. Manetti, F. Annunziato, C. Livi, S. Romagnani, and E. Maggi. 1995. Progesterone favors the development of human T helper cells producing Th2-type cytokines and promotes both IL-4 production and membrane CD30 expression in established Th1 cell clones. *J. Immunol.* 155:128–133.

Plebanski, M., K. L. Flanagan, E. A. Lee, W. H. Reece, K. Hart, C. Gelder, G. Gillespie, M. Pinder, and A. V. Hill. 1999. Interleukin 10-mediated immunosuppression by a variant CD4 T cell epitope of *Plasmodium falciparum*. *Immunity* 10:651–660.

Reiner, S. L., S. Zheng, Z. E. Wang, L. Stowring, and R. M. Locksley. 1994. *Leishmania* promastigotes evade interleukin 12 (IL-12) induction by macrophages and stimulate a broad range of cytokines from CD4+ T cells during initiation of infection. *J. Exp. Med.* **179:**447–456.

Reis e Sousa, C., A. Sher, and P. Kaye. 1999a. The role of dendritic cells in the induction and regulation of immunity to microbial infection. *Curr. Opin. Immunol.* **11:**392–399.

Reis e Sousa, C., G. Yap, O. Schulz, N. Rogers, M. Schito, J. Aliberti, S. Hieny, and A. Sher. 1999b. Paralysis of dendritic cell IL-12 production by microbial products prevents infection-induced immunopathology. *Immunity* **11:**637–647.

Riviere, I., M. J. Sunshine, and D. R. Littman. 1998. Regulation of Il-4 expression by activation of individual alleles. *Immunity* **9:**217–228.

Sad, S., and T. R. Mosmann. 1994. Single IL-2-secreting precursor CD4 T cell can develop into either Th1 or Th2 cytokine secretion phenotype. *J. Immunol.* **153:**3514–3522.

Sallusto, F., D. Lenig, R. Forster, M. Lipp, and A. Lanzavecchia. 1999. Two subsets of memory T lymphocytes with distinct homing potentials and effector functions. *Nature* **401:**708–712.

Saunders, B. M., and A. M. Cooper. 2000. Restraining mycobacteria: role of granulomas in mycobacterial infections. *Immunol. Cell Biol.* **78:**334–341.

Schesser, K., A. K. Spiik, J. M. Dukuzumuremyi, M. F. Neurath, S. Pettersson, and H. Wolf-Watz. 1998. The yopJ locus is required for *Yersinia*-mediated inhibition of NF-kappaB activation and cytokine expression: YopJ contains a eukaryotic SH2-like domain that is essential for its repressive activity. *Mol. Microbiol.* **28:**1067–1079.

Sousa, C. R., S. Hieny, T. Scharton-Kersten, D. Jankovic, H. Charest, R. N. Germain, and A. Sher. 1997. In vivo microbial stimulation induces rapid CD40 ligand-independent production of interleukin 12 by dendritic cells and their redistribution to T cell areas. *J. Exp. Med.* **186:**1819–1829.

Spriggs, M. K. 1994. Cytokine and cytokine receptor genes 'captured' by viruses. *Curr. Opin. Immunol.* **6:**526–529.

Stockinger, B., T. Zal, A. Zal, and D. Gray. 1996. B cells solicit their own help from T cells. *J. Exp. Med.* **183:**891–899.

Street, N. E., J. H. Schumacher, T. A. Fong, H. Bass, D. F. Fiorentino, J. A. Leverah, and T. R. Mosmann. 1990. Heterogeneity of mouse helper T cells. Evidence from bulk cultures and limiting dilution cloning for precursors of Th1 and Th2 cells. *J. Immunol.* **144:**1629–1639.

Tao, X., S. Constant, P. Jorritsma, and K. Bottomly. 1997. Strength of TCR signal determines the costimulatory requirements for Th1 and Th2 CD4+ T cell differentiation. *J. Immunol.* **159:**5956–5963.

Vieira, P. L., E. C. de Jong, E. A. Wierenga, M. L. Kapsenberg, and P. Kalinski. 2000. Development of Th1-inducing capacity in myeloid dendritic cells requires environmental instruction. *J. Immunol.* **164:**4507–4512.

Whelan, M., M. M. Harnett, K. M. Houston, V. Patel, W. Harnett, and K. P. Rigley. 2000. A filarial nematode-secreted product signals dendritic cells to acquire a phenotype that drives development of Th2 cells. *J. Immunol.* **164:**6453–6460.

Yssel, H., S. Fasler, J. E. de Vries, and R. de Waal Malefyt. 1994. IL-12 transiently induces IFN-gamma transcription and protein synthesis in human CD4+ allergen-specific Th2 T cell clones. *Int. Immunol.* **6:**1091–1096.

Immunology of Infectious Diseases
Edited by S. H. E. Kaufmann, A. Sher, and R. Ahmed
© 2002 ASM Press, Washington, D.C.

Chapter 13

Immunological Memory and Infection

RAFI AHMED, J. GIBSON LANIER, AND ERIC PAMER

The primary function of the immune system is to defend against microbial pathogens. It accomplishes this task at two levels: first, by generating a specific immune response against the invading pathogen and controlling the infection, and second, by remembering this first encounter and mounting an accelerated immune response on reexposure to the same pathogen. This rapid recall response can either completely prevent disease or greatly lessen the severity of clinical symptoms. The first documentation of "immune memory" dates back to the time of the Greek historian Thucydides, who recorded, while describing the plague of Athens in 430 B.C., that the "same man was never attacked twice" (Finley, 1951). It is remarkable that nothing was known about the immune system or about microbes when Thucydides made his astute observations on immune memory; it was not until at least 2,000 years later that we gained an appreciation of the immune system and learned that microbes cause infectious diseases. However, it is now well established that memory and specificity constitute the two defining features of the immune response.

The focus of this chapter is on the principles of immune memory. The reader should refer to other chapters in the book (chapters 15 to 18, 29 and 30) for specific information on acquired immune responses to individual pathogens. This chapter is divided into four parts: (i) a historical perspective of vaccination, (ii) an overview of protective immunity to microbes, (iii) a discussion of the current models of memory T- and B-cell differentiation, and (iv) an overview of the mechanisms involved in maintaining immunological memory.

HISTORY OF VACCINATION

Immunological memory is the basis for vaccination; the discipline of vaccinology originated from the observation that previous exposure to the disease conferred resistance to a subsequent episode. Thus, the principle of vaccinology was that if somehow the first episode of a disease could be attenuated, one would be protected against the more severe form of the disease. The earliest recorded attempts to put this into practice were made in China and India around 1500 A.D., when pustular material from smallpox patients was inoculated into healthy people. This process, called variolation, caused smallpox, but for reasons which are not clear, the disease was often milder than naturally acquired infection. More importantly, the variolated individuals were then protected against the naturally acquired and more severe smallpox. However, this approach did not gain popularity and was eventually discontinued because the degree of morbidity and mortality associated with variolation was simply too variable and too high to be acceptable.

The major breakthrough came with the classic experiments of Edward Jenner in 1796. Jenner had noticed that milkmaids who were commonly infected with cowpox were spared the ravages of smallpox. He reasoned that inoculation of cowpox pustular material might prevent smallpox. In many ways, vaccinology was born in 1796, when Jenner inoculated young James Phipps with cowpox virus and prevented smallpox, thereby showing that exposure to an antigenically related but less pathogenic virus could confer protection against a more virulent virus. However, despite this remarkable achievement, the field of vaccinology stood still for the next 50 to 75 years. This lack of progress was due to the fact that

Rafi Ahmed and J. Gibson Lanier • Emory Vaccine Center and Department of Microbiology and Immunology, Emory University School of Medicine, Atlanta, GA 30322. **Eric Pamer** • Infectious Disease Service, Laboratory of Antimicrobial Immunity, Memorial Sloan-Kettering Cancer Center, New York, NY 10021.

it was still not proven that microbes caused smallpox or, for that matter, any disease. Thus, there was no clear scientific basis for developing vaccines.

Things changed dramatically in the second half of the 19th century due to the pioneering work of Pasteur, Koch, Ross, von Behring, Ehrlich, and others. Not only did these scientific giants prove that microbes cause infectious diseases, thus laying the foundations of immunology and microbiology, but also their work resulted in the development of successful vaccines against rabies, typhoid, cholera, plague, and diphtheria. It is only fitting that the first Nobel prize in medicine and physiology, given in 1901, was awarded to von Behring for his work on diphtheria. Several additional vaccines were developed during the first half of the 20th century including the highly effective yellow fever virus vaccine by Theiler, for which he was awarded the Nobel prize in 1951. It is interesting that his live yellow fever virus vaccine developed 65 years ago by the rather empirical method of doing serial passages for viral attenuation remains to this day one of our safest and most effective vaccines.

Until 1950, all viral vaccines were prepared in either mammalian or avian tissues. The classic work of Enders showing that viruses can be grown in vitro in cell culture marked a major breakthrough in vaccine development, changing the source of virus from infected tissues to infected cells in culture. This facilitated the development of many of our currently used vaccines (Table 1) including vaccines against poliomyelitis, for which Enders and colleagues received the Nobel prize in 1954. This technology continues to be the most common method of producing viral vaccines even to this day.

Major advances in our ability to "cut and paste" genes have occurred during the past 25 years, yet only one of our currently used vaccines, the hepatitis B vaccine, is made by recombinant DNA technology. In this case, the hepatitis B surface antigen is expressed by recombinant yeast and the purified protein is then used as a vaccine. However, this situation is certain to change. A multitude of expression vectors (bacterial, viral, naked DNA) have been developed, and considerable effort has gone into optimizing their in vivo expression and methods and routes of immunization (Table 2). It is likely that this will become the main technology for our future vaccines, and, in fact, several recombinant vaccines are currently at various stages of human clinical trials. It remains to be seen which of these vectors will prove to be the most effective. The crucial properties will be the ability to target antigen-presenting cells, the level and duration of gene expression in vivo, the

ease of constructing the vector, and issues such as the cost and safety of the vectors.

PROTECTIVE IMMUNITY

There has been great interest in determining the relative importance of humoral and cellular responses in protective immunity. This has resulted in much debate and considerable experimentation to assess the role of T- and B-cell responses in protection against reinfection. When examining this issue, one must remember that antibodies and T cells have evolved to perform entirely different functions. The business of antibodies is to deal with the microbe itself (i.e., free virus particles, bacteria, and parasites), and that of T cells is to deal with infected cells. Since T cells can recognize microbial antigens only in association with host major histocompatibility complex (MHC) molecules, the free virus particles or bacteria are invisible to them. Thus, antibody provides our only specific defense against free microbial organisms, and the importance of preexisting antibody in protective immunity against infectious diseases cannot be overemphasized. In fact, antibody is likely to be the sole mechanism of protective immunity against bacteria and parasites that have an exclusively extracellular lifestyle. However, the equation begins to change for most viruses and for bacteria and parasites that can survive or replicate intracellularly. Although antibody again provides the first line of defense against such infections, there are often situations where not all of the inoculum is neutralized by the preexisting antibody. This is where the T cells come into play, since their main function is surveillance of infected cells. T cells are divided into two subsets, CD4 and CD8 T cells, and both of these subsets play roles in protective immunity. They do this by either killing the infected cell and/or releasing cytokines that inhibit growth of the microbe or impair the ability of the pathogen to survive inside the cell. In addition to these effector functions carried out by both CD4 and CD8 T cells, CD4 T cells play an important role in providing help for antibody production and for generation of CD8 T-cell responses.

Thus, it appears that protective immunity for extracellular pathogens depends primarily on B cells and CD4 T cells (as helpers) whereas for intracellular pathogens it would require a concerted effort by B cells, CD4 T cells (as both helpers and effectors), and CD8 T cells. While this generalization is reasonably accurate, there are several examples where microbial infections have been controlled exclusively by antibody (i.e., passive antibody transfer) or by CD8 T cells (i.e., after immunization by a vaccine only con-

Table 1. General approaches for vaccines

Type of vaccine	Comments	Example	
		Viral	Bacterial
Live attenuated organism	The organism is attenuated such that it does not produce clinical disease but still retains the ability to replicate to the extent sufficient to induce immunity	Polio (Sabin), measles, mumps, rubella, yellow fever, varicella	Bacillus Calmette-Guérin (BCG), typhoid
Killed organism	The vaccine consists of the whole organism that has been inactivated to prevent any replication in vivo, but immunogenicity is preserved	Polio (Salk), influenza, Japanese encephalitis, rabies, hepatitis A	Pertussis, cholera, typhoid
Subunit vaccines	The vaccine consists of subcomponents of the organism; these subcomponents can be either surface proteins of a virus or proteins and/or polysaccharides of bacteria	Hepatitis B	*Haemophilus influenzae* B, pneumococci, meningococci, typhoid, pertussis, anthrax
Antitoxins	The vaccine consists of inactivated toxin (toxoid) that is no longer toxic but retains immunogenicity	None	Diphtheria, tetanus
Vectored vaccines	These vaccines are currently in development; the idea is to construct recombinant viral or bacterial vectors that express the antigen of interest and to use these recombinant vectors as vaccines (see Table 2 for a list of promising viral and bacterial vectors)	None licensed, but some in phase I and II clinical trials	None licensed, but several in experimental stage
Nuclei acid (DNA) vaccines	Currently a very popular approach but still at the experimental/developmental stage; the vaccine consists of plasmid DNA expressing the antigen of interest	None licensed, but some in phase I and II clinical trials	None licensed, but several in experimental stage

Table 2. Recombinant delivery systems for future vaccines

Plasmid naked DNA

Bacterial vectors[a]
  Listeria
  Mycobacterium
  Salmonella
  Shigella

Viral vectors[a]
  Adenoviruses
  Alphaviruses
  Lentiviruses
  Poxviruses
  Retroviruses

[a] This is a partial list of the many bacterial and viral vectors currently being tested.

taining the CD8 T-cell epitopes) (Ahmed and Biron, 1999). These experiments clearly show that there are situations where either humoral or cellular immunity can be sufficient for protection. The correct conclusion from such experiments is that in the given situation the CD8 T-cell response or the antibody response alone was adequate for protection. However, it is misleading to conclude from this type of experiment that the missing response does not play a role in protective immunity. The danger of drawing such a conclusion is that a potentially useful immune response may be excluded from the design of a vaccine. In the same vein, when designing a vaccine, it is prudent to look beyond the type of immunity generated during the natural infection. For example, antibody plays a minimal to no role in controlling an acute primary lymphocytic choriomeningitis virus infection in mice or in conferring protection against reinfection (CD8 T cells are the major players in both instances) (Buchmeier and Zajac, 1999). However, passive transfer of neutralizing antibody can confer a reasonable degree of protection (Buchmeier and Zajac, 1999). A similar situation exists for *Listeria monocytogenes*; this has long been considered an infection controlled exclusively by T cells, but a recent study (Edelson et al., 1999) has shown that antibody is also effective in eliminating *Listeria*. These findings have obvious implications for vaccine design. For example, although very little neutralizing antibody is generated during the course of human immunodeficiency virus (HIV) infection, there is evidence suggesting that immunization with the right form of HIV envelope protein can induce neutralizing antibody that may be useful in conferring protective immunity (LaCasse et al., 1999). Thus, the right strategy for an HIV vaccine would be to stimulate both the humoral and cellular arms of the immune system.

What is the basis of protective immunity? Is it protection from infection or from disease? In the strictest sense, protection from infection would mean that there was sufficient preexisting antibody to neutralize or opsonize all of the pathogen in the inoculum and there was no further amplification of the microbe. Does this ever happen? The precise answer is not known, but it is likely that if it does happen it may occur only when the inoculum is very low. What is more likely is that a substantial fraction of the virus is neutralized and the remaining fraction, which is able to initiate infection, is quickly controlled by the rapid anamnestic response of memory T cells (Ahmed and Gray, 1996; McChesney et al., 1997). This is in fact a pretty good scenario; first, the infection is rapidly controlled and there is no disease; second, the virus is fully eliminated, thus achieving sterilizing immunity; and third, this low-grade transient subclinical infection serves as a natural booster to the immune system. A similar situation would apply for extracellular pathogens—either all of the inoculum would be killed by preexisting antibody prior to colonization and growth or the growth would be so minimal that no disease would occur and sterilizing immunity would be achieved.

MEMORY T- AND B-CELL DIFFERENTIATION

Before considering models of memory B- and T-cell differentiation, it is important to appreciate a fundamental difference between cellular and humoral immunity. Microbial infections usually induce both T- and B-cell long-term memory. However, the natures of T- and B-cell memory are different (Fig. 1; and Table 3). B-cell memory is usually manifested by continuous antibody production, even after resolution of the disease. Prolonged antibody production, lasting for several years after infection or vaccination,

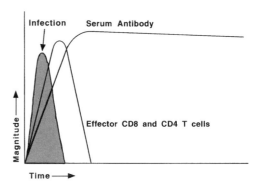

Figure 1. The natures of effector T- and B-cell responses are different. Most microbial infections induce prolonged serum antibody responses that can persist for months or years after resolution of the infection. In contrast, effector T-cell responses (i.e., active killer cells and cytokine producers) are short-lived and are seen only during the acute phase of infection.

has been observed in humans as well as in experimental systems (Cohen et al., 1994; Kjeldsen et al., 1985; Scheibel et al., 1966; Simonsen et al., 1984; Slifka et al., 1995). In contrast, the effector phase of the T-cell response is short-lived (a few weeks), and "memory" in the T-cell compartment results from the presence of memory T cells, which are found at higher frequencies and can respond faster and develop into effector cells (i.e., cytotoxic T lymphocytes [CTL] or cytokine producers) more efficiently than can naïve T cells (Bachmann et al., 1999a; Cho et al., 1999; Kedl and Mescher, 1998; Zimmermann et al., 1999). This dichotomy in the humoral and cellular responses is a feature of most acute infections (also of immunization, in general) and makes teleo-

Table 3. Distinction between effector B and T cells

Effector B cells
  Plasma cells are end-stage differentiated cells that constitutively produce antibody in the absence of antigen.[a] A proportion of plasma cells can live for extended periods in the bone marrow. These long-lived plasma cells are an important source of antibody in the serum and can also contribute to antibody in the mucosa. This preexisting antibody forms the first line of defense against infection and is a key aspect of protective immunity against microbial infections.

Effector T cells
  Effector T cells secrete cytokines and can kill infected cells. In contrast to plasma cells, T cells maintain effector functions only in the presence of antigen. In the absence of antigen, effector T cells either die or differentiate into memory T cells. This also contrasts with plasma cells, which are fully differentiated end-stage cells that do not give rise to memory B cells.

[a] Antigen is needed for differentiation of naïve or memory B cells into antibody-secreting plasma cells but is not required for maintaining antibody production by fully differentiated plasma cells.

logical sense. Sustained secretion or overproduction of cytokines can have deleterious effects, and the presence of fully active killers could result in immunopathological damage if some of these CTLs were cross-reactive with self-antigens. Thus, maintaining T-cell immunity by sustaining the effector phase carries a high price tag. Because memory T cells can rapidly develop into effectors and quickly gain access to sites of infection, it is not essential, in most instances, to have preexisting effector T cells to provide protection.

B-Cell Memory

The two critical cell types involved in B-cell memory are memory B cells and plasma cells. The major differences between naïve B cells, memory B cells, and plasma cells are summarized in Tables 4 and 5, and the lineage relationships between these three cell types are shown in Fig. 2. In this simple model, following the initial activation of naïve B cells (by antigen and T-cell help), memory B cells differentiate along a separate pathway from plasma cells. The signals that drive these two pathways appear to be distinct; for example interactions involving OX-40 (Stuber and Strober, 1996), CD23 (Kehry and Yamashita, 1989; Liu et al., 1991; Mudde et al., 1995; Pirron et al., 1990), and Blimp-1 (Lin et al., 1997; Turner et al., 1994) favor plasma cell differentiation whereas interactions with CD40L and transcription factors such as B-cell-specific activator favor memory B-cell development (Ahmed and Gray, 1996; McHeyzer-Williams and Ahmed, 1999).

An important aspect of the model described in Fig. 2 is affinity maturation of memory B cells and generation of long-lived plasma cells. Following antigenic stimulation of naïve B cells, there is clonal expansion of the activated B cells in the T-cell-rich areas of secondary lymphoid organs. During this initial phase of activation, there is minimal somatic mutation and affinity maturation of the B-cell receptor and most of the antibody-secreting plasma cells generated from these activated B cells are short-lived and tend to produce immunoglobulin M (IgM) antibody. Following the initial phase, there is a second phase

of clonal expansion of the activated B cells within the specialized microenvironment of the germinal center (GC) reaction. It is within the GCs that affinity maturation occurs and where these high-affinity memory B cells are further expanded (Berek et al., 1985; Jacob et al., 1991). GCs contain follicular dendritic cells (FDC), which can retain depots of antigen for stimulation and selection of high-affinity B cells. There is evidence suggesting that plasma cells derived from high-affinity isotype-switched B cells tend to be longer-lived and reside in the bone marrow (Manz et al., 1997, 1998; Slifka et al., 1998).

The kinetics and anatomic location of antibody production after an acute viral infection are shown in Fig. 3. The IgM response is very transient, but the serum IgG response is long-lived and can persist for several years. Antibody is initially produced by plasma cells present in GCs in the spleen and draining lymph nodes. The antibody response in these organs peaks during the first 2 weeks and then declines within 2 to 4 weeks after infection (Slifka et al., 1995). The decline in the number of plasma cells appears to be due to selection for higher-affinity plasma cells and apoptotic loss of low-affinity cells. As the numbers of splenic plasma cell populations decline, antigen-specific plasma cells begin to migrate and/or accumulate in the bone marrow compartment. After the GC reaction subsides, the bone marrow becomes the predominant site of antibody production, with 80 to 90% of the plasma cells being located in this compartment. Plasma cell longevity studies have indicated that the initial antibody response is due to short-lived plasma cells whereas long-term antibody is maintained by long-lived plasma cells. On reinfection, antibody responses once again occur in the spleen and lymph nodes, because most of the memory B cells reside in these organs. After secondary viral infection, the memory B cells in the spleen and lymph nodes proliferate and/or differentiate into plasma cells, resulting in a transient increase in the number of ASCs in the spleen. However, once the secondary infection is cleared, this response subsides and, once again, the bone marrow becomes the predominant site of antibody production. It is worth

Table 4. Differences between naïve and memory B cells

Naïve B cells	Memory B cells
No somatic mutation or affinity maturation of B cell receptor	Somatic mutation and affinity maturation of B-cell receptor
Not isotype switched; IgM$^+$ IgD$^+$	Often isotype switched (IgG$^+$ or IgA$^+$) but can also be IgM$^+$
CD27$^-$	CD27$^+$
CD148$^-$	CD148$^+$

Table 5. Differences between memory B cells and plasma cells

Property	Memory B cell	Plasma cell
Location	Reside primarily in the secondary lymphoid organs	Reside primarily in the bone marrow
Function	Important for replenishing the pool of plasma cells and memory B cells; do not actively secrete antibody but respond to antigen by rapidly dividing and giving rise to more memory B cells and also differentiating into plasma cells	Terminally differentiated cells that constitutively produce antibody; not stimulated by antigen (low to no surface B-cell receptor); do not divide
Markers[a]		
Surface Ig	++++	±
B220	++++	±
CD19	++++	±
CD21	++++	±
MHC class II	++++	±
CD138 (syndecan-1)	−	++++
Blimp-1	−	++++

[a] List of markers commonly used to distinguish between memory B cells and plasma cells (not a comprehensive listing). All of the markers listed here except for Blimp-1 are expressed at the cell surface and can be used to separate plasma cells from memory B cells.

noting the anatomic segregation between plasma cells and memory B cells. One way of looking at this is to consider the spleen and lymph nodes to be "factories" where B-cell differentiation into plasma cells occurs and to consider the bone marrow to be the storehouse where the products (i.e., plasma cells) are kept. It makes sense that the B cells should reside in the vicinity of the factories so that they can be quickly mobilized into action as the need arises and that the plasma cells are shipped out to the bone marrow to make room in the factory. Plasma cells resid-

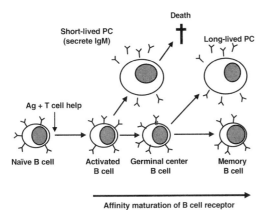

Figure 2. Model of memory B-cell differentiation. Following antigenic stimulation, naïve B cells differentiate along separate pathways into memory B cells and plasma cells (PC). In this model, low-affinity B cells differentiate into short-lived plasma cells whereas high-affinity B cells give rise to long-lived plasma cells. Memory B cells, in general, are extremely long-lived and, on reencountering antigen (Ag), can rapidly differentiate into plasma cells and also proliferate to generate more memory B cells. Plasma cells are terminally differentiated effector cells that can neither divide in response to antigen nor revert to memory B cells.

ing in the bone marrow go on with their business of making antibody, which ends up in the blood and can protect against reinfection. It should be pointed out that serum antibody (IgG) can enter the mucosa by transudation, and it is possible that plasma cells residing in the bone marrow can also contribute to the antibody present at mucosal sites.

In summary, immunological memory in the B-cell compartment consists of memory B cells and plasma cells: two distinct cell types with different anatomic locations and very different functions (Table 5). Memory B cells are located primarily in the secondary lymphoid organs and are present at much higher frequencies than naïve B cells of the same specificity. In addition to this quantitative advantage over naïve B cells, memory B cells are qualitatively different and produce antibody of much higher affinity. However, memory B cells do not actively secrete antibody (i.e., they are not effector cells). Their major function is to make rapid recall responses to infection by quickly dividing and giving rise to more memory B cells and also by differentiating into plasma cells. The rapid rise in antibody levels on reinfection is the result of memory B-cell differentiation into new antibody-secreting plasma cells. In contrast to B cells, plasma cells cannot be stimulated by antigen to either divide or increase their rate of antibody production since they contain very little to no surface immunoglobulin (i.e., B-cell receptor). These plasma cells are terminally differentiated cells that constitutively produce and secrete antibody. Plasma cells are extraordinarily efficient in their ability to make antibody; it has been estimated that they can secrete >1,000 antibody molecules per s (Helm-

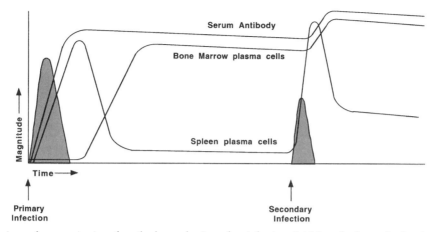

Figure 3. Kinetics and anatomic site of antibody production after infection. Initial antibody production is by plasma cells within GCs in the spleen and lymph nodes, but after the infection is resolved, the bone marrow becomes the site of long-term antibody production. On secondary infection, the spleen and lymph nodes mount a rapid but transient antibody response, and after a return to homeostasis, the bone marrow is again the predominant source of antigen-specific plasma cells.

reich et al., 1961; Hibi and Dosch, 1986). Since pre-existing antibody provides the first line of defense against infection by microbial pathogens, the importance of plasma cells in protective immunity cannot be overstated. In fact, it could be argued that plasma cells may be the single most important cell type in protective immunity to infections.

T-Cell Memory

T-cell memory does not have a plasma cell equivalent, i.e., an effector cell that can continue its effector function in the absence of antigenic stimulation. In contrast to plasma cells, effector T cells elaborate their effector functions (i.e., cytokine secretion and killing of infected cells by release of secretory granules containing perforin or granzymes) only in the presence of antigen (Fig. 1; Table 3). These cells exhibit an on-off lifestyle, with antigen regulating this switch (Badovinac et al., 2000; Slifka and Whitton, 2000). If effector T-cell responses are only transient, then what is the cellular basis of long-term T-cell immunity? It is well established that T-cell memory, as assessed by accelerated recall responses in vivo, is long-lived and is seen after most microbial infections (Ahmed and Gray, 1996; Dutton et al., 1998; Freitas and Rocha, 2000; Zinkernagel et al., 1996). These rapid recall responses to reinfection are the result of both quantitative and qualitative changes in the pathogen-specific T cells. After primary infection there is substantial expansion of the pools of naive CD8 and CD4 T cells specific to the pathogen (Fig. 4). Several studies have shown that the size of the memory T-cell pool is determined by the burst size during the expansion phase (Fig. 5)

(Busch et al., 1998; Hou et al., 1994; Murali-Krishna et al., 1998). In some acute viral infections, the increase in the number of antigen-specific T cells can be as great as 1,000- to 10,000-fold (Ahmed and Biron, 1999; Murali-Krishna et al., 1998). This numerical advantage alone can make an enormous

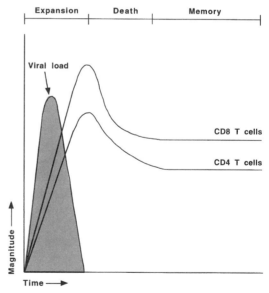

Figure 4. Antiviral CD8 and CD4 T-cell responses. The three phases of the immune response are indicated at the top. The increase in cell number during the expansion phase is due to clones of T cells undergoing cell division. Soon after the virus is cleared, there is a death phase, characterized by decreasing numbers of virus-specific T cells due to apoptosis. Following the death phase, the number of virus-specific T cells stabilizes and can be maintained for extended periods (the memory phase). The CD4 T-cell response is similar to the CD8 T-cell response, except that the magnitude of the CD4 response is lower and the death phase can be more protracted than the CD8 response.

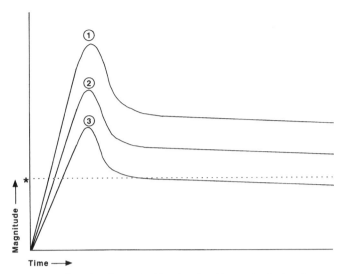

Figure 5. The size of the memory T-cell pool is determined by the clonal burst size during the expansion phase. In this figure, lines 1, 2, and 3 represent the T-cell responses induced by three different vaccines. Vaccine 1 induces the largest expansion of T cells and hence generates the largest pool of memory T cells; vaccine 2 is next; and vaccine 3 is the weakest. The asterisk denotes the minimum number of antigen-specific T cells required for protective immunity. In this scenario, vaccines 1 and 2 will confer long-term immunity whereas protective immunity induced by vaccine 3 will be of short duration. The main reason for the failure of vaccine 3 is a smaller burst size during the expansion phase. Note that the maintenance of the memory T-cell pool is similar for all three vaccines.

difference in the recall response, but recent studies have shown that memory T cells are also qualitatively distinct from naïve T cells and can respond much quicker on reexposure to antigen (Bachmann et al., 1999a, 1999b; Cho et al., 1999; Kedl and Mescher, 1998; Zimmermann et al., 1999). In fact, this faster responsiveness is clearly the defining characteristic of memory T cells (Table 6). Another important property of memory T cells is their ability to extravasate into nonlymphoid tissues, and several recent studies have shown that a subset of memory T cells (termed effector memory cells) are present in many peripheral tissues and also at mucosal sites (Marshall et al., 2001; Masopust et al., 2001; Reinhardt et al., 2001; Sallusto et al., 1999). Thus, it is the combination of increased numbers of antigen-specific T cells, their faster responsiveness, and their better location (i.e., near sites of microbial entry) that underpins T-cell memory and explains how memory T cells confer long-term protective immunity (Ahmed and Gray, 1996; Dutton et al., 1998; Freitas and Rocha, 2000; Lau et al., 1994; Zinkernagel et al., 1996).

It is well established that memory B cells and plasma cells differentiate along separate pathways, and some of the conditions and signals that direct naïve B cells into the memory versus effector pathways are being defined (McHeyzer-Williams and Ahmed, 1999). Our understanding of memory T-cell differentiation is less clear, but during the past few years there has been substantial progress in defining the lineage relationships between naïve, effector, and memory T cells (Champagne et al., 2001; Lanzavecchia and Sallusto, 2001). Also, several markers have been identified that distinguish between these three cell types (Table 7) (Ahmed and Gray, 1996; Dutton et al., 1998; Freitas and Rocha, 2000; Harrington et al., 2000; Zinkernagel et al., 1996). Possible models

Table 6. Defining characteristics of memory B and T cells

Memory B cells
  The hallmark of memory B cells is affinity maturation of the B-cell receptor. This means that the antibody produced by these cells after their differentiation into antibody secreting cells is of higher affinity. Thus, the fundamental difference between naïve and memory B cells is that the memory B cells can make a better "product."

Memory T cells
  The hallmark of memory T cells is faster responsiveness on reencountering the antigen. In some instances the response is so rapid (i.e., cytokine production in less than 4 h) that memory T cells give the illusion of being effector cells. The effector molecules (cytokines, perforin, granzymes, etc.) of naïve and memory T cells are identical. Thus, the fundamental difference between memory and naïve T cells is that the memory T cells are a much more efficient "factory" than are the naïve cells, even though the product is the same. Also, unlike naïve T cells, which are located mostly in lymphoid tissues, a subset of memory T cells (CD62L[lo] CCR7[−]) are present in nonlymphoid tissues and at mucosal sites and can immediately confront the invading pathogen.

Table 7. Markers that distinguish between naïve, effector, and memory T cells[a]

Marker[b]	Naïve	Effector	Memory
Group A			
CD44	Low	High	High
CD11a (LFA-1)	Low	High	High
Ly-6C	Low	High	High
CD122 (IL-2Rβ)	Low	High	High
Group B			
CD25 (IL-2Rα)	Low	High	Low
CD43 (high MW form)	Low	High	Low
CD80 (B7-1)	Low	High	Low
CD38	Low	High	Low
MHC class II	Low	High	Low
Group C			
CD62 L (L-selectin)	High	Low	High/Low
CCR7	High	Low	High/Low
CD45RA	High	Low	High/Low
CD45RO	Low	High	Low/High

[a] Not a comprehensive list but it illustrates the three patterns of changes seen as naïve T cells go through the naive → effector → memory transition. Some surface markers (group A) are expressed at low levels in naïve cells, upregulated on antigen activation (effector cells), and maintained at high levels in memory T cells. Other markers (group B) are only transiently upregulated in effector cells and can be useful in discriminating between memory and effector T cells. Finally, a third group of markers (group C) show a much more gradual change during the effector-to-memory transition and have turned out to be very useful in identifying different subsets of memory T cells, e.g., lymphoid versus nonlymphoid. This group of markers may also be useful in identifying the various stages of memory T-cell differentiation.

[b] IL-2, interleukin-2; MW, molecular weight.

of memory T-cell differentiation are shown in Fig. 6. It is unlikely that the "divergent-pathway" (model 1) represents a major pathway of memory T-cell differentiation since recent experimental evidence favors the linear-differentiation model (model 2). Studies using transgenic T cells or using genetic techniques to mark antigen-specific T cells have shown that memory T cells are derived from effector cells (Jacob and Baltimore, 1999; Opferman et al., 1999). However, this simple linear-differentiation model does not account for the fact that the majority of effector cells undergo apoptosis and that only a fraction (~10%) of these cells survive to become memory cells. The "decreasing-potential hypothesis" (model 3) incorporates a mechanism for discriminating between effectors that preferentially die and those that preferentially survive and differentiate into memory cells. According to this model, the balance between effector cells and memory cells is governed by the duration and level of antigenic stimulation. Cells become more and more terminally differentiated with prolonged antigenic stimulation, and this is accompanied by an increasing susceptibility to apoptosis and a decreasing potential for memory cell development. This model also explains the phenomenon of clonal deletion and exhaustion that occurs during chronic viral infections with a high antigen load (Ahmed and Biron, 1999; Moskophidis et al., 1993; Zajac et al., 1998). Finally, the last memory

differentiation model we would like to discuss incorporates the development of central and effector memory T cells (Fig. 7) (Sallusto et al., 1999). In this model a shorter duration of antigenic stimulation favors the development of central memory cells whereas a longer duration favors effector memory cells. Effector memory cells (CCR7⁻ CD62L^lo) are characterized by the rapid acquisition of effector function and are found predominantly in nonlymphoid tissues, whereas central memory cells (CCR7⁺ CD62L^hi) are located in lymphoid tissues and presumably respond more slowly than effector memory cells. However, it should be noted that even the central memory cells respond much faster than naïve T cells do. There are some interesting parallels between the decreasing-potential model and the model incorporating the development of central and effector memory T-cell subsets. In both models the duration of antigenic stimulus regulates differentiation and a more prolonged antigenic stimulus favors cells with a more effector phenotype (i.e., terminally differentiated cells).

MAINTENANCE OF IMMUNOLOGICAL MEMORY

How is immunological memory maintained? This question has fascinated immunologists, micro-

1. Divergent pathway

2. Linear differentiation pathway

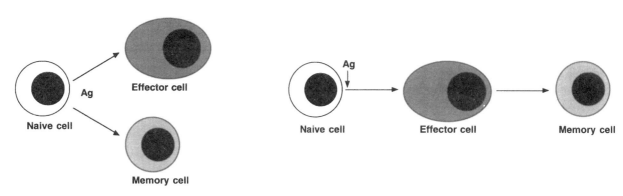

3. Decreasing potential hypothesis

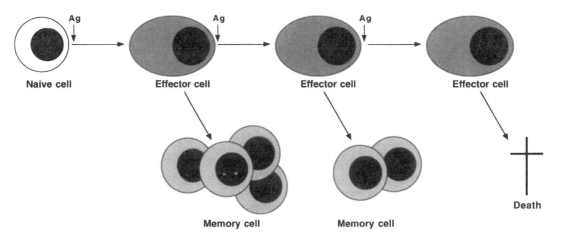

Figure 6. Models of memory T-cell differentiation. Model 1 represents the B-cell paradigm of dichotomy in memory and effector pathways. Model 2 is the more traditional view of memory T-cell differentiation representing a linear-differentiation pathway. Model 3 is a variation of model 2 and takes into account the finding that only 5 to 10% of the effector cells survive to become memory T cells. In this model, progress toward terminal differentiation (driven by antigen [Ag]) is accompanied by increased susceptibility to apoptosis and a decreased potential for memory cell development. In all of these models the effector cells represent a transient population whereas the memory cells survive for long periods. On reexposure to antigen, the memory T cells can develop into effector cells and can also generate more memory cells.

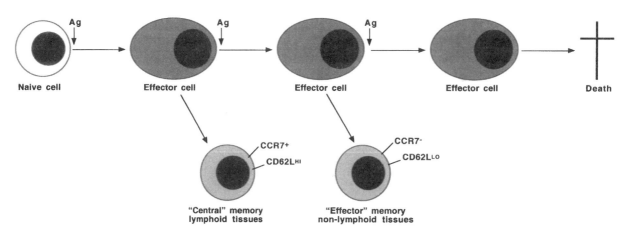

Figure 7. Model of memory T-cell differentiation incorporating the development of central and effector memory T cells. In this model, a short duration of antigenic (Ag) stimulation favors the development of central memory cells whereas a longer duration favors differentiation to effector memory T cells.

biologists, and infectious-disease specialists for many years, and there has been great interest in understanding the mechanisms that maintain long-term protective immunity. This information not only is of fundamental interest but also has important practical applications for vaccine development.

The mechanisms involved in sustaining immunological memory are listed in Table 8. These can be divided into two categories: antigen dependent and antigen independent. One of the most effective means of maintaining immunity is periodic reexposure to the pathogen. Such reinfections are usually asymptomatic or produce only mild clinical symptoms and serve as a natural booster to the immune system. The importance of this mechanism is documented by epidemiological studies showing that protective immunity is maintained for longer periods in individuals living in areas where a given disease is endemic. Having said this, it is at least as important to point out that there are several striking examples of long-term protective immunity in the absence of reexposure to the pathogen. Three such examples are given in Table 9. These observations were crucial in shaping our ideas about immunological memory because they showed that the immune system could remember an encounter that occurred many years ago and that there are inherent (endogenous) mechanisms for sustaining this long-term memory (Panum, 1847; Paul et al., 1951; Sawyer, 1931).

Among the endogenous mechanisms of maintaining immunity, two are antigen dependent: microbial persistence and antigen depots on FDC. Several microbes can persist at low levels in healthy individ-

---

Table 8. Mechanisms of maintaining immunological memory

Antigen dependent
  Reexposure to pathogen can serve as a periodic natural
    booster to the immune system.
  In low-grade chronic or latent infection, many pathogens can
    persist at low levels and provide a continuous or
    intermittent stimulus to memory T and B cells.
  Antigen-antibody complexes on FDC can persist for extended
    periods and provide a reservoir of antigen for stimulating
    memory B cells and CD4 T cells.

Antigen independent
  Long-lived plasma cells can constitutively produce antibody
    and provide a mechanism of sustaining antibody levels in
    the absence of antigen.
  Memory B and T cells can persist and maintain their numbers
    in an antigen-free environment; memory T cells can
    undergo homeostatic proliferation to replenish their pool;
    this homeostatic proliferation does not require stimulation
    with specific antigen.
  Memory CD8 and CD4 T cells can retain their rapid
    responsiveness in the absence of specific antigen and are
    able to confer protective immunity.

---

uals, and this chronicity can provide either a continuous or an intermittent antigenic stimulus to the immune system. This can be an effective mechanism of maintaining a higher frequency of antigen-specific T and B cells but requires a careful balance between pathogen levels and immune responses. This critical balance is necessary to avoid excessive immunopathology and also to avoid overstimulation of the antigen-specific T cells to such an extent that these cells are deleted or become functionally exhausted (Moskophidis et al., 1993; Zajac et al., 1998). Pathogens that cause latent infection with periodic reactivation, such as the herpes viruses (Epstein-Barr virus, herpes simplex virus, and varicella-zoster virus), exhibit a lifestyle that is perhaps most conducive to providing an antigenic stimulus for maintaining long-term immunity.

The second antigen-dependent mechanism relies on the ability of FDC to trap antigen-antibody complexes on their cell surface and retain them for extended periods (Ahmed and Gray, 1996; Dutton et al., 1998; Freitas and Rocha, 2000; MacLennan, 1994; Mandel et al., 1980; Zinkernagel et al., 1996). FDC express Fc receptors on their cell surface, and antigen-antibody complexes can bind to these Fc receptors. It appears that FDC do not internalize these antigen-antibody complexes but instead display them on their cell surface for long periods. Some studies have suggested that antigen can persist on FDC for more than 1 year (Mandel et al., 1980). It has been postulated that this trapped antigen directly stimulates the specific B cells and can also be acquired by the B cells, processed, and then presented via MHC class II molecules to CD4 T cells (MacLennan, 1994; Mandel et al., 1980). Thus, it appears that FDC-trapped antigen can be used for stimulating both memory B cells and CD4 T cells. Many interesting questions about FDC remain unanswered. What is their half-life? Do they divide? What prevents the antigen-antibody complexes from being degraded and/or internalized by the FDC? FDC are usually found only within GCs (and most probably play an important role in affinity maturation of B cells), but GCs are short-lived, and if FDC are to play a role in maintaining long-term immunity, then where are the FDC located after the GCs have receded? It will be important to study FDC in more detail to better understand their role in maintaining B- and T-cell memory.

During the past decade, major advances have been made in identifying antigen-independent mechanisms of maintaining immunological memory (Ahmed and Gray, 1996; Dutton et al., 1998; Freitas and Rocha, 2000; Lanzavecchia and Sallusto, 2001; Marrack et al., 2000; Sprent and Surh, 2001). These

Table 9. Long-term immunity in the absence of reexposure to the pathogen

Infection	Duration of immunity (yr)	Reference
Measles in the Faroe Islands	65	Panum (1847) (reprinted in 1939 in *Med. Classics* 3:829–840)
Yellow fever virus in Norfolk, Va.	75	Sawyer (1931)
Polio in remote Eskimo villages	40	Paul et al. (1951)

studies were greatly facilitated by the development of new and sensitive techniques for assessing T- and B-cell functions at the single-cell level and, even more importantly, by the ability to physically identify antigen-specific T cells using MHC class I and class II tetramers (Altman et al., 1996; Crawford et al., 1998; Murali-Krishna et al., 1998). Also, the use of transgenic T and B cells has allowed us to monitor the immune response in vivo as naïve cells are activated and differentiate into effector and memory cells (Kearney et al., 1994; Zimmermann et al., 1999). Using a combination of these approaches and analyzing immune responses to a variety of antigenic systems (both infectious and noninfectious), it is now clear that both memory CD4 and CD8 T cells, as well as memory B cells, can persist in the absence of antigen (Ahmed and Gray, 1996; Dutton et al., 1998; Freitas and Rocha, 2000; Hou et al., 1994; Lanzavecchia and Sallusto, 2001; Lau et al., 1994; Markiewicz et al., 1998; Marrack et al., 2000; Maruyama et al., 2000; Mullbacher, 1994; Murali-Krishna et al., 1999; Sprent and Surh, 2001; Swain et al., 1999; Tanchot et al., 1997). It has also been shown that memory T cells can undergo homeostatic proliferation to replenish their numbers and that this proliferative renewal does not require stimulation with antigen (Murali-Krishna et al., 1999; Swain et al., 1999; Tanchot et al., 1997). Taken together, these experimental studies done with mice have unequivocally shown that memory B and T cells can persist for extended periods ($\geq$2 years) in the absence of antigen. What about in humans? Here the results are less definitive, but there are data showing long-term memory under conditions where antigen persistence is unlikely. For example, it has been shown that vaccinia virus-specific memory CD8 T cells can be detected in individuals vaccinated more than 30 years earlier (Demkowicz et al., 1996). It is unlikely that this long-term CTL memory is due to antigenic stimulation, because vaccinia virus does not cause a chronic or latent infection in humans and there is no possibility of reexposure to it, because vaccination against smallpox virus was discontinued in 1977. There are also studies documenting the per-

sistence of memory CD4 T cells to tetanus toxoid many years after vaccination (Helms et al., 2000). Nevertheless, there is clearly a need for more detailed analysis of memory responses in humans. It would also be worthwhile to pursue such studies by using nonhuman primates.

It is clear that there are antigen-independent mechanisms for maintaining memory B and T cells, but what about antibody production? The traditional view has been that plasma cells are short-lived cells (half-life estimates ranging from 3 days to at most 2 to 3 weeks) and that continuous antigenic stimulation of memory B cells is essential to replenish the pool of rapidly dying plasma cells and thereby maintain antibody production. This view has been challenged by recent studies showing that plasma cells can live for extended periods and that some plasma cells can survive for the life of the mouse (Manz et al., 1997, 1998; Slifka et al., 1998). This finding may provide an explanation for the remarkable longevity of antibody responses seen in humans after certain acute infections and vaccinations (Ahmed and Gray, 1996; Slifka and Ahmed, 1998). Many acute viral infections induce serum antibody responses that persist for decades, but what is even more striking is that some nonreplicating antigens can also induce long-term humoral immunity. For example, people vaccinated with diphtheria or tetanus toxoid can have circulating antibody for more than 25 years (Cohen et al., 1994; Kjeldsen et al., 1985; Scheibel et al., 1966; Simonsen et al., 1984). Although antibody levels do decline over this period, it is remarkable that circulating antibody can still be detected $\geq$25 years after immunization with an inert antigen.

Not all infections and vaccines induce long-term antibody responses, and there are several instances where antibody responses decay rapidly (Plotkin and Orenstein, 1999). The underlying reasons for this are not well understood. Are there only certain conditions and/or antigen formulations that can result in the generation of long-lived plasma cells? One possibility is that T-cell help is necessary and that only high-affinity B cells can differentiate into long-lived plasma cells whereas low-affinity B cells give rise to short-lived plasma cells. What are the factors that regulate plasma cell survival? Is residence in the bone marrow essential for plasma cell survival? These issues about plasma cells need to be addressed to gain a better understanding of long-term humoral immunity.

CONCLUSION

In conclusion, in this chapter we have attempted to give an overview of the principles of immunological memory to infection. This remains one of the most exciting areas of immunology and infectious diseases, and there are many challenges ahead. Although considerable progress has been made in the past few years and some of our questions have been answered, many more remain. For example, what is the molecular definition of a memory T cell? Are there memory-specific genes? How are these cells "wired" that makes them so different from naïve cells (Bachmann et al., 1999b)? What controls the homeostasis of memory T and B cells? How many memory cells can we accommodate as we age and encounter multiple infections (Selin et al., 1999)? What signals regulate the differentiation program of memory cells (Kaech and Ahmed, 2001; Lanzavecchia and Sallusto, 2001; van Stipdonk et al., 2001; Wong and Pamer, 2001)? Answers to these and many other questions are needed to define the cellular and molecular basis of immunological memory.

REFERENCES

Ahmed, R., and C. A. Biron. 1999. Immunity to viruses, p. 1295–1335. In W. E. Paul (ed.), Fundamental Immunology. Lippincott-Raven, Philadelphia, Pa.

Ahmed, R., and D. Gray. 1996. Immunological memory and protective immunity: understanding their relation. Science 272:54–60.

Altman, J. D., P. A. Moss, P. J. Goulder, D. H. Barouch, M. G. McHeyzer-Williams, J. I. Bell, A. J. McMichael, and M. M. Davis. 1996. Phenotypic analysis of antigen-specific T lymphocytes. Science 274:94–96.

Bachmann, M. F., M. Barner, A. Viola, and M. Kopf. 1999a. Distinct kinetics of cytokine production and cytolysis in effector and memory T cells after viral infection. Eur. J. Immunol. 29:291–299.

Bachmann, M. F., A. Gallimore, S. Linkert, V. Cerundolo, A. Lanzavecchia, M. Kopf, and A. Viola. 1999b. Developmental regulation of Lck targeting to the CD8 coreceptor controls signaling in naive and memory T cells. J. Exp. Med. 189:1521–1530.

Badovinac, V. P., G. A. Corbin, and J. T. Harty. 2000. Cutting edge: OFF cycling of TNF production by antigen-specific CD8+ T cells is antigen independent. J. Immunol. 165:5387–5391.

Berek, C., G. M. Griffiths, and C. Milstein. 1985. Molecular events during maturation of the immune response to oxazolone. Nature 316:412–418.

Buchmeier, M. J., and A. J. Zajac. 1999. Lymphocytic choriomeningitis virus, p. 575–605. In R. Ahmed, and I. S. Y. Chen (ed.), Persistent Viral Infections. John Wiley & Sons, Ltd., Chichester, United Kingdom.

Busch, D. H., I. M. Pilip, S. Vijh, and E. G. Pamer. 1998. Coordinate regulation of complex T cell populations responding to bacterial infection. Immunity 8:353–362.

Champagne, P., G. S. Ogg, A. S. King, C. Knabenhans, K. Ellefsen, M. Nobile, V. Appay, G. P. Rizzardi, S. Fleury, M. Lipp, et al. 2001. Skewed maturation of memory HIV-specific CD8 T lymphocytes. Nature 410:106–111.

Cho, B. K., C. Wang, S. Sugawa, H. N. Eisen, and J. Chen. 1999. Functional differences between memory and naive CD8 T cells. Proc. Natl. Acad. Sci. USA 96:2976–2981.

Cohen, D., M. S. Green, E. Katzenelson, R. Slepon, H. Bercovier, and M. Wiener. 1994. Long-term persistence of anti-diphtheria toxin antibodies among adults in Israel. Implications for vaccine policy. Eur. J. Epidemiol. 10:267–270.

Crawford, F., H. Kozono, J. White, P. Marrack, and J. Kappler. 1998. Detection of antigen-specific T cells with multivalent soluble class II MHC covalent peptide complexes. Immunity 8:675–682.

Demkowicz, W. E., Jr., R. A. Littaua, J. Wang, and F. A. Ennis. 1996. Human cytotoxic T-cell memory: long-lived responses to vaccinia virus. J. Virol. 70:2627–2631.

Dutton, R. W., L. M. Bradley, and S. L. Swain. 1998. T cell memory. Annu. Rev. Immunol. 16:201–223.

Edelson, B. T., P. Cossart, and E. R. Unanue. 1999. Cutting edge: paradigm revisited: antibody provides resistance to Listeria infection. J. Immunol. 163:4087–4090.

Finley, J. H. 1951. The Complete Writings of Thucydides: The Peloponnesian War. Modern Library, New York, N.Y.

Freitas, A. A., and B. Rocha. 2000. Population biology of lymphocytes: the flight for survival. Annu. Rev. Immunol. 18:83–111.

Harrington, L. E., M. Galvan, L. G. Baum, J. D. Altman, and R. Ahmed. 2000. Differentiating between memory and effector CD8 T cells by altered expression of cell surface O-glycans. J. Exp. Med. 191:1241–1246.

Helmreich, E., M. Kern, and H. N. Eisen. 1961. The secretion of antibody by isolated lymph node cells. J. Biochem. 236:464–473.

Helms, T., B. O. Boehm, R. J. Asaad, R. P. Trezza, P. V. Lehmann, and M. Tary-Lehmann. 2000. Direct visualization of cytokine-producing recall antigen-specific CD4 memory T cells in healthy individuals and HIV patients. J. Immunol. 164:3723–3732.

Hibi, T., and H. M. Dosch. 1986. Limiting dilution analysis of the B cell compartment in human bone marrow. Eur. J. Immunol. 16:139–145.

Hou, S., L. Hyland, K. W. Ryan, A. Portner, and P. C. Doherty. 1994. Virus-specific CD8+ T-cell memory determined by clonal burst size. Nature 369:652–654.

Jacob, J., and D. Baltimore. 1999. Modelling T-cell memory by genetic marking of memory T cells in vivo. Nature 399:593–597.

Jacob, J., G. Kelsoe, K. Rajewsky, and U. Weiss. 1991. Intraclonal generation of antibody mutants in germinal centres. Nature 354:389–392.

Kaech, S. M., and R. Ahmed. 2001. Memory CD8+ T cell differentiation: initial antigen encounter triggers a developmental program in naive cells. Nat. Immunol. 2:415–422.

Kearney, E. R., K. A. Pape, D. Y. Loh, and M. K. Jenkins. 1994. Visualization of peptide-specific T cell immunity and peripheral tolerance induction in vivo. Immunity 1:327–339.

Kedl, R. M., and M. F. Mescher. 1998. Qualitative differences between naive and memory T cells make a major contribution to the more rapid and efficient memory CD8+ T cell response. *J. Immunol.* **161:**674–683.

Kehry, M. R., and L. C. Yamashita. 1989. Low-affinity IgE receptor (CD23) function on mouse B cells: role in IgE-dependent antigen focusing. *Proc. Natl. Acad. Sci. USA* **86:**7556–7560.

Kjeldsen, K., O. Simonsen, and I. Heron. 1985. Immunity against diphtheria 25–30 years after primary vaccination in childhood. *Lancet* **i:**900–902.

LaCasse, R. A., K. E. Follis, M. Trahey, J. D. Scarborough, D. R. Littman, and J. H. Nunberg. 1999. Fusion-competent vaccines: broad neutralization of primary isolates of HIV. *Science* **283:**357–362.

Lanzavecchia, A., and F. Sallusto. 2001. Antigen decoding by T lymphocytes: from synapses to fate determination. *Nat. Immunol.* **2:**487–492.

Lau, L. L., B. D. Jamieson, T. Somasundaram, and R. Ahmed. 1994. Cytotoxic T-cell memory without antigen. *Nature* **369:**648–652.

Lin, Y., K. Wong, and K. Calame. 1997. Repression of c-myc transcription by Blimp-1, an inducer of terminal B cell differentiation. *Science* **276:**596–599.

Liu, Y. J., J. A. Cairns, M. J. Holder, S. D. Abbot, K. U. Jansen, J. Y. Bonnefoy, J. Gordon, and I. C. MacLennan. 1991. Recombinant 25-kDa CD23 and interleukin 1 alpha promote the survival of germinal center B cells: evidence for bifurcation in the development of centrocytes rescued from apoptosis. *Eur. J. Immunol.* **21:**1107–1114.

MacLennan, I. C. 1994. Germinal centers. *Annu. Rev. Immunol.* **12:**117–139.

Mandel, T. E., R. P. Phipps, A. Abbot, and J. G. Tew. 1980. The follicular dendritic cell: long term antigen retention during immunity. *Immunol. Rev.* **53:**29–59.

Manz, R. A., M. Lohning, G. Cassese, A. Thiel, and A. Radbruch. 1998. Survival of long-lived plasma cells is independent of antigen. *Int. Immunol.* **10:**1703–1711.

Manz, R. A., A. Thiel, and A. Radbruch. 1997. Lifetime of plasma cells in the bone marrow. *Nature* **388:**133–134.

Markiewicz, M. A., C. Girao, J. T. Opferman, J. Sun, Q. Hu, A. A. Agulnik, C. E. Bishop, C. B. Thompson, and P. G. Ashton-Rickardt. 1998. Long-term T cell memory requires the surface expression of self-peptide/major histocompatibility complex molecules. *Proc. Natl. Acad. Sci. USA* **95:**3065–3070.

Marrack, P., J. Bender, D. Hildeman, M. Jordan, T. Mitchell, M. Murakami, A. Sakamoto, B. C. Schaefer, B. Swanson, and J. Kappler. 2000. Homeostasis of alpha beta TCR+ T cells. *Nat. Immunol.* **1:**107–111.

Marshall, D. R., S. J. Turner, G. T. Belz, S. Wingo, S. Andreansky, M. Y. Sangster, J. M. Riberdy, T. Liu, M. Tan, and P. C. Doherty. 2001. Measuring the diaspora for virus-specific CD8+ T cells. *Proc. Natl. Acad. Sci. USA* **98:**6313–6318.

Maruyama, M., K. P. Lam, and K. Rajewsky. 2000. Memory B-cell persistence is independent of persisting immunizing antigen. *Nature* **407:**636–642.

Masopust, D., V. Vezys, A. L. Marzo, and L. Lefrancois. 2001. Preferential localization of effector memory cells in nonlymphoid tissue. *Science* **291:**2413–2417.

McChesney, M. B., C. J. Miller, P. A. Rota, Y. D. Zhu, L. Antipa, N. W. Lerche, R. Ahmed, and W. J. Bellini. 1997. Experimental measles. I. Pathogenesis in the normal and the immunized host. *Virology* **233:**74–84.

McHeyzer-Williams, M. G., and R. Ahmed. 1999. B cell memory and the long-lived plasma cell. *Curr. Opin. Immunol.* **11:**172–179.

Moskophidis, D., F. Lechner, H. Pircher, and R. M. Zinkernagel. 1993. Virus persistence in acutely infected immunocompetent mice by exhaustion of antiviral cytotoxic effector T cells. *Nature* **362:**758–761.

Mudde, G. C., R. Bheekha, and C. A. Bruijnzeel-Koomen. 1995. Consequences of IgE/CD23-mediated antigen presentation in allergy. *Immunol. Today* **16:**380–383.

Mullbacher, A. 1994. The long-term maintenance of cytotoxic T cell memory does not require persistence of antigen. *J. Exp. Med.* **179:**317–321.

Murali-Krishna, K., J. D. Altman, M. Suresh, D. J. Sourdive, A. J. Zajac, J. D. Miller, J. Slansky, and R. Ahmed. 1998. Counting antigen-specific CD8 T cells: a reevaluation of bystander activation during viral infection. *Immunity* **8:**177–187.

Murali-Krishna, K., L. L. Lau, S. Sambhara, F. Lemonnier, J. Altman, and R. Ahmed. 1999. Persistence of memory CD8 T cells in MHC class I-deficient mice. *Science* **286:**1377–1381.

Opferman, J. T., B. T. Ober, and P. G. Ashton-Rickardt. 1999. Linear differentiation of cytotoxic effectors into memory T lymphocytes. *Science* **283:**1745–1748.

Panum, P. L. 1847. Beobachtungen uber das Maserncontagium. *Virchows Arch.* **1:**492–503.

Paul, J. R., J. T. Riordan, and J. L. Melnick. 1951. Antibodies to three different antigenic types of poliomyelitis virus in sera from North Alaskan Eskimos. *Am. J. Hyg.* **54:**275–285.

Pirron, U., T. Schlunck, J. C. Prinz, and E. P. Rieber. 1990. IgE-dependent antigen focusing by human B lymphocytes is mediated by the low-affinity receptor for IgE. *Eur. J. Immunol.* **20:**1547–1551.

Plotkin, S. A., and W. A. Orenstein. 1999. *Vaccines,* 3rd ed. The W. B. Saunders Co., Philadelphia, Pa.

Reinhardt, R. L., A. Khoruts, R. Merica, T. Zell, and M. K. Jenkins. 2001. Visualizing the generation of memory CD4 T cells in the whole body. *Nature* **410:**101–105.

Sallusto, F., D. Lenig, R. Forster, M. Lipp, and A. Lanzavecchia. 1999. Two subsets of memory T lymphocytes with distinct homing potentials and effector functions. *Nature* **401:**708–712.

Sawyer, W. A. 1931. Persistence of yellow fever immunity. *J. Prev. Med.* **5:**413–428.

Scheibel, I., M. W. Bentzon, P. E. Christensen, and A. Biering. 1966. Duration of immunity to diphtheria and tetanus after active immunization. *Acta Pathol. Microbiol. Scand.* **67:**380–392.

Selin, L. K., M. Y. Lin, K. A. Kraemer, D. M. Pardoll, J. P. Schneck, S. M. Varga, P. A. Santolucito, A. K. Pinto, and R. M. Welsh. 1999. Attrition of T cell memory: selective loss of LCMV epitope-specific memory CD8 T cells following infections with heterologous viruses. *Immunity* **11:**733–742.

Simonsen, O., K. Kjeldsen, and I. Heron. 1984. Immunity against tetanus and effect of revaccination 25–30 years after primary vaccination. *Lancet* **ii:**1240–1242.

Slifka, M. K., and R. Ahmed. 1998. Long-lived plasma cells: a mechanism for maintaining persistent antibody production. *Curr. Opin. Immunol.* **10:**252–258.

Slifka, M. K., R. Antia, J. K. Whitmire, and R. Ahmed. 1998. Humoral immunity due to long-lived plasma cells. *Immunity* **8:**363–372.

Slifka, M. K., M. Matloubian, and R. Ahmed. 1995. Bone marrow is a major site of long-term antibody production after acute viral infection. *J. Virol.* **69:**1895–1902.

Slifka, M. K., and J. L. Whitton. 2000. Activated and memory CD8+ T cells can be distinguished by their cytokine profiles and phenotypic markers. *J. Immunol.* **164:**208–216.

Sprent, J., and C. D. Surh. 2001. Generation and maintenance of memory T cells. *Curr. Opin. Immunol.* **13:**248–254.

Stuber, E., and W. Strober. 1996. The T cell-B cell interaction via OX40-OX40L is necessary for the T cell-dependent humoral immune response. *J. Exp. Med.* **183:**979–989.

Swain, S. L., H. Hu, and G. Huston. 1999. Class II-independent generation of CD4 memory T cells from effectors. *Science* **286:** 1381–1383.

Tanchot, C., F. A. Lemonnier, B. Perarnau, A. A. Freitas, and B. Rocha. 1997. Differential requirements for survival and proliferation of CD8 naive or memory T cells. *Science* **276:**2057–2062.

Turner, C. A., Jr., D. H. Mack, and M. M. Davis. 1994. Blimp-1, a novel zinc finger-containing protein that can drive the maturation of B lymphocytes into immunoglobulin-secreting cells. *Cell* **77:**297–306.

van Stipdonk, M. J., E. E. Lemmens, and S. P. Schoenberger. 2001. Naive CTLs require a single brief period of antigenic stimulation for clonal expansion and differentiation. *Nat. Immunol.* **2:**423–429.

Wong, P., and E. G. Pamer. 2001. Cutting edge: antigen-independent CD8 T cell proliferation. *J. Immunol.* **166:**5864–5868.

Zajac, A. J., J. N. Blattman, K. Murali-Krishna, D. J. Sourdive, M. Suresh, J. D. Altman, and R. Ahmed. 1998. Viral immune evasion due to persistence of activated T cells without effector function. *J. Exp. Med.* **188:**2205–2213.

Zimmermann, C., A. Prevost-Blondel, C. Blaser, and H. Pircher. 1999. Kinetics of the response of naive and memory CD8 T cells to antigen: similarities and differences. *Eur. J. Immunol.* **29:**284–290.

Zinkernagel, R. M., M. F. Bachmann, T. M. Kundig, S. Oehen, H. Pirchet, and H. Hengartner. 1996. On immunological memory. *Annu. Rev. Immunol.* **14:**333–367.

Immunology of Infectious Diseases
Edited by S. H. E. Kaufmann, A. Sher, and R. Ahmed
© 2002 ASM Press, Washington, D.C.

Chapter 14

Regional Immune Response to Microbial Pathogens

MARIAN R. NEUTRA AND JEAN-PIERRE KRAEHENBUHL

ORGANIZATION AND DISTRIBUTION OF MUCOSAL LYMPHOID TISSUES

The mucosal surfaces of the body together represent a vast surface area separated from the outside world only by delicate epithelial barriers. Thus, it is not surprising that mucosal tissues are extremely immunologically active. For example, the number of antibody-producing B cells in the lamina propria of the intestine is estimated to be greater than in any other organ in the body including the spleen, thymus, and lymph nodes (Brandtzaeg et al., 1999a). Although antigen-specific effector lymphocytes are present throughout mucosal tissues, the initial inductive events that lead to their formation occur at specific sites in the mucosa, which are recognized by the presence of organized lymphoid tissues (Kraehenbuhl and Neutra, 1992; McGhee et al., 1999).

Organized MALT

The hallmark of typical organized mucosa-associated lymphoid tissues (MALT) is the presence of lymphoid follicles. The best-known example of organized MALT is the Peyer's patches of the intestine, where follicles are aggregated in large clusters. The composition of these tissues and the variations observed in vivo have been described in detail and extensively reviewed (Brandtzaeg and Farstad, 1999; Brandtzaeg et al., 1999a; Hein, 1999; McGhee et al., 1999). Each mucosal follicle consists of an assembly of immature B cells often including a germinal center, supported by a network of follicular dendritic cells (DCs). The follicles are flanked by T-cell areas that contain a distinct population of interdigitating DCs and high endothelial venules that serve as entry and exit points for migrating cells (Kelsall and Strober, 1999). In Peyer's patches, each follicle is separated from the overlying epithelium by a subepithelial "dome" region rich in T and B cells, DCs, and macrophages (Brandtzaeg et al., 1999a). Cells of the dome function in close collaboration with the follicle-associated epithelium (FAE), which delivers antigens and microorganisms from the lumen into the subepithelial tissue. Restriction of such uptake to these sites effectively localizes antigen entry in sites where incoming foreign materials and pathogens can be processed and presented for induction of appropriate immune responses (Neutra et al., 1996).

The distribution of organized MALT in mucosal tissues of the body varies among species, but there are certain consistent patterns. Major organized mucosal lymphoid tissues appear at predictable sites before birth, and thus their assembly seems to be predetermined genetically (Hein, 1999). These MALT assemblies appear to be positioned to monitor the incoming antigens and pathogens that challenge the mucosa immediately after birth. Macroscopically visible aggregations of follicles consistently occur in the distal small intestine (Peyer's patches), the tonsils and adenoids, the appendix, and, in some species, the large intestine. In sheep, ileal Peyer's patches are sites of B-cell expansion where rearrangement and diversification of immunoglobulin (Ig) V-region genes occur, apparently regulated by antigen-independent mechanisms (Reynaud et al., 1995). In humans, the oral pharynx is monitored by a ring of mucosal lymphoid tissues including the palatine tonsils, lingual tonsils, and adenoids (Perry and White, 1998). In rodents, a strip of organized lymphoid tissue lies along the base of the nasal cavity (Sminia and Kraal, 1999). The structure of the various large MALT assemblies is complex. For example, the tonsils consist of oropharyngeal mucosa amplified and thickened by

Marian R. Neutra • Department of Pediatrics, Harvard Medical School, and GI Cell Biology Laboratory, Children's Hospital, Boston, MA 02115.   **Jean-Pierre Kraehenbuhl** • Swiss Institute for Experimental Cancer Research, Institute of Biochemistry, University of Lausanne, CH 1066 Epalinges, Switzerland.

folds and deep crypts. Along the walls of the crypts, a series of B-cell follicles, associated closely with the stratified squamous epithelium, are separated by dense interfollicular T-cell zones.

Solitary follicles and associated structures, only visible microscopically, occur in many locations and are particularly abundant throughout the gastrointestinal (GI) tract. In the human digestive tract, single lymphoid follicles occur from the cardiac region of the stomach to the rectoanal junction. The greatest frequency of individual follicles occurs in the large intestine and in dead-ended extensions of the GI lumen such as the cecum and appendix, where the microflora is abundant (O'Leary and Sweeney, 1986). Lymphoid follicles in the trachea and bronchi are usually solitary and generally sparse except under conditions of antigenic challenge, where they can become more abundant (Bienenstock et al., 1999; Pabst and Gehrke, 1990). Solitary follicles are also common at mucocutaneous transitions, such as the rectoanal junction, and near the ducts of secretory glands that empty onto mucosal surfaces.

Recently, a new type of organized MALT termed the cryptopatch has been detected in the intestines of mice (Kanamori et al., 1996). Cryptopatches are microscopic (each containing about 1,000 lymphocytes), are located in the lamina propria near the bases of crypts, and first become detectable 14 to 17 days after birth. They differ from other types of organized MALT in their histogenesis, lymphocyte phenotypes, and cell proliferative activity. It has been proposed that they represent sites of early generation of interleukin-7 (IL-7)-dependent progenitors of T- and/or B-cell lineages (Kanamori et al., 1996).

Diffuse MALT

Lamina propria as effector site

Most mucosal cells involved in immune defense are distributed diffusely throughout the subepithelial connective tissue and are directly or indirectly responsible for effector functions, i.e., preventing the entry of commensals and pathogens across the epithelial barrier and destroying pathogens and infected cells if invasion occurs (McGhee et al., 1999). These effectors include terminally differentiated B cells, helper CD4$^+$ and cytotoxic CD8$^+$ T cells, and NK cells. In addition, mucosal macrophages and dendritic cells phagocytose pathogens and macromolecular debris and monitor the mucosa for incoming antigens (Kelsall and Strober, 1999). The collective action of these cells minimizes the entry of pathogens and infection of mucosal tissues of the host.

IELs and immune surveillance

Intraepithelial lymphocytes (IELs) form a heterogeneous cell population that consists of both CD4$^+$ and CD8$^+$ cells (MacDonald, 1999). In the upper airways most IELs are CD4$^+$ cells, while in the gut most IELs are CD8$^+$ cells expressing either α/β or $\gamma\delta$ T-cell receptors (Lefrancois and Puddington, 1998). In rodents, especially young animals, $\gamma\delta$ T cells predominate, whereas in humans they are uncommon ($<5\%$) except in those with celiac disease. Two classes of IELs have been identified which have different origins, depending on whether they express the CD8 β chain. IELs expressing CD8 $\alpha\alpha$ homodimers on their surface are thymus independent, while $\alpha\beta$ heterodimeric CD8 IELs are derived from the thymus (Lefrancois and Puddington, 1998). It has been proposed that CD8 $\alpha\alpha$ IELs derive from cryptopatches (Saito et al., 1998). In humans, CD8 $\alpha\alpha$ IELs are rare and there is limited evidence for extrathymic maturation. Whether IELs migrate back into the lamina propria is not known, although they migrate in and out of a human intestinal epithelial monolayer in vitro (Shaw et al., 1998). Rodent studies indicate that IELs can be long-lived (MacDonald, 1999) and persist in the epithelium for extended periods as the enterocyte layer is renewed around them. Both $\alpha\beta$ and $\gamma\delta$ IELs are oligoclonal (Arstila et al., 2000), with highly complex T-cell receptors and extensive N-region insertions, suggesting that they have been selected by specific ligands. IELs, like skin dendritic T lymphocytes, probably recognize a limited repertoire of microbial or cellular antigens and participate in epithelial monitoring and repair processes rather than in immune defense (Boismenu et al., 1996; Boismenu and Havran, 1994).

Modulation and suppression of immune responses in mucosal tissues

It should be emphasized that the vast majority of foreign antigens in the intestine are derived from food and the commensal microbial flora and that these generally do not trigger defensive immune responses even though they regularly enter the mucosa. This is because mucosal antigen-presenting cells, lymphocytes, and even the epithelium itself play important but poorly understood roles in modulating immune responses to incoming antigens. Indeed, a major role of the mucosal immune system is the down-regulation or suppression of immune responses to food antigens and commensal bacteria. The exact sites or mechanisms of this "oral tolerance" are still controversial and have been reviewed elsewhere (Mayer, 2000; Mowat and Weiner, 1999).

SAMPLING OF ANTIGENS AND PATHOGENS AT MUCOSAL SURFACES

The sequence of events involved in processing and presentation of foreign antigens by professional antigen-presenting cells and the responses and interactions of local lymphocytes that lead to the production of effector and memory cells are likely to be similar in the mucosal and systemic branches of the immune system. However, induction of mucosal immune responses is complicated by the fact that antigens and microorganisms on mucosal surfaces are separated from cells of the mucosal immune system by epithelial barriers. To mount protective mucosal immune responses, samples of the external environment on mucosal surfaces must be delivered to the immune system without compromising the integrity and protective functions of the epithelium (Neutra et al., 1996). Strategies for antigen sampling at diverse mucosal sites are adapted to the cellular organization of the local epithelial barrier, but two major paradigms emerge (Color Plate 4). In stratified epithelia, motile DCs (or Langerhans cells) move into the narrow intraepithelial spaces and even to the outer limit of the epithelium, where they may obtain samples to carry back to local mucosal lymphoid tissues or distant lymph nodes. In simple epithelia where intercellular spaces are sealed by tight junctions, epithelial M cells transport samples of luminal material directly to MALT. Antigens and pathogens that cross epithelial barriers may be released at the basolateral side of the epithelium and taken up by intra- or subepithelial antigen-presenting cells. Then they may be carried by DCs into local organized MALT and to draining lymph nodes or spleen (Kelsall and Strober, 1999; McGhee et al., 1999).

Antigen Sampling across Stratified Epithelia

Intraepithelial DCs, equivalent in function to the Langerhans' cells originally described in skin, are present in the stratified epithelia of the oral cavity, anal mucosa, and vagina (Desvignes et al., 1998; Miller et al., 1992; Okato et al., 1989; Parr and Parr, 1994). DCs appear to capture antigens within and under stratified epithelia and then migrate out of the mucosa to draining lymph nodes, where they presumably mature and function as antigen-presenting cells (Holt et al., 1994; MacPherson and Liu, 1999; Steinman et al., 2000). Alternatively, DCs located in the epithelium over organized MALT, such as those that are abundant in the tonsils, could present antigens either in local MALT or after migration to draining lymph nodes (MacPherson and Liu, 1999).

Antigen Sampling across Simple Epithelia

The lining of the small and large intestines is formed by a single layer of epithelial cells that are protected by multiple nonimmune defense mechanisms (Madara et al., 1990). However, microbial adherence and antigen uptake are common occurrences, and this is reflected by the constant state of "immunologic alert" in the mucosa. Small amounts of intact proteins and peptides are taken up by absorptive enterocytes. Although most are transported to lysosomes and degraded, enterocytes express major histocompatibiliy complex (MHC) class I and II and can present peptides in vitro (Kaiserlian, 1999). In addition, the class I-related molecule CD1d is expressed at the basolateral surfaces of intestinal epithelial cells and appears to function as an antigen-presenting molecule by interacting with specialized populations of T cells (Blumberg et al., 1999; Campbell et al., 1999). The possible role of antigen uptake by enterocytes in induction of immune responses or immune tolerance is discussed below (Mayer, 2000).

FAE and M cells

Throughout the intestines, multiple crypts provide a continuous supply of fresh epithelial cells to each villus or intercrypt area (Gordon and Hermiston, 1994). Where mucosal lymphoid follicles occur, epithelial cells emerging from the adjacent follicle-associated crypts migrate onto the dome formed by the underlying lymphoid follicle to form the FAE (Bye et al., 1984; Gebert et al., 1999; Sierro et al., 2000). There is evidence that gene expression in cells of the FAE is strongly influenced by the lymphoid cells of the underlying follicle, with the result that the FAE differs dramatically from the villus epithelium. Whereas the villus epithelium is dominated by absorptive enterocytes, mucin-secreting goblet cells, and enteroendocrine cells, the FAE contains few or no goblet or enteroendocrine cells but contains M cells, a phenotype found only in the FAE (Kato and Owen, 1999).

The entire FAE presents a biochemical "face" to the lumen that is distinct from that of villi, and this may promote the recognition of these relatively infrequent areas by microbial pathogens (Neutra et al., 1999). Follicle-associated enterocytes differ from villus enterocytes in that their brush borders contain much lower levels of digestive hydrolases. Other FAE features tend to promote local contact of intact antigens and pathogens with the epithelial surface: there is little or no mucus production by the FAE (Kato and Owen, 1999) and few defensin- and lysozyme-producing Paneth cells in follicle-associated crypts (Giannasca et al., 1994). In addition, the FAE does not transport protective IgA into the lumen because it is devoid of polymeric Ig receptors (Pappo and Owen, 1988). The FAE may provide recognition sites for pathogens since the glycosylation patterns of its enterocytes differ from those on villi in humans, rabbits, and mice (Neutra et al., 1999). Recent experiments using transgenic mice demonstrated that a single gene could be upregulated specifically in the FAE (S. El Bahi, M. E. Caliot, A. Vandewalle, A. Kahn, J. P. Kraehenbuhl, and E. Pringault, submitted for publication), suggesting the existence of a tissue-specific transcription factor that may control the expression of multiple genes in FAE cells and not elsewhere along the gut. FAE differentiation and gene expression appear to be dependent on influences from the underlying follicle, because new sites of FAE can appear wherever mucosal lymphoid follicles assemble in response to microbial challenge (Savidge et al., 1991) or after injection of Peyer's patch cells into the mucosa (Kernéis et al., 1997).

The most striking feature of the FAE is the presence of M cells, whose function is to deliver samples of foreign material by transepithelial transport from the lumen to organized lymphoid tissues within the mucosa (Neutra et al., 1996). Unlike other epithelial cells, M cells amplify their basolateral membrane to form an intraepithelial pocket, which provides a sequestered space for special subpopulations of IELs. The pocket shortens the distance that transcytotic vesicles must travel from the apical to basolateral side of the epithelial barrier (Neutra et al., 1996) and provides for rapid delivery of luminal samples to cells of the mucosal immune system. The numbers of M cells in the FAE can increase rapidly in response to bacterial adherence, apparently by conversion of uncommitted FAE enterocytes to the M-cell phenotype (Borghesi et al., 1999). Studies using an epithelial-cell–lymphocyte coculture system suggest that this effect is mediated by interaction of B lymphocytes with the epithelium (Kernéis et al., 1997).

The apical membranes of M cells are designed to facilitate adherence and uptake of antigens and microorganisms, and these cells take up macromolecules, microorganisms, and particles by multiple mechanisms (Neutra et al., 1999). Their clathrin-coated microdomains mediate endocytosis of ligand-coated particles (Frey et al., 1996), adherent macromolecules (Bye et al., 1984), and viruses (Sicinski et al., 1990). M cells also use fluid-phase pinocytosis to take up soluble macromolecules and actin-dependent phagocytosis to take up adherent microorganisms (Neutra et al., 1995). In addition, pathogens can induce macropinocytotic engulfment involving disruption of the apical cytoskeletal orga-

nization (Jones et al., 1994). M cells display carbohydrate structures that differ from those of other epithelial-cell types. Human M cells display the sialyl Lewis A antigen (defined as Neu5Ac α(2-3) Gal β(1-3) GlcNAc [Fuc α(1-4)]. However, there are variations in M-cell glycosylation among species, between different mucosal regions, and even within the same FAE (Neutra et al., 1999). These distinct oligosaccharides may serve as recognition sites for pathogens that exploit the M-cell pathway, as described below.

Fate of antigens in organized MALT

M cells provide a pathway across the epithelial barrier through vesicular transport activity, but little is known about the fates of specific antigens and pathogens that enter this pathway. Antigens and pathogens released into the M-cell pocket would come in contact with B and T cells that display characteristic phenotypes, as shown by immunocytochemistry tests with experimental animals (Ermak and Owen, 1994) and humans (Farstad et al., 1997). M-cell pocket T cells are distinct from villus IELs: they are mostly CD4$^+$, and in humans they display the antigen CD45RO typical of memory cells (Brandtzaeg et al., 1999a). Most of the B cells in the pocket express MHC class II and IgM but not IgG or IgA, suggesting that these cells are B memory cells that are capable of antigen presentation. The presence of such phenotypes suggests that pocket B cells have positioned themselves for reexposure to incoming antigen and efficient presentation of antigen to cognate T cells and that lymphoblast traffic into the M-cell pocket may allow amplification and diversification of the immune response (Brandtzaeg et al., 1999a). However, no direct information is available concerning the interactions and events that occur in this sequestered intraepithelial space, and the purpose of the M-cell pocket is unproven. One possibility is that the pocket allows lymphocytes to interact with incoming antigens in the absence of circulating antibodies. This is suggested by the observations that injected Igs do not freely diffuse into the organized mucosal lymphoid tissues (Allan and Trier, 1991) and that protein tracers injected intravenously percolate into the mucosa but do not readily enter the M-cell pockets. However, some serum antibodies do gain access to Peyer's patches, as evidenced by the observation that B-cell infection by mouse mammary tumor virus (MMTV) in Peyer's patches or nasal associated lymphoid tissue can be prevented by passive transfer of MMTV-specific antibodies (Velin et al., 1999).

Immediately under the FAE, in the so-called dome region that caps the underlying lymphoid follicle, is an extensive network of DCs and possibly macrophages, intermingled with CD4[+] T cells and B cells that appear to be derived from the underlying follicle (Brandtzaeg et al., 1999a; Kelsall and Strober, 1999). The dome region has all the earmarks of an active immune inductive site, where endocytosis and killing of incoming pathogens, as well as processing and presentation of antigens, occur. M-cell-transported lectins, cholera toxin conjugates, protein tracers, and particles have been detected in cells of the dome. A recent confocal light microscopic study detected live, attenuated *Salmonella enterica* serovar Typhimurium in DCs of the dome region after oral administration (Hopkins et al., 2000). However, there is little information about the processing of nonliving macromolecules, particles, killed microbes, and mucosal vaccines in this tissue, and the migration patterns of antigen-containing DCs out of the dome region are in need of further investigation. It is likely that dome DCs migrate to adjacent T cell areas, but they may also enter the follicle or leave the mucosa to enter the T-cell areas of draining lymph nodes (Kelsall and Strober, 1999).

The local signals that govern the migration of cells into the subepithelial dome region or M-cell pocket are unknown, but recent studies suggest that chemokines play a role. This seems reasonable since chemokines direct immune cell migration in other systems (Baggiolini, 1998). In situ hybridization showed that the human CC chemokine macrophage inflammatory protein 3α (MIP-3α) is produced by intestinal FAE cells but not villus cells of mice (Iwasaki and Kelsall, 2000). This chemokine is therefore the first protein shown to be expressed specifically by FAE cells. The facts that MIP-3α has selective chemotactic activity for naive B and T lymphocytes and DCs that express CCR6 receptors and that CCR6[+] cells are present immediately under the FAE suggest that MIP-3α is important for maintenance of mucosal antigen-sampling functions. The observation that MIP-3α expression is transiently induced in epithelial cells in vitro by pathogenic bacteria (Izadpanah et al., 2001) suggests that this chemokine could play a role in the induction of new lymphoid follicles seen in intestines exposed to gram-negative enteropathogens such as *Salmonella*.

Hybrid antigen sampling systems

The lining of the airways, including the nasopharynx, trachea, bronchi, and bronchioles, varies from pseudostratified to simple epithelium. These epithelia have an immune surveillance system with two distinct antigen-sampling mechanisms. One mechanism is provided by DCs, which migrate into pseudostratified and simple epithelia of the airways to capture antigens. These intraepithelial DCs form a contiguous network with up to 700 DCs per mm[2] (Holt et al., 1994). Cells of the airway epithelium are sealed by apical tight junctions, and it is not known exactly how DCs gain access to luminal antigens or pathogens: do they send processes through tight junctions to obtain samples from the lumen, or do they simply endocytose antigens that have entered the lateral intercellular spaces of the epithelium? In any case, airway DCs are MHC class II-positive migratory cells, spending a short time (average, 2 days) in the respiratory mucosa (Holt et al., 1994). A second respiratory antigen-sampling mechanism occurs in the nasal cavities and bronchi in the form of isolated mucosal lymphoid follicles with overlying FAE containing M cells (Bienenstock et al., 1999) that seem to be structurally and functionally analogous to their counterparts in intestine. The intraepithelial DC network and the M cell/organized lymphoid follicle system presumably play distinct roles in induction of local and systemic immune responses to antigens and pathogens. Both DCs and M cells function in antigen transport in the tonsils and adenoids as well. At intervals along the walls of tonsillar crypts, the epithelium invaginates and thins to a single cell layer containing M cells. In addition, the entire crypt epithelium contains many intraepithelial DCs as well as migratory lymphocytes (Hein, 1999; MacPherson and Liu, 1999). The relative importance and functional implications of these alternative antigen capture systems in immune responses to specific pathogens are not clear.

EXPLOITATION OF MUCOSAL IMMUNE SAMPLING MECHANISMS BY PATHOGENS

Although transepithelial transport of antigens is a prerequisite for efficient induction of mucosal immune responses, certain pathogens use these pathways to invade mucosal tissues. For example, enteric pathogens exploit the special features of M cells that are intended to promote immunological sampling (Neutra et al., 1995; Siebers and Finlay, 1996). In general, antigens that adhere to mucosal surfaces tend to induce vigorous mucosal immune responses whereas nonadherent antigens do not. Similarly, pathogens or vaccines that can bind selectively to M cells appear most effective in mucosal invasion. The endocytic or phagocytic vesicles formed at the apical surfaces of M cells can acidify their content and contain proteases (Allan et al., 1993; Finzi et al., 1993), but endocytosed materials are rapidly released at the pocket membrane (Neutra et al., 1996). Many pathogens survive M-cell transcytosis and can go on to infect cells of the mucosa or the epithelium itself (Phalipon and Sansonetti, 1999; Siebers and Finlay, 1996).

Bacteria

The predilection of some bacteria for M cells may be due in part to the relative lack of a thick, protective brush border glycocalyx on these cells. Experiments using plant lectins and a bacterial toxin immobilized on virus-sized and bacterium-sized particles showed that specific glycolipid and oligosaccharide epitopes are more accessible on the FAE than on villus epithelium and are more accessible on M cells than on FAE enterocytes (Frey et al., 1996; Mantis et al., 2000). Diverse gram-negative bacteria bind selectively to M cells (Neutra et al., 1995; Siebers and Finlay 1996); these include *Vibrio cholerae,* some strains of *Escherichia coli, Salmonella enterica* serovars Typhi and Typhimurium, *Shigella flexneri, Yersinia enterocolitica* and *Y. pseudotuberculosis,* and *Campylobacter jejuni.* M-cell adherence and uptake seems to involve common events including initial adherence (perhaps via a lectin-carbohydrate interaction) followed by more intimate contact and activation of intracellular signaling pathways. However, each pathogen interacts with the mucosa in a distinct fashion, as exemplified by *Salmonella* and *Shigella.*

S. enterica serovar Typhimurium is capable of binding to all epithelial cells in mice, but it binds most readily to M cells in vivo, and the initial foci of infection are the Peyer's patches. Adherence of the bacteria induces dramatic host cell cytoskeletal rearrangement that results in ruffling of the apical cell surface and bacterial engulfment by a process that resembles macropinicytosis (Jones et al., 1994). This presumably involves the same bacterial gene products that are involved in invasion of cultured epithelial cells (Finlay and Cossart, 1997). The fact that strains carrying mutations in the *lpf* operon, a cluster of genes that encodes a putative fimbria, were reduced in their ability to adhere to Peyer's patch epithelium implies that pili are involved in the initial *Salmonella*–M-cell interaction (Bäumler et al., 1996). However, the M-cell receptor exploited by *Salmonella* is not known. *S. enterica* serovar Typhimurium recognizes a cell surface carbohydrate epitope containing Gal β(1-3) GalNAc on cultured epithelial Caco-2 cells (Giannasca et al., 1996), but in mice this epitope is present on all small intestinal epithelial cells (Giannasca et al., 1994). Thus the predilection

of serovar Typhimurium for M cells may be due to the greater accessibility of M-cell-binding sites. The ability of *Salmonella* to target itself to M cells makes it a promising candidate mucosal vaccine vector, and we have shown that it may function as a vector via multiple mucosal routes (Sirard et al., 1999). A live attenuated *Salmonella* vaccine expressing genes for the core and surface antigens of hepatitis B virus was administered to mice by the oral, nasal, rectal, or vaginal routes (Hopkins et al., 1995). By all four routes, the vaccine elicited both local and systemic antibody responses against the foreign antigen as well as the vaccine carrier. This indicates that *Salmonella* can gain access to inductive sites across both simple and stratified epithelia, presumably by interacting with intraepithelial DCs in vagina and airways, as well as M cells and antigen-presenting cells in organized mucosal lymphoid tissues of the nasopharynx and GI tract.

Shigella infects cells by adhering to the plasma membrane, inducing phagocytosis, disrupting the phagosome membrane, and entering the host cell cytoplasm. The bacteria proliferate in the cytoplasm, move by assembly of "tails" of actin filaments, and are extruded in cytoplasmic processes which can be phagocytosed by neighboring cells (Phalipon and Sansonetti, 1999). However, *Shigella* is unable to adhere to the apical surfaces of enterocytes. Instead, pathogenic as well as selected nonpathogenic strains of *Shigella* are transported into the mucosa by M cells, and this allows *Shigella* access to basolateral membranes of both M cells and enterocytes as well as underlying macrophages, all of which may then be invaded. In addition, the bacteria induce the release of chemotactic signals that attract inflammatory cells, whose products contribute to epithelial breakdown. Attenuated *Shigella* strains lacking key genes are attractive candidates as mucosal vaccines against *Shigella* itself or as vaccine vectors for targeting the expression of foreign antigens to mucosal lymphoid tissues (Phalipon and Sansonetti, 1999).

Viruses

Viruses also exploit antigen sampling mechanisms to invade mucosal tissues and spread to other organs. Viruses are unable to enzymatically alter epithelial cell surfaces or to use signal transduction strategies to modify host cell architecture, but they can be carried by both M cells and DCs across epithelial barriers. The ability of M cells to endocytose and transport particles suggests that many viruses could enter the mucosa via these cells, and M-cell uptake of several viruses has been documented (Siebers and Finlay, 1996). The best characterized of these is reovirus, a mouse pathogen which uses the M-cell transport pathway exclusively to gain access to its target cells. When reovirus is ingested orally, it selectively binds to mouse M cells in Peyer's patches (Amerongen et al., 1994; Wolf et al., 1981), but it also can enter via M cells in the colon and airways. In the intestinal lumen, digestive proteases remove the outermost capsid protein (σ3), modify a second outer capsid protein (μ1C), and induce extension of the viral hemagglutinin σ1, the adhesin used by the virus to bind to target neurons and fibroblasts in culture (Nibert et al., 1991). Proteolytic processing of the outer capsid is required for M-cell adherence (Amerongen et al., 1994). Reovirus binding to M cells is likely to be mediated by interaction of the extended σ1, which contains a lectin-like domain, with a specific sialic acid-containing determinant on the M cell apical surface. This determinant is present on all epithelial cells but appears to be more accessible on M cells (Mantis et al., 2000). Adherent reovirus is endocytosed by M cells in clathrin-coated pits and transcytosed to the intraepithelial pocket and subepithelial tissue, where it can infect multiple cell types and spread to the draining lymph nodes, spleen, and central nervous system in neonates.

There is evidence that human immunodeficiency virus (HIV) and simian immunodeficiency virus (SIV) may use M cells, DCs, and perhaps other transepithelial transport pathways to cross epithelial barriers during sexual transmission (Miller, 1994; Spira et al., 1996; Neutra, 1998). Studies using enterocyte-like cell lines in culture have identified galactosylceramide as an epithelial-cell component that can serve as a receptor for binding of the HIV envelope glycoprotein, and it has been proposed that this glycolipid could serve as an HIV receptor on human rectal epithelial cells (Yahi et al., 1992). Virus-infected cells can form close contacts with cultured epithelial monolayers and may bud viruses directly onto epithelial apical membranes (Phillips and Bourinbaiar, 1992). This phenomenon was shown to facilitate endocytosis and transport of virus across Caco-2 cell monolayers in vitro (Bomsel, 1997). However, recent studies in one of our laboratories failed to detect transcytosis of HIV across well-differentiated Caco-2 monolayers, although the epithelial cells themselves became infected. The CXCR4 or CCR5 chemokine receptors, together with galactosylceramide, mediated the infection of epithelial cells by syncytium- or non-syncytial-inducing HIV-1 strains, respectively (G. Fotopoulos, A. Harari, D. Trono, G. Pantaleo, and J. P. Kraehenbuhl, submitted for publication). Another potential entry route in vivo was suggested by the observation that HIV adhered to rabbit and mouse M cells and was transcytosed in mucosal ex-plants (Amerongen et al., 1991). If such M-cell-selective uptake occurs in the human rectum, it would deliver the virus directly to target cells in the M-cell pocket and MALT. In the vagina, intraepithelial DCs may be the first to encounter HIV during sexual transmission (Spira et al., 1996). Recent studies suggest that DCs may not be the first cells to become productively infected and support viral replication, however. In vitro, DCs can bind HIV via a novel mannose receptor (DC-SIGN), a surface molecule that is included in the DC–T-cell "synapse" (Geijtenbeek et al., 2000). In vivo, DCs carrying virus would migrate to the nearest lymph node, where they could readily transmit the virus to T cells (Steinman, 2000).

IMMUNE RESPONSES IN MUCOSAL TISSUES

Induction of B-Cell Responses

Following stimulation by antigens and T helper cells, naive B cells in organized MALT of the gut, the airways, or the oropharyngeal cavity move to the germinal center, where they clonally proliferate. During clonal expansion B cells undergo affinity maturation, first by somatic hypermutation, which generates variability in B-cell receptors, and then by selection of those with highest affinity for the antigen. Selection of cells bearing mutated receptors by antigen occurs on the surfaces of follicular DCs, a process which rescues cells expressing high-affinity Ig receptors from apoptosis (MacLennan et al., 1992). In MALT germinal centers, B lymphocytes undergo isotype switching and differentiate further into B cells that express IgA (Brandtzaeg et al., 1999a; McGhee et al., 1999). MALT CD4$^+$ T cells promote IgA isotype switching of IgM-bearing B cells. Cytokines produced by activated Th2 CD4$^+$ T cells, including IL-5, IL-10, and transforming growth factor β (TGF-β), play a major role in triggering the switch, but the precise molecular mechanism which mediates the recombination event has not yet been fully elucidated. Bacterial lipopolysaccharide (LPS) stimulates expression of the recombination machinery in pre-B lymphocytes, and mucosal adjuvants, including cholera toxin and E. coli heat labile toxin, are known to facilitate the switch. Subsequently, B lymphocytes differentiate into effector or memory cells following contact with T-helper lymphocytes and CD40-CD40 ligand interactions. In MALT, stimulated B and T cells acquire mucosal homing receptors. The effector and memory lymphocytes lose their adhesion to stromal cells, leave organized MALT structures, and enter the bloodstream via the lymph. Depending on the mucosal site at which priming took place, different homing receptors are expressed by B lymphocytes (Brandtzaeg et al., 1999b) (Color Plate 4). Virtually all IgA- and even IgG-antibody secreting cells detected after peroral and rectal immunization expressed $\alpha_4\beta_7$ integrin, the mucosal homing receptor, while only a minor fraction of these cells expressed L-selectin, the peripheral homing receptor. In contrast, circulating B cells induced by intranasal immunization expressed both L-selectin and $\alpha_4\beta_7$.

Effector and memory B cells are able to home to distant mucosal tissues or return to MALT structures. The lymphocytes expressing mucosal $\alpha_4\beta_7$ homing receptors interact with postcapillary venule endothelial cells bearing mucosal addressins on their luminal surfaces (Butcher and Picker, 1996). Antigen receptors (surface Igs) do not participate in the selectivity of lymphocyte binding to the vascular bed, but it has been proposed that antigen-specific plasmablasts become locally enriched in mucosal sites through retention at sites of antigen deposition (Butcher and Picker, 1996). The mucosal addressin MadCam-1 (mucosal addressin cell adhesion molecule 1) is preferentially expressed in human and mouse intestinal flat postcapillary venules of the lamina propria and high endothelial venules of organized MALT but not in other mucosal tissues (Briskin et al., 1997). The vascular addressins mediating selective binding of lymphocytes in the airways and the genital tract have not yet been identified. Extravasation of lymphocytes requires the action of chemokines (Butcher and Picker, 1996). B lymphocytes express a specific chemokine receptor, and in knockout mice lacking this receptor lymphocytes fail to reach mucosal tissues (Förster et al., 1996). A chemokine that attracts B cells has recently been identified (Gunn et al., 1998; Legler et al., 1998) and shown to be expressed by stromal cells in MALT and not by epithelial cells (Mazzucchelli et al., 1999).

After migration into the lamina propria, effector B lymphocytes differentiate into antibody-secreting plasma cells. This process is regulated by cytokines from T lymphocytes as well as epithelial cells. In the intestinal mucosa, the number of plasma cells producing IgA exceeds the number of those producing all other Ig isotypes (Brandtzaeg et al., 1999a). Maturation of IgA-bearing B cells into plasma cells is triggered by T-cell-derived IL-5 and TGF-β and epithelial IL-6 (McGhee et al., 1999). In IL-6 deficient mice, a reduced number of IgA-producing plasma cells have been observed in the respiratory tract, and targeting IL-6 DNA into bronchial epithelial cells restored the maturation of IgA B cells into plasma cells (Ramsay et al., 1994). However, this result has not been confirmed in the digestive tract,

suggesting that IL-6 is probably not the only cytokine involved in B-cell maturation (Bromander et al., 1996). In the mucosal environment, all plasma cells, irrespective of their Ig isotype, express J chain, the small polypeptide required for IgA polymerization (Brandtzaeg and Farstad, 1999).

Regulation of Immune Responses

Uptake of antigens in mucosal tissues may result in the development of immunity, tolerance, or both, depending on the physical-chemical nature of the antigen and where antigen presentation takes place. Deletion (Chen et al., 1995), anergy of antigen-specific T cells (Whitacre et al., 1991), and/or expansion of cells producing immunosuppressive cytokines (IL-4, IL-10, and TGF-β) (Khoury et al., 1992) has been linked to decreased T-cell responsiveness. Interestingly, the array of cytokines secreted by regulatory T cells that trigger systemic T-cell tolerance can elicit at the same time a secretory humoral immune response. Since both serum and cells can transfer tolerance from tolerized animals, it is possible that humoral antibodies, circulating undegraded antigens, tolerogenic protein fragments, and cytokines may act synergistically to confer T-cell unresponsiveness. Little is known about the molecular mechanisms whereby antigens administered mucosally can induce local and/or systemic tolerance (Mowat and Weiner, 1999). On mucosal surfaces, antigens encounter multiple factors including proteases, acids, salts, and detergents that can alter their native conformation and expose new epitopes. The observation that mucosally induced systemic tolerance depends on an intact epithelial barrier suggests a central role for the epithelium. Antigens sampled from the lumen by intestinal enterocytes are usually soluble molecules that can diffuse through the glycocalyx (Kaiserlian, 1999). Nonclassical MHC class I (CD1d) molecules expressed by enterocytes in the intestine may present these antigens to subsets of CD8$^+$ regulatory IELs known to induce local unresponsiveness (Blumberg et al., 1999). Epithelial enterocytes are also known to produce cytokines such as IL-10 and TGF-β which are particularly efficient at suppressing the inductive phase of CD4$^+$ T-cell-mediated responses.

In addition to epithelial cells and T cells, B cells (Czerkinsky et al., 1999), T cells (Mowat and Weiner, 1999), and DCs (Huang et al., 2000) have been proposed as important players in induction of oral tolerance. Activated B cells and tissue macrophages are known to efficiently present antigens to memory T-helper cells, while antigen presentation by resting B cells results in T-cell tolerance (Eynon and Parker, 1993; Fuchs and Matzinger, 1992). Resting B cells lack critical costimulatory molecules but are efficient at internalizing specific antigens. B cells activated in vitro with bacterial LPS, a prominent by-product of the normal mucosal microflora, are capable of inducing tolerance when injected into naïve hosts (Fuchs and Matzinger, 1992). DCs in mucosal tissues such as Peyer's patches (Kelsall and Strober, 1999) and mesenteric lymph nodes (MacPherson and Liu, 1999), the intestinal lamina propria (Pavli et al., 1990), and the airways (Nelson et al., 1994) stimulate rather than suppress immune responses. Interestingly, LPS, which is known to cause the rapid exit of DCs from mucosal tissues, has also been shown to enhance tolerance induction (Khoury et al., 1990). Transfer of immunogenic peptides from MHC class II to MHC class I molecules or to nonclassical restriction elements in a subpopulation of DCs, and the subsequent presentation of the peptides to CD8$^+$ $\gamma\delta$ T cells, has been shown to occur in the airways (Holt, 1994). Such activated cells might prevent the proliferation of CD4$^+$ T-helper cells, especially of the Th2 type, by releasing immunosuppressive cytokines. Such a mechanism could explain the suppressive effect of airborne antigens on induction of respiratory allergic responses. Recently, a distinct DC subset has been shown to endocytose apoptotic intestinal cells and transport them to T-cell areas in the draining mesenteric lymph nodes (Huang et al., 2000). This suggests a role for DCs in inducing and maintaining peripheral self-tolerance. It was recently observed that expression of ligands of the notch pathway in DCs can induce naive peripheral CD4$^+$ T cells to become regulatory cells that inhibit primary and secondary immune responses (Hoyne et al., 2000). This is the first demonstration of a molecular mechanism that may underlie the induction of tolerance.

Immunologic Memory

While systemic infections usually induce long-lasting protective immunity and prolonged serum antibody titers, mucosal antibody responses are usually relatively short-lived (Belyakov et al., 1999; Rudin et al., 1998). This may be due to differences in the maturation and selection of B cells in mucosal tissues compared to other peripheral compartments. Such differences are reflected by distinct CDR3 sequence patterns in the Ig heavy-chain genes and different mutation rates (Dunn-Walters et al., 2000). Long-lived memory B cells and plasma cells have recently been isolated from spleen and bone marrow (Manz et al., 1997; McHeyzer-Williams et al., 2000; Slifka et al., 1998). The nature of the signals and microenvironmental factors that promote the survival of specific B cells has yet not been identified,

but there is evidence that follicular DCs play a crucial role. Follicular DCs in germinal centers of MALT organs express MadCam-1, which could recruit $\alpha_4\beta_7$-expressing B lymphocytes (Szabo et al., 1997). Antigen-specific $\alpha_4\beta_7{}^{high}$ B lymphocytes, a memory phenotype, have been detected in Peyer's patches and lamina propria of mice (Williams et al., 1998), but how long these cells persist in the gut remains unclear. Additional factors such as chemokines and/or survival signals might be required for the retention and maintenance of specific B cells and antibody-secreting plasma cells in MALT compartments. Oral vaccination with cholera toxin B subunit promotes long-term antibody responses in the intestinal mucosa of mice and humans (Quiding et al., 1991; Vajdy and Lycke, 1992). This is most probably a result of an efficient priming of systemic B-cell responses along with continuous reentry of antibody-secreting B cells into mucosal tissue. There is evidence that some mucosal IgA B-cell responses are T-cell independent and represent a short-lived immune defense system in the gut (Macpherson et al., 2000). Taken together, the ability of a vaccine to induce mucosal B-cell memory responses seems to be dependent on systemic B-cell and T-helper cell priming.

Regional Nature of Mucosal Immune Responses

In both mice and humans, the secretory immune response to foreign antigens and microorganisms may be detected at the mucosal site where the antigen was initially taken up and also in distant mucosal and glandular secretions (McGhee et al., 1999). This phenomenon reflects the dissemination via the bloodstream of effector and memory cells from the site of antigen exposure into widespread mucosal and glandular connective tissues, where they differentiate into plasma cells that produce dimeric IgA. This has been termed the common mucosal immune system and has led to the idea that immunization at one mucosal site could induce protective secretory immunity in mucosal tissues throughout the body (McGhee et al., 1992). Indeed, although oral immunization results in antigen uptake only at inductive sites of the oral cavity and upper intestine, it can elicit antibodies not only in salivary and intestinal secretions but also in mammary gland and vaginal secretions (Cui et al., 1991; Holmgren et al., 1992).

However, there is increasing evidence that local exposure to antigen can result in much higher levels of specific secretory IgA (sIgA) in the region of exposure than at distant sites. Even within the GI tract, administration of antigen to the proximal small intestine, distal small intestine, colon, or rectum evokes highest levels of specific secretory IgA in the segment of antigen exposure (Haneberg et al., 1994; Ogra and Karzon, 1969; Pierce and Cray, 1982). Such observations have led to testing of rectal and vaginal immunization strategies for vaccines against sexually transmitted diseases (Lehner et al., 1992; Wassen et al., 1996). The rectum appears to be a particularly effective inductive site, consistent with the fact that M cells and lymphoid aggregates are numerous in the rectal mucosa. Rectal immunization of mice, rhesus macaques, and humans generated high levels of specific antibodies in local rectal secretions (Haneberg et al., 1994; Kozlowski et al., 1997; Lehner et al., 1993). Conversely, in rhesus macaques and humans, the vaginal immunization route effectively induced local immune responses in the female genital tract (Kozlowski et al., 1997; Lehner et al., 1992). In mice, vaginal immunization evoked local and systemic immune responses against live pathogens (McDermott et al., 1990) but not against nonliving antigens (Haneberg et al., 1994). There is great current interest in the nasal immunization route. Nasal immunization has been shown to produce impressive systemic immune responses, as well as local secretory responses in the upper respiratory tract and in the female genital tract (Hordnes et al., 1997; Rudin et al., 1998; Russell et al., 1996). Nasal immunization has been used experimentally to confer protection against vaginal mucosal challenge by herpes simplex virus type 1 (Parr and Parr, 1997) and respiratory challenge with *Bordetella pertussis* (Berstad et al., 1997).

MECHANISMS OF MUCOSAL PROTECTION

Nonspecific Mucosal Defenses

Luminal microorganisms are generally excluded from close contact with epithelial cell surfaces by the interplay of mucus and fluid secretions, antimicrobial peptides, and mucosal clearance mechanisms such as ciliary activity and peristaltic movements. Secretory mucins, the products of genes such as *muc2* (Van Klinken et al., 1995), are large, heavily glycosylated, negatively charged glycoproteins that are secreted into the crypts and onto the surfaces of the intestinal mucosa by goblet cells. Mucins form highly hydrated, loose gels that allow diffusion of large molecules including Igs (Cone, 1999). Thus, polymeric Igs that are exported into the crypts by receptor-mediated transcytosis as well as transudated serum Igs and other proteins, percolate through the mucus associated with mucosal surfaces. However, microorganisms coated with antibody are immobilized in mucus

gels, presumably due to multiple low-affinity interactions of Igs with mucins, and this promotes entrapment and clearance, preventing microbial contact with epithelial surfaces. The luminal side of the mucus layer is continually eroded and dispersed into the lumen as it is replenished from the crypts below (Forstner et al., 1995).

Defensins and other antibacterial proteins such as lysozyme are also released from epithelial cells into the lumens of the crypts and diffuse through the microenvironment associated with epithelial surfaces (Lehrer et al., 1999). In addition, IgA can interact with microorganisms nonspecifically through its carbohydrate side chains (Wold et al., 1990) or through other binding mechanisms to block adherence, entrap potential pathogens, and facilitate clearance. For example, we observed that monoclonal IgA antibodies specific for reovirus provided partial protection of mice against oral challenge with *Cryptosporidium parvum* (X. Y. Zhou, S. Tzipori, H. Ward, and M. R. Neutra, unpublished data).

Surface specializations of epithelial cells also provide mucosal protection against microorganisms. In the intestines, the apical plasma membranes of enterocytes are highly differentiated structures with closely packed microvilli (Madara et al., 1990) coated with a thick layer of membrane-associated mucins called the filamentous brush border glycocalyx (Maury et al., 1995). This coat serves as a diffusion barrier that prevents contact of most microorganisms with integral components of the enterocyte plasma membrane and impedes access to the small intermicrovillus membrane domains involved in endocytosis (Frey et al., 1996). These membrane-associated mucins are continually shed from the surfaces of enterocytes and mix with secreted goblet cell mucins in the lumen.

Epithelial "Alarm" System and Apoptosis

When microbial pathogens adhere to or invade the epithelial cells that line mucosal surfaces, the cells release proinflammatory cytokines and chemokines and upregulate chemokine receptors and adhesion molecules (Dwinell et al., 1999; Huang et al., 1996; Jung et al., 1995). These chemical alarms can lead to rapid influx of inflammatory cells as well as immune effector cells into the mucosa. In addition, epithelial cells can respond to microbial infection by apoptosis (Kim et al., 1998). Human colon epithelial cells grown in vitro as monolayers undergo apoptosis following infection with invasive enteric pathogens such as *Salmonella* or enteroinvasive *E. coli*. Induction of apoptosis requires bacterial internalization and replication. Tumor necrosis factor alpha and nitric oxide, which are produced as components of the intestinal epithelial-cell proinflammatory program in the early period after bacterial invasion (Rasmussen et al., 1997; Witthoft et al., 1998), play an important role in the later induction and regulation of the epithelial-cell apoptotic program. Onset of apoptosis in human colonic cell lines in vitro is delayed for several hours after bacterial infection. This would provide sufficient time for epithelial cells to generate proinflammatory signals, but it also may give invading bacteria enough time to activate genes that promote intracellular survival invasion of deeper mucosal cells (Kim et al., 1998). In vivo, apoptosis in response to bacterial infection may function to delete infected and damaged epithelial cells and stimulate epithelial-cell growth, thus maintaining epithelial integrity. Tumor necrosis factor alpha which is produced at sites of microbial invasion, induces apoptosis and detachment of the enterocytes at the tips of the villi, and this is preceded by an increase of caspase expression (Piguet et al., 1999).

Mucosal CTLs

The function of mucosal cytotoxic T lymphocytes (CTLs) in protection against infectious agents has been recently reviewed (Kelsall and Strober, 1999). Compelling evidence for a role of mucosal CTLs in protection against microbial pathogens was found in an experiment using immunodeficient mice, which showed that CD8$^+$ T cells are required for rapid clearance of primary rotavirus infection and for protection against reinfection (Franco et al., 1997). Protection was shown to be mediated by mucosal CTLs expressing mucosal homing receptors. Sorted CD8$^+$ T lymphocytes from rotavirus-infected mice were adoptively transferred into Rag-2 (T- and B-cell-deficient) recipients that were chronically infected with murine rotavirus. Memory $\alpha_4\beta_7^{high}$ CD8$^+$ cells were highly efficient at clearing rotavirus infection, while $\alpha_4\beta_7^-$ or CD44^{low} cells were inefficient or ineffective (Rose et al., 1998). To trigger mucosal CTLs, it is necessary to immunize by the mucosal route. Thus, immunization of monkeys with a particulate SIV vaccine by rectal and oral routes or by vaginal and oral routes or subcutaneous injection targeting the iliac lymph nodes elicited SIV-specific CTLs in the draining lymph nodes as well as in the genital or rectal mucosal tissues (Klavinskis et al., 1996). More recently, a single mucosal immunization with an attenuated vaccinia virus expressing HIV-1 gp160 elicited long-lasting, antigen-specific mucosal CTL responses in Peyer's patches and lamina propria as well as in the spleen (Belyakov et al., 1998).

IgG Antibodies

Although the presence of specific secretory IgA is generally considered to be the major factor in host defense at mucosal surfaces, it is likely that locally produced IgG antibodies also contribute to protection. In humans and nonhuman primates, secretions of the rectum and female genital tract contain significant amounts of IgG. Quantitative information about concentrations of specific antibodies and Ig isotypes in undiluted secretions associated with mucosal surfaces of humans has been obtained by using absorbent wicks or sponges to collect local secretions from the female rectum, endocervix, and vagina. This method revealed that local Ig concentrations are higher than previously appreciated: for example, an average of about 3 mg of IgA per ml was measured in secretions of the human rectal mucosa (Kozlowski et al., 1997). However, rectal IgG concentrations were also high, and in the female cervix both IgA and IgG were present in concentrations approaching 1 mg/ml.

The interstitial tissue of the mucosa may contain high concentrations of Igs (including IgG) produced by local plasma cells, and serum proteins that leak from fenestrated subepithelial capillaries (Choudari et al., 1993; Prigent-Delecourt et al., 1995). These could neutralize microorganisms that have gained entry into the mucosa or could enter secretions. IgG and albumin are generally said to enter normal secretions by "transudation," but the exact pathway involved is not clear. There is evidence for Fc gamma receptors in rectal epithelial cells (Hussain et al., 1991) and for the presence of neonatal Fc receptors on epithelial cells of the human intestine (Dickinson et al., 1999). However, there is no evidence that either IgG or albumin is selectively transported into adult intestinal secretions. Nonspecific mechanisms might be sufficient to allow IgG to cross the normal epithelial barrier; these could include fluid-phase transport in the vesicular transcytotic system that exports IgA, or leakage between epithelial cells. It is often assumed that this IgG is passively derived from serum, but a significant fraction of the B cells in the mucosa of human cervix and vagina are IgG$^+$ (Kutteh et al., 1988). Rectal or vaginal immunization results in local production of specific IgG in the mucosa of the rectum or the female genital tract. This is evidenced by the fact that after local vaginal immunization, the relative concentrations of Ig isotypes and IgG subclasses in cervical-vaginal fluids differ from those in serum (Hocini et al., 1995; Hordnes et al., 1996; Kozlowski et al., 1997).

Interaction of Secretory IgA Antibodies with M Cells

The FAE does not secrete polymeric IgA, since it does not express basolateral polymeric Ig receptors (Pappo and Owen, 1988). However, IgA that has been secreted into the lumen adheres selectively to the apical membranes of M cells in mice, rabbits, and humans (Neutra et al., 1999). The purpose of the IgA–M-cell interaction is unknown, but there is experimental evidence that IgA-mediated mucosal uptake of antigens can result in mucosal immune responses (Zhou et al., 1995). In addition, secretory IgA itself can serve as a mucosal vaccine carrier. Secretory component (SC), genetically engineered to contain a foreign epitope from the invasin of *Shigella flexneri*, was used to make SC-IgA complexes, which effectively delivered the epitope into mucosal lymphoid tissue and evoked anti-invasin immune responses (Corthésy et al., 1996). On the other hand, it is possible that IgA could have some other modulating effect on mucosal immune responses, and further work is needed to resolve the function of M-cell IgA-binding sites.

Acknowledgments. We are grateful to the current and former members of our laboratories who have contributed to the work summarized in this review. We are supported by NIH research grants HD17557 and AI34757, NIH AIDS Vaccine Development grant AI35365, and NIH Center grant DK34854 to the Harvard Digestive Diseases Center (to M.R.N.) and by Swiss National Science Foundation grant 31-56936-99 and Swiss League against Cancer grant SKL 635-2—1998 (to J.P.K.).

REFERENCES

Allan, C. H., D. L. Mendrick, and J. S. Trier. 1993. Rat intestinal epithelial M cells contain acidic endosomal-lysosomal compartments and express class II major histocompatibility complex determinants. *Gastroenterology* 104:698–708.

Allan, C. H., and J. S. Trier. 1991. Structure and permeability differ in subepithelial villus and Peyer's patch follicle capillaries. *Gastroenterology* 100:1172–1179.

Amerongen, H. M., R. A. Weltzin, C. M. Farnet, P. Michetti, W. A. Haseltine, and M. R. Neutra. 1991. Transepithelial transport of HIV-1 by intestinal M cells: a mechanism for transmission of AIDS. *J. Acquired Immune Defic. Syndr.* 4:760–765.

Amerongen, H. M., G. A. R. Wilson, B. N. Fields, and M. R. Neutra. 1994. Proteolytic processing of reovirus is required for adherence to intestinal M cells. *J. Virol.* 68:8428–8432.

Arstila, T., T. P. Arstila, S. Calbo, F. Selz, M. Malassis-Seris, P. Vassalli, P. Kourilsky, and D. Guy-Grand. 2000. Identical T cell clones are located within the mouse gut epithelium and lamina propria and circulate in the thoracic duct lymph. *J. Exp. Med.* 191:823–834.

Baggiolini, M. 1998. Chemokines and leukocyte traffic. *Nature* 392:565–568.

Bäumler, A. J., R. M. Tsolis, F. A. Bowe, J. G. Kusters, S. Hoffmann, and F. Heffron. 1996. The pef fimbrial operon of *Salmonella typhimurium* mediates adhesion to murine small intestine and is necessary for fluid accumulation in the infant mouse. *Infect. Immun.* 64:61–68.

Belyakov, I. M., B. Moss, W. Strober, and J. A. Berzofsky. 1999. Mucosal vaccination overcomes the barrier to recombinant vaccinia immunization caused by preexisting poxvirus immunity. *Proc. Natl. Acad. Sci. USA* 96:4512–4517.

Belyakov, I. M., L. S. Wyatt, J. D. Ahlers, P. Earl, C. D. Pendleton, B. L. Kelsall, W. Strober, B. Moss, and J. A. Berzofsky. 1998. Induction of a mucosal cytotoxic T-lymphocyte response by intrarectal immunization with a replication-deficient recombinant vaccinia virus expressing human immunodeficiency virus 89.6 envelope protein. *J. Virol.* 72:8264–8272.

Berstad, A. K. H., J. Holst, B. Møgster, I. L. Haugen, and B. Haneberg. 1997. A nasal whole-cell pertussis vaccine can induce strong systemic and mucosal antibody responses which are not enhanced by cholera toxin. *Vaccine* 15:1473.

Bienenstock, J., M. R. McDermott, and R. L. Clancy. 1999. Respiratory tract defenses: role of mucoal lymphoid tissues, p. 283–292. *In* R. Ogra, J. Mestecky, J. McGhee, J. Bienenstock, M. Lamm, and W. Strober (ed.), *Mucosal Immunology*. Academic Press, Inc., New York, N.Y.

Blumberg, R. S., W. I. Lencer, X. Zhu, H. S. Kim, S. Claypool, S. P. Balk, L. J. Saubermann, and S. P. Colgan. 1999. Antigen presentation by intestinal epithelial cells. *Immunol. Lett.* 69:7–11.

Boismenu, R., L. Feng, Y. Y. Xia, J. C. Chang, and W. L. Havran. 1996. Chemokine expression by intraepithelial gamma delta T cells. Implications for the recruitment of inflammatory cells to damaged epithelia. *J. Immunol.* 157:985–992.

Boismenu, R., and W. L. Havran. 1994. Modulation of epithelial cell growth by intraepithelial gamma delta T cells. *Science* 266:1253–1255.

Bomsel, M. 1997. Transcytosis of infectious human immunodeficiency virus across a tight human epithelial cell line barrier. *Nat. Med.* 3:42–47.

Borghesi, C., M. J. Taussig, and C. Nicoletti. 1999. Rapid appearance of M cells after microbial challenge is restricted at the periphery of the follicle-associated epithelium of Peyer's patch. *Lab. Investig.* 79:1393–1401.

Brandtzaeg, P., E. S. Baekkevold, I. N. Farstad, F. L. Jahnsen, F. E. Johansen, E. M. Nilsen, and T. Yamanaka. 1999a. Regional specialization in the mucosal immune system: what happens in the microcompartments? *Immunol. Today* 20:141–151.

Brandtzaeg, P., and I. N. Farstad. 1999. The human mucosal B cell system, p. 439–468. *In* R. Ogra, J. Mestecky, J. McGhee, J. Bienenstock, M. Lamm, and W. Strober (ed.), *Mucosal Immunology*. Academic Press, Inc., New York, N.Y.

Brandtzaeg, P., I. N. Farstad, and G. Haraldsen. 1999b. Regional specialization in the mucosal immune system: primed cells do not always home along the same track. *Immunol. Today* 20:267–277.

Briskin, M., D. Winsorhines, A. Shyjan, N. Cochran, S. Bloom, J. Wilson, L. M. McEvoy, E. C. Butcher, N. Kassam, C. R. Mackay, W. Newman, and D. J. Ringler. 1997. Human mucosal addressin cell adhesion molecule-1 is preferentially expressed in intestinal tract and associated lymphoid tissue. *Am. J. Pathol.* 151:97–110.

Bromander, A. K., L. Ekman, M. Kopf, J. G. Nedrud, and N. Y. Lycke. 1996. IL-6-deficient mice exhibit normal mucosal IgA responses to local immunizations and *Helicobacter felis* infection. *J. Immunol.* 156:4290–4297.

Butcher, E. C., and L. J. Picker. 1996. Lymphocyte homing and homeostasis. *Science* 272:60–66.

Bye, W. A., C. H. Allan, and J. S. Trier. 1984. Structure, distribution and origin of M cells in Peyer's patches of mouse ileum. *Gastroenterology* 86:789–801.

Campbell, N., X. Y. Yio, L. P. So, Y. Li, and L. Mayer. 1999. The intestinal epithelial cell: processing and presentation of antigen to the mucosal immune system. *Immunol. Rev.* **172**:315–324.

Chen, Y. H., J. Inobe, R. Marks, P. Gonnella, V. K. Kuchroo, and H. L. Weiner. 1995. Peripheral deletion of antigen-reactive t cells in oral tolerance. *Nature* **376**:177–180.

Choudari, C. P., S. O'Mahony, G. Brydon, O. Mwantembe, and A. Ferguson. 1993. Gut lavage fluid protein concentrations: objective measures of disease activity in inflammatory bowel disease. *Gastroenterology* **104**:1064–1071.

Cone, R. A. 1999. Mucus, p. 43–64. *In* R. Ogra, J. Mestecky, J. McGhee, J. Bienenstock, M. Lamm, and W. Strober (ed.) *Mucosal Immunology*. Academic Press, Inc., New York, N.Y.

Corthésy, B., M. Kaufmann, A. Phalipon, M. C. Peitsch, M. R. Neutra, and J.-P. Kraehenbuhl. 1996. A pathogen-specific epitope inserted into recombinant secretory immunoglobulin A is immunogenic by the oral route. *J. Biol. Chem.* **271**:33670–33677.

Cui, Z.-D., D. Tristram, L. J. LaScolea, T. J. Kwiatkovski, S. Kopti, and P. L. Ogra. 1991. Induction of antibody response to *Chlamydia trachomatis* in the genital tract by oral immunization. *Infect. Immun.* **59**:1465–1469.

Czerkinsky, C., J. B. Sun, and J. Holmgren. 1999. Oral tolerance and anti-pathological vaccines. *Curr. Top. Microbiol. Immunol.* **236**:79–92.

Desvignes, C., F. Esteves, N. Etchart, C. Bella, C. Czerkinsky, and D. Kaiserlian. 1998. The murine buccal mucosa is an inductive site for priming class I restricted CD8(+) effector T cells in vivo. *Clin. Exp. Immunol.* **113**:386–393.

Dickinson, B. L., K. Badizadegan, Z. Wu, J. C. Ahouse, X. P. Zhu, N. E. Simister, R. S. Blumberg, and W. I. Lencer. 1999. Bidirectional FcRn-dependent IgG transport in a polarized human intestinal epithelial cell line. *J. Clin. Investig.* **104**:903–911.

Dunn-Walters, D. K., M. Hackett, L. Boursier, P. J. Ciclitira, P. Morgan, S. J. Challacombe, and J. Spencer. 2000. Characteristics of human IgA and IgM genes used by plasma cells in the salivary gland resemble those used in duodenum but not those used in the spleen. *J. Immunol.* **164**:1595–1601.

Dwinell, M. B., L. Eckmann, J. D. Leopard, N. M. Varki, and M. F. Kagnoff. 1999. Chemokine receptor expression by human intestinal epithelial cells. *Gastroenterology* **117**:359–367.

Ermak, T. H., and R. L. Owen. 1994. Differential distribution of lymphocytes and accessory cells in mouse Peyer's patches. *Am. J. Trop. Med. Hyg.* **50**:S14–S28.

Eynon, E. E., and D. C. Parker. 1993. Parameters of tolerance induction by antigen targeted to B lymphocytes. *J. Immunol.* **151**:2958–2964.

Farstad, I. N., T. S. Halstensen, O. Fausa, and P. Brandtzaeg. 1994. Heterogeneity of M-cell-associated B and T cells in human Peyer's patches. *Immunology* **83**:457–464.

Farstad, I. N., J. Norstein, and P. Brandtzaeg. 1997. Phenotypes of B and T cells in human intestinal and mesenteric lymph. *Gastroenterology* **112**:163–173.

Finlay, B. B., and P. Cossart. 1997. Exploitation of mammalian host cell functions by bacterial pathogens. *Science* **276**:718–725.

Finzi, G., M. Cornaggia, C. Capella, R. Fiocca, F. Bosi, E. Solcia, and I. M. Samloff. 1993. Cathepsin E in follicle associated epithelium of intestine and tonsils: localization to M cells and possible role in antigen processing. *Histochemistry* **99**:201–211.

Förster, R., A. E. Mattis, E. Kremmer, E. Wolf, G. Brem, and M. Lipp. 1996. A putative chemokine receptor, BLR1, directs B cell migration to defined lymphoid organs and specific anatamic compartments of the spleen. *Cell* **87**:1037–1047.

Forstner, J. F., M. G. Oliver, and F. A. Sylvester. 1995. Production, structure, and biological relevance of gastrointestinal mucins, p. 71–88. *In* M. Blaser, P. D. Smith, J. I. Ravdin, H. B. Greenberg, and R. L. Guerrant (ed.), *Infections of the Gastrointestinal Tract*. Raven Press, New York, N.Y.

Franco, M. A., C. Tin, and H. B. Greenberg. 1997. CD8[+] T cells can mediate almost complete short-term and partial long-term immunity to rotavirus in mice. *J. Virol.* **71**:4165–4170.

Frey, A., K. T. Giannasca, R. Weltzin, P. J. Giannasca, H. Reggio, W. I. Lencer, and M. R. Neutra. 1996. Role of the glycocalyx in regulating access of microparticles to apical plasma membranes of intestinal epithelial cells—implications for microbial attachment and oral vaccine targeting. *J. Exp. Med.* **184**:1045–1059.

Fuchs, E. J., and P. Matzinger. 1992. B cells turn off virgin but not memory T cells. *Science* **258**:1156–1159.

Gebert, A., S. Fassbender, K. Werner, and A. Weissferdt. 1999. The development of M cells in Peyer's patches is restricted to specialized dome-associated crypts. *Am. J. Pathol.* **154**:1573–1582.

Geijtenbeek, T. B. H., D. S. Kwon, R. Torensma, S. J. van Vliet, G. C. F. van Duijnhoven, J. Middel, I. Cornelissen, H. Nottet, V. N. KewalRamani, D. R. Littman, C. G. Figdor, and Y. van Kooyk. 2000. DC-SIGN, a dendritic cell-specific HIV-1-binding protein that enhances trans-infection of T cells. *Cell* **100**:587–597.

Giannasca, K. T., P. J. Giannasca, and M. R. Neutra. 1996. Adherence of *Salmonella typhimurium* to Caco-2 cells: identification of a glycoconjugate receptor. *Infect. Immun.* **64**:135–145.

Giannasca, P. J., K. T. Giannasca, P. Falk, J. I. Gordon, and M. R. Neutra. 1994. Regional differences in glycoconjugates of intestinal M cells in mice: potential targets for mucosal vaccines. *Am. J. Physiol.* **267**:G1108–G1121.

Gordon, J. I., and M. L. Hermiston. 1994. Differentiation and self-renewal in the mouse gastrointestinal epithelium. *Curr. Opin. Cell Biol.* **6**:795–803.

Gunn, M. D., V. N. Ngo, K. M. Ansel, E. H. Ekland, J. G. Cyster, and L. T. Williams. 1998. A B-cell-homing chemokine made in lymphoid follicles activates Burkitts-lymphoma receptor-1. *Nature* **391**:799–803.

Haneberg, B., D. Kendall, H. M. Amerongen, F. M. Apter, J. P. Kraehenbuhl, and M. R. Neutra. 1994. Induction of specific immunoglobulin A in the small intestine, colon-rectum, and vagina measured by a new method for collection of secretions from local mucosal surfaces. *Infect. Immun.* **62**:15–23.

Hein, W. R. 1999. Organization of mucosal lymphoid tissue. *Curr. Top. Microbiol. Immunol.* **236**:1–15.

Hocini, H., A. Barra, L. Bélec, S. Iscaki, J.-L. Preud'homme, J. Pillot, and J.-P. Bouvet. 1995. Systemic and secretory humoral immunity in the normal human vaginal tract. *Scand. J. Immunol.* **42**:269–274.

Holmgren, J., C. Czerkinsky, N. Lycke, and A. M. Svennerholm. 1992. Mucosal immunity: implications for vaccine development. *Immunobiology* **184**:157–179.

Holt, P. G. 1994. Immunoprophylaxis of atopy: light at the end of the tunnel? *Immunol. Today* **15**:484–489.

Holt, P. G., S. Haining, D. J. Nelson, and J. D. Sedgwick. 1994. Origin and steady-state turnover of class II MHC-bearing dendritic cells in the epithelium of the conducting airways. *J. Immunol.* **153**:256–261.

Hopkins, S., J. P. Kraehenbuhl, F. Schödel, A. Potts, D. Peterson, P. De Grandi, and D. Nardelli-Haefliger. 1995. A recombinant *Salmonella typhimurium* vaccine induces local immunity by four different routes of immunization. *Infect. Immun.* **63**:3279–3286.

Hopkins, S., F. Niedergang, I. E. Corthésy-Theulaz, and J. P. Kraehenbuhl. 2000. A recombinant *Salmonella typhimurium* vaccine strain is taken up and survives within murine Peyer's patch dendritic cells. *Cell. Microbiol.* 2:56–68.

Hordnes, K., T. Tynning, T. A. Brown, B. Haneberg, and R. Jonsson. 1997. Nasal immunization with group B streptococci can induce high levels of specific IgA antibodies in cervicovaginal secretions in mice. *Vaccine* 15:1244–1251.

Hordnes, K., T. Tynning, A. I. Kvam, R. Jonsson, and B. Haneberg. 1996. Colonization in the rectum and uterine cervix with group B streptococci may induce specific antibody responses in cervical secretions of pregnant women. *Infect. Immun.* 64:1643–1652.

Hoyne, G. F., I. Le Roux, M. Corsin-Jimenez, K. Tan, J. Dunne, L. M. G. Forsyth, M. J. Dallman, M. J. Owen, D. Ish-Horowicz, and J. R. Lamb. 2000. Serrate 1-induced Notch signalling regulates the decision between immunity and tolerance made by peripheral CD4(+) T cells. *Int. Immunol.* 12:177–185.

Huang, F. P., N. Platt, M. Wykes, J. R. Major, T. J. Powell, C. D. Jenkins, and G. G. MacPherson. 2000. A discrete subpopulation of dendritic cells transports apoptotic intestinal epithelial cells to T cell areas of mesenteric lymph nodes. *J. Exp. Med.* 191:435–443.

Huang, G. T. J., L. Eckmann, T. C. Savidge, and M. F. Kagnoff. 1996. Infection of human intestinal epithelial cells with invasive bacteria upregulates apical intercellular adhesion molecule-1 (ICAM-1) expression and neutrophil adhesion. *J. Clin. Invest.* 98:572–583.

Hussain, L. A., C. G. Kelly, E. M. Hecht, R. Fellowes, M. Jourdan, and T. Lehner. 1991. The expression of Fc receptors for immunoglobulin G in human rectal epithelium. *AIDS* 5:1089–1094.

Iwasaki, A., and B. L. Kelsall. 2000. Localization of distinct Peyer's patch dendritic cell subsets and their recruitment by chemokines macrophage inflammatory protein (MIP)-3a, MIP3b, and secondary lymphoid organ chemokine. *J. Exp. Med.* 191:1381–1393.

Izadpanah, A., M. B. Dwinell, L. Eckmann, N. M. Varki, and M. F. Kagnoff. 2001. Regulated MIP-3/CCL20 production by human intestinal epithelium: mechanism for modulating mucosal immunity. *Am. J. Physiol.* 280:G710–G719.

Jones, B. D., N. Ghori, and S. Falkow. 1994. *Salmonella typhimurium* initiates murine infection by penetrating and destroying the specialized epithelial M cells of the Peyer's patches. *J. Exp. Med.* 180:15–23.

Jung, H. C., L. Eckmann, S. K. Yang, A. Panja, J. Fierer, E. Morzycka-Wroblewska, and M. F. Kagnoff. 1995. A distinct array of proinflammatory cytokines is expressed in human colon epithelial cells in response to bacterial invasion. *J. Clin. Investig.* 95:55–65.

Kaiserlian, D. 1999. Antigen sampling and presentation in mucosal tissues: epithelial cells. *Curr. Top. Microbiol. Immunol.* 236:55–78.

Kanamori, Y., K. Ishimaru, M. Nanno, K. Maki, K. Ikuta, and H. Nariuchi. 1996. Identification of novel lymphoid tissues in murine intestinal mucosa where clusters of c-kit$^+$ IL-7R$^+$ Thy1$^+$ lympho-hematopoietic progenitors develop. *J. Exp. Med.* 184:1449–1459.

Kato, T., and R. L. Owen. 1999. Structure and function of intestinal mucosal epithelium, p. 115–132. *In* R. Ogra, J. Mestecky, J. McGhee, J. Bienenstock, M. Lamm, and W. Strober (ed.), *Mucosal Immunology.* Academic Press, Inc., New York, N.Y.

Kelsall, B., and W. Strober. 1999. Gut-associated lymphois tissue: antigen handling and T cell responses, p. 293–318. *In* R. Ogra, J. Mestecky, J. McGhee, J. Bienenstock, M. Lamm, and W. Strober (ed.), *Mucosal Immunology,* Academic Press, Inc., New York, N.Y.

Kernéis, S., A. Bogdanova, J. P. Kraehenbuhl, and E. Pringault. 1997. Conversion by Peyer's patch lymphocytes of human enterocytes into M cells that transport bacteria. *Science* 277:948–952.

Khoury, S. J., W. W. Hancock, and H. L. Weiner. 1992. Oral tolerance to myelin basic protein and natural recovery from experimental autoimmune encephalomyelitis are associated with downregulation of inflammatory cytokines and differential upregulation of TGF-β, IL-4 and PGE expression in the brain. *J. Exp. Med.* 176:1355–1364.

Khoury, S. J., O. Lider, A. Al-Sabbagh, and H. L. Weiner. 1990. Suppression of experimental autoimmune encephalomyelitis by oral administration of myelin basic protein. III. Synergistic effect of lipopolysaccharide. *Cell. Immunol.* 131:302–310.

Kim, J. M., L. Eckmann, T. C. Savidge, D. C. Lowe, T. Witthoft, and M. F. Kagnoff. 1998. Apoptosis of human intestinal epithelial cells after bacterial invasion. *J. Clin. Investig.* 102:1815–1823.

Klavinskis, L. S., L. A. Bergmeier, L. Gao, E. Mitchell, R. G. Ward, G. Layton, R. Brookes, N. J. Meyers, and T. Lehner. 1996. Mucosal or targeted lymph node immunization of macaques with a particulate SIVp27 protein elicits virus-specific CTL in the genito-rectal mucosa and draining lymph nodes. *J. Immunol.* 157:2521–2527.

Kozlowski, P. A., S. Cu-Uvin, M. R. Neutra, and T. P. Flanigan. 1997. Comparison of the oral, rectal, and vaginal immunization routes for induction of antibodies in rectal and genital tract secretions of women. *Infect. Immun.* 65:1387–1394.

Kraehenbuhl, J. P., and M. R. Neutra. 1992. Molecular and cellular basis of immune protection of mucosal surfaces. *Physiol. Rev.* 72:853–879.

Kutteh, W. H., K. D. Hatch, R. E. Blackwell, and J. Mestecky. 1988. Secretory immune system of the female reproductive tract. I. Immuoglobulin and secretory component-containing cells. *Obstet. Gynecol.* 71:56–60.

Lefrancois, L., and L. Puddington. 1998. Anatomy of T-cell development in the intestine. *Gastroenterology* 115:1588–1591.

Legler, D. F., M. Loetscher, R. Stuber Roos, I. Clark-Lewis, M. Baggiolini, and B. Moser. 1998. B cell-attracting chemokine 1, a human CXC chemokine expressed in lymphoid tissues, selectively attracts B lymphocytes via BRL1/CxCR5. *J. Exp. Med.* 187:665–660.

Lehner, T., R. Brookes, C. Panagiotidi, L. Tao, L. S. Klavinskis, J. Walker, P. Walker, R. Ward, L. Hussain, A. J. H. Gearing, S. E. Adams, and L. A. Bergmeier. 1993. T- and B-cell functions and epitope expression in nonhuman primates immunized with simian immunodeficiency virus antigen by the rectal route. *Proc. Natl. Acad. Sci. USA* 90:8638–8642.

Lehner, T., C. Panagiotidi, L. A. Bergmeier, T. Ping, R. Brookes, and S. E. Adams. 1992. A comparison of the immune response following oral, vaginal, or rectal route of immunization with SIV antigens in nonhuman primates. *Vaccine Res.* 1:319–330.

Lehrer, R. I., C. L. Bevins, and T. Ganz. 1999. Defensins and other antimicrobial peptides, p. 89–100. *In* R. Ogra, J. Mestecky, J. McGhee, J. Bienenstock, M. Lamm, and W. Strober (ed.), *Mucosal Immunology.* Academic Press, Inc., New York, N.Y.

MacDonald, T. T. 1999. Effector and regulatory lymphoid cells and cytokines in mucosal sites. *Curr. Top. Microbiol. Immunol.* 236:113–135.

MacLennan, I. C., Y. J. Liu, and G. D. Johnson. 1992. Maturation and dispersal of B-cell clones during T cell-dependent antibody responses. *Immunol. Rev.* 126:143–161.

Macpherson, A. J., D. Gatto, E. Sainsbury, G. R. Harriman, H. Hengartner, and R. M. Zinkernagel. 2000. A primitive T cell-dependent mechanism of intestinal mucosal IgA responses to commensal bacteria. *Science* 288:2222–2226.

MacPherson, G. G., and L. M. Liu. 1999. Dendritic cells and Langerhans cells in the uptake of mucosal antigens. *Curr. Top. Microbiol. Immunol.* 256:33–54.

Madara, J. L., S. Nash, R. Moore, and K. Atisook. 1990. Structure and function of the intestinal epithelial barrier in health and disease. *Monogr. Pathol.* 31:306–324.

Mantis, N. J., A. Frey, and M. R. Neutra. 2000. Accessibility of glycolipid and oligosaccharide epitopes on apical surfaces of rabbit villus and follicle-associated epithelium. *Am. J. Physiol.* 278: G915–G929.

Manz, R. A., A. Thiel, and A. Radbruch. 1997. Lifetime of plasma cells in the bone marrow. *Nature* 388:133–134.

Maury, J., C. Nicoletti, L. Guzzo-Chambraud, and S. Maroux. 1995. The filamentous brush border glycocalyx, a mucin-like marker of enterocyte hyper-polarization. *Eur. J. Biochem.* 228: 323–331.

Mayer, L. 2000. Oral tolerance: new approaches, new problems. *Clin. Immunol.* 94:1–8.

Mazzucchelli, L., A. Blaser, A. Kappeler, P. Scharli, J. A. Laissue, M. Baggiolini, and M. Uguccioni. 1999. BCA-1 is highly expressed in *Helicobacter pylori*-induced mucosa-associated lymphoid tissue and gastric lymphoma. *J. Clin. Investig.* 104:R49– R54.

McDermott, M. R., L. J. Brais, and M. J. Evelegh. 1990. Mucosal and systemic antiviral antibodies in mice inoculated intravaginally with herpes simplex virus type 2. *J. Gen. Virol.* 71:1497– 1504.

McGhee, J. R., M. E. Lamm, and W. Strober. 1999. Mucosal immune responses, p. 485–506. *In* R. Ogra, J. Mestecky, J. McGhee, J. Bienenstock, M. Lamm, and W. Strober (ed.), *Mucosal Immunology*, 2nd ed. Academic Press, Inc., New York, N.Y.

McGhee, J. R., J. Mestecky, M. T. Dertzbaugh, J. H. Eldridge, M. Hirasawa, and H. Kiyono. 1992. The mucosal immune system: from fundamental concepts to vaccine development. *Vaccine* 10: 75–88.

McHeyzer-Williams, L. J., M. Cool, and M. G. McHeyzer-Williams. 2000. Antigen-specific B cell memory: expression and replenishment of a novel B220(-) memory B cell compartment. *J. Exp. Med.* 191:1149–1165.

Miller, C. J. 1994. Mucosal transmission of SIV. *Curr. Top. Microbiol. Immunol.* 188:107–122.

Miller, C. J., M. McChesney, and P. F. Moore. 1992. Langerhans cells, macrophages and lymphocyte subsets in the cervix and vagina of rhesus macaques. *Lab. Investig.* 67:628–634.

Mowat, A. M., and H. L. Weiner. 1999. Oral tolerance: physiological basis and clinical applications, p. 587–618. *In* R. Ogra, J. Mestecky, J. McGhee, J. Bienenstock, M. Lamm, and W. Strober (ed.), *Mucosal Immunology*, 2nd ed. Academic Press, Inc., New York, N.Y.

Nelson, D. J., C. McMenamin, A. S. McWilliam, M. Brenan, and P. G. Holt. 1994. Development of the airway intraepithelial dendritic cell network in the rat from class II major histocompatibility (Ia)-negative precursors: differential regulation of Ia expression at different levels of the respiratory tract. *J. Exp. Med.* 179:203–212.

Neutra, M. R. 1998. HIV transmission and immune protection at mucosal surfaces. *Adv. Exp. Med. Biol.* 452:169–176.

Neutra, M. R., P. J. Giannasca, K. T. Giannasca, and J. P. Kraehenbuhl. 1995. M cells and microbial pathogens, p. 163–178. *In* M. J. Blaser, P. D. Smith, J. I. Ravdin, H. B. Greenberg, and L. Guerrant (ed.), *Infections of the Gastrointestinal Tract*. Raven Press, New York, N.Y.

Neutra, M. R., N. J. Mantis, A. Frey, and P. J. Giannasca. 1999. The composition and function of M cell apical membranes: implications for microbial pathogenesis. *Semin. Immunol.* 11:171– 181.

Neutra, M. R., E. Pringault, and J. P. Kraehenbuhl. 1996. Antigen sampling across epithelial barriers and induction of mucosal immune responses. *Annu. Rev. Immunol.* 14:275–300.

Nibert, M. L., D. B. Furlong, and B. N. Fields. 1991. Mechanisms of viral pathogenesis. Distinct forms of reoviruses and their roles during replication in cells and host. *J. Clin. Investig.* 88:727– 734.

Ogra, P. L., and D. T. Karzon. 1969. Distribution of poliovirus antibody in serum, nasopharynx and alimentary tract following segmental immunization of lower alimentary tract with poliovaccine. *J. Immunol.* 102:1423–1430.

Okato, S., S. Magari, Y. Yamamoto, M. Sakanaka, and H. Takahashi. 1989. An immunoelectron microscopic study on interactions among dendritic cells, macrophages and lymphocytes in the human palatine tonsil. *Arch. Histol. Cytol.* 52:231–240.

O'Leary, A. D., and E. C. Sweeney. 1986. Lymphoglandular complexes of the colon: structure and distribution. *Histopathology* 10:267–283.

Pabst, R., and I. Gehrke. 1990. Is the bronchus-associated lymphoid tissue (BALT) an integral structure of the lung in normal mammals, including humans? *Am. J. Respir. Cell Mol. Biol.* 3: 132–135.

Pappo, J., and R. L. Owen. 1988. Absence of secretory component expression by epithelial cells overlying rabbit gut-associated lymphoid tissue. *Gastroenterology* 95:1173–1177.

Parr, M. B., and E. L. Parr. 1994. Mucosal immunity in the female and male reproductive tracts, p. 677–690. *In* P. L. Ogra, J. Mestecky, M. E. Lamm, W. Strober, J. R. McGhee, and J. Bienenstock (ed.), *Handbook of Mucosal Immunology*. Academic Press, Inc., New York, N.Y.

Parr, M. B., and E. L. Parr. 1997. Protective immunity against HSV-2 in the mouse vagina. *J. Reprod. Immunol.* 36:77.

Pavli, P., C. E. Woodhams, W. F. Doe, and D. A. Hume. 1990. Isolation and characterization of antigen-presenting dendritic cells from the mouse intestinal lamina propria. *Immunology* 70: 40–47.

Perry, M., and A. White. 1998. Immunology of the tonsils. *Immunol. Today* 19:414–421.

Phalipon, A., and P. J. Sansonetti. 1999. Microbial-host interactions at mucosal sites. Host response to pathogenic bacteria at mucosal sites. *Curr. Top. Microbiol. Immunol.* 236:163–190.

Phillips, D. M., and A. S. Bourinbaiar. 1992. Mechanism of HIV spread from lymphocytes to epithelia. *Virology* 186:261–273.

Pierce, N. F., and W. C. Cray, Jr. 1982. Determinants of the localization, magnitude, and duration of a specific mucosal IgA plasma cell response in enterically immunized rats. *J. Immunol.* 128:1311–1315.

Piguet, P. F., C. Vesin, Y. Donati, and C. Barazzone. 1999. TNF-induced enterocyte apoptosis and detachment in mice: induction of caspases and prevention by a caspase inhibitor, ZVAD-fmk. *Lab. Investig.* 79:495–500.

Prigent-Delecourt, L., B. Coffin, J. F. Colombel, J. P. Dehennin, J. P. Vaerman, and J. C. Rambaud. 1995. Secretion of immunoglobulins and plasma proteins from the colonic mucosa: an in vivo study in man. *Clin. Exp. Immunol.* 99:221–225.

Quiding, M., I. Nordström, A. Kilander, G. Andersson, L. A. Hanson, J. Holmgren, and C. Czerkinsky. 1991. Intestinal immune responses in humans. Oral cholera vaccination induces strong intestinal antibody responses, gamma-interferon production, and evokes local immunological memory. *J. Clin. Investig.* 88:143–148.

Ramsay, A. J., A. J. Husband, I. A. Ramshaw, S. Bao, K. I. Matthaei, G. Koehler, and M. Kopf. 1994. The role of interleukin-6 in mucosal IgA antibody responses in vivo. *Science* 264:561–563.

Rasmussen, S. J., L. Eckmann, A. J. Quayle, L. Shen, Y. X. Zhang, D. J. Anderson, J. Fierer, R. S. Stephens, and M. F. Kagnoff. 1997. Secretion of proinflammatory cytokines by epithelial cells in response to chlamydia infection suggests a central role for epithelial cells in chlamydial pathogenesis. *J. Clin. Investig.* 99:77–87.

Reynaud, C. A., C. Garcia, W. R. Hein, and J. C. Weill. 1995. Hypermutation generating the sheep immunoglobulin repertoire is an antigen-independent process. *Cell* 80:115–125.

Rose, J. R., M. B. Williams, L. S. Rott, E. C. Butcher, and H. B. Greenberg. 1998. Expression of the mucosal homing receptor alpha4beta7 correlates with the ability of CD8[+] memory T cells to clear rotavirus infection. *J. Virol.* 72:726–730.

Rudin, A., E. L. Johansson, C. Bergquist, and J. Holmgren. 1998. Differential kinetics and distribution of antibodies in serum and nasal and vaginal secretions after nasal and oral vaccination of humans. *Infect. Immun.* 66:3390–3396.

Russell, M. W., Z. Moldoveanu, P. L. White, G. J. Sibert, J. Mestecky, and S. M. Michalek. 1996. Salivary, nasal, genital, and systemic antibody responses in monkeys immunized intranasally with a bacterial protein antigen and the cholera toxin B subunit. *Infect. Immun.* 64:1272–1283.

Saito, H., Y. Kanamori, T. Takemori, H. Nariuchi, E. Kubota, H. Takahashi-Iwanaga, T. Iwanaga, and H. Ishikawa. 1998. Generation of intestinal T cells from progenitors residing in gut cryptopatches. *Science* 280:275–278.

Savidge, T. C., M. W. Smith, P. S. James, and P. Aldred. 1991. Salmonella-induced M-cell formation in germ-free mouse Peyer's patch tissue. *Am. J. Pathol.* 139:177–184.

Shaw, S. K., A. Hermanowski-Vosatka, T. Shibahara, B. A. McCormick, C. A. Parkos, S. L. Carlson, E. C. Ebert, M. B. Brenner, and J. L. Madara. 1998. Migration of intestinal intraepithelial lymphocytes into a polarized epithelial monolayer. *Am. J. Physiol.* 38:G584–G591.

Sicinski, P., J. Rowinski, J. B. Warchol, Z. Jarczabek, W. Gut, B. Szczygiel, K. Bielecki, and G. Koch. 1990. Poliovirus type 1 enters the human host through intestinal M cells. *Gastroenterology* 98:56–58.

Siebers, A., and B. B. Finlay. 1996. M cells and the pathogenesis of mucosal and systemic infections. *Trends Microbiol.* 4:22–29.

Sierro, F., E. Pringault, P. Simon Assman, J. P. Kraehenbuhl, and N. Debard. 2000. Transient expression of M-cell phenotype by enterocyte-like cells of the follicle-associated epithelium of mouse Peyer's patches. *Gastroenterology* 119:734–743.

Sirard, J. C., F. Niedergang, and J. P. Kraehenbuhl. 1999. Live attenuated *Salmonella:* a paradigm of mucosal vaccines. *Immunol. Rev.* 171:5–26.

Slifka, M. K., R. Antia, J. K. Whitmire, and R. Ahmed. 1998. Humoral immunity due to long-lived plasma cells. *Immunity* 8:363–372.

Sminia, T., and G. Kraal. 1999. Nasal-associated lymphoid tissue, p. 357–364. *In* R. Ogra, J. Mestecky, J. McGhee, J. Bienen-stock, M. Lamm, and W. Strober (ed.), *Mucosal Immunology,* 2nd ed. Academic Press, Inc., New York, N.Y.

Spira, A. I., P. A. Marx, B. K. Patterson, J. Mahoney, R. A. Koup, S. M. Wolinsky, and D. D. Ho. 1996. Cellular targets of infection and route of viral dissemination after an intravaginal inoculation of simian immunodeficiency virus into rhesus macaques. *J. Exp. Med.* 183:215–225.

Steinman, R. M. 2000. DC-SIGN: a guide to some mysteries of dendritic cells. *Cell* 100:491–494.

Steinman, R. M., S. Turley, I. Mellman, and K. Inaba. 2000. The induction of tolerance by dendritic cells that have captured apoptotic cells. *J. Exp. Med.* 191:411–416.

Szabo, M. C., E. C. Butcher, and L. M. McEvoy. 1997. Specialization of mucosal follicular dendritic cells revealed by mucosal adressin-cell adhesion molecule-1 display. *J. Immunol.* 158:5584–5588.

Vajdy, M., and N. Y. Lycke. 1992. Cholera toxin adjuvant promotes long-term immunological memory in the gut mucosa to unrelated immunogens after oral immunization. *Immunology* 75:488–492.

Van Klinken, B. N., J. Dekker, H. A. Buller, and A. W. Einerhand. 1995. Mucin gene structure and expression: protection vs. adhesion. *Am. J. Physiol.* 269:G613–G627.

Velin, D., G. Fotopoulos, J. P. Kraehenbuhl, and H. Acha Orbea. 1999. Systemic antibodies can inhibit MMTV driven superantigen response in mucosal associated lymphoid tissues. *J. Virol.* 73:1729–1733.

Wassen, L., K. Schon, J. Holmgren, M. Jertborn, and N. Lycke. 1996. Local intravaginal vaccination of the female genital tract. *Scand. J. Immunol.* 44:408–414.

Whitacre, C., C. Gienapp, I. E. Orosz, and D. Bitar. 1991. Oral tolerance in experimental autoimmune encephalomyelitis. III. Evidence for clonal anergy. *J. Immunol.* 147:2155–2163.

Williams, M. B., J. R. Rose, L. S. Rott, M. A. Franco, H. B. Greenberg, and E. C. Butcher. 1998. The memory B cell subset responsible for the secretory IgA response and protective humoral immunity to rotavirus expresses the intestinal homing receptor, alpha(4)beta(7). *J. Immunol.* 161:4227–4235.

Witthoft, T., L. Eckmann, J. M. Kim, and M. F. Kagnoff. 1998. Enteroinvasive bacteria directly activate expression of iNOS and NO production in human colon epithelial cells. *Am. J. Physiol.* 275:G564–G571.

Wold, A. E., J. Mestecky, M. Tomana, A. Kobata, H. Ohbayashi, T. Endo, and C. Svanborg-Eden. 1990. Secretory immunoglobulin A carries oligosaccharide receptors for *Escherichia coli* type 1 fimbrial lectin. *Infect. Immun.* 58:3073–3077.

Wolf, J. L., D. H. Rubin, R. Finberg, R. S. Kauffman, A. H. Sharpe, J. S. Trier, and B. N. Fields. 1981. Intestinal M cells: a pathway for entry of reovirus into the host. *Science* 212:471–472.

Yahi, N., S. Baghdiguian, C. Bolmont, and J. Fantini. 1992. Inhibition of human immunodeficiency virus infection in human colon epithelial cells by recombinant interferon-gamma. *Eur. J. Immunol.* 22:2495–2499.

Zhou, F., J.-P. Kraehenbuhl, and M. R. Neutra. 1995. Mucosal IgA response to rectally administered antigen formulated in IgA-coated liposomes. *Vaccine* 13:637–644.

Immunology of Infectious Diseases
Edited by S. H. E. Kaufmann, A. Sher, and R. Ahmed
© 2002 ASM Press, Washington, D.C.

Chapter 15

Acquired Immunity against Bacteria

HELEN L. COLLINS AND STEFAN H. E. KAUFMANN

The adaptive immune response, in contrast to innate mechanisms discussed in previous chapters, requires the specific recognition of foreign antigens (Ag). However, components of the innate immune system have a profound influence on the type of acquired immune mechanisms generated, and, reciprocally, the specific immune response executes several of its effector functions via the activation of elements of innate immunity. Principally, the specific response can be divided into cell-mediated mechanisms which focus mainly on T-cell activation and effector mechanisms, and the humoral response, consisting of B-cell maturation and antibody (Ab) production. Of course, these divergent arms of the host response to pathogens are not mutually exclusive, and T-cell help is required for Ab maturation and isotype switching, while B cells can function as Ag-presenting cells (APC) in the induction of specific T cells. This chapter will focus on the generation and maintenance of the acquired immune response against bacterial pathogens and the pathological effects that may occur if this response is left uncontrolled or actively disregulated. First we outline the general mechanisms of acquired immunity, and then, using specific examples, we discuss how various bacterial pathogens induce and modulate this response.

GENERATION AND EFFECTOR FUNCTIONS OF THE ACQUIRED IMMUNE RESPONSE

Cell-Mediated Immune Responses

The specific T-cell response to bacterial antigens can be broadly divided into two distinct stages: (i) induction (Ag recognition and T-cell activation) and (ii) effector functions (cytokine production and cytolytic activity). Induction occurs mostly within the

peripheral lymphoid organs, primarily the lymph nodes and spleen, where circulating naive T cells from the blood are brought into contact with Ag. Lymphocytes communicate with high endothelial venules via receptor-ligand interactions, which induce lymphocyte transmigration. These adhesion molecules include selectins, integrins, and members of the immunoglobulin (Ig) superfamily. Following stimulation with specific Ag in the lymphoid organs, T cells undergo substantial proliferation and a subsequent increase in the expression of these molecules. During T-cell differentiation, the affinity of the accessory molecules for their endothelial-cell ligands within the peripheral organ decreases, permitting the preferential homing of these cells to the sites of infection and inflammation, where their effector mechanisms are required to combat the pathogen. To further improve immune defense, pathogens which persist for long periods induce secondary lymphoid organs, such as granulomatous lesions at the sites of microbial persistence. This basic pattern of activation and expansion is identical in principle for both CD4 and CD8 T cells. In the following, the requirements for the activation of and the effector mechanisms unique to each subset will be outlined. Figure 1 and Table 1 provide an overview of the mechanisms underlying activation of the different T-cell populations involved in antibacterial defense.

CD4 T cells

For infections with intracellular bacteria in particular, CD4 T cells dominate both the induction and effector phases of the immune response. The generation of specific CD4 T cells is initiated by the recognition of peptides that are presented in the context of major histocompatibility (MHC) class II molecules

Helen L. Collins and Stefan H. E. Kaufmann • Department of Immunology, Max Planck Institute for Infection Biology, 10117 Berlin, Germany.

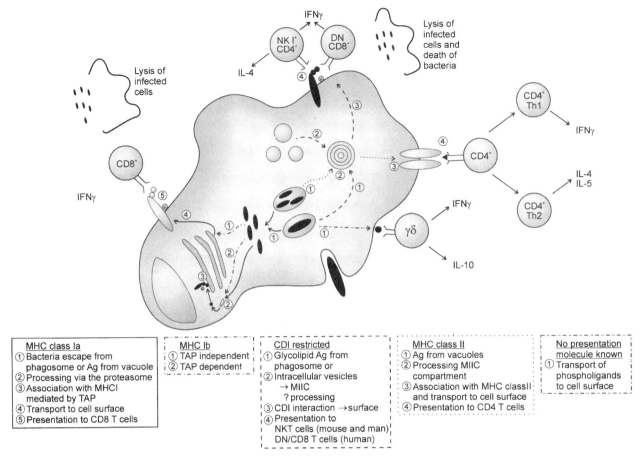

Figure 1. Pathways of Ag processing and presentation. A schematic representation of the pathways of processing of bacterially derived Ag for recognition by T cells is shown.

on the surface of specialized APC, such as macrophages and dendritic cells (DC) (Fig. 1). Typically, but not exclusively, these peptides are derived from Ag of exogenous origin which have been processed in acidified late endosomal or lysosomal compartments prior to presentation. Resting macrophages express low levels of MHC class II molecules and require stimulation by cytokines, in particular gamma interferon (IFN-γ), to reach full processing capacity. In contrast, DC represent the dominant APC for initial T-cell activation since they constitutively express high levels of MHC class II and costimulatory mol-

Table 1. T-cell populations involved in host resistance to bacterial infections

T-cell population	MHC restriction	Ligand	Effector function
CD4$^+$ $\alpha\beta$	MHC class II	Peptides (12–20 aa)	Cytokine secretion (IFN-γ, TNF-β, IL-4, IL-5, IL-13)
CD8$^+$ $\alpha\beta$	MHC class Ia	Peptides (9 aa)	Cytokine secretion (IFN-γ), cytolysis, bacterial killing
CD8$^+$ $\alpha\beta$	MHC class Ib (H2-M3, Qa-1)	N-fMet (murine)	Cytokine secretion (IFN-γ)
DN/CD8$^+$ $\alpha\beta$	Group I CD1	Glycolipids (human)	Cytokine secretion (IFN-γ), cytolysis, bacterial killing
DN/CD4$^+$ NK1$^+$ $\alpha\beta$	Group II CD1	Ceramides, GPI (murine)	Cytokine secretion (IL-4, IFN-γ)
DN/CD8$^+$ $\gamma\delta$	Unknown	Phospholigands (human)	Cytokine secretion (IFN-γ, IL-10)

ecules. The processing of antigenic proteins into peptide fragments occurs as a result of cleavage by intracellular proteases. Such proteases include cathepsins B, D, E, H, L, and S as well as aminopeptidases, some of which are upregulated by IFN-γ activation. The loading of antigenic peptides onto MHC class II molecules occurs in a compartment of the cell termed the MIIC. MHC class II molecules in a monomeric complex are diverted to this compartment from the normal secretory pathway by the invariant chain (Ii), which is subsequently cleaved by cathepsins S and L, resulting in the 23-amino-acid (aa) class II-associated invariant chain peptide (CLIP), which occupies the peptide binding groove. The association of this complex with HLA-DM facilitates the exchange of CLIP for a foreign peptide of 15 to 22 aa. The peptide-loaded MHC molecule is then transported to the cell surface where it is available for recognition by CD4 T cells (reviewed by Pieters [1999]).

Following MHC-restricted recognition of antigen, CD4 T cells differentiate into effector cells, termed T helper (Th) cells, which are distinguished by their ability to produce the maximum level of cytokines. A critical part of the differentiation process is the commitment of CD4 T cells to a polarized, distinct cytokine pattern, i.e., Th1 cells, characterized by the production of IFN-γ and tumor necrosis factor beta (TNF-β), and Th2 cells, which typically secrete interleukin-4 (IL-4), IL-5, IL-6, and IL-13. Multiple factors influence the development of these T-cell subsets, including antigen dose, MHC and peptide density, and the expression of different levels of costimulatory molecules. However, by far the most critical determining factor is the cytokine milieu present during Ag activation (Seder and Paul, 1994). Thus, CD4 T cells absolutely require IL-4 to become committed to the Th2 cell subset. While the necessity of this cytokine has been unequivocally demonstrated, to date the initial cellular source remains unclear. Various candidate cells have been proposed, including NK T cells and basophils (Paul, 1997). Obviously, once effector Th2 cells are generated, autocrine secretion of IL-4 can further drive Th2-cell differentiation. In contrast, the generation of Th1 cells depends centrally on the production of IL-12 and IL-18, which are produced by macrophages and DC during the initial interaction with antigen. Thus, in the absence of these Th1-promoting cytokines, Th2 cells preferentially develop. However, due to the diverse components that are abundant within bacterial cell walls, such as lipoarabinomannan from mycobacteria, lipoteichoic acid from gram-positive bacteria, and lipopolysaccharides (LPS) from gram-negative bacteria, as well as methylated bacterial

DNA sequences (CpG) (Fig. 2), which can induce the production of IL-12 and probably IL-18, the Th1 subset is generally strongly activated by bacterial infection. Once fully committed to the Th1 or Th2 effector phenotype, these T cells do not revert. This is partly because the conditions that promote one phenotype are inhibitory to the development of the other (Morel and Oriss, 1998). Thus, Th2 cells downregulate the expression of the IL-12 receptor β chain and are no longer able to respond to this cytokine. Furthermore, the expression of the Th1-specific transcription factor, T-bet, and the equivalent Th2-cell molecule, GATA3, are mutually exclusive, further illustrating the stable polarization of these subsets (Szabo et al., 2000). Additionally, surface markers distinguishing the two T-cell subsets have been identified. In mice, T1/ST2 is exclusively expressed on Th2 cells and is critical for Th2 cell effector functions (Xu et al., 1998a; Lohning et al., 1998) and the IL-18 receptor is present only on Th1 cells (Xu et al., 1998b). In humans, it is the preferential expression of chemokine receptors that distinguish between the subsets, with CXCR3 and CCR5 found on Th1 cells and CCR3 and CCR4 on Th2 cells (Sallusto et al., 1998).

Obviously this dichotomy of cytokine secretion patterns influences the subsequent immune response (Abbas et al., 1996). The production of IL-4 and IL-5 by Th2 cells directs the development of the humoral immune response by controlling the differentiation of B cells into Ig-producing plasma cells and promoting class switching to IgE and IgA, respectively (see below). The induction of a Th1 response results in the production of IFN-γ which is critical in the activation of macrophages for microbicidal mechanisms such as the production of NO and O radicals and is therefore the response that is considered central in the control of infections with intracellular bacteria. Moreover, at least in mice, the opsonizing Ab isotypes (IgG2a and IgG3) are produced by plasma cells which have been activated by IFN-γ.

CD8 T cells

Generally, the development of CD8 T cells requires the recognition of antigenic peptides in the context of conventional MHC class Ia molecules (Fig. 1). In contrast to MHC class II molecules, these peptide-loaded, MHC class Ia molecules noncovalently complexed with β_2-microglobulin (β_2m) are expressed on the surface of virtually every nucleated cell. The MHC class I-restricted peptides are generated via the proteasome, which is a proteolytic complex consisting of 28 subunits that is located in the

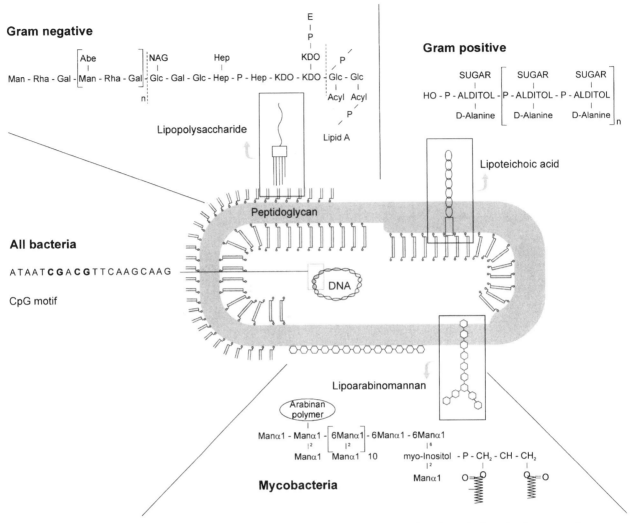

Figure 2. Bacterial components that stimulate the host immune response. Structures from bacteria that stimulate macrophages to release cytokines that have a direct impact on the development of the acquired T-cell response are shown. P, phosphate groups.

cytoplasm. Peptides produced by the proteasome are 5 to 15 aa in length and are precursors of the final MHC class Ia binding peptides, which have a required length of 8 to 9 aa. Peptides are transported via the transporters associated with Ag processing (TAP 1 and TAP 2) to the endoplasmic reticulum, where they associate with newly synthesized MHC class Ia molecules in a process involving TAP, tapasin, and various molecular chaperones including calnexin and the heat shock protein gp96 (Pamer and Cresswell, 1998). Peptides that are presented by MHC class I molecules are generated from endogenous proteins or proteins that are secreted into the cytoplasm. In light of this, CD8 T-cell responses are central to the immune response to viruses. Bacteria that can enter and reside within the cytoplasm of host cells, such as *Listeria monocytogenes*, also introduce their Ag into the MHC class I pathway. How-

ever, some intracellular pathogens can elicit a CD8 T-cell response despite their phagosomal location within the cell, and these include *Salmonella enterica* and *Mycobacterium tuberculosis*. Various mechanisms have been proposed to explain how and where such Ag encounter MHC class I molecules (Schaible et al., 1999) and will be discussed in more detail below.

A small subset of CD8 T cells recognize Ag presented by the nonclassical MHC class Ib molecules H2-M3 and Qa-1 in mice. H2-M3 presents short peptides that contain *N*-formylmethionine (N-fMet). Since N-fMet-containing peptides are commonly found in bacteria but are restricted to the few mitochondrial proteins in eukaryotes, it is postulated that these Ag-presenting molecules are specialized for the presentation of bacterial peptides. Indeed, to date, the only peptides which have been found to elicit N-fMet-restricted CD8 T-cell responses are of listerial origin, and this T-cell population confers a degree of protection against listerial infection in mice (Lenz and Bevan, 1997). To date there is no direct human homologue for H2-M3, and N-fMet-reactive T cells have not been isolated from humans. Qa-1-restricted CD8 T-cell responses have been implicated in infections with both *L. monocytogenes* and *S. enterica*, and this molecule has a functional human homologue, HLA-E (Stevens and Flaherty, 1996). Due to the nonpolymorphic nature of the MHC class Ib molecules and the limited diversity of the peptides that they present, there is a degree of cross-reactivity in the responses. For example, T cells raised against N-fMet-containing peptides of *L. monocytogenes* also respond to formylated peptides from *Staphylococcus aureus* (Nataraj et al., 1998). Additionally, nonclassical MHC class I-restricted CD8 T cells have been isolated from mice immunized with heat-killed mycobacteria, although the peptides responsible have not been identified. These MHC class Ib-restricted CD8 T cells may represent an intermediate between the natural, innate immune response and the specific acquired response.

Regardless of the MHC class I molecule utilized, the process of Ag recognition, together with appropriate costimulation, is the critical step in the transition from a precursor to an effector cytotoxic T lymphocyte. Costimulation is provided by costimulatory molecules on the surface of APC and by cytokines such as IL-2 and IFN-γ produced by CD4 T cells. Effector CD8 T cells can exert antimicrobial effects in two major ways: (i) via the secretion of cytokines such as IFN-γ and TNF, which contribute to macrophage activation in the same way as CD4 T cells, and (ii) by lysis of pathogen-infected cells either via the perforin/granzyme pathway or by the Fas/Fas-ligand pathway. Although it was once thought that these pathways were redundant, evidence has now been presented that the granule exocytosis-dependent pathway is more involved in the lysis of pathogen-infected cells while the Fas-dependent pathway is required to control lymphocyte activation and to prevent autoreactivity. Perforin itself can induce cell death, but its major function is to introduce granzymes and other molecules into the target cell, where they can induce death via the initiation of the caspase cascade resulting in apoptosis. More recently, a molecule with direct bactericidal activity, granulysin, has been identified, and this molecule is introduced into the bacterium-containing phagosome by means of perforin (Stenger et al., 1998, 1999).

CD1-controlled T cells

CD1 molecules are a group of nonpolymorphic MHC molecules encoded for by genes located outside of the MHC loci. They have some sequence homology to both MHC class I and II and, like MHC class I, are noncovalently bound to β2m at the cell surface. In contrast to protein-derived peptides presented via conventional processing pathways, these molecules present glycolipid Ag to T cells (Burdin and Kronenberg, 1999) (Fig. 1). The CD1 molecules are further subdivided into two groups—group I molecules comprise human CD1a (hCD1a), hCD1b, and hCD1c and are not present in mice, while the group II subset consists of hCD1d and murine CD1.1 (mCD1.1) and mCD1.2, although mCD1.2 is encoded by a pseudogene, which is not expressed. hCD1a, hCD1b, and hCD1c have been demonstrated to bind a variety of glycolipid moieties derived from mycobacteria, including lipoarabinomannan and glucose monomycolate (reviewed by Prigozy and Kronenberg [1998]) and more recently an evolutionarily conserved family of isoprenoid glycolipids with essential functions in protein glycosylation and cell wall synthesis (Branch Moody et al., 2000). Additionally, Ag derived from the gram-negative bacterium *Haemophilus influenzae* can be presented by these molecules (Fairhurst et al., 1998). Relatively little is known about the processing requirements for glycolipid Ag. Initial experiments studying CD1b-mediated Ag presentation revealed similarities to MHC class II processing in that the prevention of vesicular acidification by the lysosomotropic agent chloroquine reduced Ag presentation. However, a cell line deficient in invariant chain and HLA-DM could efficiently present mycolic acid when transfected with hCD1b, suggesting that the accessory molecules required for MHC class II processing are not necessary (Prigozy and Kronenberg, 1998). Exactly where CD1 molecules encounter their Ag is not fully understood, although recent evidence has underlined differences in the intracellular distribution of CD1 molecules. Whereas CD1b and CD1c molecules are trafficked through endosomal compartments, CD1a is found mainly at the cell surface and within the recycling pathway of the early endocytic pathway (Sugita et al., 1999; Schaible et al., 2000). The cells that respond to group 1 CD1 molecules are T cells expressing the αβ T-cell receptor (TCR) and are either double negative or CD8 positive. These T cells are capable of Ag-specific IFN-γ secretion and cytolytic activity. Recently it has been shown that CD8[+] CD1-restricted T cells not only lyse mycobacterium-infected cells but subsequently also reduce the viability of the intracellular organisms via a perforin- and granulysin-dependent mechanism (see above).

The crystal structure for the group II CD1d molecule has been solved and reveals similarity to the

MHC class I molecule with a deep, highly hydrophobic antigen-binding groove. The T-cell populations that recognize this molecule are either double negative or CD4$^+$ cells. The latter cells are distinguished by their invariant TCR Vα14Jα281 in mice and the homologous combination Vα24JαQ in humans and the expression of NK1.1; in short, they are NK T cells (Bendelac et al., 1997). Although the majority of these cells appear to be autoreactive, more recently ceramides derived from marine sponges have been identified as ligands (Kawano et al., 1997). Tentative evidence has been presented that NK T cells can recognize glycosylphosphatidylinositol (GPI) moieties of parasites (Schofield et al., 1999), although what role this plays in disease is still somewhat controversial (Molano et al., 2000). Regardless of the uncertainty of the exact Ag recognition, it has been clearly established that these cells have important functions since they rapidly produce large quantities of cytokines on stimulation. Although IL-4 was often found to be the predominant cytokine produced, following infection with bacteria such as *L. monocytogenes* and *Mycobacterium bovis* BCG, there is a preponderance of IFN-γ which is promoted via IL-12 and IL-18 (Emoto et al., 1999). This rapid cytokine burst occurs without tight control, and whereas it may help to ensure a rapid defense, it may also result in harmful sequelae when the host is confronted with an overload of pathogens.

$\gamma\delta$ T cells

In both mice and humans there is a minor population of T cells (1 to 5%) which express the $\gamma\delta$ TCR (Hayday, 2000), and such cells isolated from healthy donors respond to bacterially derived, nonprotein, phosphate-containing compounds such as isopentenyl pyrophosphate. In adult humans, 50% of the $\gamma\delta$ T-cell population expresses Vγ2δ2, and in vitro, mycobacterial phospholigands rapidly stimulate all T cells expressing this TCR combination. Thus, extrapolating these data to the in vivo situation, 1 to 2% of the T-cell population of an adult human can rapidly respond to mycobacterial infection, and, indeed, $\gamma\delta$ T cells have been shown to accumulate in the lesions of leprosy patients. The process of Ag recognition by this T-cell population appears to be independent of any known Ag-presenting molecules and requires no distinct processing step (Fig. 1). Thus, it is assumed that there is direct recognition of the antigenic ligand by the TCR (Kaufmann, 1996). In mice, these cells do not recognize phospholigands but, rather, recognize peptides, and although to date there is not an exhaustive list of known ligands, it has been shown that murine $\gamma\delta$ T cells can identify

a heptamer from HSP60, potentially via a Qa-1-dependent mechanism.

In terms of effector functions, $\gamma\delta$ T cells can produce cytokines including IFN-γ and IL-10, and it has been proposed that this T-cell population primarily plays a regulatory role in bacterial infections by controlling conventional Th-cell responses and limiting tissue damage. In the absence of $\gamma\delta$ T cells, mice infected with *L. monocytogenes* develop abscesses rather than granulomas in the liver (Mombaerts et al., 1993), and in experimental models of tuberculosis, the cellular composition of the granuloma is altered in the absence of $\gamma\delta$ T cells, resulting in a greater influx of neutrophils, in contrast to the usual lymphocytic infiltrate (D'Souza et al., 1997). Additionally, the $\gamma\delta$ T-cell population probably plays a compensatory role if $\alpha\beta$ T cells are absent. Thus, mice deficient in both $\alpha\beta$ and $\gamma\delta$ T cells are more susceptible to *Listeria* infection than are either of the single-knockout strains alone. Furthermore, in a high-dose intravenous challenge with *M. tuberculosis*, δ TCR knockout mice succumbed to infection with doses that were not lethal for wild-type mice (Ladel et al., 1995). This is in contrast to a low-dose aerosol challenge, where no differences were observed between $\gamma\delta$ T-cell-deficient mice and controls (D'Souza et al., 1997), suggesting that if bacterial growth can be contained until $\alpha\beta$ T cells are sufficiently activated, the infection can be controlled independently of $\gamma\delta$ T cells.

Humoral Immune Responses

Whereas the cell-mediated immune response is the major effector mechanism against intracellular bacteria, humoral immunity, mediated by Ab produced by activated B lymphocytes (plasma cells), provides the most effective response against extracellular bacteria (Nahm et al., 1999). Similar to T-cell responses, specific Ab responses are initiated by the interaction of Ag with a subset of mature IgM- or IgD-expressing B cells within peripheral lymphoid organs. Ag that stimulate Ab production can be divided into two categories which require different conditions of initiation and result in distinct isotype production. Bacteria express both types of Ag.

T-dependent antigens

T-dependent Ag comprise protein antigens that can be processed and presented by APC, including B cells, to CD4 Th cells. The Ag binds to the surface of its specific B cell via membrane Ig and is internalized into endosomal vesicles, processed, and presented on the cell surface in the context of MHC class II molecules as previously described. However, Ag uptake via Ig imposes specificity on the Ag presentation; i.e., the APC focuses on the pathogen of importance. An additional consequence of the binding and cross-linking of the Ig receptor is B-cell activation and the upregulation of costimulatory molecules including B7-1, B7-2, and CD40. Thus, via recognition of Ag and MHC, Th cells are activated for cytokine secretion. Cytokines in turn play two critical roles in humoral immunity: (i) T-cell-derived cytokines IL-2, IL-4, and IL-5 act in synergy to promote the expansion and differentiation into activated Ab-secreting plasma cells, and (ii) the cytokine milieu influences Ig heavy-chain class switching and hence the isotype of Ab produced (Table 2). The different isotypes perform distinct functions, and therefore the class of Ab produced will directly influence the response to a specific pathogen. Thus, both IgM and IgG2a activate the complement cascade to generate C3b and iC3b, which can opsonize bacteria for phagocytosis, and IgG2a production is promoted by a Th1 cytokine, IFN-γ, consistent with its production in infections with many bacteria. Additionally, some isotypes such as IgG1, IgG2b, and IgA can bind directly to specific high-affinity receptors (FcR) on cells including macrophages, monocytes, and neutrophils and can promote internalization of bacteria in this manner. In contrast, the isotypes induced by Th2 cytokines cannot fix complement or bind to FcR on macrophages and are more important in the response to extracellular pathogens, where they act to block the adhesion of bacteria to host cells and also to neutralize harmful bacterial toxins. The production of IgA, which is the major class of Ab at mucosal sites and therefore important in the response to respiratory and intestinal pathogens, is controlled by IL-4, IL-5, and transforming growth factor β (TGF-β).

T-independent antigens

T-independent Ag comprise nonprotein compounds which directly stimulate B-cell production independently of Ag-specific T-cell help. Bacterial capsules, which are composed of polysaccharides and glycolipids, are often highly immunogenic. They are generally polymeric and include repetitive epitopes, which results in the cross-linking of multiple surface Ig receptors on B cells, which is sufficient to activate these cells independently from T cells. Characteristically, the Ab produced as a result of interaction with these Ag are low-affinity IgM with little or no heavy-chain class switching. It is this isotype that provides the initial Ab response to all bacterial infections, and the subsequent class switching to IgG can be of diagnostic value in infections such as those with *Treponema pallidum*, where the presence of IgM Ab indicates acute or congenital disease and IgG isotypes signify secondary syphilis. For bacterial infections such as *H. influenzae* and *Neisseria meningitidis*, the capsule elicits significant Ab production but only after 2 years of age. Accordingly, the capsular polysaccharide vaccine initially used against *H. influenzae* elicited strong Ab-mediated protection only in children older than 2 years. This obstacle could be resolved by conjugation of the polysaccharide to a T-cell-dependent carrier protein, a so-called conjugate vaccine. Some T-independent Ag are directly mitogenic for B cells and induce them to differentiate into Ab-secreting plasma cells, although this process results in nonspecific activation. Such compounds are abundant in bacterial cell walls and include peptidoglycan, LPS, and lipoproteins.

ACQUIRED IMMUNE RESPONSE AND BACTERIAL INFECTIONS

Now that we have outlined the components of the acquired immune response and discussed how they are induced, we will change focus and discuss this host response with regard to specific bacterial pathogens. We have divided the infections into three groups: acute infections, either extra- or intracellular, and chronic infections. Using specific examples of organisms within each category, we will discuss which components of the specific host response are required to counteract each infection and the mechanisms developed by pathogens to manipulate the host response to their own advantage. MHC class I- and II-restricted CD8 and CD4 T cells are central to antibacterial protection. This feature is shared with defense against viral infections. However, in contrast to viral pathogens, immunity to bacteria involves additional presentation elements and T-cell populations. This evolution is probably a consequence of the higher complexity of bacterial pathogens.

Extracellular Infections

As the name implies, extracellular bacteria replicate outside host cells in tissue spaces such as intestinal, urogenital, and respiratory tracts and within selected tissue sites. The major goal of these bacteria is to avoid internalization and subsequent killing by neutrophils, monocytes, and macrophages. Consequently, the host relies on the production of complement and specific Ab, rather than T cells, to counteract these pathogens (reviewed by Nahm et al. [1999]). This is well illustrated by the fact that patients suffering from Bruton's agammaglobulinemia,

Table 2. Murine Ab isotypes important in bacterial infections

Isotype	Properties	Factor promoting class switching	Factor inhibiting class switching	Effector function in bacterial infections
IgG1	FcγRI binding (macrophages, neutrophils, DC)	IL-4, LPS, anti-CD40L/CD40	IFN-γ	Promotion of phagocytosis; activation of microbicidal mechanisms; toxin neutralization
IgG2a	C'^{a} fixation; FcγRI binding (see above)	IFN-γ, LPS + IL-12	IL-4	Promotion of phagocytosis; toxin neutralization
IgG2b	C' fixation; FcγRII/III binding (macrophages, neutrophils, eosinophils, B cells, mast cells, NK cells)	TGF-β	IL-4	Promotion of phagocytosis; granule release in eosinophils; Ab-dependent cytotoxicity
IgG3	C' fixation	IFN-γ	IFN-γ, IL-4	Promotion of phagocytosis
IgA	C' fixation (alternative); FcαRI binding (macrophages, neutrophils, eosinophils)	TGF-β, IL-4, IL-5	IL-10	Promotion of phagocytosis; blocking of adhesion; toxin neutralization

^{a} C', complement.

who have no serum Ab but have normal T-cell function are infected primarily with extracellular bacteria. Many such bacteria possess a polysaccharide capsule, which is in itself antiphagocytic, preventing uptake by host cells. However, capsular components such as polysaccharides are also highly immunogenic, leading to the production of IgM and in some cases, such as the pneumococcal polysaccharide, IgG2. The production of IgM and IgG can activate complement components to generate C3b and iC3b, which opsonize bacteria, thus promoting phagocytosis via specific complement receptors (Table 2). Additionally, IgG, but not IgM, binds to Fc receptors on host phagocytes and hence has direct opsonizing activities. To avoid complement opsonization, the pneumolysin of *Streptococcus pyogenes* as well as the lipoteichoic acid of *Staphylococcus aureus* can bind complement at a site remote from the bacteria, thus counteracting this host defense mechanism. The production of IgM and IgG leads to the activation of the C5-9 membrane attack complex of complement, which kills certain bacteria such as neisseriae by direct lysis. Consequently, patients deficient in the late complement components, C5-8, are highly susceptible to infections with neisseriae, while people with a lack of C3 are especially prone to infections with the pyogenic bacteria, e.g., streptococci and staphylococci. To avoid the deleterious effects of host Ab, many extracellular bacteria exhibit antigenic variation of their cell walls and capsules. This process permits them to escape recognition by specific Ab that were generated in response to previous infections. Examples of such variation include *S. pyogenes,* in which there are over 100 distinct serotypes of M proteins and in which Ab generated to one serotype fail to protect against infection with another.

Principally, extracellular bacteria cause disease by two primary mechanisms, which do not have to be mutually exclusive. The first occurs via the production of toxins. Toxins produced by extracellular bacteria can be divided into exotoxins, which are secreted by the bacteria (Balfanz et al., 1996), and endotoxins (Ulevitch and Tobias, 1999), which form an integral part of the outer membrane of gram-negative bacteria and which are released on bacterial lysis. These toxins have the potential to damage the host in a variety of ways and require a rapid response to neutralize their effects. In its extreme form, a single toxin is responsible for the disease, e.g., the toxin produced by *Clostridium botulinum*, while others, such as diphtheria toxin and cholera toxin, are assisted by other virulence factors that promote colonization and invasion of the causative agents. Following infection with *Vibrio cholerae*, the bacteria attach to the intestinal mucosa and the enterotoxin is produced. The excreted toxin attaches to host GM1 gangliosides and the active A subunit is translocated into the cell, where it disregulates the control of cyclic AMP via the ADP-ribosylation of a host cell protein. This results in the copious production of diarrhea, the hallmark of this disease, and the subsequent spreading of the bacteria from host to host. The exotoxin of *Corynebacterium diphtheriae* is produced following the colonization of the mucosa of the upper respiratory tract. In contrast to cholera toxin, diphtheria toxin exerts its effects at a site remote from colonization. The toxin enters the circulation, and once bound to its receptor, heparin-binding epidermal growth factor (HB-EGF), it ADP-ribosylates host elongation factor 2, which inhibits protein synthesis, resulting in cell damage. The HB-EGF receptor is abundantly expressed on heart and nerve cells, explaining why heart failure and neurological complications are frequent consequences of severe disease. For both cholera and diphtheria, a person who has recovered from an infection is immune to reinfection. This is due to the production of high-affinity IgG and IgA Ab, which are directed against the receptor-binding domain of the toxin and prevent it from binding to the host cell surface. Indeed, it is this principle that underlies the successful vaccination against diphtheria where infants are immunized with modified toxin molecules (toxoids) which lack toxic activity but retain the receptor-binding site and therefore the ability to induce blocking Ab (Burnette, 1996). Endotoxins, in contrast to exotoxins, are released in large amounts only following the destruction of the bacteria. Lipopolysaccharides from gram-negative bacteria induce indirect tissue damage and pathologic changes via the stimulation of proinflammatory cytokines such as IL-1, TNF, macrophage inhibitory factor, IFN-γ, and IL-8. If this response is not regulated or if the bacterial burden is too high, septic shock can result.

The second mechanism used by extracellular bacteria to cause disease involves the induction of inflammation and tissue destruction at the site of infection. Typically, purulent lesions develop, which can result in the penetration of the bacteria into deeper tissues and the establishment of a chronic infection state. For this to occur, the bacteria must first colonize the host by adhering to a tissue surface and then promote invasion into the host tissues. Adherence is mediated by a variety of cell wall structures such as the pili of *N. gonorrhoeae* and *V. cholerae* and the polysaccharide of *Streptococcus pneumoniae*. Obviously, a host response targeted against such structures would prevent the attachment of these bacteria and subsequent disease, and at mucosal surfaces especially, IgA production can block adhesion. The importance of IgA production at these sites is highlighted by the fact that people suffering from a relatively common selective deficiency in the IgA isotype are particularly susceptible to respiratory infections. To evade this type of immune defense, *Neisseria* spp., *S. pneumoniae,* and *H. influenzae* produce an IgA protease which can cleave human IgA, rendering it more susceptible to proteolytic degradation (Mulks and Shoberg, 1994). Furthermore, *Neisseria* spp. possess the genetic machinery to rapidly alter the antigenic composition of the pili, evading the binding of specific Ab (Meyer et al., 1994). Once the host surface is colonized, many bacteria, including *Staphylococcus aureus,* can produce tissue-destroying enzymes such as hyaluronidases and lipases, which further promote bacterial spreading.

In some cases extracellular bacteria can establish a chronic, persistent infection. This generally occurs after invasion of the underlying tissues and the formation of purulent abscesses which can be the result of unresolved or untreated staphylococcal infections. Alternatively, approximately 30% of the population can be symptomless carriers of *S. aureus*. Most of these people harbor the organism only transiently for a few weeks, but some may become persistent carriers. A similar situation is seen for *Neisseria meningitidis*, where although up to 70% of the population harbor organisms in their upper respiratory tract, only very few of these develop disease.

Intracellular Infections

The hallmark of intracellular bacteria is their ability to reside within host cells, either permanently or transiently; following the entry of the bacteria into the host, there is a period of coexistence which may or may not result in disease. The occurrence of clinical symptoms depends on several factors including whether the host immune response can control the infection and what mechanisms the bacteria have developed to evade or manipulate this reaction (Schaible et al., 1999).

Acute infections

One of the best-studied intracellular bacteria is *L. monocytogenes,* which, in the immunocompetent mouse, causes an acute infection which is rapidly controlled and eradicated by the host immune response. From various murine experimental systems, it has been unequivocally shown that T cells are required to achieve sterilizing immunity, although, as discussed in the chapters dealing with innate immunity, the cytokines IFN-γ and TNF produced by NK cells and macrophages can control early infection. However, this innate response is insufficient in the long term to control the disease, and, accordingly, T-cell-deficient mice will die of listeria infection eventually. Although *L. monocytogenes* was extensively used to define the mechanisms of processing of bacterial Ag for presentation by MHC class II molecules, experimental evidence from infections with mice deficient in components required for MHC class I processing or in CD8 T cells have demonstrated that it is the CD8 T-cell response that is central to the successful resolution of infection (Harty and Bevan, 1999). The reason for this lies in the ability of *L. monocytogenes* to escape from its intraphagosomal location into the cytoplasm by means of the secretion of the pore-forming enzyme listeriolysin O (LLO). This molecule, in addition to other secreted proteins, is readily accessible to the MHC class I presentation pathway in the cytoplasm. Indeed, in BALB/c mice, peptides derived from p60 and LLO form the immunodominant peptides in the CD8 T-cell response to listeriae. Elegant studies using MHC class I tetramers specific for these peptides have shown that CD8 T cells dominate both the primary and secondary T-cell responses to this organism (Busch et al., 1998), and to date CD8 T-cell epitopes from nonsecreted listerial proteins have not been identified. However, experiments with recombinant listeriae which express a viral epitope as either a secreted fusion protein or retained within the bacteria revealed that CD8 T-cell priming against the nonsecreted epitope did occur and was only slightly reduced in comparison to that in the nonsecreted form (Shen et al., 1998).

In apparent contrast to these findings, auxotrophic (AroA⁻), *Salmonella enterica* serovar Typhimurium, when made recombinant for listerial proteins, could elicit protective immunity against listerial challenge only when the protein was secreted (Hess et al., 1996). This pathogen also resides intracellularly and thus underlines a fundamental difference between these two bacteria. The majority of *L. monocytogenes* organisms escape from the membrane-bound phagosome, and those that remain are rapidly killed, exposing somatic antigens to the cellular Ag-processing machinery. In contrast to this, even auxotrophic salmonellae remain within the phagosome for prolonged periods, and thus theoretically only secreted proteins are available in the cytoplasm for interaction with MHC class I molecules. Thus, in experimental models, a deficiency of CD4 T cells has a more profound effect on the outcome of salmonella infection than does a depletion of CD8 T cells, consistent with the potent induction of CD4 cells by phagosomal Ags which are presented by MHC class II molecules.

There is now evidence that many intracellular bacteria that remain vacuole bound can elicit CD8 T-cell responses. Indeed, results from a variety of experimental systems clearly support a role for transfer of antigens from the phagosome to the cytosol. In light of this, it has been shown that CD8 T cells also play a role in salmonella infections. However, a large proportion of the CD8 T cells elicited in vitro recognize infected target cells in an MHC class Ib-restricted manner, with the dominant restricting element being Qa-1b (Lo et al., 1999). For infections with both listeriae and salmonellae, the achievement of sterilizing immunity is definitively dependent on the generation of a specific T-cell response.

Chronic infections

Perhaps the best examples of intracellular bacteria that persist for long periods within the host are the pathogenic members of the *Mycobacterium* species, namely, *M. tuberculosis* and *M. leprae*. This is best illustrated by the fact that although one-third of the worldwide population (2 billion people) are infected with *M. tuberculosis*, more than 90% of these people remain healthy and free of clinical disease. Therefore, although host immune mechanisms are effective in controlling this bacterial infection, they fail to achieve sterile eradication and hence are suboptimal. As described for all intracellular infections, the primary protective immune response is T-cell rather than Ab mediated. The tubercle bacilli reside within macrophages and appear to be relatively resistant to microbicidal mechanisms, which may in part be due to their ability to prevent their host cells from being adequately activated by IFN-γ. The critical importance of this cytokine is underlined by the fact that in both mice and humans, a deficiency in IFN-γ or its receptor renders the individual more susceptible to mycobacterial infections (Jouanguy et al., 1999). Therefore, the induction of a Th1-type immune response affords the host the greatest protective capacity.

The phagosomal location of mycobacteria within the macrophage should facilitate the interaction of mycobacterial Ag with MHC class II and the subsequent induction of a protective CD4 Th1-cell response. Consistent with this is the fact that mice deficient in either MHC class II or CD4 T cells are more susceptible to *M. tuberculosis* infection. Moreover, humans coinfected with HIV who suffer a depletion in CD4 T cells are considerably more susceptible to both primary infection and reactivation of existing infection. However, in apparent contradiction to this, it has been reported that *M. tuberculosis*-infected cells have a diminished capacity for MHC class II-restricted Ag presentation. There are several potential explanations for this. The first is that mycobacteria can modify the phagosomal compartment in which they reside. The bacillus-containing vacuole is maintained at a pH of 6.5 due to a paucity of the vacuolar proton ATPase (Russell et al., 1997), and this may partially impede the actions of the proteolytic enzymes required for antigen processing, which have an optimal pH requirement of pH 5 to 6. The second explanation is that there is defective transport and processing of MHC class II molecules through the lysosomal-endosomal pathway in mycobacterium-infected cells (Hmama et al., 1998). The third explanation is that infection of macrophages with *M. bovis* BCG severely impairs the presentation of exogenous protein Ag to a T-cell hybridoma, and this is mediated by IL-6 production (Russell et al., 1997).

In addition to the obligate requirement for CD4 T cells in control of mycobacterial infections, experimental infections of gene-deficient mice have strongly indicated an additional role for CD8 T cells. Mice that lack the β_2m gene and that have no functional MHC class I molecules and thus no conventional CD8 $\alpha\beta$ T cells suffer from increased susceptibility to *M. tuberculosis* infection (Flynn et al., 1992). However, it should be noted that these mice also lack other Ag-presenting molecules such as CD1d, which also require β_2m for their surface expression. In both murine and human infections, CD8 T cells recognizing specific mycobacterial Ag in the context of MHC class I have been isolated. In light of the fact that the mycobacteria remain inside the phagosomal compartment throughout their intracellular life, the mechanism by which mycobacterium-derived Ag interact with MHC class I molecules remains unclear. There are several potential mechanisms that may facilitate the induction of MHC class I-restricted CD8 T cells, some of which are not restricted only to *Mycobacterium* spp. but also apply to other phagosomal bacteria such as *Salmonella* spp. The first is that a specific secretion apparatus (type III) facilitates the translocation of secreted Ag into the cytoplasm. This has been shown to be the case for salmonellae (Jones and Falkow, 1996; Russman et al., 1998). The second mechanism is that bacteria may possess molecules with membranolytic activity, permitting the leakage of Ag from the phagosome. This has been suggested for *M. tuberculosis* following the observation that MHC class I presentation of ovalbumin occurred after its engulfment with the tubercle bacilli (Mazzacaro et al., 1996). The third mechanism is that, as shown for several intracellular bacteria, apoptosis is induced on infection of the host cell. Macrophages and DC can take up Ag from apoptotic cells and induce an Ag-specific CD8 T-cell response (Albert et al., 1998). Recently this has been demonstrated to occur following *Salmonella*-induced apoptosis (Yrlid and Wick, 2000).

The cytolytic effector functions of CD8 T cells could directly lyse target cells and inhibit the growth of the bacteria or could facilitate the lysis of infected cells that are refractory to activation by IFN-γ, thereby releasing the bacteria and exposing them to Ab and complement, facilitating uptake by more competent phagocytes. Additionally, CD8 T cells are a potent source of IFN-γ production, as evidenced by the fact that the CD4 T-cell-deficient mouse exhibits only a transient decrease in IFN-γ production upon infection with *M. tuberculosis* and that the compensatory IFN-γ was produced by CD8 T cells (Caruso et al., 1999).

In addition to conventional MHC class I- and II-restricted T-cell responses, unconventional T-cell subsets have been suggested to play a role in the control of mycobacterial infections. In humans, T cells controlled by group I CD1 molecules have been isolated that respond to mycobacterial glycolipid Ag. These T cells are either CD4$^-$ CD8$^-$ or CD8$^+$. They produce IFN-γ on antigen stimulation, and lysis of infected macrophages by CD1-restricted CD8 T cells results in a reduction in the viability of the mycobacteria (Stenger et al., 1998). In mice, the lack of group 2 CD1 molecules has no apparent impact on the ability to control experimental tuberculosis infection, which leaves open the question of exactly what role these cells play in the immune response (Behar et al., 1999).

Perhaps the most important hallmark of the host response to chronic intracellular infections is the formation of granulomas. Granulomas are critical to protection since they restrict bacterial replication and confine pathogens to discrete foci and prevent dissemination. This process is achieved by the recruitment and organization of T cells, predominantly CD4 T cells, and macrophages to the site of infection. Cytokines, predominantly T-cell-derived IFN-γ, then activate macrophage microbicidal mechanisms, resulting in the inhibition of bacterial growth. Eventually, the granuloma becomes encapsulated via fibrosis and calcification, leading to necrosis of the center of the foci and presumably to reduced nutrient and oxygen supply for the bacteria. Cytokines such as TNF and IFN-γ are critical in granuloma formation, and recent evidence has strongly indicated an important role for $\gamma\delta$ T cells. In mice deficient in $\gamma\delta$ T cells, the primary lymphocytic infiltration into the granuloma is replaced by neutrophil influx, resulting in a pyogenic granuloma resembling an abscess. Therefore, it has been proposed that the primary role of $\gamma\delta$ T cells is to regulate cell traffic by promoting the influx of macrophages and lymphocytes and inhibiting potentially detrimental neutrophil infiltration (Orme and Cooper, 1999). This is most probably achieved via the production of chemokines such as monocyte chemoattractant protein 1 or the production of inhibitory cytokines such as TGF-β.

Potential Role of Antibodies in Intracellular Bacterial Infections

Despite the unequivocal requirement for T-cell-mediated immunity in the control of acute intracellular infections, there has recently been renewed interest in the role of Ab. It has been assumed that because of their intracellular location, these bacteria are not exposed to Ab. However, at the initiation of infection and for most bacteria, with the notable exception of *L. monocytogenes,* which can infect adjacent cells without leaving the intracellular environment, for short periods during infection they will be extracellular. Under these circumstances, Ab may provide important functions such as prevention of entry of bacteria at mucosal surfaces, Ab-dependent cytotoxicity, and/or complement-mediated lysis. Furthermore, Ab can opsonize bacteria, facilitating increased phagocytosis by macrophages, which then kill the organism. Recent experiments have revealed that in the murine listerial infection model, passive immunization with a monoclonal Ab generated against LLO protected mice from a lethal challenge and resulted in a decrease in bacterial load within the first 6 to 48 h of infection. This passive protection was independent of T or B cells, since equivalent results were seen in the SCID mouse, which lacks these cells. Despite these results, it should be noted that the experiments were performed with a defined Ab and that the titers of anti-LLO Ab during natural listerial infection are low to negligible (Edelson et al., 1999). Similarly, in vitro coating of *M. tuberculosis* with Ab prior to the infection of mice ameliorated the course of the disease (Teitelbaum et al., 1998). In *Salmonella* infections, B-cell-deficient mice were more susceptible to oral infection with wild-type bacteria in both primary and secondary responses, and following vaccination with attenuated *S. enterica* serovar Typhimurium, B-cell-deficient mice were more susceptible to an intravenous challenge (Mittrücker et al., 2000). Taken together, these data suggest that Ab contribute to the control of intracellular bacterial infections, although they are rarely able to accomplish this in the absence of cell-mediated mechanisms.

Immunopathology

Although the host response to an infectious organism is critical in preventing disease, it must be tightly regulated to prevent the immune mechanisms from directly contributing to pathologic responses. Both uncontrolled humoral and cell-mediated responses have been implicated in disease states. Antibody-mediated pathologic changes generally occur due to the formation of immune complexes which are deposited at various tissue sites remote from the bacteria themselves. An example of this is post-streptococcal glomerulonephritis, which can develop 1 to 3 weeks after a streptococcal throat or skin infection. In this case, lysis of the bacteria releases cell wall components, which provoke an intense Ab response. Ag-Ab complexes are deposited in the kidneys, and this induces local complement activation and tissue damage (Norstrand et al., 1999). Similarly, immune complexes generated following infections with gram-negative bacteria as well as meningococci can result in reactive arthritis or, in rare cases, endocarditis. A further complication of the humoral response to pathogens is the generation of autoreactive Ab. Ab generated against the M protein of *Streptococcus pyogenes* cross-react with cardiac myosin and sarcolemmal proteins. These cross-reactive Ab induce inflammation and damage to the heart valves, resulting in rheumatic fever in approximately 3% of patients following streptococcal infection that is left untreated (Gibofsky et al., 1998). For reasons that are not well understood, strains that induce glomerulonephritis do not induce rheumatic fever and vice versa. Not only can cross-reactive Ab result in immunopathology, but also T cells can be generated against bacterial components that cross-react with host molecules, resulting in tissue damage. Such components can include conserved Ag such as heat shock proteins (hsp). These proteins are ubiquitous and are present in many species. Hence, the response to hsp is not tissue specific but can promote or exacerbate a tissue-specific response (Zügel and Kaufmann, 1999). This mechanism is illustrated by the observation that a CD8 T-cell clone specific for mycobacterial hsp60 cross-reacts with host hsp, resulting in intestinal inflammation resembling inflammatory bowel disease (Steinhoff et al., 1999). Previously, hsp cross-reactive CD4 T cells have been implicated in adjuvant-induced arthritis in rats (Van Eden et al., 1998). Additionally, there is coincidental cross-reactivity between unrelated proteins of microbial and host origin. Recently it has been demonstrated that T cells reactive against peptides derived from the outer membrane protein of *Chlamydia* spp. induced autoimmune inflammatory heart disease in mice due to cross-reactivity with a heart muscle-specific protein, α-myosin (Bachmaier et al., 1999).

Most bacterial infections provoke an inflammatory response mediated by T cells and macrophages, and if this is not adequately controlled it will lead to tissue damage. Thus, regulatory mechanisms occur, mostly mediated by cytokines, such as IL-10 and TGF-β, to keep this response in check. A notable example where this does not occur is in the activation of the host T-cell response by the enterotoxins of staphylococci and streptococci. These toxins can function as superantigens in that they activate a larger T-cell population than processed Ag do (Michie and Cohen, 1998). These Ag bind to the outer surface of the MHC molecule, outside the peptide binding site, and additionally to the Vβ region of the TCR. Hence, superantigens can stimulate 2 to 20% of all T cells in a response that is independent of their fine Ag specificity. Accordingly, the response is not specific for the causative pathogen. The consequences of this massive unrestricted T-cell stimulation are the overproduction of T-cell-derived cytokines and the uncontrolled activation of bystander cells such as macrophages, as well as the downregulation of the specific immune response, resulting in an anergic state. Superantigen production has been implicated in a variety of clinical conditions, including the potentially lethal toxic shock syndrome which occurs following the production of *Staphylococcus aureus* toxic shock syndrome toxin, which activates T cells bearing Vβ2. Experimental studies have shown that the majority of individuals develop protective Ab to this toxin by the time they have reached adolescence, which further underlines the importance of host humoral responses in the neutralization of this toxin/superantigen. In a similar way, overzealous cytokine production is stimulated by LPS in septic shock, leading to organ failure and high fatalities.

For infections with *M. tuberculosis,* the host inflammatory processes cause the pathologic changes associated with the disease. The formation of granulomas within lung tissue reduces the capacity of the lung per se, and the excessive secretion of fibrogenic cytokines such as TNF and TGF-β leads to lung fibrosis. Thus, production of cytokines such as TNF must be highly balanced. Its production is critically required for the formation of the granuloma and hence for bacterial containment, but its overproduction promotes further damage to host tissues. Similarly, trachoma caused by *Chlamydia trachomatis* is due to scarring which results from a continuous antibacterial cell-mediated immune response in the eyes, which represent a particularly vulnerable site.

It is not only the uncontrolled activation of the immune response but also the induction of inappropriate effector mechanisms that result in pathologic consequences for the host. One of the most stringent examples of this occurs in infections with *M. leprae.* Toward the tuberculoid pole of leprosy, a Th1 CD4 T-cell response is induced, leading to potent macrophage activation. This cell-mediated response can control but not eradicate disease, and although few viable organisms can be detected within the tissues, the symptoms of the disease are caused by local inflammatory responses to the persistent bacteria and generally result in localized nerve damage. Conversely, in lepromatous leprosy, a Th2-type response is generated, leading to the suppression of T-cell-mediated responses and to a subsequent uncontrolled

proliferation of the bacilli. A state of anergy develops in which the T-cell responses to many Ag of *M. leprae* are inhibited, and this is a more severe form of the disease since, in the absence of macrophage activation, the infection becomes widely disseminated, leading to widespread damage of the peripheral nervous system (Lucey et al., 1996). In contrast to the situation in leprosy, the induction of a Th1 response by the extracellular bacterium *Borrelia burgdorferi* leads to inflammation of joints and to Lyme arthritis. Protection is associated with Ab production, which is promoted by a Th2 response. However, *Borrelia*-induced arthritis develops in SCID mice that are devoid of functional T and B cells. It is therefore assumed that the local activation of macrophages by the bacteria directly induces pathologic changes, which are potentiated by a Th1 response which can be downregulated by a Th2 response (Hu and Klempner, 1997).

CONCLUDING REMARKS

Immunologists frequently tend to view the immune system as a weapon that developed to combat foreign intruders in the most efficient way. Microbiologists often place the bacteria in the center when they state that pathogens have developed highly successful evasion strategies to outwit host defenses. In fact, the two strategies evolved hand-in-hand, and the two standpoints rather reflect the investigators' bias. Given the fast replication of bacteria compared with that of humans (a difference of several hundredfold), we should appreciate that our immune system did quite well in keeping pace with the pathogens. This is even more astounding when we realize how much the acquired immune response to bacterial pathogens had to diversify. Virus immunology has shown that T lymphocytes are peptide specific and MHC restricted. Specificity for antigenic polypeptides comprising 8 to 20 aa guaranteed sufficient specificity to avoid autoaggression against the individual. At the same time, MHC restriction allowed broad enough Ag coverage to prevent the pathogen from evading the immune response through mutation. Principally, viruses are composed of proteins and nucleic acids. In contrast, bacteria—the smallest living entities on this planet—encompass a vast array of other physicochemical entities in addition to nucleic acids and proteins. In particular, their cell wall is rich in a variety of glycolipids. To counter bacterial complexity, the antigen spectrum for T cells had to be broadened to include nonproteinacious entities. Thus, we are increasingly aware that the Ag recognition pattern in the antibacterial T-cell response is as broad as that of Ab (the breadth of this response having been known to us for a long time). Apparently, this diversification of both the humoral and cellular immune responses has helped us to coexist along side the most successful inhabitants of Earth—the bacteria. As a corollary, understanding antibacterial immunity provides us with deeper insights into the versatility and complexity of the immune system. Both basic and applied immunology will profit from this. Several bacterial pathogens, such as *M. tuberculosis, Shigella* spp., and *S. enterica* serovar Typhi to name the major culprits, significantly contribute to worldwide morbidity and mortality. In the current absence of effective vaccines against these pathogens a better understanding of the acquired immune response may contribute to the rational design of novel preventative measures.

Acknowledgment. We thank Diane Schad for excellent assistance with the figures.

REFERENCES

Abbas, A. K., K. M. Murphy, and A. Sher. 1996. Functional diversity of helper T lymphocytes. *Nature* 383:787–793.

Albert, M. L., B. Sauter, and N. Bhardwaj. 1998. Dendritic cells acquire antigen from apoptotic cells and induce class I restricted CTLs. *Nature* 392:86–89.

Bachmaier, K., N. Neu, L. M. de la Maza, S. Pal, A. Hessel, and J. M. Penninger. 1999. Chlamydia infections and heart disease linked through antigenic mimicry. *Science* 283:1335–1339.

Balfanz, J., P. Rautenberg, and U. Ullmann. 1996. Molecular mechanisms of action of bacterial exotoxins. *Zentbl. Bakteriol.* 284:170–206.

Behar, S. M., C. C. Dascher, M. J. Grusby, C. R. Wang, and M. B. Brenner. 1999. Susceptibility of mice deficient in CD1D or TAP1 to infection with *Mycobacterium tuberculosis*. *J. Exp. Med.* 189:1973–1980.

Bendelac, A, M. N. Rivera, S. H. Park, and J. H. Roark. 1997. Mouse CD1-specific NK1 T cells: development, specificity and function. *Annu. Rev. Immunol.* 15:535–562.

Branch Moody, D., T. Ullrichs, W. Mühlecker, D. C. Young, S. S. Gurcha, E. Grant, J.-P. Rosat, M. B. Brenner, C. E. Costello, G. S. Besra, and S. A. Porcelli. 2000. CD1c-mediated T-cell recognition of isoprenoid glycolipids in *Mycobacterium tuberculosis* infection. *Nature* 404:884–888.

Burdin, N., and M. Kronenberg. 1999. CD1-mediated immune responses to glyolipids. *Curr. Opin. Immunol.* 11:326–331.

Burnette, W. N. 1996. Parameters for the rational design of genetic toxoid vaccines. *Adv. Exp. Med. Biol.* 397:61–67.

Busch, D. H., I. M. Pilip, S. Vijh, and E. G. Pamer. 1998. Coordinate regulation of complex T cell populations responding to bacterial infection. *Immunity* 8:353–362.

Caruso, A. M., N. Serbina, E. Klein, K. Triebold, B. R. Bloom, and J. L. Flynn. 1999. Mice deficient in CD4 T cells have only transiently diminished levels of IFN-γ, yet succumb to tuberculosis. *J. Immunol.* 162:5407–5416.

D'Souza, C., A. M. Cooper, A. A. Frank, R. J. Mazzaccaro, B. R. Bloom, and I. M. Orme. 1997. An inflammatory role for γδ T lymphocytes in acquired immunity to *Mycobacterium tuberculosis*. *J. Immunol.* 158:1217–1221.

Edelson, B. T., P. Cossart, and E. R. Unanue. 1999. Cutting edge: paradigm revisited: antibody provides resistance to *Listeria* infection. *J. Immunol.* 163:4087–4090.

Emoto, M., Y. Emoto, B. Buchwalow, and S. H. Kaufmann. 1999. Induction of IFNγ producing CD4+ natural killer T cells by *Mycobacterium bovis* bacillus Calmette Guerin. *Eur. J. Immunol.* 29:650–659.

Fairhurst, R. M., C. X. Wang, P. A. Sieling, R. L. Modlin, and J. Braun. 1998. CD1 presents antigens from a gram-negative bacterium, *Haemophilus influenzae* type b. *Infect. Immun.* 66:3523–3526.

Flynn, J. L., M. M. Goldstein, K. J. Triebold, B. Koller, and B. R. Bloom. 1992. Major histocompatibility complex class I-restricted T cells are required for resistance to *Mycobacterium tuberculosis* infection. *Proc. Natl. Acad. Sci. USA* 89:12013–12017.

Gibofsky, A., S. Kerwar, and J. B., Zabriskie. 1998. Rheumatic fever. The relationships between host, microbe and genetics. *Rheum. Dis. Clin. North Am.* 24:237–259.

Harty, J. T., and M. J. Bevan. 1999. Responses of CD8+ T cells to intracellular bacteria. *Curr. Opin. Immunol.* 11:89–93.

Hayday, A. C. 2000. γδ cells: a right time and a right place for a conserved third way of protection. *Annu. Rev. Immunol.* 18:709–737.

Hess, J., I. Gentschev, D. Miko, M. Welzel, C. Ladel, W. Goebel, and S. H. Kaufmann. 1996. Superior efficacy of secreted over somatic antigen display in recombinant Salmonella vaccine induced protection against listeriosis. *Proc. Natl. Sci. Acad. USA* 93:1458–1463.

Hmama, Z., R. Gabathuler, W. A. Jeffries, G. de Jong, and N. E. Reiner. 1998. Attenuation of HLA-DR expression by mononuclear phagocytes infected with *Mycobacterium tuberculosis* is related to intracellular sequestration of immature class II heterodimers. *J. Immunol.* 161:4882–4893.

Hu, L. T., and M. S. Klempner. 1997. Host-pathogen interactions in the immunopathogenesis of Lyme disease. *J. Clin. Immunol.* 17:354–365.

Jones, B. D., and S. Falkow. 1996. Salmonellosis: Host immune responses and bacterial virulence determinants. *Annu. Rev. Immunol.* 14:533–561.

Jouanguy, E., R. Doffinger, S. Dupuis, A. Pallier, F. Altare, and J. L. Casanova. 1999. IL-12 and IFN-gamma in host defense against mycobacteria and salmonella in mice and men. *Curr. Opin. Immunol* 11:346–351.

Kaufmann, S. H. E. 1996. γδ T cells and other unconventional T lymphocytes: what do they see and what do they do? *Proc. Natl. Acad. Sci. USA* 93:2272–2279.

Kawano T., J. Q. Cui, Y. Koezuka, I. Toura, Y. Kaneko, K. Motoki, H. Ueno, R. Nakagawa, H. Sato, E. Kondo, H. Koseki, and M. Taniguchi. 1997. CD1d-restricted and TCR-mediated activation of V(alpha)14 NKT cells by glycosylceramides. *Science* 278:1626–1629.

Ladel, C. H., C. Blum, A. Dreher, K. Reifenberg, and S. H. E. Kaufmann. 1995. Protective role of γδ T cells and αβ T cells in tuberculosis. *Eur. J. Immunol.* 25:2877–2881.

Lenz, L., and M. J. Bevan. 1997. CTL responses to H2-M3 restricted Listeria epitopes. *Immunol. Rev.* 158:115–121.

Lo, W.-F., H. Ong, E. S. Metcalf, and M. J. Soloski. 1999. T cell responses to Gram-negative intracellular bacterial pathogens: A role for CD8+ T cells in immunity to *Salmonella* infection and the involvement of MHC class Ib molecules. *J. Immunol.* 162:5398–5406.

Lohning, M., A. Stroehmann, A. J. Coyle, J. L. Grogan, S. Lin, J. C. Guttierez-Ramos, D. Levinson, A. Radbruch, and T. Kamradt. 1998. T1/ST2 is preferentially expressed on murine Th2 cells, independent of IL-4, IL-5 and IL-10, and important for

Th2 effector functions. *Proc. Natl. Acad. Sci. USA* 95:6930–6935.

Lucey, D. R., M. Clerici, and G. M. Shearer. 1996. Type 1 and type 2 cytokine dysregulation in human infectious, neoplastic and inflammatory diseases. *Clin. Microbiol. Rev.* 9:532–562.

Mazzacarro, R. J., M. Gedde, E. R. Jensen, H. M. van Santen, H. M. Ploegh, K. L. Rock, and B. R. Bloom. 1996. Major histocompatibility class I presentation of soluble antigen facilitated by *Mycobacterium tuberculosis* infection. *Proc. Natl. Acad. Sci. USA* 93:11786–11791.

Meyer, T. F., J. Pohlner, and J.P. van Putten. 1994. Biology of the pathogenic neisseriae. *Curr. Top. Microbiol. Immunol.* 192:283–317.

Michie, C. A., and J. Cohen. 1998. The clinical significance of T-cell superantigens. *Trends Microbiol.* 6:61–65.

Mittrücker, H.-W., B. Raupach, A. Kohler, and S. H. Kaufmann. 2000. Cutting edge: role of B lymphocytes in protective immunity against *Salmonella typhimurium* infection. *J. Immunol.* 164:1648–1652.

Molano, A., S. H. Park, Y. H. Chiu, S. Nosseir, A. Bendelac, and M. Tsuji. 2000. Cutting edge: the IgG response to the circumsporozoite protein is MHC class II-dependent and CD1d independent: exploring the role of GPIs in NK T cell activation and antimalarial responses. *J. Immunol.* 164:5005–5009.

Mombaerts, P., J. Arnoldi, F. Russ, S. Tonegawa, and S. H. E. Kaufmann. 1993. Different roles of αβ and γδ T cells in immunity against an intracellular bacterial pathogen. *Nature* 365:53–56.

Morel, P. A., and T. B. Oriss. 1998. Cross regulation between Th1 and Th2 cells. *Crit. Rev. Immunol.* 18:275–303.

Mulks, M. H., and R. J. Shoburg. 1994. Bacterial immunoglobulin A1 proteases. *Methods Enzymol.* 235:543–554.

Nahm, M. H., M. A. Apicella, and D. E. Briles. 1999. Immunity to extracellular bacteria, p. 1373–1386. *In* W. E. Paul (ed.), *Fundamental Immunology*, 4th ed. Lippincott-Raven, New York, N.Y.

Nataraj, C., G. R. Huffman, and R. J. Kurlander. 1998. H2M3 (wt)-restricted, *Listeria monocytogenes*-immune CD8 T cells respond to multiple formylated peptides and to a variety of Gram positive and Gram negative bacteria. *Int. Immunol.* 10:7–15.

Norstrand, A., M. Norgren, and S. E. Holm. 1999. Pathogenic mechanisms of acute post-streptococcal glomerulonephritis. *Scand. J. Infect. Dis.* 31:523–537.

Orme, I. M., and A. M. Cooper. 1999. Cytokine and chemokine cascades in immunity to tuberculosis. *Immunol. Today* 20:307–312.

Pamer, E., and P. Cresswell. 1998. Mechanisms of MHC class I restricted antigen processing. *Annu. Rev. Immunol.* 16:323–358.

Paul, W. E. 1997. Interleukin-4: signalling mechanisms and control of T cell differentiation. *Ciba Found. Symp.* 204:208–216.

Pieters, J. 1999. Processing and presentation of phagocytosed antigens to the immune system. *Adv. Cell Mol. Biol. Membr. Organs* 5:379–406.

Prigozy, T. I., and M. Kronenberg. 1998. Presentation of bacterial lipid antigens by CD1 molecules. *Trends Microbiol.* 6:454–459.

Russell, D. G., S. Sturgill-Koszycki, T. K. VanHeyningen, H. L. Collins, and U. E. Schaible. 1997. Why intracellular parasitism need not be a degrading experience for *Mycobacterium*. *Philos. Trans. R. Soc. Lond. Ser. B* 352:1303–1310.

Russman, H., H. Shams, F. Poblete, Y. Fu, J. E. Galan, and R. O. Donis. 1998. Delivery of epitopes by the salmonella type III secretion system for vaccine development. *Science* 281:565–568.

Sallusto, F., A. Lanzavecchia, and C. R. Mackay. 1998. Chemokines and chemokine receptors in T-cell priming and Th1/Th2 mediated responses. *Immunol. Today* 19:568–574.

Schaible, U. E., H. L. Collins, and S. H. E. Kaufmann. 1999. Confrontation between intracellular bacteria and the immune system. *Adv. Immunol.* 71:267–377.

Schaible, U. E., K. Fischer, K. Hagens, H. L. Collins, and S. H. E. Kaufmann. 2000. Intersection of group I CD1 molecules and mycobacteria in different intracellular compartments of dendritic cells. *J. Immunol.* 164:4843–4852.

Schofield, L., M. J. McConville, D. Hansen, A. S. Campbell, B. Fraser-Reid, M. J. Grusby, and M. D. Tachado. 1999. CD1d-restricted immunoglobulin G formation to GPI anchored antigens mediated by NKT cells. *Science* 283:225–229.

Seder, R. A., and W. E. Paul. 1994. Acquisition of lymphokine-producing phenotype by CD4+ T cells. *Annu. Rev. Immunol.* 12:635–673.

Shen, H., J. F. Miller, X. Fan, D. Kolwyck, R. Ahmed, and J. T. Harty. 1998. Compartmentalization of bacterial antigens: differential effects on priming of CD8+ T cells and protective immunity. *Cell* 92:535–545.

Steinhoff, U., V. Brinkmann, U. Klemm, P. Aichele, P. Seiler, U. Brandt, P. W. Bland, I. Prinz, U. Zügel, and S. H. E. Kaufmann. 1999. Autoimmune intestinal pathology indiced by hsp60-specific CD8 T cells. *Immunity* 11:349–355.

Stenger, S., D. A. Hanson, R. Teitelbaum, P. Dewan, K. R. Niazi, C. J. Froelich, T. Ganz, S. Thoma-Uszynski, A. Melian, C. Bogdan, S. A. Porcelli, B. R. Bloom, A. M. Krensky, and R. L. Modlin. 1998. An antimicrobial activity of cytolytic T cells mediated by granulysin. *Science* 282:121–125.

Stenger, S., J. P. Rosat, B. R. Bloom, A. M. Krensky, and R. L. Modlin. 1999. Granulysin: a lethal weapon of cytolytic T cells. *Immunol. Today* 20:390–394.

Stevens, C., and L. Flaherty. 1996. Evidence for antigen presentation by the class Ib molecule Qa-1. *Res. Immunol.* 147:286–290.

Sugita, M., E. P. Grant, E. van Donselaar, V. W. Hsu, R. A. Rogers, P. J. Peters, and M. J. Brenner. 1999. Separate pathways for antigen presentation by CD1 molecules. *Immunity* 11:743–750.

Szabo, S. J., S. T. Kim, G. L. Costa, X. K. Zhang, C. G. Fathman, and L. H. Glimcher. 2000. A novel transcription factor, T-bet, directs Th1 lineage commitment. *Cell* 100:655–669.

Teitelbaum, R., A. Glatman-Freedman, B. Chen, J. B. Robbins, E. Unanue, A. Casadavell, and B. R. Bloom. 1998. A mAb recognising a surface antigen of *Mycobacterium tuberculosis* enhances host survival. *Proc. Natl. Acad. Sci. USA* 95:15688–15693.

Ulevitch, R. J., and P. S. Tobias. 1999. Recognition of Gram-negative bacteria and endotoxin by the innate immune system. *Curr. Opin. Immunol.* 11:19–22.

Van Eden, W., R. van der Zee, L. S. Taams, A. B. Praaken, J. van Roon, and M. H. Wauben. 1998. Heat shock protein T cell epitopes trigger a spreading regulatory control in a diversified arthritogenic T cell response. *Immunol. Rev.* 164:169–174.

Xu, D., W. L. Chan, B. P. Leung, F.-P. Huang, R. Wheeler, D. Piedrafita, J. H. Robinson, and F. Y. Liew. 1998a. Selective expression of a stable cell surface molecule on type 2 but not type 1 helper T cells. *J. Exp. Med.* 187:787–794.

Xu, D., W. L. Chan, B. P. Leung, D. Hunter, K. Schulz, R. W. Carter, I. B. McInnes, J. H. Robinson, and F. Y. Liew. 1998b. Selective expression and functions of interleukin 18 receptor on T helper (Th) type 1 but not Th2 cells. *J. Exp. Med.* 188:1485–1492.

Yrlid, U., and M. J. Wick. 2000. Salmonella-induced apoptosis of infected macrophages results in presentation of a bacteria encoded antigen after uptake by bystander dendritic cells. *J. Exp. Med.* 191:613–624.

Zügel, U., and S. H. E. Kaufmann. 1999. Role of heat shock proteins in protection from and pathogenesis of infectious disease. *Clin. Microbiol. Rev.* 12:19–39.

Immunology of Infectious Diseases
Edited by S. H. E. Kaufmann, A. Sher, and R. Ahmed
© 2002 ASM Press, Washington, D.C.

Chapter 16

Acquired Immunity against Fungi

ARTURO CASADEVALL

Of the more than 100,000 fungal species known, only about 150 are pathogenic in humans, and of these, only a few are common pathogens (Table 1). With the exception of *Candida* spp., the overwhelming majority of fungal infections are acquired from the environment. Most fungal pathogens are free-living organisms that cause disease primarily in hosts with impaired immune function. As a class, fungal pathogens represent a remarkably diverse group of organisms which pose several unique problems for host defense mechanisms. Fungi are antigenically complex, and many species produce powerful hydrolytic enzymes that can destroy tissue. Several fungal pathogens are capable of yeast-hypha transitions in tissue (dimorphism). Since yeast and hyphal cells can differ in antigenic composition, size, shape, and invasive potential, fungi capable of dimorphism provide a formidable challenge for the immune system. Despite an impressive arsenal of virulence characteristics that can subvert host defense mechanisms (Hogan et al., 1996), invasive fungal infections are relatively rare in individuals with normal immune function. This in turn implies that normal host defense mechanisms are highly effective against fungal pathogens.

Acquired immunity consists of two arms: humoral and cellular. Humoral immunity is mediated by B lymphocytes, which protect the host by making antibodies that opsonize pathogens, neutralize toxins, mediate antibody-dependent cellular cytotoxicity, and activate the classical complement pathway. Cell-mediated immunity is mediated by T lymphocytes, which protect the host by promoting inflammatory responses, by activating effector cells through cytokine production, and possibly by exerting direct antifungal effects. There is general consensus in the field of medical mycology that cell-mediated immunity is critical for protection against most fungal in-

fections (Romani and Howard, 1995; Murphy, 1991). In contrast, the role of humoral immunity against fungi has been less certain, but recent data indicate that antibody can also make a decisive contribution to host defense.

Serological responses and skin delayed-hypersensitivity testing have provided conclusive evidence that fungal infection can elicit humoral and cellular acquired immune responses to fungal antigens. Candidiasis, blastomycosis, coccidioidomycosis, cryptococcosis, and histoplasmosis are each associated with strong antibody responses to fungal antigens (Matthews and Burnie, 1998). Similarly, delayed-hypersensitivity responses can be elicited by injection of fungal antigens in patients with a history of infection with *Candida albicans, Blastomyces dermatitidis, Coccidioides immitis, Cryptococcus neoformans,* and *Histoplasma capsulatum* (Bennett, 1981; Salvin, 1959). In vitro, lymphocytes from patients with these fungal infections often demonstrate proliferation when challenged with fungal antigens consistent with acquired cellular immunity.

Among the fungi, the contribution of the acquired immune response has been most extensively studied for four organisms, *C. albicans, C. immitis, C. neoformans,* and *H. capsulatum.* For each of these organisms there is conclusive evidence that acquired immune responses can make a critical contribution to host defense. This chapter will focus primarily on these four fungi but will also consider examples from other fungal pathogens. Given the enormous breadth of the subject and the size limitation of this review, the primary goal in this chapter is to focus on the general principles involved in the acquired immune response to fungi. Whenever possible, citations are made to recent reviews which cover the subject in greater depth. Table 1 includes references to author-

---

Arturo Casadevall • Albert Einstein College of Medicine, 1300 Morris Park Ave., Bronx, NY 10461.

Table 1. Major human fungal pathogens and medical conditions predisposing to invasive disease

Fungus	Infection	Source of infection	Predisposing conditions	Review(s) on acquired immunity
Aspergillus spp.	Aspergillosis	Environment	Neutropenia, immunosuppressive therapy, AIDS	Latge (1999)
Blastomyces dermatitidis	Blastomycosis	Environment	Hematological malignancy, immunosuppressive therapy, AIDS	Di Salvo (2000)
Candida spp.	Candidiasis	Endogenous	Neutropenia, surgery, antibiotic treatment	Vazquez-Torres and Balish (1997), Ashman (1997), Ashman and Papadimitriou (1995), Fidel et al. (1999)
Coccidioides immitis	Coccidioidomycosis	Environment	Hematological malignancies, pregnancy, immunosuppressive therapy, AIDS	Cox and Magee (1998)
Cryptococcus neoformans	Cryptococcosis	Environment	Hematological malignancies, immunosuppressive therapy, AIDS	Lipscomb et al. (1993), Murphy (1998), Vecchiarelli and Casadevall (1998)
Histoplasma capsulatum	Histoplasmosis	Environment	Immunosuppressive therapy, AIDS	Deepe and Seder (1998)
Paracoccidioides brasiliensis	Paracoccidioidomycosis	Environment	Alcoholism, malnutrition, AIDS	Calich et al. (1998)

itative reviews on the immunology of several fungal pathogens.

ESTABLISHING THE IMPORTANCE OF ACQUIRED IMMUNITY AGAINST FUNGAL INFECTIONS

The most direct method for establishing the importance of acquired immune mechanisms in host protection is to demonstrate that infection and recovery provide protection against a subsequent infection (e.g., that a state of immunity follows recovery from infection). For many bacterial and viral pathogens the importance of acquired immunity is evident from the observation that recovery from symptomatic infection results in long-lasting immunity. Obtaining similar information for fungal infections is more difficult because primary fungal infections are often unrecognized. Nevertheless, for several fungal pathogens, serological skin reactivity surveys indicate that infections are common but clinical disease is rare, consistent with the development of acquired immunity. For *C. immitis* and *H. capsulatum,* there is evidence that initial infection either is asymptomatic or results in mild disease and that confers immunity (Kong and Levine, 1967). Similar criteria may apply to *C. neoformans* infections, where a high prevalence of antibodies to cryptococcal antigens (Chen et al., 1999; DeShaw and Pirofski, 1995; Fleuridor et al., 1999) in normal individuals suggests that primary infection is followed by containment and lifelong immunity.

Association of Invasive Fungal Infections with Disorders of T-Cell Function

One method for ascertaining the importance of an immune component in host protection is to associate deficits in the function of that component with increased susceptibility to disease. Extensive clinical experience indicates that medical conditions that impair T-cell function can dramatically increase the risk of invasive fungal infections. For example, the incidences of mucosal candidiasis, histoplasmosis, coccidioidomycosis, and cryptococcosis are markedly higher in patients with advanced human immunodeficiency virus infection, a condition associated with profound derangements of T-cell function (Wheat, 1995; Dixon et al., 1996). In contrast, disorders of the humoral immune system are not classically associated with increased susceptibility to fungal infections. However, recent studies have associated AIDS-related cryptococcosis with qualitative deficiencies in the antibody response to capsular polysaccharide, suggesting that subtle humoral deficiencies may predispose to certain fungal infections (Fleuridor et al., 1999). The fact that AIDS patients are significantly more susceptible to most fungal infections than are individuals with normal immune function is commonly cited as evidence for the importance of cellular immunity in protection against fungi. Although there is no question that intact T-cell function is critical for protection, it is noteworthy that T-cell deficits produce a global dysfunction in immune responses and may result in impaired innate and humoral immunity. Disorders of T-cell function such as those that occur in patients with AIDS are associated with some types of infection and not others. For example, patients with AIDS are highly susceptible to mucosal but not systemic *C. albicans* infections. Furthermore, not all mucosal sites are comparable. Oropharyngeal candidiasis is common in women with AIDS, but vaginal candidiasis is not. In fact, local immune responses and not systemic immunity appear to be the most important factors in determining susceptibility for vaginal candidiases (Fidel and Sobel, 1998). Finally, it is worth noting that with the exception of mucosal candidiasis, only a small fraction of AIDS patients at risk suffer invasive fungal infections. For example, only 6 to 8% of AIDS patients in New York City develop cryptococcosis (Currie and Casadevall, 1994) despite serological evidence for widespread exposure (Chen et al., 1999; DeShaw and Pirofski, 1995; Fleuridor et al., 1999; Deepe and Seder, 1998). This suggests the existence of other defense mechanisms in the setting of profound T-cell dysfunction.

Animal Experimentation in T- and B-Cell-Deficient Animals

Mice with defects in T-cell function are more susceptible to fungal pathogens than are mice without these defects (Table 2). This is consistent with clinical experience indicating a critical role for cell-mediated immunity. In contrast, it has been more difficult to demonstrate a role for humoral immunity using B-cell-deficient mice. For example, antibody-deficient mice are not more susceptible to *C. albicans* (Wagner et al., 1996), *C. neoformans* (Aguirre and Johnson, 1997; Monga et al., 1979), or *H. capsulatum* (Allendoerfer et al., 1999) infection than are wild-type mice. For *C. neoformans* there is considerable evidence that humoral immunity can be important, and the lack of enhanced susceptibility in B-cell-deficient mice appears, at first look, perplexing. However, normal mice seldom mount significant antibody responses to the capsular polysaccharide during infection (Casadevall and Scharff, 1991). Hence, for *C. neoformans* the comparable susceptibility of B-cell-sufficient and B-cell-deficient mice may be explained because B-cell-sufficient mice seldom mount a strong antibody response to the polysaccharide (Casadevall and Scharff, 1991; Casadevall et al., 1992) whereas B-cell-deficient mice are unable to mount a response. Hence, the response in B-cell-sufficient and B-cell-deficient mice against *C. neoformans* may be functionally comparable. Furthermore, there is evidence that qualitative aspects of the humoral response could influence the outcome of cryptococcal infection in mice (Lovchik et al., 1999). Comparisons of susceptible and resistant mouse strains suggest that immunoglobulin heavy-chain genes are associated with increased susceptibility to infection (Lovchik et al., 1999). For *C. albicans,* the susceptibility of B-cell-deficient mice varies with the infection model, such that B-cell-deficient mice are more susceptible to systemic infection but not mucosal candidiasis (Wagner et al., 1996). For *H. capsulatum,* no difference has been demonstrated for infection in B-cell-sufficient and B-cell-deficient mice (Allendoerfer et al., 1999).

Fungal Vaccines Can Elicit Protective Responses

Demonstration that vaccination elicits a protective immune response to a particular pathogen provides direct evidence for the potential usefulness of acquired immune responses in host defense against such pathogens. For the fungi, certain vaccines can elicit protective immune responses in experimental animals (for reviews spanning several decades of experimentation, see Kong and Levine [1967], Segal [1987], and Deepe [1997]). In general, immunization by infection with attenuated strains or sublethal inocula elicits protective responses against *B. dermatitidis, C. immitis, C. neoformans,* and *H. capsulatum* in experimental animals (Kong and Levine, 1967; Segal, 1987). In contrast, immunization with killed cells has elicited little or no protection (Kong and Levine, 1967). For *C. neoformans,* careful studies have shown that although CD4$^+$ and CD8$^+$ T cells are induced in response to the inoculation of live and heat-killed yeasts in mice, protection is elicited only by infection with small inocula or immunization with a culture filtrate preparation in adjuvant (reviewed by Murphy [1998]). Some success has been obtained using partially purified fractions of fungal cells as vaccines. For example, immunization of mice with ribosomes or ribosomal proteins of *H. capsulatum* protected against a subsequent lethal challenge (reviewed by Tewari et al. [1998]). Similarly, immunization of mice with a concentrated culture filtrate known as CneF in complete Freund's adjuvant results in partial protection against lethal cryptococcal infection (reviewed by Murphy [1998]).

In recent years, vaccines based on defined antigens have been shown to elicit protective immunity against several fungal pathogens in mice. Deepe and collaborators have shown that an *H. capsulatum* protein with homology to the heat shock protein hsp60 family conferred protection against lethal experimental histoplasmosis (Gomez et al., 1995). Devi and collaborators have generated a polysaccharide-protein conjugate vaccine that elicits an antibody response protecting mice against lethal challenge with *C. neoformans* (Devi et al., 1991; Devi, 1996). For *B. der-*

Table 2. Examples of mouse experiments that indicate the importance of the acquired immune system

Pathogen	Mouse phenotype	Outcome	Reference(s)
Aspergillus spp.	IL-4$^{-/-}$	↓ Susceptibility	Cenci et al. (1999)
	IL-10$^{-/-}$	↑ Susceptibility	Grunig et al. (1997)
	IL12$^{-/-}$	↑ Susceptibility	Cenci et al. (1999)
	IFN-$\gamma^{-/-}$	↑ Susceptibility	Cenci et al. (1999)
	BALB/c + IFN-γ	↓ Susceptibility	Nagai et al. (1995)
	BALB/c + TNF-α	↓ Susceptibility	Nagai et al. (1995)
Candida albicans	β2-Microglobulin$^{-/-}$	No difference (systemic)	Balish et al. (1996)
	β2-Microglobulin$^{-/-}$	↑ Susceptibility (mucosal)	Balish et al. (1996)
	IL-4$^{-/-}$	↑ Fungal burden (systemic)	Vazquez-Torres et al. (1999)
	IL6$^{-/-}$	↓ Fungal burden (systemic)	Vazquez-Torres et al. (1999)
	IL-10$^{-/-}$	↑ Susceptibility	van Enckevort et al. (1999)
	IFN-$\gamma^{-/-}$	↑ Susceptibility	Balish et al. (1998)
	IFN-$\gamma^{-/-}$	No difference	Qian and Cutler (1997)
	TNF$^{-/-}$	↑ Susceptibility	Marino et al. (1997)
	BALB/c + anti-CD4	↑ Tissue damage	Ashman et al. (1999)
	BALB/c + anti-CD8	↑ Tissue damage	Ashman et al. (1999)
Coccidioides immitis	DBA/2 + anti-IL-12	↑ Fungal burden	Magee and Cox (1996)
	BALB/c + IFN-γ	↓ Fungal burden	Magee and Cox (1995)
	BALB/c + anti-IL-4	↓ Fungal burden	Magee and Cox (1995)
Cryptococcus neoformans	Anti-IL-4	↓ Susceptibility	Kawakami et al. (1999a)
	Anti-IFN-γ	↑ Susceptibility	Kawakami et al. (1999b), Hoag et al. (1997)
	Anti-IL-12	↑ Susceptibility	Hoag et al. (1997)
	Anti-TNF-α	↑ Susceptibility	Aguirre et al. (1995)
	SCID	↑ Susceptibility	Hill (1992)
	SCID + T cells	↓ Susceptibility	Huffnagle et al. (1991a)
	BALB/c + anti-CD4	↑ Fungal burden	Huffnagle et al. (1991b)
	BALB/c + anti-CD8	↑ Fungal burden	Huffnagle et al. (1991b)
	CD4$^{-/-}$	↑ Susceptibility	Yuan et al. (1997)
	CD8$^{-/-}$	↑ Susceptibility	Yuan et al. (1997)
	IFN-$\gamma^{-/-}$	↑ Susceptibility	Yuan et al. (1997)
	IL-4$^{-/-}$	↓ Susceptibility	Decken et al. (1998)
	IL-12$^{-/-}$	↑ Susceptibility	Decken et al. (1998)
	IL-18$^{-/-}$	↓ Fungal clearance	Kawakami et al. (2000)
Histoplasma capsulatum	Anti-IFN-γ	↑ Susceptibility	Zhou et al. (1995)
	Anti-TNF-α	↑ Susceptibility	Zhou et al. (1995), Allendoerfer and Deepe (1998)
	Anti-IL-12	↑ Susceptibility	Zhou et al. (1995)
	Anti-IL-4	↓ Susceptibility	Zhou et al. (1995)
	β_2-Microglobulin$^{-/-}$	↑ Fungal burden	Deepe (1994)
	C57BL/6 + anti-Vβ4$^+$	↑ Fungal burden	Gomez et al. (1998)
	CD40$^{-/-}$	No difference	Zhou and Seder (1998)
	CD40L$^{-/-}$ + anti-CD4	↑ Susceptibility	Zhou and Seder (1998)
	CD40L$^{-/-}$ + anti-CD8	↑ Susceptibility	Zhou and Seder (1998)

matitidis, serological and lymphocyte proliferation studies have identified a 120-kDa antigen known as WI-1 as a major target of the acquired immune response (Klein et al., 1992; Wuthrich et al., 1998). Immunization of mice with WI-1 antigen elicits immune responses that confer significant protection against lethal pulmonary infection (Wuthrich et al., 1998). Similarly, several *Coccidioides immitis* antigens have been demonstrated to elicit strong immune responses (Zhu et al., 1997; Yang et al., 1997; Jiang et al., 1999; Kirkland et al., 1998b; Hung et al., 2000). Immunization of mice with a spherule cell wall proline-rich antigen (also known as antigen 2) induces strong lymphoproliferative responses, and vaccinated mice have a substantially reduced organ fungal burden relative to nonvaccinated controls (Kirkland et al., 1998a). Genetic immunization with DNA expressing antigen 2 also elicits protective immune responses to lethal infection with *C. immitis* (Jiang et al., 1999). For *Candida albicans,* immunization with mannan extract-protein conjugates has been demonstrated to elicit a protective antibody response in mice against lethal experimental candidiasis (Han et al., 1999).

In summary, immunization with certain defined antigen preparations will protect against some fungal infections. For *H. capsulatum, B. dermatitidis,* and *C. immitis,* the available evidence suggests that the protective immune response to immunization is the result of cell-mediated immunity. For *C. neoformans* and *C. albicans,* the protection observed after immunization with polysaccharide conjugate vaccines is antibody mediated. Hence, the experience with experimental vaccines against fungi indicates that acquired immunity can be protective against fungi and that both arms of the immune system can be effective depending on the antigen used and the fungal pathogen in question.

Requirement for Th1 Responses and Granulomatous Inflammation in Control of Certain Fungal Infections

For many fungal pathogens, the effective tissue response to invasion is granulomatous inflammation. For example, control of *C. neoformans* and *H. capsulatum* infections is associated with the development of granuloma formation in infected tissue (Deepe and Bullock, 1992; Goldman et al., 2000). Since granulomatous inflammation is a tissue hallmark of cell-mediated immunity, this implies that acquired immunity is required for an effective host response to some fungal pathogens.

In response to infection, CD4$^+$ T helper cells differentiate into two types, which differ in the types of cytokines produced (reviewed by Fresno et al. [1997] and Romagnani [1996]). Type 1 (Th1) cells produce gamma interferon (IFN-γ), interleukin 2 (IL-2), and tumor necrosis factor beta (TNF-β). Type 2 (Th2) cells produce IL-4, IL-5, IL-6, and IL-10. For many fungal pathogens, depletion of Th1-associated cytokines has consistently been associated with enhanced host susceptibility to infection (Table 2). Conversely, administration of Th1-associated cytokines or depletion of Th2-associated cytokines has often been associated with enhanced host resistance to infection. This has led to the view that Th1-polarized responses are generally protective against fungal pathogens. Although this paradigm is almost certainly an oversimplification of a very complex response (Allen and Maizels, 1997), it provides a useful conceptual approach to dissection of the immune response to various pathogens. The observation that administration of Th1-associated cytokines or depletion of Th2-associated cytokines is often associated

with increased resistance to fungal infection (Table 2) has led to the view that Th1-polarized responses are generally protective. Analysis of cytokine responses in murine models of candidiasis strongly supports the view that Th1 responses are required for protection against *C. albicans* (reviewed by Ashman and Papadimitriou [1995]). Depletion of the Th1-associated cytokine IFN-γ enhances susceptibility to *C. albicans,* whereas depletion of the Th2-associated cytokines IL-4 and IL-10 is associated with increased resistence (Romani et al., 1992a, 1992b). For *C. albicans,* the contribution of T-cell immunity may differ for systemic and mucosal infection. For example, IL-10- and IL-4-deficient mice are more resistant and susceptible, respectively, to systemic candidiasis but no difference is apparent against mucosal infection (Vazquez-Torres et al., 1999).

For both *H. capsulatum* and *C. neoformans* pulmonary infections, a predominance of Th1-associated cytokines appears to be necessary for control and clearance of infection (Allendoerfer et al., 1999; Deepe and Seder, 1998; Hoag et al., 1995, 1997; Huffnagle, 1996). A variety of studies have shown that the Th1-associated cytokine IFN-γ is essential for control of both *H. capsulatum* and *C. neoformans* infection, presumably because of its critical role in activating macrophage antifungal activity (Hoag et al., 1997; Lovchik et al., 1995; Deepe and Seder, 1998). For *Coccidioides immitis,* analysis of cytokine profiles in mouse strains in response to infection also strongly suggests that resistance is associated with a shift from a Th2 to a Th1 response (Magee and Cox, 1996). Consistent with this observation, the susceptibility of mouse strains to *C. immitis* infection has been associated with increased levels of IL-4 and IL-10 production in response to infection (Fierer et al., 1998).

Establishment of Latency and Reactivation of Latent Infection

Some fungal pathogens, such as *H. capsulatum* and *C. neoformans,* can establish latent infections that persist in tissue and can reactivate if the host becomes immunosuppressed. For both *H. capsulatum* and *C. neoformans,* establishment of latency is accompanied by granuloma formation that contains the infection (Deepe and Bullock, 1992; Goldman et al., 2000). Recently, a rat model of *C. neoformans* latent infection has been described which provides insight into the mechanism by which fungal infections persist in immunocompetent hosts (Goldman et al., 2000). Intratracheal infection in rats results in acute pneumonia, which rapidly resolves as the host mounts a strong granulomatous response, but some foci of infection remain in the form of subpleural granulomas where yeast cells are found inside macrophages (Goldman et al., 2000). Persistence of infection is accompanied by down regulation of both cellular and humoral immune responses (Goldman et al., 2000). Although latency represents an inability to clear the infection from the host, this state is an example of a successful acquired immune response because it contains the infection.

Passive Immunization and T-Cell Transfer Studies

A direct method for establishing the efficacy of acquired immune mechanisms in protection is to transfer either immune sera or sensitized T cells to a native host and then challenge it with the infectious agent. Historically, it has been difficult to demonstrate antibody-mediated protection against fungal infections by passive transfer of immune sera (reviewed by Casadevall [1995]). In recent years, various groups have shown that passive immunization with immune sera generated against defined antigens or with certain monoclonal antibodies (MAbs) can mediate protection against two fungal pathogens: *C. albicans* and *C. neoformans* (reviewed by Casadevall [1995] and Casadevall et al. [1998]). For both fungi, studies with MAbs have demonstrated that protective and nonprotective antibodies exist. Antibodies to the *C. neoformans* capsular glucuronoxylomannan are protective (reviewed by Vecchiarelli and Casadevall [1998]). For *C. neoformans* the structure-function relationship between protective and nonprotective MAbs has been extensively studied and both isotype and epitope specificities have been shown to contribute to antibody efficacy. For *C. albicans,* antibodies to cell wall mannan (Han and Cutler, 1995; Han et al., 2000), hsp90 (Matthews and Burnie, 1996; Matthews et al., 1991), and proteases (De Bernardis et al., 1997) have been shown to mediate protection. Interestingly, anti-idiotypic antibodies to an antibody that binds killer toxin can also mediate protection against *C. albicans* (Magliani et al., 1997; Polonelli et al., 1994). The emerging view is that humoral immune responses to fungal pathogens are complex and that, consequently, the efficacy of the response reflects the composition of protective and nonprotective antibodies.

In contrast to the difficulties encountered in consistently transferring protection by immune sera, adoptive transfer experiments using sensitized T cells have consistently been shown to confer protection against several fungal infections. Transfer of T cells from immunized mice to naive mice confers protection against *C. immitis* (Beaman et al., 1977), *H. capsulatum* (Allendoerfer et al., 1993), and *C.*

neoformans (Hill, 1992; Huffnagle et al., 1991a; Lim and Murphy, 1980). Both CD4$^+$ and CD8$^+$ T cells are important in protection against *C. immitis* (Cox and Magee, 1998), *C. neoformans* (Hill, 1992; Huffnagle et al., 1991b), and *H. capsulatum* (Allendoerfer et al., 1993; Deepe, 1994). In *C. neoformans* pulmonary infection, CD4$^+$ T cells appear necessary for recruitment of an inflammatory cell infiltrate whereas CD8$^+$ T cells may be involved in lysing infected macrophages (Huffnagle et al., 1991b). Other studies have suggested that CD8$^+$ T cells also contribute to recruiting inflammatory cells (Huffnagle et al., 1994). For *H. capsulatum*, adoptive transfer of CD4$^+$ T cells in mice protects against infection but CD8$^+$ T cells are also needed for clearance of infection (Allendoerfer et al., 1999; Deepe, 1994). Furthermore, *H. capsulatum* infection is associated with clonal amplification of the Vβ4$^+$ T-cell subset, which is essential for containment of the infection (Gomez et al., 1998).

MECHANISMS BY WHICH ACQUIRED IMMUNITY CONTRIBUTES TO PROTECTION

Humoral Immune Mechanisms

Antibody specificity and affinity are a function of the variable region, which is assembled by rearrangement of immunoglobulin variable gene elements. The isotype (constant region) determines the antibody pharmacokinetics, ability to activate complement, and the interaction with Fc receptors. The typical antibody response to fungal infections includes antibodies to protein and polysaccharide antigens of various isotypes. The potential of humoral immune mechanisms in host defense has been most extensively studied for *Candida albicans* and *Cryptococcus neoformans*. For both fungi, studies with MAbs indicate that protective and nonprotective antibodies exist (Pirofski and Casadevall, 1996; Casadevall, 1995; Han and Cutler, 1995). For *C. neoformans,* the antibody isotype has been shown to be a critical determinant of whether the antibody is effective (Mukherjee et al., 1992; Yuan et al., 1995, 1998; Sanford et al., 1990). Hence, negative conclusions regarding the existence of protective antibodies cannot be made on the bases of protection experiments using polyclonal serum preparations since the overall efficacy of such preparations reflects the antibody composition of the humoral response.

Passive administration of MAbs to *C. albicans* prolongs survival and reduces CFU in the organs (Han and Cutler, 1995, 1997; Han et al., 1999). Similarly, administration of MAb recognizing the capsular polysaccharide of *C. neoformans* has been shown to prolong survival and to reduce CFU in the organs in intraperitoneal (Mukherjee et al., 1992), intracerebral (Mukherjee et al., 1993), intravenous (Dromer et al., 1987), and intratracheal (Feldmesser and Casadevall, 1997) murine models of cryptococcosis. Although the exact mechanism of antibody-mediated protection is not understood, MAbs to *C. neoformans* are opsonic (Mukherjee et al., 1996), clear antigen (Lendvai et al., 1998), promote fungal killing by effector cells in vitro (Mukherjee et al., 1995b; Monari et al., 1999), alter cytokine production (Lendvai et al., 2000; Vecchiarelli et al., 1998c), enhance macrophage CD4 expression (Monari et al., 1999; Pietrella et al., 1998), enhance costimulatory molecule expression (Vecchiarelli et al., 1998a), and activate complement (Kozel et al., 1998a, 1998b; Vecchiarelli et al., 1998b). Administration of immunoglobulin G1 MAbs to mice prior to intratracheal infection results in enhanced granulomatous inflammation (Feldmesser and Casadevall, 1997). This observation suggests that antibody mediates protection against *C. neoformans* by enhancing the cell-mediated response (reviewed by Vecchiarelli and Casadevall [1998]).

Antibody to *C. neoformans* does not mediate antifungal effects directly. Instead, humoral immunity mediates protection by enhancing the efficacy of immune effector cells. This could be accomplished directly through opsonization or direct cells or indirectly through the removal of polysaccharide and alterations in the expression of cytokines and other immune molecules. However, antibody efficacy against *C. neoformans* appears to be critically dependent on the presence of T lymphocytes since protective antibodies are unable to prolong survival in mice that lack CD4$^+$ T cells (Yuan et al., 1997). This observation may reflect a requirement for T-cell activation of effector cells to kill ingested *C. neoformans* since administration of IFN-γ to CD4$^+$ T-cell-deficient mice restores antibody efficacy (Yuan et al., 1997).

Cell-Mediated Immunity

The importance of Th1-polarized responses for the control of fungal infections has been discussed above. T cells play a critical role in defense against fungi by producing cytokines which are essential for facilitating inflammatory responses and stimulating effector cell antifungal activity. Th1 cells produce IFN-γ and IL-2, which activate macrophages for antifungal activity. Cell-mediated immunity is believed to play a critical role in stimulating macrophages for phagocytic and fungicidal activity against *C. albicans*

(Vazquez-Torres and Balish, 1997). CD4$^+$ T cells promote the formation of multinucleated cells in the lung, which are essential for control of *C. neoformans* infection (Hill, 1992) and possibly other fungal pathogens. Furthermore, there is evidence that T cells can directly inhibit *C. albicans* and *C. neoformans*, suggesting the possibility that they function as direct antifungal effector cells (Levitz et al., 1995). Direct antimicrobial activity of T cells involves cell contact and the release of granules onto the fungal cell (Levitz et al., 1995). CD4$^+$ T cells are essential for antibody-mediated protective effects against *C. neoformans* (Yuan et al., 1997). Finally, T cells are important for the generation of antibody responses including isotype switching and possibly somatic mutation. In this regard, both isotype and somatic mutations have been shown to be important elements in antibody efficacy against *C. neoformans* (Mukherjee et al., 1995a; Yuan et al., 1998). For *H. capsulatum*, murine experiments have shown that CD4$^+$ T cells are the primary cells responsible for the production of IFN-γ in the lungs, and this cytokine is essential for the control of infection (Allendoerfer et al., 1999).

CAVEATS, PERSPECTIVES, AND SUMMARY

Given that an extensive body of evidence indicates an important role for acquired immunity in host defense against fungal pathogens, it is nevertheless important to consider certain caveats with regard to the studies performed in this field. Much of what we know about the relative efficacy of cellular and humoral immune responses is based on murine studies, but the degree to which observations made in mice are generalizable to other species including humans is unknown. Mice are often selected for studies of fungal infections because they are susceptible and relatively cheap and we have available many reagents for the study of immunological phenomena. The experience with *C. neoformans* studies in mice provides an illustration of the limitations of murine studies. Analysis of the relative contribution of cellular and humoral immune responses in mice has provided overwhelming evidence that control of infection relies on cellular immunity (reviewed by Casadevall and Perfect [1998]). However, this information has been gathered in a species that seldom mounts significant antibody responses to *C. neoformans* polysaccharide during infection (reviewed by Casadevall and Perfect [1998]). This in turn raises a type of circular logic which can be stated as follows: cellular immunity must be the essential mechanism for host defense because humoral immunity is not effective, even though significant humoral responses against the polysaccharide are seldom made. Interestingly, when humoral immunity is provided in mice by polysaccharide conjugate vaccination (Devi, 1996) or passive antibody administration (Dromer et al., 1987), then it is possible to demonstrate that antibody contributes to host defense. In contrast to mice, rats and rabbits are both relatively resistant to *C. neoformans* infection and mount both strong cellular and humoral responses (Goldman et al., 1994; Hobbs et al., 1990). Humans also appear to be highly resistant, given the paucity of cryptococcal infections in normal individuals, and humans mount both cellular and humoral responses (Bennett, 1981; DeShaw and Pirofski, 1995). Hence, the conclusions made in the mouse with regard to the relative efficacy of the two arms of the acquired immune response may not be generally applicable.

Many of our notions of the effective immune response are derived from experiments in mice which have been made deficient in some type of cytokine or cell type by administration of specific serum or by gene disruption technology (knockout mice). With regard to antibody-mediated depletion experiments, it is important to note that such experiments lead to the formation of antigen-antibody complexes which have protean effects on the immune system through their effects on immune cells. For example, antigen-antibody complexes can elicit IL-10 (Tripp et al., 1995) and various chemokines (Lendvai et al., 2000). Hence, neutralization experiments are likely to change more variables than causing a simple depletion of the molecule or cell in question. Routine controls for such experiments involve the administration of isotype-matched irrelevant antibody, but this cannot control for the formation of antigen-antibody complexes and their secondary effects through stimulation of Fc receptors. Experiments in gene-deficient (knockout) mice avoid the problem of depletion experiments but introduce a new concern: immune systems that develop in the absence of a particular cell type or immunological molecule may not be comparable to those of normal mice.

The problems with the relevance of mouse models, the controls for depletion experiments, and the ontogeny of the immune system in knockout mice raise the question of what approach should be taken to study the role of acquired immunity. It is my view that currently we have no choice but to rely on existing systems of experimentation but care should be taken whenever possible to obtain independent confirmation for an effect. Hence, it is probably wise to confirm results from depletion experiments in knockout mice and vice versa. Furthermore, whenever possible, reversal of the effect by complementation of the deficit should be attempted. Lastly, conclusions made in mice should be validated in other species.

Several themes emerge from reviewing the literature: (i) fungal infections invariably induce acquired immunity in the form of delayed-type hypersensitivity and humoral responses; (ii) T-cell function is critical for the control of most if not all fungal infections; (iii) Th1 responses are generally associated with protection against fungal infections; (iv) demonstrating a role for humoral immunity by attempting to show that B-cell-deficient mice are more susceptible or by transferring immune sera is difficult; and (v) passive administration of certain MAbs protects against some fungal pathogens. These observations in turn raise the following questions for future investigation. What is the relationship between delayed hypersensitivity to fungal antigens and protection against infection? Why is it so difficult to protect against fungi with immune sera? What is the nature of the fungal antigens that elicit protective immunity? What is the structure-function relationship between protective and nonprotective antibodies? What are the mechanisms by which humoral immunity and cellular immunity cooperate in protection against fungal pathogens? Rapid progress is being made in the field of medical mycology, and there is optimism that answers to these questions will be forthcoming in the future. In the meantime, the difficulty in treating fungal infections has stimulated a search for vaccines against fungal pathogens, and several candidate vaccines are in advanced preclinical development (Deepe, 1997; Dixon et al., 1998).

In summary, there is overwhelming evidence that acquired immune responses are essential for the control and eradication of fungal infections. For most fungi, there is conclusive evidence that cellular immunity is essential for host defense. With regard to cell-mediated immunity, it is remarkable how all lines of evidence are consistent and complementary. For example, the importance of cell-mediated immunity can be deduced from clinical experience, T-cell transfer studies, T-cell depletion studies, and the analysis of cytokine expression. The evidence for an important contribution for humoral immunity is less consistent. For two fungi, *Candida albicans* and *Cryptococcus neoformans,* the ability of antibody to contribute to host defense has also been demonstrated by passive-transfer experiments using MAbs. However, efforts to establish the efficacy of humoral immunity by transfer of immune sera or attempts to associate deficits in antibody production with enhanced susceptibility have been less rewarding. Nevertheless, there is sufficient evidence to state that both the cellular and humoral arms of acquired immune responses can make important contributions to host protection against fungal pathogens.

REFERENCES

Aguirre, K., E. A. Havell, G. W. Gibson, and L. L. Johnson. 1995. Role of tumor necrosis factor and gamma interferon in acquired resistance to *Cryptococcus neoformans* in the central nervous system of mice. *Infect. Immun.* 63:1725–1731.

Aguirre, K. M., and L. L. Johnson. 1997. A role for B cells in resistance to *Cryptococcus neoformans* in mice. *Infect. Immun.* 65:525–530.

Allen, J. E., and R. M. Maizels. 1997. Th1-Th2: reliable paradigm or dangerous dogma. *Immunol. Today* 18:387–392.

Allendoerfer, R., G. D. Brunner, and G. S. Deepe, Jr. 1999. Complex requirements for nascent and memory immunity in pulmonary histoplasmosis. *J. Immunol.* 162:7389–7396.

Allendoerfer, R., and G. S. Deepe, Jr. 1998. Blockade of endogenous TNF-alpha exacerbates primary and secondary pulmonary histoplasmosis by differential mechanisms. *J. Immunol.* 160: 6072–6082.

Allendoerfer, R., D. M. Magee, G. S. Deepe, Jr., and J. R. Graybill. 1993. Transfer of protective immunity in murine histoplasmosis by a CD4$^+$ T-cell clone. *Infect. Immun.* 61:714–718.

Ashman, R. B. 1997. Genetic determination of susceptibility and resistance in the pathogenesis of *Candida albicans* infection. *FEMS Immunol. Med. Microbiol.* 19:183–189.

Ashman, R. B., A. Fulurija, and J. M. Papadimitriou. 1999. Both CD4$^+$ and CD8$^+$ lymphocytes reduce the severity of tissue lesions in murine systemic cadidiasis, and CD4$^+$ cells also demonstrate strain-specific immunopathological effects. *Microbiology* 145:1631–1640.

Ashman, R. B., and J. M. Papadimitriou. 1995. Production and function of cytokines in natureal and acquired immunity to *Candida albicans* infection. *Microbiol. Rev.* 59:646–672.

Balish, E., F. A. Vazquez-Torres, J. Jones-Carson, R. D. Wagner, and T. Warner. 1996. Importance of β_2-microglobulin in murine resistance to mucosal and systemic candidiasis. *Infect. Immun.* 64:5092–5097.

Balish, E., R. D. Wagner, A. Vazquez-Torres, C. Pierson, and T. Warner. 1998. Candidiasis in interferon-gamma knockout (IFN-gamma-/-) mice. *J. Infect. Dis.* 178:478–487.

Beaman, L., D. Pappagianis, and E. Benjamini. 1977. Significance of T cells in resistance to experimental murine coccidioidomycosis. *Infect. Immun.* 17:580–585.

Bennett, J. E. 1981. Cryptococcal skin test antigen: preparation variables and characterization. *Infect. Immun.* 32:373–380.

Calich, V. L., C. A. Vaz, and E. Burger. 1998. Immunity to *Paracoccidioides brasiliensis* infection. *Res. Immunol.* 149:407–417.

Casadevall, A. 1995. Antibody immunity and invasive fungal infections. *Infect. Immun.* 63:4211–4218.

Casadevall, A., A. Cassone, F. Bistoni, J. E. Cutler, W. Magliani, J. W. Murphy, L. Polonelli, and L. Romani. 1998. Antibody and/or cell-mediated immunity, protective mechanisms in fungal disease: an ongoing dilemma or an unnecessary dispute? *Med. Mycol.* 36:95–105.

Casadevall, A., J. Mukherjee, S. J. N. Devi, R. Schneerson, J. B. Robbins, and M. D. Scharff. 1992. Antibodies elicited by a *Cryptococcus neoformans* glucuronoxylomannan-tetanus toxoid conjugate vaccine have the same specificity as those elicited in infection. *J. Infect. Dis.* 65:1086–1093.

Casadevall, A., and J. R. Perfect. 1998. *Cryptococcus neoformans.* American Society for Microbiology. Washington, D.C.

Casadevall, A., and M. D. Scharff. 1991. The mouse antibody response to infection with *Cryptococcus neoformans*: V$_H$ and V$_L$ usage in polysaccharide binding antibodies. *J. Exp. Med.* 174: 151–160.

Cenci, E., A. Mencacci, G. Del Sero, A. Bacci, C. Montagnoli, C. F. d'Ostiani, P. Mosci, M. Bachmann, F. Bistoni, M. Kopf, and L. Romani. 1999. Interleukin-4 causes susceptibility to invasive pulmonary aspergillosis through suppression of protective type I responses. *J. Infect. Dis.* 180:1957–1968.

Chen, L.-C., D. L. Goldman, T. L. Doering, L. Pirofski, and A. Casadevall. 1999. Antibody response to *Cryptococcus neoformans* proteins in rodents and humans. *Infect. Immun.* 67: 2218–2224.

Cox, R. A., and D. M. Magee. 1998. Protective immunity in coccidioidomycosis. *Res. Immunol.* 148:417–428.

Currie, B. P., and A. Casadevall. 1994. Estimation of the prevalence of cryptococcal infection among HIV infected individuals in New York City. *Clin. Infect. Dis.* 19:1029–1033.

De Bernardis, F., M. Boccanera, D. Adriani, E. Spreghini, G. Santoni, and A. Cassone. 1997. Protective role of antimannan and anti-aspartyl proteinase antibodies in an experimental model of *Candida albicans* vaginitis in rats. *Infect. Immun.* 65: 3399–3405.

Decken, K., G. Kohler, K. Palmer-Lehmann, A. Wunderlin, F. Mattner, J. Magram, M. K. Gately, and G. Alber. 1998. Interleukin-12 is essential for a protective Th1 response in mice infected with *Cryptococcus neoformans.* *Infect. Immun.* 66: 4994–5000.

Deepe, G. S., Jr. 1994. Role of CD8$^+$ T cells in host resistance to systemic infection with *Histoplasma capsulatum* in mice. *J. Immunol.* 152:3491–3500.

Deepe, G. S., Jr. 1997. Prospects for the development of fungal vaccines. *Clin. Microbiol. Rev.* 10:585–596.

Deepe, G. S., Jr., and W. E. Bullock. 1992. Histoplasmosis. A granulomatous inflammatory response, p. 943–958. *In* J. I. Gallin, I. M. Goldstein, and R. Snyderman (ed.), *Inflammation: Basic Principles and Clinical Correlates.* Raven Press, New York, N.Y.

Deepe, G. S., Jr., and R. A. Seder. 1998. Molecular and cellular determinants of immunity to *Histoplasma capsulatum.* *Res. Immunol.* 149:397–406.

DeShaw, M., and L.-A. Pirofski. 1995. Antibodies to the *Cryptococcus neoformans* capsular glucuronoxylomannan are ubiquitous in serum from HIV+ and HIV− individuals. *Clin. Exp. Immunol.* 99:425–432.

Devi, S. J. N. 1996. Preclinical efficacy of a glucuronoxylomannan-tetanus toxoid conjugate vaccine of *Cryptococcus neoformans* in a murine model. *Vaccine* 14:841–842.

Devi, S. J. N., R. Schneerson, W. Egan, T. J. Ulrich, D. Bryla, J. B. Robbins, and J. E. Bennett. 1991. *Cryptococcus neoformans* serotype A glucuronoxylomannan-protein conjugate vaccines: synthesis, characterization, and immunogenicity. *Infect. Immun.* 59:3700–3707.

Di Salvo, A. F. 2000. *Blastomyces dermatitidis*, p. 337–355. *In* L. Ajello and R. J. Hay (ed.), *Topley & Wilson's Microbiology and Microbial Infections.* Edward Arnold, London, United Kingdom.

Dixon, D. M., A. Casadevall, B. Klein, L. R. Travassos, and G. Deepe. 1998. Development of vaccines and their use in the prevention of fungal infections. *Med. Mycol.* 36(Suppl.):57–67.

Dixon, D. M., M. M. McNeil, M. L. Cohen, B. G. Gellin, and J. R. LaMontagne. 1996. Fungal infections. A growing threat. *Public Health Rep.* 111:226–235.

Dromer, F., J. Charreire, A. Contrepois, C. Carbon, and P. Yeni. 1987. Protection of mice against experimental cryptococcosis by anti-*Cryptococcus neoformans* monoclonal antibody. *Infect. Immun.* 55:749–752.

Feldmesser, M., and A. Casadevall. 1997. Effect of serum IgG1 against murine pulmonary infection with *Cryptococcus neoformans*. *J. Immunol.* **158**:790–799.

Fidel, P. L., Jr., and J. D. Sobel. 1998. Protective immunity in experimental *Candida* vaginitis. *Res. Immunol.* **149**:361–373.

Fidel, P. L., Jr., J. A. Vazquez, and J. D. Sobel. 1999. *Candida glabrata:* review of epidemiology, pathogenesis, and clinical disease with comparison to *C. albicans*. *Clin. Microbiol. Rev.* **12**:80–96.

Fierer, J., L. Walls, L. Eckmann, T. Yamamoto, and T. N. Kirkland. 1998. Importance of interleukin-10 in genetic susceptibility of mice to *Coccidioides immitis*. *Infect. Immun.* **66**:4397–4402.

Fleuridor, R., R. H. Lyles, and L. Pirofski. 1999. Quantitative and qualitative differences in the serum antibody profiles of human immunodeficiency virus-infected persons with and without *Cryptococcus neoformans* meningitis. *J. Infect. Dis.* **180**:1526–1535.

Fresno, M., M. Kopf, and L. Rivas. 1997. Cytokines and infectious diseases. *Immunol. Today* **18**:56–58.

Goldman, D., S. C. Lee, and A. Casadevall. 1994. Pathogenesis of pulmonary *Cryptococcus neoformans* infection in the rat. *Infect. Immun.* **62**:4755–4761.

Goldman, D. L., S. C. Lee, A. J. Mednic, L. Montell, and A. Casadevall, 2000. Persistent *Cryptococcus neoformans* infection in the rat is associated with intracellular parasitism, decreased inducible nitric oxide synthase expression, and altered antibody responsiveness. *Infect. Immun.* **68**:832–838.

Gomez, F. J., R. Allendoerfer, and G. S. Deepe, Jr. 1995. Vaccination with recombinant heat shock protein 60 from *Histoplasma capsulatum* protects mice against pulmonary histoplasmosis. *Infect. Immun.* **63**:2587–2595.

Gomez, F. J., J. A. Cain, R. Gibbons, R. Allendoerfer, and G. S. Deepe, Jr. 1998. Vbeta4(+) T cells promote clearance of infection in murine pulmonary histoplasmosis. *J. Clin. Investig.* **102**:984–995.

Grunig, G., D. B. Corry, M. W. Leach, B. W. Seymour, V. P. Kurup, and D. M. Rennick. 1997. Interleukin-10 is a natural suppressor of cytokine production and inflammation in a murine model of allergic bronchopulmonary aspergillosis. *J. Exp. Med.* **185**:1089–1099.

Han, Y., and J. E. Cutler. 1995. Antibody response that protects against disseminated candidiasis. *Infect. Immun.* **63**:2714–2719.

Han, Y., and J. E. Cutler. 1997. Assessment of a mouse model of neutropenia and the effect of an anti-candidiasis monoclonal antibody in these animals. *J. Infect. Dis.* **175**:1169–1175.

Han, Y., M. H. Riesselman, and J. E. Cutler, 2000. Protection against candidiasis by an immunoglobulin G3 (IgG3) monoclonal antibody specific for the same mannotriose as an IgM protective antibody. *Infect. Immun.* **68**:1649–1654.

Han, Y., M. A. Ulrich, and J. E. Cutler. 1999. *Candida albicans* mannan extract-protein conjugates induce a protective immune response against experimental candidiasis. *J. Infect. Dis.* **179**:1477–1484.

Hill, J. O. 1992. CD4+ T cells cause multinucleated giant cells to form around *Cryptococcus neoformans* and confine the yeast within the primary site of infection in the respiratory tract. *J. Exp. Med.* **175**:1685–1695.

Hoag, K. A., M. F. Lipscomb, A. A. Izzo, and N. E. Street. 1997. IL-12 and IFN-gamma are required for initiating the protective Th1 response to pulmonary cryptococcosis in resistant C.B-17 mice. *Am. J. Respir. Cell Mol. Biol.* **17**:733–739.

Hoag, K. A., N. E. Street, G. B. Huffnagle, and M. F. Lipscomb. 1995. Early cytokine production in pulmonary *Cryptococcus neoformans* infections distinguishes susceptible and resistant mice. *Am. J. Respir. Cell Mol. Biol.* **13**:487–495.

Hobbs, M. M., J. R. Perfect, D. L. Granger, and D. T. Durack. 1990. Opsonic activity of cerebrospinal fluid in experimental cryptococcal meningitis. *Infect. Immun.* **58**:2115–2119.

Hogan, L. H., S. M. Levitz, and B. S. Klein. 1996. Virulence factors of medically important fungi. *Clin. Microbiol. Rev.* **9**:469–488.

Huffnagle, G. B.. 1996. Role of cytokines in T cell immunity to a pulmonary *Cryptococcus neoformans* infection. *Biol. Signals* **5**:215–222.

Huffnagle, G. B., M. F. Lipscomb, J. A. Lovchik, K. A. Hoag, and N. E. Street. 1994. The role of CD4+ and CD8+ T-cells in protective inflammatory response to a pulmonary cryptococcal infection. *J. Leukoc. Biol.* **55**:35–42.

Huffnagle, G. B., J. L. Yates, and M. F. Lipscomb. 1991a. T cell-mediated immunity in the lung: a *Cryptococcus neoformans* pulmonary infection model using SCID and athymic nude mice. *Infect. Immun.* **59**:1423–1433.

Huffnagle, G. B., J. L. Yates, and M. F. Lipscomb. 1991b. Immunity to pulmonary *Cryptococcus neoformans* infection requires both CD4+ and CD8+ T cells. *J. Exp. Med.* **173**:793–800.

Hung, C. Y., N. M. Ampel, L. Christian, K. R. Seshan, and G. T. Cole, 2000. A major cell surface antigen of *Coccidioides immitis* which elicits both humoral and cellular immune responses. *Infect. Immun.* **68**:584–593.

Jiang, C., D. M. Magee, T. N. Quitugua, and R. A. Cox. 1999. Genetic vaccination against *Coccidioides immitis:* comparison of vaccine efficacy of recombinant antigen 2 and antigen 2 cDNA. *Infect. Immun.* **67**:630–635.

Kawakami, K., Q. M. Hossain, T. Zhang, Y. Koguchi, Q. Xie, M. Kurimoto, and A. Saito. 1999a. Interleukin-4 weakens host resistance to pulmonary and disseminated cryptococcal infection caused by combined treatment with interferon-gamma-inducing cytokines. *Cell Immunol.* **197**:55–61.

Kawakami, K., Y. Koguchi, M. H. Qureshi, Y. Kinjo, S. Yara, A. Miyazato, M. Kurimoto, K. Takeda, S. Akira, and A. Saito, 2000. Reduced host resistance and Th1 response to *Cryptococcus neoformans* in interleukin-18 deficient mice. *FEMS Microbiol. Lett.* **186**:121–126.

Kawakami, K., M. H. Qureshi, T. Zhang, Y. Koguchi, K. Shibuya, S. Naoe, and A. Saito. 1999b. Interferon-gamma (IFN-gamma)-dependent protection and synthesis of chemoattractants for mononuclear leucocytes caused by IL-12 in the lungs of mice infected with *Cryptococcus neoformans*. *Clin. Exp. Immunol.* **117**:113–122.

Kirkland, T. N., F. Finley, K. I. Orsborn, and J. N. Galgiani. 1998a. Evaluation of the proline-rich antigen of *Coccidioides immitis* as a vaccine candidate in mice. *Infect. Immun.* **66**:3519–3522.

Kirkland, T. N., P. W. Thomas, F. Finley, and G. T. Cole. 1998b. Immunogenicity of a 48-kilodalton recombinant T-cell-reactive protein of *Coccidioides immitis*. *Infect. Immun.* **66**:424–431.

Klein, B. S., P. M. Sondel, and J. M. Jones. 1992. WI-1, a novel 120-kilodalton surface protein on *Blastomyces dermatitidis* yeast cells, is a target antigen of cell-mediated immunity in human blastomycosis. *Infect. Immun.* **60**:4291–4300.

Kong, Y., and H. B. Levine. 1967. Experimentally induced immunity in the mycoses. *Bacteriol. Rev.* **31**:35–53.

Kozel, T. R., B. C. H. deJong, M. M. Grinsell, R. S. MacGill, and K. K. Wall. 1998a. Characterization of anti-capsular monoclonal antibodies that regulate activation of the complement system by *Cryptococcus neoformans*. *Infect. Immun.* **66**:1538–1546.

Kozel, T. R., R. S. MacGill, and K. K. Wall. 1998b. Bivalency is required for anticapsular monoclonal antibodies to optimally suppress activation of the alternative complement pathway by the *Cryptococcus neoformans* capsule. *Infect. Immun.* **66:** 1547–1553.

Latge, J. P. 1999. *Aspergillus fumigatus* and aspergillosis. *Clin. Microbiol. Rev.* **12:**310–350.

Lendvai, N., A. Casadevall, Z. Liang, D. L. Goldman, J. Mukherjee, and L. Zuckier. 1998. Effect of immune mechanisms on the pharmacokinetics and organ distribution of cryptococcal polysaccharide. *J. Infect. Dis.* **177:**1647–1659.

Lendvai, N., X. Qu, W. Hsueh, and A. Casadevall, 2000. Mechanism for the isotype dependence of antibody-mediated toxicity in *Cryptococcus neoformans* infected mice. *J. Immunol.* **164:** 4367–4374.

Levitz, S. M., H. L. Mathews, and J. W. Murphy. 1995. Direct antimicrobial activity by T cells. *Immunol. Today* **16:**387–391.

Lim, T. S., and J. W. Murphy. 1980. Transfer of immunity to cryptococcosis by T-enriched splenic lymphocytes from *Cryptococcus neoformans*-sensitized mice. *Infect. Immun.* **30:**5–11.

Lipscomb, M. F., G. B. Huffnagle, J. A. Lovchik, C. R. Lyons, A. M. Pollard, and J. L. Yates. 1993. The role of T lymphocytes in pulmonary microbial defense mechanisms. *Arch. Pathol. Lab. Med.* **117:**1225–1232.

Lovchik, J. A., C. R. Lyons, and M. F. Lipscomb. 1995. A role for gamma interferon-induced nitric oxide in pulmonary clearance of *Cryptococcus neoformans*. *Am. J. Respir. Cell Mol. Biol.* **13:**116–124.

Lovchik, J. A., J. A. Wilder, G. B. Huffnagle, R. Riblet, C. R. Lyons, and M. F. Lipscomb. 1999. Ig heavy chain complex-linked genes influence the immune response in a murine cryptococcal infection. *J. Immunol.* **163:**3907–3913.

Magee, D. M., and R. A. Cox. 1995. Roles of gamma interferon and interleukin-4 in genetically determined resistance to *Coccidioides immitis*. *Infect. Immun.* **63:**3514–3519.

Magee, D. M., and R. A. Cox. 1996. Interleukin-12 regulation of host defenses against *Coccidioides immitis*. *Infect. Immun.* **64:** 3609–3613.

Magliani, W., S. Conti, F. De Bernardis, M. Gerloni, D. Bertolotti, P. Mozzoni, A. Cassone, and L. Polonelli. 1997. Therapeutic potential of antiidiotypic single chain antibodies with yeast killer toxin activity. *Nat. Biotechnol.* **15:**155–158.

Marino, M. W., A. Dunn, D. Grail, M. Inglese, Y. Noguchi, E. Richards, A. Jungbluth, H. Wada, M. Moore, B. Williamson, S. Basu, and L. J. Old. 1997. Characterization of tumor necrosis factor-deficient mice. *Proc. Natl. Acad. Sci. USA* **94:**8093–8098.

Matthews, R., and J. Burnie. 1998. Mycoserology, p. 89–109. *In* L. Ajello and R. J. Hay (ed.), *Topley & Wilson's Microbiology and Microbial Infections*, vol. 4. Edward Arnold, London, United Kingdom.

Matthews, R. C., and J. P. Burnie. 1996. Antibodies and *Candida*: potential therapeutics. *Trends Microbiol.* **4:**354–358.

Matthews, R. C., J. P. Burnie, D. Howat, T. Rowland, and F. Walton. 1991. Autoantibody to heat shock protein 90 can mediate protection against systemic candidosis. *Immunology* **74:** 20–24.

Monari, C., A. Casadevall, C. Retini, F. Baldelli, F. Bistoni, and A. Vecchiarelli. 1999. Antibody to capsular polysaccharide enhances the function of neutrophils from patients with AIDS against *Cryptococcus neoformans*. *AIDS* **13:**653–660.

Monga, D. P., R. Kumar, L. N. Mahapatra, and A. N. Malaviya. 1979. Experimental cryptococcosis in normal and B-cell deficient mice. *Infect. Immun.* **26:**1–3.

Mukherjee, J., G. Nussbaum, M. D. Scharff, and A. Casadevall. 1995a. Protective and non-protective monoclonal antibodies to *Cryptococcus neoformans* originating from one B-cell. *J. Exp. Med.* **181:**405–409.

Mukherjee, J., L. Pirofski, M. D. Scharff, and A. Casadevall. 1993. Antibody mediated protection in mice with lethal intracerebral

Cryptococcus neoformans infection. *Proc. Natl. Acad. Sci. USA* **90:**3636–3640.

Mukherjee, J., M. D. Scharff, and A. Casadevall. 1992. Protective murine monoclonal antibodies to *Cryptococcus neoformans*. *Infect. Immun.* **60:**4534–4541.

Mukherjee, S., M. Feldmesser, and A. Casadevall. 1996. J774 murine macrophage-like cell interactions with *Cryptococcus neoformans* in the presence and absence of opsonins. *J. Infect. Dis.* **173:**1222–1231.

Mukherjee, S., S. C. Lee, and A. Casadevall. 1995b. Antibodies to *Cryptococcus neoformans* glucuronoxylomannan enhance antifungal activity of murine macrophages. *Infect. Immun.* **63:** 573–579.

Murphy, J. W. 1991. Mechanisms of natural resistance to human pathogenic fungi. *Annu. Rev. Microbiol.* **45:**509–538.

Murphy, J. W. 1998. Protective cell-mediated immunity against *Cryptococcus neoformans*. *Res. Immunol.* **149:**373–386.

Nagai, H., J. Guo, H. Choi, and V. Kurup. 1995. Interferon-gamma and tumor necrosis factor-alpha protect mice from invasive aspergillosis. *J. Infect. Dis.* **172:**1554–1560.

Pietrella, D., C. Monari, C. Retini, B. Palazzetti, T. R. Kozel, and A. Vecchiarelli. 1998. *Cryptococcus neoformans* and *Candida albicans* regulate CD4 expression on human monocytes. *J. Infect. Dis.* **178:**1464–1471.

Pirofski, L., and A. Casadevall. 1996. Antibody immunity to *Cryptococcus neoformans*: paradigm for antibody immunity to the fungi? *Zentbl. Bakteriol.* **284:**475–495.

Polonelli, L., F. De Bernardis, M. Boccanera, M. Gerloni, G. Morace, W. Magliani, C. Chezzi, and A. Cassone. 1994. Idiotypic intravaginal vaccination to protect against candidal vaginitis by secretory, yeast killer toxin-like anti-idiotypic antibodies. *J. Immunol.* **152:**3175–3181.

Qian, Q., and J. E. Cutler. 1997. Gamma interferon is not essential in host defense against disseminated candidiasis in mice. *Infect. Immun.* **65:**1748–1753.

Romagnani, S. 1996. Understanding the role of the Th1/Th2 cells in infection. *Trends Microbiol.* **4:**470–473.

Romani, L., E. Cenci, A. Mencacci, R. Spaccapelo, U. Grohmann, P. Puccetti, and F. Bistoni. 1992a. Gamma interferon modifies CD4+ subset expression in murine candidiasis. *Infect. Immun.* **60:**4950–4952.

Romani, L., and D. H. Howard. 1995. Mechanisms of resistance to fungal infections. *Curr. Opin. Immunol.* **7:**517–523.

Romani, L., A. Mencacci, U. Grohmann, S. Mocci, P. Mosci, P. Puccetti, and F. Bistoni. 1992b. Neutralizing antibody to interleukin 4 induces systemic protection and T helper type 1-associated immunity in murine candidiasis. *J. Exp. Med.* **176:** 19–25.

Salvin, S. B. 1959. Current concepts of diagnostic serology and skin hypersensitivity in the mycoses. *Am. J. Med.* **27:**97–114.

Sanford, J. E., D. M. Lupan, A. M. Schlagetter, and T. R. Kozel. 1990. Passive immunization against *Cryptococcus neoformans* with an isotype-switch family of monoclonal antibodies reactive with cryptococcal polysaccharide. *Infect. Immun.* **58:** 1919–1923.

Segal, E. 1987. Vaccines against fungal infections. *Crit. Rev. Microbiol.* **14:**229–273.

Tewari, R., L. J. Wheat, and L. Ajello. 1998. Agents of histoplasmosis, p. 373–393. *In* L. Ajello and R. J. Hay (ed.), *Topley & Wilson's Microbiology and Microbial Infections*, vol. 4. Edward Arnold, London, United Kingdom.

Tripp, C. S., K. P. Beckerman, and E. R. Unanue. 1995. Immune complexes inhibit antimicrobial responses through interleukin-10 production. *J. Clin. Investig.* **95:**1628–1694.

van Enckevort, F. H., M. G. Netea, A. R. Hermus, C. G. Sweep, J. F. Meis, J. W. Van der Meer, and B. J. Kullberg. 1999. Increased susceptibility to systemic candidiasis in interleukin-6 deficient mice. *Med. Mycol.* **37:**419–426.

Vazquez-Torres, A., and E. Balish. 1997. Macrophages in resistance to candidiasis. *Microbiol. Mol. Biol. Rev.* **61:**170–192.

Vazquez-Torres, A., J. Jones-Carson, R. D. Wagner, T. Warner, and E. Balish. 1999. Early resistance of interleukin-10 knockout mice to acute systemic candidiasis. *Infect. Immun.* **67:**670–674.

Vecchiarelli, A., and A. Casadevall. 1998. Antibody-mediated effects against *Cryptococcus neoformans:* evidence for interdependency and collaboration between humoral and cellular immunity. *Res. Immunol.* **149:**321–333.

Vecchiarelli, A., C. Monari, C. Retini, D. Pietrella, B. Palazzetti, L. Pitzurra, and A. Casadevall. 1998a. *Cryptococcus neoformans* differently regulates B7-1 (CD80) and B7-2 (CD86) expression on human monocytes. *Eur. J. Immunol.* **28:**114–121.

Vecchiarelli, A., C. Retini, A. Casadevall, C. Monari, D. Pietrella, and T. R. Kozel. 1998b. Involvement of C3a and C5a in Interleukin-8 secretion by human polymorphonuclear cells in response to capsular polysaccharide material of *Cryptococcus neoformans*. *Infect. Immun.* **66:**4324–4330.

Vecchiarelli, A., C. Retini, C. Monari, and A. Casadevall. 1998c. Specific antibody to *Cryptococcus neoformans* alters human leukocyte cytokine synthesis and promotes T cell proliferation. *Infect. Immun.* **66:**1244–1247.

Wagner, R. D., A. Vazquez-Torres, J. Jones-Carson, T. Warner, and E. Balish. 1996. B cell knockout mice are resistant to mucosal and systemic candidiasis of endogenous origin but susceptible to experimental systemic candidiasis. *J. Infect. Dis.* **174:**589–597.

Wheat, J. 1995. Endemic mycoses in AIDS: a clinical review. *Clin. Microbiol. Rev.* **8:**146–159.

Wuthrich, M., W. L. Chang, and B. S. Klein. 1998. Immunogenicity and protective efficacy of the WI-1 adhesin of *Blastomyces dermatitidis*. *Infect. Immun.* **66:**5443–5449.

Yang, M. C., D. M. Magee, and R. A. Cox. 1997. Mapping of a *Coccidioides immitis*-specific epitope that reacts with complement-fixing antibody. *Infect. Immun.* **65:**4068–4074.

Yuan, R., A. Casadevall, J. Oh, and M. D. Scharff. 1997. T cells cooperate with passive antibody to modify *Cryptococcus neoformans* infection in mice. *Proc. Natl. Acad. Sci. USA* **94:**2483–2488.

Yuan, R., A. Casadevall, G. Spira, and M. D. Scharff. 1995. Isotype switching from IgG3 to IgG1 converts a non-protective murine antibody to *C. neoformans* into a protective antibody. *J. Immunol.* **154:**1810–1816.

Yuan, R., G. Spira, J. Oh, M. Paizi, A. Casadevall, and M. D. Scharff. 1998. Isotype switching increases antibody protective efficacy to *Cryptococcus neoformans* infection in mice. *Infect. Immun.* **66:**1057–1062.

Zhou, P., and R. A. Seder. 1998. CD40 ligand is not essential for induction of type 1 cytokine responses or protective immunity after primary or secondary infection with histoplasma capsulatum. *J. Exp. Med.* **187:**1315–1324.

Zhou, P., M. C. Sieve, J. Bennett, K. J. Kwon-Chung, R. P. Tewari, R. T. Gazzinelli, A. Sher, and R. A. Seder. 1995. IL-12 prevents mortality in mice infected with *Histoplasma capsulatum* through induction of IFN-gamma. *J. Immunol.* **155:**785–795.

Zhu, Y., V. Tryon, D. M. Magee, and R. A. Cox. 1997. Identification of a *Coccidioides immitis* antigen 2 domain that expresses B-cell-reactive epitopes. *Infect. Immun.* **65:**3376–3380.

Immunology of Infectious Diseases
Edited by S. H. E. Kaufmann, A. Sher, and R. Ahmed
© 2002 ASM Press, Washington, D.C.

Chapter 17

Adaptive Immune Effector Mechanisms against Intracellular Protozoa and Gut-Dwelling Nematodes

PHILLIP SCOTT AND RICHARD K. GRENCIS

The immune response to pathogens is initiated in most cases because pathogens contain conserved motifs not found in higher eukaryotes, which are recognized by pattern recognition receptors on a variety of cells (Medzhitov and Janeway, 2000). Ligation of these receptors leads to cell activation and sets into motion a series of innate immune responses. These early responses play an important role in alerting the host to the presence of an invading organism and in shaping the subsequent adaptive immune response. However, they rarely provide long-term control of parasitic infections. Rather, control of these diseases depends on the development and maintenance of specific effector mechanisms, which requires recognition of pathogen-derived epitopes by B and T cells and selection of the appropriate types of T cells to orchestrate such effector responses. The effector mechanisms required for protection against any given infection are quite varied and will depend on specific characteristics of the parasite, such as the location of the parasites within the host, the number of life cycle stages within the host, and the evasion strategies developed by the parasite.

Immunologic effector mechanisms have historically been divided into two categories, termed cell-mediated immunity and humoral immunity. With advances in our understanding of the cellular and molecular basis of immune responses, we can now separate effector responses into two slightly different categories based on the CD4$^+$ T cells that regulate them. The two major T-cell subsets, termed Th1 and Th2, produce a large number of cytokines but are defined by a smaller, unique set. Thus, CD4$^+$ Th1 cells produce interleukin-2 (IL-2) and gamma interferon (IFN-γ), while CD4$^+$ Th2 cells produce IL-4,

IL-5, IL-10, and IL-13 (Mosmann et al., 1986). The responses mediated by these cells are referred to as type 1 and type 2 responses, respectively. Type 1 responses are associated with the activation of cells by IFN-γ, the induction of cytolytic activity by CD8$^+$ T cells, and the production of complement-fixing antibodies. Type 2 responses are associated with high levels of neutralizing and cell-bound antibodies, mast cell activation, eosinophilia, and suppression of type 1 responses. An examination of the immune responses associated with parasitism indicates that multiple effector mechanisms—at times including both type 1 and type 2 responses—may be used to eliminate the same parasite. These different effector responses may be operating at the same time, during different stages of the life cycle, or in different locations. Understanding the complexity of effector mechanisms elicited during a parasitic infection and determining which of them are crucial for control are essential in the development of effective therapies for parasitic diseases.

In this chapter, we will cover the acquired immune responses to two types of parasites. The first is the immune response associated with intracellular protozoa, and our principal examples will be *Leishmania, Toxoplasma,* and *Trypanosoma cruzi.* Although these organisms can be found outside cells, they spend a substantial portion of their life in the mammalian host within cells, and type 1 immune responses are crucial in their control. We will then discuss the immune responses associated with control of helminth infections, particularly focusing on gut-dwelling nematodes. Because of their location and perhaps their size, the host has developed a different

Phillip Scott • Department of Pathobiology, School of Veterinary Medicine, University of Pennsylvania, 3800 Spruce St., Philadelphia, PA 19104. **Richard K. Grencis** • Immunology Group, School of Biological Sciences, University of Manchester, Manchester, United Kingdom.

repertoire of effector mechanisms to eliminate these multicellular parasites.

ACQUIRED IMMUNITY AND CONTROL OF INTRACELLULAR PARASITES

Although *Leishmania, T. cruzi,* and *Toxoplasma* are all intracellular, they differ substantially in their life cycles. *Leishmania* exists in two major forms, the promastigote, which is a flagellated organism found in the sand fly, and the amastigote, which multiplies within macrophages of the host. Once inoculated into the mammalian host, the promastigotes rapidly invade cells—primarily macrophages, although other cells may also be infected—and transform to amastigotes, which multiply within the cell. *T. cruzi* is transmitted by reduviid bugs, and, similar to *Leishmania,* once they gain access to the skin, these parasites invade cells and transform to an amastigote form. However, *T. cruzi* can invade almost all cells, and after several rounds of division the organisms transform to a trypomastigote form that is released from the infected cells and can circulate in the blood. The trypomastigotes can reinvade other cells and again transform to amastigotes that will multiply intracellularly. *Toxoplasma* has a more complicated life cycle than either *Leishmania* or *T. cruzi.* Within the gut epithelial cells of the cat, the organisms undergo sexual multiplication, resulting in the production of oocytes, which become infective after being shed in the feces. While *Toxoplasma* can multiply sexually only in the cat, many vertebrate species can be infected, and in these animals the parasites invade the intestinal epithelium and transform to tachyzoites, a rapidly multiplying form of the parasite. The parasites can then disseminate and are able to invade any cell in the body. Once an effective immune response is established, a slowly multiplying form, termed bradyzoites, is able to survive within cysts. Thus, *Toxoplasma* infection is often viewed as having an acute phase, associated with rapid tachyzoite multiplication, and a chronic phase, where cysts containing bradyzoites persist for the life of the host.

In addition to differences in their life cycle, these intracellular parasites use different strategies to survive within cells (Bogdan and Rollinghoff, 1999). For example, *T. cruzi* parasites secrete a lysin that releases the parasites into the cytoplasm, thus escaping fusion of the phagosome with the toxic environment of the lysosome. *Toxoplasma* creates its own parasitophorous vacuole, which does not fuse with lysosomes. In contrast, *Leishmania* can survive after the phagosome has fused with the lysosomes. The immunologic consequences of these differences are that

proteins from both *T. cruzi* and *Toxoplasma* appear to more readily enter the class I pathway, leading to generation of a CD8$^+$ T-cell response that contributes to protection. However, even with *Leishmania,* class I presentation occurs, although the role that leishmania-specific CD8$^+$ T cells play in leishmaniasis is not well defined (discussed in more detail below) (Kima et al., 1997). All of these infections are associated with CD4$^+$ T-cell activation, which is required for resistance (Denkers and Gazzinelli, 1998; Reed, 1998; Solbach and Laskay, 2000). The antigen-presenting cells could be infected macrophages or dendritic cells (DCs) or class II-expressing cells that have taken up parasite antigens or dead parasites. The possibility that much of the antigen presentation may not be from infected cells is supported by in vitro studies showing that macrophages infected with *Leishmania* are poor antigen-presenting cells (Prina et al., 1996).

Initiation and Maintenance of Immunity

IL-12 plays a central role in initiating protective immune responses against intracellular parasites, by promoting IFN-γ production and the development of type 1 responses. Increased IL-12 production is measurable after infection of mice with these parasites. Macrophages and DCs are the main sources of IL-12, and parasite infection or exposure to products of the parasites is thought to induce IL-12 production (Trinchieri, 1998). Interestingly, however, following in vitro infection with *Leishmania* metacyclic promastigotes or with amastigotes, macrophages fail to produce IL-12, although DCs can produce IL-12 after *Leishmania* infection (Carrera et al., 1996). Moreover, infection of macrophages can suppress IL-12 production stimulated by other microbial products (Carrera et al., 1996). This led to studies to define other pathways that would lead to IL-12 production. Chief among these may be the stimulation of IL-12 production through ligation of CD40 by T cells expressing CD40 ligand (CD40L). That this is a critical pathway is suggested by the findings that CD40- or CD40L-deficient mice (on a normally resistant background) are susceptible to infection and that this susceptibility can be reversed by IL-12 treatment (Campbell et al., 1996; Kamanaka et al., 1996; Soong et al., 1996). More recently, another critical pathway leading to IL-12 production was found to involve chemokines. Thus, *Toxoplasma* lysates were found to stimulate the production of ligands (such as MIP1a and MIP1b) for the chemokine receptor CCR5 and ligation of CCR5 on DCs was found to lead to IL-12 production (Aliberti et al., 2000). The importance of this pathway in initiating protective immunity was demonstrated by the finding that CCR5$^{-/-}$ mice were more susceptible to *Toxoplasma* infection.

Since each of these organisms can infect antigen-presenting cells, activation of naïve CD4$^+$ T cells may be due to interactions with such infected cells, although it may be as likely that priming of CD4$^+$ T cells occurs by interactions with macrophages or dendritic cells that have taken up dead parasites. In either case, efficient priming for a CD4$^+$ T-cell response requires that the antigen get to the lymph nodes to contact naïve, recirculating T cells. DCs facilitate this process by taking up parasites or parasite antigens and migrating from the site of infection to the draining lymph nodes. Chemokines play a key role in this migration. Monocyte chemoattractant protein 1 (MCP-1) is produced early after *Leishmania* infection (Vester et al., 1999; C. Zaph and P. Scott, unpublished data) and may contribute to DC migration, since it was recently shown that in CCR2$^{-/-}$ mice DC migration is impaired and that associated with this impairment was enhanced susceptibility to *L. major* infection (Sato et al., 2000). Following intravenous injection of *Toxoplasma* antigen, DCs can also be seen to move from the red pulp and marginal zones of the spleen to the T-cell regions of the periarterial lymphoid sheath (Sousa et al., 1997), and this migration is dependent on expression of the CCR5 chemokine receptor (Aliberti et al., 2000).

Activation of Infected Cells

The activation of macrophages to be microbicidal or static is a primary effector mechanism that leads to the control of intracellular pathogens. Activated macrophages exhibit a large number of physiologic changes, including increased expression of cell surface molecules (such as class II), increased phagocytosis, and generation of highly reactive toxic molecules. While reactive oxygen intermediates (ROIs) and reactive nitrogen intermediates (RNIs), such as nitric oxide, are effective microbicidal agents, nitric oxide appears to be particularly important for controlling intracellular parasites. Nitric oxide is derived from the nitrogen donated by L-arginine in a reaction catalyzed by the enzyme inducible nitric oxide synthase (iNOS). Infection of iNOS$^{-/-}$ mice with either *L. major* or *T. cruzi* indicates that iNOS is required for resistance (Holscher et al., 1998; Wei et al., 1995). Furthermore, a direct comparison of the relative importance of ROIs and RNIs in control of *L. donovani* indicates that although ROIs may contribute to parasite control early after infection, the critical effector molecule for *L. donovani* control is nitric

oxide (Murray and Nathan, 1999). In contrast, a more complicated picture emerges following *Toxoplasma* infection of iNOS$^{-/-}$ mice. *Toxoplasma* infections are associated with both iNOS-dependent and -independent mechanisms of parasite control. Thus, iNOS knockout mice are able to control *Toxoplasma* during the acute phase of the disease, but they succumb during the chronic phase (Scharton-Kersten et al., 1997). Moreover, following vaccination with an avirulent strain of *Toxoplasma*, iNOS knockout mice were found to be as resistant as control mice to a challenge with virulent parasites (Khan et al., 1998). Thus, the relative importance of nitric oxide as an effector molecule associated with resistance is dependent on which intracellular parasite is examined, and which stage of the infection is being studied.

The most important macrophage-activating cytokine is IFN-γ, although several other cytokines may facilitate this process. Infection of mice depleted of IFN-γ by administration of anti-IFN-γ monoclonal antibodies or infection of IFN-γ knockout mice leads to enhanced susceptibility to *Leishmania*, *Toxoplasma*, and *T. cruzi* (Denkers and Gazzinelli, 1998; Reed, 1998; Solbach and Laskay, 2000). The current model for macrophage activation is that IFN-γ primes cells, and that additional signals, such as tumor necrosis factor (TNF), trigger activation of the cell. The importance of TNF in control of parasites was observed following infection of TNF receptor (TNFR)-deficient mice with either *Leishmania* or *Toxoplasma,* where in both cases the mice exhibited increased susceptibility (Nashleanas et al., 1998; Yap et al., 1998). However, TNFRp55 knockout mice and TNFRp55p75 knockout mice were able to eventually control and eliminate most of the parasites after *L. major* infection (Nashleanas et al., 1998), suggesting that other signals, such as CD40-CD40L interactions, may compensate for the absence of TNF. A critical role for TNF in parasite control is also evident following infection of IFN-γ knockout mice with *L. donovani* (Taylor and Murray, 1997). As expected, these mice are initially much more susceptible to *L. donovani* infection. However, after 8 weeks of infection, parasite replication is partially controlled. Early control can be induced in these IFN-γ knockout mice by administration of IL-12 but not of IL-12 plus anti-TNF (Taylor and Murray, 1997).

While most studies of intracellular parasite killing have focused on the macrophage, it is evident that for *Toxoplasma* and *T. cruzi*, cells other than phagocytes will need to eliminate the parasites in order to control the infection. It has been suggested that nitric oxide from nearby activated macrophages may kill parasites in nonhematopoietic cells. This issue was directly addressed by the creation of bone marrow chimeras between wild-type (WT) and IFN-γ receptor (IFN-γR)-deficient mice (Yap and Sher, 1999). The results indicate that resistance in *Toxoplasma* is dependent on expression of IFN-γR on both hematopoietic and nonhematopoietic cells. However, the mechanism(s) by which IFN-γ mediates its effects in nonhematopoetic cells is unclear. It has been shown that IFN-γ can increase indoleamine dioxygenase activity in *Toxoplasma*-infected fibroblasts, which results in the degradation of tryptophan, which is required for replication of the parasites (Pfefferkorn, 1984), although this pathway does not operate in human macrophages (MacKenzie et al., 1999) or in *T. cruzi* infection (Ceravolo et al., 1999). Thus, the iNOS-independent mechanism that operates to control *Toxoplasma* or *T. cruzi* remains undefined. However, some insight into this issue may come from studies with mice lacking the IFN-γ-regulated GTP-binding protein (IGTP). Mice lacking this molecule are able to control infections with the intracellular bacterium *Listeria monocytogenes* and cytomegalovirus, but are unable to control *Toxoplasma* infections (Taylor et al., 2000). Whether IGTP is a pivotal factor in a mechanism of *Toxoplasma* control by nonhematopoietic cells must await further studies.

CD8 T-Cell Activation

The importance of CD8$^+$ T cells in resistance to *T. cruzi* and *Toxoplasma* is well established, since enhanced susceptibility to these pathogens is observed following infection of mice deficient in CD8$^+$ T cells (Denkers and Gazzinelli, 1998; Reed, 1998). CD8$^+$ T cells recognize antigen in the context of class I, which is expressed on almost all cells. This allows CD8$^+$ T cells to survey intracellular infections in any cell in the body, which would be particularly important for control of *T. cruzi* and *Toxoplasma*. CD8$^+$ T cells secrete cytokines, such as IFN-γ, and can also lyse target cells through the release of molecules such as perforin. The in vivo importance of the lytic pathway for CD8$^+$ T-cell effector function in toxoplasmosis was shown in studies with perforin knockout mice, which exhibited increased susceptibility to *Toxoplasma* infection during the chronic phase of infection (Denkers et al., 1997). Interestingly, however, perforin knockout mice vaccinated with an avirulent *Toxoplasma* strain were as resistant to challenge infection as were WT control mice, suggesting that cytolytic T cells may be important for control of the chronic phase of toxoplasmosis, when cysts are present in the brain, but less important during the acute

phase, when tachyzoites are rapidly multiplying. A different result is obtained with *T. cruzi* infection, where it was found that even after immunization with an avirulent *T. cruzi* strain, CD8$^+$ T cells were still required for protection (Kumar and Tarleton, 1998). Moreover, perforin and granzyme B knockout mice were as resistant as wild-type mice, indicating that for CD8$^+$ T cells to be protective against *T. cruzi*, lytic pathways involving either perforin or granzyme B are not required.

The role that CD8$^+$ T cells play in leishmaniasis is less clear, since CD8$^+$-deficient mice are able to resolve a primary infection with *L. major* (Wang et al., 1993). Since *Leishmania* resides within the phagolysosome, one might predict that CD8$^+$ T cells are not activated during infection. However, in both human and experimental leishmanial infections, the numbers of antigen-specific CD8$^+$ T cells are expanded (Solbach and Laskay, 2000), and in vitro studies have shown that infected cells can present antigen to CD8$^+$ T cells (Kima et al., 1997). The importance of the CD8$^+$ T cells in leishmaniasis was demonstrated by studies indicating that they contribute to resistance to a secondary challenge infection and to vaccine-induced resistance (Farrell et al., 1989; Gurunathan et al., 2000; Muller et al., 1994). The way CD8$^+$ T cells influence *Leishmania* infection is not well established. However, in vitro studies indicate that infected macrophages do not act as targets for cytolysis by CD8$^+$ T cells (Russell et al., 1991), making it likely that they protect by providing an additional source of IFN-γ, rather than by acting as cytolytic cells. In summary, it would appear that the role of CD8$^+$ T cells in resistance to leishmaniasis needs to be further investigated.

The Role of Antibody in Controlling Intracellular Pathogens

Infection with *T. cruzi*, *Toxoplasma*, or *Leishmania* is associated with the production of antibodies, which have the potential to play a variety of roles in controlling these parasites. For example, antibodies may coat the parasites as they move from one cell to another or, for *T. cruzi*, when nondividing trypomastigotes circulate in the blood. These antibodies may be lytic or opsonic, may promote antibody-dependent cell-mediated cytotoxicity, and/or may block or modulate invasion. While many in vitro studies have indicated some role for each of these mechanisms, the in vivo role of antibodies has been more difficult to establish. However, the use of B-cell- and Fc receptor (FcR)-deficient mice has unequivocally indicated that B cells and antibodies may be required for protection against *T. cruzi* and *Toxoplasma*.

B-cell-deficient mice infected with *Toxoplasma* die during the chronic phase of infection, with large numbers of tachyzoites in the brain and lungs, and an increase in the number of cysts (Kang et al., 2000). These data indicate that antibodies are not required for protection during the acute phase of infection. Other studies have shown that *Toxoplasma*-immunized B-cell-deficient mice are much more susceptible than control immunized mice, and further studies with FcR- and C5-deficient mice indicate that neither Fc-mediated uptake nor complement-mediated lysis is required for the protective effects of antibodies (Sayles et al., 2000). B cells are also required for long-term control of *T. cruzi,* although B-cell-deficient mice survive longer than mice lacking either CD4 or CD8 T cells (Kumar and Tarleton, 1998).

In contrast, recent studies with B-cell-deficient mice infected with *L. major* indicate that B cells are not required for susceptibility or resistance (Brown and Reiner, 1999). However, studies with *L. amazonensis* indicate that in the absence of B cells or FcR, *L. amazonensis* infections are less severe (Kima et al., 2000). These results suggest that ligation of the FcR may contribute to enhanced uptake (and survival) of the parasites or that FcR signaling modulates the host cell response to infection. Interestingly, it has been found that FcR ligation enhances IL-10 production, which could downregulate protective immune responses (Sutterwala et al., 1998).

ACQUIRED IMMUNITY TO GASTROINTESTINAL NEMATODES

As a group of infectious agents, the gastrointestinal nematodes are one of the most successful, with current estimates of one in five of the human population harboring at least one species (Chan, 1997). Infection by these pathogens is not usually fatal but insidious, often with a high degree of morbidity, particularly in children. A particularly important feature of this type of infection, which is dramatically different from most other infections, is that the level of infection harbored by the host is a reflection of the number of infection events encountered. Gut nematodes do not, in general, multiply within the host. Moreover, the worm burden is usually acquired in the field by multiple infection events, not through a single bolus of infective stages. This will have important consequences for how the host immune system deals with antigen.

Due to the difficulty in studying infection in the field, most of our current understanding of gut nematode infection comes from investigations of model systems in rodents, including most notably *Nippostrongylus brasiliensis, Trichinella spiralis, Trichuris muris, Heligmosomoides polygyrus,* and *Strongyloides* spp. Most work has concentrated on systems which naturally involve expulsion of the parasites from the gastrointestinal tract following a primary infection (*N. brasiliensis, T. spiralis,* and *Strongyloides*), although interesting new data are being generated in systems in which natural chronic primary infection can occur (*T. muris* and *H. polygyrus*).

Type 2 Cytokine Responses and Host Protective Responses to Intestinal Nematodes

It is very clear from many studies that worm expulsion from the intestine is primarily a CD4$^+$ T-cell-mediated phenomenon and is associated with the secretion of type 2 cytokines (Finkelman et al., 1997) although it is interesting that the IL-1 receptor-related protein T1, thought to be a marker for Th2 cells, is not essential for type 2-mediated resistance to *N. brasiliensis* (Senn et al., 2000) or *T. muris* (R. K. Grencis and A. N. McKenzie, unpublished observations). In accordance with a role for Th2 cells, Urban et al. (1991) first demonstrated that IL-4 was a key cytokine in the response that cleared *H. polygyrus* from the small intestine in the challenge infection model of resistance. This observation has been extended to other systems including *T. muris,* a parasite of the large bowel (Else et al., 1994). However, an essential role for IL-4 was not observed for *N. brasiliensis,* with anti-IL-4 treated or IL-4 knockout (IL-4KO) mice clearing infection similar to WT mice (Lawrence et al., 1998; Madden et al., 1991). Anti-CD4-treated mice or SCID mice could be induced to clear infection, however, following injection of IL-4 in the form of a long-acting complex (Urban et al., 1995). For *T. spiralis,* IL-4 KO mice generally show little alteration in expulsion kinetics from WT mice, suggesting a nonessential role for IL-4 in mediating worm expulsion (Urban et al., 2000). In this model, injection of IL-4 complexes could induce worm expulsion only in WT mice, not in immunodeficient mice (e.g., RAG2 mice [Urban et al., 2000]).

Most interestingly, it has now been clearly demonstrated that the closely related cytokine IL-13 plays a more substantial role in mediating the expulsion of many of these species. IL-13KO mice show delayed worm expulsion and depressed intestinal goblet cell hyperplasia following *N. brasiliensis* infection (McKenzie et al., 1999). IL-4/IL-13 double KO mice show even slower worm expulsion than do single-

KO mice (McKenzie et al., 1999). Moreover, IL-4Ra KO mice show a marked susceptibility to infection by *N. brasiliensis;* IL-4 and IL-13 both utilize the IL-4Ra subunit (Barner et al., 1998), as do IL-4KO mice in which IL-13 is blocked by treatment with soluble IL-13Ra2 fusion protein (Urban et al., 1998). Similarly, *T. spiralis* expulsion is delayed in IL-4KO mice in which IL-13 is blocked (Urban et al., 2000). These observations are supported by studies showing that IL-13KO mice do not exhibit a marked delay in *T. spiralis* expulsion compared to WT mice whereas IL-13/IL-4 double KO mice do (R. K. Grencis, A. N. McKenzie, and J. L. Pennock, unpublished observations). The relative importance of IL-4 and IL-13 in resistance is also influenced by host genetic background and highlighted by studies in the *T. muris* system. Here, IL-4KO mice on a C57BL/6 background are uniformly susceptible and develop chronic infections whereas WT mice expel their worm burden. IL-4KO mice on a BALB/c background, however, show a split responsiveness in that while males develop chronic infection, females expel their parasites. Expulsion from female mice is mediated through IL-13, as can clearly be shown by administration of sIL-13Ra2 fusion protein. The corollary is that delivery of IL-13 to male mice induces worm expulsion; this cannot be achieved in IL-4Ra KO mice on a BALB/c background (Bancroft et al., 2000).

The importance of IL-4/IL-13 and IL-4Ra in responses to gut nematodes suggests a centrally important role for the signaling molecule STAT6 in the generation of the protective response. Indeed, STAT6KO mice are more susceptible to *T. spiralis* than are WT mice and exhibit depressed intestinal mast cell responses, depressed type 2 cytokine responses, and suppressed parasite-specific immunoglobulin G1 (IgG1) production (Urban et al., 2000). STAT6KO mice also show a delayed expulsion of *N. brasiliensis,* although their cytokine and mast cell responses were not depressed (Urban et al., 1998). In the challenge model of *H. polygyrus* infection, STAT6 also appears to play a role in protection. This correlates with a depression of the type 2 cytokine response following challenge infection in STAT6KO mice. Interestingly, this was in contrast to responses observed following primary infection, in which cytokine responses were comparable to those in WT mice despite an inability to expel the primary worm burden. Finkleman et al. (2000) have suggested that while STAT6 enhances primary type 2 responses, its requirement is not absolute, whereas STAT6 is required for the development or maintenance of the type 2 memory response.

While IL-4 and IL-13 dominate the cytokines which mediate protection, other cytokines may play important roles. A role for IL-3 has been implicated in *Strongyloides* and *T. spiralis* infections following administration of recombinant cytokine (Abe et al., 1992; Korenaga et al., 1996; Lantz et al., 1998). Surprisingly, however, IL-5 does not seem to be critical for protection against the intestinal phases of *T. spiralis* (Herndon and Kayes, 1992), *N. brasiliensis* (Coffman et al., 1989), *T. muris* (Betts and Else, 1999), or *Strongyloides* spp. (Korenaga et al., 1994). In the challenge model of *H. polygyrus*, IL-5 appears to play only a small role (Urban et al., 1991), although recent work has suggested that *H. polygyrus* worm fecundity during primary infection may be elevated in animals depleted of the IL-5 gene (Behm and Ovington, 2000).

A more definite role has been suggested for IL-9, a cytokine that is assuming increasing importance in mechanisms of allergy. Studies using IL-9 transgenic mice (which greatly overexpress IL-9) have clearly shown enhanced expulsion of *T. spiralis* (Faulkner et al., 1997), *T. muris* (Faulkner et al., 1998), *N. brasiliensis,* and *H. polygyrus* (J. C. Renauld, J. Van Snick, and N. Humphrey, unpublished observations). In the *T. spiralis* model, resistance is manifested through enhanced intestinal mastocytosis, although other aspects of the type 2 mediated response are generally enhanced (Faulkner et al., 1997, 1998). Studies in the *T. muris* model utilized the technique of autoanticytokine antibody production to demonstrate that neutralization of IL-9 in vivo during infection induced chronic infection in normally resistant mice (Richard et al., 2000). Most recently, studies with IL-9KO mice (Townsend et al., 2000) indicate that this cytokine was not essential for expulsion of *N. brasiliensis* although other type 2 cytokine responses were enhanced, perhaps suggesting that compensatory mechanisms were operating or were influenced by the genetic background of the mice (129 × C57BL/6). Recent work with several systems has also identified interesting roles for cytokines which are not usually associated with type 2 responses. In the *T. spiralis* model, which mounts a very strong type 2 cytokine response, TNF-α profoundly influences the changes in gut architecture (crypt hyperplasia and villous atrophy) that occur during infection (Lawrence et al., 1998), probably through the action of NO (Lawrence et al., 2000), although no effect on the kinetics of worm expulsion was observed. In the *T. muris* system, however, a clear effect of TNF-α involvement in worm expulsion has been shown, with a strong link to the overall IL-13-mediated expulsion process (Artis et al., 1999). Overall, the current data strongly support a role for type 2-mediated responses to intestinal dwelling helminths, with a dominance for the cytokines IL-4 and IL-13. Signaling mechanisms remain undefined, and the variation in STAT6 involvement may reflect the variation in effector mechanisms required to expel the parasites from their different niches within the intestinal environment.

Type 2-Mediated Effector Mechanisms of Resistance to Gastrointestinal Nematodes

Whilst the type 2 cytokine response underlying the expulsion of intestinal nematodes is well established, the effector mechanisms that they control to regulate parasite clearance remain to be defined. One of the most surprising observations is the lack of evidence implicating eosinophils, often a hallmark of infection, in host protection. Studies from many model systems in which eosinophil responses are abrogated (e.g., in IL-5KO mice or in animals treated with neutralizing anti-IL-5 monoclonal antibodies) fail to support an essential role for these granulocytes (Betts and Else, 1999; Coffman et al., 1989; Herndon and Kayes, 1992; Urban et al., 1991). Moreover, there are few studies which support an important or critical role for parasite-specific antibody (including IgE) in resistance (at least with regard to expulsion of primary infections). There are notable exceptions, such as the transfer of IgG1 from hyperimmune animals to H. polygyrus-infected mice (Pritchard et al., 1983) and the T. spiralis model (Ahmad et al., 1991; Appleton and McGregor, 1987; Dessein et al., 1981; Love et al., 1976). Studies have also suggested that immune serum transfer could enhance resistance to infection by T. muris (Else et al., 1990; Roach et al., 1991) and that the resistance is associated with peak numbers of IgG1- and IgA-producing B cells in the draining lymph nodes (Koyama et al., 1999). However, in all cases, high levels of the immunoglobulins are transferred before or during the early stages of infection—a time when natural levels of antibody would not be expected to be present following infection. It is interesting that in the T. muris model, expulsion can occur in the complete absence of antibody, as shown by adoptive transfer of resistance by CD4$^+$ T cells to SCID mice (Else and Grencis, 1996). The notion of antibody-dependent cell-mediated cytotoxicity as a major effector mechanism against gastrointestinal nematodes is therefore doubtful. This conclusion is strengthened by studies from several systems using mice lacking Fc receptors (Betts and Else, 1999).

The importance of the role of the intestinal mast cell in resistance has also been controversial over the years. Recent work has, however, demonstrated an important role for this cell type in resistance to at least some species of nematode. Arguably, the most convincing evidence comes from the T. spiralis system, where abrogation of the mast cell response in immunocompetent mice clearly delays the expulsion of the parasite from the intestine (Donaldson et al., 1996), supporting earlier work demonstrating a delayed expulsion from mast cell-deficient (WW^v) mice (Alizadeh and Murrell, 1984). Mast cell function in vivo is reflected by the secretion of mucosal mast cell-specific proteases (especially mouse mast cell protease 1 [MMCP1]) during infection (Huntley et al., 1990). Most recently, it has been shown that MMCP1KO mice exhibit delayed expulsion of T. spiralis from the intestine. Although the function of MMCP1 remains to be defined, it has been suggested that a target for this and other mast cell-specific proteases may be the tight junctions between intestinal epithelial cells.

Mast cell-dependent effects may operate through alterations in smooth muscle contractility. Such changes are observed following challenge infections with H. polygyrus (Grencis, 1997). Expulsion of T. spiralis is also accompanied by increases in smooth muscle contractility and is shown to be depressed in WW^v mice, indicating a link with the mast cell (Vallance et al., 1997, 1998; Weisbrodt et al., 1994). Associated changes in increased intestinal permeability and decreased fluid absorption often accompany worm expulsion and have been noted following H. polygyrus and T. spiralis challenge infections (Castro et al., 1979; Grencis, 1997).

Despite the strong intestinal mast cell response, there is little evidence to support a protective role of mast cells against N. brasiliensis. For example, mast cell-deficient (Crowle and Reed, 1981) or depleted (Urban et al., 1995) animals do not show expulsion kinetics different from those of control mice. However, in situations where goblet cells are altered, worm expulsion is delayed; e.g., IL-13KO mice show a greatly reduced goblet cell hyperplasia and delayed worm expulsion (McKenzie et al., 1999). IL-9KO mice also show a defect in the intestinal goblet cell response, but the defect is not sufficiently different from that of WT animals to affect worm expulsion (Townsend et al., 2000). It is noteworthy that defined changes in the glycosylation of intestinal mucins following N. brasiliensis infection in the rat have been observed (Karlsson et al., 2000), and thus subtle changes in the goblet cell/mucin axis may contribute to their role in worm expulsion (Khan et al., 1995).

Overall, it appears that multiple type 2 cytokine-mediated effector mechanisms are likely to operate against intestinal nematodes, and to date few have been precisely defined. It is increasingly clear that novel mechanisms of protection are coming to the fore, reflecting the mucosal site of habitation and the distinct niches within this environment in which the different species of nematode live. A general theme that is finally becoming established involves generating an intestinal environment which is unsuitable for worm survival and reproduction (Else and Finkelman, 1998; Grencis, 1997; Wakelin, 1978), with multiple potential effector mechanisms operating in combination.

Type 1 Responses to and Susceptibility to Infection by Intestinal Nematodes

While it is clear that resistance to infection is dominated by type 2 cytokine-mediated responses, in the wild most natural intestinal nematode infections are chronic. Relatively few studies have investigated the underlying mechanisms of chronicity and susceptibility (Behnke et al., 1992), although it is certainly apparent that when type 2 responses are depressed, worm expulsion is delayed. It is also clear that this occurs following the promotion of type 1 responses, e.g., via administration of IL-12 (Finkelman et al., 1994). In the field situation, a variety of factors could be envisaged to influence the development of resistance, including coinfection and host nutrition. Interestingly, a recent study in the *H. polygyrus* challenge system clearly shows the importance of dietary protein on resistance to infection, with hosts exposed to a low-protein diet exhibiting depressed type 2 cytokine responses and severely delayed worm expulsion compared to animals on a higher-protein diet (Ing et al., 2000).

Two models of infection, however, naturally exhibit chronic infection, and observations with these models have identified key factors involved in susceptibility. In the *T. muris* system, while most inbred strains of mouse expel a moderate to high worm burden, a few strains fail to expel the worms and exhibit high-level chronic infection (Else and Finkelman, 1998). It is now clear that in these animals, a dominant type 1 cytokine (IFN-γ-mediated) response develops. Neutralization of IFN-γ (Else et al., 1994) or IL-12 (A. J. Bancroft and R. K. Grencis, unpublished observations) in susceptible strains induces worm expulsion, with a coincident rise in type 2 responses. Moreover, administration of IL-12 to resistant animals induces susceptibility which is IFN-γ dependent (Bancroft et al., 1997). IL-12KO mice are highly resistant to infection, as are IFN-γRKO mice (Helmby et al., in press; D. Artis and A. J. Bancroft, unpublished observations). More recently, work has identified IL-18 as a major factor involved in the induction of susceptibility. Susceptible strains show a strong early upregulation of IL-18 mRNA in the in-

fected intestine compared to resistant strains, and this is followed by IL-12 and IFN-γ upregulation. Caspase 1 mRNA upregulation is coincident with IL-18 mRNA upregulation, and active protein is produced. IL-18KO mice are highly resistant to infection, and administration of IL-18 to resistant strains induces chronicity. Interestingly, the data suggest that rather than by inducing higher levels of IFN-γ, IL-18 may mediate its effects through regulation of IL-13 production (Helmby and Grencis, submitted). The actions of IL-18 may be very sensitive to the influence of the cytokine melieu, since recent data clearly show that IL-18 can also promote IL-4 production (Yoshimoto et al., 2000) and the development of type 2 responses (Xu et al., 2000).

In the *H. polygyrus* system, most strains of mice harbor chronic primary infections, although some strains do begin to lose worms several weeks after infection. Chronic primary infection is associated with many facets of a type 2 cytokine response and not a major shift to a dominant type 1 cytokine response. Interestingly, however, chronic infection may be associated with a selective downregulation of certain type 2 cytokines (most notably IL-9 and IL-10), which is reflected by a downregulation of intestinal mastocytosis (Behnke et al., 1992). The basis for downregulation of the cytokine response in both *T. muris* and *H. polygyrus* remains to be completely defined but is thought to involve immunomodulatory factors produced by the parasite. In the *T. muris* system, there is evidence to suggest the parasite may produce a cytokine (IFN-γ) mimic (Grencis and Entwistle, 1997). The concept that gut nematodes produce and secrete immunomodulatory molecules has also been recently shown for *N. brasiliensis*, where parasite extracts can induce strong type 2 responses in the absence of infection (Ehigiator et al., 2000; Holland et al., 2000; Uchikawa et al., 2000).

The *T. muris* system also adds another interesting facet to the induction of chronic infection that is related to exposure to different levels of infection. Mouse strains, which normally expel a moderate to large bolus infection (resistant), do not expel low-level infections (10 to 20 worms) and develop long-lived chronic parasite burdens. In this case, the host generates a dominant type 1 cytokine response. Moreover, priming by such an infection leads to susceptibility to a challenge with a low-level infection or a high-level infection. Repeated low-level infections can build up to levels whereby the host expels parasites from the intestine coincident with the development of a more robust type 2 cytokine response. The levels of infection that need to be built up before expulsion occurs vary among host strains. Furthermore, priming with a high-level infection generates a strong type 2 response and resistance to challenge, as may be expected, and this secondary response is very difficult to alter even after treatment of the animals with IL-12, which normally induces a strong type 1 response and susceptibility (Bancroft et al., 2000). Taken together, the data from such experiments using infection levels which more closely reflect those seen in the field suggest that low-level infection leads to susceptibility, repeated low-level challenge can lead to resistance, and it is difficult to alter this response once resistance is achieved. This bears more than a passing resemblance to the epidemiological observations made in field studies, and although it is an oversimplification, it does suggest that laboratory model systems can inform about similar infections in humans.

CONCLUSION

This chapter has reviewed the effector mechanisms associated with resistance to a select group of parasites, particularly focusing on parasites that illustrate the diversity of effector mechanisms contributing to protective immunity. The immune responses required for eliminating intracellular protozoa are quite different from those required to control gut-dwelling nematodes and can be divided into type 1 and type 2 responses. However, while type 1 or type 2 responses may dominate following infection with intracellular protozoa or gut-dwelling nematodes, respectively, the effector mechanisms required for resistance to any one particular parasite are often tailored to the biological characteristics of that parasite, which in some cases remain to be defined.

REFERENCES

Abe, T., H. Sugaya, K. Yoshimura, and Y. Nawa. 1992. Induction of the expulsion of *Strongyloides ratti* and retention of *Nippostrongylus brasiliensis* in athymic nude mice by repetitive administration of recombinant interleukin-3. *Immunology* **76:**10–14.

Ahmad, A., C. H. Wang, and R. G. Bell. 1991. A role for IgE in intestinal immunity. Expression of rapid expulsion of *Trichinella spiralis* in rats transfused with IgE and thoracic duct lymphocytes. *J. Immunol.* **146:**3563–3570.

Aliberti, J., C. Reis e Sousa, M. Schito, S. Hieny, T. Wells, G. B. Huffnagel, and A. Sher. 2000. CCR5 provides a signal for microbial induced production of IL-12 by CD8a+ dendritic cells. *Nat. Immunol.* **1:**83–87.

Alizadeh, H., and K. D. Murrell. 1984. The intestinal mast cell response to *Trichinella spiralis* infection in mast cell-deficient w/wv mice. *J. Parasitol.* **70:**767–773.

Appleton, J. A., and D. D. McGregor. 1987. Characterization of the immune mediator of rapid expulsion of *Trichinella spiralis* in suckling rats. *Immunology* **62:**477–484.

Artis, D., N. E. Humphreys, A. J. Bancroft, N. J. Rothwell, C. S. Potten, and R. K. Grencis. 1999. Tumor necrosis factor alpha is a critical component of interleukin 13-mediated protective T helper cell type 2 responses during helminth infection. *J. Exp. Med.* **190:**953–962.

Bancroft, A. J., D. Artis, D. D. Donaldson, J. P. Sypek, and R. K. Grencis. 2000. Gastrointestinal nematode expulsion in IL-4 knockout mice is IL-13 dependent. *Eur. J. Immunol.* **30:**2083–2091.

Bancroft, A. J., K. J. Else, J. P. Sypek, and R. K. Grencis. 1997. Interleukin-12 promotes a chronic intestinal nematode infection. *Eur. J. Immunol.* **27:**866–870.

Barner, M., M. Mohrs, F. Brombacher, and M. Kopf. 1998. Differences between IL-4R alpha-deficient and IL-4-deficient mice reveal a role for IL-13 in the regulation of Th2 responses. *Curr. Biol.* **8:**669–672.

Behm, C. A., and K. S. Ovington. 2000. The role of eosinophils in parasitic helminth infections: insights from genetically modified mice. *Parasitol. Today* **16:**202–209.

Behnke, J. M., C. J. Barnard, and D. Wakelin. 1992. Understanding chronic nematode infections: evolutionary considerations, current hypotheses and the way forward. *Int. J. Parasitol.* **22:**861–907.

Betts, C. J., and K. J. Else. 1999. Mast cells, eosinophils and antibody-mediated cellular cytotoxicity are not critical in resistance to *Trichuris muris*. *Parasite Immunol.* **21:**45–52.

Bogdan, C., and M. Rollinghoff. 1999. How do protozoan parasites survive inside macrophages? *Parasitol. Today* **15:**22–28.

Brown, D. R., and S. L. Reiner 1999. Polarized helper-T-cell responses against *Leishmania major* in the absence of B cells. *Infect. Immun.* **67:**266–270.

Campbell, K. A., P. J. Ovendale, M. K. Kennedy, W. C. Fanslow, S. G. Reed, and C. R. Maliszewski. 1996. CD40 ligand is required for protective cell-mediated immunity to *Leishmania major*. *Immunity* **4:**283–290.

Carrera, L., R. T. Gazzinelli, R. Badolato, S. Hieny, W. Muller, R. Kuhn, and D. L. Sacks. 1996. Leishmania promastigotes selectively inhibit interleukin 12 induction in bone marrow-derived macrophages from susceptible and resistant mice. *J. Exp. Med.* **183:**515–526.

Castro, G. A., J. J. Hessel, and G. Whalen. 1979. Altered intestinal fluid movement in response to *Trichinella spiralis* in immunized rats. *Parasite Immunol.* **1:**259–266.

Ceravolo, I. P., A. C. Chaves, C. A. Bonjardim, D. Sibley, A. J. Romanha, and R. T. Gazzinelli. 1999. Replication of *Toxoplasma gondii*, but not *Trypanosoma cruzi*, is regulated in human fibroblasts activated with gamma interferon: requirement of a functional JAK/STAT pathway. *Infect. Immun.* **67:**2233–2240.

Chan, M. S. 1997. The global burden of intestinal nematode infections—fifty years on. *Parasitol. Today* **13:**438–443.

Coffman, R. L., B. W. Seymour, S. Hudak, J. Jackson, and D. Rennick. 1989. Antibody to interleukin-5 inhibits helminth-induced eosinophilia in mice. *Science* **245:**308–310.

Crowle, P. K., and N. D. Reed. 1981. Rejection of the intestinal parasite *Nippostrongylus brasiliensis* by mast cell-deficient W/Wv anemic mice. *Infect. Immun.* **33:**54–58.

Denkers, E. Y., and R. T. Gazzinelli. 1998. Regulation and function of T-cell-mediated immunity during *Toxoplasma gondii* infection. *Clin. Microbiol. Rev.* **11:**569–588.

Denkers, E. Y., G. Yap, T. Scharton-Kersten, H. Charest, B. A. Butcher, P. Caspar, S. Hieny, and A. Sher. 1997. Perforin-mediated cytolysis plays a limited role in host resistance to *Toxoplasma gondii*. *J Immunol.* **159:**1903–1908.

Dessein, A. J., W. L. Parker, S. L. James, and J. R. David. 1981. IgE antibody and resistance to infection. I. Selective suppression of the IgE antibody response in rats diminishes the resistance and the eosinophil response to *Trichinella spiralis* infection. *J. Exp. Med.* **153:**423–436.

Donaldson, L. E., E. Schmitt, J. F. Huntley, G. F. Newlands, and R. K. Grencis. 1996. A critical role for stem cell factor and c-kit in host protective immunity to an intestinal helminth. *Int. Immunol.* **8:**559–567.

Ehigiator, H. N., A. W. Stadnyk, and T. D. Lee. 2000. Modulation of B-cell proliferative response by a soluble extract of *Nippostrongylus brasiliensis*. *Infect Immun.* **68:**6154–6161.

Else, K. J., and F. D. Finkelman. 1998. Intestinal nematode parasites, cytokines and effector mechanisms. *Int. J. Parasitol.* **28:** 1145–1158.

Else, K. J., F. D. Finkelman, C. R. Maliszewski, and R. K. Grencis. 1994. Cytokine-mediated regulation of chronic intestinal helminth infection. *J. Exp. Med.* **179:**347–351.

Else, K. J., and R. K. Grencis. 1996. Antibody-independent effector mechanisms in resistance to the intestinal nematode parasite *Trichuris muris*. *Infect. Immun.* **64:**2950–2954.

Else, K. J., D. Wakelin, D. L. Wassom, and K. M. Hauda. 1990. MHC-restricted antibody responses to *Trichuris muris* excretory/secretory (E/S) antigen. *Parasite Immunol.* **12:**509–527.

Farrell, J. P., I. Muller, and J. A. Louis. 1989. A role for Lyt2+ T cells in resistance to cutaneous leishmaniasis in immunized mice. *J. Immunol.* **142:**2052–2056.

Faulkner, H., N. Humphreys, J. C. Renauld, J. Van Snick, and R. Grencis. 1997. Interleukin-9 is involved in host protective immunity to intestinal nematode infection. *Eur. J. Immunol.* **27:** 2536–2540.

Faulkner, H., J. C. Renauld, J. Van Snick, and R. K. Grencis. 1998. Interleukin-9 enhances resistance to the intestinal nematode *Trichuris muris*. *Infect Immun.* **66:**3832–3840.

Finkelman, F. D., K. B. Madden, A. W. Cheever, I. M. Katona, S. C. Morris, M. K. Gately, B. R. Hubbard, W. C. Gause, and J. F. Urban, Jr. 1994. Effects of interleukin 12 on immune responses and host protection in mice infected with intestinal nematode parasites. *J. Exp. Med.* **179:**1563–1572.

Finkelman, F. D., S. C. Morris, T. Orekhova, M. Mori, D. Donaldson, S. L. Reiner, N. L. Reilly, L. Schopf, and J. F. Urban, Jr. 2000. Stat6 regulation of in vivo IL-4 responses. *J. Immunol.* **164:**2303–2310.

Finkelman, F. D., T. Shea-Donohue, J. Goldhill, C. A. Sullivan, S. C. Morris, K. B. Madden, W. C. Gause, and J. F. Urban, Jr. 1997. Cytokine regulation of host defense against parasitic gastrointestinal nematodes: lessons from studies with rodent models. *Annu. Rev. Immunol.* **15:**505–533.

Grencis, R. K. 1997. Enteric helminth infection: immunopathology and resistance during intestinal nematode infection. *Chem. Immunol.* **66:**41–61.

Grencis, R. K., and G. M. Entwistle. 1997. Production of an interferon-gamma homologue by an intestinal nematode: functionally significant or interesting artefact? *Parasitology* **115:** S101–S106.

Gurunathan, S., L. Stobie, C. Prussin, D. L. Sacks, N. Glaichenhaus, D. J. Fowell, R. M. Locksley, J. T. Chang, C. Y. Wu, and R. A. Seder. 2000. Requirements for the maintenance of Th1 immunity in vivo following DNA vaccination: a potential immunoregulatory role for CD8+ T cells. *J. Immunol.* **165:**915–924.

Helmby, H., K. Takeda, S. Akira, and R. K. Grencis. Interleukin (IL)-18 promotes the development of chronic gastrointestinal helminth infection by down-regulating IL-13. *J. Exp. Med.*, in press.

Herndon, F. J., and S. G. Kayes. 1992. Depletion of eosinophils by anti-IL-5 monoclonal antibody treatment of mice infected with *Trichinella spiralis* does not alter parasite burden or immunologic resistance to reinfection. *J. Immunol.* **149:**3642–3647.

Holland, M. J., Y. M. Harcus, P. L. Riches, and R. M. Maizels. 2000. Proteins secreted by the parasitic nematode *Nippostrongylus brasiliensis* act as adjuvants for Th2 responses. *Eur. J. Immunol.* **30:**1977–1987.

Holscher, C., G. Kohler, U. Muller, H. Mossmann, G. A. Schaub, and F. Brombacher. 1998. Defective nitric oxide effector functions lead to extreme susceptibility of *Trypanosoma cruzi*-infected mice deficient in gamma interferon receptor or inducible nitric oxide synthase. *Infect. Immun.* **66:**1208–1215.

Huntley, J. F., C. Gooden, G. F. Newlands, A. Mackellar, D. A. Lammas, D. Wakelin, M. Tuohy, R. G. Woodbury, and H. R. Miller. 1990. Distribution of intestinal mast cell proteinase in blood and tissues of normal and *Trichinella*-infected mice. *Parasite Immunol.* **12:**85–95.

Ing, R., Z. Su, M. E. Scott, and K. G. Koski. 2000. Suppressed T helper 2 immunity and prolonged survival of a nematode parasite in protein-malnourished mice. *Proc. Natl. Acad. Sci. USA* **97:**7078–7083.

Kamanaka, M., P. Yu, T. Yasui, K. Yoshida, T. Kawabe, T. Horii, T. Kishimoto, and H. Kikutani. 1996. Protective role of CD40 in *Leishmania major* infection at two distinct phases of cell-mediated immunity. *Immunity* **4:**275–282.

Kang, H., J. S. Remington, and Y. Suzuki. 2000. Decreased resistance of B cell-deficient mice to infection with *Toxoplasma gondii* despite unimpaired expression of IFN-gamma, TNF-alpha, and inducible nitric oxide synthase. *J. Immunol.* **164:**2629–2634.

Karlsson, N. G., F. J. Olson, P. A. Jovall, Y. Andersch, L. Enerback, and G. C. Hansson. 2000. Identification of transient glycosylation alterations of sialylated mucin oligosaccharides during infection by the rat intestinal parasite *Nippostrongylus brasiliensis*. *Biochem. J.* **350:**805–814.

Khan, I. A., T. Matsuura, and L. H. Kasper. 1998. Inducible nitric oxide synthase is not required for long-term vaccine-based immunity against *Toxoplasma gondii*. *J. Immunol.* **161:**2994–3000.

Khan, W. I., T. Abe, N. Ishikawa, Y. Nawa, and K. Yoshimura. 1995. Reduced amount of intestinal mucus by treatment with anti-CD4 antibody interferes with the spontaneous cure of *Nippostrongylus brasiliensis* infection in mice. *Parasite Immunol.* **17:**485–491.

Kima, P. E., S. L. Constant, L. Hannum, M. Colmenares, K. S. Lee, A. M. Haberman, M. J. Shlomchik, and D. McMahon-Pratt. 2000. Internalization of *Leishmania mexicana* complex amastigotes via the Fc receptor is required to sustain infection in murine cutaneous leishmaniasis. *J. Exp. Med.* **191:**1063–1068.

Kima, P. E., N. H. Ruddle, and D. McMahon-Pratt. 1997. Presentation via the class I pathway by *Leishmania amazonensis*-infected macrophages of an endogenous leishmanial antigen to CD8+ T cells. *J. Immunol.* **159:**1828–1834.

Korenaga, M., T. Abe, and Y. Hashiguchi. 1996. Injection of recombinant interleukin 3 hastens worm expulsion in mice infected with *Trichinella spiralis*. *Parasitol. Res.* **82:**108–113.

Korenaga, M., Y. Hitoshi, K. Takatsu, and I. Tada. 1994. Regulatory effect of anti-interleukin-5 monoclonal antibody on intestinal worm burden in a primary infection with strongyloides venezuelensis in mice. *Int. J. Parasitol.* **24:**951–957.

Koyama, K., H. Tamauchi, M. Tomita, T. Kitajima, and Y. Ito. 1999. B-cell activation in the mesenteric lymph nodes of resistant BALB/c mice infected with the murine nematode parasite *Trichuris muris*. *Parasitol Res.* **85:**194–199.

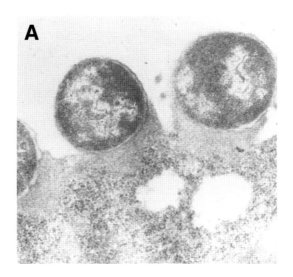

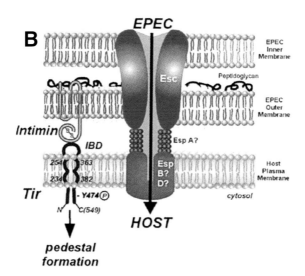

Color Plate 1 (chapter 1). (A) Electron micrograph of an A/E lesion caused by EPEC. (B) Model of protein secretion and Tir-intimin binding. The LEE-encoded Esc proteins form the secretion apparatus, and EspA-containing filaments form a channel through which secreted proteins are translocated into the host cytosol. EspB and EspD are thought to form a translocation pore in the host plasma membrane. Tir is one effector protein translocated into the host, where it is phosphorylated on tyrosine. It is then inserted into the plasma and serves as the receptor for the EPEC outer membrane protein, intimin, through its extracellular intimin binding domain (IBD). The Tir-intimin interaction triggers pedestal formation and A/E lesion induction. Electron micrograph courtesy of F. Ebel, Institut Pasteur, Paris, France. Model reproduced from Celli et al. (2000) with permission.

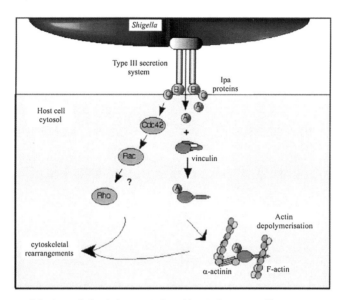

Color Plate 2 (chapter 1). Model of cytoskeletal changes induced by *S. flexneri*. Following contact with the host cell, the Ipa proteins IpaB and IpaC are inserted into the host plasma membrane by the type III secretion apparatus. These proteins form a pore through which IpaA is secreted into the host cytosol. IpaA interacts with vinculin, resulting in its unfolding and thus mediating the interaction between vinculin and actin. IpaC can activate the small GTPases Cdc42 and Rac, whereas Rho is activated by Rac. These changes culminate in the actin rearrangements that are required to form the macropinocytotic structure that mediates *Shigella* entry. Model courtesy of R. Bourdet-Sicard, Institut Pasteur, Paris, France.

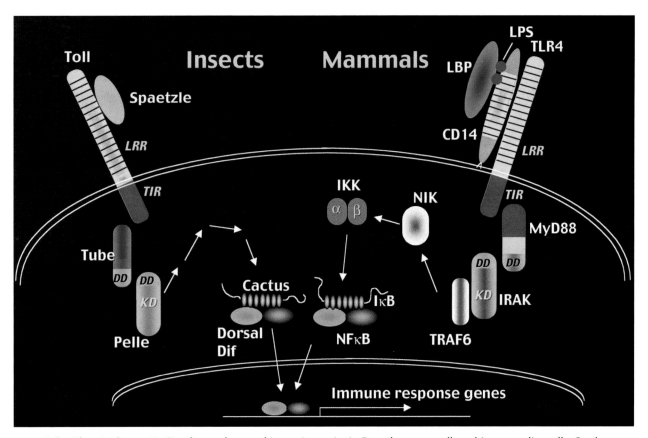

Color Plate 3 (chapter 7). Signaling pathways of innate immunity in *D. melanogaster* cells and in mammalian cells. On the left are the pathways involved in the induction of the antifungal gene drosomycin when the processed Spaetzle protein binds to Toll. On the right are similar pathways that take place in mammalian cells when the bacterial product LPS interacts with TLR4, leading to activation of costimulatory genes. DD, death domains; KD, kinase domain; LRR, leucine-rich repeat domain. For details, see Hoffman et al. (1999) and Medzhitov et al. (1997). Reproduced from Hoffman et al. (1999) with permission of the American Association for the Advancement of Science.

Inductive sites

Effector sites

Dendritic cells

M cells

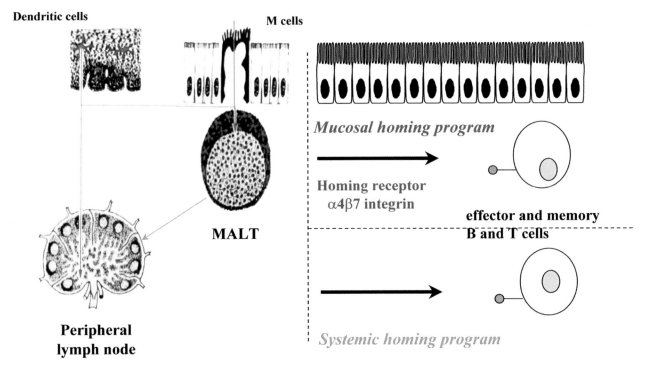

MALT

Peripheral lymph node

Mucosal homing program

Homing receptor α4β7 integrin

effector and memory B and T cells

Systemic homing program

Color Plate 4 (chapter 14). Inductive and effector sites in mucosal tissues. Different strategies are used to sample antigens across epithelial barriers and deliver them to inductive sites. In stratified epithelia (oral cavity and vagina), circulating monocytes are recruited that differentiate within the epithelial microenvironment into Langerhans' cells or DCs. These cells capture and internalize antigenic macromolecules and microorganisms and subsequently migrate into local MALT or, via lymphatics, into the draining lymph nodes. In simple epithelia, M cells transport antigens into MALT, where they are taken up by DCs. If induction of the immune response occurs in MALT and lymph nodes associated with mucosal tissues, the effector and memory immune cells acquire a mucosal homing program ($\alpha_4\beta_7$ integrin) and return to mucosal effector sites. If induction occurs in distant organized lymphoid tissues, the resulting effector and memory cells express a systemic homing program.

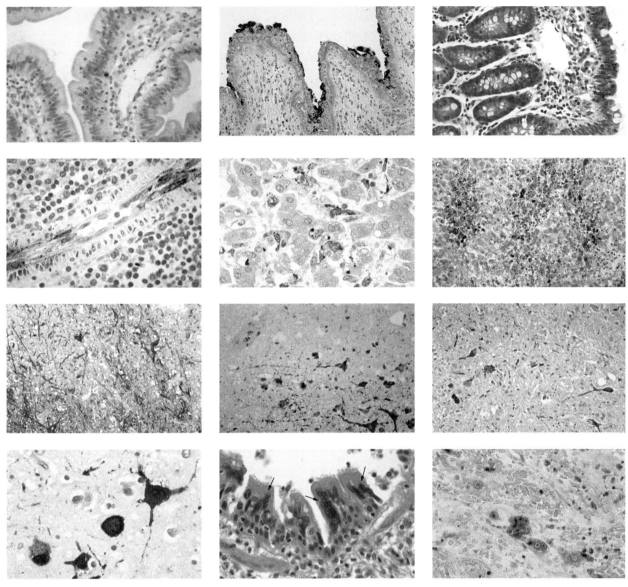

Color Plate 5 (chapter 22). (Row 1, left) SIV in a naturally infected sooty mangabey. In situ hybridization for viral RNA shows an infected lymphocyte in the lamina propria of the jejunum. Nitroblue tetrazolium–5-bromo-4-chloro-3-indolyl phosphate chromogen (blue) with nuclear fast red counterstain. Magnification, ×368. (Row 1, middle) Influenza A virus infection in the lung of a human. Viral antigens are present in lining bronchial epithelial cells. Immunoalkaline phosphatase staining, naphthol fast red substrate with light hematoxylin counterstain. Magnification, ×46. (Row 1, right) Rotavirus infection in the small intestine of a human. Viral antigens are present in superficial epithelial cells of small intestine and cellular debris. Immunoalkaline phosphatase staining, naphthol fast red substrate with light hematoxylin counterstain. Magnification, ×92. (Row 2, left) Dengue virus infection in the spleen of a human. Viral antigens are present in endothelial cells of a large vessel. Immunoalkaline phosphatase staining, naphthol fast red substrate with light hematoxylin counterstain. Magnification, ×145. (Row 2, middle) Dengue virus infection in the liver of a human. Viral antigens are present in Kupffer cells and sinusoidal lining cells of the liver. Immunoalkaline phosphatase staining, naphthol fast red substrate with light hematoxylin counterstain. Magnification, ×145. (Row 2, right) Rift Valley fever virus infection in the liver of a human. Viral antigens are present in hepatocytes, Kupffer cells, and sinusoidal lining cells of the liver. Immunoalkaline phosphatase staining, naphthol fast red substrate with light hematoxylin counterstain. Magnification, ×92. (Row 3, left) Eastern equine encephalitis virus infection in the brain of a human. Most cells were infected, as evidenced by the presence of viral antigens in neurons and neuronal processes. Immunoalkaline phosphatase staining, naphthol fast red substrate with light hematoxylin counterstain. Magnification, ×46. (Row 3, middle) Nipah virus infection in the brain of a human. Viral antigens are present in neurons and neuronal processes. Immunoalkaline phosphatase staining, naphthol fast red substrate with light hematoxylin counterstain. Magnification, ×46. (Row 3, right) West Nile virus infection in the brain of a human. Viral antigens are present in neurons and neuronal processes. Immunoalkaline phosphatase staining, naphthol fast red substrate with light hematoxylin counterstain. Magnification, ×46. (Row 4, left) Adenovirus infection in the brain of a human. Viral antigens are present in neurons and neuronal processes. Immunoalkaline phosphatase staining, naphthol fast red substrate with light hematoxylin counterstain. Magnification, ×145. (Row 4, middle) Measles virus infection in the lung of a human. Multinucleated syncytial cells (arrows) are seen in the bronchial epithelium. Hematoxylin and eosin stain. Magnification, ×145. (Row 4, right) Measles virus infection in the lung of a human. Viral antigens are present in intranuclear inclusions of multinucleated syncytial cells. Immunoalkaline phosphatase staining, naphthol fast red substrate with light hematoxylin counterstain. Magnification, ×145.

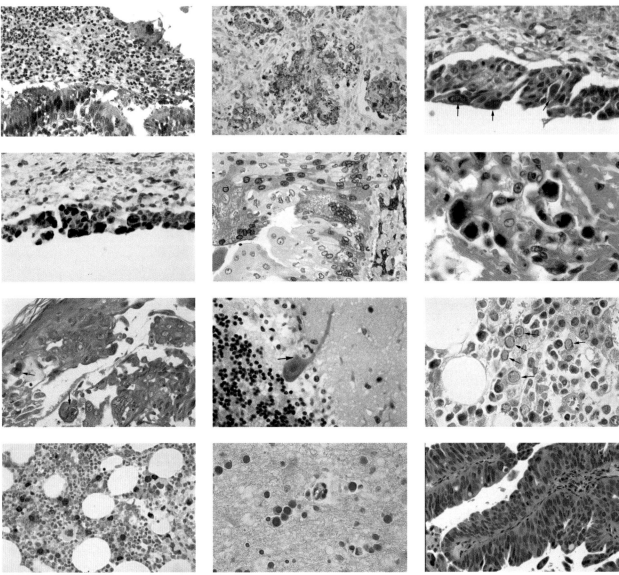

Color Plate 6 (chapter 22). (Row 1, left) Nipah virus infection in the lung of a pig. Viral antigens are present in bronchial epithelial cells and sloughing cellular debris. Immunoalkaline phosphatase staining, naphthol fast red substrate with light hematoxylin counterstain. Magnification, ×145. (Row 1, middle) Respiratory syncytial virus infection in the lung of a human. Viral antigens are present in the nuclei and cytoplasm of multinucleated syncytial cells. Immunoalkaline phosphatase staining, naphthol fast red substrate with light hematoxylin counterstain. Magnification, ×46. (Row 1, right) BK polyomavirus infection in the urinary bladder of a human. Multiple viral inclusions (arrows) are present in epithelial cells. Hematoxylin and eosin stain. Magnification, ×145. (Row 2, left) BK polyomavirus infection in the urinary bladder of a human. Viral antigens are present in epithelial cells. Immunoalkaline phosphatase staining, naphthol fast red substrate with light hematoxylin counterstain. Magnification, ×92. (Row 2, middle) Nipah virus infection in the urinary bladder of a pig. Viral antigens are present in epithelial cells and multinucleated syncytial cells. Immunoalkaline phosphatase staining, naphthol fast red substrate with light hematoxylin counterstain. Magnification, ×92. (Row 2, right) Adenovirus infection in the lung of a human. Viral inclusions and smudge cells are present in the interstitium and alveolar space. Hematoxylin and eosin stain. Magnification, ×230. (Row 3, left) Varicella-zoster virus infection in the skin of a human. Large intranuclear inclusions (arrows) are present in the epidermis. Hematoxylin and eosin stain. Magnification, ×145. (Row 3, middle) Rabies virus infection in the cerebellum of a human. An intracytoplasmic inclusion body (Negri body [arrow]) is present in a Purkinje cell. Hematoxylin and eosin stain. Magnification, ×145. (Row 3, right) Human parvovirus infection in the bone marrow of a human. Intranuclear inclusions (arrows) are present in nucleated red blood cells. Hematoxylin and eosin stain. Magnification, ×230. (Row 4, left) Human parvovirus infection in the bone marrow of a human. Viral antigens are present in nucleated red blood cells. Immunoalkaline phosphatase staining, naphthol fast red substrate with light hematoxylin counterstain. Magnification, ×92. (Row 4, middle) Measles virus infection in the brain of a human with subacute sclerosing panencephalitis. Viral antigens are present in intranuclear inclusions in neurons. Immunoalkaline phosphatase staining, naphthol fast red substrate with light hematoxylin counterstain. Magnification, ×145. (Row 4, right) Human papillomavirus infection in the cervix of a human with cervical papillary adenocarcinoma. Hematoxylin and eosin stain. Magnification, ×92.

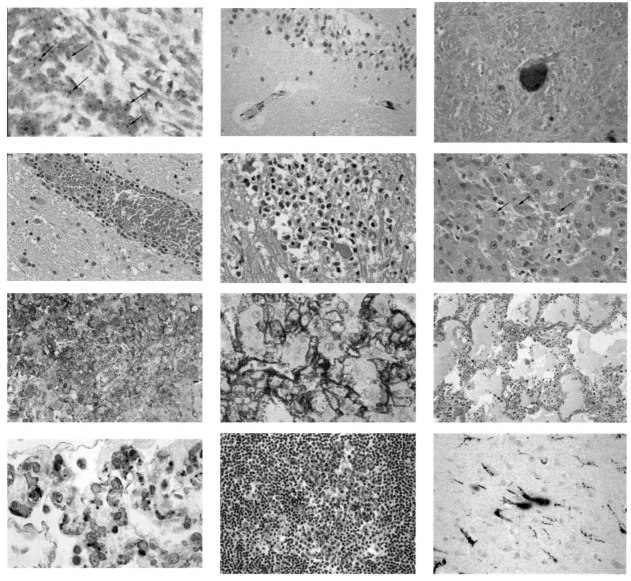

Color Plate 7 (chapter 22). (Row 1, left) Human papillomavirus infection in the cervix of a human showing an integrated HPV genome (arrows) in carcinoma cells. In situ hybridization. Magnification, ×92. (Row 1, middle) Nipah virus infection in the brain of a human. Viral antigens are present in endothelial cells and syncytial cells of cerebral vasculature. Immunoalkaline phosphatase staining, naphthol fast red substrate with light hematoxylin counterstain. Magnification, ×145. (Row 1, right) SIV infection in the brain of a pig-tailed macaque monkey. In situ hybridization for viral RNA, showing an infected perivascular multinucleated giant cell within the parenchyma of the brain. Nitroblue tetrazolium–5-bromo-4-chloro-3-indolyl phosphate chromogen (blue) with nuclear fast red counterstain. Magnification, ×368. (Row 2, left) West Nile virus infection in the brain of a human. Perivascular "cuffs" of inflammatory cells, as shown here, are a common feature of viral encephalitides and are not specific for a particular viral agent. Hematoxylin and eosin stain. Magnification, ×92. (Row 2, middle) Japanese encephalitis virus infection in the brain of a human. Neuronal necrosis, neuronophagia, and parenchymal inflammation are major histopathologic features. Hematoxylin and eosin stain. Magnification, ×92. (Row 2, right) Ebola virus infection in the liver of a human. This section shows severe hepatocellular necrosis and multiple inclusions (arrows) in hepatocytes. Hematoxylin and eosin stain. Magnification, ×145. (Row 3, left) Ebola virus infection in the liver of a human. Viral antigens are present in hepatocytes, Kupffer cells, and the cells lining the hepatic sinusoids. Immunoalkaline phosphatase staining, naphthol fast red substrate with light hematoxylin counterstain. Magnification, ×92. (Row 3, middle) Lassa fever virus infection in the liver of a human. Viral antigens are present in hepatocytes, Kupffer cells, and cells lining the hepatic sinusoids. Immunoalkaline phosphatase staining, naphthol fast red substrate with light hematoxylin counterstain. Magnification, ×145. (Row 3, right) Hantavirus infection in the lung of a human. Pulmonary edema and hyaline membrane formation are present. Hematoxylin and eosin stain. Magnification, ×46. (Row 4, left) Hantavirus infection in the lung of a human. Viral antigens are present in endothelial cells of the pulmonary microvasculature. Immunoalkaline phosphatase staining, naphthol fast red substrate with light hematoxylin counterstain. Magnification, ×230. (Row 4, middle) Human immunodeficiency virus type 1 (HIV-1) infection in a chimpanzee. Immunohistochemistry for the major viral capsid antigen, p24, in a section of lymph node is shown. Note the reticular pattern of intercellular p24 reactivity within the germinal center, typical of dendritic cell trapping of virions. Immunoperoxidase reaction, with diaminobenzidine chromogen (brown) and hematoxylin counterstain. Magnification, ×368. (Row 4, right) SIV infection in the brain of a pig-tailed macaque. Most of the productively infected cells in the brain are macrophages, as revealed by the dual-label technique, using in situ hybridization to localize viral RNA (blue) and immunohistochemistry to localize the macrophage phenotype marker, Ham-56 (black). Nitroblue tetrazolium–5-bromo-4-chloro-3-indolyl phosphate chromogen (ISH) plus immunogold (IHC); counterstain was omitted. Magnification, ×368.

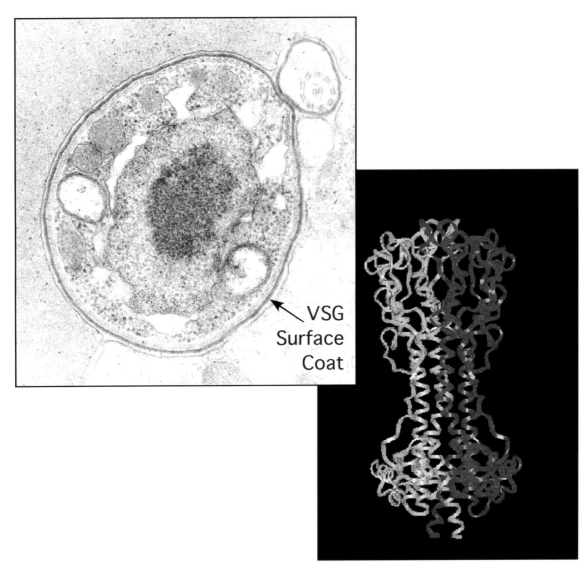

Tbr LouTat 1 VSG Homodimer

Color Plate 8 (chapter 25). VSG coat of African trypanosomes. An electron photomicrograph of *Trypanosoma brucei rhodesiense* (*Tbr*) LouTat 1 reveals the dense molecular packing of VSG molecules on the plasma membrane. Also shown is a structural model of the LouTat 1 VSG homodimer in an orientation that it assumes on the membrane with other identical homodimers to form the surface coat.

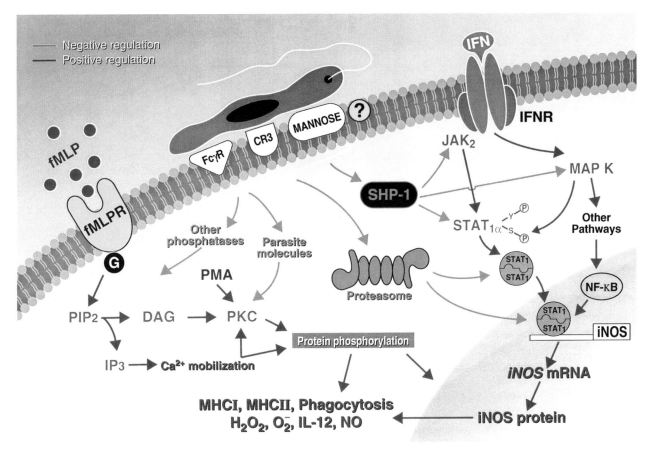

Color Plate 9 (chapter 25). *Leishmania*-induced macrophage signaling alteration. Binding of *Leishmania* to host cell receptors is potentially responsible for the induction of deactivating events involving proteasome and SHP-1 activation. SHP-1 negatively affects JAK2 kinase and Erk1/Erk2 mitogen-activated protein kinase (MAP K) conducting to the inhibition of IFNγ-inducible macrophage functions. Proteolysis of signaling molecules such as STAT1 contributes to this inactivation process. Other phosphatases (e.g., IP3 phosphatase and calcineurin) and surface parasite molecules (i.e., LPG) are recognized for their role in the alteration of various second messengers (i.e., PKC, Ca^{2+}, inositol lipids, and inositol phosphates) necessary for the induction of important phagocyte functions in response to chemotactic peptide (f-Met-Leu-Phe) and phorbol ester (PMA).

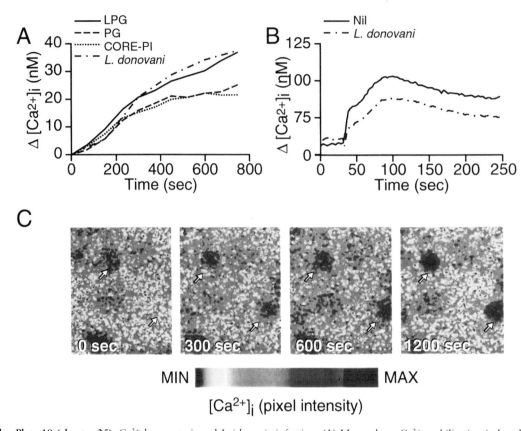

Color Plate 10 (chapter 25). Ca²⁺ homeostasis and *Leishmania* infection. (A) Macrophage Ca²⁺ mobilization induced by *L. donovani* and its surface molecule LPG (PG + CORE-PI; LPG structural components). (B) Thapsigargin-mediated intracellular Ca²⁺ stores emptying in uninfected and *L. donovani*-infected cells. Reduced levels of Ca²⁺ released from intracellular stores in *Leishmania*-infected cells suggests partial Ca²⁺ store depletion which could contribute to the activation of the capacitative mechanism responsible for the sustained Ca²⁺ influx. (C) *Leishmania*-induced Ca²⁺ mobilization observed by confocal microscopy.

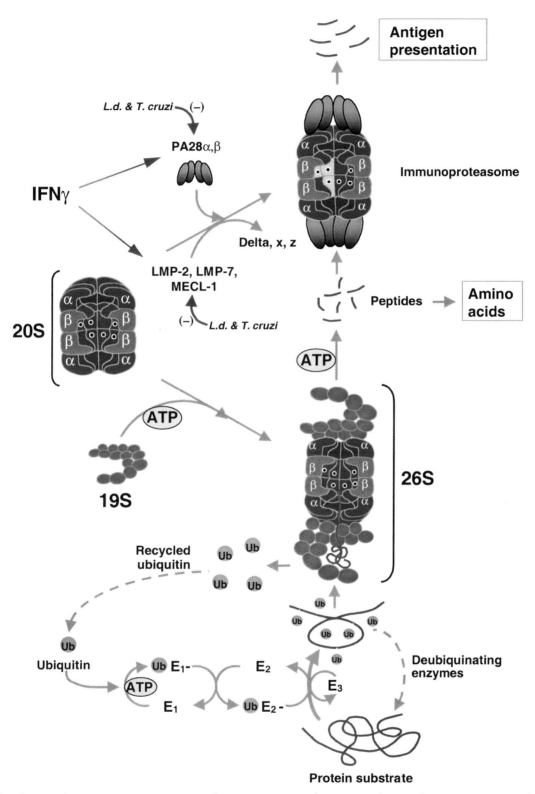

Color Plate 11 (chapter 25). Proteasome (26S) and immunoproteasome formation. Both types of proteasomes originate from the cylindrical 20S proteasome. The 26S proteasome is involved in the proteolysis of diverse proteins, which require ubiquitination for their recognition and degradation. IFN-γ-inducible immunoproteasome is formed by the addition of immunoproteasome (LMP-2, LMP-7, and MECL-1) and catalytic (PA28α and PA28β) subunits to the 20S proteasome. Immunoproteasome is necessary for the generation of peptides to be presented in an MHC class I context. Infection of macrophages by *L. donovani* and *T. cruzi* parasites leads to abnormal immunoproteasome formation.

Kumar, S., and R. L. Tarleton. 1998. The relative contribution of antibody production and CD8+ T cell function to immune control of *Trypanosoma cruzi*. *Parasite Immunol.* 20:207–216.

Lantz, C. S., J. Boesiger, C. H. Song, N. Mach, T. Kobayashi, R. C. Mulligan, Y. Nawa, G. Dranoff, and S. J. Galli. 1998. Role for interleukin-3 in mast-cell and basophil development and in immunity to parasites. *Nature* 392:90–93.

Lawrence, C. E., J. C. Paterson, L. M. Higgins, T. T. MacDonald, M. W. Kennedy, and P. Garside. 1998. IL-4-regulated enteropathy in an intestinal nematode infection. *Eur. J. Immunol.* 28: 2672–2684.

Lawrence, C. E., J. C. Paterson, X. Q. Wei, F. Y. Liew, P. Garside, and M. W. Kennedy. 2000. Nitric oxide mediates intestinal pathology but not immune expulsion during *Trichinella spiralis* infection in mice. *J. Immunol.* 164:4229–4234.

Love, R. J., B. M. Ogilvie, and D. J. McLaren. 1976. The immune mechanism which expels the intestinal stage of *Trichinella spiralis* from rats. *Immunology* 30:7–15.

MacKenzie, C. R., R. Langen, O. Takikawa, and W. Daubener. 1999. Inhibition of indoleamine 2,3-dioxygenase in human macrophages inhibits interferon-gamma-induced bacteriostasis but does not abrogate toxoplasmastasis. *Eur. J. Immunol.* 29:3254–3261.

Madden, K. B., J. F. Urban, Jr., H. J. Ziltener, J. W. Schrader, F. D. Finkelman, and I. M. Katona. 1991. Antibodies to IL-3 and IL-4 suppress helminth-induced intestinal mastocytosis. *J. Immunol.* 147:1387–1391.

McKenzie, G. J., P. G. Fallon, C. L. Emson, R. K. Grencis, and A. N. McKenzie. 1999. Simultaneous disruption of interleukin (IL)-4 and IL-13 defines individual roles in T helper cell type 2-mediated responses. *J. Exp. Med.* 189:1565–1572.

Medzhitov, R., and C. Janeway, Jr. 2000. Innate immune recognition: mechanisms and pathways. *Immunol. Rev.* 173:89–97.

Mosmann, T. R., H. Cherwinski, M. W. Bond, M. A. Giedlin, and R. L. Coffman. 1986. Two types of murine helper T cell clone. Definition according to profiles of lymphokine activities and secreted proteins. *J. Immunol.* 126:2348–2357.

Muller, I., P. Kropf, J. A. Louis, and G. Milon. 1994. Expansion of gamma interferon-producing CD8+ T cells following secondary infection of mice immune to *Leishmania major*. *Infect. Immun.* 62:2575–2581.

Murray, H. W., and C. F. Nathan. 1999. Macrophage microbicidal mechanisms in vivo: reactive nitrogen versus oxygen intermediates in the killing of intracellular visceral *Leishmania donovani*. *J. Exp. Med.* 189:741–746.

Nashleanas, M., S. Kanaly, and P. Scott. 1998. Control of *Leishmania major* infection in mice lacking TNF receptors. *J. Immunol.* 160:5506–5513.

Pfefferkorn, E. R. 1984. Interferon gamma blocks the growth of *Toxoplasma gondii* in human fibroblasts by inducing the host cells to degrade tryptophan. *Proc. Natl. Acad. Sci. USA* 81:908–912.

Prina, E., T. Lang, N. Glaichenhaus, and J. C. Antoine. 1996. Presentation of the protective parasite antigen LACK by *Leishmania*-infected macrophages. *J. Immunol.* 156:4318–4327.

Pritchard, D. I., D. J. Williams, J. M. Behnke, and T. D. Lee. 1983. The role of IgG1 hypergammaglobulinaemia in immunity to the gastrointestinal nematode *Nematospiroides dubius*. The immunochemical purification, antigen-specificity and in vivo anti-parasite effect of IgG1 from immune serum. *Immunology* 49:353–365.

Reed, S. G. 1998. Immunology of *Trypanosoma cruzi* infections. *Chem. Immunol.* 70:124–143.

Richard, M., R. K. Grencis, N. E. Humphreys, J. C. Renauld, and J. Van Snick. 2000. Anti-IL-9 vaccination prevents worm expulsion and blood eosinophilia in *Trichuris muris*-infected mice. *Proc. Natl. Acad. Sci. USA* 97:767–772.

Roach, T. I., K. J. Else, D. Wakelin, D. J. McLaren, and R. K. Grencis. 1991. *Trichuris muris*: antigen recognition and transfer of immunity in mice by IgA monoclonal antibodies. *Parasite Immunol.* 13:1–12.

Russell, D. G., E. Medina-Acosta, and A. Golubev. 1991. The interface between the Leishmania-infected macrophage and the host's immune system. *Behring Inst. Mitt.* 88:68–79.

Sato, N., S. K. Ahuja, M. Quinones, V. Kostecki, R. L. Reddick, P. C. Melby, W. A. Kuziel, and S. S. Ahuja. 2000. CC chemokine receptor (CCR)2 is required for Langerhans cell migration and localization of T helper cell type 1 (Th1)-inducing dendritic cells. Absence of CCR2 shifts the *Leishmania major*-resistant phenotype to a susceptible state dominated by Th2 cytokines, B cell outgrowth, and sustained neutrophilic inflammation. *J. Exp. Med.* 192:205–218.

Sayles, P. C., G. W. Gibson, and L. L. Johnson. 2000. B cells are essential for vaccination-induced resistance to virulent *Toxoplasma gondii*. *Infect. Immun.* 68:1026–1033.

Scharton-Kersten, T. M., G. Yap, J. Magram, and A. Sher. 1997. Inducible nitric oxide is essential for host control of persistent but not acute infection with the intracellular pathogen *Toxoplasma gondii*. *J. Exp. Med.* 185:1261–1273.

Senn, K. A., K. D. McCoy, K. J. Maloy, G. Stark, E. Frohli, T. Rulicke, and R. Klemenz. 2000. T1-deficient and T1-Fc-transgenic mice develop a normal protective Th2- type immune response following infection with *Nippostrongylus brasiliensis*. *Eur. J. Immunol.* 30:1929–1938.

Solbach, W., and T. Laskay. 2000. The host response to *Leishmania* infection. *Adv. Immunol.* 74:275–317.

Soong, L., J.-C. Su, I. S. Grewal, P. Kima, J. Sun, B. J. Longley, N. H. Ruddle, D. McMahon-Pratt, and R. A. Flavell. 1996. Disruption of CD40-CD40 ligand interactions results in enhanced susceptibility to *Leishmania amazonensis* infection. *Immunity* 4:263–274.

Sousa, C. R., S. Hieny, T. Scharton-Kersten, D. Jankovic, H. Charest, R. N. Germain, and A. Sher. 1997. In vivo microbial stimulation induces rapid CD40 ligand-independent production of interleukin 12 by dendritic cells and their redistribution to T cell areas. *J. Exp. Med.* 186:1819–1829.

Sutterwala, F. S., G. J. Noel, P. Salgame, and D. M. Mosser. 1998. Reversal of proinflammatory responses by ligating the macrophage Fcgamma receptor type I. *J. Exp. Med.* 188:217–222.

Taylor, A. P., and H. W. Murray. 1997. Intracellular antimicrobial activity in the absence of interferon-gamma: effect of interleukin-12 in experimental visceral leishmaniasis in interferon-gamma gene-disrupted mice. *J. Exp. Med.* 185:1231–1239.

Taylor, G. A., C. M. Collazo, G. S. Yap, K. Nguyen, T. A. Gregorio, L. S. Taylor, B. Eagleson, L. Secrest, E. A. Southon, S. W. Reid, L. Tessarollo, M. Bray, D. W. McVicar, K. L. Komschlies, H. A. Young, C. A. Biron, A. Sher, and G. F. Vande Woude. 2000. Pathogen-specific loss of host resistance in mice lacking the IFN-gamma-inducible gene IGTP. *Proc. Natl. Acad. Sci. USA* 97:751–755.

Townsend, M. J., P. G. Fallon, D. J. Matthews, P. Smith, H. E. Jolin, and A. N. McKenzie 2000. IL-9-deficient mice establish fundamental roles for IL-9 in pulmonary mastocytosis and goblet cell hyperplasia but not T cell development. *Immunity* 13: 573–583.

Trinchieri, G. 1998. Interleukin-12: a cytokine at the interface of inflammation and immunity. *Adv. Immunol.* 70:83–243.

Uchikawa, R., S. Matsuda, and N. Arizono. 2000. Suppression of gamma interferon transcription and production by nematode excretory-secretory antigen during polyclonal stimulation of rat lymph node T cells. *Infect. Immun.* 68:6233–6239.

Urban, J. F., Jr., I. M. Katona, W. E. Paul, and F. D. Finkelman. 1991. Interleukin 4 is important in protective immunity to a gastrointestinal nematode infection in mice. *Proc. Natl. Acad. Sci. USA* **88:**5513–5517.

Urban, J. F., Jr., C. R. Maliszewski, K. B. Madden, I. M. Katona, and F. D. Finkelman. 1995. IL-4 treatment can cure established gastrointestinal nematode infections in immunocompetent and immunodeficient mice. *J. Immunol.* **154:**4675–4684.

Urban, J. F., Jr., N. Noben-Trauth, D. D. Donaldson, K. B. Madden, S. C. Morris, M. Collins, and F. D. Finkelman. 1998. IL-13, IL-4Ralpha, and Stat6 are required for the expulsion of the gastrointestinal nematode parasite *Nippostrongylus brasiliensis*. *Immunity.* **8:**255–264.

Urban, J. F., Jr., L. Schopf, S. C. Morris, T. Orekhova, K. B. Madden, C. J. Betts, H. R. Gamble, C. Byrd, D. Donaldson, K. Else, and F. D. Finkelman 2000. Stat6 signaling promotes protective immunity against *Trichinella spiralis* through a mast cell- and T cell-dependent mechanism. *J. Immunol.* **164:**2046–2052.

Vallance, B. A., P. A. Blennerhassett, and S. M. Collins. 1997. Increased intestinal muscle contractility and worm expulsion in nematode-infected mice. *Am. J. Physiol.* **272:**G321–G327.

Vallance, B. A., K. Croitoru, and S. M. Collins. 1998. T lymphocyte-dependent and -independent intestinal smooth muscle dysfunction in the *T. spiralis*-infected mouse. *Am. J. Physiol.* **275:** G1157–G1165.

Vester, B., K. Muller, W. Solbach, and T. Laskay. 1999. Early gene expression of NK cell-activating chemokines in mice resistant to *Leishmania major*. *Infect Immun.* **67:**3155–3159.

Wakelin, D. 1978. Immunity to intestinal parasites. *Nature* **273:** 617–620.

Wang, Z. E., S. L. Reiner, F. Hatam, F. P. Heinzel, J. Bouvier, C. W. Turck, and R. M. Locksley. 1993. Targeted activation of CD8 cells and infection of beta-2-microglobulin-deficient mice fail to confirm a primary protective role for CD8 cells in experimental leishmaniasis. *J. Immunol.* **151:**2077–2086.

Wei, X.-Q., I. G. Charles, A. Smith, J. Ure, G.-J. Feng, F.-P. Huang, X. Damo, W. Muller, S. Moncada, and F. Y. Liew. 1995. Altered immune responses in mice lacking inducible nitric oxide synthase. *Nature* **375:**408–411.

Weisbrodt, N. W., M. Lai, R. L. Bowers, Y. Harari, and G. A. Castro. 1994. Structural and molecular changes in intestinal smooth muscle induced by *Trichinella spiralis* infection. *Am. J. Physiol.* **266:**G856–G862.

Xu, D., V. Trajkovic, D. Hunter, B. P. Leung, K. Schulz, J. A. Gracie, I. B. McInnes, and F. Y. Liew. 2000. IL-18 induces the differentiation of Th1 or Th2 cells depending upon cytokine milieu and genetic background. *Eur. J. Immunol.* **30:**3147–3156.

Yap, G. S., T. Scharton-Kersten, H. Charest, and A. Sher. 1998. Decreased resistance of TNF receptor p55- and p75-deficient mice to chronic toxoplasmosis despite normal activation of inducible nitric oxide synthase in vivo. *J. Immunol.* **160:**1340–1345.

Yap, G. S., and A. Sher. 1999. Effector cells of both nonhemopoietic and hemopoietic origin are required for interferon (IFN)-gamma- and tumor necrosis factor (TNF)-alpha-dependent host resistance to the intracellular pathogen, *Toxoplasma gondii*. *J. Exp. Med.* **189:**1083–1092.

Yoshimoto, T., H. Mizutani, H. Tsutsui, N. Noben-Trauth, K. Yamanaka, M. Tanaka, S. Izumi, H. Okamura, W. E. Paul, and K. Nakanishi. 2000. IL-18 induction of IgE: dependence on CD4 T cells, IL-4 and STAT 6. *Nat. Immunol.* **1:**132–137.

Immunology of Infectious Diseases
Edited by S. H. E. Kaufmann, A. Sher, and R. Ahmed
© 2002 ASM Press, Washington, D.C.

Chapter 18

Acquired Immunity against Viral Infections

EVA SZOMOLANYI-TSUDA, MICHAEL A. BREHM, AND RAYMOND M. WELSH

Viral infections activate both the humoral and cellular arms of the antigen-specific acquired immune system, and the combined action of B and T lymphocytes acts to clear virus and to provide protective immunity against subsequent infections. The importance of acquired immunity against viruses is demonstrated by the fatal outcome of infections with many viruses (such as vaccinia virus, polyomavirus, and influenza virus) in mice with severe combined immunodeficiency (SCID mice), which lack functional T and B cells. Infection of immunocompetent mice with the same viruses under the same conditions (viral dose and route of infection) does not result in apparent disease or mortality. Viruses such as lymphocytic choriomeningitis virus (LCMV) that are not highly cytopathic and do not kill SCID mice establish persistent infections in the host. Therefore, the acquired immune system is required for the efficient control of virus infections.

The relative contributions of the cellular and humoral arms to viral clearance vary with the particular virus. Viruses have evolved by interacting with components of the innate and adaptive immune systems and, as a consequence, have developed diverse strategies for replication, spread, and survival in the host. To counter these strategies, the vertebrate immune system has a wide range of effector mechanisms employed by B and T lymphocytes to control viral infections. The humoral and cellular arms collaborate with each other, enhancing or modulating these effector mechanisms. The multiple ways to clear virus provide redundant systems that become apparent in individuals with partial immunodeficiency.

Most of our present understanding of antiviral immune mechanisms comes from experiments performed with inbred laboratory mice. Different components of the immune system can be easily manipulated in mice by the depletion of specific cell types, by blocking of specific interactions with monoclonal antibodies, or by adoptive transfer of cell populations into hosts. In addition, the use of genetically targeted mutant knockout or transgenic strains of mice allows one to address fundamental questions that had not been accessible for experimentation previously. The data obtained with mice, however, must be carefully interpreted and compared with clinical observations in order for us to understand the human immune functions operating in virus-infected patients.

Viruses encode immunogenic protein antigens, but the immune responses to live viruses and inert proteins are fundamentally different. Most inert proteins are poorly immunogenic and have to be administered with adjuvants to generate detectable responses. In contrast, live viruses elicit strong immune responses. Because viruses interact with components of the innate and acquired immune systems and actively replicate in certain cell types, they may generate many signals that act as costimulatory or "danger" signals and contribute to the efficient activation of adaptive immune responses. Very high doses of antigens from rapidly replicating viruses can be reached locally. In addition, the repetitive surface structure of many viruses may enable them to cross-link B-cell receptors and thereby enhance their efficiency to induce antibody responses.

In this chapter we will describe the dynamics of the T- and B-cell responses elicited by virus infections and illustrate the functions and importance of these cells with examples from well-studied viral models.

T-CELL RESPONSES

Virus-specific T lymphocytes are important for the immunologic control of viral infections. Studies

Eva Szomolanyi-Tsuda, Michael A. Brehm, and Raymond M. Welsh • Department of Pathology, University of Massachusetts Medical School, Worcester, MA 01655.

with numerous viruses in murine systems have laid the foundation for our current understanding of the functionality of T lymphocytes, including major histocompatibility complex (MHC) restriction (Zinkernagel and Doherty, 1974), the nature of T-cell epitopes (Townsend et al., 1986), and the hierarchies of epitope recognition (Gairin et al., 1995; Mylin et al., 1995). The T-lymphocyte response elicited by an antigenic challenge is generally composed of two cell types: the MHC class II-restricted CD4[+] T cells and the MHC class I-restricted CD8[+] T cells. T lymphocytes recognize antigen derived from either exogenous or endogenous protein antigens (Fig. 1). This duality enables T lymphocytes to recognize antigens derived from viral proteins that have been internalized by professional antigen-presenting cells (APC) and to detect other types of virus-infected cells throughout the body. In addition to the differences in target recognition, the two T-cell subsets generally have distinct functions during the response to the infection. The CD4[+] T cells serve as regulators of the antiviral immune response by providing help to both CD8[+] T cells and B cells by secreting cytokines and by making direct contact via costimulatory molecules in the

case of B cells. In contrast, a main role of CD8[+] T cells is to eliminate virus-infected cells through cytotoxic mechanisms, and these cells are generally referred to as cytotoxic T lymphocytes (CTL). These distinctions are not absolute, since cytotoxic CD4[+] T-cell lines have been isolated from the peripheral blood of herpes simplex virus (HSV)-infected and measles virus-infected humans (Jacobson et al., 1984; Yasukawa and Zarling, 1984), and CD8[+] T cells have been demonstrated to synthesize a wide range of cytokines including interleukin-2 (IL-2), gamma interferon (IFN-γ), and tumor necrosis factor alpha (TNF-α). While much emphasis has been placed on ascertaining the relative contributions of either T-cell subset to the resolution of viral infections, the optimal control of infection in vivo usually occurs with cooperation between both sets.

Virus-Specific T-Lymphocyte Epitopes

T-cell recognition of antigen is mediated by the T-cell receptor (TCR), which is structurally similar to immunoglobulins (Ig) (Davis et al., 1998). As described in Fig. 1, CD8[+] CTL recognize short peptides presented by MHC class I molecules. Proteins con-

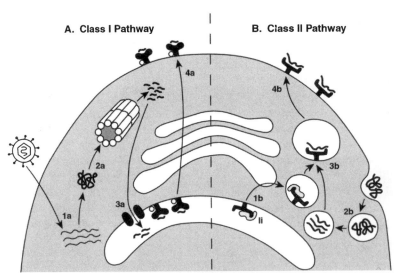

Figure 1. Presentation of viral antigens. (A) Processing and presentation of MHC class I-restricted peptides. (Step 1a) Following virus infection, viral gene products are synthesized. (Step 2a) Viral proteins are degraded via cellular proteasomes to produce short peptide fragments. (Step 3a) The viral peptides are transported into the endoplasmic reticulum (ER) by the transporters associated with antigen processing. Within the ER, peptides associate with class I molecules that are complexed with the β_2-microglobulin. (Step 4a) This newly formed tripartite complex is then shuttled to the cell surface for recognition by virus-specific CTL. (B) Processing and presentation of MHC class II-restricted peptides. (Step 1b) Newly synthesized MHC class II molecules are localized within the ER and are complexed with the invariant chain (Ii), which obstructs the peptide-binding site. The invariant chain also participates in the folding of class II molecules and in their transport to the endocytic pathway. The class II complex is shuttled out of the ER into an endosomal compartment (MIIC), where the invariant chain is degraded by proteases, revealing the peptide-binding site. (Step 2b) APC internalize exogenous viral proteins by endocytosis. The proteins are localized to the endocytic pathway, where they are degraded by proteases into peptides. (Step 3b) As peptide-containing endosomes enter the MIIC, the virus-derived peptides bind to class II molecules. (Step 4b) The class II-peptide complexes migrate to the cell surface for presentation.

tain numerous peptide sequences that conform to binding motifs for MHC class I molecules, but relatively few peptides elicit CTL responses. For the virus-derived peptides that serve as epitopes, distinct hierarchies for their recognition by CTL have been demonstrated in numerous viral models (Chen et al., 2000; Gallimore et al., 1998; Mylin et al., 1995; Salvucci et al., 1995). Epitopes can be categorized as either immunodominant or subdominant, and this classification is dictated by the immunogenicity of a given epitope (Yewdell and Bennink, 1999). Immunodominant epitopes are highly immunogenic and therefore elicit CTL responses that are easily detectable, whereas CTL specific for weakly immunogenic, subdominant epitopes are often difficult to detect. A number of factors influence the hierarchy of CTL epitopes, including peptide affinity for the presenting class I molecule, the efficiency of peptide processing and presentation, the availability of reactive T cells within the repertoire, and the ability of immunodominant peptides to negatively influence the induction of CTL specific for weaker epitopes (Chen et al., 2000).

The hierarchies of virus-derived CTL epitopes have been defined in numerous viral systems. Six H-2^b-restricted CTL epitopes have been defined for LCMV; four are contained within the glycoprotein (GP33–41, GP34–41, GP92–101, and GP276–286) and two are within the nucleoprotein (NP396–404 and NP205–212) (Gairin et al., 1995; Hudrisier et al., 1997; van der Most et al., 1998; Whitton et al., 1988). The NP396, GP33, GP34, and GP276 epitopes are considered immunodominant, whereas NP205 and GP92 are subdominant. CTL responses directed against any individual immunodominant or subdominant epitope provide protection against an LCMV challenge. In the HSV model, three H-2K^b-restricted epitopes have been identified: one is contained within glycoprotein B (gB498–505) (Bonneau et al., 1993); one is contained within ICP6, which is the large subunit of ribonucleotide reductase (RR1-822–829) (Salvucci et al., 1995); and one is contained within ICP27 (ICP27-445–452) (Nugent et al., 1995). These three H-2^b-restricted epitopes are derived from proteins that are expressed early during infection (Roizman and Sears, 1996). The early processing and presentation of HSV epitopes allow CTL to contribute to the elimination of infected cells prior to the rampant spread of infectious particles. The gB498 epitope is immunodominant and has been demonstrated to protect against HSV challenge (Blaney et al., 1998), while the RR1-822 and ICP27-445 epitopes are subdominant and their role in protection has yet to be evaluated.

CD4$^+$ T-cell epitopes are generally longer than class I-restricted peptides, and the binding motifs for MHC class II-restricted peptides have not been as completely delineated. LCMV infection elicits a marked increase in activated CD4$^+$ T cells during the acute response to the virus (Varga and Welsh, 1996) and results in relatively high frequencies of LCMV-specific CD4$^+$ T cells (~10% of the total CD4 T cells) (Varga and Welsh, 1998a, 1998b). Following this peak in the CD4 response, the frequency of LCMV-specific CD4 T cells decreases to approximately 2% of the total CD4 cells, and this frequency is maintained into memory (Varga and Welsh, 1998a; Whitmire et al., 1998). Two I-A^b-restricted peptides have been identified as targets for LCMV-induced CD4$^+$ T cells: one within GP, spanning amino acid residues 61 to 80, and one within NP, spanning residues 309 to 328 (Oxenius et al., 1995). Stimulation of CD4$^+$ T cells from LCMV-infected mice with either of these peptides induces the production of IFN-γ, IL-2, and TNF-α (Varga and Welsh, 1998a, 2000).

Kinetics of the T-Cell Response

Recent technologic advances have furthered our understanding of the dynamics of T-cell responses elicited by virus infection. Innovative techniques that stain epitope-specific T cells (MHC tetramers [Altman et al., 1996] and dimeric MHC-IgG chimeras [Dal Porto et al., 1993]) and that examine the functionality of individual T cells (intracellular cytokine stains and enzyme-linked immunospot (ELISPOT) assays [reviewed by Doherty and Christensen, 2000]), have demonstrated that studies utilizing limiting-dilution analysis had, not unexpectedly, often underestimated the magnitude of virus-specific responses. In agreement with previous studies demonstrating minimal virus-induced bystander expansion of T-cell populations (Zarozinski and Welsh, 1997), these novel approaches have shown that the majority of the proliferating CD8$^+$ T cells elicited by virus infection are virus specific (Butz and Bevan, 1998; Murali-Krishna et al., 1998). A generalized schematic depicting the kinetics of the T-cell response to a viral infection is shown in Fig. 2. The response is divided into three segments, beginning with the activation and proliferation of the T lymphocytes, continuing with the effector phase, and ending with the silencing of the response.

Activation of Virus-Specific T Cells

Prior to encountering antigen, T cells are in a naïve state and must be activated in order to contrib-

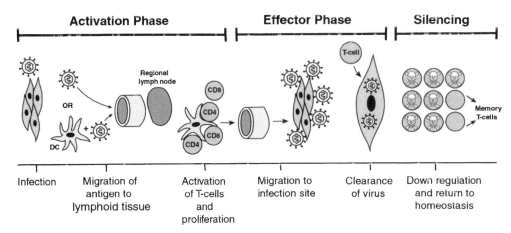

Figure 2. Kinetics of virus-induced T-cell responses. The T-lymphocyte response to virus infection can be divided into three segments: activation, effector phase, and silencing. After a virus infection at a peripheral site, viral antigens accumulate within draining lymphoid tissue, where they are processed and presented to virus-specific T cells. Following the activation and proliferation of the T-cell population, the activated lymphocytes migrate to the site(s) of infection to eliminate virus-infected cells. Once the host is cleared of viral antigens, the immune system restores homeostasis by deleting a large portion of the T cells. The remaining virus-specific T cells can acquire a memory phenotype.

ute to the resolution of a viral infection. The first step in this activation is the recognition of specific peptides processed from viral proteins and presented in the context of MHC molecules. Professional APC, such as dendritic cells (DC), B cells, and macrophages, are all efficient at processing and presenting peptide antigens to T cells. T-cell activation is also greatly enhanced by costimulatory signals delivered through the CD40 and CD28 pathways. The recognition of antigen in the absence of costimulation may result in an unresponsive or an anergic T-cell population. Following activation, the lymphocytes proliferate extensively, at three to four cell divisions per day, to produce the cell numbers required to eliminate the infection. Cytokines, such as IL-2, and antigen triggering of the TCR provide the stimulus needed for the dividing lymphocytes. The magnitude of this primary T-cell response, i.e, the burst size, directly correlates with the size of the virus-specific memory pool after antigen is cleared (Hou et al., 1994).

Antigen Presentation

Virus-infected cells synthesize large quantities of viral proteins at the peripheral infection site, but the T-cell response does not develop there. Draining lymphoid tissue is the preferred site for T-cell activation, largely due to the compartmentalization of both cells and factors important to the induction of the response. Thus, viral antigens must be available within the lymphoid organs draining the site of infection for optimal T-cell stimulation. Viruses with the ability to replicate in many different tissues may

reach lymphoid organs during the normal course of infection by the spread of replicating virus. Viruses may also have the ability to infect professional APC and then be transported by these cells into lymph nodes. Finally, uninfected professional APC may internalize viral antigens from the site of infection and traffic into draining lymphoid tissue for presentation.

DC are thought to be the primary APC for the stimulation of virus-specific T lymphocytes, due to their abilities to process and present antigen from the periphery and to provide costimulation and cytokine help (Klagge and Schneider-Schaulies, 1999). DC originate from bone marrow progenitors, enter the circulation, and home to peripheral tissues to await the opportunity to capture foreign antigen (Reis e Sousa et al., 1999). The distribution of DC throughout the body makes them ideal sentinels for the immune system. Generally, DC in the periphery are in an immature state that is characterized by the low expression of MHC and costimulatory molecules and by an increased phagocytic activity. Immature DC are attracted to infection sites by the release of chemokines during the innate response to virus and then begin to internalize antigen by several pathways, including macropinocytosis, receptor-mediated endocytosis, and phagocytosis. Inflammatory cytokines and the internalization of antigen can both provide the signals that initiate the transition of DC to maturity. Mature DC are the prototypical professional APC with high expression of MHC and costimulatory molecules (such as B7), a decreased ability to capture antigen, and the ability to synthesize cytokines and chemokines (Banchereau et al., 2000). DC that are undergoing maturation will migrate to draining lymphoid tissue, such as the regional lymph nodes, where mature DC can efficiently activate both CD4[+] and CD8[+] T cells.

The pathways of viral antigen presentation to T cells vary for different viruses. LCMV either can infect DC (Barchet et al., 2000) and be transported to the T-cell-rich lymphoid tissue or can reach these sites during the normal spread of infection. Within the lymphoid tissue, LCMV can replicate to high levels, providing ample antigen to stimulate the massive T-cell proliferation observed during infection. Influenza virus also infects DC, but in contrast to LCMV, the infected DC do not produce infectious viral particles (Bender et al., 1998). A block in influenza virus replication prevents the death of the DC, allowing the infected DC to continue presenting viral antigens to T cells. HSV also infects DC, but the infection blocks the maturation of human DC, as is shown by the lack of costimulatory molecule up-regulation, decreased cytokine expression, and a diminished capacity to stimulate T cells in vitro (Salio et al., 1999). This should help HSV escape immune surveillance, yet HSV is cleared during the acute response. This result suggests that in addition to the classical antigen presentation pathway, the peptides stimulating virus-specific T cells may be derived from alternative pathways. Recent evidence has indicated that virus-specific CD8[+] CTL can also recognize peptides derived from exogenous proteins (Sigal et al., 1999).

Costimulation

Costimulatory molecules are vital for the efficient induction of T-cell responses to many antigens. Two interactions that have been extensively examined for their contribution to the stimulation of T cells are CD40-CD40L and B7-1,B7-2–CD28. Whereas the engagement of CD40 and CD40L provides an indirect signal mediated through the up-regulation of costimulatory molecules such as B7 on the surface of APC, interactions between B7 molecules and CD28 deliver a direct activation stimulus for T cells. Costimulatory signals can also decrease the antigen levels necessary to activate T lymphocytes, thus making the immune system much more sensitive to pathogens that elicit these signals.

CD40-CD40L

CD40L expressed on activated CD4[+] T cells interacts with CD40 expressed on a variety of APC, including B cells, activated macrophages, and DC (Grewal and Flavell, 1998). Whereas CD40-CD40L engagement plays a direct role in the induction of B-cell responses, this interaction has an indirect in-

fluence on developing T-cell responses, since it contributes to the completion of the maturation of antigen-bearing DC (Toes et al., 1998). As described above, this maturation is manifested by an enhanced capacity to present antigens, up-regulation of costimulatory molecules such as B7 and CD40, and induction of cytokine secretion. Studies with CD40[−/−] and CD40L[−/−] mice demonstrated that the CD40-CD40L interaction is essential for the induction of CD4[+] Th cells, but the involvement in the activation of CD8[+] CTL is still being investigated. In the LCMV model, the induction of primary LCMV-specific CTL was only marginally reduced in CD40L knockout mice (Borrow et al., 1998) but the CD4[+] T-cell response was dramatically diminished (Whitmire et al., 1999). These CD40L knockout mice were unable to control infections with high doses of highly virulent LCMV strains (Thomsen et al., 1998; Whitmire et al., 1999). LCMV is a natural murine pathogen with the ability to replicate extensively in vivo without down-regulating class I expression or lysing infected cells, and the consequential abundance of antigenic stimulation may allow for the generation of LCMV-specific CTL in the absence of costimulatory signals. Thus, the generation of CTL responses by LCMV infection may not be representative of the T-cell responses evoked by other viral infections. This conclusion is consistent with studies on vesicular stomatitis virus (VSV), which has a limited capacity to replicate in mice and stimulates a CTL response that is dependent on CD40L (Andreasen et al., 2000).

B7-1,B7-2–CD28

The engagement of CD28 on T cells with B7 molecules on the surface of the activated APC (Harris et al., 1995), coupled with TCR signaling, enhances T-cell activation by stimulating the synthesis of cytokines (including IL-2) and antiapoptotic proteins (including Bcl$_{xL}$), and by up-regulating the expression of the α and β chains of the IL-2 receptor (McAdam et al., 1998). The B7-CD28 interaction is crucial for the activation of CD4[+] Th responses (Harris and Ronchese, 1999), but its importance for CTL stimulation appears to be dependent on the characteristics of the immunizing antigen. The activation of CD8[+] CTL that have a high affinity for their specific peptide is less dependent on CD28 signaling than is the activation of T cells with lower-affinity interactions (Bachmann et al., 1996; Wang et al., 2000). Sustained or repeated antigenic stimulation may also alleviate the need for CD28 signaling in CTL induction. Studies with TCR-transgenic, CD28 knockout mice indicated that a single injection with the peptide targeted by the transgenic TCR induced unresponsiveness in the CTL population but that repeated immunizations with the peptide generated CTL activity (Kundig et al., 1996). The importance of the duration and/or intensity of antigenic stimulation on CTL activation was suggested by studies that compared the induction of CTL following infection with two vaccinia virus strains that differed only in the expression of the thymidine kinase virulence gene, which prolongs replication and enhances virus spread. Whereas the two viruses elicited comparable vaccinia virus-specific CTL in wild-type mice, the less virulent thymidine kinase-lacking strain did not elicit CTL in CD28 knockout animals (Kundig et al., 1996). Therefore, a large antigenic load or the persistence of antigen in vivo may override the requirement for B7 interaction with CD28. In agreement, the induction of virus-specific CTL by infection with viruses that replicate to high levels in mice, such as LCMV (Andreasen et al., 2000), does not require CD28 signaling whereas viruses with limited replication capacity, such as VSV (Kundig et al., 1996) and influenza (Lumsden et al., 2000), do require CD28 signaling for the CTL activation. These observations suggest that the role of the B7-CD28 interaction in the activation of virus-specific CTL may be less important with viruses that present high levels of antigenic stimulation.

T-Cell Help

CD4$^+$ Th cells usually orchestrate the production of cytokines that will shape the profile of the developing T-cell response. As discussed in a previous chapter, the CD4$^+$ response can be typically categorized as Th1 (favoring cell-mediated immunity) or Th2 (favoring antibody production) on the basis of the cytokine production. During the generation of virus-specific T-cell responses, CD4$^+$ T cells produce cytokines such as IL-2 that will drive the optimal proliferation of lymphocytes. In the LCMV model, CD4$^+$ T cells are not required for the generation of virus-specific CTL during an infection, demonstrating that induction of LCMV-specific CTL occurs in the absence of cytokines produced by CD4 cells. However, CD4-deficient mice are unable to control infections with high doses of more virulent LCMV strains (Matloubian et al., 1994). The generation of CTL in the absence of CD4$^+$ T-cell help may be attributed to the ability of CD8$^+$ T cells to secret low levels of IL-2 during an LCMV infection (Su et al., 1998). Although the IL-2 production by CD8 T cells may be sufficient for the short-term maintenance of CTL, it seems to be insufficient to resolve infections with highly virulent LCMV strains. This hypothesis is consistent with the finding that IL-2-deficient mice

mount a weak LCMV-specific CTL response following infection (Cousens et al., 1995). The need for T-cell help in the induction of influenza virus-specific CTL is dependent on the subtype of virus (Wu and Liu, 1994). An influenza virus subtype that induces costimulatory molecules (e.g., B7-2) on APC elicits CTL without a need for CD4$^+$ T cells. However, a subtype that requires CD4 help to evoke influenza virus-specific CTL failed to up-regulate costimulatory molecules on infected APC. During HSV infection, mice lacking CD4$^+$ T cells generate frequencies of HSV-specific CTL precursors that are similar to that in wild-type mice but only low cytolytic activity is detectable ex vivo (Jennings et al., 1991). Thus, CD4$^+$ T-cell help may be necessary to sustain the expansion of CTL following the initial activation. In agreement, the addition of exogenous IL-2 restores the HSV-specific CTL response to wild-type levels in the absence of CD4$^+$ T cells. While the role of CD4$^+$ T cells in the generation of virus-specific CTL is variable, depending on the particular virus, the optimal stimulation of CTL appears to require T-cell help.

Specificity of Virus-Induced CTL

A substantial enlargement of the CD8$^+$ CTL compartment is characteristic of the immune response to viral infections. It is now known that the majority of the T cells expanding during infection are virus specific (Butz and Bevan, 1998; Murali-Krishna et al., 1998; Zarozinski and Welsh, 1997), but many virus-specific CTL also cross-react with unrelated antigens (Alexander-Miller et al., 1993; Braciale et al., 1981; Sheil et al., 1987; Nahill and Welsh, 1993; Selin et al., 1994). The cross-reactive nature of T cells may be attributed to the degeneracy of the TCR in antigen recognition (Boesteanu et al., 1998). Recent predictions have estimated that a single TCR has the potential to interact or cross-react with approximately 10^6 different peptide sequences (Mason, 1998).

The degenerate nature of antigen recognition by CTL is evident in the LCMV model. Virus-specific CTL generated during an LCMV infection recognize and lyse allogeneic cells by targeting the foreign MHC class I molecules (Yang and Welsh, 1986; Yang et al., 1989). Approximately 10% of the LCMV-specific, CD8$^+$ CTL generated in C57BL/6 (H-2^b) mice recognize H-2^k-expressing target cells (Nahill and Welsh, 1993). The induction of allospecific responses by virus infection may have detrimental effects for allogeneic transplants, since these cross-reactive T cells may enhance rejection (Welsh et al., 2000). LCMV-specific CTL can also recognize syngeneic cells infected with heterologous viruses such as Pichinde virus, vaccinia virus, and murine cytomegalovirus (Selin et al., 1994; Yang et al., 1989). Following infection of LCMV-immune mice with heterologous viruses, a large number of LCMV-specific memory CTL are reactivated. In the specific case of Pichinde virus infection, about one-third of the Pichinde virus-specific T cells elicited early in infection were shown clearly to cross-react with LCMV (Selin et al., 1994). Cross-reactive CTL have also been demonstrated between variant influenza virus strains (Haanen et al., 1999) and between divergent peptides derived from polyomavirus-expressed proteins (Wilson et al., 1999). The effect of this CTL promiscuity can be variable. Cross-reactivity between heterologous viruses may enhance protective immune responses or, alternatively, result in damaging immunopathology (Selin et al., 1998).

T-Cell Repertoire

The frequency of CTL specific for a given viral epitope in the naive T-cell repertoire is extremely low. Following the expansion of T cells induced by viral infection, the frequencies of virus-specific T lymphocytes increase, and the repertoire is significantly altered (Lin and Welsh, 1998; Bousso and Kourilsky, 1999). As the T cells proliferate, populations expressing distinct TCR Vβ chains often dominate the antiviral response. During an LCMV infection of an H-2^b mouse strain, approximately 30 to 35% of the CD8$^+$ T cells utilized Vβ8 (Lin and Welsh, 1998), and in an H-2^d strain the usage included Vβ8 (40%) and Vβ10 (30%) (Sourdive et al., 1998). A dominant Vβ usage has been observed in H-2^b mice following an HSV infection, where approximately 40% of the activated CD8$^+$ T cells utilized Vβ10 (Cose et al., 1997). To further analyze the diversity in the TCR repertoire following virus infection, the CDR3 lengths within the CD8$^+$ Vβ8$^+$ population of H-2^b mice infected with LCMV were examined (Lin and Welsh, 1998). The CDR3 region is a region of hypervariability within the variable domain of the TCR and is critical for the recognition of peptide presented by MHC molecules. The CDR3 length profile or "spectratype" was diverse between animals, suggesting a stochastic process in the selection of dominant T-cell clones. Within an individual, however, the profile was maintained through the primary response and underwent minimal changes during the silencing phase of the antiviral T-cell responses following virus clearance (Lin and Welsh, 1998). The unique CDR3 spectratype utilized during the primary CTL response also left its imprint on the memory T-cell repertoire (Lin and Welsh, 1998; Sourdive et al., 1998).

Effector Phase

Homing

After the priming of virus-specific T cells within secondary lymphoid organs, these activated lymphocytes must migrate to the infection site to eliminate the viral challenge. This homing of activated T cells to peripheral sites is an essential feature of the antiviral immune response. Chemokines and chemokine receptors are believed to play an integral role in the trafficking of effector T cells (Price et al., 1999). Chemokines are small (8- to 10-kDa) chemotactic cytokines that are classified either into structural categories or into two functional classes: (i) inflammatory chemokines, which are produced during inflammatory responses at peripheral sites, and (ii) lymphoid chemokines, which are produced in lymphoid tissue to regulate the cellular organization and trafficking within these organs (Sallusto et al., 2000). Naive T cells express an array of chemokine receptors that recognize lymphoid chemokines, resulting in the migration of naive cells into lymphoid tissues (Butcher and Picker, 1996). It is thought that following activation, T cells adjust their migratory patterns by altering the expression of chemokine receptors. This modified expression allows the activated T lymphocyte to leave the lymphoid tissue and home to peripheral infection sites, where inflammatory chemokines are being synthesized (Ward et al., 1998). Once the activated T cells have localized to the infection site, the elimination of the viral pathogen commences.

T-cell effector mechanisms

When activated T cells migrate into an infection site, they hunt for infected cells by scanning the MHC class I molecules displayed on the surface. Upon encountering an infected cell, the T cells will initiate steps to eliminate the infection. Both CD4$^+$ and CD8$^+$ T cells can induce an inflammatory response at the infection site, similar to a delayed-type hypersensitivity (DTH) reaction (Galli and Lantz, 1999). This term is normally used to describe the delayed rather than the immediate inflammation that occurs on reexposure of a host to a T-cell immunogen, but a similar reaction can occur during a primary virus infection. The DTH reaction involves the attraction of effector cells to the infection site and the release of proinflammatory cytokines. These reactions sometimes lead to severe damage of host tissue. Virus can be cleared by either direct cytolytic mechanisms or the secretion of cytokines with antiviral properties. The effectiveness of each pathway can be dependent on the nature of the viral agent and the tissues infected. However, the optimal control of a majority of viral infections most probably requires the combined action of both effector measures. Ironically, a potent immune response that efficiently clears virus may also destroy uninfected tissue, resulting in immunopathology at the infection site.

Direct cytotoxicity. CTL have two separate systems that mediate cytolytic function. The first is the granule exocytosis pathway, and the second is the interaction of Fas ligand (FasL, expressed on T cells) and Fas (expressed on targets) (Shresta et al., 1998). The granule exocytosis pathway is dependent on perforin and on granzymes A and B (Kagi et al., 1996). These three components are expressed in T cells following activation and are then stored in membrane-bound, cytotoxic granules within the cytoplasm. After the recognition of an infected cell, the granules migrate to the membrane region, interact with the target cell, and fuse with the T-cell membrane, releasing perforin and granzymes. The free perforin will polymerize, forming a complex that creates pores in the target's plasma membrane. The channels created by perforin allow the passage of granzymes into the cytosol of the target cell. The granzymes will induce apoptotic pathways that result in the eventual death of the infected cell. The granule exocytosis pathway is thought to be utilized predominantly by CD8[+] CTL, but perforin has been detected in some CD4[+] T cell clones (Nakata et al., 1992). Perforin-dependent cytotoxity associated with the granule exocytosis pathway is the primary mechanism for the control of LCMV (Kagi et al., 1994), ectromelia virus (Mullbacher et al., 1999), and influenza virus (Topham et al., 1997), since perforin-deficient mice are severely impaired in the ability to clear these viruses.

The ligation of Fas with FasL expressed on activated T cells triggers a well-characterized apoptotic pathway in the Fas-expressing target cell (Ashkenazi and Dixit, 1998). This pathway involves the aggregation of Fas activation death domains, which leads to the activation of caspases and ultimately to apoptosis. An important consideration for FasL-mediated cytotoxicity is that the expression of Fas is not ubiquitous and that only Fas-expressing cells would be sensitive to the FasL-induced cell death (Shresta et al., 1998). The specificity of Fas-mediated cell death is enhanced by the fact that FasL expression is up-regulated following TCR triggering, so that an infected cell expressing viral antigens would more probably receive the death signal than would an uninfected cell. It is thought that CD4[+] effector T cells preferentially utilize FasL-mediated cytotoxicity, but

the ability of CD8[+] CTL to induce Fas-dependent apoptosis has been demonstrated in the influenza virus model (Harty et al., 2000). CTL cleared influenza virus from the lungs of Fas-deficient (*lpr*) mice with delayed kinetics (Topham et al., 1997). Interestingly, optimal clearance of influenza virus required both Fas and perforin, implying that the two mechanisms can have an additive effect in the appropriate environment.

Antiviral cytokines. Activated T lymphocytes have the ability to produce large quantities of antiviral cytokines, such as IFN-γ and TNF-α. Both CD4[+] and CD8[+] T cells synthesize IFN-γ and TNF-α, suggesting that both T-cell populations contribute to the resolution of infections with viruses that are sensitive to these effector cytokines (Guidotti and Chisari, 1999). The interaction of these cytokines with their receptors dramatically alters gene expression in the target cells and impedes the progression of the viral infection process. IFN-γ increases the expression of MHC molecules and antiviral proteins, such as protein kinase R, 2′-5′ oligoadenylate synthetase, and double-stranded RNA-specific adenosine deaminase (Boehm et al., 1997). A major effect of IFN-γ may also be to up-regulate nitric oxide synthase, whose metabolic product, NO, may have antiviral properties against viruses such as HSV, murine cytomegalovirus, VSV, and poxvirus family members (Karupiah et al., 1993; MacMicking et al., 1997; Tay and Welsh, 1997; van den Broek et al., 2000). The expression of IFN-γ and TNF-α by T cells is tightly regulated and is restricted to the period of contact with antigen (Slifka et al., 1999). Removal of antigen induces the rapid shutdown of cytokine expression by the virus-specific T cells, which can be turned on again by the addition of antigen. This cyclic expression confines the secretion of cytokines to the infection site and reduces the impact on uninfected tissues.

The antiviral effects of cytokines like IFN-γ and TNF-α can occur without lysis of the targeted cells (Guidotti and Chisari, 1999). Noncytolytic mechanisms may be useful for the resolution of infections in vital organ systems, where a large amount of tissue destruction is not desirable. In agreement with this hypothesis, studies have demonstrated the noncytolytic control of hepatitis B virus infections in hepatocytes by IFN-γ and TNF-α (Guidotti et al., 1996). Cytokine-mediated antiviral protection has also been observed with vaccinia virus (Harris et al., 1995) and adenovirus (Zhang et al., 1998). IFN-γ contributes to the control of HSV infections at mucosal surfaces but is minimally involved at cutaneous and neuronal sites (Holterman et al., 1999). IFN-γ is not required for the control of LCMV infections, but a limited role for the cytokine has been observed in studies evaluating the ability of IFN-γ-deficient T cells to control an LCMV infection in newborn mice (Tishon et al., 1995). Infection of newborn mice with LCMV establishes a lifelong infection that can be cleared by the transfer of LCMV-specific memory T cells (Harty et al., 2000). The adoptive transfer of IFN-γ-deficient memory T cells did not resolve this LCMV infection. Thus, protective effects of cytokines produced by effector T cells appear to be dependent on many factors, including the site of the viral infection.

Silencing Phase of the T-Cell Responses

Following clearance of viral antigen, the immune system begins turning off the antiviral response and establishing a virus-specific memory pool. The development of memory is discussed in another chapter. A key aspect of the return of the immune system to homeostasis is the reduction of the activated T-cell population. During the virus infection, the number of T lymphocytes has expanded dramatically, and following the elimination of viral antigen, the population must be thinned. The mechanisms involved in the silencing of the virus-specific T-cell responses have not been completely elucidated, but the process is thought to involve the induction of apoptosis in the T-lymphocyte population (Razvi et al., 1995). This down-regulation of the T-cell response following the clearance of an LCMV infection appears to occur independently of Fas signaling. T cells surviving these apoptotic processes appear to express slightly more Bcl2 than do naive T cells (Grayson et al., 2000).

B-CELL RESPONSES

Importance of Antibody Responses to Viruses

Sustained high levels of virus-specific antibody following primary infection provide the main mechanism to prevent reinfection for most viruses, but in many acute virus infections, such as with VSV, Sindbis virus, or rotavirus, humoral immune responses are also important for the resolution of acute infection and recovery (Bachmann and Zinkernagel, 1997; Griffin et al., 1997; Feng et al., 1994). In humans, a comparison of fatal cases of Ebola virus infection with cases in which the patients survived indicated a lack of virus-specific antibodies in the former group and an early and robust IgG response in the latter, suggesting that quick and efficient IgG se-

cretion may play an essential role in the survival from this viral disease (Baize et al., 1999). In virus infections that are cleared mainly by CTL responses during the acute phase, humoral immunity can play an important role in long-term control. Antibodies can control reactivation or recrudescence of viruses that establish latency or persistence. Examples of this include persistent mouse hepatitis virus infection in the central nervous system (Lin et al., 1999) or mouse gammaherpesvirus 68 reactivation from latently infected macrophages and B cells (Virgin and Speck, 1999) in studies using B-cell-deficient mice. In addition, antibody-mediated clearance can serve as a backup mechanism of defense in a partially immunocompromised host. For example, T cells can control polyomavirus in normal and B-cell-deficient mice. However, T-cell-deficient mice also recover from acute polyomavirus infection, and in this case B cells provide protection by secreting virus-specific antibodies in a T-cell-independent fashion (Szomolanyi-Tsuda and Welsh, 1998). The control of very high dose LCMV infection that is overwhelming for the virus-specific T-cell responses also is dependent on intact humoral immunity, because mice deficient in B cells cannot clear this infection (Brundler et al., 1996).

Recognition of Viral Antigens by B Cells

In contrast to T cells, which recognize processed antigens presented as peptides on the MHC molecules of APC, B cells recognize epitopes on the unprocessed antigen. The specificity of the membrane-bound surface immunoglobulin B-cell receptors (BCR) is directed against the three-dimensional structure of viral antigenic determinants on virus particles or on the surface of infected cells. Most of the viral epitopes recognized by B cells are nonlinear. These epitopes (also called conformational epitopes) consist of amino acids derived from different regions of the linear polypeptide chain, and they are formed as a result of the three-dimensional folding of the molecule. Denaturation of these proteins leads to loss of binding with the antibodies. In contrast, linear or nonconformational epitopes represent contiguous amino acid sequences on the polypeptide chain, and they are not destroyed by denaturation. The contact surface between the binding site of the antigen and antibody is approximately 700 Å² (Wilson and Cox, 1990). Three-dimensional structural studies of viral antigen-antibody complexes revealed that 15 to 20 residues on each molecule are in close contact (Davies et al., 1990; Berzofsky et al., 1999). A change in only one residue can drastically reduce the affinity of antibody binding and result in the appearance of viral escape mutants that are resistant to neutralizing antibodies (Knossow et al., 1984).

B cells function not only as antigen-specific effector cells activated by viruses but also as APC. After capturing antigens through their BCR, they internalize and process the viral antigens and present them on MHC class II molecules. Therefore, by activating CD4$^+$ Th cells, B cells, together with other professional APC (e.g., DC) contribute to the recruitment of their T-cell helpers.

Kinetics of Antibody Responses

The interaction of DC, CD4$^+$ T cells, and B cells in the secondary lymphoid organs activates the humoral responses. These responses start with IgM secretion (Fig. 3). In mice infected with LCMV or polyomavirus, antibody-secreting cells appear in the spleen (detectable by ELISPOT assays) and virus-specific IgM can be measured in the serum by enzyme-linked immunosorbent assay (ELISA) by day 3 to 4 postinfection (Slifka and Ahmed, 1996a; Szomolanyi-Tsuda et al., 1998). The IgM molecules form pentamers via disulfide bonds. This structure greatly increases the avidity of the complexes to the antigen by linking 10 binding sites that may otherwise be of low affinity.

Isotype switching occurs after the initial phase of antibody responses. The activated B cells reacting to cytokine signals start to produce antibodies with the same antigen binding domains and specificity but combined with another constant-region backbone. This change has important consequences, because the biological function of antibodies depends largely on the constant region of the heavy (H) chain. In mice, IgM, IgG2a and IgG2b are very efficient at complement fixation, followed by IgG3. The constant regions of IgG subclasses also differ in their binding affinities to Fcγ receptors (FcγRI to FcγRIII) expressed on various cell types. In mice, FcγRI and FcγRII on monocytes and macrophages bind both IgG2a and IgG2b antibodies and mediate the phagocytosis of antibody-coated viral particles. FcγRIII, which are expressed on natural killer (NK) cells in addition to monocytes and macrophages, bind mainly IgG2a, IgG2b, and IgG1 antibodies, and have the potential to mediate antibody-dependent cell-mediated cytotoxicity (ADCC) of virus-infected cells (Frazer and Capra, 1999). IFN-γ, a cytokine known to promote isotype switching to IgG2a, is induced during many virus infections. It is not surprising, therefore, that most antiviral IgG responses are predominantly of the IgG2a isotype in mice during acute infection. In contrast to the acute infection, however, mice persistently infected from birth with LCMV

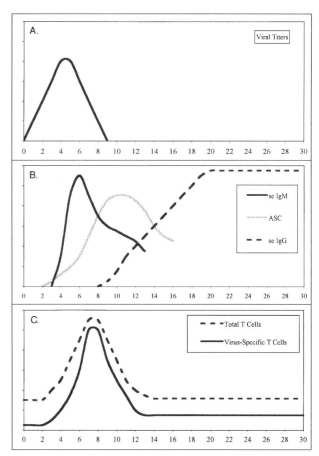

Figure 3. Kinetics of antiviral immune responses. (A) Viral replication and clearance. Time is given as days postinfection. (B) Antiviral humoral immune responses. ASC, antibody (IgG)-secreting cells in the spleen; se IgM, virus-specific serum IgM; se IgG, virus-specific serum IgG. (C) Virus-specific and total T-cell responses. The frequency of virus-specific T cells before infection is very low. After infection, the majority of the expanding T-cell population is virus specific, and after the down-regulation of T-cell responses, the host is left with an elevated frequency of the virus-specific T cells.

produce predominantly antiviral IgG1 (Courtelier et al., 1987, 1988; Thomsen et al., 1985; Tishon et al., 1991). In humans, IgG1 and IgG3 are the good complement-fixing IgG isotypes and also bind efficiently to FcγRIII on NK cells and mediate ADCC (Frazer and Capra, 1999). IgG1 is the predominant antiviral isotype in patients with acute human immunodeficiency virus (HIV) or hepatitis B virus infections (Tishon et al., 1991).

B cells that complete isotype switching and secrete IgG start to accumulate in the spleen on days 4 to 5, and their numbers reach a peak on days 9 to 10 in LCMV-infected mice and in polyomavirus-infected mice. Virus-specific serum IgG levels reach peak values on day 15 in LCMV-infected and on day 21 in polyomavirus-infected mice (Slifka and Ahmed,

1996a; Szomolanyi-Tsuda et al., 1998). The serum IgG levels do not decrease substantially for the rest of the life of the mouse in the presence of a systemic (intravenous or intraperitoneal) infection (Fig. 3). Many systemic virus infections in humans lead to high antibody levels that are sustained for several decades or even for life. Continuous antigenic stimulation of naive and memory B cells and their consequential differentiation into antibody-secreting plasma cells have been thought to be the mechanisms responsible for maintaining the high antibody levels. However, recent findings implicate long-lived antibody-secreting plasma cells localized mainly in the bone marrow as sources of the sustained serum antibody levels (Slifka and Ahmed, 1998). Interestingly, antibody responses to localized mucosal infections are much more short-lived, since they wane in a few months in humans (reviewed by Slifka and Ahmed [1996b]).

Antibody responses to most virus infections are detectable by ELISA starting on day 3 to 5 postinfection. Some of these early antibodies may already have neutralizing activity, such as in infections with VSV, rotavirus, yellow fever virus, or influenza virus (Roost et al., 1995; Franco and Greenberg, 1999; Tomori, 1999; Gerhard et al., 1997). In contrast, LCMV, hepatitis B virus, and HIV infection induce neutralizing antibodies only at a later phase, after 50 to 150 days postinfection (Bachmann and Zinkernagel, 1997). It has been suggested that cytotoxic T cells in LCMV-infected mice interfere with the appearance of neutralizing antibodies in the serum. B lymphocytes specific for neutralizing surface epitopes of LCMV bind to the virus, become infected, and, as a consequence, become targets for CTL activity. Supporting this hypothesis are the observations that in vivo depletion of CD8$^+$ T cells results in an earlier appearance of neutralizing antibodies in the serum and that neutralizing-antibody-secreting hybridomas can be generated from spleens of LCMV-infected mice on day 4 (before the CTL response develops), but not on day 10 postinfection (Planz et al., 1996).

The maturation of antiviral antibody responses, involving somatic hypermutation and selection, leading to a significant increase in the average affinity of the antibodies has been investigated only in a few studies. In influenza virus-infected mice there is evidence for hypermutation in the VDJ regions of the hemagglutinin-specific antibodies and for affinity maturation of the antiviral antibodies (Clarke et al., 1990). In contrast, the average affinity of IgG antibodies to VSV G glycoprotein is quite high early (on day 6) postinfection and does not further increase with time (Roost et al., 1995).

T-Cell-Independent and T-Cell-Dependent Antiviral Antibody Responses

The induction of antiviral antibody responses in immunocompetent normal mice involves complex interactions of antigen-specific activated CD4 T cells and B cells. The delivery of this "cognate" T-cell help includes signaling via costimulatory molecules (e.g., CD28 and CD40L on activated T cells and B7-1, B7-2, and CD40 on B cells) and cytokines secreted by T cells (Kehry and Hodgkin, 1993). Because most viral antigens are proteins and because antibody responses to proteins usually depend on T-cell help, antibody responses to viruses had initially been assumed to be strictly T-cell dependent. Studies on polyomavirus infection in mice lacking both $\alpha\beta$ and $\gamma\delta$ T cells (TCR $\beta\times\delta^{-/-}$) clearly indicated, however, that a virus can behave as a T-cell-independent antigen and induce antibody synthesis without T-cell help (Szomolanyi-Tsuda and Welsh, 1996). These T-cell-deficient mice synthesized virus-specific IgM and IgG that controlled virus infection and did not develop an acute myeloproliferative disease that led to 100% mortality in SCID mice. The T-cell-independent IgG responses were elicited only by live polyomavirus infection, not by immunization with viral proteins or virus-like particles, which are empty viral capsids assembled from VP1 capsomeres. Therefore, the repetitive nature of the viral capsid is not sufficient to induce isotype-switched T-cell-independent antibody secretion (Szomolanyi-Tsuda et al., 1998). These findings suggest that live viruses activate components of the innate immune system, which then provide signals that "help" T-cell-independent B-cell responses. The T-cell-independent IgG titers to polyomavirus amount to approximately 10% of the T-cell-dependent responses in immunocompetent mice and lack the IgG1 isotype. Several recent studies suggest that other viruses, such as VSV, rotavirus, LCMV, Pichinde virus, murine cytomegalovirus, and vaccinia virus, can also induce IgM and isotype-switched IgG and IgA antibody responses in the absence of CD4 T-cell help (Table 1).

Whereas T-cell-independent antibody responses can be essential for the survival of virus infection in T-cell-deficient mice, an important question is whether T-cell-independent antibody responses to viruses play any significant role in normal, immunocompetent hosts that have intact T-cell functions. T-cell-independent responses probably start earlier than T-cell-dependent antibody synthesis that requires T-cell activation (deVinuesa et al., 1999). Therefore, this early control by T-cell-independent antibodies may inhibit virus spread and replication, could limit the damage of host tissues caused by cy-

Table 1. Antiviral antibody responses in mice with targeted mutations affecting T-cell helper function

Virus	Route[a]	Mouse strain	Ig produced	Reference
Polyomavirus	i.p.	TCR $\beta \times \delta^{-/-}$ [b]	IgM, IgG	Szomolanyi-Tsuda et al. (1998)
Polyomavirus	i.p.	CD3Etg[c]	IgM, IgG	Szomolanyi-Tsuda et al. (2001)
Polyomavirus	i.n.	TCR $\beta \times \delta^{-/-}$ [b]	IgM, IgG, IgA	E. Szomolanyi-Tsuda, unpublished data
Polyomavirus	i.p.	CD40$^{-/-}$	IgM, IgG	Szomolanyi-Tsuda et al. (2000)
VSV	i.v.	TCR$\beta^{-/-}$ [d]	IgM, IgG	Maloy et al. (1998)
VSV	i.v.	TCR $\beta \times \delta^{-/-}$ [b]	IgM	Maloy et al. (1998)
VSV	i.v.	CD40L$^{-/-}$	IgM, IgG	Borrow et al. (1996)
VSV	i.v.	CTLA4Tg[e]	IgM, IgG	Zimmermann et al. (1997)
Rotavirus	p.o.	TCR $\beta \times \delta^{-/-}$ [b]	IgA	Franco and Greenberg (1997)
Influenza virus	i.m., i.p.	CD4$^{-/-}$	IgM, IgG	Sha and Compans (2000)
Pichinde virus	i.p.	CD40L$^{-/-}$	IgG	Borrow et al. (1996)
LCMV	i.p.	CD40L$^{-/-}$	IgG	Whitmire et al. (1996)

[a] i.p., intraperitoneal; i.n., intranasal; i.v., intravenous; p.o., oral; i.m. intramuscular.
[b] TCR $\beta \times \delta^{-/-}$ mice have targeted mutations in their T-cell receptor β and δ genes; therefore, they lack all $\alpha\beta$ T cells and $\gamma\delta$ T cells.
[c] CD3ETg mice lack all $\alpha\beta$ and $\gamma\delta$ T cells and NK cells.
[d] TCR$\beta^{-/-}$ mice have a targeted mutation in their T-cell receptor β gene; therefore they lack $\alpha\beta$ T cells.
[e] CTLA4Tg mice are transgenic for soluble CTLA4, and the expression of this molecule blocks B7-CD28 costimulatory interactions.

topathic viruses, and could reduce the virus load that the T-cell-dependent responses subsequently need to handle.

Mechanisms of the Control of Virus Infections by Antibodies

Antibodies exert their antiviral effects by a wide variety of mechanisms, acting at various stages of the viral life cycle (Fig. 4). Antibodies can neutralize viral particles before they reach permissive cells by inhibiting their attachment to cells. This is most commonly achieved by direct binding of the antibody to the viral attachment site, blocking its interaction with receptors on the cell surface. Antibody binding to a viral determinant distinct from the attachment site may also lead to conformational changes of the attachment site, preventing virus adsorption. Virus neutralization can also occur by aggregation or agglutination of the virus particles by antibodies, resulting in a reduction of infectious units. After the attachment of viral particles to the cell, neutralizing antibodies can interfere with virus penetration and uncoating by inhibiting the endocytotic internalization of virions and the fusion of the viral envelope with the cell membrane, respectively (Dimmock, 1993).

Complement activation by virus-antibody complexes can further enhance the efficiency of antibody-mediated control of virus infections. Enveloped viruses can be lysed by antibody and complement. Moreover, both opsonization of virus-antibody-complement complexes by macrophages via complement receptors and direct lysis of virus-infected cells displaying viral antigen determinants on the cell membrane by antibodies and complement are potent antiviral mechanisms (Dimmock, 1993).

Antibodies binding to viral antigenic determinants on the surface of infected cells can be targeted to NK cells or macrophages via Fc receptors on these cells. This may lead to lysis of the infected cells via ADCC. ADCC, mediated mostly by NK cells, has been demonstrated in vitro in several human viral systems (reviewed by Welsh and Vargas-Cortes [1992]). Very little is known, however, of the in vivo contribution of ADCC to the control of virus infections in mice or in humans.

Antibodies can also disrupt the viral life cycle inside the infected cells. Measles virus-specific antibodies were shown to suppress viral protein and RNA synthesis in measles virus-infected cells in vitro (Fujinami and Oldstone, 1979). More recently, in vivo studies have demonstrated that antibodies specific for the surface glycoprotein E2 of Sindbis virus protected mice from lethal central nervous system infection and cleared infectious virus from neurons. This process did not involve complement or mononuclear cells, and it was not cytolytic. Cross-linking of the E2 viral glycoproteins displayed on the infected cell surface by the bivalent antibodies in vitro resulted in an inhibition of budding and release of the new virions. Subsequently, viral RNA and protein synthesis gradually decreased and the infected cells recovered. Although the exact molecular mechanisms participating in antibody-mediated intracellular clearance have not yet been characterized, restoration of the cellular Na$^+$K$^+$ATPase function, which had been severely inhibited in the virus-infected neurons, and a subsequent switch from transcription of viral mRNAs and translation of viral proteins to cellular

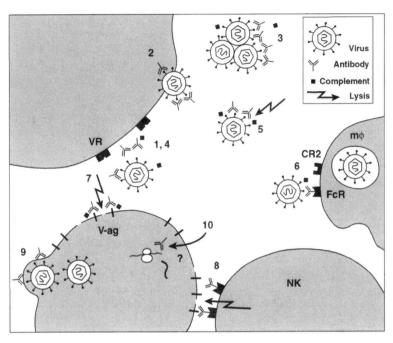

Figure 4. Antibody-mediated antiviral effector mechanisms. (1) Prevention of viral attachment by blocking the viral attachment site. (2) Prevention of uncoating. (3) Aggregation of viral particles. (4) Blocking of virus absorption by inducing conformational changes in the attachment site. (5) Lysis of virion-antibody-complement complexes. (6) Opsonization. (7) Lysis of virus-infected cells by antibody and complement. (8) ADCC. (9) Inhibition of the release of virus particles. (10) Intracellular inhibition of the viral life cycle. VR, virus receptor; V-ag, viral antigen; mf, macrophage; CR2, complement receptor.

ones are thought to be involved in this process (Griffin et al., 1997).

In a given host, a wide variety of antibodies are produced with different specificities, affinities, and isotypes, and only some of these antibodies have a potent antiviral effect. Therefore it would be important to determine the essential characteristics of the antibodies that are capable of providing protection to virus infections. Studies with monoclonal antibodies generated during various virus infections (such as reovirus, VSV, influenza virus, and LCMV) concluded that in vitro characteristics of the antibodies, such as neutralizing ability or affinity, could not predict their utility in preventing or resolving virus infection in vivo (Tyler et al., 1993; Lefrançois, 1984; Mozdzanowska et al., 1997; Balridge and Buchmeier, 1992). These findings suggest that some of the antiviral mechanisms mediated by antibodies in vivo may be different from the mechanisms studied in vitro.

Natural infections with several important human pathogens elicit mostly weak, nonprotective antibody responses. Because convalescent-phase sera transferred from survivors of these infections into naive hosts does not protect or help recovery after virus challenge in experimental models, antibodies are thought to have little or no protective value in these infections. However, new findings indicate that monoclonal antibodies generated from convalescent donors or raised by experimental immunization protocols can be effective in limiting or preventing these infections, which previously were regarded relatively insensitive to antibodies (Burton and Parren, 2000). An important example is HIV-1 infection, which induces typically low neutralizing-antibody titers in seropositive individuals; polyclonal serum antibody preparations do not give protection in rhesus macaques infected with simian immunodeficiency virus /HIV-1 chimeric viruses that carry HIV-1 env. Human monoclonal env-specific antibodies, however, have a protective effect in these models, particularly against mucosal challenge (Shibata et al., 1999; Igarashi et al., 1999; Mascola et al., 2000; Baba et al., 2000). These data and similar findings with other viruses (e.g., Ebola virus) suggest that the efficacy of antiviral antibodies in providing protection or facilitating recovery should be reassessed.

Influence of Memory T and B Cells on the Acute Responses to Heterologous Viruses

In most experimental models, immune responses to a virus are studied by infecting immunologically naive animals. In nature, however, a host encounters numerous consecutive virus infections. Recent findings demonstrated that a history of prior virus infections can have a profound effect on the host's primary response to a heterologous virus. Mice immune to LCMV clear Pichinde virus or vaccinia virus infection faster than naive mice do, and this enhanced clearance is in part mediated by cross-reactive CD8 T cells (Selin et al., 1998). Previously acquired humoral immunity to a heterologous dengue virus serotype may lead to a more severe form of dengue virus infection, dengue hemorrhagic fever. This antibody-dependent "immune enhancement" is mediated by complexes of virions and nonneutralizing cross-reactive antibodies. These complexes are adsorbed to and internalized with increased efficiency by Fc receptor-bearing monocytes and macrophages, resulting in a major increase in virus replication. The increased viral load is a potent stimulus for the reactivation of cross-reactive memory T cells that can mediate the immunopathologic changes contributing to the severity of dengue hemorrhagic fever (Littana et al., 1990; Kurane and Ennis, 1992). Antibody-dependent immune enhancement has also been observed in Rous sarcoma virus and HIV infection (Morens, 1994; Osiowy et al., 1994).

Transient Immune Deficiency in Virus Infections

The acute T-cell response during infections with many viruses, including measles virus, Epstein-Barr virus, and cytomegalovirus in humans and LCMV in the mouse, is paradoxically associated with a transient period of immune deficiency (Razvi and Welsh, 1993; Welsh and McNally, 1999). This is characterized by impaired lymphocyte responsiveness to T- and B-cell mitogens and impaired antigen-specific memory cell recall responses to previously encountered antigens. For example, patients infected with measles virus have reduced tuberculin-specific DTH responses, which recover in part after resolution of the infection (von Pirquet, 1908). It also is difficult to initiate new primary immune responses in a host with an ongoing immune response for several days. There can be damage to cellular immune mechanisms as a direct consequence of virus infection, but several immunoregulatory mechanisms can account for much of this transient immunodeficiency. Immunosuppressive prostaglandins and cytokines, such as IL-10 and transforming growth factor β, are produced at high levels at late stages of the immune response and can interfere with antigen presentation and lymphocyte proliferation. These act as part of a complex regulatory scheme to prevent the immune system from getting overstimulated and to shut down the acute immune response as soon as the antigen has cleared. Stimulation of T cells by overwhelming doses of antigen can lead to their clonal exhaustion, which may be the preferred alternative to the massive

cytokine bath that might otherwise ensue (Moskophidis et al., 1993).

A major mechanism for controlling the overstimulation of T cells relates to the fact that highly activated T cells will express both Fas and FasL. Strong signaling through their TCR can, under appropriate conditions, drive these cells into a suicidal apoptotic pathway (Russell et al., 1993), since ligand-bound Fas will interact with Fas activation death domains, which activates a caspase that initiates the cell death program (Ashkenazi and Dixit, 1998). Hence, stimulation of these highly activated cells with T-cell mitogens may drive them into apoptosis instead of into division. A host with an abundance of FasL-expressing T cells creates an environment hostile to the development of antigen-specific memory recall responses or to newly initiated primary responses. Studies have shown that FasL$^+$ but not FasL$^-$ virus-specific T cells can sensitize non-virus-specific "bystander" T cells to undergo apoptosis instead of proliferation on signaling of their TCR (Zarozinski et al., 2000). This mechanism of immune deficiency may have implications in persistent infections, such as with HIV, where T cells are chronically stimulated, as well as in autoimmune diseases, which often are associated with concurrent immunodeficiencies.

Redundancy of the Antiviral Immune Responses

Studies with virus-infected genetically engineered "knockout" mice have revealed a remarkable degree of redundancy within the antiviral immune responses. Infection of mice defective in genes thought to be important for protection often did not cause the expected pathologic responses. For example, infections of CD8$^+$ T-cell-deficient mice with vaccinia virus or Sendai virus (viruses known to be controlled by CD8$^+$ CTL) were cleared by compensating CD4$^+$ T cells (Spriggs et al., 1992; Hou et al., 1992). Polyomavirus and influenza virus infections were cleared efficiently by T cells, but in the absence of functional T cells, B-cell responses provided protection (Szomolanyi-Tsuda and Welsh, 1996; Mozdzanowska et al., 2000). LCMV infection is mostly controlled by a perforin-dependent CTL response, but it is also cleared in LCMV-NP transgenic BALB/c mice that lack high-affinity CTL responses to the virus. In this case, however, IFN-γ is required for LCMV clearance, even though the lack of this cytokine does not impair virus clearance in mice with a normal CTL repertoire (Von Herrath et al., 1997). Thus, the immune system has components with overlapping functions, and this redundancy allows protection in case of partial immunodeficiency. At the same time, the existence of multiple antiviral effector mechanisms ensures control in different organs and at different stages of the virus infection. For example, in mice infected with neurotropic mouse hepatitis virus the acute disease is controlled mostly by T cells and viral clearance during acute infection is similar in normal mice and in mice deficient in humoral immunity (IgM$^{-/-}$). Long-term control of virus persisting in the central nervous system, however, requires humoral immunity, and the lack of antibody responses leads to recrudescence of infectious virus in the brains and spinal cords (Lin et al., 1999). Thus, the prognosis of viral infections is the best in a host with a fully intact acquired immune system, which can employ diverse antiviral mechanisms at various anatomical sites and at different phases of a virus infection to tip the balance of virus-host interactions in favor of the host.

REFERENCES

Alexander-Miller, M. A., K. Burke, U. H. Koszinowski, T. H. Hansen, and J. M. Connolly. 1993. Alloreactive cytotoxic T lymphocytes generated in the presence of viral-derived peptides show exquisite peptide and MHC specificity. *J. Immunol.* 151: 1–10.

Altman, J. D., P. A. H. Moss, P. J. R. Goulder, D. H. Barouch, M. G. McHeyzer-Williams, J. I. Bell, A. J. McMichael, and M. M. Davis. 1996. Phenotypic analysis of antigen-specific T lymphocytes. *Science* 274:94–96.

Andreasen, S. O., J. E. Christensen, O. Marker, and A. R. Thomsen. 2000. Role of CD40 ligand and CD28 in induction and maintenance of antiviral CD8+ effector T cell responses. *J. Immunol.* 164:3689–3697.

Ashkenazi, A., and V. M. Dixit. 1998. Death receptors: signaling and modulation. *Science* 281:1305–1308.

Baba, T. W., V. Liska, R. Hofmann-Lehmann, J. Vlasak, W. Xu, S. Ayehunie, L. A. Cavacini, M. R. Posner, H. Katinger, G. Stiegler, B. J. Bernacky, T. A. Rizvi, R. Schmidt, L. R. Hill, M. E. Keeling, Y. Lu, J. E. Wright, T.-C. Chou, and R. M. Ruprecht. 2000. Human neutralizing monoclonal antibodies of the IgG1 subtype protect against mucosal simian-human immunodeficiency virus infection. *Nat. Med.* 6:200–206.

Bachmann, M. F., E. Sebzda, T. M. Kundig, A. Shahinian, D. E. Speiser, T. W. Mak, and P. S. Ohashi. 1996. T cell responses are governed by avidity and co-stimulatory thresholds. *Eur. J. Immunol.* 26:2017–2022.

Bachmann, M. F., and R. M. Zinkernagel. 1997. Neutralizing antiviral B cell responses. *Annu. Rev. Immunol.* 15:235–270.

Baize, S., E. M. Leroy, M.-C. Georges-Courbot, M. Capron, J. Lansoud-Soukate, P. Debre, S. P. Fisher-Hoch, J. B. McCormick, and A. J. Georges. 1999. Defective humoral responses and extensive intravascular apoptosis are associated with fatal outcome in Ebola virus-infected patients. *Nat. Med.* 5:423–426.

Balridge, J. R., and M. J. Buchmeier. 1992. Mechanism of antibody-mediated protection against lymphocytic choriomeningitis virus infection: mother-to-baby transfer of humoral protection. *J. Virol.* 66:4252–4257.

Banchereau, J., F. Briere, C. Caux, J. Davoust, S. Lebecque, Y. J. Liu, B. Pulendran, and K. Palucka. 2000. Immunobiology of dendritic cells. *Annu. Rev. Immunol.* 18:767–811.

Barchet, W., S. Oehen, P. Klenerman, D. Wodarz, G. Bocharov, A. L. Lloyd, M. A. Nowak, H. Hengartner, R. M. Zinkernagel, and S. Ehl. 2000. Direct quantitation of rapid elimination of viral antigen-positive lymphocytes by antiviral CD8(+) T cells in vivo. *Eur. J. Immunol.* 30:1356–1363.

Bender, A., M. Albert, A. Reddy, M. Feldman, B. Sauter, G. Kaplan, W. Hellman, and N. Bhardwaj. 1998. The distinctive features of influenza virus infection of dendritic cells. *Immunobiology* 198:552–567.

Berzofsky, J. A., I. J. Berkower, and S. L. Epstein. 1999. Antigen-antibody interactions and monoclonal antibodies, p. 75–110. *In* W. E. Paul (ed.), *Fundamental Immunology*, 4th ed. Lippincott-Raven, Philadelphia, Pa.

Blaney, J. E., Jr., E. Nobusawa, M. A. Brehm, R. H. Bonneau, L. M. Mylin, T. M. Fu, Y. Kawaoka, and S. S. Tevethia. 1998. Immunization with a single major histocompatibility complex class I-restricted cytotoxic T-lymphocyte recognition epitope of herpes simplex virus type 2 confers protective immunity. *J. Virol.* 72:9567–9574.

Boehm, U., T. Klamp, M. Groot, and J. C. Howard. 1997. Cellular responses to interferon-gamma. *Annu. Rev. Immunol.* 15: 749–795.

Boesteanu, A., M. Brehm, L. M. Mylin, G. J. Christianson, S. S. Tevethia, D. C. Roopenian, and S. Joyce. 1998. A molecular basis for how a single TCR interfaces multiple ligands. *J. Immunol.* 161:4719–4727.

Bonneau, R. H., L. A. Salvucci, D. C. Johnson, and S. S. Tevethia. 1993. Epitope specificity of H-2Kb-restricted, HSV-1-, and HSV-2-cross-reactive cytotoxic T lymphocyte clones. *Virology* 195:62–70.

Borrow, P., A. Tishon, S. Lee, J. Xu, I. S. Grewal, M. B. A. Oldstone, and R. A. Flavell. 1996. CD40L-deficient mice show deficits in antiviral immunity and have an impaired memory CD8+ CTL response. *J. Exp. Med.* 183:2129–2142.

Borrow, P., D. F. Tough, D. Eto, A. Tishon, I. S. Grewal, J. Sprent, R. A. Flavell, and M. B. Oldstone. 1998. CD40 ligand-mediated interactions are involved in the generation of memory CD8+ cytotoxic T lymphocytes (CTL) but are not required for the maintenance of CTL memory following virus infection. *J. Virol.* 72:7440–7449.

Bousso, P., and P. Kourilsky. 1999. A clonal view of alphabeta T cell responses. *Semin. Immunol.* 11:423–431.

Braciale, T. J., M. E. Andrew, and V. L. Braciale. 1981. Simultaneous expression of H-2-restricted and alloreactive recognition by a cloned line of influenza virus-specific cytotoxic T lymphocytes. *J. Exp. Med.* 153:1371–1376.

Brundler, M.-A., P. Aichele, M. Bachmann, D. Kitamura, K. Rajewsky, and R. M. Zinkernagel. 1996. Immunity to viruses in B cell-deficient mice: influence of antibodies on virus persistence and on T cell memory. *Eur. J. Immunol.* 26:2257–2262.

Burton, D. R., and P. W. H. I. Parren. 2000. Vaccines and the induction of functional antibodies: time to look beyond the molecules of natural infection? *Nat. Med.* 6:123–125.

Butcher, E. C., and L. J. Picker. 1996. Lymphocyte homing and homeostasis. *Science* 272:60–66.

Butz, E. A., and M. J. Bevan. 1998. Massive expansion of antigen-specific CD8+ T cells during an acute virus infection. *Immunity* 8:167–175.

Chen, W., L. C. Anton, J. R. Bennink, and J. W. Yewdell. 2000. Dissecting the multifactorial causes of immunodominance in class I-restricted T cell responses to viruses. *Immunity* 12:83–93.

Clarke, S. H., L. M. Staudt, J. Kavaler, D. Schwartz, W. U. Gerhard, and M. G. Weigert. 1990. V region usage and somatic mutation in the primary and secondary responses to influenza virus hemagglutinin. *J. Immunol.* 144:2795–2801.

Cose, S. C., C. M. Jones, M. E. Wallace, W. R. Heath, and F. R. Carbone. 1997. Antigen-specific CD8[+] T cell subset distribution in lymph nodes draining the site of herpes simplex virus infection. *Eur. J. Immunol.* **27:**2310–2316.

Courtelier, J. P., J. T. Van der Logt, F. W. Hessen, A. Vink, and J. Van Snick. 1988. Virally induced modulation of murine IgG antibody subclasses. *J. Exp. Med.* **168:**2373–2378.

Courtelier, J. P., J. T. Van der Logt, F. W. Hessen, G. Warnier, and J. Van Snick. 1987. IgG2a restriction of murine antibodies elicited by viral infections. *J. Exp. Med.* **165:**64–69.

Cousens, L. P., J. S. Orange, and C. A. Biron. 1995. Endogenous IL-2 contributes to T cell expansion and IFN-gamma production during lymphocytic choriomeningitis virus infection. *J. Immunol.* **155:**5690–5699.

Dal Porto, J., T. E. Johansen, B. Catipovic, D. J. Parfiit, D. Tuveson, U. Gether, S. Kozlowski, D. T. Fearon, and J. P. Schneck. 1993. A soluble divalent class I major histocompatibility complex molecule inhibits alloreactive T cells at nanomolar concentrations. *Proc. Natl. Acad. Sci. USA* **90:**6671–6675.

Davies, D. R., E. A. Padlan, and S. Sheriff. 1990. Antibody-antigen complexes. *Annu. Rev. Biochem.* **59:**439–473.

Davis, M. M., J. J. Boniface, Z. Reich, D. Lyons, J. Hampl, B. Arden, and Y. Chien. 1998. Ligand recognition by alpha beta T cell receptors. *Annu. Rev. Immunol.* **16:**523–544.

deVinuesa, G., P. O'Leary, D. M.-Y. Sze, K.-M. Toellner, and I. C. M. MacLennan. 1999. T-independent type 2 antigens induce B cell proliferation in multiple splenic sites, but exponential growth is confined to extrafollicular foci. *Eur. J. Immunol.* **29:**1314–1327.

Dimmock, N. J. 1993. Neutralization of animal viruses. *Curr. Top. Microbiol. Immunol.* **183:**1–149.

Doherty, P. C., and J. P. Christensen. 2000. Accessing complexity: the dynamics of virus-specific T cell responses. *Annu. Rev. Immunol.* **18:**561–592.

Feng, N., J. W. Burns, L. Bracy, and H. B. Greenberg. 1994. Comparison of mucosal and systemic humoral immune responses and subsequent protection in mice orally inoculated with a homologous or a heterologous rotavirus. *J. Virol.* **68:**7766–7773.

Franco, M. A., and H. B. Greenberg. 1997. Immunity to rotavirus in T cell-deficient mice. *Virology* **238:**169–179.

Franco, M. A., and H. B. Greenberg. 1999. Immunity to rotavirus infection in mice. *J. Infect. Dis.* **179**(Suppl. 3)**:**S466–S469.

Frazer, J. K., and J. D. Capra. 1999. Immunoglobulins: structure and function, p. 37–74. *In* W. E. Paul (ed.), *Fundamental Immunology,* 4th ed. Lippincott-Raven, Philadelphia, Pa.

Fujinami, R. S., and M. B. Oldstone. 1979. Antiviral antibody reacting on the plasma membrane alters measles virus expression inside the cell. *Nature* **279:**529–530.

Gairin, J. E., H. Mazarguil, D. Hudrisier, and M. B. Oldstone. 1995. Optimal lymphocytic choriomeningitis virus sequences restricted by *H-2D^b* major histocompatibility complex class I molecules and presented to cytotoxic T lymphocytes. *J. Virol.* **69:**2297–2305.

Galli, S. J., and C. S. Lantz. 1999. Allergy, p. 1127–1174. *In* W. E. Paul (ed.), *Fundamental Immunology,* 4th ed. Lippincott-Raven, Philadelphia, Pa.

Gallimore, A., H. Hengartner, and R. Zinkernagel. 1998. Hierarchies of antigen-specific cytotoxic T-cell responses. *Immunol. Rev.* **164:**29–36.

Gerhard, W., K. Mozdzanowska, M. Furchner, G. Wasko, and K. Maiese. 1997. Role of the B-cell response in recovery of mice from primary influenza virus infection. *Immunol. Rev.* **159:**95–103.

Grayson, J. M., A. J. Zajac, J. D. Altman, and R. Ahmed. 2000. Increased expression of Bcl-2 in antigen-specific memory CD8[+] T cells. *J. Immunol.* **164:**3950–3954.

Grewal, I. S., and R. A. Flavell. 1998. CD40 and CD154 in cell-mediated immunity. *Annu. Rev. Immunol.* **16:**111–135.

Griffin, D., B. Levine, W. Tyor, S. Ubol, and P. Despres. 1997. The role of antibody in recovery from alphavirus encephalitis. *Immunol. Rev.* **159:**155–161.

Guidotti, L. G., and F. V. Chisari. 1999. Cytokine-induced viral purging—role in viral pathogenesis. *Curr. Opin. Microbiol.* **2:**388–391.

Guidotti, L. G., T. Ishikawa, M. V. Hobbs, B. Matzke, R. Schreiber, and F. V. Chisari. 1996. Intracellular inactivation of the hepatitis B virus by cytotoxic T lymphocytes. *Immunity* **4:**25–36.

Haanen, J. B., M. C. Wolkers, A. M. Kruisbeek, and T. N. Schumacher. 1999. Selective expansion of cross-reactive CD8(+) memory T cells by viral variants. *J. Exp. Med.* **190:**1319–1328.

Harris, N., R. M. Buller, and G. Karupiah. 1995. Gamma interferon-induced, nitric oxide-mediated inhibition of vaccinia virus replication. *J. Virol.* **69:**910–915.

Harris, N. L., and F. Ronchese. 1999. The role of B7 costimulation in T-cell immunity. *Immunol. Cell Biol.* **77:**304–311.

Harty, J. T., A. R. Tvinnereim, and D. W. White. 2000. CD8+ T cell effector mechanisms in resistance to infection. *Annu. Rev. Immunol.* **18:**275–308.

Holterman, A. X., K. Rogers, K. Edelmann, D. M. Koelle, L. Corey, and C. B. Wilson. 1999. An important role for major histocompatibility complex class I-restricted T cells, and a limited role for gamma interferon, in protection of mice against lethal herpes simplex virus infection. *J. Virol.* **73:**2058–2063.

Hou, S., P. C. Doherty, M. Zijlstra, R. Jaenish, and M. J. Katz. 1992. Delayed clearance of Sendai virus in mice lacking class I MHC-restricted CD8+ T cells. *J. Immunol.* **149:**1319–1325.

Hou, S., L. Hyland, K. W. Ryan, A. Portner, and P. C. Doherty. 1994. Virus-specific CD8+ T-cell memory determined by clonal burst size. *Nature* **369:**652–654.

Hudrisier, D., M. B. Oldstone, and J. E. Gairin. 1997. The signal sequence of lymphocytic choriomeningitis virus contains an immunodominant cytotoxic T cell epitope that is restricted by both H-2D(b) and H-2K(b) molecules. *Virology* **234:**62–73.

Igarashi, T., C. Brown, A. Azadegan, D. Dimitrov, M. A. Martin, and R. Shibata. 1999. Human immunodeficiency virus type 1 neutralizing antibodies accelerate clearance of cell-free virions from blood plasma. *Nat. Med.* **5:**211–216.

Jacobson, S., J. R. Richert, W. E. Biddison, A. Satinsky, R. J. Hartzman, and H. F. McFarland. 1984. Measles virus-specific T4+ human cytotoxic T cell clones are restricted by class II HLA antigens. *J. Immunol.* **133:**754–757.

Jennings, S. R., R. H. Bonneau, P. M. Smith, R. M. Wolcott, and R. Chervenak. 1991. CD4-positive T lymphocytes are required for the generation of the primary but not the secondary CD8-positive cytolytic T lymphocyte response to herpes simplex virus in C57BL/6 mice. *Cell. Immunol.* **133:**234–252.

Kagi, D., B. Ledermann, K. Burki, P. Seiler, B. Odermatt, K. J. Olsen, E. R. Podack, R. M. Zinkernagel, and H. Hengartner. 1994. Cytotoxicity mediated by T cells and natural killer cells is greatly impaired in perforin-deficient mice. *Nature* **369:**31–37.

Kagi, D., B. Ledermann, K. Burki, R. M. Zinkernagel, and H. Hengartner. 1996. Molecular mechanisms of lymphocyte-mediated cytotoxicity and their role in immunological protection and pathogenesis in vivo. *Annu. Rev. Immunol.* **14:**207–232.

Karupiah, G., Q. W. Xie, R. M. Buller, C. Nathan, C. Duarte, and J. D. MacMicking. 1993. Inhibition of viral replication by interferon-gamma-induced nitric oxide synthase. *Science* **261:**1445–1448.

Kehry, M. R., and P. D. Hodgkin. 1993. Helper T cells: delivery of cell contact and lymphokine-dependent signals to B cells. *Semin. Immunol.* 5:393–400.

Klagge, I. M., and S. Schneider-Schaulies. 1999. Virus interactions with dendritic cells. *J. Gen. Virol.* 80:823–833.

Knossow, M., R. S. Daniels, A. R. Douglas, J. J. Skehel, and D. C. Wiley. 1984. Three-dimensional structure of an antigenic mutant of the influenza virus. *Nature* 311:678–680.

Kundig, T. M., A. Shahinian, K. Kawai, H. W. Mittrucker, E. Sebzda, M. F. Bachmann, T. W. Mak, and P. S. Ohashi. 1996. Duration of TCR stimulation determines costimulatory requirement of T cells. *Immunity* 5:41–52.

Kurane, I., and F. E. Ennis. 1992. Immunity and immunopathology in dengue virus infections. *Semin. Immunol.* 4:121–127.

Lefrançois, L. 1984. Protection against lethal viral infection by neutralizing and nonneutralizing monoclonal antibodies: distinct mechanisms of action in vivo. *J. Virol.* 51:208–214.

Lin, M. T., D. R. Hinton, N. W. Marten, C. C. Bergmann, and S. A. Stohlman. 1999. Antibody prevents virus reactivation within the central nervous system. *J. Immunol.* 162:7358–7368.

Lin, M. Y., and R. M. Welsh. 1998. Stability and diversity of T cell receptor repertoire usage during lymphocytic choriomeningitis virus infection of mice. *J. Exp. Med.* 188:1993–2005.

Littana, R., I. Kurane, and F. A. Ennis. 1990. Human IgG Fc receptor II mediates antibody-dependent enhancement of Dengue virus infection. *J. Immunol.* 144:3183–3186.

Lumsden, J. M., J. M. Roberts, N. L. Harris, R. J. Peach, and F. Ronchese. 2000. Differential requirement for CD80 and CD80/CD86-dependent costimulation in the lung immune response to an influenza virus infection. *J. Immunol.* 164:79–85.

MacMicking, J., Q. W. Xie, and C. Nathan. 1997. Nitric oxide and macrophage function. *Annu. Rev. Immunol.* 15:323–350.

Maloy, K. J., B. Odermatt, H. Hengartner, and R. M. Zinkernagel. 1998. Interferon γ-producing γδ T cell-dependent antibody isotype switching in the absence of germinal center formation during virus infection. *Proc. Natl. Acad. Sci. USA* 95:1160–1165.

Mascola, J. R., G. Stiegler, T. C. VanCott, H. Katinger, C. B. Carpenter, C. E. Hanson, H. Beary, D. Hayes, S. S. Frankel, D. L. Birx, and M. G. Lewis. 2000. Protection of macaques against vaginal transmission of a pathogenic HIV-1/SIV chimeric virus by passive infusion of neutralizing antibodies. *Nat. Med.* 6:207–210.

Mason, D. 1998. A very high level of crossreactivity is an essential feature of the T-cell receptor. *Immunol. Today* 19:395–404.

Matloubian, M., R. J. Concepcion, and R. Ahmed. 1994. CD4+ T cells are required to sustain CD8+ cytotoxic T-cell responses during chronic viral infection. *J. Virol.* 68:8056–8063.

McAdam, A. J., A. N. Schweitzer, and A. H. Sharpe. 1998. The role of B7 co-stimulation in activation and differentiation of CD4+ and CD8+ T cells. *Immunol. Rev.* 165:231–247.

Morens, D. M. 1994. Antibody-dependent enhancement of infection and the pathogenesis of viral disease. *Clin. Infect. Dis.* 19:500–512.

Moskophidis, D., F. Lechner, H. Pircher, and R. M. Zinkernagel. 1993. Virus persistence in acutely infected immunocompetent mice by exhaustion of antiviral cytotoxic effector cells. *Nature* 362:758–761.

Mozdzanowska, K., M. Furchner, G. Washko, J. Mozdzanowski, and W. Gerhard. 1997. A pulmonary influenza virus infection in SCID mice can be cured by treatment with hemagglutinin-specific antibodies that display very low virus-neutralizing activity in vitro. *J. Virol.* 71:4347–4355.

Mozdzanowska, K., K. Maiese, and W. Gerhard. 2000. Th cell-deficient mice control influenza virus infection more effectively than Th- and B cell-deficient mice: evidence for a Th-

independent contribution by B cells to virus clearance. *J. Immunol.* 164:2635–2643.

Mullbacher, A., R. T. Hla, C. Museteanu, and M. M. Simon. 1999. Perforin is essential for control of ectromelia virus but not related poxviruses in mice. *J. Virol.* 73:1665–1667.

Murali-Krishna, K., J. D. Altman, M. Suresh, D. J. Sourdive, A. J. Zajac, J. D. Miller, J. Slansky, and R. Ahmed. 1998. Counting antigen-specific CD8 T cells: a reevaluation of bystander activation during viral infection. *Immunity* 8:177–187.

Mylin, L. M., R. H. Bonneau, J. D. Lippolis, and S. S. Tevethia. 1995. Hierarchy among multiple H-2^b-restricted cytotoxic T-lymphocyte epitopes within simian virus 40 T antigen. *J. Virol.* 69:6665–6677.

Nahill, S. R., and R. M. Welsh. 1993. High frequency of cross-reactive cytotoxic T lymphocytes elicited during the virus-induced polyclonal cytotoxic T lymphocyte response. *J. Exp. Med.* 177:317–327.

Nakata, M., A. Kawasaki, M. Azuma, K. Tsuji, H. Matsuda, Y. Shinkai, H. Yagita, and K. Okumura. 1992. Expression of perforin and cytolytic potential of human peripheral blood lymphocyte subpopulations. *Int. Immunol.* 4:1049–1054.

Nugent, C. T., J. M. McNally, R. Chervenak, R. M. Wolcott, and S. R. Jennings. 1995. Differences in the recognition of CTL epitopes during primary and secondary responses to herpes simplex virus infection in vivo. *Cell. Immunol.* 165:55–64.

Osiowy, C., D. Horne, and R. Anderson. 1994. Antibody-dependent enhancement of respiratory syncytial virus infection by sera from young infants. *Clin. Diagn. Lab. Immunol.* 1:670–677.

Oxenius, A., M. F. Bachmann, P. G. Ashton-Rickardt, S. Tonegawa, R. M. Zinkernagel, and H. Hengartner. 1995. Presentation of endogenous viral proteins in association with major histocompatibility complex class II: on the role of intracellular compartmentalization, invariant chain and the TAP transporter system. *Eur. J. Immunol.* 25:3402–3411.

Planz, O., P. Seiler, H. Hengartner, and R. M. Zinkernagel. 1996. Specific cytotoxic T cells eliminate cells producing neutralizing antibodies. *Nature* 382:726–729.

Price, D. A., P. Klenerman, B. L. Booth, R. E. Phillips, and A. K. Sewell. 1999. Cytotoxic T lymphocytes, chemokines and antiviral immunity. *Immunol. Today* 20:212–216.

Razvi, E. S., Z. Jiang, B. A. Woda, and R. M. Welsh. 1995. Lymphocyte apoptosis during the silencing of the immune response to acute viral infections in normal, lpr, and Bcl-2-transgenic mice. *Am. J. Pathol.* 147:79–91.

Razvi, E. S., and R. M. Welsh. 1993. Programmed cell death of T lymphocytes during acute viral infection: a mechanism for virus-induced immune deficiency. *J. Virol.* 67:5754–5765.

Reis e Sousa, C., A. Sher, and P. Kaye. 1999. The role of dendritic cells in the induction and regulation of immunity to microbial infection. *Curr. Opin. Immunol.* 11:392–399.

Roizman, B., and A. E. Sears. 1996. Herpes simplex viruses and their replication, p. 2231–2295. *In* B. N. Fields, D. M. Knipe, and P. M. Howley (ed.), *Fields Virology*, 3rd ed., vol. 2. Lippincott-Raven Publishers, Philadelphia, Pa.

Roost, H.-P., M. F. Bachmann, A. Haag, U. Kalinke, V. Pliska, H. Hengartner, and R. M. Zinkernagel. 1995. Early high-affinity neutralizing anti-viral IgG responses without further improvements of affinity. *Proc. Natl. Acad. Sci. USA* 92:1257–1261.

Russell, J. H., B. Rush, C. Weaver, and R. Wang. 1993. Mature T cells of autoimmune lpr/lpr mice have a defect in antigen-stimulated suicide. *Proc. Natl. Acad. Sci. USA* 90:4409–4413.

Salio, M., M. Cella, M. Suter, and A. Lanzavecchia. 1999. Inhibition of dendritic cell maturation by herpes simplex virus. *Eur. J. Immunol.* 29:3245–3253.

Sallusto, F., C. R. Mackay, and A. Lanzavecchia. 2000. The role of chemokine receptors in primary, effector, and memory immune responses. *Annu. Rev. Immunol.* 18:593–620.

Salvucci, L. A., R. H. Bonneau, and S. S. Tevethia. 1995. Polymorphism within the herpes simplex virus (HSV) ribonucleotide reductase large subunit (ICP6) confers type specificity for recognition by HSV type 1-specific cytotoxic T lymphocytes. *J. Virol.* 69:1122–1131.

Selin, L. K., S. R. Nahill, and R. M. Welsh. 1994. Cross-reactivities in memory cytotoxic T lymphocyte recognition of heterologous viruses. *J. Exp. Med.* 179:1933–1943.

Selin, L. K., S. M. Varga, I. C. Wong, and R. M. Welsh. 1998. Protective heterologous antiviral immunity and enhanced immunopathogenesis mediated by memory T cell populations. *J. Exp. Med.* 188:1705–1715.

Sha, Z., and R. W. Compans. 2000. Induction of CD4+ T-cell-independent immunoglobulin responses by inactivated influenza virus. *J. Virol.* 74:4999–5005.

Sheil, J. M., M. J. Bevan, and L. Lefrancois. 1987. Characterization of dual-reactive H2kb-restricted anti-vesicular stomatitis virus and alloreactive cytotoxic T cells. *J. Immunol.* 138:3654–3660.

Shibata, R., T. Igarashi, N. Haigwood, A. Buckler-White, R. Ogert, W. Ross, R. Willey, M. W. Cho, and M. A. Martin. 1999. Neutralizing antibody directed against the HIV-1 envelope glycoprotein can completely block HIV-1/SIV chimeric virus infections of macaque monkeys. *Nat. Med.* 5:204–210.

Shresta, S., C. T. Pham, D. A. Thomas, T. A. Graubert, and T. J. Ley. 1998. How do cytotoxic lymphocytes kill their targets? *Curr. Opin. Immunol.* 10:581–587.

Sigal, L. J., S. Crotty, R. Andino, and K. L. Rock. 1999. Cytotoxic T-cell immunity to virus-infected non-haematopoietic cells requires presentation of exogenous antigen. *Nature* 398:77–80.

Slifka, M. K., and R. Ahmed. 1996a. Limiting dilution analysis of virus-specific memory B cells by an ELISPOT assay. *J. Immunol. Methods* 199:37–46.

Slifka, M. K., and R. Ahmed. 1996b. Long-term humoral immunity against viruses: revisiting the issue of plasma cell longevity. *Trends Microbiol.* 4:394–400.

Slifka, M. K., and R. Ahmed. 1998. Long-lived plasma cells: a mechanism for maintaining persistent antibody production. *Curr. Opin. Immunol.* 10:252–258.

Slifka, M. K., F. Rodriguez, and J. L. Whitton. 1999. Rapid on/off cycling of cytokine production by virus-specific CD8+ T cells. *Nature* 401:76–79.

Sourdive, D. J., K. Murali-Krishna, J. D. Altman, A. J. Zajac, J. K. Whitmire, C. Pannetier, P. Kourilsky, B. Evavold, A. Sette, and R. Ahmed. 1998. Conserved T cell receptor repertoire in primary and memory CD8 T cell responses to an acute viral infection. *J. Exp. Med.* 188:71–82.

Spriggs, M. K., B. H. Koller, T. Sato, P. J. Morrissey, W. C. Fanslow, O. Smithies, R. F. Voice, M. B. Widmer, and C. R. Maliszewski. 1992. B2 microglobulin, CD8+ T cell-deficient mice survive inoculation with high doses of vaccinia virus and exhibit altered IgG responses. *Proc. Natl. Acad. Sci. USA* 89:6070–6074.

Su, H. C., L. P. Cousens, L. D. Fast, M. K. Slifka, R. D. Bungiro, R. Ahmed, and C. A. Biron. 1998. CD4+ and CD8+ T cell interactions in IFN-gamma and IL-4 responses to viral infections: requirements for IL-2. *J. Immunol.* 160:5007–5017.

Szomolanyi-Tsuda, E., J. D. Brien, J. E. Dorgan, R. L. Garcea, R. T. Woodland, and R. M. Welsh. 2001. Antiviral T cell-independent type 2 antibody responses induced in vivo in the absence of T and NK cells. *Virology* 280:160–168.

Szomolanyi-Tsuda, E., J. D. Brien, J. E. Dorgan, R. M. Welsh, and R. L. Garcea. 2000. The role of CD40-CD154 interaction

in antiviral T cell-independent IgG responses. *J. Immunol.* 164:5877–5882.

Szomolanyi-Tsuda, E., Q. P. Le, R. L. Garcea, and R. M. Welsh. 1998. T cell-independent immunoglobulin G responses in vivo are elicited by live-virus infection but not by immunization with viral proteins or virus-like particles. *J. Virol.* 72:6665–6670.

Szomolanyi-Tsuda, E., and R. M. Welsh. 1996. T cell-independent antibody-mediated clearance of polyoma virus in T cell-deficient mice. *J. Exp. Med.* 183:403–411.

Szomolanyi-Tsuda, E., and R. M. Welsh. 1998. T cell-independent antiviral antibody responses. *Curr. Opin. Immunol.* 10:431–435.

Tay, C. H., and R. M. Welsh. 1997. Distinct organ-dependent mechanisms for the control of murine cytomegalovirus infection by natural killer cells. *J. Virol.* 71:267–275.

Thomsen, A. R., A. Nansen, J. P. Christensen, S. O. Andreasen, and O. Marker. 1998. CD40 ligand is pivotal to efficient control of virus replication in mice infected with lymphocytic choriomeningitis virus. *J. Immunol.* 161:4583–4590.

Thomsen, A. R., M. Volkert, and O. Marker. 1985. Different isotype profiles of virus-specific antibodies in acute and persistent lymphocytic choriomeningitis virus infection in mice. *Immunology* 55:213–223.

Tishon, A., H. Lewicki, G. Rall, M. Von Herrath, and M. B. Oldstone. 1995. An essential role for type 1 interferon-gamma in terminating persistent viral infection. *Virology* 212:244–250.

Tishon, A., A. Salmi, R. Ahmed, and M. B. A. Oldstone. 1991. Role of viral strains and host genes in determining levels of immune complexes in a model system—implications for HIV infection. *AIDS Res.* 7:963–969.

Toes, R. E. M., S. P. Schoenberger, E. I. H. van der Voort, R. Offringa, and C. J. M. Melief. 1998. CD40-CD40Ligand interactions and their role in cytotoxic T lymphocyte priming and anti-tumor immunity. *Semin. Immunol.* 10:443–448.

Tomori, O. 1999. Impact of yellow fever on the developing world. *Adv. Virus Res.* 53:5–34.

Topham, D. J., R. A. Tripp, and P. C. Doherty. 1997. CD8+ T cells clear influenza virus by perforin- or Fas-dependent processes. *J. Immunol.* 159:5197–5200.

Townsend, A. R., J. Rothbard, F. M. Gotch, G. Bahadur, D. Wraith, and A. J. McMichael. 1986. The epitopes of influenza nucleoprotein recognized by cytotoxic T lymphocytes can be defined with short synthetic peptides. *Cell* 44:959–968.

Tyler, K. L., M. A. Mann, B. N. Fields, and H. W. Virgin IV. 1993. Protective anti-reovirus monoclonal antibodies and their effects on viral pathogenesis. *J. Virol.* 67:3446–3453.

van den Broek, M., M. F. Bachmann, G. Kohler, M. Barner, R. Escher, R. Zinkernagel, and M. Kopf. 2000. IL-4 and IL-10 antagonize IL-12-mediated protection against acute vaccinia virus infection with a limited role of IFN-gamma and nitric oxide synthetase 2. *J. Immunol.* 164:371–378.

van der Most, R. G., K. Murali-Krishna, J. L. Whitton, C. Oseroff, J. Alexander, S. Southwood, J. Sidney, R. W. Chesnut, A. Sette, and R. Ahmed. 1998. Identification of Db- and Kb-restricted subdominant cytotoxic T-cell responses in lymphocytic choriomeningitis virus-infected mice. *Virology* 240:158–167.

Varga, S. M., and R. M. Welsh. 1996. The CD45RB-associated epitope defined by monoclonal antibody CZ-1 is an activation and memory marker for mouse CD4 T cells. *Cell. Immunol.* 167:56–62.

Varga, S. M., and R. M. Welsh. 1998a. Stability of virus-specific CD4+ T cell frequencies from acute infection into long term memory. *J. Immunol.* 161:367–374.

Varga, S. M., and R. M. Welsh. 1998b. Detection of a high frequency of virus-specific CD4+ T cells during acute infection with lymphocytic choriomeningitis virus. *J. Immunol.* **161:** 3215–3218.

Varga, S. M., and R. M. Welsh. 2000. High frequency of virus-specific interleukin-2-producing CD4⁺ T cells and Th1 dominance during lymphocytic choriomeningitis virus infection. *J. Virol.* **74:**4429–4432.

Virgin, H. W., IV, and S. H. Speck. 1999. Unraveling immunity to γ-herpesviruses: a new model for understanding the role of immunity in chronic virus infection. *Curr. Opin. Immunol.* **11:** 371–379.

Von Herrath, M. G., B. Coon, and M. B. A. Oldstone. 1997. Low-affinity cytotoxic T-lymphocytes require IFNg to clear an acute viral infection. *Virology* **229:**349–359.

von Pirquet, C. 1908. Das Verhalten der kurtanen Tuberkulin-Reakton wahrend der Masern. *Dtsch. Med. Wochenschr.* **34:** 1297–1300.

Wang, B., R. Maile, R. Greenwood, E. J. Collins, and J. A. Frelinger. 2000. Naive CD8+ T cells do not require costimulation for proliferation and differentiation into cytotoxic effector cells. *J. Immunol.* **164:**1216–1222.

Ward, S. G., K. Bacon, and J. Westwick. 1998. Chemokines and T lymphocytes: more than an attraction. *Immunity* **9:**1–11.

Welsh, R. M., T. G. Markees, B. A. Woda, K. A. Daniels, M. A. Brehm, J. P. Mordes, D. L. Greiner, and A. A. Rossini. 2000. Virus-induced abrogation of transplantation tolerance induced by donor-specific transfusion and anti-CD154 antibody. *J. Virol.* **74:**2210–2218.

Welsh, R. M., and J. M. McNally. 1999. Immune deficiency, immune silencing, and clonal exhaustion of T cell responses during viral infections. *Curr. Opin. Microbiol.* **2:**382–387.

Welsh, R. M., and M. Vargas-Cortes. 1992. Natural killer cells in viral infection, p. 107–150. *In* C. E. Lewis and J. O. McGee (ed.), *The Natural Killer Cell. The Natural Immune System.* IRL Press, Ltd., Oxford, United Kingdom.

Whitmire, J. K., M. S. Asano, K. Murali-Krishna, M. Suresh, and R. Ahmed. 1998. Long-term CD4 Th1 and Th2 memory following acute lymphocytic choriomeningitis virus infection. *J. Virol.* **72:**8281–8288.

Whitmire, J. K., R. A. Flavell, I. S. Grewal, C. P. Larsen, T. C. Pearson, and R. Ahmed. 1999. CD40-CD40 ligand costimulation is required for generating antiviral CD4 T cell responses but is dispensable for CD8 T cell responses. *J. Immunol.* **163:** 3194–3201.

Whitmire, J. K., M. K. Slifka, I. S. Grewal, R. A. Flavell, and R. Ahmed. 1996. CD40-ligand-deficient mice generate a normal primary cytotoxic T-lymphocyte response but a defective humoral response to a viral infection. *J. Virol.* **70:**8375–8381.

Whitton, J. L., P. J. Southern, and M. B. Oldstone. 1988. Analyses of the cytotoxic T lymphocyte responses to glycoprotein and nucleoprotein components of lymphocytic choriomeningitis virus. *Virology* **162:**321–327.

Wilson, C. S., J. M. Moser, J. D. Altman, P. E. Jensen, and A. E. Lukacher. 1999. Cross-recognition of two middle T protein epitopes by immunodominant polyoma virus-specific CTL. *J. Immunol.* **162:**3933–3941.

Wilson, I. A., and N. J. Case. 1990. Structural basis of immune recognition of influenza virus hemagglutinin. *Annu. Rev. Immunol.* **8:**737–771.

Wu, Y., and Y. Liu. 1994. Viral induction of co-stimulatory activity on antigen-presenting cells bypasses the need for CD4+ T-cell help in CD8+ T-cell responses. *Curr. Biol.* **4:**499–505.

Yang, H., and R. M. Welsh. 1986. Induction of alloreactive cytotoxic T cells by acute virus infection of mice. *J. Immunol.* **136:** 1186–1193.

Yang, H. Y., P. L. Dundon, S. R. Nahill, and R. M. Welsh. 1989. Virus-induced polyclonal cytotoxic T lymphocyte stimulation. *J. Immunol.* **142:**1710–1718.

Yasukawa, M., and J. M. Zarling. 1984. Human cytotoxic T cell clones directed against herpes simplex virus-infected cells. I. Lysis restricted by HLA class II MB and DR antigens. *J. Immunol.* **133:**422–427.

Yewdell, J. W., and J. R. Bennink. 1999. Immunodominance in major histocompatibility complex class I-restricted T lymphocyte responses. *Annu. Rev. Immunol.* **17:**51–88.

Zarozinski, C. C., J. M. McNally, B. L. Lohman, K. A. Daniels, and R. M. Welsh. 2000. Bystander sensitization to activation-induced cell death as a mechanism of virus-induced immune suppression. *J. Virol.* **74:**3650–3658.

Zarozinski, C. C., and R. M. Welsh. 1997. Minimal bystander activation of CD8 T cells during the virus-induced polyclonal T cell response. *J. Exp. Med.* **185:**1629–1639.

Zhang, X., S. Sun, I. Hwang, D. F. Tough, and J. Sprent. 1998. Potent and selective stimulation of memory-phenotype CD8+ T cells in vivo by IL-15. *Immunity* **8:**591–599.

Zimmermann, C., P. Seiler, P. Lane, and R. M. Zinkernagel. 1997. Antiviral immune response in CTLA4 transgenic mice. *J. Virol.* **71:**1802–1807.

Zinkernagel, R. M., and P. C. Doherty. 1974. Restriction of in vitro T cell-mediated cytotoxicity in lymphocytic choriomeningitis within a syngeneic or semiallogeneic system. *Nature* **248:** 701–702.

V. PATHOLOGY

Immunology of Infectious Diseases
Edited by S. H. E. Kaufmann, A. Sher, and R. Ahmed
© 2002 ASM Press, Washington, D.C.

Chapter 19

Autoimmunity as a Consequence of Infection

KAI W. WUCHERPFENNIG AND NILUFER P. SETH

GENERAL FEATURES OF AUTOIMMUNE DISEASES

In autoimmune diseases, the immune system plays a key role in pathogenesis. The ability of T cells and B cells to recognize a vast variety of linear peptide sequences or complex structures is beneficial during an anti-infective immune response but can become detrimental when such a response is directed against host antigens. This chapter focuses on the basic mechanisms by which infectious agents can trigger or exacerbate autoimmune diseases. Several examples of human diseases for which there is strong evidence of involvement of infectious agents will also be discussed.

Despite obvious differences in clinical presentation, autoimmune diseases have certain common features that reflect basic biological mechanisms. In all human diseases and animal models that have been examined to date, genetic susceptibility is due to multiple loci (Vyse and Todd, 1996). Due to the involvement of multiple genes, only a relatively small fraction of the population appears to be genetically susceptible to a given autoimmune disease. In the context of infection and autoimmunity, this means that a relatively small fraction of individuals who encounter a certain infectious agent may be susceptible to the development of a particular autoimmune disease. The epidemiology of several human autoimmune diseases that are associated with defined infectious agents supports this concept, as discussed in the clinical examples.

The major histocompatibility complex (MHC) is an important susceptibility locus in many human autoimmune diseases, as well as in a number of experimental models. The role of the MHC was first observed in studies that compared the frequency of particular MHC alleles in patient and control populations. More recently, a genetic linkage to the MHC has been formally shown in genome-wide analyses of families with certain autoimmune diseases. In the majority of autoimmune diseases, alleles of MHC class II genes show the strongest association. Since MHC class II molecules present peptides to $CD4^+$ T cells, these disease associations indicate that antigen presentation to $CD4^+$ T cells is likely to be important in the initiation and/or progression of these diseases. Notable exceptions are ankylosing spondylitis and reactive arthritis, which show a striking association with the MHC class I molecule HLA-B27 (Nepom, 1993; Wucherpfennig and Strominger, 1995a).

Tissue damage can be mediated either by autoantibodies or by cellular effector mechanisms. In many autoimmune diseases, $CD4^+$ T cells are thought to represent critical effector cells, but $CD8^+$ T cells have received renewed attention based on studies in the NOD mouse model of type I diabetes. A number of antibody-mediated autoimmune diseases also show an association with MHC class II genes, indicating that activation of autoantigen-specific $CD4^+$ T cells that provide help for autoantigen-specific B cells is likely to be important in the pathogenesis (Nepom, 1993; Wucherpfennig and Strominger, 1995a; Zamvil and Steinman, 1990; Wong et al., 1999).

AUTOIMMUNITY AND INFECTION: BASIC MECHANISMS

Activation of autoreactive T cells is a critical step in the development of autoimmune diseases. In experimental models of autoimmunity, disease can only be transferred by activated but not resting autoreac-

Kai W. Wucherpfennig and Nilufer P. Seth • Department of Cancer Immunology and AIDS, Dana-Farber Cancer Institute and Harvard Medical School, Boston, MA 02115.

tive T cells (Zamvil and Steinman, 1990). Autoreactive T cells can be activated by the following mechanisms:

1. Viral and bacterial antigens that have sufficient structural similarity to self-antigens (molecular mimicry)
2. Viral and bacterial superantigens
3. Release of autoantigens during inflammation in the target organ
4. Infection of lymphocytes with a lymphotropic virus

First, we will discuss these basic mechanisms, including studies in relevant animal models (Table 1). Then we will analyze several human autoimmune diseases which have a strong association with defined infectious agents (Table 2).

Structural Similarity between Microbial Antigens and Self-Antigens: Molecular Mimicry

T cells were previously considered to be highly specific for single foreign peptides. Numerous studies over the last several years have, however, demonstrated that the same T-cell receptor (TCR) can recognize a number of peptides with limited primary sequence homology (Wucherpfennig and Strominger, 1995b). This degeneracy in TCR recognition can result in TCR cross-reactivity between microbial peptides and self-peptides (molecular mimicry) (Fig. 1).

TCRs recognize peptides bound to MHC class I or class II molecules. Crystal structures of MHC-peptide-TCR complexes have provided general insights into the structural basis of TCR specificity and cross-reactivity. The TCR contact surface with the MHC-peptide complex was found to be remarkably flat, except for a central pocket created by the CDR3 loops of TCR α and β. Also, the TCR makes substantial contacts with the MHC helices, such that the bound peptide represents only a relatively small fraction of the total contact surface with the TCR (approximately 22 to 33%) (Garboczi et al., 1996; Garcia et al., 1996). In addition, peptide binding by MHC class II molecules is highly degenerate. Peptide elution studies have demonstrated that several hundred different peptides are bound by MHC class II molecules (Rammensee et al., 1993).

TCR specificity and cross-reactivity has been examined using human T-cell clones specific for the complex of HLA-DR2 and an immunodominant myelin basic protein (MBP) peptide (residues 85 to 99). These T-cell clones were isolated from multiple sclerosis patients with the disease-associated HLA-DR2 haplotype. Peptide binding studies demonstrated that two hydrophobic residues of the MBP peptide (V89 and F92) were critical for HLA-DR2 binding and that each anchor residue could be replaced by other hydrophobic amino acids. In the crystal structure of the HLA-DR2–MBP peptide complex, these peptide residues occupy the hydrophobic P1 and P4 pockets of the binding site. Only a limited number of MBP peptide residues (H90, F91, and K93), which are located in the center of the HLA-DR2–MBP peptide surface in the crystal structure, were critical for TCR recognition (Wucherpfennig et al., 1994; Smith et al., 1998).

The HLA-DR2 binding/TCR recognition motif was used to identify peptides from human pathogens through a protein database search. Based on this search, seven viral peptides and one bacterial peptide were found that stimulated at least one of seven MBP-specific T-cell clones. The microbial peptides were quite distinct in their sequence from the MBP peptide and from each other since only primary TCR contact residues were conserved. Only one of these peptides had obvious sequence similarity and could have been identified by sequence alignment (Wucherpfennig and Strominger, 1995b; Hausmann et al., 1999).

Microbial peptides that activate a human MBP-specific T-cell clone were also identified when the T-cell recognition motif was defined with combinatorial peptide libraries. Using this strategy, the same MBP peptide residues were found to be important for T-cell recognition. Peptide recognition by this T-cell clone was highly degenerate because the clone was stimulated by random peptide libraries, which contained large numbers of different peptides (2×10^{14} different sequences for an X11 library) (Hemmer et al., 1997). Several other relevant examples of TCR

Table 1. Mechanisms for the induction of autoimmunity by infectious agents

Molecular mimicry
    TCR and antibody cross-reactivity due to structural similarity between microbial antigens and self-antigens

Superantigens
    Activation of T cells that express particular Vβ segments, including autoreactive T cells with such TCR Vβ segments

Release of autoantigen during an infection
    Uptake of autoantigens by antigen presenting cells recruited to an inflammatory site and priming of autoreactive T cells and B cells

Activation of lymphocytes by lymphotropic viruses
    B-cell activation, enhanced antibody production, and formation of circulating immune complexes (hepatitis C virus)

Table 2. Human inflammatory diseases induced by defined infectious agents

Diseases	Major target organ(s)	Pathogen(s)	MHC association(s)
Postinfectious syndromes			
Guillain-Barré syndrome	Peripheral nerves	*C. jejuni*, Epstein-Barr virus, cytomegalovirus	
Rheumatic fever, glomerulonephritis	Heart, heart valves, kidneys, CNS	Group A streptococci	
Acute and chronic inflammatory diseases			
Lyme arthritis	Large joints	*B. burgdorferi*	HLA-DR4, HLA-DR1
Reactive arthritis	Axial skeleton	*Yersinia, Shigella, Salmonella, Chlamydia trachomatis*	HLA-B27
Immune complex-mediated disease			
Mixed cryoglobulinemia	Blood vessels, kidneys, lungs	Hepatitis C virus	

crossreactivity have been described and will be discussed in the section on human autoimmune diseases.

Induction of Experimental Autoimmune Diseases by Molecular Mimicry

The induction of an autoimmune disease by microbial antigens has been studied by immunization with microbial peptides that have sequence homology to immunodominant self-peptides. The first of these studies examined the induction of experimental autoimmune encephalomyelitis (EAE) with a hepatitis B virus polymerase peptide in which six amino acids were identical to the encephalitogenic region of rabbit MBP. Following immunization with this peptide, T-cell reactivity to MBP was observed and 4 of 11 rabbits showed histological signs of EAE (Fujinami and Oldstone, 1985).

An important issue regarding the molecular mimicry hypothesis has been whether autoimmunity can also be induced by infection with a viral or bacterial pathogen. Infection-based experiments have been performed in a murine model of herpes simplex keratitis in which tissue destruction is mediated by CD4$^+$ T cells. In humans, herpes simplex virus type 1 (HSV-1) infection causes destruction of corneal tissue and is a leading cause of blindness. In the mouse model, disease can be induced by keratogenic T-cell clones that cross-react with a peptide from the HSV-1 UL6 protein. T cells specific for this HSV-1 peptide are important in the pathogenesis because tolerance induction with soluble UL6 peptide protects from keratitis. A virus with a mutation in the UL6 gene was also generated and found to be greatly impaired in its ability to induce herpes simplex keratitis. The failure of this mutant virus to induce disease was not associated with its replication deficiency, since replication-deficient control viruses were able to induce disease under these experimental conditions (Zhao et al., 1998).

Another example of molecular mimicry is the murine myocarditis model in which disease can be induced with cross-reactive peptides from *Chlamydia*. In BALB/c mice, immunization with a 30-amino-acid peptide from the cardiac myosin heavy chain induces a severe inflammatory heart disease. Based on the recognition motif for these myosin-specific T cells, cross-reactive peptides from the 60-kDa cysteine-rich outer membrane protein of *Chlamydia trachomatis* and other chlamydiae were identified. These *Chlamydia*-derived peptides in-

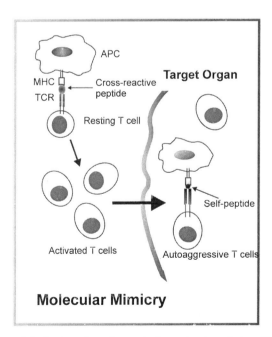

Figure 1. Induction of autoimmunity by molecular mimicry. Viral and bacterial peptides that have sufficient structural similarity to a self-peptide can activate autoreactive T cells during an infection. These activated T cells can migrate to the target organ and initiate an autoimmune process following TCR recognition of the self-peptide bound to MHC molecules.

duced inflammatory heart disease at a frequency similar to that for the myosin peptide, although with a significantly lower severity. T cells from mice immunized with the *Chlamydia* peptide showed a strong proliferative response to the myosin peptide, and *Chlamydia*-reactive T-cell lines induced myocarditis with a moderate severity. Infection of mice with *Chlamydia* resulted in the production of antibodies that cross-reacted with myosin, but the authors did not report whether such an infection induced myocarditis (Bachmaier et al., 1999).

The majority of animal models that have examined TCR cross-reactivity have focused on the role of CD4$^+$ T cells. The role of CD8$^+$ T cells was investigated in a mouse model of inflammatory bowel disease, using CD8$^+$ T-cell clones specific for mycobacterial hsp60, which cross-reacted with murine hsp60. These T cells also recognized a self-epitope presented by gamma interferon (IFN-γ) stressed target cells. After adoptive transfer of hsp60-specific T cells into TCR $\beta^{-/-}$ mice, massive infiltration could be detected in the small intestine and the liver. Transfer of hsp60-specific T cells into wild-type mice did not lead to expansion of CD8$^+$ T cells and pathologic responses. Disease was mediated by TCR recognition of the hsp60 self-antigen, because a non-cross-reactive T-cell clone that reacted only with mycobacterial hsp60 did not cause disease. The incidence of disease was similar in germ-free animals, indicating that recognition of bacterial hsp60 was not required in this adoptive-transfer model. These results demonstrate TCR cross-reactivity between murine and bacterial hsp60 for CD8$^+$ T cells and illustrate the potential involvement of such cross-reactivity in autoimmune pathology (Steinhoff et al., 1999).

Viral and Bacterial Superantigens

Superantigens activate T cells through the variable domain of the TCR β chain. This distinctive mode of T-cell activation, together with the ability of superantigens to bind to a wide variety of MHC class II molecules, leads to activation of large numbers of T cells irrespective of their MHC and peptide specificity (Fig. 2). Superantigens are involved in several human diseases, including food poisoning and toxic shock syndrome (Scherer et al., 1993).

Experiments with murine models of autoimmunity have clearly demonstrated that superantigens can induce relapses and exacerbations of a T-cell-mediated autoimmune process. EAE can be induced in PL/J mice with the N-terminal peptide of MBP (Ac1–11). The majority of T cells specific for this peptide express Vβ8, allowing activation of such T cells by the superantigen staphylococcal enterotoxin

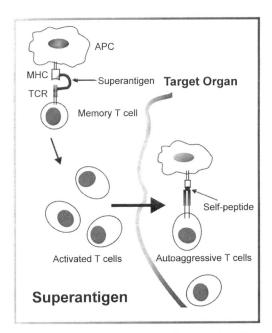

Figure 2. Reactivation of memory T cells by viral and bacterial superantigens. Superantigens can activate T cells that express certain TCR Vβ segments. In experimental models of autoimmunity, such superantigens can induce relapses of autoimmunity by reactivation of memory T cells specific for autoantigens.

B. Administration of this superantigen induced relapses and exacerbation of EAE (Brocke et al., 1993).

Superantigens also reactivate bacterial cell wall-induced arthritis and collagen-induced arthritis. The *Mycoplasma arthritidis* superantigen, MAM, is derived from a naturally occurring murine arthritogenic mycoplasma. MAM is a potent superantigen that activates T cells expressing Vβ5.1, Vβ6, and Vβ8. As in EAE, T cells expressing Vβ8 play a major role in murine type II collagen-induced arthritis. MAM caused a severe exacerbation of arthritis that persisted for at least 40 days when administered during the chronic stage of the disease. The arthritis flare that was induced by MAM was more severe than the initial arthritis induced by type II collagen. The superantigen could also trigger arthritis in mice that had previously been immunized with type II collagen but had failed to develop clinical disease (Cole and Griffiths, 1993).

Superantigens can therefore reactivate autoreactive T cells that express particular TCR Vβ chains. However, it is not clear whether superantigens can also initiate an autoimmune process. Naive T cells are deleted or become anergic following superantigen administration, explaining why injection of superantigen prior to immunization with MBP prevented the development of EAE in PL/J mice (Soos et al., 1993). Viral and bacterial superantigens may therefore contribute to established autoimmune processes and induce relapses and exacerbations of disease.

Release of Autoantigens during an Infection

A T-cell response directed against a single self-peptide can diversify during an inflammatory process by priming of T cells that are specific for other self-peptides (Fig. 3). This concept of "epitope spreading" was first delineated in a murine EAE model. At an early time point following immunization with MBP (day 9), the T-cell response in both draining lymph nodes and spleen was focused on the N-terminal peptide of MBP (Ac1-11). However, at a later stage (day 40), T-cell responses to several other MBP epitopes (residues 35 to 47, 81 to 100, and 121 to 140) were also detected. Importantly, this epitope spreading was also observed in mice that had been immunized with only the Ac1–11 peptide, indicating that endogenous priming to the self-antigen was responsible for the diversification of the T-cell response (Lehmann et al., 1992).

The role of epitope spreading in chronic viral infections has been examined using the Theiler's virus model. Theiler's murine encephalomyelitis virus, a natural mouse pathogen, is a picornavirus that induces a chronic, CD4$^+$ T-cell-mediated demyelinat-

ing disease. Virus-specific CD4$^+$ T cells initiate the demyelinating process and target virus that persists in the central nervous system (CNS). Clinical disease begins approximately 30 days after infection and displays a chronic-progressive course, with 100% of animals being affected by 40 to 50 days. T-cell proliferative responses to UV-inactivated virus could be detected in the spleen at the onset of clinical signs. At later stages of the disease, T-cell responses to myelin antigens were also observed. T-cell responses to an immunodominant peptide from proteolipid protein (residues 139 to 151) were detected first, followed by responses to other peptides derived from proteolipid protein, MBP, and myelin oligodendrocyte glycoprotein. Induction of tolerance with Theiler's murine encephalomyelitis virus peptides, but not with myelin peptides, inhibited disease induction, indicating that virus-specific T cells are key effector cells in this model. Nevertheless, these data demonstrate that a chronic CNS infection can result in priming to self-antigens (Miller et al., 1997). Priming of autoreactive T cells may be important in human diseases caused by a persisting pathogen.

Activation of Lymphocytes by Lymphotropic Viruses

Infection of human B cells by hepatitis C virus can cause a lymphoproliferative disease termed mixed cryoglobulinemia. Infection of B cells results in B-cell proliferation, enhanced antibody production, and the formation of circulating immune complexes (Ferri and Zignego, 2000). The clinical features and pathophysiology of this disease are described in detail in the following section. This example illustrates how a persistent virus infection of lymphocytes can result in an autoimmune process.

The different mechanisms by which infectious agents can be involved in autoimmunity are not mutually exclusive. Molecular mimicry has been proposed as an initiating event in autoimmune diseases. As discussed above, superantigens can reactivate autoreactive T cells that were previously primed and can thereby induce relapses in experimental models of autoimmunity. Epitope spreading has been detected in the chronic stages of CNS disease mediated by Theiler's murine encephalomyelitis virus. Taken together, these results suggest that infectious agents can affect an autoimmune process at different stages of disease initiation and progression.

INFECTIOUS AGENTS AND HUMAN AUTOIMMUNE DISEASES

The concept of infectious triggers for human autoimmune diseases has attracted considerable

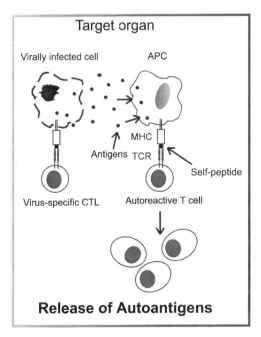

Figure 3. Activation of autoreactive T cells by release of autoantigens in the course of an infection. Virus-specific T cells can kill infected cells in the target organ, resulting in uptake of autoantigens by antigen-presenting cells (APC). These antigen-presenting cells can activate autoreactive T cells. CTL, cytotoxic T lymphocytes.

interest. Despite its potential importance, this is a challenging field for research and clear-cut criteria are required for establishing a causative role for infectious agents in such disease processes (Table 3). A role for an infectious agent in the development of an autoimmune disease can be established by isolation of the infectious agent from patients with the disease and by documenting the development of antibodies to the pathogen, in particular immunoglobulin M (IgM) antibodies, which are indicative of recent exposure. In examining infection with a pathogen in an autoimmune disease, it is very important to analyze appropriate control groups. For acute infections, household and community controls are critical, as described below.

For direct isolation of an infectious agent from patients with an autoimmune disease, it is essential that the clinical diagnosis be made while the infectious agent is still present. This requirement can be met in acute autoimmune diseases that bring the disease to immediate attention and in chronic diseases caused by a persisting pathogen. However, isolation of an infectious agent can be difficult when the disease onset is slow and insidious, allowing clearance of an infectious agent prior to clinical diagnosis of the autoimmune disease. For example, type I diabetes is preceded for months or years by a prediabetic state, during which destruction of the insulin-producing β cells in the pancreas occurs. When insulin deficiency becomes clinically apparent, the majority of β cells have already been lost. Due to the long delay between disease onset and clinical diag-

nosis, the temporal relationship between an infection and the development of autoimmunity can be lost.

Since autoimmune diseases are defined by mechanisms of disease pathogenesis, it is also important to determine how the autoimmune disease is initiated or amplified by an infectious agent. For that purpose, the creation of relevant animal models is important.

For many autoimmune diseases, much speculation still surrounds the potential involvement of infectious agents in the disease process. The following examples will therefore focus on diseases in which a definitive association with one or several infectious agents has been established.

Autoimmune Diseases Triggered by Acute Infection

Guillain-Barré syndrome (GBS) and rheumatic fever are classic examples of autoimmune diseases with an acute onset that follow infection with defined microorganisms. GBS is an acute peripheral neuropathy that can follow infection with *Campylobacter jejuni,* Epstein-Barr virus, cytomegalovirus, or *Mycoplasma pneumoniae.* Rheumatic fever is triggered by infection with group A streptococci and affects multiple organs, principally the heart, joints, kidneys, and CNS. Both examples highlight general principles of autoimmunity triggered by infection.

Triggering of GBS by bacterial and viral pathogens

GBS is a striking neurologic condition that is usually serious enough to require medical attention at an early stage. The onset is sudden, and limb weakness typically progresses to maximum disability within 1 week of onset. In ~25% of patients, artificial ventilation is required because the respiratory muscles are severely affected. The seriousness of this condition is reflected by a mortality rate of ~10%. GBS is a prototypic "postinfectious disease," and approximately two-thirds of patients report antecedent illnesses. Respiratory infections are most frequently reported, followed by gastrointestinal infections. The acute onset and the severity of the illness have greatly facilitated the isolation of infectious organisms from patients with GBS (Hughes and Rees, 1997).

C. jejuni is the principal infectious agent that has been associated with the development of GBS. Campylobacters are gram-negative bacilli that have a propensity to invade the intestinal mucosa and are considered to be the most common cause of bacterial diarrhea in the United States. In GBS, the involvement of *C. jejuni* has been shown not only by serological methods but, more importantly, also by direct isolation of the bacterium from GBS patients. In a well-controlled study that compared the frequency of

---

Table 3. Criteria for establishing the role of infectious agents in autoimmune diseases

Identification of the pathogen(s) in patients with autoimmune disease
    Isolation of pathogen
        Autoimmune process must be diagnosed at the time of infection
        Appropriate control groups are critical
        Isolation of pathogen is difficult in autoimmune diseases with a slow, insidious onset since some infectious agents can be cleared prior to clinical diagnosis

Identification of antibodies specific for pathogen
    IgM antibodies indicate recent infection with pathogen

Determination of the mechanism(s) by which the pathogen(s) induces autoimmunity
    Isolation of T cells and/or antibodies from patients with the disease

Development of an animal model that recapitulates essential features of the disease process

positive cultures from patients and household controls, C. jejuni was found in 26% of GBS patients and 2% of control subjects (Rees et al., 1995). Since such culture methods tend to underestimate the frequency of infection, a larger fraction of cases may be caused by this pathogen. Importantly, the association of C. jejuni with GBS has been found in four different continents, based on studies from the United States, Europe, South Africa, China, and Japan. C. jejuni is therefore an important worldwide cause of GBS (Hughes and Rees, 1997).

Summer epidemics of GBS occur among children and young adults in northern China and are particularly likely to be associated with C. jejuni infection (McKhann et al., 1993). In Japan, a high prevalence of a certain serotype of C. jejuni (O:19) was observed among GBS patients. In that study, 45% of patients showed evidence of a recent C. jejuni infection, based on elevated antibody titers. Of 16 isolates, 12 (75%) had the O:19 serotype, compared to 2.3% of control isolates from the region and 1.1% of isolates from the rest of Japan (Saida et al., 1997). Different serotypes have been observed in GBS patients in other countries.

Infection with C. jejuni correlates with clinical features and the specificity of cross-reactive autoantibodies. Specifically, GBS following infection with C. jejuni is associated with a more severe clinical course, prominent motor symptoms, and the presence of antibodies to the GM_1 ganglioside (Rees et al., 1995; Ang et al., 1999). In contrast, infection with cytomegalovirus is associated with a more pronounced sensory involvement, a milder clinical course, and cross-reactive antibodies that bind to the GM_2 ganglioside (Visser et al., 1996). GBS can also follow infection with Epstein-Barr virus and M. pneumoniae. These infections have been reported at the following frequencies: C. jejuni, 32%; cytomegalovirus, 13%; Epstein-Barr virus, 10%; and M. pneumoniae, 5% (Jacobs et al., 1998). The microorganisms that trigger GBS are therefore highly diverse (viral or bacterial) and have very distinct life cycles. A common denominator of these infections may be the specificity of the immune response that results in GBS in susceptible individuals.

Infection with C. jejuni triggers antibodies that cross-react with peripheral nerve antigens. A number of studies have demonstrated that patients with GBS develop antibodies specific for lipopolysaccharides (LPS) of certain strains of C. jejuni which cross-react with gangliosides from peripheral nerves. Gangliosides are glycosphingolipids that have a ceramide moiety in the lipid bilayer and an extracellular sialylated oligosaccharide. The outer polysaccharide moieties of LPS from certain strains of Campylo-

bacter bear striking structural similarities to gangliosides found in peripheral nerves. For example, the Campylobacter O:19 serotype shares an identical tetrasaccharide with the GM_1 ganglioside and a pentasaccharide with the GD_{1a} ganglioside. Serotypes O:23 and O:36 share a branched tetrasaccharide with the GM_2 ganglioside (Moran, 1997).

Cross-reactivity (molecular mimicry) between peripheral nerve gangliosides and LPS from Campylobacter has been demonstrated using a variety of different experimental approaches, including analysis of sera from patients with GBS and generation of murine monoclonal antibodies. IgM monoclonal antibodies specific for LPS from the O:19 serotype bound to gangliosides GQ_{1b}, GT_{1a}, and GD_3, which have related oligosaccharide structures. Immunofluorescence experiments demonstrated strong staining of peripheral nerves. In the presence of complement, the IgM antibodies induced a temporary increase in spontaneous neurotransmitter release from the murine peripheral nerves, which was followed by a block that resulted in paralysis (Goodyear et al., 1999).

The specificity of ganglioside antibodies also correlates with clinical manifestations of the disease. A striking association is observed between a clinical variant of GBS (Miller-Fisher syndrome) and antibodies specific for gangliosides GQ_{1b} and GT_{1a}. In Miller-Fisher syndrome, ocular muscles and the cerebellum are also affected. GQ_{1b} is concentrated in extraocular nerves, a principal motor site affected in patients with this syndrome. Antibodies to the GM_1 ganglioside are associated with a form of GBS that is characterized by primary motor involvement (Carpo et al., 1999; Hughes and Rees, 1997; Rees et al., 1995).

Taken together, these data demonstrate a strong association between preceding infection with C. jejuni and the development of GBS. Nevertheless, susceptibility of the host must play an important role in the development of this disease. The Centers for Disease Control and Prevention estimate that there are ~1,000 cases of C. jejuni infection per 100,000 population per year, and only a small fraction of these patients develop GBS (incidence of approximately 1 per 100,000) (Blaser, 1997). This situation is similar in other autoimmune diseases triggered by infection, such as rheumatic fever triggered by group A streptococci. It would therefore be of great interest to define the genes that confer susceptibility to GBS and to determine how they affect the immune response to the infectious agent and to self-antigens.

Also, very little is known about the T-cell response to C. jejuni in GBS. In particular, it will be important to determine whether bacterial antigens activate T cells that cross-react with peripheral nerve antigens. CD1 molecules can present bacterial glycolipid antigens to T cells, raising the question whether peripheral-nerve gangliosides are recognized by CD1-restricted T cells (Porcelli et al., 1998). It will also be important to develop an animal model in which key aspects of the pathogenesis are recapitulated. Defining the specificity of the T-cell response in this disease may be critical to such efforts.

Triggering of rheumatic fever by group A streptococci

Rheumatic fever following pharyngeal infection with group A streptococci is another classic example of a postinfectious autoimmune disease. The association of group A streptococci with rheumatic fever is strong, since outbreaks of rheumatic fever closely follow epidemics of streptococcal sore throats and because adequate treatment of documented streptococcal pharyngitis markedly reduces the incidence of subsequent rheumatic fever. In addition, recurrence of the disease can be prevented by antimicrobial prophylaxis. Due to widespread use of antibiotics, the disease has become rare in the United States, but it is still common in developing countries (Gibofsky and Zabriskie, 1995; Stollerman, 1997).

Typically, after an acute streptococcal pharyngitis there is a latent period of 2 to 3 weeks, which is followed by an acute febrile illness that can involve the heart, joints, and/or CNS. Involvement of the heart valves is the most serious aspect of the disease and can result in severe functional impairment. Apparently due to differences between streptococcal strains that colonize mucous membranes and the skin, rheumatic fever follows only streptococcal pharyngitis, not streptococcal skin infections. Streptococci can also trigger a postinfectious glomerulonephritis in which immune complexes are deposited in the kidneys. It has been suggested that different strains of streptococci are responsible for these different clinical outcomes (Gibofsky and Zabriskie, 1995; Stollerman, 1997).

The streptococcal M protein is thought to play a role in the pathogenesis of rheumatic fever. M protein has an extended, α-helical structure and has significant sequence homology to human proteins of similar structure, such as the myosin heavy chain, tropomyosin, laminin, and keratin. Antibody cross-reactivity between M protein and cardiac myosin has been most extensively examined, but cross-reactivity with the other structurally related proteins may also be relevant. Human and murine antibodies that are specific for streptococcal M protein cross-react with cardiac myosin. Murine monoclonal antibodies generated by immunization with M protein were found to bind to myosin, and the major epitope was localized to the segment of the M protein from residues 184 to 197. Myosin-specific antibodies have also been affinity purified from sera of patients with rheumatic fever. These antibodies cross-react with streptococcal M protein; their binding to myosin is partially inhibited by the streptococcal M protein peptide from residues 184 to 197 (Cunningham et al., 1989; Dell et al., 1991).

As in GBS, little is known about the specificity of T cells to streptococcal antigens in rheumatic fever and there is no good animal model for the disease at present. Despite these gaps in our mechanistic understanding, rheumatic fever is a relevant example of a postinfectious autoimmune disease. Particularly compelling are the epidemiological association of the pathogen with the disease, the isolation of the pathogen from patients with rheumatic fever, and the fact that this postinfectious syndrome can be prevented by early use of antibiotics (Gibofsky and Zabriskie, 1995; Stollerman, 1997).

Acute and Chronic Inflammatory Diseases Induced by Bacterial Infection

Two rheumatological diseases, Lyme arthritis and reactive arthritis, have been the subjects of intensive investigation because of a strong association with defined bacterial agents. Susceptibility is associated with particular alleles of MHC class I and class II genes, respectively, indicating that antigen presentation to T cells is important in the pathogenesis of these diseases. Two major hypotheses have been proposed: (i) disease is mediated by T cells that respond to persisting bacterial antigens, and (ii) bacterial infection activates T cells that recognize joint-specific self-antigens.

CD4$^+$ T cells in the pathogenesis of Lyme arthritis

Lyme disease is caused by the spirochete *Borrelia burgdorferi* and is the most common tick-borne disease in the United States. The disease occurs worldwide, with most cases being found in temperate regions. The earliest manifestation is an erythema migrans, which appears at the site of the deer tick bite. In some untreated individuals, the spirochete disseminates hematogenously to multiple sites. Symptoms of hematogenous dissemination include secondary skin lesions, mild hepatitis, cardiac disease, and neurological abnormalities. Arthritis and neurological disease dominate the later phases of the illness (Evans, 1999).

In the United States, arthritis is the dominant feature of late Lyme disease, being reported in ~70% of untreated individuals. In adults, symptoms range from intermittent to chronic arthritis, primarily in large joints. In the majority of patients, the arthritis can be successfully treated with antibiotics. However, ~10% of patients develop a treatment-resistant chronic arthritis that lasts for months or even years (Carlson et al., 1999; Chen et al., 1999; Evans, 1999; Steere et al., 1990).

The development of treatment-resistant arthritis could be due to persistent bacteria or bacterial antigens or could be due to the development of autoimmunity. Patients with persistent arthritis have negative findings for *B. burgdorferi* on PCR testing of joint fluid after >2 months of oral antibiotic therapy. Symptoms therefore persist after the apparent eradication of live spirochetes from joints by antibiotic therapy (Carlson et al., 1999).

Susceptibility to the treatment-resistant form of Lyme arthritis is associated with particular alleles of MHC class II genes, suggesting that CD4$^+$ T cells play a critical role in the pathogenesis. An increased frequency of HLA-DR4 (DRB1*0401) and HLA-DR1 (DRB1*0101 and DRB1*0102) is found in patients who have had arthritis for 1 to 4 years (Steere et al., 1990). Interestingly, the same MHC class II alleles are associated with susceptibility to rheumatoid arthritis, a common inflammatory joint disease that is not triggered by *B. burgdorferi* infection.

The severity and duration of Lyme arthritis correlate with the IgG antibody response to the outer surface proteins A and B (OspA and OspB) of *B. burgdorferi*. These findings also support the hypothesis that CD4$^+$ T cells are involved in the pathogenesis. A direct analysis of the T-cell response to OspA demonstrated that treatment-resistant patients had an increased responsiveness to five different OspA peptides, compared to patients who responded to treatment with antibiotics. Increased T-cell responses were observed in blood and synovial fluid, indicating that both systemic and local immune responses to the bacteria differ between the two groups (Chen et al., 1999).

This information was used to identify a candidate autoantigen that is recognized by *B. burgdorferi*-specific CD4$^+$ T cells. The immunodominant OspA epitope that is presented by HLA-DR4 was determined by immunization of HLA-DR4 transgenic mice. A search of protein sequence databases with this OspA peptide (residues 164 to 183) showed that it had significant homology to human LFA-1. When 12 patients with treatment-resistant Lyme arthritis were tested, 6 had a strong T-cell response to this OspA peptide. T cells from four of these patients showed strong cross-reactivity with LFA-1. LFA-1 is not a joint-specific antigen, but the chronic inflammatory process results in the recruitment of large numbers of lymphocytes, which express LFA-1 (Gross et al., 1998).

In a separate study, molecular mimicry of OspA was examined in HLA-DR4 transgenic mice. A large number of T-cell hybridomas ($n = 118$) were generated from OspA-primed mice, allowing the identification of OspA (residues 164 to 175 and 235 to 246) as immunodominant T-cell epitopes. A set of single-amino-acid analog peptides was used to determine the T-cell recognition motif, as described above for human MBP-specific T-cell clones. Using this strategy, a total of 28 self-peptides were identified that stimulated T cells specific for OspA residues 164 to 175 or OspA residues 235 to 246 (Maier et al., 2000). These results suggest that additional cross-reactive self-peptides remain to be identified for human OspA-specific T cells.

CD8$^+$ T cells in the pathogenesis of reactive arthritis

Reactive arthritis follows genitourinary or enteric infection with certain intracellular bacteria, including *Chlamydia*, *Salmonella*, *Shigella*, and *Yersinia* species. The association of these bacteria with reactive arthritis is well established, based on isolation of these bacteria and analysis of antibody responses. These bacteria enter the body through mucosal surfaces and are capable of invading living cells. *Yersinia enterocolitica* is taken up by M cells in Peyer's patches through an interaction between the bacterial invasin and host β_1-integrins. *Yersinia* can use phagocytes to translocate through endothelial monolayers, allowing it to enter the bloodstream and reach synovial tissue. In nonprofessional antigen-presenting cells, *Yersinia* replicates intracellularly (Märker-Hermann and Höhler, 1998).

In reactive arthritis and ankylosing spondylitis, the axial skeleton is primarily affected. Ankylosing spondylitis is a chronic disease and can follow reactive arthritis. Initial symptoms are lower back pain and morning stiffness, which progress, often with exacerbations and remissions, over the years to a fixed rigidity of the spine caused by bony fusion of the vertebral and paravertebral joints. Ankylosing spondylitis can also show extraskeletal manifestations, such as acute anterior uveitis, aortic valve disease, and enteric mucosal inflammatory lesions. In most cases, ankylosing spondylitis is not associated with any other disorders, but secondary ankylosing spondylitis sometimes occurs in association with reactive arthritis, psoriasis, ulcerative colitis, or Crohn's disease (López-Larrea et al., 1998).

Reactive arthritis and ankylosing spondylitis have a striking association with the MHC class I allele HLA-B27. HLA-B27 is found in ~80% of patients with reactive arthritis, >95% of patients with primary ankylosing spondylitis, and ~9% of the general population. In Caucasian populations, ankylosing spondylitis is a relatively common disease, with a prevalence ranging from 0.1 to 0.8% (López-Larrea et al., 1998; Märker-Hermann and Höhler, 1998).

Several lines of evidence indicate that bacteria and/or bacterial antigens persist in patients with reactive arthritis. Patients with reactive arthritis have persisting antibody responses against the triggering microorganisms, in particular IgA responses. Mononuclear phagocytes that carry antigens of arthritogenic microorganisms (LPS, heat shock proteins) can enter the peripheral circulation. It is thought that monocytes harboring such bacteria are the major source of microbial antigens that reach the synovium. In patients with *Yersinia*-induced arthritis, LPS, the 60-kDa heat shock protein, and the urease β subunit have been detected in the joints by immunohistochemistry or immunoblotting. However, DNA from *Yersinia* has not been detected by PCR in joints. In contrast, chlamydial DNA and RNA are often detectable in the synovial membrane or synovial fluid (Märker-Hermann and Höhler, 1998).

The bacteria associated with reactive arthritis are all invasive, and their antigens can therefore be presented by the MHC class I pathway. HLA-B27-specific T-cell responses have been demonstrated in the synovial fluid from patients with reactive arthritis, and HLA-B27-restricted peptide epitopes have been identified for the 60-kDa heat shock protein and the urease β subunit of *Yersinia*. Integrin $\alpha_4\beta_7$, which is known to be involved in the specific homing of T cells to the intestinal lamina propria and to the Peyer's patches, is also expressed by cells from synovial tissue (Hermann et al., 1993; Ugrinovic et al., 1997; Märker-Hermann and Höhler, 1998).

An interesting animal model of reactive arthritis has been generated by overexpression of HLA-B27. Such HLA-B27 transgenic mice and rats develop a chronic inflammatory arthritis. Interestingly, the development of disease is dependent on the intestinal flora, since no arthritis is observed in animals kept under germ-free housing conditions. Therefore, disease development in this model may also be dependent on intestinal infection by certain bacteria (Hammer et al., 1990; Taurog et al., 1994).

However, the hypothesis that reactive arthritis is due to a T-cell response to persistent bacterial antigens in the joint does not readily explain the strong association of disease susceptibility with HLA-B27. If the disease is mediated solely by presentation of bacterial peptides by this MHC class I antigen, other MHC class I molecules should be able to perform a similar function. A major question in the field is therefore whether an autoimmune response to synovial antigens plays an important role in the disease process. Several alternative hypotheses have been proposed, which have been the subjects of excellent reviews (López-Larrea et al., 1998; Märker-Hermann and Höhler, 1998).

Hepatitis C Virus-Induced Lymphoproliferative Disease

Mixed cryoglobulinemia (MC) is a systemic autoimmune disease caused by vascular deposition of circulating immune complexes and complement. The name is based on the in vitro observation that immune complexes precipitate from the serum when it is cooled below 37°C; these precipitates redissolve when the sample is brought back to 37°C. The fact that a chronic hepatitis is observed in almost two-thirds of the patients led to the identification of hepatitis C virus as a causative agent in 70 to 100% of patients with MC (Ferri and Zignego, 2000).

Hepatitis C virus infects both hepatocytes and B cells, due to binding of the E2 envelope protein to CD81 on the surface of hepatocytes and B cells (Pileri et al., 1998). Infection of B cells by hepatitis C virus results in a lymphoproliferative disease with clonal expansion of B cells. Hepatitis C virus RNA is markedly more concentrated in the cryoprecipitate than in the supernatant, suggesting a direct involvement of hepatitis C virus antigens in the immune-complex-mediated vasculitis. Patients with MC also develop autoantibodies, due to B-cell activation by the virus. Vascular deposition of these circulating immune complexes causes a vasculitis of small to medium-sized blood vessels and a nonerosive arthritis. Glomerulonephritis and alveolitis result from deposition of immune complexes on basement membranes in the kidneys and the lungs. These data demonstrate how a virus causes a systemic autoimmune disease, due to virus-induced B-cell expansion and formation of circulating immune complexes (Ferri and Zignego, 2000).

These clinical examples illustrate the relationship between infectious agents and the development of autoimmune diseases. For many of these diseases, further work must be done on the mechanisms, based on the principles outlined at the beginning of this chapter. Also, there are a number of common autoimmune diseases for which little is known about a role of infectious triggers. A better understanding of the relationship between infection and autoimmunity may allow the prevention of autoimmune sequelae in at least some of these conditions. The example of rheumatic fever caused by group A streptococci demonstrates that early intervention can prevent the development of postinfectious autoimmunity.

REFERENCES

Ang, C. W., N. Yuki, B. C. Jacobs, M. Koga, P. A. Van Doorn, P. I. Schmitz, and F. G. Van Der Meche. 1999. Rapidly progressive, predominantly motor Guillain-Barré syndrome with anti-GalNAc-GD1a antibodies. *Neurology* 53:2122–2127.

Bachmaier, K., N. Neu, L. M. de la Maza, S. Pal, A. Hessel, and J. M. Penninger. 1999. Chlamydia infections and heart disease linked through antigenic mimicry. *Science* 283:1335–1339.

Blaser, M. J. 1997. Epidemiologic and clinical features of *Campylobacter jejuni* infections. *J. Infect. Dis.* 176(Suppl. 2):S103–S105.

Brocke, S., A. Gaur, C. Piercy, A. Gautam, K. Gijbels, C. G. Fathman, and L. Steinman. 1993. Induction of relapsing paralysis in experimental autoimmune encephalomyelitis by bacterial superantigen. *Nature* 365:642–644.

Carlson, D., J. Hernandez, B. J. Bloom, J. Coburn, J. M. Aversa, and A. C. Steere. 1999. Lack of *Borrelia burgdorferi* DNA in synovial samples from patients with antibiotic treatment-resistant Lyme arthritis. *Arthritis Rheum.* 42:2705–2709.

Carpo, M., R. Pedotti, S. Allaria, F. Lolli, S. Mata, G. Cavaletti, A. Protti, S. Pomati, G. Scarlato, and E. Nobile-Orazio. 1999. Clinical presentation and outcome of Guillain-Barré and related syndromes in relation to anti-ganglioside antibodies. *J. Neurol. Sci.* 168:78–84.

Chen, J., J. A. Field, L. Glickstein, P. J. Molloy, B. T. Huber, and A. C. Steere. 1999. Association of antibiotic treatment-resistant Lyme arthritis with T cell responses to dominant epitopes of outer surface protein A of *Borrelia burgdorferi*. *Arthritis Rheum.* 42:1813–1822.

Cole, B. C., and M. M. Griffiths. 1993. Triggering and exacerbation of autoimmune arthritis by the *Mycoplasma arthritidis* superantigen MAM. *Arthritis Rheum.* 36:994–1002.

Cunningham, M. W., J. M. McCormack, P. G. Fenderson, M. K. Ho, E. H. Beachey, and J. B. Dale. 1989. Human and murine antibodies cross-reactive with streptococcal M protein and myosin recognize the sequence GLN-LYS-SER-LYS-GLN in M protein. *J. Immunol.* 143:2677–2683.

Dell, A., S. M. Antone, C. J. Gauntt, C. A. Crossley, W. A. Clark, and M. W. Cunningham. 1991. Autoimmune determinants of rheumatic carditis: localization of epitopes in human cardiac myosin. *Eur. Heart J.* 12(Suppl. D):158–162.

Evans, J. 1999. Lyme disease. *Curr. Opin. Rheumatol.* 11:281–288.

Ferri, C., and A. L. Zignego. 2000. Relation between infection and autoimmunity in mixed cryoglobulinemia. *Curr. Opin. Rheumatol.* 12:53–60.

Fujinami, R. S., and M. B. Oldstone. 1985. Amino acid homology between the encephalitogenic site of myelin basic protein and virus: mechanism for autoimmunity. *Science* 230:1043–1045.

Garboczi, D. N., P. Ghosh, U. Utz, Q. R. Fan, W. E. Biddison, and D. C. Wiley. 1996. Structure of the complex between human T-cell receptor, viral peptide and HLA-A2. *Nature* 384:134–141.

Garcia, K. C., M. Degano, R. L. Stanfield, A. Brunmark, M. R. Jackson, P. A. Peterson, L. Teyton, and I. A. Wilson. 1996. An αβ T cell receptor structure at 2.5 Å and its orientation in the TCR-MHC complex. *Science* 274:209–219.

Gibofsky, A., and J. B. Zabriskie. 1995. Rheumatic fever and poststreptococcal reactive arthritis. *Curr. Opin. Rheumatol.* 7:299–305.

Goodyear, C. S., G. M. O'Hanlon, J. J. Plomp, E. R. Wagner, I. Morrison, J. Veitch, L. Cochrane, R. W. Bullens, P. C. Molenaar, J. Conner, and H. J. Willison. 1999. Monoclonal antibodies raised against Guillain-Barré syndrome-associated *Campylobacter jejuni* lipopolysaccharides react with neuronal gangliosides and paralyze muscle-nerve preparations. *J. Clin. Investig.* 104:697–708.

Gross, D. M., T. Forsthuber, M. Tary-Lehmann, C. Etling, K. Ito, Z. A. Nagy, J. A. Field, A. C. Steere, and B. T. Huber. 1998. Identification of LFA-1 as a candidate autoantigen in treatment-resistant Lyme arthritis. *Science* 281:703–706.

Hammer, R. E., S. D. Maika, J. A. Richardson, J. P. Tang, and J. D. Taurog. 1990. Spontaneous inflammatory disease in transgenic rats expressing HLA-B27 and human β_2m: an animal model of HLA-B27-associated human disorders. *Cell* 63:1099–1112.

Hausmann, S., M. Martin, L. Gauthier, and K. W. Wucherpfennig. 1999. Structural features of autoreactive TCR that determine the degree of degeneracy in peptide recognition. *J. Immunol.* 162:338–344.

Hemmer, B., B. T. Fleckenstein, M. Vergelli, G. Jung, H. McFarland, R. Martin, and K. H. Wiesmüller. 1997. Identification of high potency microbial and self ligands for a human autoreactive class II-restricted T cell clone. *J. Exp. Med.* 185:1651–1659.

Hermann, E., D. T. Yu, K. H. Meyer zum Büschenfelde, and B. Fleischer. 1993. HLA-B27-restricted CD8 T cells derived from synovial fluids of patients with reactive arthritis and ankylosing spondylitis. *Lancet* 342:646–650.

Hughes, R. A., and J. H. Rees. 1997. Clinical and epidemiologic features of Guillain-Barré syndrome. *J. Infect. Dis.* 176(Suppl. 2):S92–S98.

Jacobs, B. C., P. H. Rothbarth, F. G. van der Meche, P. Herbrink, P. I. Schmitz, M. A. de Klerk, and P. A. van Doorn. 1998. The spectrum of antecedent infections in Guillain-Barré syndrome: a case-control study. *Neurology* 51:1110–1115.

Lehmann, P. V., T. Forsthuber, A. Miller, and E. E. Sercarz. 1992. Spreading of T-cell autoimmunity to cryptic determinants of an autoantigen. *Nature* 358:155–157.

López-Larrea, C., S. González, and J. Martínez-Borra. 1998. The role of HLA-B27 polymorphism and molecular mimicry in spondylarthropathy. *Mol. Med. Today* 4:540–549.

Maier, B., M. Molinger, A. P. Cope, L. Fugger, J. Schneider-Mergener, G. Sonderstrup, T. Kamradt, and A. Kramer. 2000. Multiple cross-reactive self-ligands for *Borrelia burgdorferi*-specific HLA-DR4-restricted T cells. *Eur. J. Immunol.* 30:448–457.

Märker-Hermann, E., and T. Höhler. 1998. Pathogenesis of human leukocyte antigen B27-positive arthritis. Information from clinical materials. *Rheum. Dis. Clin. North Am.* 24:865–881.

McKhann, G. M., D. R. Cornblath, J. W. Griffin, T. W. Ho, C. Y. Li, Z. Jiang, H. S. Wu, G. Zhaori, Y. Liu, L. P. Jou, et al. 1993. Acute motor axonal neuropathy: a frequent cause of acute flaccid paralysis in China. *Ann. Neurol.* 33:333–342.

Miller, S. D., C. L. Vanderlugt, W. S. Begolka, W. Pao, R. L. Yauch, K. L. Neville, Y. Katz-Levy, A. Carrizosa, and B. S. Kim. 1997. Persistent infection with Theiler's virus leads to CNS autoimmunity via epitope spreading. *Nat. Med.* 3:1133–1136.

Moran, A. P. 1997. Structure and conserved characteristics of *Campylobacter jejuni* lipopolysaccharides. *J. Infect. Dis.* 176(Suppl. 2):S115–S121.

Nepom, G. T. 1993. MHC and autoimmune diseases. *Immunol. Ser.* **59**:143–164.

Pileri, P., Y. Uematsu, S. Campagnoli, G. Galli, F. Falugi, R. Petracca, A. J. Weiner, M. Houghton, D. Rosa, G. Grandi, and S. Abrignani. 1998. Binding of hepatitis C virus to CD81. *Science* **282**:938–941.

Porcelli, S. A., B. W. Segelke, M. Sugita, I. A. Wilson, and M. B. Brenner. 1998. The CD1 family of lipid antigen-presenting molecules. *Immunol. Today* **19**:362–368.

Rammensee, H. G., K. Falk, and O. Rötzschke. 1993. MHC molecules as peptide receptors. *Curr. Opin. Immunol.* **5**:35–44.

Rees, J. H., S. E. Soudain, N. A. Gregson, and R. A. Hughes. 1995. *Campylobacter jejuni* infection and Guillain-Barré syndrome. *N. Engl. J. Med.* **333**:1374–1379.

Saida, T., S. Kuroki, Q. Hao, M. Nishimura, M. Nukina, and H. Obayashi. 1997. *Campylobacter jejuni* isolates from Japanese patients with Guillain-Barré syndrome. *J. Infect. Dis.* **176**(Suppl. 2):S129–S134.

Scherer, M. T., L. Ignatowicz, G. M. Winslow, J. W. Kappler, and P. Marrack. 1993. Superantigens: bacterial and viral proteins that manipulate the immune system. *Annu. Rev. Cell Biol.* **9**:101–128.

Smith, K. J., J. Pyrdol, L. Gauthier, D. C. Wiley, and K. W. Wucherpfennig. 1998. Crystal structure of HLA-DR2 (DRA*0101, DRB1*1501) complexed with a peptide from human myelin basic protein. *J. Exp. Med.* **188**:1511–1520.

Soos, J. M., J. Schiffenbauer, and H. M. Johnson. 1993. Treatment of PL/J mice with the superantigen, staphylococcal enterotoxin B, prevents development of experimental allergic encephalomyelitis. *J. Neuroimmunol.* **43**:39–43.

Steere, A. C., E. Dwyer, and R. Winchester. 1990. Association of chronic Lyme arthritis with HLA-DR4 and HLA-DR2 alleles. *N. Engl. J. Med.* **323**:219–223.

Steinhoff, U., V. Brinkmann, U. Klemm, P. Aichele, P. Seiler, U. Brandt, P. W. Bland, I. Prinz, U. Zugel, and S. H. Kaufmann. 1999. Autoimmune intestinal pathology induced by hsp60-specific CD8 T cells. *Immunity* **11**:349–358.

Stollerman, G. H. 1997. Rheumatic fever. *Lancet* **349**:935–942.

Taurog, J. D., J. A. Richardson, J. T. Croft, W. A. Simmons, M. Zhou, J. L. Fernandez-Sueiro, E. Balish, and R. E. Hammer. 1994. The germfree state prevents development of gut and joint inflammatory disease in HLA-B27 transgenic rats. *J. Exp. Med.* **180**:2359–2364.

Ugrinovic, S., A. Mertz, P. Wu, J. Braun, and J. Sieper. 1997. A single nonamer from the *Yersinia* 60-kDa heat shock protein is the target of HLA-B27-restricted CTL response in *Yersinia*-induced reactive arthritis. *J. Immunol.* **159**:5715–5723.

Visser, L. H., F. G. van der Meche, J. Meulstee, P. P. Rothbarth, B. C. Jacobs, P. I. Schmitz, and P. A. van Doorn. 1996. Cytomegalovirus infection and Guillain-Barré syndrome: the clinical, electrophysiologic, and prognostic features. *Neurology* **47**:668–673.

Vyse, T. J., and J. A. Todd. 1996. Genetic analysis of autoimmune disease. *Cell* **85**:311–318.

Wong, F. S., J. Karttunen, C. Dumont, L. Wen, I. Visintin, I. M. Pilip, N. Shastri, E. G. Pamer, and C. A. Janeway, Jr. 1999. Identification of an MHC class I-restricted autoantigen in type 1 diabetes by screening an organ-specific cDNA library. *Nat. Med.* **5**:1026–1031.

Wucherpfennig, K. W., A. Sette, S. Southwood, C. Oseroff, M. Matsui, J. L. Strominger, and D. A. Hafler. 1994. Structural requirements for binding of an immunodominant myelin basic protein peptide to DR2 isotypes and for its recognition by human T cell clones. *J. Exp. Med.* **179**:279–290.

Wucherpfennig, K. W., and J. L. Strominger. 1995a. Selective binding of self peptides to disease-associated major histocompatibility complex (MHC) molecules: a mechanism for MHC-linked susceptibility to human autoimmune diseases. *J. Exp. Med.* **181**:1597–1601.

Wucherpfennig, K. W., and J. L. Strominger. 1995b. Molecular mimicry in T cell-mediated autoimmunity: viral peptides activate human T cell clones specific for myelin basic protein. *Cell* **80**:695–705.

Zamvil, S. S., and L. Steinman. 1990. The T lymphocyte in experimental allergic encephalomyelitis. *Annu. Rev. Immunol.* **8**:579–621.

Zhao, Z. S., F. Granucci, L. Yeh, P. A. Schaffer, and H. Cantor. 1998. Molecular mimicry by herpes simplex virus-type 1: autoimmune disease after viral infection. *Science* **279**:1344–1347.

Immunology of Infectious Diseases
Edited by S. H. E. Kaufmann, A. Sher, and R. Ahmed
© 2002 ASM Press, Washington, D.C.

Chapter 20

Pathology and Pathogenesis of Bacterial Infections

STEFFEN STENGER AND ROBERT MODLIN

Humoral and cellular immune reactions play critical roles in host defense against infectious agents. The immune response is generally considered to provide protection against infection. However, many clinical conditions are now known to be caused by an inappropriate response of the immune system. In its attempt to protect the host from the microorganism, the immune response can cause local tissue destruction as well as life-threatening systemic reactions. The armamentarium of the host immune system includes a large repertoire of B-cell receptors and T-cell receptors with the ability to recognize a broad spectrum of foreign invaders. Antibodies can affect microbial invaders that remain in the extracellular compartment or can neutralize their toxic products in the bloodstream. Many microorganisms have adapted to survive intracellularly. Successful elimination of these pathogens requires the activation of T-cell-mediated immunity. In this case, protection may require sacrifice of the infected cell. Immunity to infections, therefore, often includes immunopathological features, since the mechanism which is necessary to clear the infectious agent may require the destruction of the infected host cells. Any immune response to microorganisms therefore requires a finely tuned balance between the basic necessity to eliminate the pathogen and the threat of causing harm to the host. This balance may shift depending on the extent and duration of infection and the damaging effects of the pathogen. Thus, immune mechanisms represent a double-edged sword combating the exogenous enemies with one edge and causing damage in the host with the other edge. To appreciate the concept of immunological mechanisms as pathological processes, the paradigm of the immune system as a beneficial event has to be reconsidered and will be the focus of this chapter. In many im-

munopathological reactions, the initiating agent may no longer be detected but may persist in small numbers. The hallmark of such processes is that they become self-perpetuating by the initiation of an immunological cascade, which continues to mediate tissue damage way beyond the original insult. Immunopathology in this context is thus very closely linked to the four patterns of tissue injury (hypersensitivity reactions). In this chapter, we will provide a classification of relevant immunopathological reactions depending on the underlying mechanisms leading to tissue damage. Because the alterations in different organ systems caused by the same process have pathologic similarities, the lesions caused by allergic reactions are best classified by the particular type of immunopathological effector mechanism involved. The most widespread classification was put forward by Coombs and Gell (1963), who defined four different types of hypersensitivity reactions which tend to follow known clinical disease patterns. We will adapt this scheme in our attempt to classify the various immunopathological reactions of the immune system.

ANAPHYLACTIC REACTIONS

Anaphylactic reactions depend on the reactions of antigens with immunoglobulin E (IgE) antibodies attached to mast cells and basophilic neutrophils. This results in a rapidly developing immunological response, which occurs in minutes; longstanding changes such as tissue destruction are uncommon. The release of mediators such as histamine, leukotrienes, and heparin from mast cells accounts for the anaphylactic reactions to horse serum or to penicillin

Steffen Stenger • Institut für Klinische Mikrobiologie, Immunologie und Hygiene, Friedrich-Alexander Universität Erlangen-Nürnberg, D-91054 Erlangen, Germany. **Robert Modlin** • Division of Dermatology and Department of Microbiology and Immunology, UCLA School of Medicine, Los Angeles, CA 90095.

but is usually not important in the immunopathology of bacterial infections.

CYTOLYTIC REACTIONS

Cytolytic reactions are triggered by the interaction of antibodies with antigen on the surface of a tissue cell. The Fc part of the antibody can then be recognized by phagocytes (killer cells) bearing an Fc receptor. This results in lysis of the antibody-labeled cell carrying the microbial antigen. This form of cytolysis is referred to as antibody-dependent cellular cytotoxicity and needs to be distinguished from T-cell mediated cytotoxicity, in which antibodies are not involved. Fc receptors of phagocytes can also interact with antibodies on the surface of a microorganism. This kind of opsonization leads to the destruction of the microorganism and therefore constitutes an important part of antimicrobial defenses, especially against extracellular pathogens. Lysis of infected cells by this mechanism will not only contribute to the elimination of pathogens but also result in tissue damage. One example of host damage mediated by the action of antibody-dependent cellular cytotoxicity is the lysis of erythrocytes by antibodies induced in patients infected with the bacterium *Mycoplasma pneumoniae* (Feizi, 1967) or several viruses (cytomegalovirus and Epstein-Barr virus) (Horwitz et al., 1977). The majority of these naturally occurring antibodies are directed against carbohydrate structures of group 0 erythrocytes. They are referred to as cold agglutinins since optimal binding occurs at 4°C. Cold agglutinins are almost always IgM class and are transient. Receptors on host cells to which the mycoplasmas adhere are sialo-oligosaccharide sequences, which contain sequences which are similar to the Ii antigen of red blood cells (Loomes et al., 1984). It seems likely that the selective production of high-titer anti-I (i.e., anti-receptor antibodies) following *M. pneumoniae* infection is related to these interactions. Possibly the lipid-rich mycoplasma serves as an adjuvant, overcoming tolerance to self antigen. Clinically, lysis of red blood cells mediated by the action of cold agglutinins causes symptoms dominated by cyanosis with impaired circulation at the extremities on exposure to the cold. In severe cases, lysis of erythrocytes results in hemolytic anemia. There is no evidence for a protective effect of cold agglutinins in host defense against microorganisms.

IMMUNE COMPLEX REACTIONS

General Immunopathology

The combination of antibody and antigen is an important event, initiating inflammatory phenomena that are inevitably involved in host defense against the plethora of microbial pathogens. Complexes are formed between circulating antigen and specific antibody, especially of the IgG class. The subsequent inflammatory response involving the activation of the complement cascade and the recruitment of antibacterial effector cells is crucial for the resolution of infection. To prevent harmful accumulation of immune complexes, the immune system has evolved mechanisms to warrant their clearance from the circulation. One major mechanism involves the fixation of complement to immune complexes. Complement fixation will intervene in the processing of immune complexes in two ways. First, the binding of C4 and C3 to the antigen-antibody network alters the size of the immune complex, giving rise to a large number of small complexes as opposed to a small number of large ones. The latter may precipitate locally and cause Arthus reactions (see below) or immune complex disease. Thus, complement helps to solubilize immune complexes, a mechanism which is referred to as the detergent-like effect. Second, the presence of C4b and C3b in the immune complex facilitates transport predominantly via complement receptor 1 (CR1) on red blood cells in the circulation. Under physiological conditions, erythrocyte-bound immune complexes are sequestered in the liver, where antigenic material can be removed by reticulohistiocytic cells. If adequate complement fixation on these complexes fails, they can be taken up by endothelial cells and sequestered at peripheral sites, giving rise to further inflammation and immune complex formation (Cooper, 1999).

Despite the presence of mechanisms to prevent the accumulation of immune complexes, they are frequently the major pathophysiological correlates of immunopathological phenomena. When the antigen-antibody reaction takes place in the extravascular compartment, inflammation and edema occur, with infiltration of polymorphonuclear leukocytes. If soluble antigen is injected intradermally into an individual with large amounts of circulating IgG antibody, the antigen-antibody reaction takes place in the walls of skin blood vessels and causes an inflammatory response. The complement cascade is activated, causing local infiltration by neutrophils. The extravasating neutrophils degenerate, and their lysosomal enzymes cause extensive vascular damage. Experimentally this is known as the Arthus reaction, which is a necrotizing vasculitis in the skin, induced by local injection of antigen in a sensitized animal (Claudy, 1998). Immune complex vasculitis in the skin can occur in a number of clinical conditions, such as serum sickness, autoimmune diseases (systemic lupus erythematosus, rheumatoid arthritis), drug reactions, and infections. Most diseases of this type that affect the skin result from complex deposition in vessel walls of the dermis and subcutaneous fat, although some (notably erythema nodosum leprosum) are caused by extra-vascular complex formation. Circulating immune complexes are believed to localize at a specific vessel site because of the action of vasoactive amines, which alter vascular permeability; endothelial cell surface receptors are also important, and in some diseases clearing of complexes by the mononuclear phagocyte system may be defective (Claudy, 1998). Allergic vasculitis is a common condition, characterized clinically by the development of a purpuric rash over the lower limbs, buttocks, and forearms, which may lead to ulceration. The joints and kidneys may also be involved, and kidney involvement may lead to renal failure. Histological examination shows a prominent swelling, intense polymorphonuclear and lymphocyte infiltration, and disintegration of the polymorphonuclear cells (leukcytoclasis). The vessels may be thrombosed, with fibrinoid change and epidermal necrosis.

Immune Complex-Mediated Diseases

We will now outline specific clinical entities in which immune complexes are the major mediators of tissue damage. The focus is on diseases in which the immunopathological cascade is known or suspected to be initiated by bacterial or fungal antigens. Due to the complexity of the interactions involved in the development of these diseases, it cannot be excluded that additional independent mechanisms are also involved in the pathophysiology.

Poststreptococcal glomerulonephritis

The occurrence of acute glomerulonephritis in humans is associated with strains of group A beta-hemolytic streptococci. Such streptococcal strains have been termed nephritogenic. The acute infection usually presents as sore throat and fever. There is a characteristic latent period following the onset of infection, during which no significant renal symptoms are observed. Acute poststreptococcal glomerulonephritis is characterized by the onset of proteinuria and hematuria. The onset of clinical symptoms corresponds in time to the appearance of host antibodies to streptococcal antigens. Although several immune mechanisms have been invoked to explain the pathogenesis of acute glomerulonephritis, the findings are most consistent with an immune complex-mediated inflammatory reaction (Zabriskie, 1971). Immunofluorescence examination of affected kidneys reveals a morphologic alteration typical of immune complex glomerulonephritis. Complement, immunoglobulins, and streptococcal antigens are found in the glomeruli. One hypothesis about the pathogenesis suggests that streptococcal M protein may have a high affinity to the glomerulus (Nordstrand et al., 1999). If an appropriate antigen-antibody complex between streptococcal M protein and host antibody could be produced, this complex would be selectively bound to the glomerulus. This could be followed by the binding of complement and the attraction of polymorphonuclear leukocytes, leading to glomerular infiltration.

Henoch-Schönlein purpura

Henoch-Schönlein purpura is an allergic vasculitis with an infectious basis. It is an important example of this type of vasculitis, and it affects both children and adults. The immune complexes which are deposited in affected tissue are dominated by IgA antibodies (Levinsky and Barratt, 1979; C. C. Tsai, J. Giangiacomo, and J. Zuckner, Letter, *Lancet* i: 342–343, 1975). Henoch-Schönlein purpura usually follows a viral infection or a respiratory infection with *Streptococcus pyogenes*. The purpura is accompanied by proteinuria and hematuria, gastrointestinal hemorrhage, and arthralgia. The course of allergic vasculitis is variable. It may last for 2 to 3 weeks or several years (Magro and Crawson, 1999).

Erythema nodosum

Erythema nodosum is a common condition, characterized clinically by tender, erythematous nodules on the shin and, less commonly, on the thighs and forearms. The lesions tend to resolve after 6 weeks. Histological examination shows evidence of vasculitis, but unlike in allergic vasculitis, the vessels involved are in the subcutaneous fat and hence the clinical picture is different. The most common infectious causes are *Streptococcus, Mycobacterium* (the species causing tuberculosis and leprosy), *Mycoplasma, Chlamydia,* and bacteria that cause infectious gastroenteritis (*Yersinia* and *Campylobacter*) (Cribier et al., 1998).

Exogenic allergic alveolitis

When certain antigens are inhaled by sensitized individuals and reach the terminal bronchioli of the lungs, an antigen-antibody reaction takes place locally and results in the formation of immune complexes (Mygind et al., 1996). More recent studies also indicate that T cells participate in this type of hypersensitivity alveolitis (Ando et al., 1999). The pathological reaction is mixed, but inflammation of the alveolar wall, usually consisting of plasma cells, lymphoid cells, and epithelioid cell granulomas, is the primary feature. The significance of a type III-like reaction in the pathogenesis of allergic alveolitis is supported by the pathological analysis of lung biopsy specimen, which reveals antigen, antibody, and complement deposition. The bronchial wall is thickened by cellular infiltration and fibrosis, while the parenchyma often shows consolidation due to granulomas consisting of eosinophils and mononuclear cells. Such exposures, by inhalation of the conidia and mycelia of various antigens originating from moldy grain, result 4 to 8 h later in extrinsic allergic alveolitis. Characteristic symptoms include wheezing and respiratory distress. Persistent inhalation of the specific antigen leads to chronic pathological changes with fibrosis and respiratory disease. A number of microorganisms cause allergic alveolitis, including bacteria and various molds. The first, and probably the most frequent antigen source, is *Micropolyspora faeni*. It was previously considered to be a fungus, but it has been accepted as a bacterium since it has no nuclear membrane. It thrives at 50 to 60°C, a temperature commonly reached during the decay of vegetable matter, at which it produces significant amounts of enzymes responsible for the decay process. *M. faeni* is abundant in hay and grain stored under damp conditions. It is a common cause of allergic alveolitis among farmers, so that this disease is known as farmer's lung. In this disease, farm workers who are repeatedly exposed to moldy hay develop respiratory disease resulting from immune complex formation. Besides the actinomycete *M. faeni*, antigens derived from *Thermoactinomyces vulgaris* also cause farmer's lung. A fungus parasitizing the bark of maple trees causes a similar clinical entity in workers in the United States employed in the extraction of maple syrup (maple bark stripper's disease). Other molds implicated in extrinsic allergic alveolitis are *Aspergillus fumigatus* and *Aspergillus clavatus* (malt worker's lung), *Sitophilus granarius* (wheat weevil disease), and *Penicillium* species (cheese washer's lung) (Sell, 1987).

A. fumigatus is unusual in its ability to cause a variety of additional airway diseases, each with its own distinct immunopathogenesis and clinical presentation (Sharma and Chwogule, 1998). These range from diseases causing direct damage by multiplication of the mold (growth in preformed pulmonary cavities [aspergilloma], invasive pneumonia, abscesses, and septicemia in immunocompromised patients) to allergic reactions against its antigens such as IgE-mediated allergic asthma in atopic subjects and allergic bronchopulmonary aspergillosis. The immune reaction in allergic pulmonary aspergillosis is referred to as type III-like, since a typical type III reaction with immune complex vasculitis does not occur. The formation of precipitating IgG antibodies, which form immune complexes with the antigen, is characteristic. This results in complement activation, which is largely responsible for the inflammation and tissue destruction. Immune complexes can also stimulate alveolar macrophages to produce proinflammatory cytokines (e.g., interleukin-1 and tumor necrosis factor [TNF]), chemokines (macrophage inflammatory protein 1), and a variety of enzymes (leukotriene B_4 and prostaglandins). These products, along with the influx of neutrophils, contribute to early alveolar damage following acute exposure to dust containing *Aspergillus* antigens.

CELL-MEDIATED IMMUNE REACTIONS

The expression of cell-mediated immunity induces inflammation due to the recruitment and activation of immune cells and can therefore pose a risk of immunopathological tissue damage. The cell-mediated response to various chronic microbial diseases such as mycobacterial infection, listeriosis, brucellosis, syphilis, actinomycosis, and histoplasmosis involves granulomas as characteristic pathological features. The hallmarks of a granulomatous reaction include mononuclear infiltration, degeneration of infected macrophages, and formation of giant cells, all of which are surrounded by a lymphocytic cuff. Tuberculosis is a prototypic disease in which the granuloma not only serves to contain the microbial invader but also marks the origin of immunopathological tissue damage. We will therefore discuss the immunopathology induced by cell-mediated immunity in the context of an infection with the intracellular pathogen *Mycobacterium tuberculosis*.

Immunopathology in Tuberculosis

Bacteria that are inhaled deeply into the lungs are phagocytosed by alveolar macrophages and either are immediately killed or survive to initiate an infection. If the alveolar macrophages are not sufficiently activated to eliminate the inhaled bacilli, caseous lesions may develop that grow locally or liquefy and introduce bacilli and their products into the bronchial tree. Successful elimination of virulent mycobacteria requires the activation of infected alveolar macrophages. This is accomplished by a cell-mediated reaction enabling macrophages to kill and digest the ingested bacilli. The cell-mediated immune response has two apparently contradictory functions, namely, to destroy macrophages unable to eliminate the bacteria and to activate infected macrophages to kill the microbial invader. This requires a finely tuned balance between the distinct effector mechanisms of lymphocytes, e.g., exerting cytolytic activity versus secreting immunoprotective cytokines such as gamma interferon (IFN-γ) (Rook and Bloom, 1994). Both the lysis of infected cells and the macrophage-activating immune responses can stop the growth of tubercle bacilli, because these bacilli do not multiply appreciably in nonliquefied caseous necrotic tissue. Inevitably, the destruction of nonactivated macrophages will result in tissue damage and, particularly in tuberculosis, will cause typical pathological changes, such as caseous necrosis and cavity formation (Dannenberg and Rook, 1994). Further progression of infection will attract circulating monocytes, lymphocytes, and neutrophils, none of which are equipped with antimycobacterial effector mechanisms to eliminate the bacteria very efficiently. Enhanced production of monocytes and their early release from bone marrow can be observed clinically. The battle observed at the cellular level, as the T cells both activate and destroy infected macrophages, is also occurring at a macroscopic level in tissues, as evidenced by granulomas. Granulomas present a typical T-cell-mediated delayed-type hypersensitivity reaction within parenchymal tissues. Granulomatous focal lesions, composed of macrophage-derived epithelioid giant cells and antigen-specific T cells, begin to form to wall off the pathogen and prevent its spread. Therefore, the pulmonary damage pathognomonic for tuberculosis appears to be almost entirely due to the tissue-damaging response. Granulomas are thought to afford the close T-cell–macrophage contact and cooperation necessary for an effective antimycobacterial defense (Fenton and Vermeulen, 1996; Schluger and Rom, 1998). On the other hand, granulomas displace and destroy adjacent tissue and may necrotize at the center, leading to cavity formation. Progressive infection is characterized by the enlargement and coalescence of granulomas. This results in relatively large areas of necrotic debris, each surrounded by a layer of epithelioid histiocytes and multinucleated giant cells. These granulomas, or tubercles, are surrounded by a cellular zone of fibroblasts, lymphocytes, and blood-derived monocytes. The acidic pH, in conjunction with the lack of essential nutrients, prevents the multiplication of mycobacteria, but a few organisms may

remain dormant and persist for decades (Rook and Stanford, 1996). This is illustrated by the clinical observation that immunosuppression (e.g., human immunodeficiency virus infection, cancer, malnutrition, advanced age) frequently results in a relapse of tuberculosis due to endogenous reactivation of dormant bacilli. Similarly, patients show a high relapse rate if chemotherapy is discontinued after 4 months, when the majority of bacilli have been killed. Generally, the process of granuloma formation is an effective means of containing pathogens and hence preventing their continued growth and dissemination (Rook and Stanford, 1996). However, the formation of cavities may facilitate the spread of the bacilli via the respiratory route to a new host.

The initial resistance to *M. tuberculosis* infection is directly proportional to the strength of the granulomatous response. Where the cell mediated immune response is inadequate, the host will continuously battle against the multiplying bacteria, but, concomitantly, lung tissue is destroyed, leading to both pulmonary damage and spread of the organisms via the lymphatics and the blood. Immunity against *M. tuberculosis* is therefore a long-term battle against a persistent organism, requiring a filigree balance between protective effector mechanisms and the loss of parenchymal tissue induced by chronic inflammation. In the course of a protective immune response, the beneficial effects of containing the bacterial growth should clearly outweigh the damage caused by the limited destruction of affected tissue.

Immunopathology of a Cytolytic T-Cell Response

There is ample evidence implicating CD8$^+$ T cells in immunity against intracellular pathogens, including viruses, bacteria, and parasites (Kaufmann, 1988; Stenger and Modlin, 1998). Gene-targeted mice with disrupted expression of key immunologic functions have provided convincing evidence for the role of CD8$^+$ cytolytic T cells in host defense. For example, β$_2$-microglobulin knockout mice generally fail to transport major histocompatibility complex class I or class I-like molecules to the cell surface and therefore cannot generate CD8$^+$ T cells, NK1.1 T cells, or CD1-restricted T cells. Infection of β$_2$-microglobulin knockout mice with *Trypanosoma cruzi* (Rottenberg et al., 1993), *Listeria monocytogenes* (Gazzinelli et al., 1991; Ladel et al., 1994), or *M. tuberculosis* (Flynn et al., 1992) results in decreased immunity to infection. These studies indicate a substantial role for CD8$^+$ T cells in complementing other components of the immune system to mount an efficient and long-lasting immune response to intracellular microbes. It should be pointed out, however, that a critical role for CD8$^+$ T cells does not hold for all intracellular pathogens (for example, *Leishmania major*) (Wang et al., 1993; Huber et al., 1998).

CD8$^+$ T cells may contribute to host resistance by at least four mechanisms: (i) release of IFN-γ, (ii) lysis of the target cell, (iii) induction of apoptosis of the target cells, and (iv) mediation of direct antimicrobial activity. We will briefly outline the immunoprotective and immunopathological features of these mechanisms, using tuberculosis as an example.

IFN-γ is clearly of paramount importance for the resolution of murine (Dalton et al., 1993; Cooper et al., 1993) and human (Newport et al., 1996; Jouanguy et al., 1996) tuberculosis. However, the paradigm holds that the major contribution of CD8$^+$ T cells to immunity against intracellular pathogens is their capacity to induce the lysis of infected host cells. Upon lysis of infected host cells, bacteria are released and can be taken up at low multiplicity by freshly activated macrophages, which then can effectively kill the pathogen (Kaufmann, 1988). On the other hand, there is in vitro evidence suggesting that cytotoxic T-lymphocyte (CTL)-mediated lysis of the target cells can result in release of the viable pathogen into the extracellular environment (Stenger et al., 1997). The bacteria could then reach lymphatic or blood vessels and spread to remote tissues, resulting in disseminated disease. In fact, studies of mice with defects in perforin or granzymes indicate that perforin-mediated lytic activity is not required for effective immunity during the initial stages of infection (Laochumroonvorapong et al., 1997; Cooper et al., 1997), suggesting that this mechanism is not beneficial for host defense against intracellular pathogens. Lysis of infected target cells by CTL could be a potential hazard for the host via an additional mechanism besides the release of the viable pathogen. Cell death could be accompanied by tissue destruction and inflammation aimed at clearing bacterial and cellular debris. In some cases, this will lead to functional impairment of the affected organ. Depending on the mode of cell death, the bystander effect on surrounding tissue may be more or less intense. Necrosis is a consequence of an acute and intense insult to the cell. This is followed by the influx of inflammatory cells. The attempt to clear necrotic tissue is accompanied by the secretion of cytokines and the recruitment of an inflammatory infiltrate. Inevitably, this process results in damage of the surrounding parenchymal tissue. The tissue-damaging effects of CTL might be restricted by a mechanism which has been described for cytokine production by antigen-specific T cells (Slifka and Whitton, 2000). Specifically, it was demonstrated that CD8$^+$ T cells exert their effector functions only while in direct contact with the target cell; termination of cell-to-cell contact is paralleled by termination of the cytokine production (Slifka et al., 1999). A similar scenario is conceivable for cytolytic CD8$^+$ cells, which can terminate their function after lysis of the target and thus avoid killing bystander cells while limiting the destruction of unaffected tissue.

A third mechanism by which CD8$^+$ CTL could contribute to an antimicrobial mechanism is by induction of target cell apoptosis. In contrast to necrosis, apoptosis is a deliberately induced process during which a cascade of specific enzymatic reactions results in programmed cell death. Despite causing cell death, apoptosis is usually not accompanied by an inflammatory reaction (Green and Ware, 1997). Instead, apoptotic bodies develop and are removed by cells of the reticuloendothelial system. Therefore, apoptosis is a physiological process to allow the maintenance of cellular homeostasis without causing tissue damage. It is not clear whether CTL-mediated lysis will cause apoptotic or necrotic cell death. Ongoing studies will shed light on this issue to clarify whether the lytic activity of T cells is more likely to be beneficial or harmful to the host.

Apoptosis can also be an immediate effect of the invasion of intracellular pathogens (Liles, 1997). In this case, activation of caspases is induced by the pathogen and occurs independently of the action of CTL. Several bacterial pathogens, including *M. tuberculosis*, *Salmonella enterica*, and *L. monocytogenes*, are capable of inducing apoptosis of their host cells. It remains to be established whether the host or the pathogen is the primary beneficiary of apoptosis. A recent study suggests that apoptosis of human monocytes induced by *M. tuberculosis* in the absence of T cells does not reduce the viability of the pathogen (Santucci et al., 2000).

A fourth mechanism by which CTL contribute to host defense involves their ability to directly kill microbial pathogens. Direct killing has been proposed as a CTL effector mechanism based on findings that CTL were able to directly mediate antimicrobial activity against parasites, fungi, and bacteria (Levitz et al., 1995). More recently, the human cytolytic granule protein granulysin, present in natural killer cells and CD8$^+$ CTL granules, has been characterized (Pena et al., 1997), and investigations have demonstrated that granulysin has a direct antimicrobial activity against a broad spectrum of pathogens (Stenger et al., 1998). Since this effector mechanism of CTL involves lysis of the host cells, the same immunopathological consequences as discussed above may act on the host tissue. However, the benefits of the direct antimicrobial activity should clearly outweigh the possible harm to the host.

Role of Cytokines in Immunopathology

Overview

Cells involved in the immune response to microbial pathogens secrete soluble mediators which generally act locally. Cytokine production is initiated only on antigen contact, and synthesis is terminated almost immediately after this contact is broken (Slifka et al., 1999). Thus, T cells secrete cytokines specifically at sites of infection and do not continuously produce these potentially toxic molecules while migrating through uninfected tissues or the bloodstream. The local effects tend to benefit the host, but under certain circumstances cytokines may gain access to the circulation and act systemically. The biological effects of circulating cytokines on the host cells are often responsible for the typical symptoms associated with infection (e.g., fever, myalgia, malaise, hypotension, and vascular leakage syndrome). At high concentrations, cytokines can potentially be life-threatening since they can mediate an uncontrolled activation of the immune system. Cytokines therefore play an important role in immune defense but also contribute to immunopathology and disease. This hypothesis is underlined by clinical trials revealing that treatment of systemic inflammatory diseases and cancer with interleukin-2, TNF, or INF-γ is thwarted by their inherent toxicity. The best example of the deleterious effects of cytokines is septic shock. Most pathological consequences of bacterial septic shock are due to the biological activity of lipopolysaccharide, derived from the cell wall of gram-negative bacteria. Lipopolysaccharide-induced acute activation of mononuclear phagocytes will result in overproduction of inflammatory cytokines, of which TNF, interleukin-1, and interleukin-6 are the most prominent. The biological effects of these cytokines will eventually cause tissue damage, organ failure, and, in many cases, death. In the following section, we will illustrate the bifunctional role of cytokines by describing the impact of TNF during the course of tuberculosis. This will allow us to depict the beneficial and harmful effects of TNF in the local and systemic response to a pathogen and may therefore serve as an example of many other infections.

Role of TNF in immunpathology to tuberculosis

TNF is a pleiotropic cytokine, produced mainly by macrophages and monocytes but also by lymphocytes and natural killer cells. It plays a central part in the immune response to many infections, including tuberculosis. Mice genetically deficient in TNF or TNF receptor p55 show increased susceptibility to tuberculosis (Flynn et al., 1995; Bean et al., 1999), and in vitro experiments indicate a role of TNF in the activation of human macrophages to kill the intracellular invader (Hirsch et al., 1994), as well as in the formation of granulomas, which are required for the demarcation of tuberculous foci (Kindler et al., 1989). Although TNF is crucial to the protective immune response, it also plays a part in the immunopathology of tuberculosis. The initiation of antimycobacterial chemotherapy often leads to a deterioration of the clinical condition, which involves fever, malaise, decompensation of pulmonary dysfunction, or even death. The typical clinical syndrome, in conjunction with knowledge about the pathophysiology of septic shock, has supported the hypothesis that TNF is released at the onset of antimycobacterial therapy and mediates immunopathology (Bekker et al., 1998). Stimulating bacterial components, including the major component of the cell wall lipoarabinomannan, could be derived from dying bacteria and could induce systemic TNF secretion by mononuclear phagocytes. This observation is reminiscent of the Koch phenomenon described in 1890 by Robert Koch, in which tuberculous guinea pigs developed local and remote tissue necrosis after intradermal challenge with M. tuberculosis culture filtrate. The involvement of the remote original lesion suggests the participation of soluble mediators in the development of necrosis.

These theoretical and experimental considerations are supported by the observation that the clinical deterioration after the initiation of antituberculous therapy is accompanied by an increase in plasma TNF concentrations (Bekker et al., 1998). To ameliorate the pathology resulting from TNF in these clinical settings, strategies for the inhibition of this cytokine have been developed. One approach put forward by Kaplan and colleagues was to alleviate the immunopathology induced by TNF by the application of the synthetic drug thalidomide, which is an immunomodulatory substance that inhibits TNF production by monocytes (but not T cells) in vivo and in vitro (Sampaio et al., 1991). The drug also acts as a costimulator of human T cells in vitro, resulting in increased production of Th1 cytokines (Haslett et al., 1998). The effect of thalidomide in tuberculosis patients was evident since it reduced the plasma TNF levels and was associated with clinical improvement, indicated by accelerated weight gain (Tramontana et al., 1995). Reduction in TNF levels has also been linked with a significant reduction of clinical symptoms in leprosy patients with erythema leprosum nodusum, including fever, malaise, and arthritic and neuritic pain. These experimental observations have prompted clinical trials and finally the approval of thalidomide for the therapy of erythema leprosum nodosum. The harmful effects of TNF were also demonstrated in a rabbit model of tuberculous meningitis (Tsenova et al., 1999). The susceptibility of rabbits to intrathecal infection with *M. tuberculosis* could be reversed by the coapplication of antituberculous drugs and thalidomide. The beneficial effect of thalidomide was associated with reduced meningeal TNF production and an attenuation of the inflammatory response. This therapeutic approach implicating TNF in local tissue damage was confirmed by experiments showing that TNF-transfected *M. bovis* BCG was more virulent than vector-transfected BCG when injected intrathecally. Taken together, these results demonstrate that the level of TNF produced during mycobacterial infection of the central nervous system determines, at least in part, the extent of pathogenesis. Mechanistically, one could argue that these effects may be ascribed to the biological activity of TNF in affecting vascular endothelium by inducing procoagulant activity, formation of thrombi, and production of nitric oxide synthase, thus causing endarteritis (Tsenova et al., 1999).

MOLECULAR MIMICRY

Many bacteria express epitopes that are cross-reactive with host antigens. This may result in neglect by the immune system as a consequence of self-tolerance which has developed during lymphocyte ontogeny or it may result in the production of an immune response directed against host tissue. Antibodies and/or T cells that recognize self epitopes are commonly found in patients after resolution of infectious diseases. The idea that disease symptoms persist even after pathogen eradication, due to cross-reactivity between the host immune response and self antigens that mimic microbial antigens, is the theoretical foundation of epitope mimicry as the basis of some autoimmune diseases. For instance, the group B antigen of the polysaccharide capsule of *Neisseria meningitidis* mimics epitopes expressed in the central nervous system (Finne et al., 1983), such as *N*-acetylneuramic acid, an epitope in the embryonic neuronal cell adhesion molecule. To prevent damage of host tissue, the immune system does not mount an immune response to this autoantigen, a property which is acquired during negative selection in the thymus. This, in conjunction with the poor immunogenicity of the capsular B antigen, has so far precluded the development of an efficient vaccine against *N. meningitidis* group B, which is a frequent cause of bacterial meningitis (Moe et al., 1999). Another example of molecular mimicry was demonstrated by Steinhoff et al. (1999), who showed that CD8[+] T cells specific for a bacterial antigen, mycobacterial heat shock protein 60 (Hsp60), can provide a link between infection and autoimmune intestinal inflammation. Since Hsp60 is highly conserved throughout evolution, T cells recognizing heat shock proteins of bacterial pathogens are at high risk of cross-reacting with self proteins, thereby causing immunopathology. Finally, studies with experimental animals found that immunizations with *Streptococcus pneumoniae* can elicit antibodies to the capsular C-polysaccharide that can react with mouse kidney glomerulus and cause proteinuria (Limpanasithikul et al., 1995). These autoimmune phenomena are believed to occur if the immune system fails to clear the plasma cells that produce the autoreactive antibodies by apoptosis (Ray et al., 1996). The presence of hyaluronic acid on some strains of streptococci may explain this phenomenon, since hyaluronic acid is a common constituent of mammalian tissue. The capsule thus permits the streptococcus to delude the immune system of the host.

In the following sections we will specify some prevalent clinical entities in which molecular mimicry of bacterial pathogens is believed to cause immunopathogenetic tissue damage after the successful elimination of the eliciting agent. In all cases, direct proof of the pathophysiological association between infection and tissue destruction is lacking. Nevertheless, epidemiological and experimental evidence for an association is striking, and it seems justified to discuss these diseases.

Rheumatic Fever

Rheumatic fever is the most commonly cited example of molecular mimicry in humans. Cheadle (1889) originally reported the association between throat infection and rheumatic fever. Although the incidence of acute rheumatic fever and its sequel, chronic rheumatic heart disease, has declined in developed countries, it remains the single most important cause of valvular heart disease worldwide. There is little doubt of the epidemiological association of this disease with group A streptococci. During the past decade, considerable progress has been made in understanding the possible basis of this association (Cunningham, 1996). Group A streptococcal pharyngitis is a necessary precondition for triggering of the autoimmune phenomena, which becomes clinically overt after a 2- to 3-week symptom-free interval after the primary infection. *S. pyogenes* can be divided into two classes depending on the antigenic properties of the antiphagocytic M protein (Bessen et al., 1989). Rheumatogenic streptococci carry the class I M protein, which expresses the epitopes that are highly cross-reactive with epitopes of cardiac myosin, tropomyosin, vimentin, laminin, and keratin (Kaplan and Meyeserian, 1962; Cunningham et al., 1988; Gulizia et al., 1991; Barnett and Cunningham, 1992). Streptococcal somatic constituents can be disseminated and diffuse through the human body. These give rise to cross-reactions and inflammatory responses including heart valve damage. Humoral and cellular immune reactions can be triggered in this way and probably take place concomitantly. The humoral phase dominates during the acute episode of rheumatic fever, whereas the cellular phase is initiated during the acute phase and leaves traces in the chronic phase. In addition to antibodies, $CD4^+$ and $CD8^+$ T cells are found at the rheumatic heart valves, and the T cells proliferate in response to M protein peptides and heart proteins (Guilherme et al., 1995, 2000). CD4-cell clones have strong cross-reactivity with sequences of M protein, especially in valvular tissues, and this is much more marked in the valvular tissue than in the remainder of the myocardium. This cellular response, which is present from the acute phase, has long-term consequences, resulting in the persistence of chronic valvular lesions especially at the mitral level (Olivier, 2000). These observations suggest that the T cells which recognize shared epitopes between M protein and myosin are involved in the pathogenesis of rheumatic fever.

Reactive Arthritis

The term "reactive arthritis" refers to an inflammatory arthropathy following infections with a broad spectrum of microbes. The most frequent form of reactive arthritis is termed Reiter's disease and often includes inflammation of the genitourinary tract and the eyes. Reiter's syndrome most frequently follows urinary tract infections with *Chlamydia trachomatis* or infectious gastroenteritis caused by *Yersinia, Shigella, Campylobacter,* or *Salmonella.* A remarkable feature of postinfectious arthritis is its association with the HLA B27 class I MHC allele. Approximately 90% of afflicted individuals have the B27 haplotype, compared with 7% of the normal population. Recent investigations have detected chlamydial DNA and, more importantly, mRNA in the affected joints of patients with reactive arthritis (Gerard et al., 1998). Similar studies attempting to demonstrate bacterial DNA in patients suffering from reactive arthritis after gastroenteritis have failed

(Nikkari et al., 1992). The pathophysiology of reactive arthritis is still poorly understood, but its association with the above-mentioned pathogens is undisputable. The antibody response to the triggering agent is of diagnostic significance, but T cells play a central role in the pathogenesis of reactive arthritis. The involvement of $CD4^+$ T-helper cells and of $CD8^+$ CTL has been implied in the pathology of reactive arthritis. In the early stage of reactive arthritis, $CD4^+$ T cells accumulate at the site of inflammation. Among the $CD4^+$ T cells, the IFN-γ-secreting Th1 cells are predominantly involved in the initiation of the inflammatory reaction. $CD8^+$ cells, which become involved later in the course of disease, are able to maintain the inflammatory process even after the bacterial pathogen itself has been eradicated by antibacterial immune responses. One hypothesis suggests that a pathogen-derived arthritogenic peptide is presented by HLA B27 to $CD8^+$ T cells. These cells are attracted into the joint, where they are activated to proliferate and secrete inflammatory mediators such as interleukin-1 and TNF. This chain of events ultimately results in local inflammation and, in severe cases, destruction of the cartilage. Alternatively, cross-reactivity between bacterial and self antigens in the joint leads to autodestruction of host tissue in accordance with the molecular mimicry hypothesis detailed above. The association with self-reactive $CD8^+$ T cells is supported by the occurrence of Reiter's disease in human immunodeficiency virus-infected individuals with severely depressed CD4 counts yet relative preservation of $CD8^+$ T cells (Altman et al., 1994).

Guillain-Barré Syndrome

Guillain-Barré syndrome (GBS) is an acute autoimmune polyradiculoneuropathy with a clinical presentation of flaccid paralysis with areflexia, variable sensory disturbance, and elevated levels of cerebrospinal fluid protein without pleocytosis. The most significant antecedent event is an infection with *Campylobacter jejuni* (4 to 66%), although cytomegalovirus (5 to 15%), Epstein-Barr virus (2 to 10%), and *Mycoplasma pneumoniae* (1 to 5%) infections have also been associated with GBS (Vedeler, 2000). *C. jejuni,* a leading cause of acute gastroenteritis, can be serotyped based on differences in the polysaccharide structure of the lipopolysaccharide of the bacterium. Isolates obtained from the stools of patients who presented with a diarrheic episode prior to the onset of GBS were frequently serotyped as O:19, which is an uncommon cause of gastroenteritis. Autoreactive antibodies to gangliosides, especially GM_1 ganglioside, are found in 14 to 50% of patients with GBS, particularly after *C. jejuni* infection (Hao et al., 1998). Experimentally it could be demonstrated that these antibodies paralyze muscle-nerve preparations (Goodyear et al., 1999). Ganglioside epitopes exist in the bacterial cell wall of *C. jejuni*. The pathophysiological link between the occurrence of GM_1 ganglioside antibodies and autoimmune disease is supported by the cross-reaction of GM_1 antibody-containing sera with the lipopolysaccharide of *C. jejuni* (Yuki et al., 1993). It is thus currently hypothesized that antiganglioside antibodies are elicited as a result of molecular mimicry between peripheral nerve gangliosides and the structurally similar *C. jejuni* lipopolysaccharide. T cells, including unconventional subsets like $\gamma\delta$ T-cell receptor-expressing cells, are also involved in the pathogenesis of most forms of GBS (Borsellino et al., 2000). T-cell responses to myelin proteins induce experimental autoimmune neuritis (Khalili-Shirazi et al., 1992). Identification of the fine specificity of the T cells is currently under investigation.

Lyme Disease

Lyme disease is an infectious disease caused by the bacterium *Borrelia burgdorferi*, which is transmitted to humans by the bite of a tick. The acute disease manifestations are caused by the spirochete itself and include the characteristic skin rash (erythema migrans), meningitis, neuritis, encephalitis, and myocarditis. However, some patients develop recurring episodes of arthritis despite succesful antibiotic therapy and resolution of all symptoms of acute disease. At this stage of the disease, bacterial DNA has not been detected reliably in afflicted synovial fluid. Antibiotic-resistant arthritis has been associated with an increased frequency of HLA DRB1 0401, suggesting that autoimmune reactions may be involved. This is bolstered by recent studies reporting T-cell cross-reactivity between an epitope of *B. burgdorferi* outer surface protein A (OspA) and an epitope of human leukocyte function-associated antigen 1 (LFA 1) (Hemmer et al., 1999). This suggests a scenario in which the *Borrelia* organisms enter the host via a tick bite and disseminate to various sites of the body. Months later, an inflammatory response is initiated in the joints, which is dominated by $CD4^+$ Th1 cells, which secrete IFN-γ. A small fraction of these cells bear a T-cell receptor specifically recognizing the bacterial surface protein OspA. The high local concentration of IFN-γ will induce upregulation of intercellular cell adhesion molecule 1 (ICAM-1) and antigen-presenting molecules on synovial cells. High expression of ICAM-1 will attract LFA-1-expressing T cells, which may consequently support antigen presentation of this molecule. These interactions induce a self perpetuation of the local inflammatory response, so that even after elimination of the spirochetes by chemotherapy, the OspA-primed cells maintain the tissue-destructive inflammation (Klempner and Huber, 1999). Lyme disease therefore presents a typical example of how epitope mimicry of pathogens can induce a vicious circle of autodestructive inflammatory reactions.

REFERENCES

Altman, E. M., L. V. Centeno, M. Mahal, and L. Bielory. 1994. AIDS-associated Reiter's syndrome. *Ann. Allergy* 72:307–316.

Ando, M., M. Suga, and H. Kohrogi. 1999. A new look at hypersensitivity pneumonitis. *Curr. Opin. Pulm. Med.* 5:299–304.

Barnett, L. A., and M. W. Cunningham. 1992. Evidence for actinlike proteins in an M protein-negative strain of *Streptococcus pyogenes*. *Infect. Immun.* 60:3932–3936.

Bean, A. G., D. R. Roach, H. Briscoe, M. P. France, H. Körner, J. D. Sedgwick, and W. J. Britton. 1999. Structural deficiencies in granuloma formation in TNF-gene targeted mice underlie the hightened susceptibility to aerosol *Mycobacterium tuberculosis* infection, which is not compensated for by lymphotoxin. *J. Immunol.* 162:3504–3511.

Bekker, L. G., G. Maartens, L. Steyn, and G. Kaplan. 1998. Selective increase in plasma tumor necrosis factor alpha and concomitant clinical deterioration after initiating therapy in patients with severe tuberculosis. *J. Infect. Dis.* 178:580–584.

Bessen, D., K. F. Jones, and V. A. Fischetti. 1989. Evidence for two distinct classes of streptococcal M protein and their relationship to rheumatic fever. *J. Exp. Med.* 169:269–283.

Borsellino, G., O. Koul, R. Placido, D. Tramonti, S. Lucchetti, S. Galgani, M. Salvetti, C. Gasperini, G. Ristori, B. Bonetti, S. Bach, B. Cipriani, and L. Battistini. 2000. Evidence for a role of gammadelta T cells in demyelinating diseases as determined by activation states and responses to lipid antigens. *J. Neuroimmunol.* 107:124–129.

Cheadle, W. B. 1889. Harveian lectures on the various manifestations of the rheumatic disease state as exemplified in childhood and early life. *Lancet* i:821–827.

Claudy, A. 1998. Pathogenesis of leukocytoclastic vasculitis. *Eur. J. Dermatol.* 8:75–79.

Coombs, R. R. A., and P. G. H. Gell. 1963. The classification of allergic reactions underlying disease, p. 317–337. *In* P. G. H. Gell and R. R. A. Coombs (ed.), *Clinical Aspects of Immunology*. Blackwell Scientific Publications, Oxford, United Kingdom.

Cooper, A. M., D. K. Dalton, T. A. Stewart, J. P. Griffin, D. G. Russell, and I. M. Orme. 1993. Disseminated tuberculosis in interferon-gamma gene-disrupted mice. *J. Exp. Med.* 178:2243–2247.

Cooper, A. M., C. D'Souza, A. A. Frank, and I. M. Orme. 1997. The course of *Mycobacterium tuberculosis* infection in the lungs of mice lacking expression of either perforin- or granzyme-mediated cytolytic mechanisms. *Infect. Immun.* 65:1317–1320.

Cooper, N. R. 1999. Biology of the complement system, p. 281–315. *In* D. T. Fearon, B. F. Haynes, C. Nathan, J. G. Gallin, and R. Snyderman (ed.), *Inflammation. Basic Principles and Clinical Correlates*, 3rd ed. Lippincott Williams & Wilkins, Philadelphia, Pa.

Cribier, B., A. Caille, E. Heid, and E. Grosshans. 1998. Erythema nodosum and associated diseases. A study of 129 cases. *Int. J. Dermatol.* 37:667–672.

Cunningham, M. W. 1996. Streptococci and rheumatic fever, p. 13–66. *In* H. N. Friedman, R. Rose, and M. Bendinelli (ed.), *Microorganisms and Autoimmune Disease.* Plenum Press, New York, N.Y.

Cunningham, M. W., J. M. McCormack, L. R. Talaber, J. B. Harley, E. M. Ayoub, R. S. Muneer, L. T. Chun, and D. V. Reddy. 1988. Human monoclonal antibodies reactive with antigens of the group A *Streptococcus* and human heart. *J. Immunol.* **141:** 2760–2766.

Dalton, D. K., S. Pitts-Meek, S. Keshav, I. S. Figari, A. Bradley, and T. A. Stewart. 1993. Multiple defects of immune cell function in mice with disrupted interferon gamma genes. *Science* **259:**1739–1742.

Dannenberg, A. M., Jr., and G. A. W. Rook. 1994. Pathogenesis of pulmonary tuberculosis: an interplay of tissue damaging and macrophage-activating immune responses—dual mechanisms that control bacillary multiplication, p. 459–483. *In* B. R. Bloom (ed.), *Tuberculosis: Pathogenesis, Protection and Control.* American Society for Microbiology, Washington, D.C.

de Libero, G., I. Flesch, and S. H. E. Kaufmann. 1988. Mycobacteria-reactive Lyt-2+ T cell lines. *Eur. J. Immunol.* **18:**59–66.

Feizi, T. 1967. Cold agglutinins, the direct Coomb's test and serum immunoglobulins in *Mycoplasma pneumoniae* infection. *Ann. N. Y. Acad. Sci.* **143:**801–812.

Fenton, M. J., and M. W. Vermeulen. 1996. Immunopathology of tuberculosis: roles of macrophages and monocytes. *Infect. Immun.* **64:**683–690.

Finne, J., M. Leinonen, and P. H. Makela. 1983. Antigenic similarities between brain components and bacteria causing meningitis. Implications for vaccine development and pathogenesis. *Lancet* **ii:**355–357.

Flynn, J. L., M. M. Goldstein, J. Chan, K. J. Triebold, K. Pfeffer, C. J. Lowenstein, R. Schreiber, T. W. Mak, and B. R. Bloom. 1995. Tumor necrosis factor alpha is required for the protective immune response against *Mycobacterium tuberculosis* in mice. *Immunity* **2:**561–572.

Flynn, J. L., M. M. Goldstein, K. J. Triebold, B. Koller, and B. R. Bloom. 1992. Major histocompatibility complex class I restricted T cells are required for resistance to *Mycobacterium tuberculosis* infection. *Proc. Natl. Acad. Sci. USA* **89:**12013–12017.

Gazzinelli, R. T., F. T. Hakim, S. Hieny, G. M. Shearer, and A. Sher. 1991. Synergistic role of CD4+ and CD8+ T-lymphocytes in IFN gamma production and protective immunity induced by an attenuated *Toxoplasma gondii* vaccine. *J. Immunol.* **146:**286–292.

Gerard, H. C., P. J. Branigan, T. Arayssi, J. H. Klippel, H. R. Schumacher, and A. P. Hudson. 1998. Synovial *Chlamydia trachomatis* in patients with reactive arthritis/Reiter's syndrome are viable but show aberrant gene expression. *J. Rheumatol.* **24:** 1092–1100.

Goodyear, C. S., G. M. O'Hanlon, J. J. Plomp, E. R. Wagner, I. Morrison, J. Veitch, L. Cochrane, R. W. Bullens, P. C. Molenaar, J. Conner, and H. J. Willison. 1999. Monoclonal antibodies raised against Guillain-Barre syndrome-associated *Campylobacter jejuni* lipopolysaccharides react with neuronal gangliosides and paralyze muscle-nerve preparations. *J. Clin. Investig.* **104:**697–708.

Green, D. G., and C. F. Ware. 1997. Fas-ligand: privilege and peril. *Proc. Natl. Acad. Sci. USA* **94:**5986–5990.

Guilherme, L., E. Cunha-Neto, V. Coelho, R. Snitcowsky, P. M. Pomerantzeff, R. V. Assis, F. Pedra, J. Neumann, A. Goldberg, M. E. Pattaroyo, F. Pileggi, and J. Kalil. 1995. Human heart-infiltrating T-cell clones from rheumatic heart disease patients recognize both streptococcal and cardiac proteins. *Circulation* **92:**415–420.

Guilherme, L., N. Dulphy, C. Douay, V. Coelho, E. Cunha-Neto, S. E. Oshiro, R. V. Assis, A. C. Tanaka, P. M. Alberto Pomerantzeff, D. Charron, A. Toubert, and J. Kalil. 2000. Molecular evidence for antigen-driven immune responses in cardiac lesions of rheumatic heart disease patients. *Int. Immunol.* **12:** 1063–1074.

Gulizia, J. M., M. W. Cunningham, and B. M. McManus. 1991. Immunoreactivity of anti-streptococcal monoclonal antibodies to human heart valves. Evidence for multiple cross-reactive epitopes. *Am. J. Pathol.* **138:**285–301.

Hao, Q., T. Saida, S. Kuroki, M. Nishimura, M. Nukina, H. Obayashi, and K. Saida. 1998. Antibodies to gangliosides and galactocerebroside in patients with Guillain-Barre syndrome with preceding *Campylobacter jejuni* and other identified infections. *J. Neuroimmunol.* **81:**116–126.

Haslett, P. A., L. G. Corral, M. Albert, and G. Kaplan. 1998. Thalidomide costimulates primary human T lymphocytes, preferentially inducing proliferation, cytokine production, and cytotoxic responses in the CD8+ subset. *J. Exp. Med.* **187:**1885–1892.

Hemmer, B., B. Gran, Y. Zhao, A. Marques, J. Pascal, A. Tzou, T. Kondo, I. Cortese, B. Bielekova, S. E. Straus, H. F. McFarland, R. Houghton, R. Simon, C. Pinilla, and R. Martin. 1999. Identification of candidate T cell epitopes and molecular mimics in chronic Lyme disease. *Nat. Med.* **5:**1375–1382.

Hirsch, C. S., J. J. Ellner, D. G. Russell, and E. A. Rich. 1994. Complement receptor-mediated uptake and tumor necrosis factor alpha-mediated growth inhibition of *Mycobacterium tuberculosis* by human alveolar macrophages. *J. Immunol.* **152:**743–753.

Horwitz, C. A., J. Moulds, W. Henle, G. Henle, H. Polesky, H. H. Balfour, Jr., B. Schwartz, and T. Hoff. 1977. Cold agglutinins in infectious mononucleosis and heterophil-antibody-negative mononucleosis-like syndromes. *Blood* **50:**195–202.

Huber, M., E. Timms, T. W. Mak, M. Röllinghoff, and M. Lohoff. 1998. Effective and longlasting immunity against the parasite *Leishmania major* in CD8-deficient mice. *Infect. Immun.* **66:**3968–3970.

Jouanguy, E., F. Altare, S. Lamhamedi, P. Revy, J. Emile, M. Newport, M. Levin, S. Blanche, E. Seboun, A. Fischer, and J. Casanova. 1996. Interferon-gamma receptor deficiency in an infant with fatal bacille Calmette Guerin infection. *N. Engl. J. Med.* **335:**1956–1961.

Kaplan, M. H., and M. Meyeserian. 1962. An immunological cross-reaction between group A streptococcal cells and human heart tissue. *Lancet* **i:**706–710.

Kaufmann, S. H. E. 1988. CD8+ T lymphocytes in intracellular microbial infections. *Immunol. Today* **9:**168–174.

Khalili-Shirazi, A., R. A. Hughes, S. W. Brostoff, C. Linington, and N. Gregson. 1992. T cell responses to myelin proteins in Guillain-Barre syndrome. *J. Neurol. Sci.* **111:**200–203.

Kindler, V., A. P. Sappino, G. E. Grau, P. F. Piguet, and P. Vassalli. 1989. The inducing role of tumor necrosis factor in the development of bactericidal granulomas during BCG infection. *Cell* **56:**731–740.

Klempner, M. S., and B. T. Huber. 1999. Is it thee or me? Autoimmunity in Lyme disease. *Nat. Med.* **5:**1346–1347.

Ladel, C. H., I. E. Flesch, J. Arnoldi, and S. H. E. Kaufmann. 1994. Studies with MHC-deficient knock out mice reveal impact of both MHC-I and MHC-II-dependent T cell responses on *Listeria monocytogenes* infection. *J. Immunol.* **153:**3116–3122.

Laochumroonvorapong, P. J. Wang, C. C. Liu, W. Ye, A. L. Moreira, K. B. Elkon, V. H. Freedman, and G. Kaplan. 1997. Perforin, a cytotoxic molecule which mediates cell necrosis, is not required for the early control of mycobacterial infection in mice. *Infect. Immun.* **65:**127–132.

Levinsky, R. J., and T. M. Barratt. 1979. IgA immune complexes in Henoch-Schoenlein purpura. *Lancet.* ii:1100–1103.

Levitz, S. M., H. L. Mathews, and J. W. Murphy. 1995. Direct antimicrobial activity of T cells. *Immunol. Today* 16:387–391.

Liles, W. C. 1997. Apoptosis: role in infection and inflammation. *Curr. Opin. Infect. Dis.* 10:165–170.

Limpanasithikul, W., S. Ray, and B. Diamond. 1995. Cross-reactive antibodies have both protective and pathogenic potential. *J. Immunol.* 155:967–973.

Loomes, L. M., K. Uemura, R. A. Childs, J. C. Paulson, G. N. Rogers, P. R. Scudder, J. C. Michalski, E. F. Hounsell, D. Taylor-Robinson, and T. Feizi. 1984. Erythrocyte receptors for *Mycoplasma pneumoniae* are sialylated oligosaccharides of Ii antigen type. *Nature* 307:560–563.

Magro, C. M., and A. N. Crawson. 1999. A clinical and histological study of 37 cases of IgA associated vasculitis. *Am. J. Dermatopathol.* 21:234–240.

Moe, G. R., S. Tan, and D. M. Granhoff. 1999. Molecular mimetics of polysaccharide epitopes as vaccine candidates for prevention of *Neisseria meningitidis* serogroup B disease. *FEMS Immunol. Med. Microbiol.* 26:209–226.

Mygind, N., R. Dahl, S. Pedersen, and K. Thestrup-Pedersen. 1996. Other allergic lung diseases, p. 400–408. *In* N. Mygind, R. Dahl, S. Pedersen, and K. Thestrup-Pedersen (ed.), *Essential Allergy*, 2nd ed. Blackwell Science, Cambridge, Mass.

Newport, M. J., C. M. Huxley, S. Huston, C. M. Hawrylowicz, B. A. Oostra, R. Williamson, and M. Levin. 1996. A mutation in the interferon-gamma-receptor gene and susceptibility to mycobacterial infection. *N. Engl. J. Med.* 335:1941–1949.

Nikkari, S., R. Merilahti, R. Saario, K. O. Soderstrom, K. Granfors, M. Skurnik, and P. Toivanen. 1992. Yersinia-triggered reactive arthritis: use of polymerase chain reaction and immunocytochemical staining in the detection of bacterial components from synovial specimens. *Arthritis Rheum.* 35:682–687.

Nordstrand, A., M. Norgren, and S. E. Holm. 1999. Pathogenic mechanisms of acute post-streptococcal glomerulonephritis. *Scand. J. Infect. Dis.* 31:523–537.

Olivier, C. 2000. Rheumatic fever—is it still a problem? *J. Antimicrob. Ther.* 45:13–21.

Pena, S. V., D. A. Hanson, B. A. Carr, T. J. Goralski, and A. M. Krensky. 1997. Processing, subcellular localization, and function of 519 (granulysin), a human late T cell activation molecule with homology to small, lytic, granule proteins. *J. Immunol.* 158:2680–2688.

Ray, S. K., C. Putterman, and B. Diamond. 1996. Pathogenic autoantibodies are routinely generated during the response to foreign antigen: a paradigm for autoimmune disease. *Proc. Natl. Acad. Sci. USA* 93:2019–2024.

Rook, G. A. W., and B. R. Bloom. 1994. Mechanisms of pathogenesis in tuberculosis, p. 485–501. *In* B. R. Bloom (ed.), *Tuberculosis: Pathogenesis, Protection, and Control.* American Society for Microbiology, Washington, D.C.

Rook, G. A. W., and J. L. Stanford. 1996. The Koch phenomenon and the immunopathology of tuberculosis, p. 239–262. *In* T. M. Shinick (ed.), *Tuberculosis.* Springer-Verlag KG, Berlin, Germany.

Rottenberg, M. E., M. Bakhiet, T. Olsson, K. Kristensson, T. Mak, H. Wigzell, and A. Orn. 1993. Differential susceptibilities of mice genomically deleted of CD4 and CD8 to infections with *Trypanosoma cruzi* and *Trypanosoma brucei. Infect. Immun.* 61:5129–5133.

Sampaio, E. P., E. N. Sarno, R. Galilly, Z. A. Cohn, and G. Kaplan. 1991. Thalidomide selectively inhibits tumor necrosis factor alpha production by stimulated human monocytes. *J. Exp. Med.* 173:699–703.

Santucci, M. B., M. Amicosante, R. Cicconi, C. Montesano, M. Casarini, S. Giosue, A. Bisetti, and M. Fraziano. 2000. *Mycobacterium tuberculosis*-induced apoptosis in monocytes/macrophages: early membrane modifications and intracellular mycobacterial viability. *J. Infect. Dis.* 181:1506–1509.

Schluger, N. W., and W. N. Rom. 1998. The host immune response to tuberculosis. *Am. J. Respir. Crit. Care Med.* 157:679–691.

Sell, S. 1987. *Immunology, Immunopathology and Immunity*, 4th ed., p. 373–412. Elsevier Science Publishing Co., New York, N.Y.

Sharma, O. P., and R. Chwogule. 1998. Many faces of pulmonary aspergillosis. *Eur. Respir. J.* 12:705–715.

Slifka, M. K., F. Rodriguez, and J. L. Whitton. 1999. Rapid on/off cycling of cytokine production by virus-specific CD8+ T cells. *Nature* 401:76–79.

Slifka, M. K., and J. L. Whitton. 2000. Antigen-specific regulation of T cell-mediated cytokine production. *Immunity* 12:451–457.

Steinhoff, U., V. Brinkmann, U. Klemm, P. Aichele, P. Seiler, U. Brandt, P. W. Bland, I. Prinz, U. Zügel, and S. H. Kaufmann. 1999. Autoimmune intestinal pathology induced by hsp60-specific CD8 T cells. *Immunity* 11:349–358.

Stenger, S., D. A. Hanson, R. Teitelbaum, P. Dewan, K. R. Niazi, C. J. Froelich, T. Ganz, S. Thoma-Uszynski, A. Melian, C. Bogdan, S. A. Porcelli, B. R. Bloom, A. M. Krensky, and R. L. Modlin. 1997. An antimicrobial activity of cytolytic T-cells mediated by granulysin. *Science* 282:121–125.

Stenger, S., R. J. Mazzaccaro, K. Uyemura, S. Cho, P. F. Barnes, J. P. Rosat, A. Sette, M. B. Brenner, S. A. Porcelli, B. R. Bloom, and R. L. Modlin. 1997. Differential effects of cytolytic T cell subsets on intracellular infection. *Science* 276:1684–1687.

Stenger, S., and R. Modlin. 1998. Cytotoxic T cell responses to intracellular pathogens. *Curr. Opin. Immunol.* 10:471–477.

Tramontana, J. M., U. Utaipat, A. Molloy, P. Akarasewi, M. Burroughs, S. Makonkawkeyoon, B. Johnson, J. D. Klausner, W. Rom, and G. Kaplan. 1995. Thalidomide treatment reduces tumor necrosis factor alpha production and enhances weight gain in patients with pulmonary tuberculosis. *Mol. Med.* 1:384–387.

Tsenova, L., A. Bergtold, V. H. Freedman, R. A. Young, and G. Kaplan. 1999. Tumor necrosis factor alpha is a determinant of pathogenesis and disease progression in mycobacterial infection in the central nervous system. *Proc. Natl. Acad. Sci. USA* 96:5657–1662.

Vedeler, C. A. 2000. Inflammatory neuropathies: update. *Curr. Opin. Neurol.* 13:305–309.

Wang, Z.-E., S. L. Reiner, F. Hatam, F. P. Heinzel, J. Bouvier, C. W. Turck, and R. M. Locksley. 1993. Targeted activation of CD8+ cells and infection of β2-microglobulin-deficient mice fail to confirm a protective role for CD8 cells in experimental leishmaniasis. *J. Immunol.* 151:2077–2086.

Yuki, N., T. Taki, F. Inagaki, T. Kasama, M. Takahashi, K. Saito, S. Handa, and T. Miyatake. 1993. A bacterium lipopolysaccharide that elicits Guillain-Barre syndrome has a GM1 ganglioside-like structure. *J. Exp. Med.* 178:1771–1775.

Zabriskie, J. B. 1971. The role of streptococci in human glomerulonephritis. *J. Exp. Med.* 134(Suppl.):180S.

Immunology of Infectious Diseases
Edited by S. H. E. Kaufmann, A. Sher, and R. Ahmed
© 2002 ASM Press, Washington, D.C.

Chapter 21

Pathology and Pathogenesis of Parasitic Disease

THOMAS A. WYNN AND DOMINIC KWIATKOWSKI

Immune pathology is generally viewed as the result of an inappropriate or excessive host response, but in many parasitic infections it may be an inevitable consequence of impossible circumstances. Nonspecific immune responses such as fever and inflammation provide an essential first line of host defense against a variety of infectious pathogens. In ideal circumstances, this is a transient phase, which terminates as soon as the host has acquired specific effector mechanisms such as antibodies or cytotoxic T lymphocytes. If specific effector mechanisms do not develop or if they are not effective in eradicating the infection, persistent inflammation and other nonspecific responses may be the only way of containing the infection. This is the case for many parasitic infections, and it carries an inevitable risk of side effects.

This does not mean that all infections with the same parasite species lead to the same immune pathology. One of the most striking features of human parasitic infection is great variability in clinical outcome, ranging from asymptomatic carriage to fatal disease. Esophageal disease due to *Trypanosoma cruzi*, portal hypertension due to *Schistosoma mansoni,* and nephrotic syndrome due to *Plasmodium malariae* are a few examples of the many immunopathological complications that occur in some infected individuals but not others. Part of this variability is determined by host genetics, while other potential determinants include parasite virulence factors, infectious dose, and the individual's prior level of immunity. The picture may be complicated by coinfection with other infectious agents: for example, the severity of *Plasmodium falciparum* malaria appears to be increased by concomitant bacteremia but reduced by concomitant *P. vivax* infection, although the underlying mechanisms remain poorly understood (Berkley et al., 1999; Luxemburger et al., 1997).

In experimental models of infection, host genotype, parasite genotype, and other variables are selected to obtain a constant disease outcome. The great value of experimental models is that radical interventions such as gene disruption may be used to investigate the molecular causation of specific pathological changes. However, when interpreting these data it is important to recognize that they apply to a specific scenario and that an intervention which is beneficial in a selected experimental context could possibly be deleterious in natural infection in humans, where the underlying genetic and environmental parameters may be highly variable.

It is impossible in a single chapter to do justice to the remarkably broad range of immunological mechanisms that contribute to the pathology of parasitic disease. Twenty years ago, much of the research in this field concerned the role of immune complexes, complement, and anaphylaxis. These areas remain important, but the focus has shifted to the molecular basis of cellular processes such as inflammation, granuloma formation, and fibrosis. An important issue is how the host maintains the fine balance between a protective immune response and one that is liable to cause pathological complications. It is becoming increasingly clear that this is one of the most critical determinants of a successful host-parasite relationship and, as such, is of considerable importance for vaccinologists. Interestingly, in many parasitic infections, this balance appears to be regulated by the coordinated actions of a few essential immunoregulatory cytokines.

This chapter focuses primarily on the question of how the balance between immune protection and immune pathology is regulated. The issue is both

---

Thomas A. Wynn • Immunobiology Section, Laboratory of Parasitic Diseases, National Institutes of Health, Bldg. 4, Rm. 126, Bethesda, MD 20892. **Dominic Kwiatkowski** • Molecular Infectious Diseases Group, Institute of Molecular Medicine, John Radcliffe Hospital, Oxford OX3 9DS, United Kingdom.

quantitative (e.g., the optimal amount of proinflammatory cytokines required when a parasite is first encountered by the immune system) and qualitative (e.g., the optimal balance between the Th1 response, which promotes cell-mediated immunity, and the Th2 response, which promotes antibody generation). A fundamental biological dilemma is that the host has to deal with many different infectious pathogens and, even for a single species of parasite, with different strains. For example, a strain of *P. falciparum* that replicates slowly, releasing highly proinflammatory factors, may require a different regulatory response from a fast-replicating strain with little proinflammatory activity (Kwiatkowski, 1995). In such circumstances, there may be no single optimal response and, however well the system is regulated, a certain proportion of natural infections will have a pathological outcome.

HOMEOSTASIS IN THE ANTI-INFECTIVE IMMUNE RESPONSE

CD4[+] T cells can be divided into two major subsets, Th1 and Th2, based on the specific cytokines produced and the functional activities exhibited by each cell type. Th1 cells produce gamma interferon (IFN-γ), interleukin-2 (IL-2), and lymphotoxin, which promote macrophage activation and the generation of cell-mediated immunity. Th2 cells produce a variety of cytokines, including IL-4, IL-5, IL-10, and IL-13, and provide help for the maturation of B cells to immunoglobulin-secreting cells, thereby primarily activating humoral defense mechanisms. Central to the concept of Th1 and Th2 subset generation is the tendency for these responses to become polarized. Thus, a Th1 or Th2 cytokine-producing profile will often dominate during an immune response by preferentially amplifying one Th subset and down-regulating the opposing response. This polarized response appears to be critical for host defense against many pathogenic organisms. Resistance to intracellular pathogens often requires a predominantly Th1 response, while Th2 responses are typically needed to fight extracellular parasites. Thus, T-cell-derived cytokines produced by the host in response to an infectious agent determine the outcome of infection in many infectious-disease models (Abbas et al., 1996). A primary goal of immunological research over the past decade has been to understand the various mechanisms that influence the polarization of the immune response following infection and to exploit those mechanisms in vaccine design.

Whereas a proinflammatory Th1 response is usually required to control intracellular infections,

there is also a need to balance the response (Taylor-Robinson, 1998). The various effector molecules, particularly those associated with the Th1 pathway, are nonspecific in their action and can be detrimental if produced for too long, in excess, or in the wrong place. The potentially harmful molecules include nitric oxide (NO), reactive oxygen intermediates, IL-1, IFN-γ, and tumor necrosis factor (TNF), and these factors often operate in a synergistic fashion. Therefore, it is important to produce a sufficiently potent type 1 response to keep the infection under control while producing at the same time just enough of a type 2 or immunosuppressive response to prevent the protective response from causing damage to the host. IL-10, transforming growth factor β (TGF-β), and, to a lesser extent, IL-4 appear to be important in preventing the Th1 response from overshooting during parasitic infection.

There are also several examples where Th2 responses appear to be detrimental. Strong antibody responses may lead to the formation of antigen-antibody complexes or complement activation, resulting in bystander lysis (Infante-Duarte and Kamradt, 1999). Eosinophils, typically associated with the Th2 response, are involved in immediate hypersensitivity reactions to the filarial worm *Onchocerca volvulus* (Ottesen, 1995). Th2 responses appear to be the primary cause of hepatic fibrosis, portal hypertension, and chronic morbidity in *Schistosoma mansoni*-infected mice (Hoffmann et al., 2000) and, outside the sphere of parasitic infection, are largely responsible for the chronic pathology of asthma (Wills-Karp, 1999). The available data suggest that IFN-γ, IL-12, and IL-10 cooperate to keep the Th2 response in check. In summary, a successful outcome following an infection requires precise titration of Th1 and Th2 responses, appropriate to the type of infection. This is not just in terms of amount but also covers where, when, and for how long these responses occur.

BENEFITS AND RISKS OF THE Th1 RESPONSE

The classical paradigm of Th1-Th2 polarization arose from studies of resistance to *Leishmania major* infection in mice (Heinzel et al., 1989; Scott et al., 1988), discussed in more detail in chapters 3 and 17. The mammalian host cells for *Leishmania* spp. are macrophages, and in this situation an adequate Th1 response is vital for protective immunity whereas mouse strains with a dominant Th2 response suffer severe disease. Humans with visceral leishmaniasis have high circulating levels of IL-10, which may partly explain their inability to control the infection (Holaday et al., 1993; Karp et al., 1993).

Many intracellular pathogens such as *Toxoplasma gondii* and *Listeria monocytogenes* initiate cell-mediated immunity by stimulating dendritic cells and/or macrophages to produce IL-12. This stimulates IFN-γ production by NK cells and T cells, and IFN-γ-activated antigen-presenting cells secrete more IL-12 in a positive feedback loop, which promotes Th1-cell development and activation of essential antimicrobial effector mechanisms. Control of *L. monocytogenes, T. gondii,* and *Trypanosoma cruzi* requires the coordinated activation of both antigen-specific cells (T lymphocytes) and less specific responses (NK cells, neutrophils, and macrophages), with IFN-γ and TNF-α playing critical roles by up-regulating macrophage activation and nitric oxide production (Yap and Sher, 1999).

In *L. monocytogenes*-infected mice, IL-10 is induced simultaneously with IFN-γ and TNF-α and appears to favor the organism by down-regulating the host-protective cell-mediated immune response. IL-10-deficient mice are highly resistant to *L. monocytogenes,* while mice treated with exogenous IL-10 succumb to infection (Dai et al., 1997). Bacterial burdens were reduced as much as 50-fold in IL-10-deficient mice early after infection, suggesting a very effective innate immune response. Proinflammatory cytokine expression was increased, and the rapid elimination of the organism in the mutant mice decreased the number and size of granulomatous lesions in the liver and spleen, thus reducing the marked tissue destruction that is typically seen late in the infection. The IL-10-deficient mice were also more resistant to a secondary infection. Thus, in this model, an increased type 1 cytokine response acts to augment innate and acquired immunity during primary and secondary *L. monocytogenes* infection (Fig. 1).

In contrast, IL-10-deficient mice inoculated with a normally avirulent *T. gondii* strain or with a virulent strain of *T. cruzi* succumbed to infection within the first 2 weeks of infection (Gazzinelli et al., 1996; Holscher et al., 2000; Hunter et al., 1997). In both infections, animals lacking IL-10 showed increased suppression of parasite growth, and in those infected with *T. cruzi,* inflammation and necrosis within the endocardium and interstitium of the myocardium were reduced (Hunter et al., 1997). The increase in mortality appears to have been caused by high systemic levels of IFN-γ, TNF-α, and IL-12, produced in large part by activated CD4$^+$ lymphocytes and macrophages. The livers of both *T. gondii*- and *T. cruzi*-infected mice showed numerous prominent foci of necrosis and increased cellular infiltration, com-

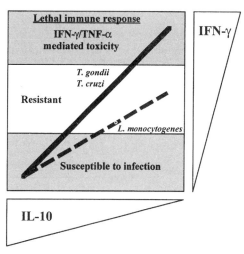

Figure 1. Resistance versus susceptibility to many intracellular organisms is regulated by a delicate balance between IFN-γ and IL-10. The type, magnitude, location, and duration of the host response dictate a susceptible or resistant outcome following infection with *T. gondii, T. cruzi,* and *L. monocytogenes.* With all three intracellular pathogens, IFN-γ is required to induce resistance. Nevertheless, the protective response must also be carefully down-regulated in a timely manner to prevent the development of immune-mediated and potentially lethal tissue pathology. Here, the immunosuppressive cytokine IL-10 appears to play a dominant role. Because of the systemic nature of *T. cruzi* and *T. gondii* infections, dysregulation in the type 1 response is more dangerous during these infections (bold line) than during an *L. monocytogenes* infection (dotted line), which tends to remain localized within granulomatous foci.

posed of lymphocytes, macrophages, and necrotic cellular debris. Levels of IL-12 and IFN-γ in sera of infected IL-10-deficient animals were four- to sixfold higher than in sera from control mice, as were mRNA levels of several proinflammatory cytokines (Gazzinelli et al., 1996). Similarly, macrophages from the mutant mice activated in vitro or in vivo with *T. gondii* secreted higher levels of TNF-α, IL-12, and inducible NO than did macrophages from control animals. The clinical manifestations of weight loss, hypothermia, hypoglycemia, and increased levels of liver-derived enzymes in the blood, together with hepatic necrosis, suggested that the IL-10 knockout (KO) mice died in response to an overwhelming systemic immune response, resembling that observed during septic shock. In support of this conclusion, administration of anti-CD4, anti-IL-12, or anti-TNF-α antibodies reduced mortality in IL-10 KO mice (Gazzinelli et al., 1996; Holscher et al., 2000; Hunter et al., 1997). Mutant mice perorally infected with *T. gondii* also succumbed rapidly to infection, but in this situation the mortality was attributed to the development of type 1-mediated intestinal rather than hepatic pathology (Suzuki et al., 2000). Thus, in these models, IL-10 plays a major role in protecting the host against an excessive and lethal type 1 cytokine response (Fig. 1).

The above findings indicate that IL-10 can be either protective or detrimental. A possible explanation for the somewhat unexpected lethal outcome observed with *T. gondii*- or *T. cruzi*-infected IL-10-deficient mice is that both pathogens infect virtually all nucleated cells and are characterized by an acute phase in which the parasites disseminate throughout the body. This induces an overwhelming systemic immune response in the absence of the immunoregulatory cytokine IL-10. In contrast, when wild-type (WT) or IL-10-deficient mice are infected with *L. monocytogenes,* macrophages serve as the primary host cells and the infection is localized within granulomatous foci. Under these circumstances, systemic cytokine levels remain relatively low (Holscher et al., 2000) and the absence of IL-10 boosts the protective type 1 cytokine response, but not to the extent that it induces damage to host tissues. Thus, depending on the timing and dose, the production of a particular set of cytokines can be either protective or detrimental, and this may be dictated largely by the nature of the host-parasite interaction.

Interestingly, death of *T. gondii*-infected IL-10-deficient mice was prevented by either systemically priming mice with soluble *T. gondii* antigens prior to infection (Reis e Sousa et al., 1999) or simultaneously blocking the CD28-B7- and CD40-CD40L-costimulatory pathways (Villegas et al., 2000). In both situations, the mutant mice mounted impaired type 1 cytokine responses and were protected from infection-induced immunopathology. The production of IL-12 was markedly decreased in the antigen-sensitized IL-10-deficient mice. These findings suggest that the immunoprotective effect of IL-10 in this model is mediated through its ability to regulate the functional activity of dendritic cells or other antigen-presenting cells.

Much has been written about the pathological consequences of excessive proinflammatory cytokine production in malaria (Clark et al., 1981, 1992b; Grau et al., 1987; Kwiatkowski and Perlmann, 1999), and a later section of the chapter will consider this from a clinical perspective. In experimental murine models of malaria, the proinflammatory response may be either protective or pathological, depending on the circumstances. During the pre-erythrocytic stage in the liver, when the parasite burden is relatively low and the infection is clinically asymptomatic, there is evidence that IL-12, IFN-γ, and NO each play an important role in preventing the infection from progressing further (Schofield et al., 1987; Sedegah et al., 1994). Once the parasites invade erythrocytes and grow to large numbers, the

risk-benefit equation is less clear. Although TNF, IL-12, and IFN-γ inhibit blood stage parasites and thereby exert a protective function (Clark et al., 1987b; Stevenson and Ghadirian, 1989; Stevenson et al., 1995), at this stage the cytokine response is systemic and some pathological side effects are perhaps inevitable. The commonest clinical consequence in humans is fever, while life-threatening complications such as profound anemia and cerebral malaria occur in a proportion of infections due to *P. falciparum* but not other *Plasmodium* species. Mice with malaria do not develop fever, but, depending on the specific host-parasite combination, they may develop profound anemia, fatal neurological symptoms, or multiorgan failure, and TNF has been the cytokine most consistently associated with severe pathology in most of these models (Clark et al., 1987a; Grau et al., 1987; Miller et al., 1989). One interpretation is that a strong early proinflammatory cytokine response is protective while a strong late response is pathological (Kwiatkowski, 1995; Taylor-Robinson, 1998).

Recent experimental studies suggest that IL-10 and TGF-β cooperate to down-regulate potentially pathogenic proinflammatory cytokine responses in malaria (Linke et al., 1996; Omer and Riley, 1998). IL-10-deficient mice infected with *P. chabaudi chabaudi* showed increased mortality compared to their normal WT littermates, although peak parasitemias did not differ markedly. Instead, acute infection was characterized by an enhanced type 1 cytokine response (Li et al., 1999). The IFN-γ response was retained in the chronic phase of infection, whereas control mice ultimately developed a dominant type 2 cytokine response. The authors concluded that the susceptibility of IL-10-deficient mice to an otherwise nonlethal infection resulted not from fulminant parasitemia but from a sustained and enhanced proinflammatory cytokine response.

Evidence for a protective role for TGF-β in blood stage infection comes from a murine model of *P. berghei* infection, where susceptible strains of mice showed increased IFN-γ and reduced TGF-β mRNA expression compared to resistant strains (Omer and Riley, 1998). Treatment of infected mice with a neutralizing antibody to TGF-β exacerbated the virulence of *P. berghei* and caused *P. c. chabaudi* infection, which normally resolves spontaneously, to become lethal. Although administration of recombinant TGF-β (rTGF-β) to *P. berghei*-infected mice slowed the parasite proliferation, this was accompanied by a marked decrease in serum TNF-α levels, and it was concluded that the protective effects of this cytokine are due less to parasite growth than to down-regulation of inflammatory responses (Omer et al., 2000). These observations are consistent with the role of TGF-β as an immunosuppressive cytokine. TGF-β was shown to directly induce IL-10 expression in macrophages (Maeda et al., 1995), and it has been proposed that this may explain its protective effects, down-regulating potentially pathogenic type 1 responses in favor of a Th2-type profile (Fig. 2).

BENEFITS AND RISKS OF THE Th2 RESPONSE

Schistosomiasis is caused by one of three major species of helminth parasites, *S. mansoni*, *S. haematobium*, and *S. japonicum*. On infection, adult parasites of *S. mansoni* migrate to the mesenteric veins, where they live for 10 years or more, laying hundreds of eggs per day. Some of the eggs become entrapped in the microvasculature of the liver and, once there, induce a granulomatous response (Wynn and Cheever, 1995). Subsequently, fibrosis and portal hypertension may develop; this is the primary cause of morbidity in infected individuals and in some cases is lethal. Consequently, much of the symptomology of schistosomiasis is attributed to the egg-induced granulomatous inflammatory response and associated pathology (hepatosplenomegaly, portal hypertension, and development of collateral blood circulation through esophageal varices, leading to internal hemorrhage). Thus, schistosomiasis is primarily an immunologic disease, and it has been suggested that "if granuloma formation could be suppressed, particularly in the early stage of the disease, the develop-ment of hepatosplenic disease might be averted" (Warren, 1982).

Nevertheless, while granulomas are widely believed to be detrimental to the infected host, evidence suggests that the egg-induced lesions also serve a requisite host protective function during infection, particularly in *S. mansoni* infections. In chronically infected hosts, schistosome eggs provide a continuous antigenic stimulus for the immune response. If these antigens are not sequestered or neutralized effectively, they can damage host tissues, with the liver being particularly sensitive. In support of this conclusion, T-cell-deprived, nude, SCID, and egg-tolerized mice infected with *S. mansoni* die earlier than do comparably infected, immunologically intact control mice because they are unable to satisfactorily mount a granulomatous response (Cheever and Yap, 1997; Fallon and Dunne, 1999; Fallon et al., 2000b). Widespread microvesicular hepatic damage induced by toxic egg products contributes to the poorer survival of infected immunosuppressed mice.

During granuloma development, the dominant CD4$^+$ T-cell response changes from a Th1 response of short duration to a sustained Th2 response that is most prominent at the height of granulomatous activity. The development of the Th2 response is highly dependent on IL-4; therefore, it was expected that IL-4-deficient mice might develop less severe disease (Wynn and Cheever, 1995). Nevertheless, consistent with the requirement to form granulomas, studies with IL-4-deficient mice indicate that Th2 responses play an essential host-protective role during infection with *S. mansoni* (Brunet et al., 1997; Pearce et al., 1998). Unlike WT mice, which develop a chronic disease when infection intensities are moderate, infected Th2 response-defective C57BL/6 IL-4-deficient mice suffer from an acute disease, which is characterized by cachexia and significant mortality. The primary cause of morbidity in the infected IL-4$^{-/-}$ animals appears to be the formation of numerous nonhemorrhagic lesions on the mucosal surface of the small intestine (Brunet et al., 1997). Little change in hepatic pathology was detected in these mice. Evidence suggests that IL-4 is required for the efficient passage of eggs through the intestinal wall (Fallon et al., 2000a). Consequently, eggs are trapped in the intestine, causing significant intestinal inflammation and ultimately systemic lipopolysaccharide leakage. This, combined with the decreased Th2-type response and the enhanced Th1-type response, results in a marked increase in proinflammatory cytokine expression, which contributes to the significant weight loss and death of the IL-4-deficient mice (Brunet et al., 1997; Fallon et al., 2000a).

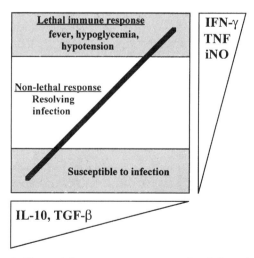

Figure 2. The proinflammatory response, mediated through IFN-γ, TNF-α, and NO, is important for acute resistance to murine malaria infection, but in the absence of IL-10 or TGF-β these responses can induce severe pathology. It is postulated that an early proinflammatory cytokine response mediates protective immunity whereas a late or uncontrolled response contributes to the development of lethal pathology.

These observations suggest that development of the egg-specific Th2 response is required to prevent the deleterious effects of sustained proinflammatory cytokine expression. Indeed, neutralization of TNF-α was shown to significantly delay the onset of severe morbidity in the IL-4-deficient mice (Brunet et al., 1997). Interestingly, IL-10 was recently shown to play a similar role during murine *S. mansoni* infection (Hoffmann et al., 2000). Here, marked increases in IFN-γ, TNF-α, and inducible nitric oxide synthase expression were detected in infected IL-10-deficient mice, and this correlated with significant morbidity and mortality between 8 and 16 weeks postinfection. Even higher mortality was observed in mice exhibiting deficiencies in both IL-4 and IL-10. These animals uniformly died between weeks 7 and 9 postinfection and did so at a rate far exceeding the mortality observed in their single-cytokine-deficient counterparts. The double-cytokine-deficient animals also developed the strongest and most highly polarized Th1-type response, and elevated serum aspartate transaminase levels suggested that mortality was in part attributable to acute hepatotoxicity. Together, these observations demonstrate that IL-4 and IL-10 are both required to prevent Th1 responses from overshooting during infection with *S. mansoni*.

While the studies described above confirm a protective role for Th2-associated cytokines, related studies indicate that they may also contribute to the development of hepatic fibrosis, the primary cause of chronic morbidity in schistosomiasis. Specifically, the Th2-associated cytokine IL-13 was shown to act as the dominant fibrogenic mediator in this disease (Chiaramonte et al., 1999). Indeed, although IL-13 production decreases in infected IL-4-deficient mice, a residual IL-13 response is apparently sufficient to maintain a significant granulomatous and fibrogenic response in the absence of IL-4. Perhaps even more striking was the recent observation that *S. mansoni*-infected IL-13-deficient mice survive longer than WT control animals (Fallon et al., 2000a). These observations confirmed that IL-13 contributes to the morbidity of the infected host. Recombinant IL-13 was shown to stimulate collagen synthesis in fibroblasts; therefore, the detrimental effects of IL-13 may be mediated directly through its profibrogenic activity (Chiaramonte et al., 1999). These results, combined with the findings from IL-4-deficient mice, suggest that IL-4 is host protective while IL-13 is host damaging during murine schistosome infection. This conclusion is supported by recent studies conducted with IL-10- plus IL-12-deficient mice, which develop a highly polarized Th2-type response (Hoffmann et al., 2000). These animals develop 10 times as many parasite-specific IL-4- and IL-13-producing cells than

do similarly infected WT controls, and hepatic fibrosis is consequently increased significantly. The double-cytokine-deficient mice also show significant morbidity and mortality in the chronic stages of the infection. It is important to point out, however, that the pathology found in infected IL-10- plus IL-12-deficient mice is completely distinct from the acute hepatotoxic tissue reaction observed in infected Th1-polarized IL-10- plus IL-4-deficient mice (Hoffmann et al., 2000). Indeed, blood was frequently found in the intestines of moribund or recently deceased IL-10- plus IL-12-deficient mice, suggesting that these animals were developing portal hypertension and collateral blood circulation, which ultimately contributed to their death. These observations demonstrate that IL-10 and IL-12 are both required to prevent the overshooting of Th2 responses during infection with *S. mansoni* (Fig. 3). Thus, in schistosomiasis, distinct but equally detrimental forms of lethal tissue pathology develop when the immune response is biased toward an extreme Th1- or Th2-type phenotype. Therefore, a mixed Th1-Th2 response may provide the best protection from severe egg-induced immunopathology.

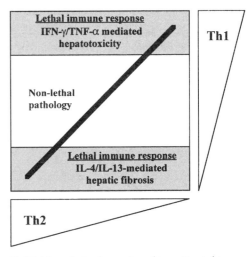

Figure 3. Highly polarized type 1 and type 2 cytokine responses induce distinct but equally detrimental forms of immunopathology in murine schistosomiasis. A mixed Th1-Th2-type cytokine response protects chronically *S. mansoni*-infected mice from the development of lethal egg-induced tissue pathology. Mice deficient in IL-4 and IL-10 develop highly polarized Th1-type cytokine responses following *S. mansoni* infection. Consequently, these mice suffer acute mortality, which is linked to overexpression of the proinflammatory mediators IFN-γ, TNF-α, and inducible NO and the formation of nonfibrotic granulomas. In contrast, mice deficient in IL-12 and IL-10 develop highly polarized Th2-type cytokine responses and show signs of chronic morbidity. These mice form large eosinophil-rich granulomas and develop severe hepatic fibrosis, causing portal hypertension, portal-systemic shunts, and fatal hematemesis.

IMMUNE DEVIATION AS A VACCINE STRATEGY FOR PARASITIC DISEASE

In schistosomiasis, the development of egg-induced hepatic fibrosis can be significantly ameliorated by sensitizing mice to egg antigens in the presence of IL-12 prior to infection (Wynn et al., 1995). These animals develop smaller and less fibrotic granulomas than do control infected mice and show markedly increased Th1-type and decreased Th2-type cytokine expression. Importantly, however, there is no evidence that mortality increases in these mice, even through the chronic stages of infection, despite the establishment of a relatively dominant type 1 cytokine response. Nevertheless, unlike the susceptible Th1-polarized IL-10- plus IL-4-deficient mice, which are incapable of producing IL-10, the egg- and IL-12-sensitized WT mice develop a significantly elevated IL-10 response, which is sustained at least through week 12 postinfection (Wynn et al., 1995). Thus, these findings suggest that the egg- and IL-12-immunized animals benefit from an increased IFN-γ (antifibrotic) and reduced IL-13 (profibrogenic) response but that, perhaps even more importantly, the immunomodulatory activity of IL-10 spares them from the potentially harmful and toxic effects of sustained proinflammatory cytokine production. However, similar IL-12-based immune deviation experiments conducted with IL-10-deficient animals would be needed to confirm this hypothesis. Regardless, these findings suggest that a highly polarized type 1 IFN-γ response, while beneficial in terms of preventing damaging tissue fibrosis, is potentially harmful, particularly if established in an IL-10-deficient setting (Hoffmann et al., 2000). Thus, the coexpression of IL-12 plus IFN-γ and IL-10 would probably provide the best protection from immunopathology in chronic schistosomiasis. This conclusion is in agreement with the poor survival of schistosome-infected IL-10- plus IL-12-deficient mice and is consistent with the pattern of cytokine expression that is often found in chronic infectious disease (Karp et al., 1993; Montenegro et al., 1999; Vanham et al., 1997).

Such approaches, however, need to be tempered with caution. River blindness, caused by the filarial parasite *Onchocerca volvulus*, is also associated with polarized Th2 responses and can be induced in mice following subcutaneous immunization and intracorneal injection of soluble *O. volvulus* antigens (Hall and Pearlman, 1999). The development of corneal pathology is dependent on T cells and IL-4. Indeed, studies in IL-4-deficient mice demonstrated that IL-4 is required for the recruitment of inflammatory cells to the cornea. It was therefore anticipated that administration of rIL-12 would reduce onchocercal keratitis. However, while expression of the Th1 cytokine IFN-γ increased and production of the Th2-associated cytokines IL-4, IL-5, IL-10, and IL-13 decreased in the corneas of the rIL-12-treated mice, corneal pathology actually worsened. Histological examination of the corneas revealed increased neutrophil, eosinophil, and mononuclear cell infiltration into the corneal stroma. Production of several chemotactic factors was augmented in the rIL-12-treated mice, and this was suggested as a possible explanation for the exacerbated pathology (Pearlman et al., 1997).

Thus, while IL-12 exhibits marked beneficial effects on the host by reducing certain types of Th2-driven immunopathology, it remains unclear whether similar immune deviation strategies will be successful for all types of Th2-mediated diseases. Indeed, results from the onchocercal keratitis model clearly demonstrate that polarized Th1-type responses can also trigger serious pathological changes in the cornea. Therefore, while IL-12 could conceivably be used as a form of therapy to modulate immunopathology resulting from established infections, or as part of an "anti-disease" vaccine, the potential to induce pathology on the opposite pole must not be overlooked when designing vaccines based on immune deviation.

INTERACTION OF THE IMMUNE RESPONSE WITH OTHER PATHOPHYSIOLOGICAL PROCESSES

In this section, we use malaria as an example of how the immune response may interact with other physiological processes to cause severe pathology that lacks typical immunological hallmarks such as inflammation or granuloma formation. Malarial infection provokes high levels of TNF and other proinflammatory cytokines (Kwiatkowski et al., 1990; Scuderi et al., 1986), as well as causing markedly elevated immunoglobulin production (Greenwood, 1974), activation of complement (Greenwood and Brueton, 1974), and redistribution of lymphocytes from the peripheral circulation to the spleen and other organs (Hviid et al., 1991). However, the tissues of individuals who die of cerebral malaria or severe malarial anemia show relatively little evidence of inflammation or other immune pathology.

The major pathological finding in cerebral malaria is that *P. falciparum*-infected erythrocytes are sequestered within small cerebral blood vessels. This is due to the ability of this species of parasite to bind endothelial adhesion molecules including CD-36, intercellular cell adhesion molecule 1 (ICAM-1), and

E-selectin (Newbold et al., 1999). Autopsy data indicate that parasites tend to sequester in cerebral blood vessels that express ICAM-1, while children who die of cerebral malaria show markedly elevated TNF levels (Grau et al., 1989; Kwiatkowski et al., 1990; Turner et al., 1994). TNF up-regulates ICAM-1 expression and the cytoadherence of ICAM-1 binding parasite strains to human endothelial cells in vitro (Berendt et al., 1989). Taken together, these observations suggest that high TNF levels may cause high levels of ICAM-1 expression and that if a significant number of the parasites are of the ICAM-1 binding phenotype, this leads to dense parasite sequestration in cerebral blood vessels.

A related phenomenon is observed in BALB/c mice, which develop fatal neurological complications of *P. berghei* ANKA infection. In this model, leukocytes rather than parasitized erythrocytes aggregate in cerebral blood vessels, and this can be prevented by blocking of the TNF pathway (with anti-TNF antibodies or by gene disruption of TNF receptor) or by antibody inhibition of LFA-1, the leukocyte ligand for ICAM-1 (Grau et al., 1987, 1991; Lucas et al., 1997). A recently described variant of the model, using young (BALB/c × C57BL/6)F$_1$ mice, shows parasite sequestration and an intrinsic variability (i.e., only a proportion of the affected animals succumb), which make it more similar to human cerebral malaria (Hearn et al., 2000).

How do the above events lead to the syndrome of cerebral malaria? This is a complex clinical entity whose cardinal features are coma and convulsions but which is often associated with hypoglycemia and lactic acidosis. There is surprisingly little histopathological evidence of inflammatory lesions in the brain, apart from tiny hemorrhages that sometimes form around blood vessels containing sequestered parasites. One hypothesis is that TNF and other inflammatory cytokines lead to the generation of NO, which diffuses into the surrounding brain where it inhibits glutamate-induced calcium entry in postsynaptic neurons, thereby suppressing excitatory neurotransmission such that the individual is effectively anesthetized (Clark et al., 1992a). This would elegantly explain how malaria can cause deep yet transient coma, but the available clinical evidence is conflicting (Al Yaman et al., 1996; Anstey et al., 1996) and the hypothesis remains controversial. It has also been speculated that TNF may contribute to the hypoglycemia which often accompanies cerebral malaria, but this is clearly not the primary cause of the coma in most cases (Brewster et al., 1990; Clark et al., 1997; Krishna et al., 1994; Kwiatkowski et al., 1990). A large proportion of deaths due to cerebral malaria are accompanied by lactic acidosis and

associated respiratory abnormalities (English et al., 1997; Krishna et al., 1994). This is probably multifactorial in origin, with a large component being generalized microcirculatory obstruction due to widespread parasite sequestration, and there is experimental evidence that systemic TNF may act to increase lactate generation (Clark et al., 1997; Krishna et al., 1994). Thus, there are a number of ways in which excessive TNF production may contribute to the clinical syndrome of cerebral malaria, both by promoting the central phenomenon of parasite sequestration and by exacerbating the pathophysiological consequences that follow.

The above observations make TNF an obvious therapeutic target in cerebral malaria, and a randomized double-blind placebo-controlled trial of a murine monoclonal anti-TNF antibody has been conducted with 600 Gambian children with cerebral malaria. The results were disappointing, since the antibody failed to reduce mortality and possibly increased the risk of neurological sequelae (van Hensbroek et al., 1996). There are several potential explanations. The underlying hypothesis may have been entirely wrong or only partly correct; e.g., it may not apply if other mediators are involved. Alternatively, the hypothesis may be correct but the treatment may have been given too late, and perhaps monoclonal antibody is not the best way to inhibit TNF in this clinical context. It is also possible that this result reflects the dual protective and pathological roles of TNF, such that the overall balance of benefits and risks for this particular therapy was unfavorable. We highlight these uncertainties about the therapeutic relevance of TNF in cerebral malaria because they illustrate a much more general problem in proceeding from experimental observation to clinical intervention. As discussed in our concluding section, it is the need for more precise information about the molecular causation of human disease that has led to growing interest in genetic epidemiology as a tool for investigating the role of specific mediators in the disease process.

Severe anemia is another complication of *P. falciparum* malaria. An individual can have both cerebral malaria and severe anemia, but they are entirely distinct disease entities. Anemia appears to predominate when there are constantly high levels of malaria transmission, and cerebral malaria predominates when transmission occurs more sporadically or in seasonal epidemics. This may say something (although it is unclear exactly what) about underlying immunological causes (Snow et al., 1997). Together, these two complications cause 1 million to 2 million deaths annually in African children.

Malaria parasites destroy the erythrocytes that they invade, but this does not adequately account for the profound anemia seen in many infections with low parasite density. Uninfected erythrocytes may be destroyed by antibody- and complement-mediated mechanisms, but, based on disease association studies, this also does not appear to be a major factor in the causation of severe malarial anemia in African children (Abdalla and Weatherall, 1982; Facer et al., 1979).

The spleen enlarges during malarial infection and is thought to play an important role in host defense (Oster et al., 1980); indeed, it is thought that parasite sequestration is an immune evasion strategy to prevent mature parasites from passing through the spleen. Splenic clearance of heat-damaged erythrocytes is increased during malarial infection (Looareesuwan et al., 1987), probably at least in part due to erythrophagocytosis stimulated by high TNF levels (Kitagawa et al., 1996). Transgenic mice in which TNF was constitutively overexpressed developed anemia due to increased clearance of autologous erythrocytes, but they also had an enhanced ability to suppress malaria parasite density when infected with *P. yoelii* or *P. berghei* (Taverne et al., 1994). Taken together, these observations suggest that increased erythrophagocytosis induced by proinflammatory cytokines is a host defensive strategy to maximize the clearance of parasitized erythrocytes but that the survival of uninfected erythrocytes may be reduced in the process.

An additional factor in malarial anemia is reduced production of new erythrocytes, and African children with chronic malaria have marked dyserythropoietic changes in the bone marrow (Abdalla et al., 1980). TNF inhibits proliferation of human erythroid progenitor cells (Roodman et al., 1987), and chronic expression of the human TNF gene in nude mice inhibits erythropoiesis (Johnson et al., 1989). As well as the systemic TNF production that accompanies acute malarial infection, large quantities of malarial pigment are taken up by splenic and bone marrow macrophages, and this may provide a chronic stimulus for TNF production at the site of erythropoiesis (Pichyangkul et al., 1994). Experimental *P. berghei* infection in mice has been reported to reduce the number of erythroid progenitors and erythrocyte iron incorporation, both of which were partially prevented by anti-TNF antibodies (Miller et al., 1989). It is unclear whether the bone marrow-suppressive effects of proinflammatory cytokines serve any biological purpose, although there is some evidence from mathematical models (Gravenor et al., 1995) and experimental studies (Yap and Stevenson, 1994) to suggest that by reducing the supply of erythrocytes, the host might achieve a reduction of the chronic parasite burden.

Thus, in severe anemia, as in cerebral malaria, the proinflammatory response appears to act in concert with various other pathophysiological processes. It has been observed that African children with severe malarial anemia have a significantly depressed plasma IL-10-to-TNF ratio compared to uncomplicated malaria, raising the possibility that IL-10 might be important in suppressing the proinflammatory pathways that lead to severe anemia (Kurtzhals et al., 1998; Othoro et al., 1999). Genetic studies may help resolve this issue since the IL-10 promoter region contains polymorphic variants that are associated with the levels of IL-10 production by peripheral blood mononuclear cells (Turner et al., 1997).

CONCLUSIONS

In this chapter, we have tried to given an overview of some major themes of current research on the immune pathology of parasitic infection. In most cases, the root of the problem is the parasite's resistance to eradication by specific immune mechanisms and the consequent need to attack the infection over a long timescale with a battery of immune responses that risk damaging the host. In recent years much has been learned about the role of the Th1-Th2 system in regulating this response. In this concluding section, we discuss some of the challenges that lie ahead in applying this information to the development of new strategies for the treatment and prevention of parasitic disease in humans.

Clinical and epidemiological studies have identified many immunological features of parasitic disease, but in relatively few cases do we understand precisely which immunological processes are truly necessary or sufficient for clinical disease to occur. This stems from a number of fundamental obstacles. The starting point of most clinical studies is an individual who has already succumbed to the disease, by which time the root cause may be inapparent. The diseased tissues are often impossible to investigate in the living subject: for example, our knowledge of the histopathology of human cerebral malaria is confined to postmortem findings, which may be unrepresentative of what happened before the individual died. The opportunities for experimental therapeutic interventions in humans are limited, not only for ethical reasons but also because of logistical obstacles such as quality control and sample size requirements. For these reasons, experimental models are essential and will become increasingly useful as conditional gene knockouts allow the immunopathological roles of specific mediators to be analyzed in different cell types and at different time points in the evolution of disease.

Although our knowledge of cytokines and other immunological mediators has grown enormously in the last 15 years, the current list is undoubtedly a small fraction of the total number of host molecules involved in the pathogenesis of parasitic disease. This represents a major limitation for experimental models as well as for clinical investigation. The situation will change dramatically as whole-genome sequence data come online: this will generate many new candidate genes, and in the long term it will allow investigators to survey the full range of genes that are expressed in a diseased tissue or by a specific type of immune cell. Microarray expression screening technology is already available for a growing number of known immunological mediators, making it much easier to obtain an overview of patterns of gene expression in immune cells and affected organs and to assess how these patterns vary with time and location as the disease progresses (Hoffmann et al., 2001). Knowing exactly when and where different immunological genes are expressed and how this relates to the stage of the disease will greatly assist efforts to identify efficient targets for drug or vaccine development.

Once causal mechanisms have been established in experimental systems, how can we gauge whether a particular vaccine strategy or immunological intervention is likely to be safe and effective in humans? The issue is not just the difference between mice and humans but also the difference between individuals, since the balance between protective benefits and pathological risks may vary across the wide range of epidemiological contexts in which human disease can occur. This is a fundamental problem for the field of pathogenesis and immunity as a whole, and it has led to growing interest in the use of molecular genetics as a tool for assessing the impact of specific immunological processes in different epidemiological settings. Over 100,000 single-nucleotide polymorphisms have already been identified in humans, and this is probably only 1% of the total (Cargill et al., 1999) (http://snp.cshl.org). By identifying common DNA polymorphisms that alter the regulation or function of candidate genes and by analyzing their association with disease susceptibility, it may be possible to gain a better insight into the genes that are critical for immunity or pathogenesis in different epidemiological settings. For example, polymorphisms of the promoter regions of TNF (Knight et al., 1999; McGuire et al., 1994, 1999) and NOS2 (D. Burgner, W. Xu, K. Rockett, M. Gravenor, I. G. Charles, A. V. Hill, and D. Kwiatkowski, Letter, *Lancet* 352:1193–1194,

1998; J. F. Kun, B. Mordmuller, B. Lell, L. G. Lehman, D. Luckner, and P. G. Kremsner, Letter, *Lancet* 351:265–266, 1998) and the coding regions of ICAM-1 (Fernandez-Reyes et al., 1997) and CD36 (Aitman et al., 2000) have been associated with susceptibility to severe complications of *P. falciparum* malaria in African children, and mucocutaneous leishmaniasis has also been associated with TNF promoter polymorphism (Cabrera et al., 1995). In *S. mansoni* infection, parasite intensity appears to be determined by an unknown genetic factor in the region of chromosome 5 that contains the IL-4, IL-5, and IL-13 genes and several other important immunological genes, while susceptibility to hepatic fibrosis has been linked to a region of chromosome 6 close to an IFN-γ receptor gene (Dessein et al., 1999; Marquet et al., 1996). Most of these observations require further work to establish reproducibility and functional significance, but these are very early days (see chapter 26), and the forthcoming human genomic blueprint, combined with a rapidly enlarging database of human genetic diversity and novel technologies for high-throughput genotyping, is likely to have a profound impact. It has been argued that parasitic infection is one of the major evolutionary driving forces for genetic diversity (Hamilton et al., 1990): if this is true, the next decade will be an exciting time to be investigating the immune pathology of parasitic disease.

REFERENCES

Abbas, A. K., K. M. Murphy, and A. Sher. 1996. Function diversity of helper T lymphocytes. *Nature* 383:787–793.

Abdalla, S., and D. J. Weatherall. 1982. The direct antiglobulin test in *P. falciparum* malaria. *Br. J. Haematol.* 51:415–425.

Abdalla, S., D. J. Weatherall, S. N. Wickramasinghe, and M. Hughes. 1980. The anaemia of *P. falciparum* malaria. *Br. J. Haematol.* 46:171–183.

Aitman, T. J., L. D. Cooper, P. J. Norsworthy, F. N. Wahid, J. K. Gray, B. R. Curtis, P. M. McKeigue, D. Kwiatkowski, B. M. Greenwood, R. W. Snow, A. V. Hill, and J. Scott. 2000. Malaria susceptibility and CD36 mutation. *Nature* 405:1015–1016.

Al Yaman, F. M., D. Mokela, B. Genton, K. A. Rockett, M. P. Alpers, and I. A. Clark. 1996. Association between serum levels of reactive nitrogen intermediates and coma in children with cerebral malaria in Papua New Guinea. *Trans. R. Soc. Trop. Med. Hyg.* 90:270–273.

Anstey, N. M., J. B. Weinberg, M. Y. Hassanali, E. D. Mwaikambo, D. Manyenga, M. A. Misukonis, D. R. Arnelle, D. Hollis, M. I. McDonald, and D. L. Granger. 1996. Nitric oxide in Tanzanian children with malaria: inverse relationship between malaria severity and nitric oxide production/nitric oxide synthase type 2 expression. *J. Exp. Med.* 184:557–567.

Berendt, A. R., D. L. Simmons, J. Tansey, C. I. Newbold, and K. Marsh. 1989. Intercellular adhesion molecule-1 is an endothelial cell adhesion receptor for *Plasmodium falciparum*. *Nature* 341:57–59.

Berkley, J., S. Mwarumba, K. Bramham, B. Lowe, and K. Marsh. 1999. Bacteraemia complicating severe malaria in children. *Trans. R. Soc. Trop. Med. Hyg.* 93:283–286.

Brewster, D. R., D. Kwiatkowski, and N. J. White. 1990. Neurological sequelae of cerebral malaria in children. *Lancet* 336: 1039–1043.

Brunet, L. R., F. D. Finkelman, A. W. Cheever, M. A. Kopf, and E. J. Pearce. 1997. IL-4 protects against TNF-alpha-mediated cachexia and death during acute schistosomiasis. *J. Immunol.* 159:777–785.

Cabrera, M., M. A. Shaw, C. Sharples, H. Williams, M. Castes, J. Convit, and J. M. Blackwell. 1995. Polymorphism in tumor necrosis factor genes associated with mucocutaneous leishmaniasis. *J. Exp. Med.* 182:1259–1264.

Cargill, M., D. Altshuler, J. Ireland, P. Sklar, K. Ardlie, N. Patil, N. Shaw, C. R. Lane, E. P. Lim, N. Kalyanaraman, J. Nemesh, L. Ziaugra, L. Friedland, A. Rolfe, J. Warrington, R. Lipshutz, G. Q. Daley, and E. S. Lander. 1999. Characterization of single-nucleotide polymorphisms in coding regions of human genes. *Nat. Genet.* 22:231–238. (Erratum, 23:373, 1999.)

Cheever, A. W., and G. S. Yap. 1997. Immunologic basis of disease and disease regulation in schistosomiasis. *Chem. Immunol.* 66:159–176.

Chiaramonte, M. G., D. D. Donaldson, A. W. Cheever, and T. A. Wynn. 1999. An IL-13 inhibitor blocks the development of hepatic fibrosis during a T-helper type 2-dominated inflammatory response. *J. Clin. Investig.* 104:777–785.

Clark, I. A., F. M. al Yaman, and L. S. Jacobson. 1997. The biological basis of malarial disease. *Int. J. Parasitol.* 27:1237–1249.

Clark, I. A., W. B. Cowden, G. A. Butcher, and N. H. Hunt. 1987a. Possible roles of tumor necrosis factor in the pathology of malaria. *Am. J. Pathol.* 129:192–199.

Clark, I. A., N. H. Hunt, G. A. Butcher, and W. B. Cowden. 1987b. Inhibition of murine malaria (*Plasmodium chabaudi*) in vivo by recombinant interferon-gamma or tumor necrosis factor, and its enhancement by butylated hydroxyanisole. *J. Immunol.* 139:3493–3496.

Clark, I. A., K. A. Rockett, and W. B. Cowden. 1992a. Possible central role of nitric oxide in conditions clinically similar to cerebral malaria. *Lancet* 340:894–896.

Clark, I. A., K. A. Rockett, and W. B. Cowden. 1992b. *TNF in Malaria.* Raven Press, New York, N.Y.

Clark, I. A., J. L. Virelizier, E. A. Carswell, and P. R. Wood. 1981. Possible importance of macrophage-derived mediators in acute malaria. *Infect. Immun.* 32:1058–1066.

Dai, W. J., G. Kohler, and F. Brombacher. 1997. Both innate and acquired immunity to *Listeria monocytogenes* infection are increased in IL-10-deficient mice. *J. Immunol.* 158:2259–2267.

Dessein, A. J., D. Hillaire, N. E. Elwali, S. Marquet, Q. Mohamed-Ali, A. Mirghani, S. Henri, A. A. Abdelhameed, O. K. Saeed, M. M. Magzoub, and L. Abel. 1999. Severe hepatic fibrosis in *Schistosoma mansoni* infection is controlled by a major locus that is closely linked to the interferon-gamma receptor gene. *Am. J. Hum. Genet.* 65:709–721.

English, M., R. Sauerwein, C. Waruiru, M. Mosobo, J. Obiero, B. Lowe, and K. Marsh. 1997. Acidosis in severe childhood malaria. *Q. J. Med.* 90:263–270.

Facer, C. A., R. S. Bray, and J. Brown. 1979. Direct Coombs antiglobulin reactions in Gambian children with *Plasmodium falciparum* malaria. I. Incidence and class specificity. *Clin. Exp. Immunol.* 35:119–127.

Fallon, P. G., and D. W. Dunne. 1999. Tolerization of mice to *Schistosoma mansoni* egg antigens causes elevated type 1 and diminished type 2 cytokine responses and increased mortality in acute infection. *J. Immunol.* 162:4122–4132.

Fallon, P. G., E. J. Richardson, G. J. McKenzie, and A. N. McKenzie. 2000a. Schistosome infection of transgenic mice defines distinct and contrasting pathogenic roles for IL-4 and IL-13: IL-13 is a profibrotic agent. *J. Immunol.* 164:2585–2591.

Fallon, P. G., E. J. Richardson, P. Smith, and D. W. Dunne. 2000b. Elevated type 1, diminished type 2 cytokines and impaired antibody response are associated with hepatotoxicity and mortalities during Schistosoma mansoni infection of CD4-depleted mice. *Eur. J. Immunol.* 30:470–480.

Fernandez-Reyes, D., A. G. Craig, S. A. Kyes, N. Peshu, R. W. Snow, A. R. Berendt, K. Marsh, and C. I. Newbold. 1997. A high frequency African coding polymorphism in the N-terminal domain of ICAM-1 predisposing to cerebral malaria in Kenya. *Hum. Mol. Genet.* 6:1357–1360.

Gazzinelli, R. T., M. Wysocka, S. Hieny, T. Scharton-Kersten, A. Cheever, R. Kuhn, W. Muller, G. Trinchieri, and A. Sher. 1996. In the absence of endogenous IL-10, mice acutely infected with *Toxoplasma gondii* succumb to a lethal immune response dependent on CD4+ T cells and accompanied by overproduction of IL-12, IFN-gamma and TNF-alpha. *J. Immunol.* 157:798–805.

Grau, G. E., L. F. Fajardo, P. F. Piguet, B. Allet, P. H. Lambert, and P. Vassalli. 1987. Tumor necrosis factor (cachectin) as an essential mediator in murine cerebral malaria. *Science* 237: 1210–1212.

Grau, G. E., P. Pointaire, P. F. Piguet, C. Vesin, H. Rosen, I. Stamenkovic, F. Takei, and P. Vassalli. 1991. Late administration of monoclonal antibody to leukocyte function-antigen 1 abrogates incipient murine cerebral malaria. *Eur. J. Immunol.* 21: 2265–2267.

Grau, G. E., T. E. Taylor, M. E. Molyneux, J. J. Wirima, P. Vassalli, M. Hommel, and P. H. Lambert. 1989. Tumor necrosis factor and disease severity in children with falciparum malaria. *N. Engl. J. Med.* 320:1586–1591.

Gravenor, M. B., A. R. McLean, and D. Kwiatkowski. 1995. The regulation of malaria parasitaemia; parameter estimates for a population model. *Parasitology* 110:115–122.

Greenwood, B. M. 1974. Possible role of a B-cell mitogen in hypergammaglobulinaemia in malaria and trypanosomiasis. *Lancet* i:435–436.

Greenwood, B. M., and M. J. Brueton. 1974. Complement activation in children with acute malaria. *Clin. Exp. Immunol.* 18: 267–272.

Hall, L. R., and E. Pearlman. 1999. Pathogenesis of onchocercal keratitis (river blindness). *Clin. Microbiol. Rev.* 12:445–453.

Hamilton, W. D., R. Axelrod, and R. Tanese. 1990. Sexual reproduction as an adaptation to resist parasites. *Proc. Natl. Acad. Sci. USA* 87:3566–3573.

Hearn, J., N. Rayment, D. N. Landon, D. R. Katz, and J. B. de Souza. 2000. Immunopathology of cerebral malaria: morphological evidence of parasite sequestration in murine brain microvasculature. *Infect. Immun.* 68:5364–5376.

Heinzel, F. P., M. D. Sadick, B. J. Holaday, R. L. Coffman, and R. M. Locksley. 1989. Reciprocal expression of interferon gamma or interleukin 4 during the resolution or progression of murine leishmaniasis. Evidence for expansion of distinct helper T cell subsets. *J. Exp. Med.* 169:59–72.

Hoffmann, K. F., A. W. Cheever, and T. A. Wynn. 2000. IL-10 and the dangers of immune polarization: excessive type 1 and type 2 cytokine responses induce distinct forms of lethal immunopathology in murine schistosomiasis. *J. Immunol.* 164: 6406–6416.

Hoffmann, K. F., T. C. McCarty, D. H. Segal, M. G. Chiaramonte, M. Hesse, E. M. Davis, A. W. Cheever, P. S. Meltzer, H. C. Morse III, and T. A. Wynn. Disease fingerprinting with cDNA microarrays reveals distinct gene expression profiles in lethal type-1 and type-2 cytokine-mediated inflammatory reactions. *FASEB J.*, in press.

Holaday, B. J., M. M. Pompeu, S. Jeronimo, M. J. Texeira, A. de Sousa, A. W. Vasconcelos, R. D. Pearson, J. S. Abrams, and R. M. Locksley. 1993. Potential role for interleukin-10 in the immunosuppression associated with kala azar. *J. Clin. Investig.* 92:2626–2632.

Holscher, C., M. Mohrs, W. J. Dai, G. Kohler, B. Ryffel, G. A. Schaub, H. Mossmann, and F. Brombacher. 2000. Tumor necrosis factor alpha-mediated toxic shock in *Trypanosoma cruzi*-infected interleukin 10-deficient mice. *Infect. Immun.* 68:4075–4083.

Hunter, C. A., L. A. Ellis-Neyes, T. Slifer, S. Kanaly, G. Grunig, M. Fort, D. Rennick, and F. C. Araujo. 1997. IL-10 is required to prevent immune hyperactivity during infection with *Trypanosoma cruzi*. *J. Immunol.* 158:3311–3316.

Hviid, L., T. G. Theander, N. H. Abdulhadi, Y. A. Abu-Zeid, R. A. Bayoumi, and J. B. Jensen. 1991. Transient depletion of T cells with high LFA-1 expression from peripheral circulation during acute *Plasmodium falciparum* malaria. *Eur. J. Immunol.* 21:1249–1253.

Infante-Duarte, C., and T. Kamradt. 1999. Th1/Th2 balance in infection. *Springer Semin. Immunopathol.* 21:317–338.

Johnson, R. A., T. A. Waddelow, J. Caro, A. Oliff, and G. D. Roodman. 1989. Chronic exposure to tumor necrosis factor in vivo preferentially inhibits erythropoiesis in nude mice. *Blood* 74:130–138.

Karp, C. L., S. H. el-Safi, T. A. Wynn, M. M. Satti, A. M. Kordofani, F. A. Hashim, M. Hag-Ali, F. A. Neva, T. B. Nutman, and D. L. Sacks. 1993. In vivo cytokine profiles in patients with kala-azar. Marked elevation of both interleukin-10 and interferon-gamma. *J. Clin. Investig.* 91:1644–1648.

Kitagawa, S., A. Yuo, M. Yagisawa, E. Azuma, M. Yoshida, Y. Furukawa, M. Takahashi, J. Masuyama, and F. Takaku. 1996. Activation of human monocyte functions by tumor necrosis factor: rapid priming for enhanced release of superoxide and erythrophagocytosis, but no direct triggering of superoxide release. *Exp. Hematol.* 24:559–567.

Knight, J. C., I. Udalova, A. V. Hill, B. M. Greenwood, N. Peshu, K. Marsh, and D. Kwiatkowski. 1999. A polymorphism that affects OCT-1 binding to the TNF promoter region is associated with severe malaria. *Nat. Genet.* 22:145–150.

Krishna, S., D. W. Waller, F. ter Kuile, D. Kwiatkowski, J. Crawley, C. F. Craddock, F. Nosten, D. Chapman, D. Brewster, P. A. Holloway, et al. 1994. Lactic acidosis and hypoglycemia in children with severe malaria: pathophysiological and prognostic significance. *Trans. R. Soc. Trop. Med. Hyg.* 88:67–73.

Kurtzhals, J. A., V. Adabayeri, B. Q. Goka, B. D. Akanmori, J. O. Oliver-Commey, F. K. Nkrumah, C. Behr, and L. Hviid. 1998. Low plasma concentrations of interleukin 10 in severe malarial anaemia compared with cerebral and uncomplicated malaria. *Lancet* 351:1768–1772. (Errata, 352:242, 1998, and 353:848, 1999.)

Kwiatkowski, D. 1995. Malarial toxins and the regulation of parasite density. *Parasitol. Today* 11:206–212.

Kwiatkowski, D., A. V. Hill, I. Sambou, P. Twumasi, J. Castracane, K. R. Manogue, A. Cerami, D. R. Brewster, and B. M. Greenwood. 1990. TNF concentration in fatal cerebral, nonfatal cerebral, and uncomplicated *Plasmodium falciparum* malaria. *Lancet* 336:1201–1204.

Kwiatkowski, D., and P. Perlmann. 1999. *Inflammatory Processes in the Pathogenesis of Malaria.* Harwood Academic Publishers.

Li, C., I. Corraliza, and J. Langhorne. 1999. A defect in interleukin-10 leads to enhanced malarial disease in *Plasmodium chabaudi* chabaudi infection in mice. *Infect. Immun.* 67:4435–4442.

Linke, A., R. Kuhn, W. Muller, N. Honarvar, C. Li, and J. Langhorne. 1996. *Plasmodium chabaudi chabaudi*: differential susceptibility of gene-targeted mice deficient in IL-10 to an erythrocytic-stage infection. *Exp. Parasitol.* 84:253–263.

Looareesuwan, S., M. Ho, Y. Wattanagoon, N. J. White, D. A. Warrell, D. Bunnag, T. Harinasuta, and D. J. Wyler. 1987. Dynamic alteration in splenic function during acute falciparum malaria. *N. Engl. J. Med.* 317:675–679.

Lucas, R., P. Juillard, E. Decoster, M. Redard, D. Burger, Y. Donati, C. Giroud, C. Monso-Hinard, T. De Kesel, W. A. Buurman, M. W. Moore, J. M. Dayer, W. Fiers, H. Bluethmann, and G. E. Grau. 1997. Crucial role of tumor necrosis factor (TNF) receptor 2 and membrane-bound TNF in experimental cerebral malaria. *Eur. J. Immunol.* 27:1719–1725.

Luxemburger, C., F. Ricci, F. Nosten, D. Raimond, S. Bathet, and N. J. White. 1997. The epidemiology of severe malaria in an area of low transmission in Thailand. *Trans. R. Soc. Trop. Med. Hyg.* 91:256–262.

Maeda, H., H. Kuwahara, Y. Ichimura, M. Ohtsuki, S. Kurakata, and A. Shiraishi. 1995. TGF-beta enhances macrophage ability to produce IL-10 in normal and tumor-bearing mice. *J. Immunol.* 155:4926–4932.

Marquet, S., L. Abel, D. Hillaire, H. Dessein, J. Kalil, J. Feingold, J. Weissenbach, and A. J. Dessein. 1996. Genetic localization of a locus controlling the intensity of infection by *Schistosoma mansoni* on chromosome 5q31-q33. *Nat. Genet.* 14:181–184.

McGuire, W., A. V. Hill, C. E. Allsopp, B. M. Greenwood, and D. Kwiatkowski. 1994. Variation in the TNF-alpha promoter region associated with susceptibility to cerebral malaria. *Nature* 371:508–510.

McGuire, W., J. C. Knight, A. V. Hill, C. E. Allsopp, B. M. Greenwood, and D. Kwiatkowski. 1999. Severe malarial anemia and cerebral malaria are associated with different tumor necrosis factor promoter alleles. *J. Infect. Dis.* 179:287–290.

Miller, K. L., P. H. Silverman, B. Kullgren, and L. J. Mahlmann. 1989. Tumor necrosis factor alpha and the anemia associated with murine malaria. *Infect. Immun.* 57:1542–1546.

Montenegro, S. M., P. Miranda, S. Mahanty, F. G. Abath, K. M. Teixeira, E. M. Coutinho, J. Brinkman, I. Goncalves, L. A. Domingues, A. L. Domingues, A. Sher, and T. A. Wynn. 1999. Cytokine production in acute versus chronic human schistosomiasis mansoni: the cross-regulatory role of interferon-gamma and interleukin-10 in the responses of peripheral blood mononuclear cells and splenocytes to parasite antigens. *J. Infect. Dis.* 179:1502–1514.

Newbold, C., A. Craig, S. Kyes, A. Rowe, D. Fernandez-Reyes, and T. Fagan. 1999. Cytoadherence, pathogenesis and the infected red cell surface in *Plasmodium falciparum*. *Int. J. Parasitol.* 29:927–937.

Omer, F. M., J. A. Kurtzhals, and E. M. Riley. 2000. Maintaining the immunological balance in parasitic infections: a role for TGF-beta? *Parasitol. Today* 16:18–23.

Omer, F. M., and E. M. Riley. 1998. Transforming growth factor beta production is inversely correlated with severity of murine malaria infection. *J. Exp. Med.* 188:39–48.

Oster, C. N., L. C. Koontz, and D. J. Wyler. 1980. Malaria in asplenic mice: effects of splenectomy, congenital asplenia, and splenic reconstitution on the course of infection. *Am. J. Trop. Med. Hyg.* 29:1138–1142.

Othoro, C., A. A. Lal, B. Nahlen, D. Koech, A. S. Orago, and V. Udhayakumar. 1999. A low interleukin-10 tumor necrosis factor-alpha ratio is associated with malaria anemia in children residing in a holoendemic malaria region in western Kenya. *J. Infect. Dis.* 179:279–282.

Ottesen, E. A. 1995. Immune responsiveness and the pathogenesis of human onchocerciasis. *J. Infect. Dis.* 171:659–671.

Pearce, E. J., A. La Flamme, E. Sabin, and L. R. Brunet. 1998. The initiation and function of Th2 responses during infection with *Schistosoma mansoni*. *Adv. Exp. Med. Biol.* **452**:67–73.

Pearlman, E., J. H. Lass, D. S. Bardenstein, E. Diaconu, F. E. Hazlett, Jr., J. Albright, A. W. Higgins, and J. W. Kazura. 1997. IL-12 exacerbates helminth-mediated corneal pathology by augmenting inflammatory cell recruitment and chemokine expression. *J. Immunol.* **158**:827–833.

Pichyangkul, S., P. Saengkrai, and H. K. Webster. 1994. *Plasmodium falciparum* pigment induces monocytes to release high levels of tumor necrosis factor-alpha and interleukin-1 beta. *Am. J. Trop. Med. Hyg.* **51**:430–435.

Reis e Sousa, C., G. Yap, O. Schulz, N. Rogers, M. Schito, J. Aliberti, S. Hieny, and A. Sher. 1999. Paralysis of dendritic cell IL-12 production by microbial products prevents infection-induced immunopathology. *Immunity* **11**:637–647.

Roodman, G. D., A. Bird, D. Hutzler, and W. Montgomery. 1987. Tumor necrosis factor-alpha and hematopoietic progenitors: effects of tumor necrosis factor on the growth of erythroid progenitors CFU-E and BFU-E and the hematopoietic cell lines K562, HL60, and HEL cells. *Exp. Hematol.* **15**:928–935.

Schofield, L., J. Villaquiran, A. Ferreira, H. Schellekens, R. Nussenzweig, and V. Nussenzweig. 1987. Gamma interferon, CD8+ T cells and antibodies required for immunity to malaria sporozoites. *Nature* **330**:664–666.

Scott, P., P. Natovitz, R. L. Coffman, E. Pearce, and A. Sher. 1988. Immunoregulation of cutaneous leishmaniasis. T cell lines that transfer protective immunity or exacerbation belong to different T helper subsets and respond to distinct parasite antigens. *J. Exp. Med.* **168**:1675–1684.

Scuderi, P., K. E. Sterling, K. S. Lam, P. R. Finley, K. J. Ryan, C. G. Ray, E. Petersen, D. J. Slymen, and S. E. Salmon. 1986. Raised serum levels of tumour necrosis factor in parasitic infections. *Lancet* **ii**:1364–1365.

Sedegah, M., F. Finkelman, and S. L. Hoffman. 1994. Interleukin 12 induction of interferon gamma-dependent protection against malaria. *Proc. Natl. Acad. Sci. USA* **91**:10700–10702.

Snow, R. W., J. A. Omumbo, B. Lowe, C. S. Molyneux, J. O. Obiero, A. Palmer, M. W. Weber, M. Pinder, B. Nahlen, C. Obonyo, C. Newbold, S. Gupta, and K. Marsh. 1997. Relation between severe malaria morbidity in children and level of *Plasmodium falciparum* transmission in Africa. *Lancet* **349**:1650–1654.

Stevenson, M. M., and E. Ghadirian. 1989. Human recombinant tumor necrosis factor alpha protects susceptible A/J mice against lethal *Plasmodium chabaudi* AS infection. *Infect. Immun.* **57**:3936–3939.

Stevenson, M. M., M. F. Tam, S. F. Wolf, and A. Sher. 1995. IL-12-induced protection against blood-stage *Plasmodium chabaudi* AS requires IFN-gamma and TNF-alpha and occurs via a nitric oxide-dependent mechanism. *J. Immunol.* **155**:2545–2556.

Suzuki, Y., A. Sher, G. Yap, D. Park, L. E. Neyer, O. Liesenfeld, M. Fort, H. Kang, and E. Gufwoli. 2000. IL-10 is required for prevention of necrosis in the small intestine and mortality in both genetically resistant BALB/c and susceptible C57BL/6 mice following peroral infection with *Toxoplasma gondii*. *J. Immunol.* **164**:5375–5382.

Taverne, J., N. Sheikh, J. B. de Souza, J. H. Playfair, L. Probert, and G. Kollias. 1994. Anaemia and resistance to malaria in transgenic mice expressing human tumour necrosis factor. *Immunology* **82**:397–403.

Taylor-Robinson, A. W. 1998. Immunoregulation of malarial infection: balancing the vices and virtues. *Int. J. Parasitol.* **28**:135–148.

Turner, D. M., D. M. Williams, D. Sankaran, M. Lazarus, P. J. Sinnott, and I. V. Hutchinson. 1997. An investigation of polymorphism in the interleukin-10 gene promoter. *Eur. J. Immunogenet.* **24**:1–8.

Turner, G. D., H. Morrison, M. Jones, T. M. Davis, S. Looareesuwan, I. D. Buley, K. C. Gatter, C. I. Newbold, S. Pukritayakamee, B. Nagachinta, et al. 1994. An immunohistochemical study of the pathology of fatal malaria. Evidence for widespread endothelial activation and a potential role for intercellular adhesion molecule-1 in cerebral sequestration. *Am. J. Pathol.* **145**:1057–1069.

Vanham, G., Z. Toossi, C. S. Hirsch, R. S. Wallis, S. K. Schwander, E. A. Rich, and J. J. Ellner. 1997. Examining a paradox in the pathogenesis of human pulmonary tuberculosis: immune activation and suppression/anergy. *Tubercle Lung Dis.* **78**:145–158.

van Hensbroek, M. B., A. Palmer, E. Onyiorah, G. Schneider, S. Jaffar, G. Dolan, H. Memming, J. Frenkel, G. Enwere, S. Bennett, D. Kwiatkowski, and B. Greenwood. 1996. The effect of a monoclonal antibody to tumor necrosis factor on survival from childhood cerebral malaria. *J. Infect. Dis.* **174**:1091–1097.

Villegas, E. N., U. Wille, L. Craig, P. S. Linsley, D. M. Rennick, R. Peach, and C. A. Hunter. 2000. Blockade of costimulation prevents infection-induced immunopathology in interleukin-10-deficient mice. *Infect. Immun.* **68**:2837–2844.

Warren, K. W. 1982. The secret of the immunopathogenesis of schistosomiasis: in vivo models. *Immunol. Rev.* **61**:189–213.

Wills-Karp, M. 1999. Immunologic basis of antigen-induced airway hyperresponsiveness. *Annu. Rev. Immunol.* **17**:255–281.

Wynn, T. A., and A. W. Cheever. 1995. Cytokine regulation of granuloma formation in schistosomiasis. *Curr. Opin. Immunol.* **7**:505–511.

Wynn, T. A., A. W. Cheever, D. Jankovic, R. W. Poindexter, P. Caspar, F. A. Lewis, and A. Sher. 1995. An IL-12-based vaccination method for preventing fibrosis induced by schistosome infection. *Nature* **376**:594–596.

Yap, G. S., and A. Sher. 1999. Cell-mediated immunity to *Toxoplasma gondii*: initiation, regulation and effector function. *Immunobiology* **201**:240–247.

Yap, G. S., and M. M. Stevenson. 1994. Blood transfusion alters the course and outcome of *Plasmodium chabaudi* AS infection in mice. *Infect. Immun.* **62**:3761–3765.

Immunology of Infectious Diseases
Edited by S. H. E. Kaufmann, A. Sher, and R. Ahmed
© 2002 ASM Press, Washington, D.C.

Chapter 22

Pathology and Pathogenesis of Virus Infections

SHAWN P. O'NEIL, WUN-JU SHIEH, AND SHERIF R. ZAKI

Viruses have been responsible for some of the great scourges that have occurred throughout the course of human history, ranging from such afflictions as smallpox and rabies, recognized since ancient times, to more modern outbreaks, like the current human immunodeficiency virus (HIV) pandemic. Viral pathogens are also among the most feared of the etiologic agents responsible for emerging infectious diseases, including Ebola hemorrhagic fever, Rift Valley fever, hantavirus pulmonary syndrome, and Nipah virus infection, and also cause human and animal diseases of great economic importance, like influenza and foot-and-mouth disease.

An understanding of viral pathogenesis requires knowledge of the anatomy and physiology of the surfaces that serve as portals of virus entry into the host, as well as an appreciation of the innate and specific antimicrobial protection mechanisms that are present at the interfaces between the host and its environment. We will begin this chapter by reviewing the cycle of virus infection, paying particular attention to the anatomic and physiologic defense mechanisms that are situated at each of the common portals of virus entry. The concepts of cell and tissue tropism are also central to an understanding of viral pathogenesis, since the lesions and, subsequently, the clinical features resulting from viral infections typically reflect the cellular and tissue localization of these obligate intracellular parasites. Thus, examples of viral receptors and attachment proteins will be introduced throughout this discussion as well. We will conclude with a discussion of virus-induced cellular injury, with emphasis on morphologic features of infection, followed by an organ system-based presentation of virologic syndromes.

INFECTION AND TRANSMISSION

Viral Reservoirs

As obligate intracellular parasites, viruses must establish and maintain infection in an animal or insect reservoir in order to survive (Table 1) (Fraenkel-Conrat et al., 1988; Nathanson, 1996). In some instances, the reservoir and host species are the same; for example, many viral pathogens of humans are maintained exclusively in human populations, without an extrinsic animal reservoir. Viruses that are typically cleared following acute infection (e.g., measles) are maintained by continuous transmission from acutely infected "reservoir" hosts to immunologically naïve hosts, which demands a large population with a steady supply of susceptible individuals (e.g., children). Alternatively, viruses may be maintained within a species by establishing persistent infection, followed by either continuous shedding, as is the case for chronic infections like HIV, or periodic shedding, as occurs during reactivation of latent herpes simplex virus or Epstein-Barr virus (EBV) infections.

Some human viral pathogens are maintained in nature in wild- or domestic-animal reservoirs with or without an arthropod vector. Arthropod-borne viruses (arboviruses) are transmitted to a vertebrate reservoir species during a blood meal by an arthropod vector, usually a mosquito or tick. After undergoing mandatory maturation and amplification in the arthropod vector, the virus is introduced into the subcutaneous tissues of the vertebrate host as the arthropod feeds. Once in the vertebrate host, the virus often undergoes amplification, which facilitates infection of additional arthropods (Fenner et al., 1987; Weaver, 1997).

Shawn P. O'Neil • Division of Microbiology and Immunology, Yerkes Regional Primate Research Center, Emory University School of Medicine, Atlanta, GA 30329.   **Wun-Ju Shieh** • Infectious Disease Pathology Activity, Division of Viral and Rickettsial Diseases, National Center for Infectious Diseases, Centers for Disease Control and Prevention, 1600 Clifton Road, N.E., Mail Stop G-32, Atlanta, GA 30333.   **Sherif R. Zaki** • Infectious Disease Pathology, National Center for Infectious Diseases, Centers for Disease Control and Prevention, 1600 Clifton Road, N.E., Mail Stop G-32, Atlanta, GA 30345.

Table 1. Natural reservoirs of selected human viral pathogens

Agent	Virus family	Natural reservoir	Arthropod vector	Host(s)
Influenza viruses	*Orthomyxoviridae*	Birds, pigs	None	Humans, horses
Rabies virus	*Rhabdoviridae*	Wild mammals and birds	None	All warm-blooded animals
EBV	*Herpesviridae*	Humans	None	Humans
Measles virus	*Paramyxoviridae*	Humans	None	Humans
EEE virus	*Togaviridae*	Passerine birds	Mosquito	Humans, horses, pheasants
HIV-1, HIV-2	*Retroviridae*	Old World monkeys and apes	None	Humans

In many instances, members of the natural reservoir species suffer little or no pathogenic consequence as a result of infection, whereas infection of humans or other "accidental" hosts can result in disease. Eastern equine encephalitis (EEE) virus, an alphavirus, produces an asymptomatic infection in passerine birds; however, occasional mosquito-borne transmission to people or horses can result in severe encephalitis (Johnston and Peters, 1996). Chimpanzees and sooty mangabey monkeys are among several species of Old World nonhuman primates that serve as natural reservoirs for simian immunodeficiency viruses (SIV) (Color Plate 5, row 1, left). Despite persistent viremia, these adapted hosts suffer no pathogenic consequences of infection; however, zoonotic transmission of SIV from chimpanzees to nonadapted human hosts in West Equatorial Africa is believed to have spawned the HIV pandemic (Hahn et al., 2000). Fatal infection of accidental wildlife hosts can sometimes facilitate the diagnosis of an outbreak, as recently demonstrated during an outbreak of West Nile virus encephalitis in New York (Shieh et al., 2000). Fatal infection of crows and other birds implicated West Nile virus as the causative agent of the outbreak rather than the closely related flavivirus, St. Louis encephalitis virus.

Virus Entry

The primary routes that viruses use to initiate infection in mammalian hosts include the skin and mucous membranes, the conjunctiva, and the mucosal surfaces of the alimentary, respiratory, and urogenital tracts (Mims et al., 2001). Each of these "external" surfaces is protected by a specialized epithelium that possesses physical, chemical, and immunological properties designed to provide protection against invasion by pathogenic microbes. Nevertheless, viruses have evolved mechanisms for initiating infection at or across each of these surfaces (Table 2). In most instances, the initial stages of viral infection are asymptomatic and produce neither

gross nor microscopic lesions that are of any consequence.

To initiate infection, viruses must first adsorb to target cells in the face of the host's innate and virus-specific defense mechanisms. To increase the efficiency of adsorption, viruses have evolved envelope or capsid attachment proteins that establish high-affinity interactions with viral receptors, molecules located on the surface of target cells (Table 3) (Knipe, 1996; Tyler and Fields, 1996; Holmes, 1997). Virus receptors are cellular surface proteins, carbohydrates, or glycolipids that have normal cellular functions as receptors or ligands for biologically active proteins. Some viruses, like HIV-1 and herpes simplex virus, use multiple receptor molecules to accomplish adsorption and entry (Doms and Peiper, 1997; Rajcani and Vojvodova, 1998; Campadelli-Fiume et al., 2000). The specific interaction between virus attachment proteins and virus receptors accounts for the species specificity, cell tropism, and tissue tropism of any given virus.

Skin and mucous membranes

Viruses that enter the host through the skin must overcome several physical and chemical barriers to initiate infection. The surface of the skin is dry and acidic, due to fatty acids that are present in oils secreted by sebaceous glands and to metabolites produced by the commensal microflora that inhabit the skin surface (Mims et al., 2001). The skin is composed of a multilayered epidermis and a subjacent dermis. The outermost component of the epidermis, the stratum corneum, consists of a highly organized layer of dead, keratinized cells, which provide a tough external barrier while being devoid of the cellular machinery necessary for viral replication (Monteiro-Riviere, 1998).

Many viruses bypass the skin's protective surface by initiating infection through macroscopic or microscopic breaks in the epidermis, which occur as the result of trauma. This provides access to the viable

Table 2. Routes and methods of viral infection

Route of infection	Method of infection	Selected examples	
		Virus family	Virus
Skin	Contact	*Poxviridae*	Variola (smallpox) virus
	Insect bite	*Togaviridae*	EEE virus
	Animal bite	*Rhabdoviridae*	Rabies virus
	Iatrogenic	*Hepadnaviridae*	Hepatitis B virus
Conjunctiva	Contact	*Adenoviridae*	Adenoviruses
Respiratory tract	Inhalation	*Orthomyxoviridae*	Influenza viruses
Gastrointestinal tract	Ingestion	*Reoviridae*	Rotavirus
Urogenital tract	Sexual intercourse	*Retroviridae*	HIV

and mitotically active keratinocytes in the stratum germinativum, the basilar layer of the epidermis, as well as to phagocytes, fibroblasts, and other cells in the dermis and subcutis. Viruses that replicate locally in the stratum germinativum include papillomaviruses, alphaherpesviruses (e.g., herpes simplex viruses), and certain poxviruses (e.g., molluscum contagiosum virus) (Tyler and Fields, 1996; Nathanson and Tyler, 1997). Several molecules present on the surface of keratinocytes have been implicated as viral receptors. The glycosaminoglycan heparan sulfate is used as a receptor for herpes simplex virus, while both heparan and chondroitin sulfate have been proposed as putative receptors for vaccinia virus (WuDunn and Spear, 1989; Chung et al., 1998; Hsiao et al., 1999).

Viruses that replicate locally in the stratum germinativum can produce spectacular lesions. Cytolytic infection of epidermal cells results in the vesicular, erosive, and ulcerative lesions of mucous membranes that are typical of infection with herpesviruses and vesicular stomatitis virus (Barker and Van Dreumel, 1985; Fenner et al., 1987; Khalifa and Lack, 1997). Warts are proliferative lesions that result from local papillomavirus replication and the resulting immortalization of infected epidermal cells (Yager and Scott, 1993; Hines and Jenson, 1997). Many other viruses produce lesions of the skin and mucous membranes after systemic dissemination and relocalization in the epidermis, including those that cause smallpox and foot-and-mouth disease.

Like certain bacterial, rickettsial, and protozoal parasites, arboviruses take advantage of the life cycle of hematophagous arthropods to initiate infection across the host's skin (Weaver, 1997). A taxonomically diverse group of viruses use arthropods as vectors to infect mammals in this manner, most notably members of the *Togaviridae, Flaviviridae, Bunyaviridae, Reoviridae,* and *Rhabdoviridae* families. An equally diverse group of arthropods serve as vectors, including insects of the order Diptera (most commonly mosquitoes, sand flies, midges, and blackflies) and acarid ticks and mites of the class Arachnida. True arboviruses are not simply transmitted mechanically by the mouthparts of the arthropod from a viremic mammalian host to a susceptible one but must first replicate within the gastrointestinal tract of the arthropod vector before the vector becomes capable of transmitting the virus to a new host. Dissemination to the salivary gland epithelium results in the release of infectious virions into the saliva of the arthropod, which are deposited into the dermis or subcutaneous tissues of the reservoir host as the arthropod feeds.

Table 3. Selected examples of cell surface receptors used for viral entry

Agent	Virus family	Virus attachment protein	Virus receptor (cell surface)	Target cell population(s)
HIV-1	*Retroviridae*	gp120/gp41	CD4 and chemokine receptor	CD4$^+$ T lymphocytes, macrophages
Influenza viruses	*Orthomyxoviridae*	HA	Sialic acid	Respiratory epithelium
Measles virus	*Paramyxoviridae*	HA	CD46	Lymphocytes, macrophages, respiratory epithelium
Rabies virus	*Rhabdoviridae*	G	Acetylcholine receptor, NCAM (CD56)	Neurons
EBV	*Herpesviridae*	gp350/220	CD21	B lymphocytes
Poliovirus	*Picornaviridae*	VP1	CD155 (PVR)	Nasopharyngeal epithelum, enterocytes, neurons
Rhinovirus	*Picornaviridae*	VP1	CD54 (ICAM-1)	Nasopharyngeal epithelium

Rabies virus traverses the skin barrier of a new host through the bite of an infected animal. This is also one way in which herpes B virus can be zoonotically transmitted from Asian macaques to humans. Still other viruses circumvent the skin barrier as "passengers" on contaminated hypodermic, acupuncture, or tattoo needles. Hepatitis B virus, hepatitis C virus, and HIV are readily transmitted in this fashion. The staggering seroprevalence of hepatitis B and hepatitis C viruses among intravenous drug users is a testament to the efficiency of this form of viral entry (Hwang et al., 2000).

Conjunctiva

The cornea and conjunctiva would seem to be easily accessible portals for viral entry; however, the continual cleansing action of the eyelids and the presence of immunoglobulin A (IgA) in tears provide protection against infection (Mims et al., 2001). Lymphoid tissue located in the conjunctiva and sclera may provide additional protection in the form of local cellular immunity. Despite these protective mechanisms, certain viruses, adenoviruses and enteroviruses in particular, are capable of initiating infection via the conjunctival route (Tyler and Fields, 1996). Rather than entering by aerosol transmission, viral infection of the conjunctiva is usually accomplished by contact of conjunctival tissue with contaminated fingers, foreign objects, or pool water. Generally speaking, conjunctival infections remain localized, producing vascular engorgement and edema of and discharge from conjunctival membranes (i.e., conjunctivitis), visible as "pink eye." On rare occasions, viral infections of the conjunctiva cause severe or even lethal systemic infections, as evidenced by paralytic infection with enterovirus 70 (Kono et al., 1977), as well as a case of fatal human herpes B virus infection that was acquired through conjunctival exposure (Centers for Disease Control and Prevention, 1998).

Respiratory tract

The primary mission of the respiratory tract is that of exchanging oxygen, an absolute requirement for respiration, for CO_2, a waste product of metabolism. This process requires a large surface area, a delicate mucosal surface for gaseous exchange, and intimate contact with the vasculature, all of which place the host in great jeopardy of microbial invasion. Thus, the mucosal surfaces of the respiratory tract are armed with an array of protective mechanisms for combating infection (Dungworth, 1985; Fenner et al., 1987; Tyler and Fields, 1996; Mims et

al., 2001). The temperature of the upper respiratory tract is maintained at 33°C, which is suboptimal for efficient replication of many viruses. However, human rhinoviruses, the causative agents of the common cold, replicate maximally at this temperature, having evolved to fill an obvious niche in the competitive microenvironment of the mammalian respiratory tract. The upper respiratory tract possesses a filtration system composed of hairs, which line the entry to the nasal passages, and ciliated respiratory epithelial cells, which line the airways and sinuses. This system effectively filters inhaled air, such that only particles smaller than 5 μm are able to gain entry into the alveoli of the lungs (Tyler and Fields, 1996). Filtration is facilitated by the presence of mucus, a secretion of the goblet cells of the nasopharynx and respiratory mucosa, which helps trap inhaled particles, including microorganisms. Through the continuous beating movement of cilia, the mucus and its trapped content are then propelled to the nasopharynx and swallowed. IgA, IgM, and IgG antibodies and effector cytotoxic T lymphocytes (CTL), which are induced within mucosa-associated lymphoid tissue (MALT), further protect the respiratory tract against microbial invasion. MALT is found throughout the mucosa of the respiratory tract and is particularly abundant within the nasopharynx of higher mammals (Wright, 1997; Imaoka et al., 1998; McGhee and Kiyono, 1999). Alveolar macrophages, the resident phagocytes of pulmonary alveoli, provide additional protection at the level of the lower respiratory tract.

Despite its well developed defenses, the respiratory tract is the most common portal of viral entry. The etiologic agents for several very important diseases of humans initiate infection via the respiratory tract, including viruses that are primarily pathogens of the respiratory tract, like rhinoviruses and influenza virus, as well as viruses that cause systemic diseases, such as measles, varicella, and hantavirus pulmonary syndrome (Wright, 1997). Respiratory viruses usually enter the host by inhalation of aerosolized virions; however, in some instances, virus particles or infected cells can be transmitted by contact, entering via the oropharynx and spreading to the respiratory epithelium via saliva. The primary cellular targets for viral infection of the respiratory tract include ciliated pseudostratified columnar epithelial cells, which line the nasopharyngeal, tracheobronchial, and pulmonary airways; alveolar epithelial cells; mucosal and luminal macrophages; and immune cells at inductive sites in the nasopharyngeal and bronchus-associated lymphoid tissues.

As at other portals of entry, viruses use cell surface molecules as receptors to promote high-affinity contact with target cells. Most rhinoviruses bind to intercellular adhesion molecule 1 (ICAM-1), which is expressed on the surface of nasal epithelial cells (Greve et al., 1989; Staunton et al., 1989; Olson et al., 1993). The hemagglutinating envelope glycoproteins of influenza and parainfluenza viruses, HA and HN, respectively, bind to sialic acid residues present on glycoproteins and glycolipids which are expressed on the apical surface of respiratory epithelial cells (Color Plate 5, top row, middle) (Weis et al., 1988; Ah-Tye et al., 1999). In contrast, the hemagglutinin protein (H) of measles virus recognizes the complement regulatory protein CD46, expressed on respiratory epithelial cells, lymphocytes, and macrophages (Dorig et al., 1993; Naniche et al., 1993; Manchester et al., 2000). Recent studies suggest that β_3-integrins on platelets and endothelial cells may serve as the cellular receptor for hantaviruses that infect the respiratory tract (Gavrilovskaya et al., 1998).

Alimentary tract

The mucosal surfaces of the oral cavity, pharynx, and esophagus are protected by a complex stratified squamous epithelium that is several cell layers thick and is keratinized in some sites (Ham and Cormack, 1979; Frappier, 1998). The tissues of the oral cavity are bathed with saliva, which possesses several nonspecific antiviral properties beneficial to the oropharynx (Mims et al., 2001). Saliva irrigates the oral cavity, diluting potential pathogens and flushing them into the gastrointestinal tract. In addition, saliva contains mucins, phagocytes, complement, defensins, and enzymes (e.g., amylases) that may inactivate virions or lyse virus-infected cells (Boackle, 1991; Su and Boackle, 1991; Wu et al., 1994; Tenovuo, 1998; Mathews et al., 1999; Goebel et al., 2000). Other factors in saliva may exhibit nonspecific antiviral activity; for example, recently saliva has been shown to contain endogenous inhibitors of HIV-1 infectivity, including thrombospondin-1 and secretory leukocyte protease inhibitor (Shugars, 1999). Saliva also serves as a vehicle for mediators of specific antiviral immunity in the form of antibodies (particularly secretory IgA) and effector CTL, which are induced in MALT (see below).

The most conspicuous components of the oropharyngeal MALT are the lingual, pharyngeal, and palatine tonsils, which are strategically situated at the entrance to both the respiratory and alimentary tracts. These tissues provide an inductive environment for the generation of antigen-specific antibodies (IgA and IgE) and CTL, which provide mucosal immunity against viral epitopes for which the host has been previously sensitized (Komada et al., 1989;

McGhee and Kiyono, 1999). In certain anatomic sites (e.g., the crypts of the palatine tonsils), the oropharyngeal epithelium is attenuated to form a specialized lymphoepithelium that is one to three cell layers thick and contains M cells (Claeys et al., 1996; Fujimura, 2000). M cells are specialized epithelial cells of mucosal lymphoid organs that are involved in antigen surveillance, uptake, and processing. In some instances, they might also serve as portals for microbial invasion (Heel et al., 1997; Neutra, 1999; Neutra et al., 1999).

Important viral pathogens known to initiate infection in the oropharynx include EBV, herpes simplex virus, foot-and-mouth disease virus, and papillomaviruses. The target cells of viral infection in the oropharynx include epithelial cells and mucosal leukocytes. Tonsillar B lymphocytes are presumed to be an early target of EBV infection, and they serve as a reservoir for persistent infection (Rickinson and Kieff, 1996; Ahmed et al., 1997). Adsorption and entry of EBV into B cells is known to occur through binding of the viral attachment glycoprotein gp350/220 to CD21 on the surface of B cells. Oropharyngeal epithelial cells may also serve as targets for EBV infection, which may explain the relationship between EBV and nasopharyngeal carcinoma (Bayliss and Wolf, 1980; Sixbey et al., 1984). In addition to initiating infection via the respiratory tract in the form of aerosolized droplets, foot-and-mouth disease virus can infect ruminants via the oropharynx (Prato Murphy et al., 1999), possibly by binding to epithelial cells through an integrin expressed on the epithelial cell surface (Jackson et al., 2000).

The gastrointestinal tract, composed of the stomach, small intestine, large intestine, rectum, and anal canal, is a particularly hostile microenvironment. Here, potential viral pathogens encounter ingesta, wide fluxes in pH, digestive enzymes, bile, mucous, microbes, and microbial toxins. In the stomach, mucosal epithelial cells lining the gastric glands secrete hydrochloric acid, which can reduce the pH of the gastric lumen to 2.0, while pancreatic juice contains bicarbonate ions, which impart a slightly alkaline pH to the intestinal lumen. Digestive enzymes (proteases, amylases, and lipases) are supplied by the pancreas and by the gastrointestinal epithelial cells themselves. Bile salts, which emulsify fats, are produced in the liver, stored in the gallbladder, and delivered to the small intestine through the bile duct.

The mucosal surface of the gastrointestinal tract is covered by a simple columnar epithelium that is composed largely of enterocytes and goblet cells but includes other specialized epithelial cells, such as M cells, enteroendocrine cells, and Paneth cells. The gastrointestinal mucosa is protected from the effects of enzymes, microbes, microbial toxins, and variation from neutral pH by a blanket of mucus produced by mucosal and submucosal glands and by goblet cells at the mucosal surface. Mucus also provides a physical barrier against microbial invasion and contains secretory IgA, which provides immunologic protection against viral infection. Further mucosal protection is provided by the glycocalyx, an extracellular mat of carbohydrate side chains that are anchored to integral membrane proteins and lipids at the apical surface of the plasma membrane (Ham and Cormack, 1979; Frappier, 1998).

The gut-associated lymphoid tissue includes Peyer's patches, which are focal aggregates of organized lymphoid tissue found throughout the length of the gastrointestinal mucosa. Each Peyer's patch consists of lymphoid follicles (which contain B lymphocytes and follicular dendritic cells), perifollicular accumulations of T lymphocytes and interdigitating dendritic cells, and an overlying lymphoepithelial dome composed of follicle-associated epithelium and M cells (Debard et al., 1999; McGhee and Kiyono, 1999). The glycocalyx is absent over M cells within the lymphoepithelium, which facilitates the process of antigen surveillance but further targets M cells as a portal for viral invasion (Neutra, 1999). In addition, macrophages, lymphocytes, plasma cells, and other immune cells are found throughout the length of the intestinal lamina propria. Collectively, the GALT provides the gastrointestinal mucosa with phagocytes and with antigen-specific protection in the form of IgA antibody and effector CTL.

A large number of viruses use the gastrointestinal tract as a portal for infection, despite the brutal microenvironment present in the gastrointestinal lumen. In many cases these infections remain localized and are asymptomatic; however, agents known to initiate infection and cause disease within the alimentary tract include adenoviruses, parvoviruses, picornaviruses, reoviruses, and coronaviruses (Connor and Ramig, 1997). Not surprisingly, viruses that are successful at initiating infection in the gut are typically resistant to the effects of digestive enzymes and to extremes of pH. Enteric picornaviruses, including enteroviruses and hepatitis A virus, remain infectious at acidic pH and are resistant to the action of digestive enzymes as well (Fenner et al., 1987; Melnick, 1992). Indeed, certain viruses, most notably members of the *Reoviridae,* have evolved mechanisms for exploiting the action of digestive enzymes to facilitate entry into host cells. For example, proteolytic alteration of the VP4 capsid protein enhances the infectivity of rotaviruses (Konno et al., 1993). The emulsifying action of bile salts probably contributes to the inactivation of most enveloped viruses within

the intestine; however, coronaviruses, which are enveloped RNA viruses, are important enteric pathogens of pigs and cattle.

As is the case in the oropharynx, epithelial cells and mucosal leukocytes serve as the primary targets for infection in the gastrointestinal tract. Parvoviruses require rapidly dividing cells for replication; therefore, canine and feline parvoviruses preferentially infect undifferentiated crypt epithelial cells. The resulting disruption in enterocyte maturation temporarily denudes the intestinal mucosa and can produce severe and often fatal diarrhea (Barker and Von Dreumel, 1985). Other viral pathogens of the gastrointestinal tract, including rotaviruses, coronaviruses, and enteroviruses, infect mature enterocytes (Color Plate 5, row 1, right). Receptors for viral pathogens of the gastrointestinal tract include the poliovirus receptor, a member of the immunoglobulin supergene family that is expressed on a wide variety of human cells, including intestinal epithelial cells (Freistadt et al., 1990).

Urogenital tract

The mucosae of the urethra, urinary bladder, ureters, and renal pelvis do not commonly serve as portals for viral entry. This is probably due in part to the periodic voiding of urine, which flushes pathogens out of the lower urinary tract. Furthermore, urine possesses both innate and specific antiviral properties, including secretory IgA and, in carnivores and omnivores, a slightly acidic pH (Guyton, 1981; Uehling et al., 1999; Pillay et al., 2001).

In contrast, several important viral pathogens, including herpes simplex virus, HIV-1, hepatitis B virus, and human papillomavirus (HPV) types 11, 16, and 18, utilize the genital mucosa as a route of infection. The mucosal surfaces of the genital tract serve as the primary portal for HIV infection (Quinn, 1996; Vernazza et al., 1999). Virus particles and infected leukocytes are shed in cervicovaginal secretions and semen (Vernazza et al., 1997a, 1997b; Overbaugh et al., 1999) and serve as the source of contagion for mucosal infections. Studies using the SIV model suggest that infectious virions are transported from mucosal portals of entry to regional lymphoid tissues either in association with mucosal dendritic cells or as virus particles in afferent lymph (Spira et al., 1996; Zhang et al., 1999; Hu et al., 2000). Recently, investigators have identified a C-type lectin (DC-SIGN) on the surface of dendritic Langerhans' cells that associates with the gp120 envelope glycoprotein of HIV, which may explain the mechanism of HIV transmission across complex epithelial surfaces (Geijtenbeek et al., 2000).

Dissemination

Some viruses remain localized at the portal of entry, whereas others disseminate to distant sites in the host, affecting multiple organ systems and causing systemic disease. Viruses that remain localized at the portal of entry usually spread by cell-to-cell infection between epithelial cells at the mucosal surface. Virions may also be disseminated locally at the site of entry by transport in mucus or inflammatory exudates or by the movement of luminal contents, which permit access to new susceptible target cells at sites removed from the effects of locally produced inhibitors to infection, like interferon (Mims et al., 2001). Some of the viruses that cause infections that remain localized at the portal of entry are assembled and released from the apical surface of polarized epithelial cells, which may help to explain why these agents fail to penetrate beyond the mucosal surface (Blau and Compans, 1995; Compans, 1995; Ravkov et al., 1997). Other factors that may restrict viruses to the point of entry include specific temperature requirements (e.g., rhinoviruses), the need for proteolytic cleavage as a prerequisite for infection (e.g., rotaviruses), and viral receptor distribution (e.g., papillomaviruses). Viral infections that remain localized at the portal of entry can still have a devastating effect on the host. Influenza virus serves as an excellent example of a virus that usually remains localized at the portal of entry, infecting, replicating, and causing disease within the respiratory tract (Color Plate 5, row 1, middle).

There are two principal methods by which viruses accomplish dissemination, hematogenous and neural (Fenner et al., 1987; Tyler and Fields, 1996; Nathanson and Tyler, 1997; Mims et al., 2001). Hematogenous or blood-borne dissemination is the most common and efficient method of virus dispersion. It requires that infectious virions or infected cells cross the epithelial barrier to gain access to extracellular tissue fluid or mucosal blood vessels. As opposed to viruses that cause infections that remain confined to the mucosal surface, some of the viruses that cross the epithelial barrier and enter the bloodstream are assembled and released from the basolateral surface of epithelial cells directly into the subepithelial connective tissues (Tashiro et al., 1990), while others cross the epithelial barrier by transcytosis (Bomsel, 1997). As mentioned above, arboviruses are deposited directly into subepithelial connective tissues by arthropods during feeding whereas many other viruses invade subepithelial tissues at sites where the epithelial barrier has been disrupted as a result of infection, inflammation, or mechanical injury.

Once viruses arrive in the subepithelial connective tissues of the lamina propria or dermis, they usually undergo local replication before entering the bloodstream. Some viruses infect mucosal or submucosal endothelial cells and are released directly into the blood (Color Plate 5, row 2, left) (Sinzger and Jahn, 1996; Burt et al., 1997; Del Piero, 2000), while others travel as cell-free virions in the afferent lymph to regional lymph nodes. Alternatively, viruses may infect immune cells, usually phagocytes, as they migrate to regional lymph nodes. For example, recent evidence suggests that certain poxviruses may establish systemic infection by using chemokine receptors to infect migratory leukocytes located in the dermis and subcutis (Lalani et al., 1999).

Further replication may occur in lymph nodes before virions or infected cells pass through efferent lymph to the bloodstream by way of the thoracic duct. Thus, within the blood, viruses can be found (i) as cell-free virions in the plasma fraction; (ii) within infected red blood cells, leukocytes, or platelets; or (iii) associated with the surface of blood cells. Infected blood cells often play a significant role in viral dissemination; for example, the extension of lentivirus infection to the tissues of the central nervous system (CNS) is thought to occur as a result of the migration of infected blood monocytes across the blood-brain barrier (Peluso et al., 1985; Meltzer et al., 1990; Sasseville and Lackner, 1997).

Viremia is an important step in the pathogenesis of many viral infections. Initial release of virus into the bloodstream, or primary viremia, results in diffuse dissemination of virions or infected cells to many primary tissues in the host. Replication in primary tissues like the liver and spleen often occurs in sinusoidal macrophages of the reticuloendothelial system and results in a marked amplification of the virus burden (Color Plate 5, row 2, middle and right). This is often followed by the release of new virions into the blood, producing a secondary viremia of much greater magnitude than the first, which further promotes dissemination of virus to target organs. The generation of a high-titer viremia appears to be a prerequisite for the dissemination of certain viruses to tissues like the CNS (Color Plate 5, row 3, left) (Tyler and Gonzalez-Scarano, 1997).

In most cases, viremia is terminated with the onset of the antiviral immune response. Virus-producing cells are lysed by CTL, while immune-complexed virions are cleared from the circulation to lymphoid tissues, where they can be inactivated. Neutralizing antibodies prevent newly produced virus particles from infecting additional cells, and opsonized virus particles are inactivated by the complement system or by antibody-dependent cell-mediated cytotoxicity. Some viral infections are characterized by a state of persistent viremia, in which the immune response is unable to clear the virus from the host, resulting in continual replication and release of virions or infected cells into the circulation. Persistent viremia is important in the pathogenesis and transmission of hepatitis B virus and HIV infections (Ahmed et al., 1996).

The tissues of the CNS and peripheral nervous system are significant sites of productive infection for many viruses and are also strategic sites for the establishment of viral latency. The bloodstream is an important avenue for infection of neural tissues; however, the axons of peripheral nerves provide extravascular access to the CNS and to ganglia within the peripheral nervous system for several viruses, including rabies virus, poliovirus, Borna virus, and herpesviruses (Nicolau and Mateisco, 1928; Carbone et al., 1987; Ren and Racaniello, 1992; Tirabassi et al., 1998; Bale, 1999). The process of neural dissemination involves the conduction of intact virions or nucleocapsids along nerve axons by microtubule-associated fast axonal transport in either the antegrade or retrograde direction (i.e., toward or away from the neuronal cell body, respectively) (Tyler and Fields, 1996).

Infection of nerve fibers often follows local replication in epithelial cells or myocytes, however, direct infection of nerve fibers has been demonstrated experimentally and is thought to occur in vivo under certain circumstances (Conomy et al., 1977; Plakhov et al., 1995). Viruses infect nerve fibers at sensory endings in the skin, in the neuroepithelium of sensory organs like the olfactory organ and retina, and at the neuromuscular junction in the motor end plates of muscle fibers (Lentz et al., 1983; Liu et al., 1996). Thus, depending on the virus, neural dissemination may involve viral transmission from epithelial cells or myocytes to cells of the nervous system and can include passage across neuromuscular junctions and synapses as well as axonal transport (Color Plate 5, row 3 and row 4, left) (Dingwell et al., 1995).

Shedding

The last stage in the cycle of virus infection involves the release of infectious virus particles or infected cells from an infected host to the environment. Viruses can be shed in respiratory secretions, feces, or body fluids or from skin lesions (Tyler and Fields, 1996; Nathanson and Tyler, 1997; Mims et al., 2001). Viruses that replicate locally at the portal of infection are usually shed from the same mucosal surface. Many enteric viruses, including rotaviruses (Color Plate 5, row 1, right), enteroviruses, and par-

voviruses, are released from the apical surface of enterocytes and shed in feces, where they can be transmitted to new hosts by the fecal-oral route (Schwab and Shaw, 1993; Alexander et al., 1997). Similarly, many of the viruses that initiate infection via the respiratory tract, including those that cause systemic disease, are also shed from the respiratory tract. Virions that are shed from respiratory surfaces can be expelled in aerosols by coughing or sneezing or can be released in serous discharges and transmitted by contact. Important viral pathogens that are shed from the respiratory tract include rhinoviruses, influenza virus, and many members of the *Paramyxoviridae*, including measles virus (Color Plate 5, row 4, middle and right), mumps virus, Nipah virus (Color Plate 6, row 1, left), and respiratory syncytial virus (Color Plate 6, row 1, middle).

Certain viruses are shed in body fluids (including milk, saliva, urine, semen, and tears), which may serve as a vehicle for transmitting the infection to new hosts. Rabies virus spreads centrifugally from brain tissue along peripheral nerves to parenchymatous organs, including the salivary glands. In the salivary glands, the virus replicates in acinar epithelial cells and is secreted into saliva (Murphy et al., 1973). New hosts are infected on exposure to infectious virus that is present in saliva through the bite of an infected animal. Other human viral pathogens that are shed in saliva include mumps virus and EBV.

Retroviruses appear particularly adept at using milk as a vehicle for postnatal vertical transmission. Milk-borne transmission plays a role in the biology of several lentiviruses, including HIV (Van de Perre et al., 1992), feline immunodeficiency virus (O'Neil et al., 1995), and visna-maedi and caprine arthritis encephalitis viruses (Fenner et al., 1987). Milk-borne transmission has also been documented for several non-lentivirus retroviruses, including human T-cell leukemia virus (Fujino and Nagata, 2000), feline leukemia virus (Pacitti et al., 1986), and mouse mammary tumor virus (Ross, 1998). Other viruses for which milk-borne transmission may play a significant role include cytomegalovirus, which can be transmitted from infected mothers to nursing infants in breast milk and may result in symptomatic infection of preterm infants (Vochem et al., 1998).

Semen and cervicovaginal secretions from HIV-positive individuals contain virions and infected leukocytes, which are central to the transmission of HIV (Vernazza, 1997a, 1997b; Overbaugh et al., 1999). Viruses that are shed in urine following hematogenous dissemination to the kidneys or lower urinary tract include polyomaviruses (e.g., BK and JC viruses, [Color Plate 6, row 1, right, and row 2, left]) and some paramyxoviruses (e.g., Nipah virus [Color Plate

6, row 2, middle]). Human infection with certain arenaviruses (e.g., lymphocytic choriomeningitis virus) and bunyaviruses (e.g., hantavirus) results from environmental exposure to infectious virus that is shed in the urine of rodents that serve as natural reservoirs for these agents (Hart and Bennett, 1999; Barton and Hyndman, 2000).

Tear fluid may serve as a vehicle for contact-mediated transmission of viruses that cause conjunctivitis, such as adenoviruses and picornaviruses (Shulman et al., 1997). Various herpesviruses, including herpes simplex virus, varicella-zoster virus, and cytomegalovirus, are also shed in the tears of patients with herpetic ophthalmologic disease or herpetic conjunctivitis (Cox et al., 1975; Hidalgo et al., 1998). Viruses that produce a high-titer viremia, such as HIV, hepatitis B virus, and hepatitis C virus, are also found in tear fluid; however, the importance of this mode of shedding to the transmission of these agents is probably negligible (Fujikawa et al., 1986; Gastaud et al., 1989; Mendel et al., 1997).

CELLULAR INJURY

Viruses utilize, and in some cases monopolize, the structural and metabolic machinery of host cells for replication; thus, viral infections often result in injury to or death of host cells. Indeed, cell death, either as a result of virus infection or as a consequence of the accompanying inflammatory response, accounts for the loss of function that produces the clinical signs of viral diseases.

Many virus infections are cytolytic, since the invading virus induces lethal physiologic or morphologic alterations in the host cell. In some instances, viruses inhibit the synthesis of host cell DNA, RNA, and proteins, diverting the cellular biosynthetic machinery toward the production of viral nucleic acids and proteins. Viral interference in host cell metabolism can have catastrophic effects on cellular homeostasis: disrupting mitochondrial ATP production, inhibiting osmotic and ionic regulation, and inflicting membrane injury, leading to cell death (Knipe, 1996). Viruses can also cause cell death indirectly, by inducing programmed cell death pathways (Gray et al., 2000), initiating autoimmune processes (Di Rosa and Barnaba, 1998; Horwitz et al., 2000; Rose, 2000), and triggering the immune-mediated elimination of infected cells. Not all viral infections lead to cell death. Many viruses, including herpesviruses, arenaviruses, and hepatitis B virus, establish persistent infections of host cells (Ahmed et al., 1997). Finally, viruses occasionally cause nonlethal functional

impairment of cells, such as that seen in hantavirus pulmonary syndrome (Zaki et al., 1995).

Viral inclusion bodies are among the most profound morphologic changes that viruses induce in host cells. Inclusion bodies, which can be found in the cell nucleus, cytoplasm, or both, can be either "viral factories," composed of excess viral structural proteins in lattice formation, or accumulations of mature virions (Cheville, 1994). While generally not pathognomonic for infection with a specific virus, the presence of inclusion bodies provides supplemental information that can be used to support a diagnosis (Color Plate 6, row 1, right, row 2, right, row 3, and row 4, left and middle). Some common viral inclusions that assist histopathologic diagnoses are listed in Table 4. Characteristic viral inclusions can also be observed by electron microscopy, and knowledge of the ultrastructural morphology of viral particles is sometimes useful for establishing an etiologic diagnosis (Fig. 1).

Some viruses induce changes in target cells that alter the relationship of these cells with neighboring cells or with extracellular-matrix components, which can result in tissue injury. For example, many viruses, including members of the *Papillomaviridae, Adenoviridae, Herpesviridae, Hepadnaviridae,* and *Retroviridae,* are able to immortalize infected cells, and some have been implicated in the formation of tumors in infected hosts (Color Plate 6, row 4, right; Color Plate 7, row 1, left) (Nevins and Vogt, 1996). Other viruses (e.g., measles virus, HIV, and influenza virus) encode glycoproteins that induce fusion with neighboring cells, resulting in the formation of syncytia (Color Plate 5, row 4, middle and right; Color Plate 6, row 1, middle, and row 2, middle; Color Plate 7, row 1, middle and right). Viruses also cause depolymerization of microtubules and rearrangement of cytoskeletal filaments, integral components of the host cytoskeleton and intracellular transport (Knipe, 1996).

DISEASES AND SYNDROMES CAUSED BY VIRUSES

This section examines viral disease pathogenesis from the perspective of major organ systems and important disease syndromes that affect them. Selected examples of disease syndromes caused by viruses, the target cells of infection, the organ systems involved, and the lesions produced are summarized in Table 5. When considering the pathogenesis of viral disease syndromes, it is imperative that we remain ever mindful of the fact that the host immune response, which has evolved to preserve a species, can have a

Table 4. Viral inclusions useful for histopathologic evaluation

Virus	Inclusions	Description
Adenovirus	Smudge cell	Moderately enlarged nucleus and indistinct nuclear membrane
	Cowdry type A intranuclear	Amphophilic or basophilic inclusion surrounded by a halo and by marginated unbeaded chromatin
Cytomegalovirus (CMV)	Intranuclear	Sharply demarcated, large amphophilic to eosinophilic inclusion
	Intracytoplasmic	Inclusion consists of clusters of small, granular, basophilic bodies of various sizes
Herpes simplex virus (HSV)	Cowdry type A intranuclear	Amphophilic to eosinophilic inclusion surrounded by a halo and by marginated beaded chromatin
Varicella virus (chickenpox/zoster)	Intranuclear	Large cell with single, eosinophilic, hyalinized inclusion
Measles virus	Intranuclear	Round or lobulated, hyalinized, eosinophilic, and surrounded by a small halo (often present in multinucleated epithelial giant cells)
	Intracytoplasmic	Eosinophilic; vary in size (often present in multinucleated epithelial giant cells)
	Warthin-Finkeldey cells	Reticuloendothelial multinucleated giant cells (usually without inclusion bodies)
Respiratory syncytial virus	Intracytoplasmic	Multinucleated giant cells with small, irregular, eosinophilic inclusion
Rabies virus	Negri body (intracytoplasmic)	Round to oval, eosinophilic, inclusion in Purkinje cells of cerebellum and large neurons of hippocampus
Papovavirus	Intranuclear	Single or multiple small hyalinized eosinophilic to amphophilic inclusion
Ebola virus	Intracytoplasmic	Filamentous, eosinphilic inclusion in hepatocytes
Nipah virus	Intranuclear	Eosinophilic inclusion with thin peripheral rim of chromatin (in neurons)
	Intracytoplasmic	Small inclusion in neurons
	Syncytial/multinucleated giant cells	Endothelium and epithelial cells
Orthopoxvirus (variola virus)	Guarnieri's body (intracytoplasmic)	Paranuclear, round to oval, hyalinized, basophilic to eosinophilic inclusion in epithelial cells of skin, usually associated with ballooning degeneration
Poxvirus (molluscum contagiosum virus)	Henderson-Patterson body (intracytoplasmic)	Purplish to red inclusion in epithelium of adnexal structures of skin, with peripherally displaced and compressed nucleus
Parapoxvirus (orf virus)	Intranuclear and intracytoplasmic	Eosinophilic inclusions in keratinocytes; usually associated with ballooning degeneration and dense inflammation

detrimental effect on the outcome of infection for an individual.

Viral Encephalitides

Viral infections of the CNS are particularly important because many are associated with high mortality or carry the potential for causing serious and sometimes permanent neurologic damage. A wide spectrum of clinical and pathologic expression is ob-served among the various causes of viral encephalitis (Kennedy and Wanglee, 1967; Whitley, 1990).

By definition, viral encephalitis means parenchymal infection of the brain; however, infection can also involve the meninges (meningoencephalitis) or spinal cord (encephalomyelitis). The most characteristic histopathologic features of viral encephalitides are perivascular and parenchymal inflammation, glial nodules, neuronal degeneration, neuronal necrosis, and neuronophagia (Color Plate 5, row 3, right;

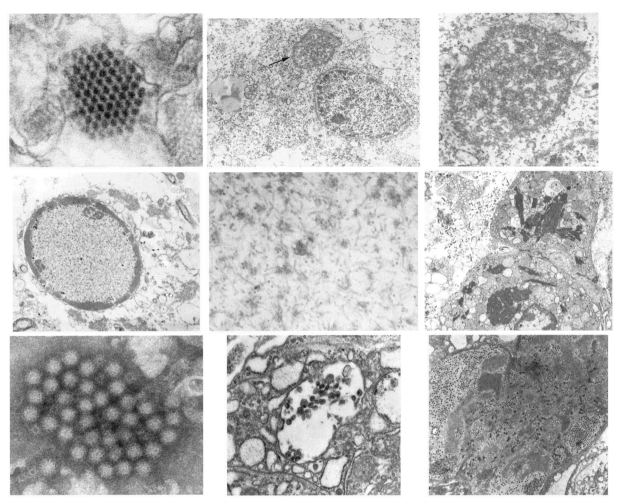

Figure 1. (Row 1, left) Enterovirus 71 infection in the brain of a human. A paracrystalline array of picornavirus particles in a neuronal cell is shown. Thin-section electron microscopy. Magnification, ×70,000. Courtesy of Cynthia Goldsmith, Centers for Disease Control and Prevention, Atlanta, Ga. (Row 1, middle and right) Nipah virus infection in the brain of a human. Inclusion of paramyxovirus nucleocapsids (arrows) is present in a neuronal cell. Thin-section electron microscopy. Magnifications, ×4,000 (middle) and 12,000 (right). Courtesy of Cynthia Goldsmith. (Row 2, left and middle) Subacute sclerosing panencephalitis, caused by measles virus infection in the brain of a human. Paramyxovirus nucleocapsids are present in the nucleus of a neuronal cell. Thin-section electron microscopy. Magnifications, ×5,000 (left) and ×40,000 (middle). Courtesy of Cynthia Goldsmith. (Row 2, right) Ebola virus infection in the liver of a human. Filovirus inclusions are present in hepatocytes and virus particles are present in the sinusoid. Thin-section electron microscopy. Magnification, ×3,000. Courtesy of Cynthia Goldsmith. (Row 3, left) Small round structured virus (Norwalk-like virus) in a stool culture. Negative-stain electron micrograph. Magnification, ×105,000. Courtesy of Charles Humphrey, Centers for Disease Control and Prevention, Atlanta, Ga. (Row 3, middle) SIV infection in the ileum of a pig-tailed macaque. Characteristic lentivirus particles are visible within an intracytoplasmic vesicle in a Peyer's patch macrophage. Thin-section electron microscopy. Magnification, ×42,000. Courtesy of Harold McClure, Yerkes Regional Primate Research Center, Atlanta, Ga. (Row 3, right) Adenovirus infection in the lung of a rhesus macaque monkey. Arrays of adenovirus particles are present within the nucleus of an alveolar epithelial cell. Thin-section electron microscopy. Magnification, ×30,000. Courtesy of Harold McClure.

Color Plate 7, row 2, left and middle). The inflammatory cell infiltrates observed in most cases of viral encephalitis are composed predominantly of mononuclear cells, including lymphocytes, plasma cells, and macrophages; however, polymorphonuclear cells may be evident during the acute stage of infection (Garcia et al., 1984; Anderson, 1988). Viral inclusion bodies are seen in a minority of viral encephalitides, including those caused by adenovirus (Color Plate 5, row 4, left), rabies virus (Color Plate 6, row 3, middle), herpesvirus, Nipah virus, and measles virus (Color Plate 6, row 4, middle). Multinucleated giant cells containing viral antigens and nucleic acid are hallmarks of HIV and SIV encephalitis (Color Plate 7, row 1, right). Examples of vascular lesions resulting from viral encephalitis include the presence of

Table 5. Syndrome presentation and major organ involvement in viral infections

Disease syndrome	Organ system	Virus family	Selected examples	General pathology description	Target cells
Encephalitis	CNS	*Togaviridae, Flaviridae, Bunyaviridae, Paramyxoviridae, Reoviridae, Rhabdoviridae, Picornaviridae, Herpesviridae, Adenoviridae*	EEE virus, Japanese encephalitis virus, West Nile virus, La Crosse virus, measles virus, Nipah virus, Colorado tick fever virus, rabies virus, enterovirus 71, herpes simplex virus, adenovirus	Perivascular and parenchymal mononuclear cell infiltrates, glial nodules, neuronal necrosis, and neuronophagia	Neurons, neuronal processes, glial cells
Pneumonitis	Respiratory	*Orthomyxoviridae, Paramyxoviridae, Herpesviridae, Adenoviridae*	Influenza A virus, parainfluenza virus, respiratory syncytial virus, cytomegalovirus, herpes simplex virus	Thickened and edematous alveolar septa with mononuclear inflammatory cell infiltrate, intra-alveolar proteinaceous material, and cellular exudate	Epithelial cells, alveolar macrophages
ARDS	Respiratory	*Bunyaviridae*	Hantavirus	Interstitial and intra-alveolar edema and mononuclear inflammatory cell infiltrate; fibrin deposition and hyaline membrane formation in the alveolar walls	Capillary endothelial cells, macrophages
Myocarditis	Cardiovascular	*Picornaviridae, Adenoviridae, Herpesviridae*	Coxsackie virus, adenovirus, EBV	Interstitial mononuclear inflammatory cell infiltrate (predominantly lymphocytic) and focal necrosis of myocytes	Myocytes
VHF	Multiple	*Flaviridae, Bunyaviridae, Filoviridae, Arenaviridae*	Yellow fever virus, Crimean Congo hemorrhagic fever virus, Ebola virus, Lassa fever virus	Various	Endothelial cells, mononuclear phagocytes
Anemia	Hematologic	*Parvoviridae*	Parvovirus	Viral inclusions in erythrocyte percursors	Nucleated red blood cells
AIDS	Multiple	*Retroviridae*	HIV	Various	CD4$^+$ T cells, macrophages
Diarrhea	Digestive	*Reoviridae, Caliciviridae, Adenoviridae*	Rotavirus, Norwalk-like virus, adenovirus	Blunting and destruction of the villus epithelial cells, secondary hyperplasia of the mucosal crypts, and a mixed inflammatory cell infiltrate of the lamina propria	Enterocytes
Hepatitis	Digestive	*Picornaviridae, Hepadnaviridae, Flaviviridae*	Hepatitis A virus, hepatitis B virus, hepatitis C virus	Acute stages show diffuse hepatocellular injury and necrosis, reactive changes in Kupffer cells, inflammatory infiltrate in portal tracts, and evidence of hepatocellular regeneration	Hepatocytes
Neoplasia	Multiple	*Papovaviridae, Herpesviridae, Hepadnaviridae, Retroviridae*	Papillomavirus, EBV, hepatitis B virus, HIV	Abnormal mass of tissue with uncoordinated growth	Various

endothelial cell syncytia (Color Plate 7, row 1, middle), vasculitis, and thrombosis, as seen in Nipah virus infection (Chua et al., 2000).

Arthropod-borne encephalitides are the prototypic viral infection of the CNS and are responsible for most outbreaks of epidemic viral encephalitis. The most important causes of arbovirus encephalitis in the Western Hemisphere include alphaviruses (e.g., EEE, Western equine encephalitis, and Venezuelan equine encephalitis viruses), flaviviruses (e.g., St. Louis encephalitis virus and West Nile virus), and bunyaviruses (e.g., California encephalitis virus and La Crosse virus) (Manz, 1997; Cotran, 1999). All have animal reservoir hosts and use mosquitoes or ticks as arthropod vectors.

The pathogenesis of viral encephalitis is largely unknown; however, a large number of factors are probably involved, including the route and mechanism of neuroinvasion, the magnitude and quality of the host immune response, the receptor interactions between the virus and the host cells, and the ability of viruses to utilize the molecular control mechanisms of host cells (Johnson, 1987). Virus-specific differences in cell and tissue tropism account for the compartmentalization of different viruses within the CNS and give rise to a wide spectrum of clinical manifestations. Some viruses infect only specific cell types after entering the CNS, while others are restricted to particular areas of the brain. Infected microglia and macrophages may affect neuronal function indirectly through the secretion of metabolites or cytokines (Smith, 1969). In addition, some viruses have the capacity to establish latent infections in neural tissues, which influences aspects of transmission and disease.

Viral Hemorrhagic Fevers

The combination of fever and hemorrhage can be caused by a diverse group of human pathogens, including viruses, rickettsiae, bacteria, protozoa, and fungi. However, the term "viral hemorrhagic fever" (VHF) is usually reserved for systemic infections characterized by fever and hemorrhage caused by a special group of viruses transmitted to humans by arthropods and rodents.

Although VHFs have many pathologic features in common, the overall changes vary among the different diseases. The pathologic findings shared by these diseases include widespread petechial hemorrhages and ecchymoses involving the skin, mucous membranes, and internal organs. Widespread, focal, and sometimes massive necrosis can be commonly observed in all organ systems and is often both ischemic and related to the cytopathic effect of the virus. Necrosis is usually most prominent in the liver, lungs,

and lymphoid tissues. The changes in the liver are similar in a number of VHFs and consist of widespread hepatocellular necrosis associated with variable degrees of hemorrhage and Councilman body formation (Color Plate 5, row 2, right; Color Plate 7, row 2, right, and row 3, left and middle). Lungs may show an interstitial pneumonitis and are usually congested, with widespread intra-alveolar edema and hemorrhage (Color Plate 7, row 3, right, and row 4, left). Although lymphoid necrosis and depletion are the general rule, proliferative changes of lymphoid tissues may be found in some diseases, such as hantavirus-related illnesses. Erythrophagocytosis is also commonly seen in the spleen, lymph nodes, and liver of patients with VHF.

Microvascular thrombosis can be seen in tissues of a small proportion of patients, and it is highly possible that disseminated intravascular coagulation is important in the pathogenesis of some VHFs. The similar pathologic and immunopathologic findings in cases of VHF suggest that microvascular involvement and instability are an important common pathogenetic pathway, leading to shock and bleeding in many instances. Infection of macrophages and other cells of the mononuclear phagocytic system is also thought to play a critical role in the pathogenesis of VHF through the secretion of physiologically active substances, including cytokines and other inflammatory mediators (Peters et al., 1997; Zaki and Peters, 1997; Zaki, 1997; Zaki and Goldsmith, 1998; Peters and Zaki, 1999; Zaki and Paddock, 1999; Nolte et al., in press).

Viral Respiratory Diseases

The respiratory tract serves as the most commonly used portal of entry for viral pathogens of humans. Viruses often affect the respiratory system in a relatively predictable pattern, producing specific clinical syndromes. A few examples of such syndromes include coryza, pharyngitis, croup, bronchiolitis, pneumonia, and acute respiratory distress syndrome (ARDS). In this section we will describe the pathogenesis of two common respiratory disease syndromes, ARDS and pneumonia.

ARDS is a clinical syndrome characterized by acute respiratory failure associated with severe arterial hypoxemia that is refractory to oxygen therapy. The causes of ARDS include infections, toxins, drugs, shock, and radiation. The pathologic changes seen in ARDS are described as diffuse alveolar damage (DAD). Two fairly distinct, but overlapping, stages of DAD are seen depending on course of disease and time following injury. The early or acute exudative stage is seen within the first few days of injury and is characterized by edema, exudation, and hyaline membrane formation. The proliferative stage follows, during which there is organization of the exudate, proliferation of interstitial cells, and fibrosis, resulting in thickening of the alveolar septa (Katzenstein, 1990; Cotran, 1999).

Viral infections that can cause ARDS include those caused by influenza virus, adenovirus, herpesviruses, and hantaviruses. Although these viruses are unrelated, they often induce the same initial type of lung injury, which consists of damage to alveolar endothelial and epithelial cells; thus, the resultant pathologic lesions are often similar. Endothelial and epithelial cell damage leads to accumulation of fluid, protein, and cellular debris in the interstitium and the alveolar spaces. In hantavirus pulmonary syndrome, acute pulmonary edema occurs as protein-rich fluid floods into the interstitium and the alveoli (Color Plate 7, row 3, right), despite the absence of an identifiable morphologic lesion in the blood-gas barrier at the light microscopic level. An abundance of hantavirus antigens (which are selectively found in pulmonary capillary endothelium) attract an inflammatory infiltrate composed of CD4$^+$ and CD8$^+$ lymphoblasts and activated macrophages (Color Plate 7, row 4, left). The combination of extremely high levels of viral antigens in the pulmonary microvasculature with antigen-specific immune responses in the lungs emphasizes the immunopathologic nature of the disease. The inflammatory cell recruitment in the lungs is thought to be the consequence of specific attraction and adherence of a selective population of inflammatory cells to the infected endothelium (Zaki et al., 1995).

Viral pneumonias often present as an interstitial pneumonitis characterized by an inflammatory reaction composed primarily of mononuclear inflammatory cells. Interstitial edema and mononuclear cell infiltration are admixed to various degrees with DAD. An influenza-like syndrome is characterized by abrupt onset of fever, nasal congestion, sore throat, cough, headache, malaise, and myalgia. Influenza A and B viruses are responsible for about half of all cases of viral pneumonia, while the remainder are caused by a number of other viruses including coronaviruses, adenoviruses, respiratory syncytial virus, and parainfluenza virus.

A wide spectrum in the severity of respiratory disease has been observed following influenza virus infection, ranging from mild upper respiratory illness to viral pneumonia, with or without complicating bacterial pneumonia. Influenza virus infection is usually confined to the ciliated epithelial cells that line the upper airways (Color Plate 5, row 1, middle). In addition to cell-to-cell spread, virions are disseminated locally in respiratory mucus, which results in a patchy pattern of epithelial cell necrosis (Dungworth, 1985; Winkler and Cheville, 1986; Cheville, 1994). The loss of infected ciliated epithelial cells from airways compromises the mucociliary apparatus, leading to an accumulation of mucus, desquamated epithelial cells, and inflammatory cells in lower airways, which impairs ventilation and predisposes the host to secondary bacterial pneumonia. Perivascular accumulations of inflammatory cells (initially neutrophils and later macrophages, lymphocytes, and plasma cells) infiltrate the regions of respiratory mucosa that have been denuded of epithelium. In severe cases, viral infection extends to the epithelial cells lining the terminal bronchioles and alveoli. Here, the accumulation of tissue fluid (pulmonary edema), fibrin, and inflammatory cells within alveoli and interstitial spaces further compromises ventilation. The majority of constitutional signs which accompany the "flu" result from the systemic effects of cytokines that are secreted by inflammatory cells in the heavily vascularized respiratory tissues; however, on rare occasions the influenza virus can achieve systemic infection, resulting in myocarditis and CNS disease (Winn, 1997).

Virus-Induced Immunodeficiency

Many viruses are known to induce transient immunosuppression of the host, by producing specific viral products that affect host immune function, altering the expression of strategic host proteins that are important for normal immune function, or "monopolizing" the host immune system during primary infection (Griffin, 1997). AIDS is a catastrophic and typically fatal form of viral immunosuppression caused by infection with HIV. AIDS is a chronic disease process that results in the progressive depletion of helper CD4$^+$ T lymphocytes, leading to immunologic impairment and the development of lethal opportunistic infections or neoplasms. HIV infection results in a state of persistent viremia, with both cell-free virions and infected leukocytes circulating in blood (Ho et al., 1989, 1995; Wei et al., 1995; Perelson et al., 1996).

The primary receptor for HIV is the CD4 molecule; thus, the principal target cells of infection are CD4-expressing helper T lymphocytes and macrophages (Klatzmann et al., 1984; Levy et al., 1985). To accomplish infection, however, HIV must bind both the primary receptor (CD4) and a coreceptor, a member of the chemokine receptor family (Doms and Peiper, 1997). Chemokine receptor usage determines the tropism of a given HIV isolate for subsets of CD4$^+$ cells. Primary macrophage-tropic isolates use the CCR5 coreceptor for entry, while dually tropic and primary T-tropic virus isolates utilize both CCR5 and CXCR4 coreceptors (Alkhatib et al., 1996; Berson et al., 1996; Deng et al., 1996; Dragic et al., 1996; Feng et al., 1996).

The fundamental lesion of AIDS is the dysfunction and depletion of helper CD4[+] T lymphocytes; however, the immunopathogenetic mechanisms that precipitate CD4[+] T-cell loss in HIV-infected individuals are complex and multifactorial (Pantaleo and Fauci, 1995; Fauci et al., 1996; Cohen et al., 1999; Cotran, 1999). Direct virolysis and elimination by virus-specific cellular and humoral immune responses are major factors contributing to the progressive depletion of infected CD4[+] T cells. However, a large body of evidence suggests that HIV infection causes a chronic state of immune activation that results in the elimination of large numbers of uninfected CD4[+] T cells as well (Pantaleo and Fauci, 1995; Copeland and Heeney, 1996). Mechanisms thought to be responsible for the elimination of uninfected CD4[+] T cells include autoimmunity and programmed cell death (Silvestris et al., 1995; Gougeon et al., 1996).

Lymphoid tissues are the principal reservoir for HIV replication throughout the course of infection (Fox et al., 1991; Pantaleo et al., 1991; Embretson et al., 1993) and are also the primary site of the HIV-specific lesions that result in the development of immunodeficiency. A complex and dynamic relationship exists between virus kinetics in blood, virus kinetics in lymphoid tissues, population kinetics of immune cells, and lymph node histomorphology (Siegel, 1997; Cohen et al., 1999; Cotran, 1999). During acute infection, as the plasma virus load peaks, the virus burden in lymphoid tissues is high and predominantly cell associated. The majority of productively infected cells are CD4[+] T lymphocytes within paracortical zones (Schacker et al., 2001). As the antiviral immune response develops, virus-specific CTL eliminate infected cells, reducing both the plasma virus load and the number of productively infected cells in lymphoid tissues. Lymph nodes then progress to a stage of follicular hyperplasia, as an aggressive humoral immune response leads to the development of large numbers of secondary lymphoid follicles. During this stage, immune complexes of antibody, virus particles, and complement are cleared from the circulation and become trapped by Fc receptors on the surface of follicular dendritic cells in lymphoid germinal centers (Color Plate 7, row 4, middle) (Fox et al., 1991). Some of the trapped virus is inactivated by complement; however, much of it remains infectious (Heath et al., 1995). The presence of infectious virus particles on the cellular processes of follicular dendritic cells facilitates new infections

of activated CD4[+] T cells and ultimately results in dendritic cell loss and the destruction of follicles. With the collapse of the dendritic cell scaffold, clearance of immune-complexed virions is impaired, resulting in an increase in circulating virus burden. At this late stage of infection, lymph nodes have barren histomorphologic features; lymphoid follicles are absent or fibrotic (i.e., follicular depletion), paracortical zones are depleted of CD4[+] T cells (i.e., lymphoid atrophy), multinucleated giant cells may be present, and medullary sinuses are infiltrated with macrophages (i.e., sinus histiocytosis) (Siegel, 1997; Cotran, 1999).

The CNS serves as an additional tissue reservoir for HIV. HIV-associated dementia is the most common and most devastating of the neurological sequelae of HIV infection. This syndrome, which affects 20 to 30% of all HIV-infected individuals, is composed of a spectrum of motor, cognitive, and behavioral disorders (Masliah et al., 1992; Glass and Johnson, 1996) and is the clinical result of HIV encephalitis (Wiley and Achim, 1994). The lesions of HIV encephalitis include microglial nodules, accumulations of perivascular and parenchymal macrophages and multinucleated giant cells, microglial and astroglial reaction, and vacuolation and demyelination of the white matter (Navia et al., 1986; Gabuzda and Hirsch, 1987; Achim et al., 1994; Rosenblum, 1997). Viral nucleic acids and antigens have been localized throughout the brains of HIV-infected individuals; however, some reports have suggested that the subcortical white matter, basal ganglia, and hippocampus harbor the greatest viral burden in demented patients (Aylward et al., 1993; Gosztonyi et al., 1994; Brew et al., 1995; Wiley et al., 1998). Macrophages and microglia are the primary targets for productive HIV infection in the brain (Color Plate 7, row 4, right) (Wiley et al., 1986; Vazeux et al., 1987; Kure et al., 1990; Gosztonyi et al., 1994; Takahashi et al., 1996), although infected astrocytes and endothelial cells have also been observed and could play an important role in HIV neuropathogenesis (Wiley et al., 1986; Takahashi et al., 1996).

Viral Enteritis and Diarrhea

Enteric viral infections usually cause acute, self-limiting diarrhea among children. The viruses that are most commonly involved include rotaviruses, Norwalk-like viruses, coronaviruses, adenoviruses, and astroviruses. Infectious diarrhea may cause severe dehydration and metabolic acidosis in infants, resulting in significant morbidity and mortality in both developed and developing countries (Cotran, 1999).

Although the enteric viruses are genetically and morphologically different from each other, the histopathologic lesions they cause in the intestinal tract are similar. During the early phase of infection, the small intestinal mucosa usually shows mild to modest shortening of villi and a mixed inflammatory cell infiltrate in the lamina propria. As infection progresses, there is vacuolization and lysis of infected villus epithelial cells or exfoliation of infected cells into the intestinal lumen, leading to progressive blunting and fusion of villi. The intestinal crypt epithelial cells undergo hyperplasia, replacing the mature villus cells lost to virus infection with poorly differentiated cells that have blunt, irregular microvillus brush borders and reduced enzyme activity. Eventually, the new enterocytes differentiate and villi regenerate (Snodgrass et al., 1979; Barker and Van Dreumel, 1985; Katyal et al., 1999). Viral particles may be present within surface epithelial cells and in stool as seen by electron microscopy, and viral antigens can also be detected by immunofluorescence or immunohistochemical staining (Color Plate 5, row 1, right) (Magar and Larochelle, 1992). In infants, rotavirus can produce a flat mucosa resembling celiac sprue.

Rotavirus is one of the major viruses causing infectious diarrhea in infants. Rotavirus is transmitted by the fecal-oral route and selectively infects and destroys mature host epithelial cells located at the tips and along the middle portions of the small intestinal villi, while sparing the crypt cells. The surface epithelium of the blunted villus is replaced with immature secretory cells (Greenberg et al., 1994). The loss of absorptive enterocytes is central to the pathogenesis of rotaviral diarrhea, since it leads to reduced absorption of sodium, water, and nutrients from the bowel lumen. The resulting osmotic diarrhea is exacerbated by the increase in the number of secretory cells, causing a net secretion of water and electrolytes into the bowel lumen, which can quickly lead to dehydration and severe metabolic acidosis in infants (Shepherd et al., 1979; Cotran, 1999). Levels of rotavirus-specific secretory IgA in the bowel lumen have been correlated with resistance to rotavirus diarrhea in older children and adults (Coulson et al., 1992); however, other immune factors are involved as well (Kuklin et al., 2001). Antirotavirus antibodies are present in breast milk; therefore, infection is most frequent at the time of weaning.

Viral Oncogenesis and Neoplasia

A large number of RNA and DNA viruses have proven to be oncogenic in a wide variety of animals. There is also strong evidence associating virus infections with certain forms of human cancer. The study of animal retroviruses has provided great insight into the molecular basis of neoplasia; however, only one human retrovirus, human T-cell leukemia virus type 1, has been firmly implicated as a cause of cancer (Lobach et al., 1985).

Several DNA viruses, including HPV (Mitchell et al., 1986), EBV (Gaffey and Weiss, 1990), and hepatitis B virus (Kim et al., 1991), have been implicated in the formation of human tumors. These transforming DNA viruses form stable associations with the host cell genome, and viral genes transcribed early in the viral life cycle are usually important for transformation (Klein, 1979).

Over 65 genetically distinct types of HPV have been identified. Some types (e.g., types 1, 2, 4, and 7) can cause benign squamous papillomas (warts) in humans. Epidemiologic studies also suggest that types 16 and 18 are associated with squamous cell carcinomas of the cervix and anogenital region. In contrast to cervical cancers, genital warts with low malignant potential are associated with distinct HPV types, predominantly types 6 and 11.

The HPV genome consists of approximately 7,900 bp. All open reading frames are arranged on one DNA strand, and all papillomaviruses have the same genetic organization. The genomes of several papillomaviruses can transform certain cell lines in tissue culture; however, the complete replicative cycle of HPV has not yet been duplicated in vitro. Molecular analyses have shown that the HPV genome is maintained in a nonintegrated form in HPV-associated benign warts. In contrast, viral DNA is usually integrated into the host cell genome in HPV-associated forms of cancer, which suggests that integration of viral DNA is important in malignant transformation.

CONCLUSIONS

In this chapter we have examined viral disease pathogenesis from three general perspectives: from the perspective of basic concepts of infection and transmission, from the perspective of morphologic aspects of cell injury, and from the perspective of major organ systems and disease syndromes that affect them. Traditional and contemporary pathologic studies provide critical information that should result in a better understanding of the pathogenesis of viral infections of historically familiar and emerging infectious diseases.

REFERENCES

Achim, C. L., R. Wang, D. K. Miners, and C. A. Wiley. 1994. Brain viral burden in HIV infection. *J. Neuropathol. Exp. Neurol.* 53:284–294.

Ahmed, R., L. A. Morrison, and D. M. Knipe. 1996. Persistence of viruses, p. 219–249. *In* B. N. Fields, D. M. Knipe, and P. M. Howley (ed.), *Fields Virology*, 3rd ed. Lippincott Williams & Wilkins, Philadelphia, Pa.

Ahmed, R., L. A. Morrison, and D. M. Knipe. 1997. Viral persistence, p. 181–205. *In* N. Nathanson (ed.), *Viral Pathogenesis*. Lippincott-Raven, Philadelphia, Pa.

Ah-Tye, C., S. Schwartz, K. Huberman, E. Carlin, and A. Moscona. 1999. Virus-receptor interactions of human parainfluenza viruses types 1, 2 and 3. *Microb. Pathog.* 27:329–336.

Alexander, J. P., H. E. Gary, and M. A. Pallansch. 1997. Duration of poliovirus excretion and its implications for acute flaccid paralysis surveillance: a review of the literature. *J. Infect. Dis.* 175(Suppl. 1):S176–S182.

Alkhatib, G., C. Combadiere, C. C. Broder, Y. Feng, P. E. Kennedy, P. M. Murphy, and E. A. Berger. 1996. CC CKR5: a RANTES, MIP-1alpha, MIP-1beta receptor as a fusion cofactor for macrophage-tropic HIV-1. *Science* 272:1955–1958.

Anderson, J. R. 1988. Viral encephalitis and its pathology. *Curr. Top. Pathol.* 76:23–60.

Aylward, E. H., J. D. Henderer, J. C. McArthur, P. D. Brettschneider, G. J. Harris, P. E. Barta, and G. D. Pearlson. 1993. Reduced basal ganglia volume in HIV-1-associated dementia: results from quantitative neuroimaging. *Neurology* 43:2099–2104.

Bale, J. F. 1999. Human herpesviruses and neurological disorders of childhood. *Semin. Pediatr. Neurol.* 6:278–287.

Barker, I. K., and A. A. Van Dreumel. 1985. The alimentary system, p. 1–237. *In* K. V. F. Jubb, P. C. Kennedy, and N. Palmer (ed.), *Pathology of Domestic Animals*, vol. 2. Academic Press, Inc., San Diego, Calif.

Barton, L. L., and N. J. Hyndman. 2000. Lymphocytic choriomeningitis virus: reemerging central nervous system pathogen. *Pediatrics* 105:E35.

Bayliss, G. J., and H. Wolf. 1980. Epstein–Barr virus-induced cell fusion. *Nature* 287:164–165.

Berson, J. F., D. Long, B. J. Doranz, J. Rucker, F. R. Jirik, and R. W. Doms. 1996. A seven-transmembrane domain receptor involved in fusion and entry of T-cell-tropic human immunodeficiency virus type 1 strains. *J. Virol.* 70:6288–6295.

Blau, D. M., and R. W. Compans. 1995. Entry and release of measles virus are polarized in epithelial cells. *Virology* 210:91–99.

Boackle, R. J. 1991. The interaction of salivary secretions with the human complement system—a model for the study of host defense systems on inflamed mucosal surfaces. *Crit. Rev. Oral Biol. Med.* 2:355–367.

Bomsel, M. 1997. Transcytosis of infectious human immunodeficiency virus across a tight human epithelial cell line barrier. *Nat. Med.* 3:42–47.

Brew, B. J., M. Rosenblum, K. Cronin, and R. W. Price. 1995. AIDS dementia complex and HIV-1 brain infection: clinical-virological correlations. *Ann. Neurol.* 38:563–570.

Burt, F. J., R. Swanepoel, W. J. Shieh, J. F. Smith, P. A. Leman, P. W. Greer, L. M. Coffield, P. E. Rollin, T. G. Ksiazek, C. J. Peters, and S. R. Zaki. 1997. Immunohistochemical and in situ localization of Crimean-Congo hemorrhagic fever (CCHF) virus in human tissues and implications for CCHF pathogenesis. *Arch. Pathol. Lab. Med.* 121:839–846.

Campadelli-Fiume, G., F. Cocchi, L. Menotti, and M. Lopez. 2000. The novel receptors that mediate the entry of herpes simplex viruses and animal alphaherpesviruses into cells. *Rev. Med. Virol.* 10:305–319.

Carbone, K. M., C. S. Duchala, J. W. Griffin, A. L. Kincaid, and O. Narayan. 1987. Pathogenesis of Borna disease in rats: evidence that intra–axonal spread is the major route for virus dissemination and the determinant for disease incubation. *J. Virol.* 61:3431–3440.

Centers for Disease Control and Prevention. 1998. Fatal cercopithecine herpesvirus 1 (B virus) infection following a mucocutaneous exposure and interim recommendations for worker protection. *Morb. Mortal. Wkly. Rep.* 47:1073–1076, 1083.

Cheville, N. F. 1994. *Ultrastructural Pathology*. Iowa State University Press, Ames.

Chua, K. B., W. J. Bellini, P. A. Rota, B. H. Harcourt, A. Tamin, S. K. Lam, T. G. Ksiazek, P. E. Rollin, S. R. Zaki, W. Shieh, C. S. Goldsmith, D. J. Gubler, J. T. Roehrig, B. Eaton, A. R. Gould, J. Olson, H. Field, P. Daniels, A. E. Ling, C. J. Peters, L. J. Anderson, and B. W. Mahy. 2000. Nipah virus: a recently emergent deadly paramyxovirus. *Science* 288:1432–1435.

Chung, C. S., J. C. Hsiao, Y. S. Chang, and W. Chang. 1998. A27L protein mediates vaccinia virus interaction with cell surface heparan sulfate. *J. Virol.* 72:1577–1585.

Claeys, S., C. Cuvelier, J. Quatacker, and P. Van Cauwenberge. 1996. Ultrastructural investigation of M-cells and lymphoepithelial contacts in naso-pharyngeal associated lymphoid tissue. (NALT). *Acta Otolaryngol. Suppl.* 523:40–42.

Cohen, O., D. Weissman, and A. S. Fauci. 1999. The immunopathogenesis of HIV infection, p. 1455–1509. *In* W. E. Paul (ed.), *Fundamental Immunology*. Lippincott-Raven, Philadelphia, Pa.

Compans, R. W. 1995. Virus entry and release in polarized epithelial cells. *Curr. Top. Microbiol. Immunol.* 202:209–219.

Connor, M. E., and R. F. Ramig. 1997. Viral enteric diseases, p. 713–743. *In* N. Nathanson (ed.), *Viral Pathogenesis*. Lippincott-Raven, Philadelphia, Pa.

Conomy, J. P., A. Leibovitz, W. McCombs, and J. Stinson. 1977. Airborne rabies encephalitis: demonstration of rabies virus in the human central nervous system. *Neurology* 27:67–69.

Copeland, K. F., and J. L. Heeney. 1996. T helper cell activation and human retroviral pathogenesis. *Microbiol. Rev.* 60:722–742.

Cotran, R. S. 1999. *Robbins Pathologic Basis of Disease*. The W. B. Saunders Co., Philadelphia, Pa.

Coulson, B. S., K. Grimwood, I. L. Hudson, G. L. Barnes, and R. F. Bishop. 1992. Role of coproantibody in clinical protection of children during reinfection with rotavirus. *J. Clin. Microbiol.* 30:1678–1684.

Cox, F., D. Meyer, and W. T. Hughes. 1975. Cytomegalovirus in tears from patients with normal eyes and with acute cytomegalovirus chorioretinitis. *Am. J. Ophthalmol.* 80:817–824.

Debard, N., F. Sierro, and J. P. Kraehenbuhl. 1999. Development of Peyer's patches, follicle-associated epithelium and M cell: lessons from immunodeficient and knockout mice. *Semin. Immunol.* 11:183–191.

Del Piero, F. 2000. Equine viral arteritis. *Vet. Pathol.* 37:287–296.

Deng, H., R. Liu, W. Ellmeier, S. Choe, D. Unutmaz, M. Burkhart, P. Di Marzio, S. Marmon, R. E. Sutton, C. M. Hill, C. B. Davis, S. C. Peiper, T. J. Schall, D. R. Littman, and N. R. Landau. 1996. Identification of a major co-receptor for primary isolates of HIV-1. *Nature* 381:661–666.

Dingwell, K. S., L. C. Doering, and D. C. Johnson. 1995. Glycoproteins E and I facilitate neuron-to-neuron spread of herpes simplex virus. *J. Virol.* 69:7087–7098.

Di Rosa, F., and V. Barnaba. 1998. Persisting viruses and chronic inflammation: understanding their relation to autoimmunity. *Immunol. Rev.* 164:17–27.

Doms, R. W., and S. C. Peiper. 1997. Unwelcomed guests with master keys: how HIV uses chemokine receptors for cellular entry. *Virology* 235:179–190.

Dorig, R. E., A. Marcil, A. Chopra, and C. D. Richardson. 1993. The human CD46 molecule is a receptor for measles virus. (Edmonston strain). *Cell* 75:295–305.

Dragic, T., V. Litwin, G. P. Allaway, S. R. Martin, Y. Huang, K. A. Nagashima, C. Cayanan, P. J. Maddon, R. A. Koup, J. P. Moore, and W. A. Paxton. 1996. HIV-1 entry into CD4+ cells is mediated by the chemokine receptor CC-CKR-5. *Nature* **381:** 667–673.

Dungworth, D. L. 1985. The respiratory system, p. 413–556. *In* K. V. F. Jubb, P. C. Kennedy, and N. Palmer (ed.), *Pathology of Domestic Animals,* vol. 2. Academic Press, Inc., San Diego, Calif.

Embretson, J., M. Zupancic, J. L. Ribas, A. Burke, P. Racz, K. Tenner-Racz, and A. T. Haase. 1993. Massive covert infection of helper T lymphocytes and macrophages by HIV during the incubation period of AIDS. *Nature* **362:**359–362.

Fauci, A. S., G. Pantaleo, S. Stanley, and D. Weissman. 1996. Immunopathogenic mechanisms of HIV infection. *Ann. Intern. Med.* **124:**654–663.

Feng, Y., C. C. Broder, P. E. Kennedy, and E. A. Berger. 1996. HIV-1 entry cofactor: functional cDNA cloning of a seventransmembrane, G protein-coupled receptor. *Science* **272:**872–877.

Fenner, F., P. A. Bachmann, E. P. J. Gibbs, F. A. Murphy, M. J. Studdert, and D. O. White. 1987. *Veterinary Virology.* Academic Press, Inc., San Diego, Calif.

Fox, C. H., K. Tenner-Racz, P. Racz, A. Firpo, P. A. Pizzo, and A. S. Fauci. 1991. Lymphoid germinal centers are reservoirs of human immunodeficiency virus type 1 RNA. *J. Infect. Dis.* **164:** 1051–1057. (Erratum, 155:1161, 1992.)

Fraenkel-Conrat, H., P. C. Kimball, and J. A. Levy. 1988. Biological consequences of viral infections on organisms and populations, p. 371–414. *In* H. Fraenkel-Contrat, P. C. Kimball, and J. A. Levy (ed.), *Virology.* Prentice Hall, Englewood Cliffs, N.J.

Frappier, B. L. 1998. Digestive system, p. 164–202. *In* H. D. Dellmann and J. Eurell (ed.), *Textbook of Veterinary Histology.* The Williams & Wilkins Co., Baltimore, Md.

Freistadt, M. S., G. Kaplan, and V. R. Racaniello. 1990. Heterogeneous expression of poliovirus receptor-related proteins in human cells and tissues. *Mol. Cell. Biol.* **10:**5700–5706.

Fujikawa, L. S., S. Z. Salahuddin, D. Ablashi, A. G. Palestine, H. Masur, R. B. Nussenblatt, and R. C. Gallo. 1986. HTLV-III in the tears of AIDS patients. *Ophthalmology* **93:**1479–1481.

Fujimura, Y. 2000. Evidence of M cells as portals of entry for antigens in the nasopharyngeal lymphoid tissue of humans. *Virchows Arch.* **436:**560–566.

Fujino, T., and Y. Nagata. 2000. HTLV-I transmission from mother to child. *J. Reprod. Immunol.* **47:**197–206.

Gabuzda, D. H., and M. S. Hirsch. 1987. Neurologic manifestations of infection with human immunodeficiency virus. Clinical features and pathogenesis. *Ann. Intern. Med.* **107:**383–391.

Gaffey, M. J., and L. M. Weiss. 1990. Viral oncogenesis: Epstein-Barr virus. *Am. J. Otolaryngol.* **11:**375–381.

Garcia, J. H., L. E. Colon, R. J. Whitley, and F. J. Wilmes. 1984. Diagnosis of viral encephalitis by brain biopsy. *Semin. Diagn. Pathol.* **1:**71–81.

Gastaud, P., C. Baudouin, and D. Ouzan. 1989. Detection of HBs antigen, DNA polymerase activity, and hepatitis B virus DNA in tears: relevance to hepatitis B transmission by tears. *Br. J. Ophthalmol.* **73:**333–336.

Gavrilovskaya, I. N., M. Shepley, R. Shaw, M. H. Ginsberg, and E. R. Mackow. 1998. Beta3 integrins mediate the cellular entry of hantaviruses that cause respiratory failure. *Proc. Natl. Acad. Sci. USA* **95:**7074–7079.

Geijtenbeek, T. B., D. S. Kwon, R. Torensma, S. J. van Vliet, G. C. van Duijnhoven, J. Middel, I. L. Cornelissen, H. S. Nottet, V. N. KewalRamani, D. R. Littman, C. G. Figdor, and Y. van Kooyk. 2000. DC-SIGN, a dendritic cell-specific HIV-1-binding protein that enhances trans-infection of T cells. *Cell* **100:**587–597.

Glass, J. D., and R. T. Johnson. 1996. Human immunodeficiency virus and the brain. *Annu. Rev. Neurosci.* **19:**1–26.

Goebel, C., L. G. Mackay, E. R. Vickers, and L. E. Mather. 2000. Determination of defensin HNP-1, HNP-2, and HNP-3 in human saliva by using LC/MS. *Peptides* **21:**757–765.

Gosztonyi, G., J. Artigas, L. Lamperth, and H. D. Webster. 1994. Human immunodeficiency virus. HIV) distribution in HIV encephalitis: study of 19 cases with combined use of in situ hybridization and immunocytochemistry. *J. Neuropathol. Exp. Neurol.* **53:**521–534.

Gougeon, M. L., H. Lecoeur, A. Dulioust, M. G. Enouf, M. Crouvoiser, C. Goujard, T. Debord, and L. Montagnier. 1996. Programmed cell death in peripheral lymphocytes from HIV-infected persons: increased susceptibility to apoptosis of CD4 and CD8 T cells correlates with lymphocyte activation and with disease progression. *J. Immunol.* **156:**3509–3520.

Gray, F., H. Adle-Biassette, F. Brion, T. Ereau, I. le Maner, V. Levy, and G. Corcket. 2000. Neuronal apoptosis in human immunodeficiency virus infection. *J. Neurovirol.* **6**(Suppl. 1):S38–S43.

Greenberg, H. B., H. F. Clark, and P. A. Offit. 1994. Rotavirus pathology and pathophysiology. *Curr. Top. Microbiol. Immunol.* **185:**255–283.

Greve, J. M., G. Davis, A. M. Meyer, C. P. Forte, S. C. Yost, C. W. Marlor, M. E. Kamarck, and A. McClelland. 1989. The major human rhinovirus receptor is ICAM-1. *Cell* **56:**839–847.

Griffin, D. E. 1997. Virus-induced immune suppression, p. 207–233. *In* N. Nathanson (ed.), *Viral Pathogenesis.* Lippincott-Raven, Phildelphia, Pa.

Guyton, A. C. 1981. *Textbook of Medical Physiology.* The W. B. Saunders Co., Philadelphia, Pa.

Hahn, B. H., G. M. Shaw, K. M. De Cock, and P. M. Sharp. 2000. AIDS as a zoonosis: scientific and public health implications. *Science* **287:**607–614.

Ham, A. W., and D. H. Cormack. 1979. *Histology.* J. B. Lippincott Co., Philadelphia, Pa.

Hart, C. A., and M. Bennett. 1999. Hantavirus infections: epidemiology and pathogenesis. *Microbes Infect.* **1:**1229–1237.

Heath, S. L., J. G. Tew, A. K. Szakal, and G. F. Burton. 1995. Follicular dendritic cells and human immunodeficiency virus infectivity. *Nature* **377:**740–744.

Heel, K. A., R. D. McCauley, J. M. Papadimitriou, and J. C. Hall. 1997. Review: Peyer's patches. *J. Gastroenterol. Hepatol.* **12:** 122–136.

Hidalgo, F., S. Melon, M. de Ona, V. Do Santos, A. Martinez, R. Cimadevilla, and M. Rodriguez. 1998. Diagnosis of herpetic keratoconjunctivitis by nested polymerase chain reaction in human tear film. *Eur. J. Clin. Microbiol. Infect. Dis.* **17:**120–123.

Hines, J. F., and A. B. Jenson. 1997. Human papillomaviruses, p. 199–208. *In* D. H. Connor, F. W. Chandler, D. A. Schwartz, H. J. Manz, and E. E. Lack (ed.), *Pathology of Infectious Diseases,* vol. 1. Appleton & Lange, Stamford, Conn.

Ho, D. D., T. Moudgil, and M. Alam. 1989. Quantitation of human immunodeficiency virus type 1 in the blood of infected persons. *N. Engl. J. Med.* **321:**1621–1625.

Ho, D. D., A. U. Neumann, A. S. Perelson, W. Chen, J. M. Leonard, and M. Markowitz. 1995. Rapid turnover of plasma virions and CD4 lymphocytes in HIV-1 infection. *Nature* **373:**123–126.

Holmes, K. V. 1997. Localization of viral infections, p. 35–53. *In* N. Nathanson (ed.), *Viral Pathogenesis.* Lippincott-Raven, Philadelphia, Pa.

Horwitz, M. S., A. La Cava, C. Fine, E. Rodriguez, A. Ilic, and N. Sarvetnick. 2000. Pancreatic expression of interferon-gamma protects mice from lethal coxsackievirus B3 infection and subsequent myocarditis. *Nat. Med.* **6:**693–697.

Hsiao, J. C., C. S. Chung, and W. Chang. 1999. Vaccinia virus envelope D8L protein binds to cell surface chondroitin sulfate and mediates the adsorption of intracellular mature virions to cells. *J. Virol.* **73:**8750–8761.

Hu, J., M. B. Gardner, and C. J. Miller. 2000. Simian immunodeficiency virus rapidly penetrates the cervicovaginal mucosa after intravaginal inoculation and infects intraepithelial dendritic cells. *J. Virol.* **74:**6087–6095.

Hwang, L. Y., M. W. Ross, C. Zack, L. Bull, K. Rickman, and M. Holleman. 2000. Prevalence of sexually transmitted infections and associated risk factors among populations of drug abusers. *Clin. Infect. Dis.* **31:**920–926.

Imaoka, K., C. J. Miller, M. Kubota, M. B. McChesney, B. Lohman, M. Yamamoto, K. Fujihashi, K. Someya, M. Honda, J. R. McGhee, and H. Kiyono. 1998. Nasal immunization of nonhuman primates with simian immunodeficiency virus p55gag and cholera toxin adjuvant induces Th1/Th2 help for virus-specific immune responses in reproductive tissues. *J. Immunol.* **161:**5952–5958.

Jackson, T., D. Sheppard, M. Denyer, W. Blakemore, and A. M. King. 2000. The epithelial integrin alphavbeta6 is a receptor for foot-and-mouth disease virus. *J. Virol.* **74:**4949–4956.

Johnson, R. T. 1987. The pathogenesis of acute viral encephalitis and postinfectious encephalomyelitis. *J. Infect. Dis.* **155:**359–364.

Johnston, R. E., and C. J. Peters. 1996. Alphaviruses, p. 843–898. *In* B. N. Fields, D. M. Knipe, and P. M. Howley (ed.), *Fields Virology*, 3rd ed. Lippincott Williams & Wilkins, Philadelphia, Pa.

Katyal, R., S. V. Rana, K. Vaiphei, S. Ohja, K. Singh, and V. Singh. 1999. Effect of rotavirus infection on small gut pathophysiology in a mouse model. *J. Gastroenterol. Hepatol.* **14:**779–784.

Katzenstein, A. A. F. 1990. Acute lung injury patterns: diffuse alveolar damage, acute interstitial pneumonia, bronchiolitis obliterans-organizing pneumonia, p. 9–57. *In* J. Bennington (ed.), *Surgical Pathology of Non-Neoplastic Lung Disease.* The W. B. Saunders Co., Philadelphia, Pa.

Kennedy, C., and P. Wanglee. 1967. Encephalitis: a variable syndrome in response to viral infection. *Pediatr. Clin. North Am.* **14:**809–817.

Khalifa, M. A., and E. E. Lack. 1997. Herpes simplex virus infection, p. 147–152. *In* D. H. Connor, F. W. Chandler, D. A. Schwartz, H. J. Manz, and E. E. Lack (ed.). *Pathology of Infectious Diseases*, vol. 1. Appleton & Lange, Stamford, Conn.

Kim, C. M., K. Koike, I. Saito, T. Miyamura, and G. Jay. 1991. HBx gene of hepatitis B virus induces liver cancer in transgenic mice. *Nature* **351:**317–320.

Klatzmann, D., E. Champagne, S. Chamaret, J. Gruest, D. Guetard, T. Hercend, J. C. Gluckman, and L. Montagnier. 1984. T-lymphocyte T4 molecule behaves as the receptor for human retrovirus LAV. *Nature* **312:**767–768.

Klein, G. 1979. The role of viral transformation and cytogenetic changes in viral oncogenesis. *Ciba Found. Symp.* **66:**335–358.

Knipe, D. M. 1996. Virus-host cell interactions, p. 273–299. *In* B. N. Fields, D. M. Knipe, and P. M. Howley (ed.), *Fields Virology*, 3rd ed. Lippincott Williams & Wilkins, Phildelphia, Pa.

Komada, H., M. Tsurudome, H. Bando, M. Nishio, M. Ueda, H. Tsumura, and Y. Ito. 1989. Immunological response of monkeys infected intranasally with human parainfluenza virus type 4. *J. Gen. Virol.* **70:**3487–3492.

Konno, T., H. Suzuki, S. Kitaoka, T. Sato, N. Fukuhara, O. Yoshie, K. Fukudome, and Y. Numazaki. 1993. Proteolytic enhancement of human rotavirus infectivity. *Clin. Infect. Dis.* **16**(Suppl. 2):S92–S97.

Kono, R., K. Miyamura, E. Tajiri, A. Sasagawa, and P. Phuapradit. 1977. Virological and serological studies of neurological complications of acute hemorrhagic conjunctivitis in Thailand. *J. Infect. Dis.* **135:**706–713.

Kuklin, N. A., L. Rott, N. Feng, M. E. Conner, N. Wagner, W. Muller, and H. B. Greenberg. 2001. Protective intestinal anti-rotavirus B cell immunity is dependent on alpha(4)beta(7) integrin expression but does not require IgA antibody production. *J. Immunol.* **166:**1894–1902.

Kure, K., W. D. Lyman, K. M. Weidenheim, and D. W. Dickson. 1990. Cellular localization of an HIV-1 antigen in subacute AIDS encephalitis using an improved double-labeling immunohistochemical method. *Am. J. Pathol.* **136:**1085–1092.

Lalani, A. S., J. Masters, W. Zeng, J. Barrett, R. Pannu, H. Everett, C. W. Arendt, and G. McFadden. 1999. Use of chemokine receptors by poxviruses. *Science* **286:**1968–1971.

Lentz, T. L., T. G. Burrage, A. L. Smith, and G. H. Tignor. 1983. The acetylcholine receptor as a cellular receptor for rabies virus. *Yale J. Biol. Med.* **56:**315–322.

Levy, J. A., J. Shimabukuro, T. McHugh, C. Casavant, D. Stites, and L. Oshiro. 1985. AIDS-associated retroviruses (ARV) can productively infect other cells besides human T helper cells. *Virology* **147:**441–448.

Liu, T., Q. Tang, and R. L. Hendricks. 1996. Inflammatory infiltration of the trigeminal ganglion after herpes simplex virus type 1 corneal infection. *J. Virol.* **70:**264–271.

Lobach, D. F., D. P. Bolognesi, and R. E. Kaufman. 1985. Retroviruses and human cancer: evaluation of T-lymphocyte transformation by human T-cell leukemia-lymphoma virus. *Cancer Investig.* **3:**145–160.

Magar, R., and R. Larochelle. 1992. Immunohistochemical detection of porcine rotavirus using immunogold silver staining (IGSS). *J. Vet. Diagn. Investig.* **4:**3–7.

Manchester, M., D. S. Eto, A. Valsamakis, P. B. Liton, R. Fernandez-Munoz, P. A. Rota, W. J. Bellini, D. N. Forthal, and M. B. Oldstone. 2000. Clinical isolates of measles virus use CD46 as a cellular receptor. *J. Virol.* **74:**3967–3974.

Manz, H. J. 1997. Arboviral encephalitides, p. 71–83. *In* D. H. Connor, F. W. Chandler, D. A. Schwartz, H. J. Manz, and E. E. Lack. *Pathology of Infectious Diseases*, vol. 1. Appleton & Lange, Stamford, Conn.

Masliah, E., C. L. Achim, N. Ge, R. DeTeresa, R. D. Terry, and C. A. Wiley. 1992. Spectrum of human immunodeficiency virus-associated neocortical damage. *Ann. Neurol.* **32:**321–329.

Mathews, M., H. P. Jia, J. M. Guthmiller, G. Losh, S. Graham, G. K. Johnson, B. F. Tack, and P. B. McCray. 1999. Production of beta-defensin antimicrobial peptides by the oral mucosa and salivary glands. *Infect. Immun.* **67:**2740–2745.

McGhee, J. R., and H. Kiyono. 1999. The mucosal immune system, p. 909–945. *In* W. E. Paul (ed.), *Fundamental Immunology.* Lippincott-Raven, Philadelphia, Pa.

Melnick, J. L. 1992. Properties and classification of hepatitis A virus. *Vaccine* **10**(Suppl. 1):S24–S26.

Meltzer, M. S., D. R. Skillman, P. J. Gomatos, D. C. Kalter, and H. E. Gendelman. 1990. Role of mononuclear phagocytes in the pathogenesis of human immunodeficiency virus infection. *Annu. Rev. Immunol.* **8:**169–194.

Mendel, I., M. Muraine, P. Riachi, F. el Forzli, C. Bertin, R. Colin, G. Brasseur, and C. Buffet-Janvresse. 1997. Detection and genotyping of the hepatitis C RNA in tear fluid from patients with chronic hepatitis C. *J. Med. Virol.* **51:**231–233.

Mims, C. A., A. Nash, and J. Stephen. 2001. *Mims' Pathogenesis of Infectious Disease*, 5th ed. Academic Press, Inc., San Diego, Calif.

Mitchell, H., M. Drake, and G. Medley. 1986. Prospective evaluation of risk of cervical cancer after cytological evidence of human papilloma virus infection. *Lancet* i:573–575.

Monteiro-Riviere, N. A. 1998. Integument, p. 303–332. *In* H. D. Dellmann, and J. Eurell (ed.), *Textbook of Veterinary Histology*. The Williams & Wilkins Co., Baltimore, Md.

Murphy, F. A., A. K. Harrison, W. C. Winn, and S. P. Bauer. 1973. Comparative pathogenesis of rabies and rabies-like viruses: infection of the central nervous system and centrifugal spread of virus to peripheral tissues. *Lab. Investig.* 29:1–16.

Naniche, D., G. Varior-Krishnan, F. Cervoni, T. F. Wild, B. Rossi, C. Rabourdin-Combe, and D. Gerlier. 1993. Human membrane cofactor protein (CD46) acts as a cellular receptor for measles virus. *J. Virol.* 67:6025–6032.

Nathanson, N. 1996. Epidemiology, p. 251–271. *In* B. N. Fields, D. M. Knipe, and P. M. Howley (ed.), *Fields Virology*, 3rd ed. Lippincott Williams & Wilkins, Philadelphia, Pa.

Nathanson, N., and K. L. Tyler. 1997. Entry, dissemination, shedding, and transmission of viruses, p. 13–33. *In* N. Nathanson (ed.), *Viral Pathogenesis*. Lippincott-Raven, Philadelphia, Pa.

Navia, B. A., E. S. Cho, C. K. Petito, and R. W. Price. 1986. The AIDS dementia complex. II. Neuropathology. *Ann. Neurol.* 19:525–535.

Neutra, M. R. 1999. Interactions of viruses and microparticles with apical plasma membranes of M cells: implications for human immunodeficiency virus transmission. *J. Infect. Dis.* 179(Suppl. 3):S441–S443.

Neutra, M. R., N. J. Mantis, A. Frey, and P. J. Giannasca. 1999. The composition and function of M cell apical membranes: implications for microbial pathogenesis. *Semin. Immunol.* 11:171–181.

Nevins, J. R., and P. K. Vogt. 1996. Cell transformation by viruses, p. 301–343. *In* B. N. Fields, D. M. Knipe, and P. M. Howley (ed.), *Fields Virology*, 3rd ed. Lippincott Williams & Wilkins, Philadelphia, Pa.

Nicolau, S., and E. Mateiesco. 1928. Septinevrites a virus rabique des rues. Preuves de la marche centrifuge du virus dans les nerfs peripheriques des lapins. *C. R. Acad. Sci.* 186:1072–1074.

Nolte, K. B., J. Guarner, W. J. Shieh., and S. R. Zaki. Emerging infectious diseases and the forensic pathologist. *In* L. R. Froede (ed.), *Handbook of Forensic Pathology*, in press. College of American Pathologists, Northfield, Ill.

O'Neil, L. L., M. J. Burkhard, L. J. Diehl, and E. A. Hoover. 1995. Vertical transmission of feline immunodeficiency virus. *AIDS Res. Hum. Retroviruses* 11:171–182.

Olson, N. H., P. R. Kolatkar, M. A. Oliveira, R. H. Cheng, J. M. Greve, A. McClelland, T. S. Baker, and M. G. Rossmann. 1993. Structure of a human rhinovirus complexed with its receptor molecule. *Proc. Natl. Acad. Sci. USA* 90:507–511.

Overbaugh, J., J. Kreiss, M. Poss, P. Lewis, S. Mostad, G. John, R. Nduati, D. Mbori-Ngacha, H. Martin, B. Richardson, S. Jackson, J. Neilson, E. M. Long, D. Panteleeff, M. Welch, J. Rakwar, D. Jackson, B. Chohan, L. Lavreys, K. Mandaliya, J. Ndinya-Achola, and J. Bwayo. 1999. Studies of human immunodeficiency virus type 1 mucosal viral shedding and transmission in Kenya. *J. Infect. Dis.* 179(Suppl. 3):S401–S404.

Pacitti, A. M., O. Jarrett, and D. Hay. 1986. Transmission of feline leukaemia virus in the milk of a non-viraemic cat. *Vet. Rec.* 118:381–384.

Pantaleo, G., and A. S. Fauci. 1995. New concepts in the immunopathogenesis of HIV infection. *Annu. Rev. Immunol.* 13:487–512.

Pantaleo, G., C. Graziosi, L. Butini, P. A. Pizzo, S. M. Schnittman, D. P. Kotler, and A. S. Fauci. 1991. Lymphoid organs function as major reservoirs for human immunodeficiency virus. *Proc. Natl. Acad. Sci. USA* 88:9838–9842.

Peluso, R., A. Haase, L. Stowring, M. Edwards, and P. Ventura. 1985. A Trojan Horse mechanism for the spread of visna virus in monocytes. *Virology* 147:231–236.

Perelson, A. S., A. U. Neumann, M. Markowitz, J. M. Leonard, and D. D. Ho. 1996. HIV-1 dynamics in vivo: virion clearance rate, infected cell life-span, and viral generation time. *Science* 271:1582–1586.

Peters, C. J., and S. R. Zaki. 1999. Viral hemorrhagic fevers: overview, p. 1182–1190. *In* R. L. Guerrant, D. J. Krogstad, J. A. Maguire, D. H. Walker, and P. F. Weller (ed.), *Tropical Infectious Diseases*. Churchill Livingstone, Inc., New York, N.Y.

Peters, C. J., S. R. Zaki, and P. E. Rollin. 1997. Viral hemorrhagic fevers, p. 10.1–10.26. *In* R. Fekety (ed.), *Current Medicine. VIII. External Manifestations of Systemic Infections*. Churchill Livingstone, Inc., Philadelphia, Pa.

Pillay, K., A. Coutsoudis, A. K. Agadzi-Naqvi, L. Kuhn, H. M. Coovadia, and E. N. Janoff. 2001. Secretory leukocyte protease inhibitor in vaginal fluids and perinatal human immunodeficiency virus type 1 transmission. *J. Infect. Dis.* 183:653–656.

Plakhov, I. V., E. E. Arlund, C. Aoki, and C. S. Reiss. 1995. The earliest events in vesicular stomatitis virus infection of the murine olfactory neuroepithelium and entry of the central nervous system. *Virology* 209:257–262.

Prato Murphy, M. L., M. A. Forsyth, G. J. Belsham, and J. S. Salt. 1999. Localization of foot-and-mouth disease virus RNA by in situ hybridization within bovine tissues. *Virus Res.* 62:67–76.

Quinn, T. C. 1996. Global burden of the HIV pandemic. *Lancet* 348:99–106.

Rajcani, J., and A. Vojvodova. 1998. The role of herpes simplex virus glycoproteins in the virus replication cycle. *Acta Virol.* 42:103–118.

Ravkov, E. V., S. T. Nichol, and R. W. Compans. 1997. Polarized entry and release in epithelial cells of Black Creek Canal virus, a New World hantavirus. *J. Virol.* 71:1147–1154.

Ren, R., and V. R. Racaniello. 1992. Poliovirus spreads from muscle to the central nervous system by neural pathways. *J. Infect. Dis.* 166:747–752.

Rickinson, A. B., and E. Kieff. 1996. Epstein-Barr virus, p. 2397–2446. *In* B. N. Fields, D. M. Knipe, and P. M. Howley (ed.), *Fields Virology*, 3rd ed. Lippincott Williams & Wilkins, Philadelphia, Pa.

Rose, N. R. 2000. Viral damage or 'molecular mimicry'—placing the blame in myocarditis. *Nat. Med.* 6:631–632.

Rosenblum, M. K. 1997. Human immunodeficiency virus infection lesions of the central nervous system, p. 183–197. *In* D. H. Connor, F. W. Chandler, D. A. Schwartz, H. J. Manz, and E. E. Lack (ed.), *Pathology of Infectious Diseases*. Appleton & Lange, Stamford, Conn.

Ross, S. R. 1998. Mouse mammary tumor virus and its interaction with the immune system. *Immunol. Res.* 17:209–216.

Sasseville, V. G., and A. A. Lackner. 1997. Neuropathogenesis of simian immunodeficiency virus infection in macaque monkeys. *J. Neurovirol.* 3:1–9.

Schacker, T., S. Little, E. Connick, K. Gebhard, Z. Q. Zhang, J. Krieger, J. Pryor, D. Havlir, J. K. Wong, R. T. Schooley, D. Richman, L. Corey, and A. T. Haase. 2001. Productive infection of T cells in lymphoid tissues during primary and early human immunodeficiency virus infection. *J. Infect. Dis.* 183:555–562.

Schwab, K. S., and R. D. Shaw. 1993. Infectious diarrhoea. Viruses. *Baillieres Clin. Gastroenterol.* 7:307–331.

Shepherd, R. W., D. G. Gall, D. G. Butler, and J. R. Hamilton. 1979. Determinants of diarrhea in viral enteritis. The role of ion transport and epithelial changes in the ileum in transmissible gastroenteritis in piglets. *Gastroenterology* **76:**20–24.

Shieh, W. J., J. Guarner, M. Layton, A. Fine, J. Miller, D. Nash, G. L. Campbell, J. T. Roehrig, D. J. Gubler, and S. R. Zaki. 2000. The role of pathology in an investigation of an outbreak of West Nile encephalitis in New York, 1999. *Emerg. Infect. Dis.* **6:**370–372.

Shugars, D. C. 1999. Endogenous mucosal antiviral factors of the oral cavity. *J. Infect. Dis.* **179**(Suppl. 3):S431–S435.

Shulman, L. M., Y. Manor, R. Azar, R. Handsher, A. Vonsover, E. Mendelson, S. Rothman, D. Hassin, T. Halmut, B. Abramovitz, and N. Varsano. 1997. Identification of a new strain of fastidious enterovirus 70 as the causative agent of an outbreak of hemorrhagic conjunctivitis. *J. Clin. Microbiol.* **35:**2145–2149.

Siegel, R. J. 1997. Human immunodeficiency virus-associated lymphoid disease, p. 161–168. *In* D. H. Connor, F. W. Chandler, D. A. Schwartz, H. J. Manz, and E. E. Lack (ed.), *Pathology of Infectious Diseases*, vol. 1. Appleton & Lange, Stamford, Conn.

Silvestris, F., R. C. Williams, and F. Dammacco. 1995. Autoreactivity in HIV-1 infection: the role of molecular mimicry. *Clin. Immunol. Immunopathol.* **75:**197–205.

Sinzger, C., and G. Jahn. 1996. Human cytomegalovirus cell tropism and pathogenesis. *Intervirology* **39:**302–319.

Sixbey, J. W., J. G. Nedrud, N. Raab-Traub, R. A. Hanes, and J. S. Pagano. 1984. Epstein-Barr virus replication in oropharyngeal epithelial cells. *N. Engl. J. Med.* **310:**1225–1230.

Smith, C. E. 1969. The role of immunological responses in the pathogenesis of encephalitis. *J. Gen. Microbiol.* **59:**17–18.

Snodgrass, D. R., A. Ferguson, F. Allan, K. W. Angus, and B. Mitchell. 1979. Small intestinal morphology and epithelial cell kinetics in lamb rotavirus infections. *Gastroenterology* **76:**477–481.

Spira, A. I., P. A. Marx, B. K. Patterson, J. Mahoney, R. A. Koup, S. M. Wolinsky, and D. D. Ho. 1996. Cellular targets of infection and route of viral dissemination after an intravaginal inoculation of simian immunodeficiency virus into rhesus macaques. *J. Exp. Med.* **183:**215–225.

Staunton, D. E., V. J. Merluzzi, R. Rothlein, R. Barton, S. D. Marlin, and T. A. Springer. 1989. A cell adhesion molecule, ICAM-1, is the major surface receptor for rhinoviruses. *Cell* **56:**849–853.

Su, H., and R. J. Boackle. 1991. Interaction of the envelope glycoprotein of human immunodeficiency virus with C1q and fibronectin under conditions present in human saliva. *Mol. Immunol.* **28:**811–817.

Takahashi, K., S. L. Wesselingh, D. E. Griffin, J. C. McArthur, R. T. Johnson, and J. D. Glass. 1996. Localization of HIV-1 in human brain using polymerase chain reaction/in situ hybridization and immunocytochemistry. *Ann. Neurol.* **39:**705–711.

Tashiro, M., M. Yamakawa, K. Tobita, J. T. Seto, H. D. Klenk, and R. Rott. 1990. Altered budding site of a pantropic mutant of Sendai virus, F1-R, in polarized epithelial cells. *J. Virol.* **64:**4672–4677.

Tenovuo, J. 1998. Antimicrobial function of human saliva—how important is it for oral health?" *Acta Odontol. Scand.* **56:**250–256.

Tirabassi, R. S., R. A. Townley, M. G. Eldridge, and L. W. Enquist. 1998. Molecular mechanisms of neurotropic herpesvirus invasion and spread in the CNS. *Neurosci. Biobehav. Rev.* **22:**709–720.

Tyler, K. L., and B. N. Fields. 1996. Pathogenesis of viral infections, p. 173–218. *In* B. N. Fields, D. M. Knipe, and P. M. Howley (ed.), *Fields Virology*, 3rd ed. Lippincott Williams & Wilkins, Philadelphia, Pa.

Tyler, K. L., and F. Gonzalez-Scarano. 1997. Viral diseases of the central nervous system: acute infections, p. 837–853. *In* N. Nathanson (ed.), *Viral Pathogenesis*. Lippincott-Raven, Philadelphia, Pa.

Uehling, D. T., D. B. Johnson, and W. J. Hopkins. 1999. The urinary tract response to entry of pathogens. *World. J. Urol.* **17:**351–358.

Van de Perre, P., P. Lepage, J. Homsy, and F. Dabis. 1992. Mother-to-infant transmission of human immunodeficiency virus by breast milk: presumed innocent or presumed guilty?" *Clin. Infect. Dis.* **15:**502–507.

Vazeux, R., N. Brousse, A. Jarry, D. Henin, C. Marche, C. Vedrenne, J. Mikol, M. Wolff, C. Michon, W. Rozenbaum, et al. 1987. AIDS subacute encephalitis. Identification of HIV-infected cells. *Am. J. Pathol.* **126:**403–410.

Vernazza, P. L., J. R. Dyer, S. A. Fiscus, J. J. Eron, and M. S. Cohen. 1997a. HIV-1 viral load in blood, semen and saliva. *AIDS* **11:**1058–1059.

Vernazza, P. L., J. J. Eron, S. A. Fiscus, and M. S. Cohen. 1999. Sexual transmission of HIV: infectiousness and prevention. *AIDS* **13:**155–166.

Vernazza, P. L., B. L. Gilliam, J. Dyer, S. A. Fiscus, J. J. Eron, A. C. Frank, and M. S. Cohen. 1997b. Quantification of HIV in semen: correlation with antiviral treatment and immune status. *AIDS* **11:**987–993.

Vochem, M., K. Hamprecht, G. Jahn, and C. P. Speer. 1998. Transmission of cytomegalovirus to preterm infants through breast milk. *Pediatr. Infect. Dis. J.* **17:**53–58.

Weaver, S. C. 1997. Vector biology in arboviral pathogenesis, p. 329–352. *In* N. Nathanson (ed.), *Viral Pathogenesis*. Lippincott-Raven, Philadelphia, Pa.

Wei, X., S. K. Ghosh, M. E. Taylor, V. A. Johnson, E. A. Emini, P. Deutsch, J. D. Lifson, S. Bonhoeffer, M. A. Nowak, B. H. Hahn, et al. 1995. Viral dynamics in human immunodeficiency virus type 1 infection. *Nature* **373:**117–122.

Weis, W., J. H. Brown, S. Cusack, J. C. Paulson, J. J. Skehel, and D. C. Wiley. 1988. Structure of the influenza virus haemagglutinin complexed with its receptor, sialic acid. *Nature* **333:**426–431.

Whitley, R. J. 1990. Viral encephalitis. *N. Engl. J. Med.* **323:**242–250.

Wiley, C. A., and C. Achim. 1994. Human immunodeficiency virus encephalitis is the pathological correlate of dementia in acquired immunodeficiency syndrome. *Ann. Neurol.* **36:**673–676.

Wiley, C. A., R. D. Schrier, J. A. Nelson, P. W. Lampert, and M. B. Oldstone. 1986. Cellular localization of human immunodeficiency virus infection within the brains of acquired immune deficiency syndrome patients. *Proc. Natl. Acad. Sci. USA* **83:**7089–7093.

Wiley, C. A., V. Soontornniyomkij, L. Radhakrishnan, E. Masliah, J. Mellors, S. A. Hermann, P. Dailey, and C. L. Achim. 1998. Distribution of brain HIV load in AIDS. *Brain Pathol.* **8:**277–284.

Winkler, G. C., and N. F. Cheville. 1986. Ultrastructural morphometric investigation of early lesions in the pulmonary alveolar region of pigs during experimental swine influenza infection. *Am. J. Pathol.* **122:**541–552.

Winn, W. C., Jr. 1997. Influenza and parainfluenza viruses, p. 221–227. *In* D. H. Connor, F. W. Chandler, D. A. Schwartz, H. J. Manz, and E. E. Lack (ed.), *Pathology of Infectious Diseases*. Appleton & Lange, Stamford, Conn.

Wright, P. F. 1997. Viral respiratory diseases, p. 703–711. *In* N. Nathanson (ed.), *Viral Pathogenesis*. Lippincott-Raven, Philadelphia, Pa.

Wu, A. M., G. Csako, and A. Herp. 1994. Structure, biosynthesis, and function of salivary mucins. *Mol. Cell. Biochem.* **137:**39–55.

WuDunn, D., and P. G. Spear. 1989. Initial interaction of herpes simplex virus with cells is binding to heparan sulfate. *J. Virol.* **63:**52–58.

Yager, J. A., and D. W. Scott. 1993. The skin and appendages, p. 531–738. *In* K. V. F. Jubb, P. C. Kennedy, and N. Palmer (ed.), *Pathology of Domestic Animals,* vol. 1. Academic Press, Inc., San Diego, Calif.

Zaki, S. R. 1997. Hantavirus-associated diseases, p. 125–136. *In* D. H. Connor, F. W. Chandler, D. A. Schwartz, H. J. Manz, and E. E. Lack (ed.), *Pathology of Infectious Diseases,* vol. 1. Appleton & Lange, Stamford, Conn.

Zaki, S. R., and C. S. Goldsmith. 1998. Pathologic features of filovirus infections in humans. *Curr. Top. Microbiol. Immunol.* **235:**97–116.

Zaki, S. R., P. W. Greer, L. M. Coffield, C. S. Goldsmith, K. B. Nolte, K. Foucar, R. M. Feddersen, R. E. Zumwalt, G. L. Miller, A. S. Khan, et al. 1995. Hantavirus pulmonary syndrome. Pathogenesis of an emerging infectious disease. *Am. J. Pathol.* **146:**552–579.

Zaki, S. R., and C. D. Paddock. 1999. The emerging role of pathology in infectious diseases, p. 181–200. *In* W. M. Scheld, W. A. Craig, and J. M. Hughes (ed.), *Emerging Infections 3.* ASM Press, Washington, D.C.

Zaki, S. R., and C. J. Peters. 1997. Viral hemorrhagic fevers, p. 347–364. *In* D. H. Connor, F. W. Chandler, D. A. Schwartz, H. J. Manz, and E. E. Lack (ed.), *Pathology of Infectious Diseases,* vol. 1. Appleton & Lange. Stamford, Conn.

Zhang, Z., T. Schuler, M. Zupancic, S. Wietgrefe, K. A. Staskus, K. A. Reimann, T. A. Reinhart, M. Rogan, W. Cavert, C. J. Miller, R. S. Veazey, D. Notermans, S. Little, S. A. Danner, D. D. Richman, D. Havlir, J. Wong, H. L. Jordan, T. W. Schacker, P. Racz, K. Tenner-Racz, N. L. Letvin, S. Wolinsky, and A. T. Haase. 1999. Sexual transmission and propagation of SIV and HIV in resting and activated CD4+ T cells. *Science* **286:**1353–1357.

VI. EVASION AND LATENCY

Immunology of Infectious Diseases
Edited by S. H. E. Kaufmann, A. Sher, and R. Ahmed
© 2002 ASM Press, Washington, D.C.

Chapter 23

Bacterial Persistence: Strategies for Survival

ERNESTO J. MUÑOZ-ELÍAS AND JOHN D. MCKINNEY

Persistent (pər–'sis–tənt), *adj.* continuing steadfastly or obstinately, especially in the face of opposition or adversity.

April 1846 was indeed the cruelest month for the denizens of the Faeroe Islands, a small Atlantic archipelago midway between Iceland and Denmark. A ship sailing from Copenhagen put into port at the Faeroes to unload cargo, which unexpectedly included an incubating case of measles. From one infected crewman, the virus jumped to the Islanders and swept through the population with devastating force. A Danish physician, Peter Ludwig Panum, was promptly dispatched from Copenhagen to lend aid and to report on the epidemic. Panum's official report highlights the epidemic's virulence: among the nearly 8,000 inhabitants of the Faeroes, there were more than 6,000 verified cases and a high rate of mortality (Panum, 1847). As is so often true for "childhood" infections like measles, the course of disease was particularly severe in exposed adults—with the exception of one group numbering a few hundreds. These individuals, all elderly, were the last survivors of an imported epidemic of measles that had briefly ravaged the Faeroes in 1781. Among these individuals, Panum found not a single case of measles. The conclusion was inescapable, if surprising—a single exposure some 65 years earlier had conferred lifelong protective immunity against reinfection.

Like the epidemic of 1781 that preceded it, the epidemic of 1846 quickly abated. With remarkable perspicacity, Panum deduced that the epidemic had burnt out because (i) an infected individual was contagious for only a brief period and (ii) the same individual was never infected twice. Panum's study laid the cornerstone for subsequent research into the epidemic dynamics of acute infections, but his tangential studies in the Faeroes were equally important, if

less famous. Motivated by the belief that each disease must be understood in the context of all, Panum dug deeper and discovered, to his astonishment, that the Faeroes harbored very few of the communicable diseases that were rife in Copenhagen. Notable among these were two bacterial infections that remain all too familiar in our own era: typhoid and tuberculosis.

Why these two diseases, and not so many others? Most bacteria cause acute infections that cannot withstand the onslaught of the host adaptive immune response. Unusually, the bacteria that cause typhoid (*Salmonella enterica* serovar Typhi) and tuberculosis (*Mycobacterium tuberculosis*) cause infections that persist, often for the lifetime of the host. Persistence is responsible for the unusual epidemic characteristics of diseases like tuberculosis. A relevant metric is the "critical community size" (CCS) required for endemicity. The theoretical and observed CCS for measles virus is a staggering 250,000 individuals; in smaller populations, measles self-extinguishes after exhausting the pool of naive susceptible hosts (Keeling and Grenfell, 1997; Keeling, 1997). Human populations on this scale have existed for only a few thousand years, suggesting that measles is a newcomer to the human niche. This view is supported by field studies by epidemiologist Francis Black, who found that imported measles was incapable of persisting in small, isolated human populations, e.g., in the South American Amazon basin (Black, 1966, 1975; Black et al., 1974). In contrast, tuberculosis was endemic in many of these "primitive" communities. Modeling studies put the CCS for tuberculosis at less than 500 individuals (McGrath, 1988), which presumably explains the antiquity of tuberculosis as a human disease (Daniel et al., 1994; Haas and Haas, 1996). Persistence is also reflected in the contrasting epidemic dynamics of diseases caused by persistent and

---

Ernesto J. Muñoz-Elías and John D. McKinney • The Rockefeller University, 1230 York Ave., New York, NY 10021.

nonpersistent pathogens; e.g., measles epidemics wax and wane over weeks or months (Fig. 1A) (Keeling, 1997), whereas tuberculosis epidemics span centuries (Fig. 1B) (Grigg, 1958; Blower et al., 1995).

   S. enterica serovar Typhi and *M. tuberculosis* are not unique in their ability to cause persistent infections. Indeed, the roster of persistent pathogens continues to lengthen as technological advances allow the identification of previously unknown species. An important example is the recognition that gastritis, gastric and duodenal ulcers, and gastric neoplasms and lymphomas are often linked to colonization of the human stomach by *Helicobacter pylori* (Dubois et al., 2000). Via mechanisms that are only partly understood, this gram-negative spiral bacterium has evolved to exploit a niche that was assumed to be devoid of microbial life. This has proven to be a remarkably successful strategy—on current estimates, the stomachs of half the global human population harbor *H. pylori*, often for the lifetime of the host (Taylor and Blaser, 1991). As the list of persistent pathogens grows, so does our appreciation of the diversity and sophistication of the mechanisms that allow these microbial invaders to survive "in the face of opposition or adversity." A comprehensive survey of persistent bacterial pathogens is beyond the scope

of this chapter, which will focus on a few organisms as paradigms of persistence strategies.

TREPONEMA PALLIDUM—WHY RUN IF YOU CAN HIDE?

   Several spirochetes of the genus *Treponema* cause persistent infections in humans, including *Treponema pallidum*, the etiologic agent of syphilis (Fig. 2). Spirochetes are a phylogenetically distinct group of prokaryotes with an outer membrane and a periplasmic space, similar to the gram-negative bacteria; however, the outer membrane of treponemes has a higher lipid-to-protein ratio and lacks the proinflammatory constituent lipopolysaccharide (LPS) (Radolf et al., 1989; Walker et al., 1989; Radolf, 1995). The periplasmic space contains the flagella of these highly motile, slender, and elongated "corkscrew" bacteria. Syphilis was first recognized in the late 15th century after the first European explorers returned from the Americas, where the disease was probably endemic (Quétel, 1990). When syphilis first erupted in Europe, it was highly virulent and usually fatal. As the spirochete spread throughout Europe it was rapidly attenuated, and a milder, more

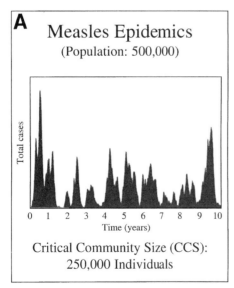

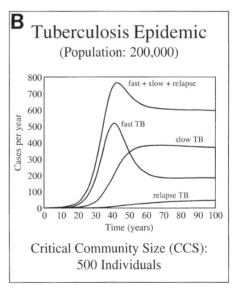

Figure 1. Contrasting epidemic dynamics of measles and TB. (A) Numerical simulation of a measles epidemic initiated by entering one infectious case at time zero into a susceptible population of 500,000. The simulation illustrates successive epidemic waves at roughly 6- to 12-month intervals. Redrawn from Keeling (1997) with permission of the American Association for the Advancement of Science. (B) Numerical simulation of a tuberculosis epidemic initiated by entering one infectious case at time zero into a population of 200,000. The simulation illustrates the relative contribution of three types of disease to the overall incidence: fast (progressive primary), slow (postprimary), and relapse tuberculosis. A fourth type, exogenous reinfection, is not included in the model but would presumably increase the peak level and duration of the epidemic. Redrawn from Blower et al. (1995) with permission of the publisher. The contrasting epidemic dynamics of measles and tuberculosis are also reflected in the CCS required for endemicity, which is roughly 250,000 for measles (Keeling, 1997) and 500 or less for tuberculosis (McGrath, 1988).

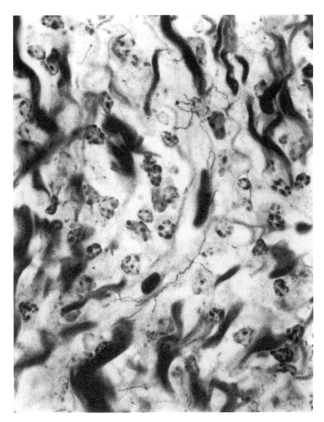

Figure 2. *T. pallidum* spirochetes visible as long, slender, spiral threads in a dermal syphilis lesion. Warthin-Starry stain. Magnification, ×695. Reprinted from Smith et al. (2000) with permission of the publisher.

chronic form of disease became dominant. Why? It may be that the attenuated strains were favored because the horrific manifestations of the early, virulent form of syphilis were a deterrent to sexual transmission. It is also tempting to speculate that attenuated treponemes enjoyed a selective advantage because prolonged survival of the infected host ensured greater opportunity for transmission. Field evidence in favor of this idea derives from the epidemic of myxomatosis that was introduced into the feral rabbit population of Australia in 1950 to 1951 (Fenner and Fantini, 1999). Following an initial period of high host mortality, attenuated strains of myxoma virus emerged and became dominant. Rabbits infected with attenuated viruses were protected against superinfection with the virulent parental virus, and because they lived longer and were more active, dissemination of the attenuated strains was favored.

The incidence of syphilis has declined steeply since the introduction of penicillin in 1943. However, the disease continues to pose a significant health problem worldwide, especially in developing countries. Syphilis is still endemic in some regions of the United States, although the disease rates reported in 1998 were the lowest ever recorded (Centers for Disease Control and Prevention, 1999). The steady decline in the incidence of syphilis from 1991 to the present should not necessarily be interpreted as a victory for public health, because syphilis epidemics display naturally periodic dynamics with approximately 10-year cycles. This means that a period of declining incidence is typically followed by a period in which case rates surge. For example, nationally reported case rates rose year by year during 1986 to 1990, such that the number of cases reported in the United States in 1990 (50,223 cases) was the highest since 1949 (Centers for Disease Control and Prevention, 1991). The periodic dynamics of syphilis epidemics underscores the need for unceasing vigilance in case detection and treatment.

Syphilis is a slowly progressing, multistage disease (Singh and Romanowski, 1999). Infection is transmitted horizontally by sexual contact and vertically by transplacental migration of treponemes. During sexual intercourse, spirochetes present in the genital tract of the donor invade the recipient through small abrasions in the mucous membranes or skin of the genitalia. Replication of the organism at the site of entry triggers massive leukocyte infiltration, blood vessel damage, and tissue necrosis, resulting in the appearance of a primary lesion or "chancre" (Fig. 3A). In most patients, the chancre heals spontaneously after a few weeks and disease progression is arrested. In the less fortunate minority, dissemination from the primary lesion occurs a few weeks after initial infection, leading to generalized infection of almost every tissue of the body, with a notable tropism for the vascular system. The onset of secondary syphilis is marked by the appearance of nodular lesions or papules at these metastatic sites of infection (Fig. 3B). In most cases of primary and secondary syphilis, infection is resolved spontaneously by the adaptive immune response. However, small populations of treponemes may persist in a few isolated lesions and eventually give rise to tertiary syphilis, a chronic disease that usually endures for the lifetime of the host (Fig. 3C). Treatment of primary or secondary syphilis with penicillin is highly effective, but once disease progresses to the tertiary or latent stages it becomes refractory (Ghinsberg and Nitzan, 1992). Tertiary syphilis is characterized by the persistence of mature granulomatous lesions (gummas) containing small numbers of spirochetes (Fig. 3D). Gummas may occur in almost any organ system, causing gradual physiological deterioration. Persistent infection of the central nervous system can lead to destruction of neural tissue, loss of motor activity, and paresthesia, as in the jerking movements

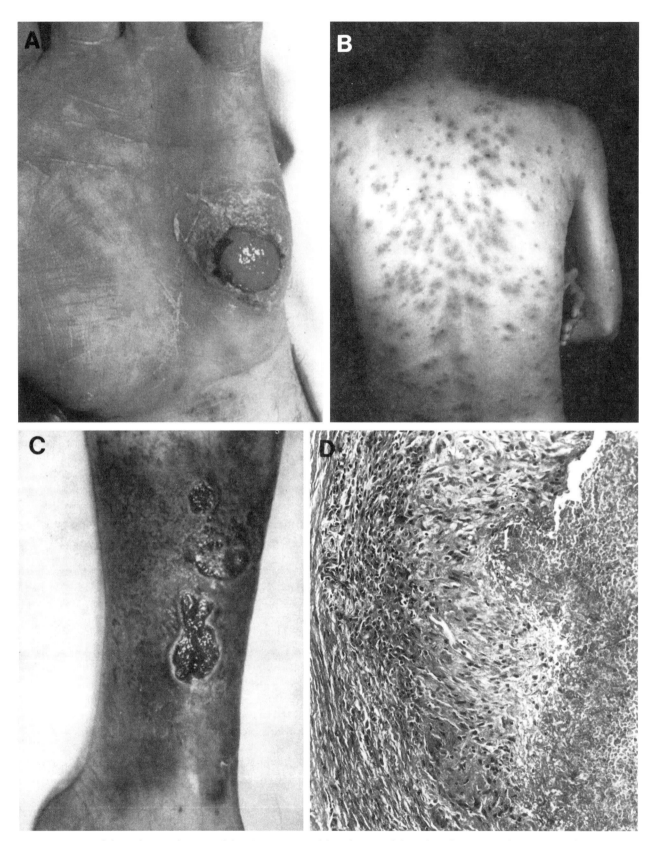

Figure 3. Stages of the multistage disease syphilis. (A) Primary syphilis. Chancre of the palm. The primary chancre most often occurs on the genitalia, but extragenital chancres are not rare. Without treatment, the chancre usually heals in 1 to 4 weeks. (B) Secondary syphilis. Generalized papulosquamous lesions. (C) Tertiary syphilis. Gummas of the leg. Ulcerative gummas can occur in multiple organ systems. The onset is usually 5 to 20 years after the primary stage. (D) Gumma of tertiary syphilis. A central region of caseation necrosis is surrounded by an epithelioid granulomatous reaction (including multinucleated giant cells) and peripheral fibrosis. H&E stain. Magnification, ×126. Panels A to C reprinted from Sauer and Hall (1996) with permission of the publisher; panel D reprinted from Smith et al. (2000) with permission of the publisher.

and paroxysmal pains that are characteristic of tabes dorsalis (sclerosis of the posterior columns of the spinal cord). Gummas occurring in other regions of the central nervous system may give rise to the most dreaded manifestations of syphilis—insanity and generalized paralysis. It is not clear how treponemes damage tissues. No bacterial toxins have been identified, and it is possible that the pathologic changes are due to chronic host responses to persistent spirochetes.

In the prechemotherapy era, longitudinal studies of untreated syphilis revealed that the great majority of patients do not progress beyond the primary stage (Gjestlaand, 1955), and reinoculation studies established that syphilitic patients were partially protected against reinfection (Fitzgerald, 1981). Both branches of the adaptive immune response (humoral and cellular) have been implicated in resistance to *T. pallidum* (Rich et al., 1933). Passive immunization of rabbits with immune serum before infection with *T. pallidum* delays the appearance of syphilitic lesions and attenuates their severity (Bishop and Miller, 1976a), and resistance to reinfection is correlated with the appearance of antitreponemal antibodies (Bishop and Miller, 1976b). Antibodies from immune rabbit serum promote complement-mediated killing of treponemes (Blanco et al., 1984) and block the interaction of *T. pallidum* with extracellular matrix components (fibronectin, laminin, and collagen), which could interfere with the invasion and dissemination of spirochetes (Fitzgerald et al., 1984). Syphilitic patients typically develop immunoglobulin M (IgM) and IgG responses to a slew of treponemal antigens (Baker-Zander et al., 1985).

A role for cellular immunity is suggested by the dramatic infiltration of lesions by mononuclear leukocytes, which occurs as early as 1 week postinfection in the rabbit model (Lukehart et al., 1980a; Sell et al., 1980). The cellular infiltration peaks by 2 weeks postinfection and is composed predominantly of mononuclear phagocytes and T cells, with *Treponema*-specific T cells emerging early in the course of infection (Lukehart et al., 1980b; Baker-Zander et al., 1988; Arroll et al., 1999). Lesions of syphilitic patients contain activated CD8$^+$ cytolytic T lymphocytes (van Voorhis et al., 1996b) and show evidence of a dominant type-1 CD4$^+$ T-cell cytokine response, i.e., gamma interferon (IFN-γ), interleukin-12 (IL-12), and IL-2, but not IL-4 (van Voorhis et al., 1996a). Activation of macrophages by type 1 cytokines is thought to be important for treponemal clearance and lesion resolution (Sell et al., 1980; Lukehart et al., 1980b; Lukehart, 1982). Degraded treponemes are found inside the phagolysosomal compartments of infiltrating macrophages in regress-

ing syphilitic lesions (Ovcinnikov and Delektorskij, 1972), and rabbit peritoneal macrophages are capable of phagocytizing and killing treponemes in vitro (Lukehart and Miller, 1978; Baker-Zander and Lukehart, 1992), particularly in the presence of opsonizing antibodies (Baker-Zander et al., 1993). However, both opsonized and nonopsonized treponemes are unusually resistant to phagocytosis by macrophages, which presumably enhances bacterial survival in inflammatory lesions (Alder et al., 1990; Lukehart et al., 1992).

In the rabbit model of syphilis, long-lasting immunity to *T. pallidum* does not develop until about 3 months postinfection and fails to develop altogether if the course of infection is interrupted by antibiotic therapy (Fitzgerald, 1981). Although adaptive immunity curtails further disease progression, sterilization does not occur, and "immune" animals continue to harbor viable treponemes indefinitely. There is a clear parallel to human disease, in which tertiary syphilis may occur years or decades after initial infection. Two key questions arise: why does acquired immunity develop so slowly in syphilis, and why is the pathogen not eliminated? Poor immunogenicity of and immune evasion by treponemes may provide partial answers.

Persistent treponemes harvested from rabbits at later stages of infection, after >99% of the bacteria have been cleared, are less susceptible to phagocytosis by macrophages (Lukehart et al., 1992), suggesting that persistent infection may be due to a subpopulation of treponemal "persisters" that evade opsonization and phagocytosis. It has been suggested that persisters adopt a "stealth" strategy in vivo, altering their surface composition to reduce their antigenicity (Radolf, 1994). Indeed, ultrastructural studies reveal that the outer membrane of *T. pallidum* is largely devoid of membrane-associated proteins (Radolf et al., 1989), and intact treponemes are poorly reactive with immune rabbit serum unless the outer membrane is removed or damaged (Cox et al., 1992). A number of cell wall-associated *T. pallidum* lipoprotein antigens have been identified, but these are apparently localized to the inner (plasma) membrane rather than the outer membrane (Radolf 1994, 1995).

T. pallidum is a highly invasive pathogen (Haake and Lovett, 1990), so the paucity of surface-exposed proteins leads to the question of what are the ligands that allow the organism to attach and invade after entering the host. These presumably surface-exposed bacterial components are likely targets of the adaptive immune response (Radolf, 1995), but few candidates have been identified to date. Two proteins termed Tromp1 and Tromp2 (for "*T. pallidum* rare outer membrane proteins") were identified by freeze-fracture electron microscopy (Blanco et al., 1997). Although localization of Tromps to the outer membrane is disputed (Akins et al., 1997), anti-Tromp antibodies are treponemicidal and correlate with protective immunity in rabbits (Lewinski et al., 1999). The sequence of the *T. pallidum* genome reveals another group of potentially surface-exposed molecules comprising a novel 12-member gene family termed *tpr* (for "*T. pallidum* repeat") (Fraser et al., 1998). The Tpr proteins contain central domains of variable length and sequence flanked by conserved N- and C-terminal domains, including conserved hypothetical transmembrane domains in some family members. One of these, TprK, is surface exposed and targeted by the protective immune response in rabbits (Centurion-Lara et al., 1999). Antisera from rabbits immunized with TprK is opsonizing for phagocytosis, and TprK-immunized animals are partially protected against challenge with virulent treponemes. The role of the Tpr proteins in treponemal pathogenesis is not known, but these studies suggest that they could be attractive subunit candidates for a vaccine. Strain differences in *tprK* copy number and sequence have been identified, suggesting that variation of TprK might contribute to immune evasion (Centurion-Lara et al., 2000). It is tempting to speculate that the advent of a subpopulation of antigenic variants during infection could account for the failure of adaptive immunity to eliminate small numbers of "persisters," resulting in the prolonged periods of latency that are characteristic of syphilis.

The sequence of the *T. pallidum* genome reveals a number of interesting features. At 1.138 Mbp, the circular chromosome is one of the smallest prokaryotic genomes yet identified, encoding just 1,041 hypothetical open reading frames (Fraser et al., 1998). Not surprisingly, the relative paucity of treponemal genes is associated with a striking reduction in the metabolic complexity of the organism (Weinstock et al., 1998; Radolf et al., 1999). Many basic metabolic pathways are missing, which may account for the failure of exhaustive efforts to cultivate the organism ex vivo. Comparison of the complete genome sequences of *T. pallidum* and *Borrelia burgdorferi* reveals more than 50 open reading frames that are (so far) unique to spirochetes (Fraser et al., 1998). Some of these proteins may determine the specific characteristics of these pathogens, including, perhaps, their unusual ability to cause persistent infections.

BORRELIA SPP.—ANTIGENIC VARIATION: A CHANGE OF FACE WINS THE RACE

Many microbial pathogens control gene expression by programmed rearrangements of specific DNA sequences (Borst and Greaves, 1987). These "contingency loci" (Moxon et al., 1994) affect processes at the interface of pathogen and host, including colonization, invasion, adaptation to different tissue environments, and evasion of immune defenses (Deitsch et al., 1997). Programmed rearrangement of genes encoding surface antigens (antigenic variation) is essential for the evasion of adaptive humoral immunity by extracellular, blood-borne pathogens such as the *Borrelia* spp. that cause relapsing fever (RF) and Lyme disease (LD).

Relapsing Fever

RF is characterized by recurrent febrile episodes, which correspond to intervals of high bacteremia (Fig. 4) (Barbour and Hayes, 1986). The causative agents are arthropod-transmitted spirochetes of the genus *Borrelia*. The RF borrelias persist at titers of up to $\sim 10^8$ bacteria per ml of blood, which ensures transmission of the pathogen to the insect vector during a blood meal. However, extracellular bacteria residing in the blood are exposed to the onslaught of the adaptive humoral immune response; survival in this perilous environment requires the pathogen to keep one step ahead of the host, which the RF borrelias accomplish by means of antigenic variation (Barbour, 1990). Referring to the spirochete-specific antibodies generated during an episode of RF, Meleney (1928) wrote: "These substances [antibodies] are specific for the strain of spirochetes which was present during the preceding attack, but have no influence on the spirochetes of the succeeding relapse. The spirochetes of the relapse give rise, in turn, to immune substances which are specific for them but not for the spirochetes of the first attack." A key question was whether a single bacterium could give rise to the observed waves of variants or whether relapses were due to simultaneous infection with a mixture of variants that were expanded and eliminated in succession. This issue was resolved by infection of rats with *B. turicatae* (one cell per rat) and recovery of antigenically distinct relapse populations (Fig. 4) (Schuhardt and Wilkerson, 1951). The population dynamics of borrelial antigenic variation were clarified by the application of serotype-specific immune sera to identify relapse isolates of *B. hermsii*, which arose at frequencies of $\sim 10^{-3}$ to 10^{-4} per generation (Stoenner et al., 1982). Only a small proportion of the spirochete population converted to other serotypes; this switch was abrupt and coincided with the clearance of the dominant (parental) population. Given the high rate at which serotype switching occurred, it was (and still is) puzzling that only one or a very small number of serotypes were found in each

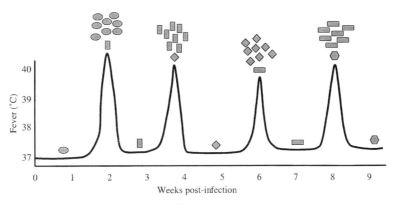

Figure 4. Relapsing fever. Spikes of fever are accompanied by waves of spirochetemia. In each successive wave, a new antigenic variant dominates (indicated by different shapes). As the bacteria are cleared by the specific humoral response, the fever subsides. However, expansion of a newly emergent variant brings about another febrile episode within a few days. Reviewed by Barbour (1990).

relapse. Inhibition of antibody production had no effect on the emergence of serotype variants, demonstrating that humoral immunity was not driving the generation of new spirochete serotypes but merely selecting against preexisting types. The serotype-specific antibodies responsible for spirochete clearance were shown by Barbour et al. (1982) to recognize a family of surface-exposed and serotype-specific lipoproteins, the variable major proteins (VMPs).

The high-frequency variation of VMPs was later shown to result from programmed rearrangements of the *vmp* genes (Meier et al., 1985). The DNA sequences encoding a serotype-specific VMP variant are present in all serotypes, including those that express a different VMP variant (Plasterk et al., 1985). However, serotypes that express a particular VMP contain not one but two DNA loci encoding that variant, i.e., duplication of a given *vmp* is associated with its expression. Duplication occurs via a nonreciprocal recombination event between a silent *vmp* cassette and a unique, unlinked expression site. Recombination between these nonhomologous loci is targeted by homologous regions flanking the expressed and silent *vmp* genes. The repertoire of *vmp* genes is carried on multicopy, linear plasmids, with silent and expressed loci being located on different plasmids (Saint Girons and Barbour, 1991; Kitten and Barbour, 1992; Wilske et al., 1992). This arrangement allows recombination to occur at high frequency without jeopardizing chromosomal integrity. Interestingly, the *vmp* expression site is linked to the telomere of the linear plasmid that carries it (Kitten and Barbour, 1990). Although the significance of telomere linkage is unclear, it is shared by the system responsible for high-frequency variation of the immunodominant variant surface glycoprotein antigen

in the protozoan parasite *Trypanosoma brucei* (Rudenko et al., 1998).

Two additional mechanisms contribute to antigenic variation in *B. hermsii*. The first involves activation of a pseudogene downstream of an expressed *vmp* by intraplasmid (rather than interplasmid) recombination (Restrepo et al., 1994). The second involves the selective hypermutation of expressed *vmp* genes by an unknown mechanism; polymorphisms in expressed *vmp* genes accumulate with time and are absent in silent *vmp* genes (Restrepo and Barbour, 1994).

None of the *vmp* genes is expressed in the insect vector, suggesting that the *vmp* system has evolved to promote bacterial survival exclusively in the vertebrate host (Schwan and Hinnebusch, 1998). What is the role of the VMP system in pathogenesis? Is it simply to offer a constantly changing face to the vertebrate immune system, or do the VMPs contribute directly to infection and dissemination within the host? Emerging evidence suggests that VMP variation may influence the organ tropism and dissemination properties of individual spirochetes (Cadavid et al., 1994, 1997; Pennington et al., 1999). It is tempting to speculate that these knock-on effects of VMP variation could promote the adaptation of *Borrelia* spp. to previously unavailable niches, possibly including new host species.

Lyme Disease

Lyme disease (LD) is a chronic syndrome caused by the tick-borne spirochete *B. burgdorferi*. The ecological cycle of the pathogen is complex, involving several small and intermediate-sized vertebrate reservoirs, which transmit bacteria to the insect vector during blood meals (Gern and Humair, 1998). Humans are thought to be a dead-end host. LD can be divided into three clinical stages (Steere, 1989; Evans, 1999). Many infections do not progress past the first stage, which is marked by a transient skin lesion at the site of inoculation (erythema migrans). In the second stage of disease, lasting up to 6 months, dissemination of the spirochetes gives rise to secondary skin lesions and other intermittent and variable pathologic responses, such as muscular and skeletal pain, meningitis, and carditis. These signs and symptoms often resolve spontaneously, leading to a subclinical or latent phase of variable duration. The third stage of disease, occurring months to years after initial infection, may be characterized by chronic arthritis, cardiomyopathy, and neurological abnormalities. Borrelial persistence has been documented in clinical studies of LD patients (Fikrig et al., 1994; Kuiper et al., 1994) and in animal models (Barthold et al., 1993; Pachner et al., 1995; Roberts et al., 1995; Gylfe et al., 2000). The mechanism(s) that allows *B. burgdorferi* to cause persistent infection—whether chronic or latent—remains poorly understood.

Although LD patients typically produce antibodies against a broad range of *B. burgdorferi* antigens, antibody production may be significantly delayed (Steere, 1989). Studies in animal models of infection also suggest that in some cases *B. burgdorferi* induces a nonprotective immune response. In different strains of mice, susceptibility seems to correlate with production of the type 1 cytokine IFN-γ, whereas resistance correlates with production of the type 2 cytokine IL-4 (Sigal, 1997). This association has also been noted in LD patients (Oksi et al., 1996) and may reflect the importance of antibody-mediated mechanisms of protection against borreliosis (Hu and Klempner, 1997), since type 2 cytokines are associated with dominant humoral immune responses. However, the association of type 1 and type 2 cytokine responses with susceptibility and resistance, respectively, may not be absolute (Brown and Reiner, 1999).

There is accumulating evidence that *B. burgdorferi* evades the humoral response by antigenic variation of surface-exposed lipoproteins encoded by *vls* genes (for "*vmp*-like sequence") (Zhang et al., 1997). The parallel to the *vmp* system of the RF borrelias is striking: the *vls* coding sequences are carried on a linear plasmid, and serotype switching occurs by nonreciprocal recombination between silent *vls* cassettes and an expressed copy (*vlsE*) that is telomere linked (Zhang and Norris, 1998a, 1998b). Because recombination between *vlsE* and segments of the silent *vls* cassettes is combinatorial, the number of unique VlsE variants that could arise by shuffling of

cassette segments is potentially enormous. Antigenic variation of VlsE in mice is associated with loss of seroreactivity, and the rate of variation is higher in immunocompetent mice than in immunodeficient SCID mice (Zhang and Norris, 1998b). These observations suggest that VlsE variation may be an important mechanism of immune evasion. However, the rate of VlsE variation in SCID mice, although relatively low, is still much higher than that observed during in vitro passage, suggesting that VlsE variation may play an adaptive role in vivo in addition to its probable role in immune evasion. This idea is supported by the observation that spirochetes lacking the *vslE* plasmid are less infective to both immunocompetent and SCID mice (Norris et al., 1995).

The genome of *B. burgdorferi* potentially encodes as many as 150 different lipoproteins (Fraser et al., 1997). Lipoproteins of the outer surface protein family (OspA through OspG) are immunodominant and elicit potent inflammatory responses (Sigal, 1997). *B. burgdorferi* does not display high-frequency variation of Osp proteins in vivo, suggesting that Osp proteins probably do not undergo antigenic variation (Barthold, 1993; Persing et al., 1994; Stevenson et al., 1994). However, selection of low-frequency spontaneous escape mutants has been observed in vivo and could account for the considerable polymorphism of Osp proteins within natural populations of spirochetes (Fikrig et al., 1993; Marconi et al., 1993; Livey et al., 1995). Strain variation in Osp serotypes could play an important role in enhancing survival during infection of a host who had previously been exposed to a different antigenic variant.

In addition to high-frequency variation and population-level heterogeneity of borrelial antigens, antigenic modulation may play a role in persistence. Expression of surface lipoproteins, e.g., OspA and OspC, fluctuates as the bacteria travel from vector to host and back again (Philipp, 1998). Spirochetes express high levels of OspA in the gut of the flat tick but precipitously downregulate its expression as they begin their migration to the salivary glands of the feeding tick (de Silva et al., 1996). While levels of OspA remain low throughout infection, expression of OspC is increased and sustained. Recent evidence suggests that antigenic modulation may enhance bacterial resistance to killing by immune sera (de Silva et al., 1998). A number of *B. burgdorferi* genes that are expressed in the host but not in the tick vector or in vitro have been identified (Suk et al., 1995; Das et al., 1997; de Silva and Fikrig, 1997), some of which are induced specifically during the persistent phases of infection (Fikrig et al., 1999).

Some late manifestations of LD may not be related to persistence of viable spirochetes. A subset of

LD patients go on to develop refractory arthritis. It is not clear whether arthritis is due to local persistent infection or to autoimmune disease initiated by infection but maintained in the absence of viable bacteria (Hu and Klempner, 1997; Evans, 1999; Hemmer et al., 1999). The controversy stems from the fact that many patients with Lyme arthritis do not respond to antibiotic therapy and may not have detectable borrelial DNA in their synovial fluid.

The persistence strategies of the RF and LD borrelias are markedly similar, but several important differences should also be noted. Both pathogens cause septicemia, but the spirochete load in blood in RF patients is much higher than in LD patients. The waves of spirochetemia and fever that are the signature of RF are not seen in LD. Antigenic variation and immune selection of variants occur at much lower rates in LD than in RF. These differences probably reflect the divergent ecologies of the causative spirochetes, their vectors, and their intermediate hosts (Barthold, 2000).

NEISSERIA GONORRHOEAE—TRAVELING INCOGNITO TO ESCAPE RECOGNITION

Gonorrhea, caused by the gram-negative diplococcus *Neisseria gonorrhoeae*, is one of the most prevalent sexually transmitted diseases of humans—every year, one million new cases are reported in the United States alone. Gonorrhea is usually a self-limiting, uncomplicated acute infection of the urethra or the cervix with localized inflammation. However, in some instances, acute infection is followed by more serious sequelae, such as epididymitis in men and pelvic inflammatory disease, salpingitis, and endometritis in women (Paavonen, 1998). Damage to the upper reproductive tract in women can lead to infertility and ectopic pregnancy. Mucosal colonization and invasion results in disseminated gonococcal infection in ca. 0.5 to 3.0% of cases, leading to arthritis, dermatitis, tenosynovitis, and (rarely) carditis or meningitis (Kerle et al., 1992). Gonoccocal arthritis is the most common type of joint infection in sexually active adults (Cucurull and Espinoza, 1998).

"Gonorrhea in the male, as well as in the female, persists for life in certain sections of the organs of generation, notwithstanding its apparent cure in a great many instances" (cited in Oriel [1991]). Thus, the persistent nature of gonorrhea was recognized by the noted veneorologist Emil Noeggerath in 1872, 7 years before Albert Neisser identified the gonococcus as the etiologic agent. Persistent infection can be symptomatic or subclinical; the high frequency of asymptomatic carriers is a major obstacle to prevention and treatment. In clinical studies, approximately half of infected males who were examined because their sexual partners were known to have gonorrhea were asymptomatic (Handsfield et al., 1974; Crawford et al., 1977), and asymptomatic infection rates may be even higher in women (McCormack et al., 1977).

Infection initiates with entry of *N. gonorrhoeae* into the lower urogenital tract. Rapid attachment to the mucosal epithelium of the genital tract is mediated by surface appendages called pili (Nassif and So, 1995). Loose attachment is followed by a more intimate association involving the surface-exposed opacity (Opa) proteins (Dehio et al., 1998). Certain Opa proteins also promote the transmigration of gonococci across the epithelial layer to the submucosa. Colonization of the (sub)mucosa is followed by extensive bacterial multiplication and shedding of bacteria into the genital secretions, triggering the massive localized inflammation that is responsible for the clinical signs and symptoms of gonorrhea. The inflammatory response begins with a massive infiltration of phagocytes, predominantly polymorphonuclear leukocytes (PMNs), in response to proinflammatory cytokines and chemokines such as IL-1, IL-6, IL-8, and tumor necrosis factor alpha (TNF-α) (Naumann et al., 1997). These are produced locally in response to factors released or triggered by the bacteria, including bacterial cell wall peptidoglycan and lipooligosaccharide (LOS), and complement component C5a.

PMNs phagocytize and kill gonococci by the oxidative burst and other mechanisms, including defensins, cathepsin G, and other cationic antimicrobial proteins (Shafer and Rest, 1989). Gonococci may, however, be able to counter these defenses. Neisserial cell wall porins inhibit phagocytosis and degranulation by PMNs (Bjerknes et al., 1995) and interfere with both the classical and alternative pathways of complement activation (Ram et al., 1999; Vogel and Frosch, 1999). The critical role of complement in host defense against *Neisseria* spp. is evidenced by the hypersusceptibility of individuals with heritable complement deficiencies (Figueroa and Densen, 1991). Virtually all patients develop specific, opsonizing antibodies to the major surface proteins of the gonococcus (Jarvis, 1995), but these do not necessarily prevent reinfection (Brooks and Lammel, 1989). In part, reinfection may reflect the ability of the gonococcus to subvert humoral immunity. Like many other mucosal pathogens, *N. gonorrhoeae* produces an IgA1-specific serine protease that cleaves the hinge region of IgA antibodies (Kilian et al., 1988, 1996). The IgA1 protease may also promote the intracellular survival of gonococci by cleaving the lysosome-associated membrane protein 1 (LAMP-1) (Lin et al., 1997), which could be important for transcytosis of gonococci across the genital epithelium (Hopper et al., 2000).

Antigenic variation also plays an important role in survival of *N. gonorrhoeae* in the face of adaptive immunity. Variation of several cell surface components of the gonococcus—notably, the pili, outer membrane Opa proteins, and LOS—is controlled by distinct and complex mechanisms. In addition to immune evasion, the ability of the organism to invade and colonize different anatomical niches may be determined by changes in surface components.

Pili

Pioneering experiments in human volunteers established the essential role of pili in infection (Kellogg et al., 1963). Pili promote the initial colonization of the urethral tract by mediating adherence to the genital epithelium (Swanson, 1973) via the CD46/MCP receptor (Kallstrom et al., 1997, 1998). Pili are immunodominant antigens, and antibodies directed against them block gonococcal adherence to epithelial cells (Rothbard et al., 1985). However, high-frequency variation of the pilin subunits that comprise pili occurs throughout the course of human infection, including early stages before the emergence of the adaptive humoral immune response (Hagblom et al., 1985; Seifert et al., 1994). These observations suggest that pilin variation might play two roles in the gonococcal life cycle: persistence in an infected individual by evasion of the adaptive immune response, and persistence at the community level by permitting transmission to individuals who had previously encountered the parental serotype. The mechanism of pilin variation in *Neisseria* is remarkably similar to the mechanisms used by *Borrelia* species to vary their surface antigens (Segal et al., 1985; Seifert, 1996). The gonococcal genome carries a large number of sequence-variable pilin genes, but only the pilin gene present at an expression locus (*pilE*) is actually transcribed and translated into protein (Fig. 5A). The silent pilin loci (*pilS*) are pseudogenes that lack the 5′-terminal coding sequences and the promoter sequences required for transcription. A pilin switch occurs when sequences stored at a *pilS* locus are transferred to a *pilE* locus by nonreciprocal recombination. Thus, the *pilE* gene that is expressed at any given time is a mosaic of sequences derived from various *pilS* cassettes, which can be endogenous or exogenous in origin, since *Neisseria* species are naturally transformable (Gibbs et al., 1989). Pili can also undergo on/off/on... phase variation by imprecise recombination between *pilS* and *pilE*, generating

aberrant forms of pilin that are not exported and assembled (Seifert, 1996). Phase variation of pili can also occur by on/off/on... switching of PilC, a minor constituent of pili that is essential for pilus assembly and maturation. Phase variation of *pilC* occurs by "slipped-strand replication" mediated by runs of G residues near the 5′ end of the gene (Fig. 5B). In addition to immune evasion, phase variation of pili might play a role in traversal of the genital epithelium, because pili interfere with invasion of epithelial cells and transcytosis of epithelial barriers (Ilver et al., 1998). If nonpiliated gonococci are responsible for mucosal invasion, reversion to the piliated state must occur rapidly, because gonococci present in the blood of patients with disseminated gonococcal infection are uniformly piliated.

Opa Proteins

The surface-exposed Opa proteins are encoded by a family of related but unlinked genes; a single isolate of *N. gonorrhoeae* may carry as many as 12 *opa* genes and may express zero, one, or multiple Opa proteins (Dehio et al., 1998; Nassif et al., 1999). Gonococci isolated from human patients or volunteers are predominantly Opa-positive, even when the initial infection was with Opa-negative bacteria, and simultaneous expression of multiple Opa proteins is apparently favored (Swanson et al., 1988; Jerse et al., 1994). The Opa repertoire expressed by a given bacterium affects invasiveness as well as tissue tropism (Kupsch et al., 1993; Dehio et al., 1998; Nassif et al., 1999). Opa proteins phase vary in vitro at a frequency of 10^{-3} to 10^{-4} (Stern et al., 1984, 1986). The *opa* genes are transcribed constitutively, but translation of an *opa* mRNA depends on the number of pentameric nucleotide repeats (CTCTT) present near the 5′ end of the gene. These vary due to strand slippage during DNA replication, and insertion or deletion of pentameric repeats can throw the downstream sequences in or out of frame, leading to on/ off/on... translation of the corresponding Opa protein. Additional variation is generated by intergenic recombination of *opa* genes, from both intra- and extragenomic sources. This promiscuous reshuffling of coding sequences is presumably responsible for the enormous repertoire of *opa* alleles observed in natural populations of gonococci (Meyer et al., 1990).

LOS

The outer membrane LOS of *Neisseria* spp. differs from the typical LPS of gram-negative bacteria in lacking the repetitive O-antigen moiety. In addition to its structural role in the cell wall, LOS is

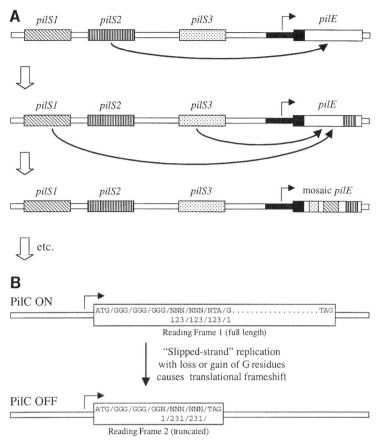

Figure 5. Antigenic and phase variation of pili in *N. gonorrhoeae*. (A) Antigenic variation. Pilin is encoded by one or two *pilE* expression loci. Variant pilin sequences are stored in silent *pilS* cassettes, which lack the 5′ coding and promoter sequences required for expression. Nonreciprocal recombination between *pilS* and *pilE* sequences gives rise to expression of variant pilin subunits. Modular recombination can generate mosaic *pilE* loci containing sequences derived from several distinct *pilS* loci. (B) Phase variation. PilC is a minor subunit that is required for proper assembly and export of pili. A run of G residues near the 5′ end of the *pilC* gene can vary in length due to slipped-strand DNA synthesis during chromosome replication. Depending on the exact number of G residues, the downstream *pilC* coding sequences may be in or out of frame for translation.

thought to facilitate mucosal invasion and survival of gonococci (Dehio et al., 2000). The resemblance of the carbohydrate moieties of LOS to host glycosphingolipids may promote immune evasion by molecular mimicry (Mandrell and Apicella, 1993; Moran et al., 1996). Extensive variation of LOS moieties can result in expression of several structurally distinct LOS molecules by a single bacterium (van Putten and Robertson, 1995; Minor and Gotschlich, 2000). LOS variation is determined by phase-variable expression of the LOS glycosyltransferases that sequentially add sugars to the LOS variable chain (Gotschlich, 1994; Minor and Gotschlich, 2000). Individual *lgt* genes contain poly(G) tracts that expand and contract by slipped-strand replication, resulting in on/off/on... expression of the corresponding LOS glycosyltransferase (Danaher et al., 1995; Yang and Gotschlich, 1996; Minor and Gotschlich, 2000).

Certain LOS variants are sialylated by a bacterial sialyltransferase using host CMP–*N*-acetylneuraminic acid (van Putten and Robertson, 1995). This modification promotes survival by blocking the bactericidal activity of normal human serum and specific antibodies against cell surface antigens such as porins or LOS itself (Parsons et al., 1989; Smith et al., 1995; Ram et al., 1999). On the other hand, LOS sialylation interferes with invasion of epithelial cells and transcytosis across mucosal barriers, suggesting that modulation of LOS sialylation could be advantageous at different stages of infection (van Putten, 1993). This idea is supported by studies in human volunteers, where sialylation levels were low during early stages of infection (facilitating mucosal invasion) but high after colonization and traversal of the mucosal barrier (conferring serum resistance) (Schneider et al., 1991). This temporal modulation of surface components in the course of infection is one of the more striking examples of the sophistication with which *Neisseria* has learned to blindside the defense mechanisms of the host.

SALMONELLA ENTERICA SEROVAR TYPHI—CHRONIC CARRIERS, A GALLING PROBLEM

Typhoid fever is a major threat to human health in many regions, particularly where treatment of sewage and drinking water is inadequate. The etiologic agent is *S. enterica* serovar Typhi, a gramnegative bacillus closely related to *Escherichia coli*. More than 16 million people worldwide suffer from the disease annually, and about 0.6 million die (Pang et al., 1998). Antibiotics are available, but resistance is increasingly prevalent—for example, some regions in India report rates of multidrug resistance in excess of 50% (Rowe et al., 1997). A vaccine based on the capsular polysaccharide antigen Vi is effective, but its application has not been sufficiently widespread to make an impact (Hessel et al., 1999). Serovar Typhi is an exclusively human pathogen, so transmission depends on contact with an infectious individual, either an acutely infected person or a chronic carrier. Because infection is acquired by the oral route, transmission is often mediated via contaminated foodstuffs, as in the infamous case of Mary Mallon ("Typhoid Mary") (Graf, 1998).

Ingested bacteria invade the intestinal wall by transcytosis of enterocytes or M cells in Peyer's patches. Bacterial replication in the submucosa is followed by entry into the bloodstream and dissemination throughout the body. Replication within macrophages in the spleen and liver leads to release of large numbers of bacteria into the bloodstream. Signs and symptoms of typhoid include enterocolitis, diarrhea, anorexia, fever, convulsions, and delirium. Much of the pathology of typhoid is attributed to the massive release of cytokines triggered by bacterial LPS. Invasion of the gallbladder leads to shedding of bacteria into the intestine, which may give rise to serious complications such as peritonitis. High fevers, accompanied by constant severe abdominal pain, persist for about 4 weeks and are followed by slow convalescence with continued shedding of bacteria in the feces (Hornick et al., 1970). Both humoral and cell-mediated immunity have been implicated in the protective immune response (Jones and Falkow, 1996; Jones, 1997). Most individuals recover fully and clear the infection; however, about 1 to 5% of those infected become asymptomatic chronic carriers and continue to shed bacteria in their stool and urine for the remainder of their lives. Although chronic carri-

ers have none of the signs and symptoms of acute typhoid, they are at increased risk of developing carcinomas of the biliary tract and other organ systems (Dutta et al., 2000; Shukla et al., 2000). This largely undetected source of contagion poses a formidable obstacle to public health efforts to eliminate typhoid, so it is unfortunate that the carrier state has received scant attention from the scientific community.

Serovar Typhi has adopted a novel strategy to evade destruction by the host immune response: by invading and adapting to an immune-privileged anatomical niche (the gallbladder), the organism puts itself out of harm's way. Little is known about the adaptive mechanisms that serovar Typhi deploys to survive and replicate within the bilious environment of the gallbladder. For reasons that are unclear, persistence of serovar Typhi in the gallbladder is more likely if gallstones are present—indeed, serovar Typhi can in many cases be cultured from gallstones that have been removed surgically. The gallbladder also seems to provide a safe haven from the onslaught of chemotherapy. Antibiotics, although generally effective in treating acute infection, show only limited success in eliminating infection from chronic carriers. About 25 to 50% of carriers are never cured despite long-term chemotherapy, and relapses are common, particularly in those with biliary or gallbladder calculi (Hornick, 1985; Gilman, 1989). In clinical studies of chronic carriers, subsets of patients had negative stool cultures for up to 2 years after chemotherapy yet eventually relapsed (Kaye et al., 1967; Johnson et al., 1973; Herzog, 1976). Most remarkable was a patient who received two full courses of chemotherapy followed by surgical removal of the gallbladder, which was unexpectedly found to contain a large calculus harboring viable, drug-sensitive serovar Typhi organisms (Kaye et al., 1967). These observations suggest that patients who have been "cured" nevertheless remain at risk for reversion to the infectious carrier state.

A major obstacle to the study of typhoid fever and the carrier state has been the lack of a suitable animal model. The related species *S. enterica* serovar Typhimurium, a significant source of food-borne gastroenteritis in humans, causes a disease in mice that resembles typhoid in humans. Although a model has not been developed that faithfully mimics the gallbladder carrier state in humans, certain strains of serovar Typhimurium are capable of causing a persistent infection in mice that involves the intestine, spleen, liver, and occasionally even the gallbladder (Sukupolvi et al., 1997). Persistence of serovar Typhimurium in mice despite chemotherapy has also been reported (Maskell and Hormaeche, 1985). Extrapolations from studies in the mouse model to human typhoid must be made with caution, since it is not yet clear whether the mechanisms of persistence are conserved between serovars Typhimurium and Typhi.

When mice are infected with serovar Typhimurium by the oral route, survival en route from the stomach to the intestine is dependent on the acid-tolerance response controlled by the alternative sigma factor RpoS (Foster, 1995; Slauch et al., 1997). The intestinal mucosa is breached by invasion of bacteria into enterocytes or M cells lining the Peyer's patches. Bacterial invasion factors are injected into the cytoplasm of the target cell by a type III secretion system encoded by *Salmonella* pathogenicity island 1 (SPI1) (Galan and Collmer, 1999; Ochman et al., 2000). Injected factors include SopE (Hardt et al., 1998) and SptP (Fu and Galan, 1999), which function as a GDP-GTP exchange factor and a GTPase-activating factor, respectively, for GTPases Cdc42 and Rac-1. The sequential activation-deactivation of Cdc42 and Rac-1 directs the transient actin cytoskeleton reorganization and membrane ruffling that accompany invasion. Once bacteria breach the mucosa, they invade and replicate within macrophages in the underlying submucosa. Alternatively, bacteria may be phagocytized on the luminal face of the intestinal wall and ferried across to the submucosa, thus bypassing the SPI1-mediated invasion pathway altogether (Vazquez-Torres et al., 1999).

Once the intestinal wall is breached, the infection is rapidly generalized throughout the reticuloendothelial system, especially in the liver and spleen. The pathogenesis of *Salmonella* hinges on the ability to survive and replicate within phagocytes of the monocyte-macrophage lineage. *Salmonella* inhabits a "loose" vacuole that acidifies to the normal phagolysosomal pH of 4.5 to 5.0 (Rathman et al., 1996), but whether this compartment is a true phagolysosome or a modified vacuole is controversial (Rathman et al., 1997; Sinai, 2000). Functions required for survival and replication within macrophages are encoded by a second *Salmonella* pathogenicity island, SPI2, which also encodes a second type III secretion system, Spi-Ssa (Ochman et al., 1996), whose expression is activated intracellularly (Valdivia and Falkow, 1997). The SPI2 type III secretion system translocates the bacterial protein SpiC from the *Salmonella* vacuole into the cytoplasm of the host cell, where it interferes with phagosome-lysosome fusion (Uchiya et al., 1999). SPI2 also encodes the PhoP-PhoQ two-component regulatory system that controls the expression of Pho-activated genes (*pag*) and Pho-repressed genes (*prg*), which are critical for intracellular survival (Groisman and Ochman, 1997). SPI2-encoded factors are responsible for evasion of

the oxidative burst via exclusion of the NADPH-dependent phagocyte oxidase complex from the membrane of the *Salmonella* vacuole (Vazquez-Torres et al., 2000).

The foregoing discussion highlights the important contributions of the mouse model of typhoid to our current understanding of the molecular basis of invasion, intracellular survival, and dissemination of *Salmonella* spp. As yet, however, the mouse typhoid model has shed little light on the asymptomatic carrier state, a key aspect of human typhoid that merits more attention. In the continued absence of strategies targeting the carrier state, elimination of typhoid as a major cause of human morbidity and mortality will remain an elusive goal.

MYCOBACTERIUM TUBERCULOSIS—AN INSIDER'S STRATEGY FOR PERSISTENCE

Persistence is the hallmark of tuberculosis (TB), which claims 2 million to 3 million lives each year worldwide (Dye et al., 1999). Persistent infection is clinical (chronic) or subclinical (latent) and is notoriously difficult to eradicate with chemotherapy. The impact of persistence on the epidemic dynamics of TB has been mentioned already. The significance of persistence for the individual patient can be illustrated with a single, well-documented clinical example (Fig. 6).

Despite the manifest importance of persistence in the pathogenesis of TB, little is known about the mechanisms that promote mycobacterial persistence in vivo. Several animal models of latent infection have been developed, but these do not provide a faithful mimic of the clinical features of latency in humans (McKinney et al., 1998; Parrish et al., 1998; Trucksis, 2000). Animals infected with *M. tuberculosis*—whether mouse, guinea pig, rabbit, or monkey—typically develop a chronic and progressive form of disease that is quite unlike latent infection in humans, where no signs or symptoms of illness may occur for many years.

Infection is initiated by the inhalation and retention in the lung alveoli of airborne "droplet nuclei" containing small numbers of tubercle bacilli, which are immediately taken up by resident alveolar macrophages (Nyka, 1962). Bacterial replication within alveolar macrophages and monocyte-derived macrophages that emigrate from the bloodstream leads to the formation of a nascent primary lesion (tubercle). Within a few weeks, infection is generalized by the dissemination of tubercle bacilli via the lymphohematogenous route. Engagement of the lymphoid organs drives the expansion of *Mycobacterium*-specific

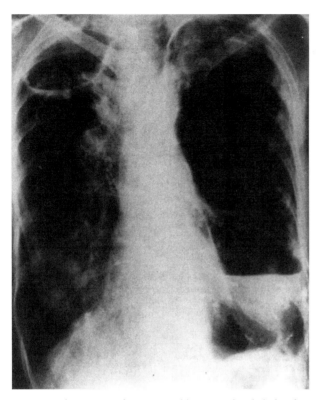

Figure 6. Chest X-ray of a 70-year-old woman shortly before her death. "A white woman had cavitary tuberculosis of 41 years' duration. She had bilateral bronchiectasis, cavitation of the right upper lobe, a collapsed left lung, pleural effusion, and an induced left pneumothorax of 36 years' duration. She had received no antituberculous drugs for 28 years from the onset of her illness, and these drugs, when finally prescribed, were taken inadequately. Pleural effusion present for 28 years required aspiration. *Mycobacterium tuberculosis* recovered by culture of sputum was resistant to all antituberculous drugs except streptomycin (which the patient had never received due to allergy)." Reprinted from Edwards et al. (1970), with permission of the American Lung Association.

T cells, which migrate to foci of infection and release macrophage-activating cytokines such as IFN-γ and TNF-α. A mature granuloma forms, consisting of a central area of necrotic tissue containing extracellular bacilli, encompassed by a mantle of macrophages harboring intracellular bacilli, surrounded in turn by a sheath of lymphocytes, consisting mainly of CD4$^+$ and CD8$^+$ T cells. Most infected humans (~90 to 95%) halt the further progression of disease at this stage, and the infection remains subclinical, or latent (McKinney et al., 1998; Parrish et al., 1998). Little is known about the physiology of persistent bacteria during latency, but it is generally assumed that bacterial metabolism and cell division rates are sluggish (Wayne, 1994). Over time, a small proportion (~5 to 10%) of latent infections reactivate and progress to clinically apparent disease. In the words of one epidemiologist, "Following infection, the incubation period of tuberculosis ranges from a few weeks to a lifetime" (Comstock et al., 1974). Whether the remainder self-sterilize or merely stabilize infection indefinitely is not known, although autopsy studies of individuals with latent TB indicate that most lesions in humans are eventually sterilized (McKinney et al., 2001). Immunosuppression increases the risk of reactivation, as evidenced by the high rates of reactivation in latently infected individuals who are coinfected with human immunodeficiency virus (Garay, 1996; Small and Selcer, 1999). However, the majority of individuals who reactivate are not obviously immunosuppressed, and the underlying cause of reactivation is unclear. It is possible that genetic factors play a determining role, but this component of host resistance to TB remains poorly understood (Hill, 1998).

Reactivation TB usually presents clinically as a slowly progressive, chronic condition; an individual with chronic, subacute TB may infect scores of contacts without realizing that he or she has the disease (Hoge et al., 1994; Valway et al., 1998). Patients with cavitary TB are particularly infectious because they shed enormous numbers of tubercle bacilli in their sputa. Cavitation is caused by the liquefaction of necrotic tuberculous tissue and its expulsion via the airways. Liquefaction is linked to a strong delayed-type hypersensitivity response and is an important example of immunopathology in TB (Dannenberg and Rook, 1994). The molecular basis of cavity formation has not been pinpointed, nor is it clear whether the immune mechanisms responsible for pathogenesis and protection are the same or different.

The protective immune response in TB is dominated by cellular immunity, with little or no contribution from antibodies. Studies with gene knockout mice point to an essential protective role for the type 1 cytokines IFN-γ, TNF-α, and IL-12 (Orme and Cooper, 1999). The importance of type 1 cytokines in human immunity has been confirmed in clinical studies of naturally occurring polymorphisms in the genes encoding type 1 cytokines and their receptors (Ottenhoff et al., 1998). The principal role of type 1 cytokines in anti-TB immunity is to activate the antimicrobial functions of macrophages. Induction of macrophage inducible nitric oxide synthase by IFN-γ and TNF-α is critical for host defense in the mouse model, and accumulating evidence points to a role for iNOS in humans as well (Chan and Flynn, 1999; Shiloh and Nathan, 2000). It is likely that additional, iNOS-independent mechanisms also contribute to host defense in both species. The phagocyte oxidase (Phox) generates reactive oxygen intermediates (ROI) and provides a key defense against many bacterial pathogens, but the tubercle bacillus is relatively resistant to ROI (Shiloh and Nathan, 2000). The intracellular environment is profoundly altered by cytokine activation (see below), but our understanding of how these changes affect intracellular bacteria remains scant. Leukocytes other than macrophages may also deploy antimycobacterial mechanisms; for example, recent studies point to a protective role for granulysin, a microbicidal component of cytotoxic T-lymphocyte granules that is released when certain CTLs lyse infected targets (Stenger et al., 1999; Stenger and Modlin, 1999).

Phagocytosis of *M. tuberculosis* by macrophages is mediated by diverse receptor-ligand interactions (Ernst, 1998; Aderem and Underhill, 1999) and requires the recruitment of cholesterol to the nascent phagosome (Gatfield and Pieters, 2000). Within non-activated macrophages, *M. tuberculosis* establishes a replication-permissive niche by inhibiting phagosome acidification, maturation, and phagosome-lysosome fusion (Gomes et al., 1999; Malik et al., 2000; Russell, 2000; Sinai, 2000). Vacuoles containing live mycobacteria exclude the vacuolar proton-ATPase and acidify slightly (to a pH of ~6.5), whereas vacuoles containing killed mycobacteria rapidly acidify to a pH of ~5.0 (Sturgill-Koszycki et al., 1994). Mycobacterial vacuoles reside within the recycling/sorting endosomal compartment—markers of early endosomes (Rab5) are retained, markers of late endosomes (Rab7) and lysosomes (LAMP-1, LAMP-2, and lgp) are largely excluded, and communication with the cytoplasmic membrane is maintained. Diversion of the mycobacterial phagosome from the normal maturation pathway correlates with retention of the actin-binding coronin TACO on the phagosomal membrane (Ferrari et al., 1999).

In macrophages activated with IFN-γ or TNF-α, reversal of the block to phagosome maturation and phagosome-lysosome fusion is correlated with inhibition of mycobacterial growth (Schaible et al., 1998; Via et al., 1998; Russell, 2000). Survival of mycobacteria in activated macrophages presumably involves phenotypic adaptation to the harsh environment of the fused phagolysosome and bombardment by ROI or reactive nitrogen intermediates (RNI). Identification of the underlying adaptive mechanisms will be key to understanding the basis of mycobacterial persistence, but there has been little progress in this area to date. A switch to fatty acid catabolism is suggested by the observation that the glyoxylate shunt enzyme isocitrate lyase is essential for survival in activated (but not resting) macrophages (McKinney et al., 2000). Isocitrate lyase is also required for late persistence (but not early growth) in mice, suggesting that fatty acids are the dominant carbon

source for persistent bacteria. Cyclopropanation of cell wall mycolic acids by the PcaA cyclopropanase also contributes to persistence and virulence in mice via an unknown mechanism (Glickman et al., 2000), possibly involving resistance to ROI or RNI. Indeed, ROI detoxification mediated by the KatG catalase is essential for bacterial persistence in mice following induction of adaptive immunity (Li et al., 1998). Other proposed mechanisms of resistance to ROI and RNI await genetic confirmation (Shiloh and Nathan, 2000; Vazquez-Torres and Fang, 2000).

Like many persistent pathogens, *M. tuberculosis* has evolved mechanisms to evade and subvert host immune responses (Samandari et al., 2000). Although activation of infected macrophages with IFN-γ or TNF-α can reverse the mycobacterium-induced blockade to phagosome maturation, *M. tuberculosis* may interfere with IFN-γ signaling (Ting et al., 1999). Down-regulation of antigen-presenting (major histocompatibility complex class II and CD1) and costimulatory (B7) molecules on infected macrophages may affect the activation of IFN-γ-secreting T cells (Samandari et al., 2000). Macrophage activation, antigen presentation, and T-cell activation may also be inhibited by cytokines secreted by infected macrophages, such as IL-10 (Murray, 1999), IL-6 (van Heyningen et al., 1997), and transforming growth factor β (Vanham et al., 1997). In addition to blocking antimicrobial signaling pathways, many pathogens prolong their survival by triggering apoptosis of leukocytes (Weinrauch and Zychlinsky, 1999). In TB, mycobacterium-induced apoptosis of γδ T cells (Egan and Carding, 2000) and macrophages could contribute to immune evasion. However, the role of macrophage apoptosis in TB is controversial; indeed, accumulating evidence suggests that mycobacteria may interfere with apoptosis of infected macrophages to perpetuate their intracellular "safe haven" (Fratazzi et al., 1999; Kornfeld et al., 1999).

Bacterial persistence also plays a critical role in chemotherapy of TB. Eradication of persistent infection requires multidrug therapy for 6 to 9 months, resulting in high rates of patient noncompliance and treatment failure. It is not clear why treatment of TB is so difficult and slow. The same antimicrobials that take months to cure a patient will sterilize a growing culture of mycobacteria in vitro within days. Penetration of drugs to sites of infection seems to be adequate (Barclay et al., 1953), and killing is not accelerated by increasing the drug dosage (McCune et al., 1957) or piling on more drugs (Jindani et al., 1980). One influential model is that persistence in the face of chemotherapy is due to physiologic heterogeneity of mycobacteria in the tissues, because slowly dividing and nondividing bacteria resist killing by antimicrobials (Mitchison, 1979, 1980). Supporting evidence for this model was provided by a remarkable clinical study in which tuberculous lung lesions from patients who had received prolonged multidrug chemotherapy were cultured (Fig. 7) (Vandiviere et al., 1956). Lesions that were "open" and active yielded colonies of drug-resistant tubercle bacilli in the normal time frame of 3 to 8 weeks; in contrast, lesions that were "closed" and inactive yielded colonies only after 3 to 10 months of incubation, and these "resurrected" bacteria were fully drug susceptible. These clinical findings parallel pioneering experiments in the mouse model of TB by McDermott and colleagues, who showed that chemotherapy induced a state of latency in which bacteria could not be cultured from the tissues unless relapse was provoked by immune suppression (McCune and Tompsett, 1956; McCune et al., 1956, 1966a, 1966b). It is tempting to speculate that the same mechanisms that allow mycobacterial persistence in the face of adaptive immunity might also explain persistence in the face of chemotherapy. Identification of these persistence factors will be critical for the development of more effective tools for the prevention and cure of TB.

BIOFILMS—STAYING ALIVE BY STAYING PUT

Pathogens persist in their hosts via phenotypic adaptation to a multitude of different tissue environments. Studies of these processes have focused on the behavior of individual cells, but accumulating evidence suggests that this is an overly reductionist view (Costerton et al., 1999). Many bacterial species fluctuate between planktonic growth and sessile growth within biofilms, which are essentially primitive multicellular superorganisms (Costerton et al., 1995). Indeed, for many prokaryotes, the biofilm mode of growth seems to be the rule rather than the exception. Biofilms are typically complex and highly structured microbial communities, often composed of several species engaged in symbiotic relationships. Bacteria living in biofilm communities are strikingly different in their physiology and metabolism from those growing planktonically (Costerton et al., 1995; Costerton and Stewart, 2000).

Biofilms begin to form when bacteria growing in nutrient-rich environments develop adhesive behavior, leading to attachment to a surface and to formation of a monolayer of cells, followed by aggregation into characteristic microcolonies (Fig. 8) (Costerton et al., 1995; Pratt and Kolter, 1999). These microcolonies secrete highly hydrated exopolysaccharides (EPS), which compose up to 80 to 90% of the mass of a mature biofilm (Lawrence et al., 1991). The architecturally complex EPS matrix is essential for biofilm formation and structure (Watnick and Kolter, 1999; Yildiz and Schoolnik, 1999), as well as resistance to environmental insults, antimicrobials, and predation by free-living protozoa—or, in the case of biofilm infection, by host phagocytes (Jensen et al., 1990; Costerton et al., 1995). The EPS matrix is penetrated by a complex system of fluid-filled channels that mediate the distribution of nutrients, elimination of metabolic waste products, and chemical communication between microcolonies in the biofilm.

Nutrient availability is an important determining factor in the early stages of biofilm formation (Cos-

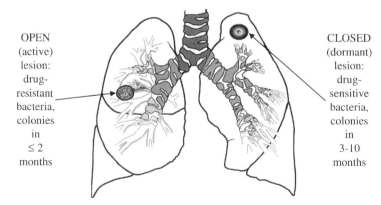

Figure 7. The treated pulmonary lesion and its tubercle bacillus: death and resurrection. Resected lung lesions from patients on chemotherapy were cultured. "Open" and active cavitary lesions, with patent connections to the airways, yielded drug-resistant tubercle bacilli in the normal time frame (less than 2 months of incubation). "Closed" and dormant encapsulated lesions, with no apparent connections to an airway, yielded drug-sensitive tubercle bacilli only after extended incubation (3 to 10 months). Derived from Vandiviere et al. (1956).

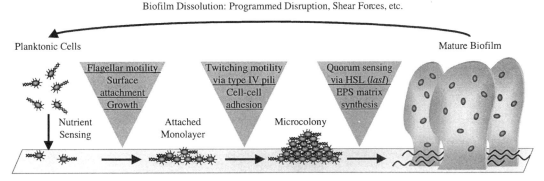

Figure 8. Biofilm biogenesis. Planktonic bacteria swim to a surface via flagellar motility and attach (mediated by flagella and nutrient sensing mechanisms). Replication on the surface leads to the formation of a monolayer of cells, which aggregate by twitching motility (mediated by type IV pili) and adhere to each other, forming surface-attached microcolonies. These microcolonies become embedded within a thick layer of secreted EPS. As the cell density increases, quorum sensing via HSLs synthesized by LasI triggers the developmental changes required for formation of the correct architecture and thickness of the fully mature biofilm. The mature biofilm is penetrated by fluid-filled channels that deliver nutrients and remove wastes. Bacteria within the biofilm are protected from destruction by antibodies, phagocytes, and antimicrobials. The steps leading to dissociation of biofilms and reversion to the planktonic form are poorly understood but may involve environmental sensing and programmed disruption or simple physical forces such as shear stress from fluid flow. Redrawn from Costerton et al. (1999) with permission of the American Association for the Advancement of Science.

terton et al., 1995; Pratt and Kolter, 1998). In *Pseudomonas aeruginosa*, the carbon metabolism sensor Crc controls the expression of functions required for biofilm genesis, such as the type IV pili that mediate twitching motility (Wall and Kaiser, 1999; O'Toole et al., 2000). Both flagellar motility and twitching motility are required for the early stages of biofilm formation by *P. aeruginosa* and *Vibrio cholerae* (O'Toole and Kolter, 1998; Watnick et al., 1999; Watnick and Kolter, 1999). Flagella are required for initial bacterium-surface contacts, while type IV pili promote the aggregation of surface-adherent bacterium into microcolonies.

The mechanisms that control the later stages of biofilm development remain largely unknown, but quorum sensing via secreted homoserine lactones (HSLs) seems to play a critical role. In *P. aeruginosa*, the *lasI* locus responsible for HSL synthesis is dispensable for the formation of a nascent and structurally simple biofilm but essential for its further maturation (Davies et al., 1998). Apparently, bacteria within the developing biofilm must talk to each other in order to coordinate the events that generate the complex architecture of the mature biofilm. Production of HSLs has been demonstrated in naturally occurring biofilms from aquatic environments (McLean et al., 1997) and from urethral catheters removed from patients (Stickler et al., 1998). The latter observation suggests the possibility that inhibitors of HSL production or function might be useful for preventing biofilm formation on indwelling medical devices. The mechanisms that mediate the dissolution of biofilms and reversion to planktonic growth are

just beginning to be explored (Costerton et al., 1999).

Biofilms are increasingly important in clinical settings. One of the most familiar and complex types of medically relevant biofilm is dental plaque, comprising hundreds of microbial species (Bloomquist and Liljemark, 2000). The heterogeneity of microenvironments within dental plaque supports the growth of metabolically diverse bacteria, including obligate aerobes, obligate anaerobes, and facultative anaerobes (Marsh, 1994; Whittaker et al., 1996). Biofilms that form on the surfaces of indwelling medical devices can cause serious complications, exacerbated by the fact that biofilm bacteria are highly resistant to killing by antimicrobials (Costerton et al., 2000). Inadequate drug penetration may contribute to the problem, as may the altered physiology of bacteria within biofilms. The heterogeneous architecture of biofilms creates chemical microenvironments that support slowly growing and nongrowing bacterial populations (Costerton et al., 1995), which are known to be less susceptible to antimicrobials (Eng et al., 1991; Evans et al., 1991). Indeed, the drug susceptibility and growth rate of biofilm bacteria are inversely related (Gilbert et al., 1990).

Among medically relevant biofilm formers, *P. aeruginosa* is the best understood. This gram-negative opportunistic pathogen afflicts immunocompromised individuals, including burn victims, neutropenic patients on cancer chemotherapy, and, particularly, cystic fibrosis (CF) patients (Govan and Deretic, 1996; Deretic, 2000). Inherited defects in the chloride ion channel CFTR (cystic fibrosis transmembrane regulator) cause CF patients to suffer from a buildup of dehydrated mucus in the respiratory tree, defective mucociliary function, and other defects in lung defenses. CF patients are unusually prone to developing chronic pulmonary infections by opportunistic pathogens, most of which respond to antibiotic therapy. However, virtually all CF patients are eventually colonized by *P. aeruginosa*, which forms biofilms that resist eradication.

Flagella are required for the early stages of *Pseudomonas* biofilm formation (see above) and for virulence in mouse models of burn wound sepsis (Drake and Montie, 1988) or pulmonary infection (Feldman et al., 1998). However, flagella can also promote nonopsonic phagocytosis of bacteria by neutrophils and macrophages (Mahenthiralingam and Speert, 1995). This conundrum might be resolved by temporal modulation of flagellar expression in the course of infection. In a prospective clinical study, bacteria isolated from CF patients at the early stages of disease were flagellum-positive, motile, and sensitive to phagocytosis whereas bacteria isolated from persistently infected patients were flagellum-negative, nonmotile, and resistant to phagocytosis (Mahenthiralingam et al., 1994). The "flagella on" state would presumably promote bacterial attachment and colonization at the early stages of infection; the "flagella off" state would promote evasion of phagocytosis and persistence at later stages, following the emergence of adaptive immunity. The rate of flagellar phase variation could be increased by the emergence of hypermutable subpopulations of *P. aeruginosa* in the lungs of CF patients (Oliver et al., 2000).

Hypermutation might also promote the replacement of nonmucoid strains, which are responsible for initial colonization, by mucoid variants, which dominate later stages of infection. Mucoid variants arise by spontaneous mutations in genes controlling the synthesis of alginate, an EPS matrix component, and their appearance is correlated with a poor prognosis for the patient. The alginate matrix shields the bacterial microcolonies from both arms of the host immune response—humoral and cellular. Most CF patients develop high levels of specific antibodies to *P. aeruginosa*, but these are ineffective against bacteria buried in the alginate matrix (Govan and Deretic, 1996; Costerton et al., 1999). Indeed, deposition of immune complexes on the surface of *Pseudomonas* biofilms is believed to contribute to lung inflammation and pathologic changes in CF. Lung damage may also result from the chronic influx of neutrophils, which are unable to clear the infection because the alginate matrix interferes with phagocytosis and killing. Bacterial communication

(quorum sensing) within the biofilm is apparently required for optimal induction of protective mechanisms, including the superoxide dismutases (Mn-SOD and Fe-SOD) and catalase (KatA) that detoxify phagocyte-generated ROI (Hassett et al., 1999).

The study of microbial biofilms and their role in persistent infections is still at an early stage. The environmental signals that promote biofilm formation and dissolution and the signals that the bacteria use to communicate with each other are just beginning to be deciphered. In addition to species-specific signals, a common language of secreted pheromones is apparently used for interspecies communication (Bassler, 1999). Elucidation of the signaling pathways that control biofilm dynamics could point the way to novel interventions targeting not individual bacterial cells but their collective behavior as biofilms.

REFERENCES

Aderem, A., and D. M. Underhill. 1999. Mechanisms of phagocytosis in macrophages. *Ann. Rev. Immunol.* **17**:593–623.

Akins, D. R., E. Robinson, D. Shevchenko, C. Elkins, D. L. Cox, and J. D. Radolf. 1997. Tromp1, a putative rare outer membrane protein, is anchored by an uncleaved signal sequence to the *Treponema pallidum* cytoplasmic membrane. *J. Bacteriol.* **179**:5076–5086.

Alder, J. D., L. Friess, M. Tengowski, and R. F. Schell. 1990. Phagocytosis of opsonized *Treponema pallidum* subsp. *pallidum* proceeds slowly. *Infect. Immun.* **58**:1167–1173.

Arroll, T. W., A. Centurion-Lara, S. A. Lukehart, and W. C. Van Voorhis. 1999. T-cell responses to *Treponema pallidum* subsp. *pallidum* antigens during the course of experimental syphilis infection. *Infect. Immun.* **67**:4757–4763.

Baker-Zander, S. A., E. W. Hook, P. Bonin, H. H. Handsfield, and S. A. Lukehart. 1985. Antigens of *Treponema pallidum* recognized by IgG and IgM antibodies during syphilis in humans. *J. Infect. Dis.* **151**:264–272.

Baker-Zander, S. A., M. J. Fohn, and S. A. Lukehart. 1988. Development of cellular immunity to individual soluble antigens of *Treponema pallidum* during experimental syphilis. *J. Immunol.* **141**:4363–4369.

Baker-Zander, S. A., and S. A. Lukehart. 1992. Macrophage-mediated killing of opsonized *Treponema pallidum*. *J. Infect. Dis.* **165**:69–74.

Baker-Zander, S. A., J. M. Shaffer, and S. A. Lukehart. 1993. Characterization of the serum requirement for macrophage-mediated killing of *Treponema pallidum* ssp. *pallidum*: relationship to the development of opsonizing antibodies. *FEMS Immunol. Med. Microbiol.* **6**:273–279.

Barbour, A. G. 1990. Antigenic variation of a relapsing fever *Borrelia* species. *Annu. Rev. Microbiol.* **44**:155–171.

Barbour, A. G., S. L. Tessier, and H. G. Stoenner. 1982. Variable major proteins of *Borrelia hermsii*. *J. Exp. Med.* **156**:1312–1324.

Barbour, A. G., and S. F. Hayes. 1986. Biology of *Borrelia* species. *Microbiol. Rev.* **50**:381–400.

Barclay, W. R., R. H. Ebert, G. V. Le Roy, R. W. Manthei, and L. J. Roth. 1953. Distribution and excretion of radioactive isoniazid in tuberculosis patients. *JAMA* **151**:1384–1388.

Barthold, S. W. 1993. Antigenic stability of *Borrelia burgdorferi* during chronic infections of immunocompetent mice. *Infect. Immun.* **61**:4955–4961.

Barthold, S. W. 2000. Lyme borreliosis, p. 281–304. *In* J. P. Nataro, M. J. Blaser, and S. Cunningham-Rundles (ed.), *Persistent Bacterial Infections.* ASM Press, Washington, D.C.

Barthold, S. W., M. S. de Souza, J. L. Janotka, A. L. Smith, and D. H. Persing. 1993. Chronic Lyme borreliosis in the laboratory mouse. *Am. J. Pathol.* **143**:959–971.

Bassler, B. L. 1999. How bacteria talk to each other: regulation of gene expression by quorum sensing. *Curr. Opin. Microbiol.* **2**:582–587.

Bishop, N. H., and J. N. Miller. 1976a. Humoral immunity in experimental syphilis. I. The demonstration of resistance conferred by passive immunization. *J. Immunol.* **117**:191–196.

Bishop, N. H., and J. N. Miller. 1976b. Humoral immunity in experimental syphilis. II. The relationship of neutralizing factors in immune serum to acquired resistance. *J. Immunol.* **117**:197–207.

Bjerknes, R., H. K. Guttormsen, C. O. Solberg, and L. M. Wetzler. 1995. Neisserial porins inhibit human neutrophil actin polymerization, degranulation, opsonin receptor expression, and phagocytosis but prime the neutrophils to increase their oxidative burst. *Infect. Immun.* **63**:160–167.

Black, F. L. 1966. Measles endemicity in insular populations: critical community size and its evolutionary implications. *J. Theor. Biol.* **11**:207–211.

Black, F. L. 1975. Infectious diseases in primitive societies. *Science* **187**:515–518.

Black, F. L., W. J. Hierholzer, F. D. Pinheiro, A. S. Evans, J. P. Woodall, E. M. Opton, J. E. Emmons, B. S. West, G. Edsall, W. G. Downs, and G. D. Wallace. 1974. Evidence for persistence of infectious agents in isolated human populations. *Am. J. Epidemiol.* **100**:230–250.

Blanco, D. R., J. N. Miller, and P. A. Hanff. 1984. Humoral immunity in experimental syphilis: the demonstration of IgG as a treponemicidal factor in immune rabbit serum. *J. Immunol.* **133**:2693–2697.

Blanco, D. R., J. N. Miller, and M. A. Lovett. 1997. Surface antigens of the syphilis spirochete and their potential as virulence determinants. *Emerg. Infect. Dis.* **3**:11–20.

Bloomquist, C. G., and W. F. Liljemark. 2000. Dental plaque, p. 409–421. *In* J. P. Nataro, M. J. Blaser, and S. Cunningham-Rundles (ed.), *Persistent Bacterial Infections.* ASM Press, Washington, D.C.

Blower, S. M., A. R. McLean, T. C. Porco, P. M. Small, P. C. Hopewell, M. A. Sanchez, and A. R. Moss. 1995. The intrinsic transmission dynamics of tuberculosis epidemics. *Nat. Med.* **1**:815–821.

Borst, P., and D. R. Greaves. 1987. Programmed gene rearrangements altering gene expression. *Science* **235**:658–667.

Brooks, G. F., and C. J. Lammel. 1989. Humoral immune response to gonococcal infections. *Clin. Microbiol. Rev.* **2**(Suppl.):S5–S10.

Brown, C. R., and S. L. Reiner. 1999. Experimental lyme arthritis in the absence of interleukin-4 or gamma interferon. *Infect. Immun.* **67**:3329–3333.

Cadavid, D., P. M. Pennington, T. A. Kerentseva, S. Bergstrom, and A. G. Barbour. 1997. Immunologic and genetic analyses of VmpA of a neurotropic strain of *Borrelia turicatae. Infect. Immun.* **65**:3352–3360.

Cadavid, D., D. D. Thomas, R. Crawley, and A. G. Barbour. 1994. Variability of a bacterial surface protein and disease expression in a possible mouse model of systemic Lyme borreliosis. *J. Exp. Med.* **179**:631–642.

Centers for Disease Control and Prevention. 1991. Primary and secondary syphilis—United States, 1981–1990. *Morb. Mortal. Wkly. Rep.* **40**:314–315, 321–323.

Centers for Disease Control and Prevention. 1999. Primary and secondary syphilis—United States, 1998. *Morb. Mortal. Wkly. Rep.* **48**:873–878.

Centurion-Lara, A., C. Castro, L. Barrett, C. Cameron, M. Mostowfi, W. C. Van Voorhis, and S. A. Lukehart, S.A. 1999. *Treponema pallidum* major sheath protein homologue TprK is a target of opsonic antibody and the protective immune response. *J. Exp. Med.* **189**:647–656.

Centurion-Lara, A., C. Godornes, C. Castro, W. C. Van Voorhis, and S. A. Lukehart. 2000. The *tprK* gene is heterogeneous among *Treponema pallidum* strains and has multiple alleles. *Infect. Immun.* **68**:824–831.

Chan, J., and J. L. Flynn. 1999. Nitric oxide in *Mycobacterium tuberculosis* infection. *In* F. C. Fang (ed.), *Nitric Oxide and Infection.* Kluwer Academic/Plenum Publishers, New York, N.Y.

Comstock, G. W., V. T. Livesay, and S. F. Woolpert. 1974. The prognosis of a positive tuberculin reaction in childhood and adolescence. *Am. J. Epidemiol.* **99**:131–138.

Costerton, J. W., Z. Lewandowski, D. E. Caldwell, D. R. Korber, and H. M. Lappin-Scott. 1995. Microbial biofilms. *Annu. Rev. Microbiol.* **49**:711–745.

Costerton, J. W., and P. S. Stewart. 2000. Biofilms and device-related infections, p. 423–439. *In* J. P. Nataro, M. J. Blaser, and S. Cunningham-Rundles (ed.), *Persistent Bacterial Infections.* ASM Press, Washington, D.C.

Costerton, J. W., P. S. Stewart, and E. P. Greenberg. 1999. Bacterial biofilms: a common cause of persistent infections. *Science* **284**:1318–1322.

Cox, D. L., P. Chang, A. W. McDowall, and J. D. Radolf. 1992. The outer membrane, not a coat of host proteins, limits antigenicity of virulent *Treponema pallidum. Infect. Immun.* **60**:1076–1083.

Crawford, C., J. S. Knapp, J. Hale, and K. K. Holmes. 1977. Asymptomatic gonorrhea in men: caused by gonococci with unique nutritional requirements. *Science* **196**:1352–1353.

Cucurull, E., and L. R. Espinoza. 1998. Gonococcal arthritis. *Rheum. Dis. Clin. North Am.* **24**:305–322.

Danaher, R. J., J. C. Levin, D. Arking, C. L. Burch, R. Sandlin, and D. C. Stein. 1995. Genetic basis of *Neisseria gonorrhoeae* lipooligosaccharide antigenic variation. *J. Bacteriol.* **177**:7275–7279.

Daniel, T. M., J. H. Bates, and K. A. Downes. 1994. History of tuberculosis, p. 13–24. *In* B. R. Bloom (ed.), *Tuberculosis: Pathogenesis, Protection, and Control.* ASM Press, Washington, D.C.

Dannenberg, A. M., Jr., and G. A. W. Rook. 1994. Pathogenesis of pulmonary tuberculosis: an interplay of tissue-damaging and macrophage-activating immune responses—dual mechanisms that control bacillary multiplication, p. 459–483. *In* B. R. Bloom (ed.), *Tuberculosis: Pathogenesis, Protection, and Control.* ASM Press, Washington, D.C.

Das, S., S. W. Barthold, S. S. Giles, R. R. Montgomery, S. R. Telford III, and E. Fikrig. 1997. Temporal pattern of *Borrelia burgdorferi* p21 expression in ticks and the mammalian host. *J. Clin. Investig.* **99**:987–995.

Davies, D. G., M. R. Parsek, J. P. Pearson, B. H. Iglewski, J. W. Costerton, and E. P. Greenberg. 1998. The involvement of cell-to-cell signals in the development of a bacterial biofilm. *Science* **280**:295–298.

Dehio, C., S. D. Gray-Owen, and T. F. Meyer. 1998. The role of neisserial Opa proteins in interactions with host cells. *Trends Microbiol.* **6**:489–495.

Dehio, C., S. D. Gray-Owen, and T. F. Meyer. 2000. Host cell invasion by pathogenic *Neisseriae. Subcell. Biochem.* **33**:61–96.

Deitsch, K. W., E. R. Moxon, and T. E. Wellems. 1997. Shared themes of antigenic variation and virulence in bacterial, protozoal, and fungal infections. *Microbiol. Mol. Biol. Rev.* **61:**281–293.

Deretic, V. 2000. *Pseudomonas aeruginosa* infections, p. 305–326. *In* J. P. Nataro, M. J. Blaser, and S. Cunningham-Rundles (ed.), *Persistent Bacterial Infections.* ASM Press, Washington, D.C.

de Silva, A. M., and E. Fikrig. 1997. Arthropod- and host-specific gene expression by *Borrelia burgdorferi. J. Clin. Investig.* **99:**377–379.

de Silva, A. M., E. Fikrig, E. Hodzic, F. S. Kantor, S. R. Telford III, and S. W. Barthold. 1998. Immune evasion by tickborne and host-adapted *Borrelia burgdorferi. J. Infect. Dis.* **177:**395–400.

de Silva, A. M., S. R. Telford III, L. R. Brunet, S. W. Barthold, and E. Fikrig. 1996. *Borrelia burgdorferi* OspA is an arthropod-specific transmission-blocking Lyme disease vaccine. *J. Exp. Med.* **183:**271–275.

Drake, D., and T. C. Montie. 1988. Flagella, motility and invasive virulence of *Pseudomonas aeruginosa. J. Gen. Microbiol.* **134:**43–52.

Dubois, A., A. Welch, D. E. Berg, and M. J. Blaser. 2000. *Helicobacter pylori,* p. 263–280. *In* J. P. Nataro, M. J. Blaser, and S. Cunningham-Rundles (ed.), *Persistent Bacterial Infections.* ASM Press, Washington, D.C.

Dutta, U., P. K. Garg, R. Kumar, and R. K. Tandon. 2000. Typhoid carriers among patients with gallstones are at increased risk for carcinoma of the gallbladder. *Am. J. Gastroenterol.* **95:**784–787.

Dye, C., S. Scheele, P. Dolin, V. Pathania, and M. C. Raviglione. 1999. Global burden of tuberculosis: estimated incidence, prevalence, and mortality by country. *JAMA* **282:**677–686.

Edwards, W. M., R. S. Cox, Jr., J. P. Cooney, and R. I. Crone. 1970. Active pulmonary tuberculosis with cavitation of forty-one years' duration. *Am. Rev. Respir. Dis.* **102:**448–455.

Egan, P. J., and S. R. Carding. 2000. Influence of $\gamma\delta$ T cells on the development of chronic disease and persistent bacterial infections, p. 165–182. *In* J. P. Nataro, M. J. Blaser, and S. Cunningham-Rundles (ed.), *Persistent Bacterial Infections,* ASM Press, Washington, D.C.

Eng, R. H., F. T. Padberg, S. M. Smith,, E. N. Tan, and C. E. Cherubin. 1991. Bactericidal effects of antibiotics on slowly growing and nongrowing bacteria. *Antimicrob. Agents Chemother.* **35:**1824–1828.

Ernst, J. D. 1998. Macrophage receptors for *Mycobacterium tuberculosis. Infect. Immun.* **66:**1277–1281.

Evans, D. J., D. G. Allison, M. R. Brown, and P. Gilbert. 1991. Susceptibility of *Pseudomonas aeruginosa* and *Escherichia coli* biofilms towards ciprofloxacin: effect of specific growth rate. *J. Antimicrob. Chemother.* **27:**177–184.

Evans, J. 1999. Lyme disease. *Curr. Opin. Rheumatol.* **11:**281–288.

Feldman, M., R. Bryan, S. Rajan, L. Scheffler, S. Brunnert, H. Tang, and A. Prince. 1998. Role of flagella in pathogenesis of *Pseudomonas aeruginosa* pulmonary infection. *Infect. Immun.* **66:**43–51.

Fenner, F., and B. Fantini. 1999. *Biological Control of Vertebrate Pests: The History of Myxomatosis—an Experiment in Evolution,* CABI Publishing, New York, N.Y.

Ferrari, G., H. Langen, M. Naito, and J. Pieters. 1999. A coat protein on phagosomes involved in the intracellular survival of mycobacteria. *Cell* **97:**435–447.

Figueroa, J. E., and P. Densen. 1991. Infectious diseases associated with complement deficiencies. *Clin. Microbiol. Rev.* **4:**359–395.

Fikrig, E., L. K. Bockenstedt, S. W. Barthold, M. Chen, H. Tao, P. Ali-Salaam, S. R. Telford, and R. A. Flavell. 1994. Sera from patients with chronic Lyme disease protect mice from Lyme borreliosis. *J. Infect. Dis.* **169:**568–574.

Fikrig, E., M. Chen, S. W. Barthold, J. Anguita, W. Feng, S. R. Telford, III, and R. A. Flavell. 1999. *Borrelia burgdorferi erpT* expression in the arthropod vector and murine host. *Mol. Microbiol.* **31:**281–290.

Fikrig, E., H. Tao, F. S. Kantor, S. W. Barthold, and R. A. Flavell. 1993. Evasion of protective immunity by *Borrelia burgdorferi* by truncation of outer surface protein B. *Proc. Natl. Acad. Sci. USA* **90:**4092–4096.

Fitzgerald, T. J. 1981. Pathogenesis and immunology of *Treponema pallidum. Annu. Rev. Microbiol.* **35:**29–54.

Fitzgerald, T. J., L. A. Repesh, D. R. Blanco, and J. N. Miller. 1984. Attachment of *Treponema pallidum* to fibronectin, laminin, collagen IV, and collagen I, and blockage of attachment by immune rabbit IgG. *Br. J. Vener. Dis.* **60:**357–363.

Foster, J. W. 1995. Low pH adaptation and the acid tolerance response of *Salmonella typhimurium. Crit. Rev. Microbiol.* **21:**215–237.

Fraser, C. M., S. Casjens, W. M. Huang, G. G. Sutton, R. Clayton, R. Lathigra, O. White, K. A. Ketchum, R. Dodson, E. K. Hickey, M. Gwinn, B. Dougherty, J. F. Tomb, R. D. Fleischmann, D. Richardson, J. Peterson, A. R. Kerlavage, J. Quackenbush, S. Salzberg, M. Hanson, R. van Vugt, N. Palmer, M. D. Adams, J. Gocayne, J. C. Venter, et al. 1997. Genomic sequence of a Lyme disease spirochaete, *Borrelia burgdorferi. Nature* **390:**580–586.

Fraser, C. M., S. J. Norris, G. M. Weinstock, O. White, G. G. Sutton, R. Dodson, M. Gwinn, E. K. Hickey, R. Clayton, K. A. Ketchum, E. Sodergren, J. M. Hardham, M. P. McLeod, S. Salzberg, J. Peterson, H. Khalak, D. Richardson, J. K. Howell, M. Chidambaram, T. Utterback, L. McDonald, P. Artiach, C. Bowman, M. D. Cotton, J. C. Venter, et al. 1998. Complete genome sequence of *Treponema pallidum,* the syphilis spirochete. *Science* **281:**375–388.

Fratazzi, C., R. D. Arbeit, C. Carini, M. K. Balcewicz-Sablinska, J. Keane, H. Kornfeld, and H. G. Remold. 1999. Macrophage apoptosis in mycobacterial infections. *J. Leukoc. Biol.* **66:**763–764.

Fu, Y., and J. E. Galan. 1999. A *Salmonella* protein antagonizes Rac-1 and Cdc42 to mediate host-cell recovery after bacterial invasion. *Nature* **401:**293–297.

Galan, J. E., and A. Collmer. 1999. Type III secretion machines: bacterial devices for protein delivery into host cells. *Science* **284:**1322–1328.

Garay, S. M. 1996. Tuberculosis and the human immunodeficiency virus infection, p. 443–465. *In* W. N. Rom, and S. Garay (ed.), *Tuberculosis.* Little, Brown & Co., Boston, Mass.

Gatfield, J., and J. Pieters. 2000. Essential role for cholesterol in entry of mycobacteria into macrophages. *Science* **288:**1647–1650.

Gern, L., and P. F. Humair. 1998. Natural history of *Borrelia burgdorferi* sensu lato. *Wien. Klin. Wochenschr.* **110:**856–858.

Ghinsberg, R. C., and Y. Nitzan. 1992. Is syphilis an incurable disease? *Med. Hypotheses* **39:**35–40.

Gibbs, C. P., B. Y. Reimann, E. Schultz, A. Kaufmann, R. Haas, and T. F. Meyer. 1989. Reassortment of pilin genes in *Neisseria gonorrhoeae* occurs by two distinct mechanisms. *Nature* **338:**651–652.

Gilbert, P., P. J. Collier, and M. P. Brown. 1990. Influence of growth rate on susceptibility to antimicrobial agents: biofilms, cell cycle, dormancy, and stringent response. *Antimicrob. Agents Chemother.* **34:**1865–1868.

Gilman, R. H. 1989. General considerations in the management of typhoid fever and dysentery. *Scand. J. Gastroenterol. Suppl.* **169:**11–18.

Gjestland, T. 1955. The Oslo study of untreated syphilis—an epidemiologic investigation of the natural course of the syphilitic infection based upon a re-study of the Boeck-Bruusgaard material. *Acta Dermatol. Vener.* 35(Suppl. 34):1–368.

Glickman, M. S., J. S. Cox, and W. R. Jacobs, Jr. 2000. A novel mycolic acid cyclopropane synthetase is required for cording, persistence, and virulence of *Mycobacterium tuberculosis. Mol. Cell* 5:717–727.

Gomes, M. S., S. Paul, A. L. Moreira, R. Appelberg, M. Rabinovitch, and G. Kaplan. 1999. Survival of *Mycobacterium avium* and *Mycobacterium tuberculosis* in acidified vacuoles of murine macrophages. *Infect. Immun.* 67:3199–3206.

Gotschlich, E. C. 1994. Genetic locus for the biosynthesis of the variable portion of *Neisseria gonorrhoeae* lipooligosaccharide. *J. Exp. Med.* 180:2181–2190.

Govan, J. R., and V. Deretic. 1996. Microbial pathogenesis in cystic fibrosis: mucoid *Pseudomonas aeruginosa* and *Burkholderia cepacia. Microbiol. Rev.* 60:539–574.

Graf, M. 1998. *Quarantine: the Story of Typhoid Mary.* Vantage Press, N.Y.

Grigg, E. R. N. 1958. The arcana of tuberculosis, with a brief epidemiologic history of the disease in the USA. *Am. Rev. Tuberc. Pulm. Dis.* 78:151–172, 426–453, 583–603.

Groisman, E. A., and H. Ochman. 1997. How *Salmonella* became a pathogen. *Trends Microbiol.* 5:343–349.

Gylfe, A., S. Bergstrom, J. Lundstrom, and B. Olsen. 2000. Reactivation of *Borrelia* infection in birds. *Nature* 403:724–725.

Haake, D. A., and M. A. Lovett. 1990. Interjunctional invasion of endothelial monolayers by *Treponema pallidum.* p. 297–315. *In* B. H. Iglewski, and V. L. Clark (ed.), *Molecular Basis of Bacterial Pathogenesis.* Academic Press Inc., San Diego, Calif.

Haas, F., and S. S. Haas. 1996. The origins of *Mycobacterium tuberculosis* and the notion of its contagiousness, p. 3–19. *In* W. N. Rom and S. Garay (ed.), *Tuberculosis.* Little, Brown & Co., Boston, Mass.

Hagblom, P., E. Segal, E. Billyard, and M. So. 1985. Intragenic recombination leads to pilus antigenic variation in *Neisseria gonorrhoeae. Nature* 315:156–158.

Handsfield, H. H., T. O. Lipman, J. P. Harnisch, E. Tronca, and K. K. Holmes. 1974. Asymptomatic gonorrhea in men. Diagnosis, natural course, prevalence and significance. *N. Engl. J. Med.* 290:117–123.

Hardt, W. D., L. M. Chen, K. E. Schuebel, X. R. Bustelo, and J. E. Galan. 1998. *S. typhimurium* encodes an activator of Rho GTPases that induces membrane ruffling and nuclear responses in host cells. *Cell* 93:815–826.

Hassett, D. J., J. F. Ma, J. G. Elkins, T. R. McDermott, U. A. Ochsner, S. E. West, C. T. Huang, J. Fredericks, S. Burnett, P. S. Stewart, G. McFeters, L. Passador, and B. H. Iglewski. 1999. Quorum sensing in *Pseudomonas aeruginosa* controls expression of catalase and superoxide dismutase genes and mediates biofilm susceptibility to hydrogen peroxide. *Mol. Microbiol.* 34:1082–1093.

Hemmer, B., B. Gran, Y. Zhao, A. Marques, J. Pascal, A. Tzou, T. Kondo, I. Cortese, B. Bielekova, S. E. Straus, H. F. McFarland, R. Houghten, R. Simon, C. Pinilla, and R. Martin. 1999. Identification of candidate T-cell epitopes and molecular mimics in chronic Lyme disease. *Nat. Med.* 5:1375–1382.

Herzog, C. 1976. Chemotherapy of typhoid fever: a review of the literature. *Infection* 4:166–173.

Hessel, L., H. Debois, M. Fletcher, and R. Dumas. 1999. Experience with *Salmonella typhi* Vi capsular polysaccharide vaccine. *Eur. J. Clin. Microbiol. Infect. Dis.* 18:609–620.

Hill, A. V. S. 1998. The immunogenetics of human infectious diseases. *Annu. Rev. Immunol.* 16:593–617.

Hoge, C. W., L. Fisher, H. D. Donnell, Jr., D. R. Dodson, G. V. Tomlinson, Jr., R. F. Breiman, A. B. Bloch, and R. C. Good. 1994. Risk factors for transmission of *Mycobacterium tuberculosis* in a primary school outbreak: lack of racial difference in susceptibility to infection. *Am. J. Epidemiol.* 139:520–530.

Hopper, S., B. Vasquez, A. Merz, S. Clary, J. S. Wilbur, and M. So. 2000. Effects of the immunoglobulin A1 protease on *Neisseria gonorrhoeae* trafficking across polarized T84 epithelial monolayers. *Infect. Immun.* 68:906–911.

Hornick, R. B. 1985. Selective primary health care: strategies for control of disease in the developing world. XX. Typhoid fever. *Rev. Infect. Dis.* 7:536–546.

Hornick, R. B., S. E. Greisman, T. E. Woodward, H. L. DuPont, A. T. Dawkins, and M. J. Snyder. 1970. Typhoid fever: pathogenesis and immunologic control. *N. Engl. J. Med.* 283:739–746.

Hu, L. T., and M. S. Klempner. 1997. Host-pathogen interactions in the immunopathogenesis of Lyme disease. *J. Clin. Immunol.* 17:354–365.

Ilver, D., H. Kallstrom, S. Normark, and A. B. Jonsson. 1998. Transcellular passage of *Neisseria gonorrhoeae* involves pilus phase variation. *Infect. Immun.* 66:469–473.

Jarvis, G. A. 1995. Recognition and control of neisserial infection by antibody and complement. *Trends Microbiol.* 3:198–201.

Jensen, E. T., A. Kharazmi, K. Lam, J. W. Costerton, and N. Hoiby. 1990. Human polymorphonuclear leukocyte response to *Pseudomonas aeruginosa* grown in biofilms. *Infect. Immun.* 58:2383–2385.

Jerse, A. E., M. S. Cohen, P. M. Drown, L. G. Whicker, S. F. Isbey, H. S. Seifert, and J. G. Cannon. 1994. Multiple gonococcal opacity proteins are expressed during experimental urethral infection in the male. *J. Exp. Med.* 179:911–920.

Jindani, A., V. R. Aber, E. A. Edwards, and D. A. Mitchison. 1980. The early bactericidal activity of drugs in patients with pulmonary tuberculosis. *Am. Rev. Respir. Dis.* 121:939–949.

Johnson, W. D., Jr, E. W. Hook, E. Lindsey, and D. Kaye. 1973. Treatment of chronic typhoid carriers with ampicillin. *Antimicrob. Agents. Chemother.* 3:439–440.

Jones, B. D., and S. Falkow. 1996. Salmonellosis: host immune responses and bacterial virulence determinants. *Annu. Rev. Immunol.* 14:533–561.

Jones, B. D. 1997. Host responses to pathogenic *Salmonella* infection. *Genes Dev.* 11:679–687.

Kallstrom, H., M. S. Islam, P. O. Berggren, and A. B. Jonsson. 1998. Cell signaling by the type IV pili of pathogenic *Neisseria. J. Biol. Chem.* 273:21777–21782.

Kallstrom, H., M. K. Liszewski, J. P. Atkinson, and A. B. Jonsson. 1997. Membrane cofactor protein (MCP or CD46) is a cellular pilus receptor for pathogenic *Neisseria. Mol. Microbiol.* 25:639–647.

Kaye, D., J. G. Merselis, Jr., S. Connolly, and E. W. Hook. 1967. Treatment of chronic enteric carriers of *Salmonella typhosa* with ampicillin. *Ann. N. Y. Acad. Sci.* 145:429–435.

Keeling, M. J. 1997. Modelling the persistence of measles. *Trends Microbiol.* 5:513–518.

Keeling, M. J., and B. T. Grenfell. 1997. Disease extinction and community size: modelling the persistence of measles. *Science* 275:65–67.

Kellogg, D. S., W. L. Peacock, W. E. Deacon, L. Brown, and C. I. Pirkle. 1963. *Neisseria gonorrhoeae.* I. Virulence genetically linked to clonal variation. *J. Bacteriol.* 85:1274–1279.

Kerle, K. K., J. R. Mascola, and T. A. Miller. 1992. Disseminated gonococcal infection. *Am. Fam. Physician* 45:209–214.

Kilian, M., J. Mestecky, and M. W. Russell. 1988. Defense mechanisms involving Fc-dependent functions of immunoglobulin A and their subversion by bacterial immunoglobulin A proteases. *Microbiol. Rev.* 52:296–303.

Kilian, M., J. Reinholdt, H. Lomholt, K. Poulsen, and E. V. Frandsen. 1996. Biological significance of IgA1 proteases in bacterial colonization and pathogenesis: critical evaluation of experimental evidence. *APMIS* 104:321–338.

Kitten, T., and A. G. Barbour. 1990. Juxtaposition of expressed variable antigen genes with a conserved telomere in the bacterium *Borrelia hermsii*. *Proc. Natl. Acad. Sci. USA* 87:6077–6081.

Kitten, T., and A. G. Barbour. 1992. The relapsing fever agent *Borrelia hermsii* has multiple copies of its chromosome and linear plasmids. *Genetics* 132:311–324.

Kornfeld, H., G. Mancino, and V. Colizzi. 1999. The role of macrophage cell death in tuberculosis. *Cell Death Differ.* 6:71–78.

Kuiper, H., A. P. van Dam, L. Spanjaard, B. M. de Jongh, A. Widjojokusumo, T. C. Ramselaar, I. Cairo, K. Vos, and J. Dankert. 1994. Isolation of *Borrelia burgdorferi* from biopsy specimens taken from healthy-looking skin of patients with Lyme borreliosis. *Clin. Microbiol.* 32:715–720.

Kupsch, E. M., B. Knepper, T. Kuroki, I. Heuer, and T. F. Meyer. 1993. Variable opacity (Opa) outer membrane proteins account for the cell tropisms displayed by *Neisseria gonorrhoeae* for human leukocytes and epithelial cells. *EMBO J.* 12:641–650.

Lawrence, J. R., D. R. Korber, B. D. Hoyle, J. W. Costerton, and D. E. Caldwell. 1991. Optical sectioning of microbial biofilms. *J. Bacteriol.* 173:6558–6567.

Lewinski, M. A., J. N. Miller, M. A. Lovett, and D. R. Blanco. 1999. Correlation of immunity in experimental syphilis with serum-mediated aggregation of *Treponema pallidum* rare outer membrane proteins. *Infect. Immun.* 67:3631–3636.

Li, Z., C. Kelley, F. Collins, D. Rouse, and S. Morris. 1998. Expression of *katG* in *Mycobacterium tuberculosis* is associated with its growth and persistence in mice and guinea pigs. *J. Infect. Dis.* 177:1030–1035.

Lin, L., P. Ayala, J. Larson, M. Mulks, M. Fukuda, S. Carlsson, C. Enns, and M. So. 1997. The *Neisseria* type 2 IgA1 protease cleaves LAMP1 and promotes survival of bacteria within epithelial cells. *Mol. Microbiol.* 24:1083–1094.

Livey, I., C. P. Gibbs, R. Schuster, and F. Dorner. 1995. Evidence for lateral transfer and recombination in OspC variation in Lyme disease *Borrelia*. *Mol. Microbiol.* 18:257–269.

Lukehart, S. A. 1982. Activation of macrophages by products of lymphocytes from normal and syphilitic rabbits. *Infect. Immun.* 37:64–69.

Lukehart, S. A., S. A. Baker-Zander, R. M. Lloyd, and S. Sell. 1980a. Characterization of lymphocyte responsiveness in early experimental syphilis. II. Nature of cellular infiltration and *Treponema pallidum* distribution in testicular lesions. *J. Immunol.* 124:461–467.

Lukehart, S. A., S. A. Baker-Zander, and S. Sell. 1980b. Characterization of lymphocyte responsiveness in early experimental syphilis. I. In vitro response to mitogens and *Treponema pallidum* antigens. *J. Immunol.* 124:454–460.

Lukehart, S. A., and J. N. Miller. 1978. Demonstration of the *in vitro* phagocytosis of *Treponema pallidum* by rabbit peritoneal macrophages. *J. Immunol.* 121:2014–2024.

Lukehart, S. A., J. M. Shaffer, and S. A. Baker-Zander. 1992. A subpopulation of *Treponema pallidum* is resistant to phagocytosis: possible mechanism of persistence. *J. Infect. Dis.* 166:1449–1453.

Mahenthiralingam, E., M. E. Campbell, and D. P. Speert. 1994. Nonmotility and phagocytic resistance of *Pseudomonas aeruginosa* isolates from chronically colonized patients with cystic fibrosis. *Infect. Immun.* 62:596–605.

Mahenthiralingam, E., and D. P. Speert. 1995. Nonopsonic phagocytosis of *Pseudomonas aeruginosa* by macrophages and polymorphonuclear leukocytes requires the presence of the bacterial flagellum. *Infect. Immun.* 63:4519–4523.

Malik, Z. A., G. M. Denning, and D. J. Kusner. 2000. Inhibition of Ca2+ signaling by *Mycobacterium tuberculosis* is associated with reduced phagosome–lysosome fusion and increased survival within human macrophages. *J. Exp. Med.* 191:287–302.

Mandrell, R. E., and M. A. Apicella. 1993. Lipo-oligosaccharides (LOS) of mucosal pathogens: molecular mimicry and host-modification of LOS. *Immunobiology* 187:382–402.

Marconi, R. T., M. E. Konkel, and C. F. Garon. 1993. Variability of *osp* genes and gene products among species of Lyme disease spirochetes. *Infect. Immun.* 61:2611–2617.

Marsh, P. D. 1994. Microbial ecology of dental plaque and its significance in health and disease. *Adv. Dent. Res.* 8:263–271.

Maskell, D. J., and C. E. Hormaeche. 1985. Relapse following cessation of antibiotic therapy for mouse typhoid in resistant and susceptible mice infected with salmonellae of differing virulence. *J. Infect. Dis.* 152:1044–1049.

McCormack, W., R. Stumacher, K. Johnson, and A. Donner. 1977. Clinical spectrum of gonococcal infection in women. *Lancet* i:1182–1185.

McCune, R. M., F. M. Feldmann, H. P. Lambert, and W. McDermott. 1966a. Microbial persistence. I. The capacity of tubercle bacilli to survive sterilization in mouse tissues. *J. Exp. Med.* 123:445–468.

McCune, R. M., F. M. Feldmann, and W. McDermott. 1966b. Microbial persistence. II. Characteristics of the sterile state of tubercle bacilli. *J. Exp. Med.* 123:469–486.

McCune, R., S. H. Lee, K. Deuschle, and W. McDermott. 1957. Ineffectiveness of isoniazid in modifying the phenomenon of microbial persistence. *Am. Rev. Tuberc. Pulm. Dis.* 76:1106–1109.

McCune, R. M., and R. Tompsett. 1956. Fate of *Mycobacterium tuberculosis* in mouse tissues as determined by the microbial enumeration technique. I. The persistence of drug-susceptible tubercle bacilli in the tissues despite prolonged antimicrobial therapy. *J. Exp. Med.* 104:737–762.

McCune, R. M., R. Tompsett, and W. McDermott. 1956. Fate of *Mycobacterium tuberculosis* in mouse tissues as determined by the microbial enumeration technique. II. The conversion of tuberculous infection to the latent state by the administration of pyrazinamide and a companion drug. *J. Exp. Med.* 104:763–801.

McGrath, J. W. 1988. Social networks of disease spread in the Lower Illinois Valley: a simulation approach. *Am. J. Phys. Anthropol.* 77:483–496.

McKinney, J. D., B. R. Bloom, and R. L. Modlin. 2001. Tuberculosis and leprosy, p. 995–1012. *In* K. F. Austen, M. M. Frank, J. P. Atkinson, and H. Cantor (ed.), *Samter's Immunologic Diseases*, 6th ed., in press. Lippincott Williams & Wilkins, Baltimore, Md.

McKinney, J. D., K. Höner zu Bentrup, E. J. Muñoz-Elías, A. Miczak, B. Chen, W. T. Chan, D. Swenson, J. C. Sacchettini, W. R. Jacobs, Jr., and D. G. Russell. 2000. Persistence of *Mycobacterium tuberculosis* in macrophages and mice requires the glyoxylate shunt enzyme isocitrate lyase. *Nature* 406:735–738.

McKinney, J. D., W. R. Jacobs, and B. R. Bloom. 1998. Persisting problems in tuberculosis, p. 51–146. *In* R. Krause, J. I. Gallin, and A. S. Fauci (ed.), *Emerging Infections*. Academic Press, New York, N.Y.

McLean, R. J., M. Whiteley, D. J. Stickler, and W. C. Fuqua. 1997. Evidence of autoinducer activity in naturally occurring biofilms. *FEMS Microbiol. Lett.* 154:259–263.

Meier, J. T., M. I. Simon, and A. G. Barbour. 1985. Antigenic variation is associated with DNA rearrangements in a relapsing fever *Borrelia*. *Cell* 41:403–409.

Meleney, H. E. 1928. Relapse phenomena of *Spironema recurrentis*. *J. Exp. Med.* **48**:65–82.

Meyer, T. F., C. P. Gibbs, and R. Haas. 1990. Variation and control of protein expression in *Neisseria*. *Annu. Rev. Microbiol.* **44**:451–477.

Minor, S. Y., and E. C. Gotschlich. 2000. The genetics of LPS synthesis by the gonococcus, p. 111–131. *In* J. B. Goldberg (ed.), *Genetics of Bacterial Polysaccharides*. CRC Press, Inc., Boca Raton, Fla.

Mitchison, D. A. 1979. Basic mechanisms of chemotherapy. *Chest* **76**(Suppl.):771–781.

Mitchison, D. A. 1980. Treatment of tuberculosis. *J. R. Coll. Physicians London* **14**:91–99.

Moran, A. P., M. M. Prendergast, and B. J. Appelmelk. 1996. Molecular mimicry of host structures by bacterial lipopolysaccharides and its contribution to disease. *FEMS Immunol. Med. Microbiol.* **16**:105–115.

Moxon, E. R., P. B. Rainey, M. A. Nowak, and R. E. Lenski. 1994. Adaptive evolution of highly mutable loci in pathogenic bacteria. *Curr. Biol.* **4**:24–33.

Murray, P. J. 1999. Defining the requirements for immunological control of mycobacterial infections. *Trends Microbiol.* **7**:366–371.

Nassif, X., and M. So. 1995. Interaction of pathogenic neisseriae with nonphagocytic cells. *Clin. Microbiol. Rev.* **8**:376–388.

Nassif, X., C. Pujol, P. Morand, and E. Eugene. 1999. Interactions of pathogenic *Neisseria* with host cells—is it possible to assemble the puzzle? *Mol. Microbiol.* **32**:1124–1132.

Naumann, M., S. Wessler, C. Bartsch, B. Wieland, and T. F. Meyer. 1997. *Neisseria gonorrhoeae* epithelial cell interaction leads to the activation of the transcription factors nuclear factor kappaB and activator protein 1 and the induction of inflammatory cytokines. *J. Exp. Med.* **186**:247–258.

Norris, S. J., J. K. Howell, S. A. Garza, M. S. Ferdows, and A. G. Barbour. 1995. High- and low-infectivity phenotypes of clonal populations of in vitro-cultured *Borrelia burgdorferi*. *Infect. Immun.* **63**:2206–2212.

Nyka, W. 1962. Studies on the infective particle in air-borne tuberculosis. I. Observations in mice infected with a bovine strain of *M. tuberculosis. Am. Rev. Respir. Dis.* **85**:33–39.

Ochman, H., J. G. Lawrence, and E. A. Groisman. 2000. Lateral gene transfer and the nature of bacterial innovation. *Nature* **405**:299–304.

Ochman, H., F. C. Soncini, F. Solomon, and E. A. Groisman. 1996. Identification of a pathogenicity island required for *Salmonella* survival in host cells. *Proc. Natl. Acad. Sci. USA* **93**:7800–7804.

Oksi, J., J. Savolainen, J. Pène, J. Bousquet, P. Laippala, and M. K. Viljanen. 1996. Decreased interleukin-4 and increased gamma interferon production by peripheral blood mononuclear cells of patients with Lyme borreliosis. *Infect. Immun.* **64**:3620–3623.

Oliver, A., R. Canton, P. Campo, F. Baquero, and J. Blazquez. 2000. High frequency of hypermutable *Pseudomonas aeruginosa* in cystic fibrosis lung infection. *Science* **288**:1251–1254.

Oriel, J. D. 1991. Noeggerath and "latent" gonorrhea. *Sex. Transm. Dis.* **18**:89–91.

Orme, I. M., and A. M. Cooper. 1999. Cytokine/chemokine cascades in immunity to tuberculosis. *Immunol. Today* **20**:307–312.

O'Toole, G. A., K. A. Gibbs, P. W. Hager, P. V. Phibbs, Jr., and R. Kolter. 2000. The global carbon metabolism regulator Crc is a component of a signal transduction pathway required for biofilm development by *Pseudomonas aeruginosa*. *J. Bacteriol.* **182**:425–431.

O'Toole, G. A., and R. Kolter. 1998. Flagellar and twitching motility are necessary for *Pseudomonas aeruginosa* biofilm development. *Mol. Microbiol.* **30**:295–304.

Ottenhoff, T. H. M., D. Kumararatne, and J. L. Casanova. 1998. Novel human immunodeficiencies reveal the essential role of type-1 cytokines in immunity to intracellular bacteria. *Immunol. Today* **19**:491–494.

Ovcinnikov, N. M., and V. V. Delektorskij. 1972. Electron microscopy of phagocytosis in syphilis and yaws. *Br. J. Vener. Dis.* **48**:227–248.

Paavonen, J. 1998. Pelvic inflammatory disease—from diagnosis to prevention. *Dermatol. Clin.* **16**:747–756.

Pachner, A. R., E. Delaney, and T. O'Neill. 1995. Neuroborreliosis in the nonhuman primate: *Borrelia burgdorferi* persists in the central nervous system. *Ann. Neurol.* **38**:667–669.

Pang, T., M. M. Levine, B. Ivanoff, J. Wain, and B. B. Finlay. 1998. Typhoid fever—important issues still remain. *Trends Microbiol.* **6**:131–133.

Panum, P. L. 1847. Iagttagelser, anstillede under Maeslinge-Epidemien paa Faeroerne i Aaret 1846. *Virch. Arch.* **1**:492–504. (Translated by Hatcher, A.S., 1939, Observations made during the epidemic of measles on the Faroe Islands in the year 1846, *Med. Classics* **3**:829–840.)

Parrish, N. M., J. D. Dick, and W. R. Bishai. 1998. Mechanisms of latency in *Mycobacterium tuberculosis*. *Trends Microbiol.* **6**:107–112.

Parsons, N. J., J. R. Andrade, P. V. Patel, J. A. Cole, and H. Smith. 1989. Sialylation of lipopolysaccharide and loss of absorption of bactericidal antibody during conversion of gonococci to serum resistance by cytidine 5′-monophospho–N-acetyl neuraminic acid. *Microb. Pathog.* **7**:63–72.

Pennington, P. M., D. Cadavid, and A. G. Barbour. 1999. Characterization of VspB of *Borrelia turicatae*, a major outer membrane protein expressed in blood and tissues of mice. *Infect. Immun.* **67**:4637–4645.

Persing, D. H., D. Mathiesen, D. Podzorski, and S. W. Barthold. 1994. Genetic stability of *Borrelia burgdorferi* recovered from chronically infected immunocompetent mice. *Infect. Immun.* **62**:3521–3527.

Philipp, M. T. 1998. Studies on OspA: a source of new paradigms in Lyme disease research. *Trends Microbiol.* **6**:44–47.

Plasterk, R. H., M. I. Simon, and A. G. Barbour. 1985. Transposition of structural genes to an expression sequence on a linear plasmid causes antigenic variation in the bacterium *Borrelia hermsii*. *Nature* **318**:257–263.

Pratt, L. A., and R. Kolter. 1998. Genetic analysis of *Escherichia coli* biofilm formation: roles of flagella, motility, chemotaxis and type I pili. *Mol. Microbiol.* **30**:285–293.

Pratt, L. A., and R. Kolter. 1999. Genetic analyses of bacterial biofilm formation. *Curr. Opin. Microbiol.* **2**:598–603.

Quétel, C. 1990. *History of Syphilis*. Johns Hopkins University Press, Baltimore, Md.

Radolf, J. D. 1994. Role of outer membrane architecture in immune evasion by *Treponema pallidum* and *Borrelia burgdorferi*. *Trends Microbiol.* **2**:307–311.

Radolf, J. D. 1995. *Treponema pallidum* and the quest for outer membrane proteins. *Mol. Microbiol.* **16**:1067–1073.

Radolf, J. D., M. V. Norgard, and W. W. Schulz. 1989. Outer membrane ultrastructure explains the limited antigenicity of virulent *Treponema pallidum*. *Proc. Natl. Acad. Sci. USA* **86**:2051–2055.

Radolf, J. D., B. Steiner, and D. Shevchenko. 1999. *Treponema pallidum*: doing a remarkable job with what it's got. *Trends Microbiol.* **7**:7–9.

Ram, S., F. G. Mackinnon, S. Gulati, D. P. McQuillen, U. Vogel, M. Frosch, C. Elkins, H. K. Guttormsen, L. M. Wetzler, M. Oppermann, M. K. Pangburn, and P. A. Rice. 1999. The contrasting mechanisms of serum resistance of *Neisseria gonor-*

rhoeae and group B *Neisseria meningitidis. Mol. Immunol.* 36: 915–928.

Rathman, M., L. P. Barker, and S. Falkow. 1997. The unique trafficking pattern of *Salmonella typhimurium*-containing phagosomes in murine macrophages is independent of the mechanism of bacterial entry. *Infect. Immun.* 65:1475–1485.

Rathman, M., M. D. Sjaastad, and S. Falkow. 1996. Acidification of phagosomes containing *Salmonella typhimurium* in murine macrophages. *Infect. Immun.* 64:2765–2773.

Restrepo, B. I., and A. G. Barbour. 1994. Antigen diversity in the bacterium *B. hermsii* through "somatic" mutations in rearranged *vmp* genes. *Cell* 78:867–876.

Restrepo, B. I., C. J. Carter, and A. G. Barbour. 1994. Activation of a *vmp* pseudogene in *Borrelia hermsii:* an alternate mechanism of antigenic variation during relapsing fever. *Mol. Microbiol.* 13:287–299.

Rich, A. R., A. M. Chesney, and T. B. Turner. 1933. Experiments demonstrating that acquired immunity in syphilis is not dependent upon allergic inflammation. *Johns Hopkins Hosp. Bull.* 52: 179–202.

Roberts, E. D., R. P. Bohm, Jr., F. B. Cogswell, H. N. Lanners, R. C. Lowrie, Jr., L. Povinelli, J. Piesman, and M. T. Philipp. 1995. Chronic Lyme disease in the rhesus monkey. *Lab. Invest.* 72:146–160.

Rothbard, J. B., R. Fernandez, L. Wang, N. N. Teng, and G. K. Schoolnik. 1985. Antibodies to peptides corresponding to a conserved sequence of gonococcal pilins block bacterial adhesion. *Proc. Natl. Acad. Sci. USA* 82:915–919.

Rowe, B., L. R. Ward, and E. J. Threlfall. 1997. Multidrug-resistant *Salmonella typhi:* a worldwide epidemic. *Clin. Infect. Dis.* 24(Suppl. 1):S106–S109.

Rudenko, G., M. Cross, and P. Borst. 1998. Changing the end: antigenic variation orchestrated at the telomeres of African trypanosomes. *Trends Microbiol.* 6:113–116.

Russell, D. G. 2000. What is the very model of a modern macrophage pathogen?, p. 107–117. *In* K. A. Brogden, J. A. Roth, T. B. Stanton, C. A. Bolin, F. C. Minion, and M. J. Wannemuehler (ed.) *Virulence Mechanisms of Bacterial Pathogens.* ASM Press, Washington, D.C.

Saint Girons, I., and A. G. Barbour. 1991. Antigenic variation in *Borrelia. Res. Microbiol.* 142:711–717.

Samandari, T., M. M. Levine, and M. B. Sztein. 2000. Mechanisms for establishing persistence: immune modulation, p. 53–78. *In* J. P. Nataro, M. J. Blaser, and S. Cunningham-Rundles (ed.), *Persistent Bacterial Infections.* ASM Press, Washington, D.C.

Sauer, G. C., and J. C. Hall. 1996. Spirochetal infections, p. 174–186. *In* G. C. Sauer and J. C. Hall (ed.), *Manual of Skin Diseases,* 7th ed., Lippincott-Raven, Philadelphia, Pa.

Schaible, U. E., S. Sturgill-Koszycki, P. H. Schlesinger, and D. G. Russell. 1998. Cytokine activation leads to acidification and increases maturation of *Mycobacterium avium*-containing phagosomes in murine macrophages. *J. Immunol.* 160:1290–1296.

Schneider, H., J. M. Griffiss, J. W. Boslego, P. J. Hitchcock, K. M. Zahos, and M. A. Apicella. 1991. Expression of paragloboside-like lipooligosaccharides may be a necessary component of gonococcal pathogenesis in men. *J. Exp. Med.* 174:1601–1605.

Schuhardt, V. T., and M. Wilkerson. 1951. Relapse phenomena in rats infected with single spirochetes (*Borrelia recurrentis* var. *turicatae*). *J. Bacteriol.* 62:215–219.

Schwan, T. G., and B. J. Hinnebusch. 1998. Bloodstream- versus tick-associated variants of a relapsing fever bacterium. *Science* 280:1938–1940.

Segal, E., E. Billyard, M. So, S. Storzbach, and T. F. Meyer. 1985. Role of chromosomal rearrangement in *N. gonorrhoeae* pilus phase variation. *Cell* 40:293–300.

Seifert, H. S. 1996. Questions about gonococcal pilus phase- and antigenic variation. *Mol. Microbiol.* 21:433–440.

Seifert, H. S., C. J. Wright, A. E. Jerse, M. S. Cohen, and J. G. Cannon. 1994. Multiple gonococcal pilin antigenic variants are produced during experimental human infections. *J. Clin. Invest.* 93:2744–2749.

Sell, S., D. Gamboa, S. A. Baker-Zander, S. A. Lukehart, and J. N. Miller. 1980. Host response to *Treponema pallidum* in intradermally-infected rabbits: evidence for persistence of infection at local and distant sites. *J. Investig. Dermatol.* 75:470–475.

Shafer, W. M., and R. F. Rest. 1989. Interactions of gonococci with phagocytic cells. *Annu. Rev. Microbiol.* 43:121–145.

Shiloh, M., and C. F. Nathan. 2000. Reactive oxygen and nitrogen intermediates in the relationship between mammalian hosts and microbial pathogens. *Proc. Natl. Acad. Sci. USA* 97:8841–8848.

Shukla, V. K., H. Singh, M. Pandey, S. K. Upadhyay, and G. Nath. 2000. Carcinoma of the gallbladder—is it a sequel of typhoid? *Dig. Dis. Sci.* 45:900–903.

Sigal, L. H. 1997. Lyme disease: a review of aspects of its immunology and immunopathogenesis. *Annu. Rev. Immunol.* 15: 63–92.

Sinai, A. P. 2000. Life on the inside: microbial strategies for intracellular survival and persistence, p. 31–51. *In* J. P. Nataro, M. J. Blaser, and S. Cunningham-Rundles (ed.), *Persistent Bacterial Infections.* ASM Press, Washington, D.C.

Singh, A. E., and B. Romanowski. 1999. Syphilis: review with emphasis on clinical, epidemiologic, and some biologic features. *Clin. Microbiol. Rev.* 12:187–209.

Slauch, J., R. Taylor, and S. Maloy. 1997. Survival in a cruel world: how *Vibrio cholerae* and *Salmonella* respond to an unwilling host. *Genes Dev.* 11:1761–1774.

Small, P. M., and U. M. Selcer. 1999. Human immunodeficiency virus and tuberculosis, p. 329–338. *In* D. Schlossberg (ed.), *Tuberculosis and Nontuberculous Mycobacterial Infections.* The W. B. Saunders Co., Philadelphia, Pa.

Smith, H., N. Parsons, and J. Cole. 1995. Sialylation of neisserial lipopolysaccharide: a major influence on pathogenicity. *Microb. Pathog.* 19:365–377.

Smith, K. J., H. G. Skelton, and E. Abell. 2000. Spirochetal infections, p. 579–601. *In* E. R. Farmer, and A. F. Hood (ed.), *Pathology of the Skin,* 2nd ed. McGraw-Hill Book Co., New York, N.Y.

Steere, A. C. 1989. Lyme disease. *N. Engl. J. Med.* 321:586–596.

Stenger, S., and R. L. Modlin. 1999. T cell mediated immunity to *Mycobacterium tuberculosis. Curr. Opin. Microbiol.* 2:89–93.

Stenger, S., J. P. Rosat, B. R. Bloom, A. M. Krensky, and R. L. Modlin. 1999. Granulysin: a lethal weapon of cytotoxic T cells. *Immunol. Today* 20:390–394.

Stern, A., M. Brown, P. Nickel, and T. F. Meyer. 1986. Opacity genes in *Neisseria gonorrhoeae:* control of phase and antigenic variation. *Cell* 47:61–71.

Stern, A., P. Nickel, T. F. Meyer, and M. So. 1984. Opacity determinants of *Neisseria gonorrhoeae:* gene expression and chromosomal linkage to the gonococcal pilus gene. *Cell* 37:447–456.

Stevenson, B., L. K. Bockenstedt, and S. W. Barthold. 1994. Expression and gene sequence of outer surface protein C of *Borrelia burgdorferi* reisolated from chronically infected mice. *Infect. Immun.* 62:3568–3571.

Stickler, D. J., N. S. Morris, R. J. McLean, and C. Fuqua. 1998. Biofilms on indwelling urethral catheters produce quorum-sensing signal molecules in situ and in vitro. *Appl. Environ. Microbiol.* 64:3486–3490.

Stoenner, H. G., T. Dodd, and C. Larsen. 1982. Antigenic variation of *Borrelia hermsii. J. Exp. Med.* 156:1297–1311.

Sturgill-Koszycki, S., P. H. Schlesinger, P. Chakraborty, P. L. Haddiz, H. L. Collins, A. K. Fok, R. D. Allen, S. L. Gluck, J. Heuser, and D. G. Russell. 1994. Lack of acidification in *Mycobacterium* phagosomes produced by exclusion of the vesicular proton-ATPase. *Science* 263:678–681.

Suk, K., S. Das, W. Sun, B. Jwang, S. W. Barthold, R. A. Flavell, and E. Fikrig. 1995. *Borrelia burgdorferi* genes selectively expressed in the infected host. *Proc. Natl. Acad. Sci. USA* 92:4269–4273.

Sukupolvi, S., A. Edelstein, M. Rhen, S. J. Normark, and J. D. Pfeifer. 1997. Development of a murine model of chronic *Salmonella* infection. *Infect. Immun.* 65:838–842.

Swanson, J. 1973. Studies on gonococcus infection. IV. Pili: their role in attachment of gonococci to tissue culture cells. *J. Exp. Med.* 137:571–589.

Swanson, J., O. Barrera, J. Sola, and J. Boslego. 1988. Expression of outer membrane protein II by gonococci in experimental gonorrhea. *J. Exp. Med.* 168:2121–2129.

Taylor, D. N., and M. J. Blaser. 1991. The epidemiology of *Helicobacter pylori* infection. *Epidemiol. Rev.* 13:42–59.

Ting, L.-M., A. C. Kim, A. Cattamanchi, and J. D. Ernst. 1999. *Mycobacterium tuberculosis* inhibits IFN-γ transcriptional responses without inhibiting activation of STAT1. *J. Immunol.* 163:3898–3906.

Trucksis, M. 2000. *Mycobacterium* infections. *In* J. P. Nataro, M. J. Blaser, and S. Cunningham-Rundles (ed.), *Persistent Bacterial Infections.* ASM Press, Washington, D.C.

Uchiya, K., M. A. Barbieri, K. Funato, A. H. Shah, P. D. Stahl, and E. A. Groisman. 1999. A *Salmonella* virulence protein that inhibits cellular trafficking. *EMBO J.* 18:3924–3933.

Valdivia, R. H., and S. Falkow. 1997. Fluorescence-based isolation of bacterial genes expressed within host cells. *Science* 277:2007–2011.

Valway, S. E., M. P. C. Sanchez, T. F. Shinnick, I. Orme, T. Agerton, D. Hoy, J. S. Jones, H. Westmoreland, and I. M. Onorato. 1998. An outbreak involving extensive transmission of a virulent strain of *Mycobacterium tuberculosis. N. Engl. J. Med.* 338:633–639.

Vandiviere, H. M., W. E. Loring, I. Melvin, and S. Willis. 1956. The treated pulmonary lesion and its tubercle bacillus. II. The death and resurrection. *Am. J. Med. Sci.* 232:30–37.

Vanham, G., Z. Toossi, C. S. Hirsch, R. S. Wallis, S. K. Schwander, E. A. Rich, and J. J. Ellner. 1997. Examining a paradox in the pathogenesis of human pulmonary tuberculosis: immune activation and suppression/anergy. *Tuberc. Lung Dis.* 78:145–158.

van Heyningen, T. K., H. L. Collins, and D. G. Russell. 1997. IL-6 produced by macrophages infected with *Mycobacterium* species suppresses T cell responses. *J. Immunol.* 158:330–337.

van Putten, J. P. 1993. Phase variation of lipopolysaccharide directs interconversion of invasive and immuno-resistant phenotypes of *Neisseria gonorrhoeae. EMBO J.* 12:4043–4051.

van Putten, J. P., and B. D. Robertson. 1995. Molecular mechanisms and implications for infection of lipopolysaccharide variation in *Neisseria. Mol. Microbiol.* 16:847–853.

van Voorhis, W. C., L. K. Barrett, D. M. Koelle, J. M. Nasio, F. A. Plummer, and S. A. Lukehart. 1996a. Primary and secondary syphilis lesions contain mRNA for Th1 cytokines. *J. Infect. Dis.* 173:491–495.

van Voorhis, W. C., L. K. Barrett, J. M. Nasio, F. A. Plummer, and S. A. Lukehart. 1996b. Lesions of primary and secondary syphilis contain activated cytolytic T cells. *Infect. Immun.* 64:1048–1050.

Vazquez-Torres, A., and F. C. Fang. 2000. Mechanisms of resistance to NO-related antibacterial activity, p. 131–142. *In* K. A. Brogden, J. A. Roth, T. B. Stanton, C. A. Bolin, F. C. Minion, and M. J. Wannemuehler (ed.), *Virulence Mechanisms of Bacterial Pathogens.* ASM Press, Washington, D.C.

Vazquez-Torres, A., J. Jones-Carson, A. J. Baumler, S. Falkow, R. Valdivia, W. Brown, M. Le, R. Berggren, W. T. Parks, and F. C. Fang. 1999. Extraintestinal dissemination of *Salmonella* by CD18-expressing phagocytes. *Nature* 401:804–808.

Vazquez-Torres, A., Y. Xu, J. Jones-Carson, D. W. Holden, S. M. Lucia, M. C. Dinauer, P. Mastroeni, and F. C. Fang. 2000. Salmonella pathogenicity island 2-dependent evasion of the phagocyte NADPH oxidase. *Science* 287:1655–1658.

Via, L. E., R. A. Fratti, M. McFalone, E. Pagan-Ramos, D. Deretic, and V. Deretic. 1998. Effects of cytokines on mycobacterial phagosome maturation. *J. Cell. Sci.* 111:897–905.

Vogel, U., and M. Frosch. 1999. Mechanisms of neisserial serum resistance. *Mol. Microbiol.* 32:1133–1139.

Walker, E. M., G. A. Zampighi, D. R. Blanco, J. N. Miller, and M. A. Lovett. 1989. Demonstration of rare protein in the outer membrane of *Treponema pallidum* subsp. *pallidum* by freeze-fracture analysis. *J. Bacteriol.* 171:5005–5011.

Wall, D., and D. Kaiser. 1999. Type IV pili and cell motility. *Mol. Microbiol.* 32:1–10.

Watnick, P. I., K. J. Fullner, and R. Kolter. 1999. A role for the mannose-sensitive hemagglutinin in biofilm formation by *Vibrio cholerae* El Tor. *J. Bacteriol.* 181:3606–3609.

Watnick, P. I., and R. Kolter. 1999. Steps in the development of a *Vibrio cholerae* El Tor biofilm. *Mol. Microbiol.* 34:586–595.

Wayne, L. G. 1994. Dormancy of *Mycobacterium tuberculosis* and latency of disease. *Eur. J. Clin. Microbiol. Infect. Dis.* 13:908–914.

Weinrauch, Y., and A. Zychlinsky. 1999. The induction of apoptosis by bacterial pathogens. *Annu. Rev. Microbiol.* 53:155–187.

Weinstock, G. M., J. M. Hardham, M. P. McLeod, E. J. Sodergren, and S. J. Norris. 1998. The genome of *Treponema pallidum*: new light on the agent of syphilis. *FEMS Microbiol. Rev.* 22:323–332.

Whittaker, C. J., C. M. Klier, and P. E. Kolenbrander. 1996. Mechanisms of adhesion by oral bacteria. *Annu. Rev. Microbiol.* 50:513–552.

Wilske, B., A. G. Barbour, S. Bergstrom, N. Burman, B. I. Restrepo, P. A. Rosa, T. Schwan, E. Soutschek, and R. Wallich. 1992. Antigenic variation and strain heterogeneity in *Borrelia* spp. *Res. Microbiol.* 143:583–596.

Yang, Q. L., and E. C. Gotschlich. 1996. Variation of gonococcal lipooligosaccharide structure is due to alterations in poly-G tracts in *lgt* genes encoding glycosyl transferases. *J. Exp. Med.* 183:323–327.

Yildiz, F. H., and G. K. Schoolnik. 1999. *Vibrio cholerae* O1 El Tor: identification of a gene cluster required for the rugose colony type, exopolysaccharide production, chlorine resistance, and biofilm formation. *Proc. Natl. Acad. Sci. USA* 96:4028–4033.

Zhang, J. R., J. M. Hardham, A. G. Barbour, and S. J. Norris. 1997. Antigenic variation in Lyme disease borreliae by promiscuous recombination of VMP-like sequence cassettes. *Cell* 89:275–285.

Zhang, J. R., and S. J. Norris. 1998a. Kinetics and in vivo induction of genetic variation of *vlsE* in *Borrelia burgdorferi. Infect. Immun.* 66:3689–3697.

Zhang, J. R., and S. J. Norris. 1998b. Genetic variation of the *Borrelia burgdorferi* gene *vlsE* involves cassette-specific, segmental gene conversion. *Infect. Immun.* 66:3698–3704.

Immunology of Infectious Diseases
Edited by S. H. E. Kaufmann, A. Sher, and R. Ahmed
© 2002 ASM Press, Washington, D.C.

Chapter 24

Viral Immune Evasion

DAVID C. JOHNSON AND GRANT MCFADDEN

Viruses have coevolved with multicellular organisms since animals developed immune systems. Rather than viruses acting as "predators," the more typical interaction between viruses and hosts is a benign infection, leading to propagation and spread of the virus to other hosts. However, host immune responses have exerted powerful selective forces on animal viruses over many millions of years. Viruses have countered by using a seemingly unlimited number of immune evasion strategies. The outcome of this coevolution can be considered in two broad categories: (i) adaptive behaviors of viruses and (ii) virus-encoded proteins that inhibit or modulate the immune system (summarized in Table 1). The effects of viral immune evasion proteins can occur outside host cells, in the case of chemokines, cytokines, or cell surface receptors, or inside cells, in the case of signal transduction and antigen presentation pathways. Both the innate and acquired immune responses are targeted, and our understanding of immune evasion tactics has largely paralleled our knowledge of the molecular details of various immune mechanisms. However, in some cases, our knowledge of the immune system has been substantially increased by studies of viral immune evasion. It has been said a number of times that viruses have had a long time to consider the host immune system, as with all aspects of host cell biology.

One central focus of this chapter will be the comparison of different animal virus families which selectively target distinct arms or facets of the host immune response. This is largely related to certain specialized replication strategies used by different viruses and to how these viruses spread to other hosts or establish latent or persistent infections. For example, influenza viruses cause acute disease, in some cases systemic infections, that are countered by rapid

and vigorous immune responses involving an important humoral component. These viruses are then largely eliminated from individual hosts and go on to infect other hosts, often of other species, where mutation of critical epitopes occurs so that a return to the original immunized host is possible. Due to space limitations, this adaptive behavior and others listed in Table 1 will not be covered extensively in this chapter. Poxviruses (large DNA viruses) also tend to cause rapid and acute lesions in epithelial tissues and must deal with a massive inflammatory response, primarily initiated by cells that are components of the innate immune response. These viruses have large coding capacities and can substantially inhibit inflammation by expressing inhibitors of cytokines, complement, intercellular and intracellular signaling, and apoptosis. Herpesviruses can also cause acute infections, and some of their immune evasion proteins function in a manner that clearly overlaps with those of poxviruses. However, herpesviruses also establish latent infections. Latency itself is one of the best strategies for immune evasion. In the latent state, virus gene expression is shut off, to wait out the immune response. However, reactivation of latent viruses in a host with fully primed immunity for that herpesvirus presents other problems. In this case, the acquired immune system, and specifically CD8 and CD4 T lymphocytes, is fully primed and robust. To deal with these T cells, all of the herpesviruses that have been studied express a panel of inhibitors that block T-cell antigen presentation pathways. Therefore, animals have adapted well to preventing the kinds of immunity that most affect their survival.

In this chapter we will attempt to summarize examples of viral immune evasion strategies, especially the facets of the immune system frequently targeted

David C. Johnson • Department of Molecular Microbiology and Immunology, Oregon Health Sciences University, Portland, OR 97201.   **Grant McFadden** • Department of Microbiology and Immunology, The University of Western Ontario and The John P. Robarts Research Institute, London, Ontario N6G 2V4, Canada.

Table 1. Summary of anti-immune strategies used by viruses

Adaptive behaviors
  Replication within immunoprivileged tissues or cells
  Antigenic variation, in some cases by hypermutation
  Infection of immune cells to directly suppress effector
    functions
  Establishment of latency (viral genes are not expressed)
  Induction of immunotolerance to viral antigens
  Skewing of Th1-versus-Th2 responses to compromise
    clearance of virus

Virus-encoded immunomodulators
  Interruption of extracellular cytokine networks
  Inhibition of the antibodies and the complement cascade
  Blockade of viral antigen presentation
  Inhibition of T- and NK-cell costimulatory molecules
  Regulation of antiviral intracellular signal transduction
    pathways
  Inhibition of immune cell killing and apoptosis

by viruses. For example, a substantial number of viruses families have independently evolved weapons against important soft targets such as tumor necrosis factor (TNF)-signaling pathway and the transporter associated with antigen presentation (TAP). We concentrate on well-characterized examples, where molecular mechanisms are better understood. However, this is a huge and ever-expanding area, and it is impossible here to cover the entire list of viral immune evasion strategies or even all the examples of a given type of inhibition. For the same reason, we have restricted the list of references to a limited number of seminal papers and reviews that cover topic areas. We apologize in advance to those whose papers were left out. Since this volume focuses on topics of host-pathogen interactions and immunity, we have attempted to reduce our discussion of molecular mechanisms of action and have, instead, focused on how various immune evasion strategies affect virus replication in animal models, allowing the virus to adjust to specific tissues or niches in the body. For more detailed listings of primary references and other mechanistic descriptions, the reader is referred to other recent comprehensive reviews on the subject (Johnson and Hill, 1998; Alcami and Koszinowski, 2000; Kotwal, 2000; McFadden and Murphy, 2000; Tortorella et al., 2000).

INHIBITION OF HUMORAL IMMUNITY

Immunoglobulin Receptors

Cells infected with herpes simplex virus (HSV), as well as a number of other alpha- and betaherpesviruses, express receptors for the Fc domain of im-

munoglobulin G (IgG) (Johnson and Hill, 1998). These receptors, and the complement receptors described below, may explain in part the lack of correlation between titers of neutralizing antibodies and severity of disease or frequency of reactivation (Corey and Spear, 1986). HSV and other alphaherpesviruses express a complex of two HSV glycoproteins, gE and gI, that binds IgG (Table 2). Extensive studies have indicated that gE and gI are predominantly or exclusively heterodimers in infected cells, there is little free gE or gI, and the complex forms quickly in the endoplasmic reticulum (ER) (Chapman et al., 1999; Johnson et al., 1988). The gE-gI heterodimer functions in two processes: (i) binding of IgG and (ii) mediating movement of the virus from infected cells to other cells (Johnson and Hill, 1998). gE-gI affects cell-to-cell spread primarily in epithelial cells, keratinocytes, and neurons, and gE⁻ or gI⁻ mutants are unable to spread both in epithelial tissues and in the nervous system in vivo. Reports that there are two distinct Fc receptors, gE (which can bind IgG weakly in the absence of gI) and gE-gI (Dubin et al., 1990; Saldanha et al., 2000), do not consider the complete absence of evidence that gE exists and/or functions without gI. Viral mutants lacking gI have not been obtained from clinical specimens. HSV gE-gI participate in a process termed bipolar bridging, in which anti-HSV antibodies bind, through their antigen-combining domain, to a viral antigen and are also mated, through their Fc domain, with gE-gI (Lehner et al., 1975; Frank and Friedman, 1989). Moreover, gE-gI inhibits complement-mediated antibody neutralization and antibody-dependent cellular cytotoxicity (Johnson and Hill, 1998).

The importance of the gE-gI IgG Fc receptor activity has been difficult to demonstrate in animal models. This relates to a number of problems: (i) HSV gE-gI plays an essential role in mediating cell-to-cell spread in epithelial and neuronal tissues, and this occurs long before there is anti-HSV IgG (Dingwell et al., 1994); (ii) HSV gE-gI does not bind mouse IgG well; and (iii) animal alphaherpesviruses, such as pseudorabies virus (which infects pigs), express Fc receptor activities that are relatively weak (Favoreel et al., 1997). Mutagenesis of HSV gE has defined a region encompassing residues 235 to 380 that is important for Fc receptor activity (Saldanha et al., 2000). The majority of mutations in this region also affect spread in epithelial cells or tissues. However, one mutation, a linker insertion at residue 399, inhibits IgG binding and does not substantially reduce epithelial-cell spread, although this mutant appears to possess defects in spread into and through the nervous system. Transfer of human anti-HSV IgG

Table 2. Viral inhibitors of humoral immunity

Strategy	Virus[a]	Mechanism
Immunoglobulin receptors	HSV	Ab neutralization, ADCC, CMCC
	PRV	Ab neutralization, ADCC, CMCC
	VZV	Ab neutralization, ADCC, CMCC
	HCMV	?
	MCMV	?
Complement inactivation	HSV	C3 binding, blocking C3 binding to C5 and properdin
	HVS	C3 convertase inhibitors
	HHV-8	C4b binding
	MHV-68	CD46, CD55
	VV	Accelerated cleavage of C3b and C4b
	CPV	Accelerated cleavage of C3b and C4b
	Variola virus	Accelerated cleavage of C3b and C4b
	HCMV	Incorporation of CD55 and CD59 into envelope
Inhibition of C9 polymerization	HVS	CD59 homolog
Factor H	HIV	Recruitment of factor H

[a] VZV, varicella-zoster virus; Ab, antibody.

into mice reduced replication and disease caused by the 399 mutant more substantially than it affected disease due to wild-type HSV. Since the concentrations of antibody were relatively low in mice, the results were consistent with protection from antibody-dependent cellular cytotoxicity or complement-mediated cytolysis rather than direct neutralization (Saldanha et al., 2000). It has also been suggested that gE-gI acts as a receptor binding glycoprotein, functioning at cell junctions, in the process of cell-to-cell spread (McMillan and Johnson, in press). Therefore, gE-gI may have several ligands, cellular proteins that are components of epithelial-cell junctions, neuronal proteins, as well as IgG, and the domains involved in binding these proteins appear to overlap.

Complement Receptors

Several members of the herpesviruses and poxvirus family express inhibitors of the complement cascade (Table 2) (Johnson and Hill, 1998; Kotwal, 2000). The best studied of the herpesvirus proteins is HSV gC, which binds to complement factor C3, C3b, and C3c (Lubinski et al., 1999). gC accelerates the decay of the alternative pathway C3 convertase and blocks the interaction of C5 and properdin with C3. gC can protect cell-free virus from complement-mediated neutralization and inhibits the lysis of HSV-infected cells by antibody and complement. However, gC also functions in virus attachment to cell surface heparan sulfate glycosaminoglycans, especially on the basolateral surfaces of epithelial cells (Sears et al., 1991). Thus, it has been difficult to in-

terpret in vivo studies with gC⁻ mutants. Skin lesions caused by an HSV gC⁻ mutant in mice were less severe than those caused by wild-type viruses, and 50-fold-higher titers of the gC⁻ mutant were required to produce disease whose severity was comparable to that caused by wild-type HSV (Lubinski et al., 1999). However, in C3 knockout mice, gC⁻ mutant disease scores were identical to those for wild-type virus, ruling out effects of gC in virus attachment, at least during limited local infections in the dermis. Therefore, gC can mediate resistance to complement in mice and may collaborate with gE-gI to mediate resistance to antibody-induced complement activation. Herpesvirus saimiri, a gammaherpesvirus that infects monkeys, encodes two homologs of complement control proteins (CCPs): CCPH, which is homologous to C3 convertase inhibitors, and HVS-15, a terminal complement inhibitor homolog that inhibits the activity of C3 convertase (Fodor et al., 1995). Human cytomegalovirus (HCMV), human retroviruses, and vaccinia virus incorporate host CCPs, CD55 and CD59, into the virion envelopes, mediating resistance to complement (Spear et al., 1995; Vanderplasschen et al., 1998). Moreover, HCMV upregulates the expression of CD55 and CD46 (Spiller et al., 1996).

The poxviruses variola virus, vaccinia virus (VV), and cowpox virus (CPV) all express CCPs, which were discovered based on sequence similarity to human and mouse CCPs (Alcami and Koszinowski, 2000; Kotwal, 2000). VV secretes an abundant 35-kDa protein similar to the human serum C4 complement binding protein, which effectively inhibits complement by blocking several steps in the complement cascade, accelerating the cleavage of C3b and C4b and increasing the decay of C3 convertase formed by either the classical or alternative pathways. A mutant VV lacking the CCP gene caused smaller and faster-healing lesions in rabbits and guinea pigs (Isaacs et al., 1992). The biological role of the CPV CCP was tested in a natural host, the mouse (Kotwal, 2000; Kotwal et al., 1998). A mutant CPV lacking the CCP gene caused substantially increased inflammation and footpad swelling compared with wild-type CPV (Kotwal et al., 1998). Similarly, there was more prolonged and substantial inflammation in C3- and C5-deficient mice. However, macrophage inflammatory protein 1α (MIP-1α)-deficient mice infected with the mutant CPV displayed markedly reduced inflammation. It was concluded that the CPV CCP can limit cellular infiltration by reducing complement-derived and non-complement-derived chemotactic agents. This is an interesting example in which the virus dampens the inflammatory response, probably so that tissue damage is reduced, allowing virus replication in host cells that would otherwise be eliminated by the immune response. Evasion of host immunity by reducing inflammation is a theme in poxvirus biology (see the following section).

Human immunodeficiency virus (HIV) gp120/gp41 interacts with complement factor H, recruiting factor H, and other CCPs to binding sites on HIV-infected cells (Stoiber et al., 1996). Factor H normally acts to inhibit complement activation, and removal of factor H from human serum augments the effects of complement on HIV-infected cells (Stoiber et al., 1996).

BLOCKADE OF INTERFERON, CHEMOKINES, AND CYTOKINES

The cytokine network constitutes the central communications circuitry that links and orchestrates both the early innate inflammatory responses and later developing acquired immune memory responses to viral infections (Biron, 1998, 1999; Biron et al., 1999; Guidotti and Chisari, 2000; Kalvakolanu, 1999; Krajcsi and Wold, 1998; Salazar-Mather et al., 2000). Here we focus particularly on the interferon (IFN) and chemokine networks as model systems for viral evasion, before considering some of the more general anticytokine strategies.

Anti-Interferon Strategies

The IFNs, primarily the IFN-α/β and IFN-γ family members, are critical for the earliest defense responses to viral infection. Consequently, it is not surprising that a wide variety of anti-IFN strategies

have been evolved by viruses to either prevent ligand function or inhibit intracellular signaling pathways downstream from the IFN-α/β and IFN-γ receptors (Cebulla et al., 1999; Goodbourn et al., 2000; Smith et al., 1998).

Many viruses induce IFN-α/β gene expression rapidly following infection, and the elaboration of soluble IFN-α/β is one of the earliest paracrine events in infected tissues. The subsequent induction within neighboring cells of the antiviral state is mediated by activation of the JAK/STAT signaling pathway, which upregulates a variety of interferon-induced genes, particularly double-stranded RNA (dsRNA)-dependent protein kinase (PKR) and the $2'$-$5'$ oligoadenylate system, which activates RNase L. The major viral anti-IFN strategies have been found to (i) prevent IFN synthesis and/or secretion from infected cells, (ii) block the ligand from reaching and signaling via IFN receptors of neighboring cells, (iii) nullify the IFN-induced intracellular signaling pathways that mediate the antiviral state, or (iv) block the activities of induced antiviral effector molecules directly (Table 3).

The ability of viruses to induce IFN gene expression via dsRNA varies greatly, and the viral proteins which have evolved to intercept this dsRNA-dependent activation can function either to block IFN-induced transcription or by neutralizing IFN-induced molecules that establish an antiviral state. The variety of intracellular inhibitors is impressive (rows 3 to 8 in Table 3), whereas extracellular viral strategies to block IFN (rows 1 and 2) are largely restricted to the expression of secreted receptor homologs (viroceptors) targeted against IFN-α/β and IFN-γ (Barry and McFadden, 1998b; McFadden et al., 1998; Nash et al., 1999; Smith, 1999, 2000). The poxvirus viroceptors for IFN-α/β and IFN-γ are efficient extracellular ligand scavengers that sequester the IFNs prior to receptor engagement, and experiments with virus mutants lacking these genes have revealed attenuated phenotypes (Mossman et al., 1996). For example, the myxomavirus (MYX) MT-7 protein binds IFN-γ. An MT-7-negative mutant displayed increased migration of inflammatory cells into lesions, whereas lesions caused by wild-type MYX showed large masses of lymphocytes in tissues underlying the lesion. Thus, MT-7 disrupts communication between inflammatory cells and antigen-presenting cells, both in the lesion and in secondary lymphoid organs (Mossman et al., 1996). This will obviously be of great advantage to a poxvirus, reducing immune recognition and reducing the immune-mediated loss of host cells that can then subsequently be used for replication.

Table 3. Viral anti-interferon strategies

Strategy	Virus examples[a]	Mechanism
Secreted homologs of vIFN-α/β receptors	B18R (VV)	Inhibits extracellular IFN-α/β
Secreted homologs of vIFN-γ receptors	B8R (VV) M-T7 (MYX)	Inhibits extracellular IFN-γ
Intracellular homologs of vIRF	vIRF-1/K9 (HHV-8) vIRF-2 (HHV-8) vIRF-3/K10.5 (HHV-8)	Represses IFN-inducible genes
Inhibition of PKR dsRNA binding	E3L (VV) σ3 (Reo) NSP3 (Rota) NS1 (IV)	Competes with PKR for binding to dsRNA
dsRNA-like analogs	VA1-RNA (Ad) EBER-1 RNA (EBV) TAR-RNA (HIV)	Binds and inactivates PKR
Substrate modifications or competition	K3L (VV) ICP 34.5 (HSV)	Homolog of eIF2α Dephosphorylation of eIF2α
Enzyme inhibition	US11 (HSV) PK2 (Bac) Tat (HIV) E2 (HCV)	Blocks PKR activity
Inhibition of RNase L	? (HSV) ? (HIV, EMCV)	Synthesis of 2′-5′ oligoadenylate analogs Induction of RNAse L inhibitors
Translation protection	γ34.5 (HSV-1)	Interferes with translational shutoff
Inhibition of IFN-induced gene expression	ElA (Ad) TP (HBV) EBNA-2 (EBV) NS1 (IV)	Represses INF-specific transcriptional responses
Interference with JAK/STAT pathway	ElA (Ad) T-Ag (Py) V (SV5) TP (HBV) Tax (HTLV) gp55 (SFFV) E7 (HPV-16) HCMV ?	Inhibits signaling downstream of IFN receptors (e.g., JAK/STAT)

[a] Reo, reovirus; Rota, rotavirus; IV, influenza virus; Bac, baculovirus; EMCV, encephalomyocarditis virus; Py, polyomavirus; SV5, simian virus 5; HBV, hepatitis B virus; HTLV, human T-cell leukemia virus; SFFV, spleen focus-forming virus.

In contrast to the apparently monolithic approach of scavenging extracellular IFN by viroceptors, there are numerous types of viral proteins that inhibit intracellular events involved in the IFN pathways. The discovery of virus-encoded homologs of IFN regulatory factors (vIRFs) within the genome of human herpesvirus 8 (HHV-8) suggested a mechanism whereby the viral homolog could outcompete cellular IRFs needed for the transcriptional activation of host cell IFN response genes (Zimring et al., 1997; Li et al., 1998; Pitha et al., 1998; Burysek et al., 1999; Lubyova and Pitha, 2000). One of the most frequent targets in the pathway mediating resistance

to IFN involves inhibition of PKR, which functions in establishing an antiviral state in cells, e.g., by shutting down translation (Clemens and Elia, 1997; Gale and Katze, 1998). As summarized in Table 1, viruses use at least four distinct strategies to defeat or evade the effects of activated PKR. These four strategies tend to focus on the PKR enzyme itself, its coactivator molecule dsRNA, or the cellular substrates of activated PKR, particularly eukaryotic initiation factor 2α (eIF2α). In contrast to the extensive literature on PKR-inhibitory mechanisms, the molecular mechanisms by which viruses block the other components that mediate this antiviral state, particularly RNase

L, remain less well defined. Nevertheless, it is likely that the neutralization of dsRNA affects many other effector molecules in addition to PKR and RNase L. Perhaps the most persuasive in vivo evidence for the key importance of PKR in the antiviral responses has come from the observation that recombinant HSV-1 with a deletion of the ICP34.5 gene (which normally blocks PKR by maintaining low phosphorylation levels of the substrate eIF2α) was attenuated in wild-type mice but had restored virulence in mice in which the PKR gene was knocked out (Leib et al., 2000). This powerful exploitation of virus genetic manipulation along with the use of knockout mice will probably prove to be invaluable in delineating antiviral pathways in vivo in the future.

Another common target of viral inhibition is the JAK/STAT pathway, which mediates IFN-receptor signaling and downstream gene activation. The mechanisms include reducing JAK/STAT levels (for example by increased degradation rates), reducing STAT phosphorylation, and forming inhibitory complexes. Inhibition of JAK/STAT signaling is also an important mechanism by which viruses block the induction of major histocompatibility complex (MHC) class II genes to avoid CD4 T cells (see "Inhibition of the MHC Class II Antigen Presentation Pathway" below). Given the widespread targeting of this pathway by viruses, it is expected that even more examples of the JAK/STAT manipulation remain to be uncovered. The reader is referred to several comprehensive reviews on this subject (Cebulla et al., 1999; Goodbourn et al., 2000).

Antichemokine Strategies

Chemokines constitute a growing superfamily of low-molecular-weight cytokines that play pivotal roles in the chemotaxis and activation of leukocytes during development, homeostasis, and the inflammatory responses to injury and infection (Baggiolini and Loetscher, 2000; Lusso, 2000; Murdoch and Finn, 2000). Over 50 chemokines have been identified, and all mediate their biological responses by binding and signaling through G-protein-coupled seven membrane-spanning chemokine receptors, which display a complex and sometimes redundant distribution on the surface of migratory immune cells. As a consequence of the critical importance of the chemokine network in response to virus infection, it is not surprising that viruses in general have evolved multiple strategies to subvert chemokines and their receptors to favor virus survival. The literature on chemokine modulation by viruses is now vast and is the subject of numerous reviews to which the reader is referred for a more comprehensive de-

tailing of primary references (Wells and Schwartz, 1998; Dairaghi et al., 1998; Pease and Murphy, 1998; Lalani and McFadden, 1999; Kotwal, 2000; Lalani et al., 2000; Mahalingam and Karupiah, 2000; McFadden and Murphy, 2000).

To date, there are three strategies by which virus-encoded proteins subvert chemokines or their receptors: (i) secreted chemokine homologs, (ii) chemokine receptor homologs, and (iii) chemokine binding proteins that do not have homology to chemokine receptors (Table 4). Viral chemokine homologs are expressed as secreted proteins that bind to one or more members of the cellular chemokine receptor family as agonists (i.e., signaling ligands) or antagonists (i.e., nonsignaling competitors of cellular ligands). Many of these viral chemokines target the CC chemokine subfamily or their receptors, suggesting the importance of this family in antiviral immune responses, but several examples of viral CXC chemokine homologs have also been described, and these may be more selective for neutrophils. The discovery of virus-encoded chemokine agonists (e.g., HHV-8 vMIP-I and -MIPIII, HHV-6 U83, HCMV UL146, and MCMV MCK-1, and MCK-2) suggested the need to revise the original view in which viruses simply inhibit chemokine functions. There are clearly situations in which these chemokines increase the recruitment of inflammatory leukocytes, and this facilitates virus infection or dissemination. For example, HCMV UL146 (also called vCXC-1) is a CXC chemokine mimic that induces the chemotaxis of neutrophils by binding and signaling with one of the two known receptors for interleukin-8 (IL-8), namely, CXCR2 (Penfold et al., 1999).

Direct evidence that a viral chemokine agonist can play a role in virus dissemination first came from experiments involving MCMV mutants lacking the m131/129 chemokine genes. An M131/129-negative MCMV exhibited reduced spread to the salivary gland, which in wild-type MCMV probably occurs within infected monocytes/macrophage (Fleming et al., 1999; Saederup et al., 1999). On the other hand, the agonistic activity of other viral chemokines, such as those encoded by HHV-8, is related not to viral dissemination but to their proangiogenic properties within Kaposi's sarcoma lesions (Boshoff et al., 1997; Stine et al., 2000).

There is, to date, only one example of a chemokine mimetic that can function in vitro as a chemoattractant for leukocytes. HIV Tat displays only very limited sequence homology to the cellular chemokine superfamily, yet it promotes migration of lymphoma cells and enhances their adhesion to endothelial cells (Albini et al., 1998a, 1998b; Chirivi et al., 1999). However, evidence for an in vivo role for

Table 4. Viral antichemokine strategies

Strategy	Virus examples[a]	Mechanism
Secreted chemokine homologs or mimetics	vMIP-I/K6 (HHV-8) vMIP-II/F4 (HHV-8) vMIP-III/K4.1 (HHV-8) U83 (HHV-6) UL146 (HCMV) UL147 (HCMV) MCK-1/m131 (MCMV) MCK-2/m129 (MCMV) MC148R/vMCC-1 (MCV)	Bind cellular chemokine receptors and function as antagonists or agonists; some are proangiogenic
	Tat (HIV)	Chemokine mimetic
Chemokine receptor homologs	orf74 (HHV-8, γ68HV, EHV-2) ECRF3/orf74 (HVS) E1 (EHV-2) UL33 (HCMV) US28 (HCMV) M33 (MCMV) U12/U51 (HHV-6) U12 (HHV-7) K2R (SPV)	Expressed at cell surface, may be capable of ligand-dependent or -independent signaling
Chemokine binding proteins		
Type I	M-T7 (MYX) S-T7 (SFV)	Nonspecific chemokine binding
Type II	M-T1 (MYX) S-T1 (SFV) C23L/B297 (VV-Lister) D1L/H5R (CPV)	CC chemokine inhibitor
Type III	M3 (MHV-68)	Broad-spectrum chemokine inhibitor

[a] SPV, swinepox virus; SFV, shape fibroma virus; see Table 3, footnote a, for other abbreviations.

Tat-induced cellular chemotaxis will be difficult to obtain.

Among the virus-encoded chemokine antagonists, HHV-8 vMIP-II and molluscum contagiosum virus (MCV) MC148R have been the best studied in vitro, but both of these viruses are difficult to study in infected hosts. Nevertheless, their potent inhibitory properties as CC chemokine antagonists in vitro suggest an in vivo role at limiting the taxis or activation of monocytes/macrophages/dendritic cells in viral lesions. Of particular note is that MCV-induced dermal lesions are generally devoid of inflammatory cells despite extensive virus replication in epidermal cells, which normally can respond robustly to injury or infection with potent proinflammatory signals (Smith et al., 1999; Mahalingam and Karupiah, 2000).

The second major category of chemokine modulators are the virus-encoded chemokine receptor homologs, which, to date, have also been detected only in members of the herpesvirus and poxvirus families (Table 4). Some of these bind only CXC chemokines (HVS orf74), others bind only CC chemokines (HHV-6 U21/U51, and equine herpesvirus 2 [EHV-2] E1), and others bind both CC and CX3C chemokines (HCMV US28) or both CC and CXC chemokines (HHV-8 orf74). Many, but not all, of these viral receptors signal in response to binding of cellular chemokines. HHV-8 orf74 can signal constitutively, although the intensity of this signal can be strongly up- or downregulated by different chemokine ligands (Arvanitakis et al., 1997). The role of HHV-8 orf74 in viral pathogenesis is controversial, and whether it is a dominant "oncogene" that mediates the transformation of cells within Kaposi's sarcomas is not yet clear (Cesarman et al., 2000). Interestingly, herpesvirus saimiri orf74/ECRF3 is not a constitutively signaling receptor, and its role in disease in primate hosts remains to be clarified. One interesting model proposes that the HCMV US28 chemokine receptor might function as a chemokine "sink" that scavenges extracellular ligands like RANTES from the extracellular compartment (Bodaghi et al., 1998). Another view suggests that US28 stimulates ligand-dependant chemotaxis of infected smooth muscle cells during development of atherosclerosis (Streblow et al., 1999).

The third major class of chemokine modulation is mediated by virus-encoded chemokine binding proteins that share the ability to bind and scavenge extracellular chemokines but do not have significant sequence homology to known chemokine receptor or other host immune molecules (Table 4). Expression of such chemokine binding proteins was originally thought to be the realm only of the poxviruses, but recently the first example of a herpesvirus-encoded version was identified in mouse herpesvirus 68 (MHV-68) (Parry et al., 2000; van Berkel et al., 2000). To date, three types of chemokine binding proteins of this class have been identified, designated types I to III. Proteins in each class are closely related to each other but not to proteins in other classes. Analysis of virus mutants lacking types I and II chemokine binding proteins has revealed that these proteins directly affect leukocyte migratory behavior within virus-infected lesions and that the purified proteins themselves inhibit inflammatory cells within nonviral models of inflammation (Mossman et al., 1996; Graham et al., 1997; Lalani et al., 1999; Alcami and Koszinowski, 2000; Liu et al., 2000).

Other Anticytokine Strategies

Beyond the viral inhibitors of interferons and chemokines, there are many other viral anticytokine strategies. Viruses have captured cellular cytokines and cytokine receptors, although this process remains poorly documented; the consequences of these capture events for viruses are profound. Other cytokine-inhibitory viral genes are summarized in Table 5. There are cytokine homologs, receptor homologs, and growth factors, as well as proteins with no obvious host counterparts. Even these orphan virus genes are suspected of having been derived from genes acquired from ancestral host species sometime during their evolutionary history, but their identities may surface only as the genomic databases continue to expand.

The first viral cytokines or growth factors, discovered in the mid-1980s, was the VV epidermal growth factor-like protein, now referred to as vaccinia growth factor (Barry and McFadden, 1997). Poxvirus growth factors are potent signaling ligands for members of the erbB receptor family (Tzahar et al., 1998), and provide a useful paradigm for other virus-encoded ligands of cellular receptors. Another of the best-studied cytokines is the Epstein-Barr virus (EBV) IL-10 homolog, which is related to other herpesviruses and poxvirus (equine herpesvirus, herpesvirus papio, HCMV, and orf virus) IL-10-like molecules. The viral IL-10 homologs bind and signal via cellular IL-10 receptors, but some possess only a subset of the biological properties of the cellular ligand. For example, in the case of EBV vIL-10, the viral protein has lost some of the immunostimulatory properties of the host cytokine while preserving the ability to inhibit IFN-γ (Barry and McFadden, 1998b; Spriggs, 1996; Stordeur and Goldman, 1998; Tortorella et al., 2000). Another example of a potent virus-encoded cytokine is the HHV-8 IL-6 homolog which acts in autocrine-like fashion in infected lymphoma cells (Jones et al., 1999). HHV-8 IL-6 activates multiple IL-6 receptor pathways but interacts with the IL-6 receptor in a different fashion from that used by cellular IL-6 (Osborne et al., 1999; Wan et al., 1999).

In contrast to viral cytokine homologs, the viral cytokine-binding proteins (Table 5) probably mimic regulatory molecules which normally function as cytokine carriers or inhibitors. The best studied of these are the IL-18 binding proteins (IL-18BPs) encoded by members of the poxvirus family (Novick et al., 1999). IL-18 is a key proinflammatory cytokine that, like IL-1β, is activated by cleavage of caspase-1 (or IL-1β-activating enzyme [ICE]), but can be inhibited extracellularly by IL-18BPs (Fantuzzi and Dinarello, 1999). The viral IL-18BPs are effective scavengers of cellular IL-18 and have excellent potential as anti-inflammatory reagents (Xiang and Moss, 1999a, 1999b; Born et al., 2000; Kim et al., 2000; Smith et al., 2000).

Other viral receptor homologs (viroceptors) have been described that bind IFN-α/β, IFN-γ, IL-1β, TNF, and colony-stimulating factor 1 (Tables 2 and 4). All of these secreted viroceptors function in the extracellular environment to bind, with high affinity, and inhibit their target cytokines (Barry and McFadden, 1997; McFadden et al., 1998; Alcami and Koszinowski, 2000; Smith, 2000). The poxvirus TNF receptors were the first viroceptors discovered (in the early 1990s) and they still provide the prototypic examples of this class of cytokine inhibitor (Cunnion, 1999; Nash et al., 1999; Xu et al., 2000). Poxvirus TNF receptor homologs generally resemble only the extracellular ligand binding domain of the cellular receptor, characterized by multiple copies of cysteine-rich domains frequently seen in members of the larger TNF receptor superfamily. Interestingly, the MYX TNF receptor, M-T2, exhibits not only the ability to inhibit extracellular TNF but also the capacity to inhibit apoptosis intracellularly in a fashion independent of TNF (Schreiber et al., 1997). This dual intracellular and extracellular activity of a viral protein of this type may well prove to be more common than is currently suspected.

Another key area of viral interference occurs at the level of signal transduction downstream from cell surface TNF and cytokine receptors. Receptors that signal to produce cell death or apoptosis are not covered extensively in this section but are covered in

Table 5. Viral anticytokine strategies

Strategy	Virus examples[a]	Mechanism[b]
Cytokine homologs	K2/vIL-6 (HHV-8)	Secreted IL-6 cytokine mimic
	ORF13/vIL-17 (HVS)	Secreted IL-17 cytokine mimic
	BCRF1/vIL-10 (EBV)	Secreted IL-10 cytokine mimic
	UL111a/cmvIL-10 (HCMV)	Secreted IL-10 cytokine mimic (see Table 3)
	OV-vIL-10 (orf)	
	v-chemokines	
Cytokine binding proteins	GIF (orf)	Binds and inhibits IL-2/GM-CSF
	MC54L/53L (MCV)	Binds and inhibits IL-18
	35-kDa (TPV)	Binds and inhibits IFN-γ, IL-2, IL-5 (see Table 3)
	Chemokine binding proteins	
Homologs of cytokine receptors	vIFNα/B-Rs (see Table 2)	Inhibits IFN-α/β
	vIFNγ-Rs (see Table 2)	Inhibits IFN-γ
	vIL-1β-R/B15R (VV)	Inhibits IL-1β
	vTNF-R/M-T2 (MYX)	Inhibits TNF
	vTNF-R/crmB, crmC, crmD, crmE (many poxviruses)	Inhibits TNF
	UL144 (HCMV)	TNF receptor homolog (see Table 3)
	v-chemokine receptors	
	vCSF-1R/BARF-1 (EBV)	Inhibits CSF-1
Growth factor homologs	VGF/C11R (VV)	EGF homolog
	MGF (MYX)	EGF homolog
	vVEGF/A2R (orf)	VEGF homolog
Intracellular signaling interference	E5 (BPV)	PDGF signaling
	gp55 (SFFV)	EPO-R signaling
	A46R/A52R (VV)	Toll/IL-1R signaling
	Tip (HVS)	pp56^{lck} signaling
	STP-C488 (HVS)	c-Ras signaling
	STP-A11 (HVS)	c-Src family signaling
	pX (HBV)	c-Src family signaling
	LMP-1 (EBV)	TNF receptor signaling (see Table 2)
	JAK/STAT inhibitors	
Cytokine secretion	crmA (CPV)	Inhibits ICE and secretion of IL-1β
	B13R (VV)	
	SERP-2 (MYX)	
Induction of cytokine inhibitors	gp350 (EBV)	Induces IL-1RA

[a] TPV, tanapoxvirus; BPV, bovine papillomavirus; see Table 3 footnote for other abbreviations.
[b] GM-CSF, granulocyte-macrophage colony-stimulating factor; EGF, epidermal growth factor; VEGF, vascular endothelial growth factor; PDGF, platelet-derived growth factor.

terms of cell-killing mechanisms in "Obstruction of Cell Killing and Apoptosis" (below). In addition, the reader is referred to recent reviews on viruses and apoptosis (Meinl et al., 1998; O'Brien, 1998; Roulston et al., 1999). As shown in Table 5, there is a diverse collection of viral proteins that activate cellular receptors in a ligand-independent fashion (e.g., bovine papillomavirus E5 and spleen focus-forming virus gp55), mimic activated cellular receptors (e.g., EBV LMP-1), or engage intracellular components of signaling pathways (e.g., HVS Tip/STP-C488/STP-A11 and EBV LMP-2). Mechanistically these strategies are very diverse, but collectively they all perturb

critical signaling molecules between activated receptors and downstream targets (DiMaio et al., 1998; Krajcsi and Wold, 1998). One of the more recent examples of this is the VV proteins A46R and A52R, which can interfere with IL-1 and Toll-like receptor signaling by virtue of the ability to mimic the TIR regulatory domains on these receptors (Bowie et al., 2000). The Toll-like receptor pathway is thought to be particularly important for the activation of NF-κB, which in turn is one of the key amplifying signals for inflammation (Janeway and Medzhitov, 2000). Interestingly, NF-κB is known to be targeted in virus-infected leukocytes by a number of strategies. For example, African swine fever virus encodes a homolog of IκB that binds calcineurin and prevents gene transcriptional upregulation dependent on the transcription factor NFAT (Miskin et al., 1998, 2000), although the in vivo significance needs to be clarified in an animal model (Neilan et al., 1997).

Another viral anticytokine strategy involves inhibition of the secretion of proinflammatory cytokines like IL-1β and IL-18 by blocking the activating enzyme caspase-1 (ICE) (Table 5). The inhibition of cellular ICE by the poxvirus crmA (SPI-2) protein proved to be the first example of a cross-class caspase inhibitor by a viral homolog of the serpin superfamily (Pickup, 1994; McFadden et al., 1998; Turner and Moyer, 1998; Zhou and Salvesen, 2000). Although attempts have been made to link the crmA/SPI-2 family to apoptosis inhibition, the most likely role for these intracellular serpins is to block ICE-dependent proinflammatory signals by ICE inhibition. However, a role in blocking cell-mediated killing pathways also remains possible (Macen et al., 1996) (see "Obstruction of Cell Killing and Apoptosis" below).

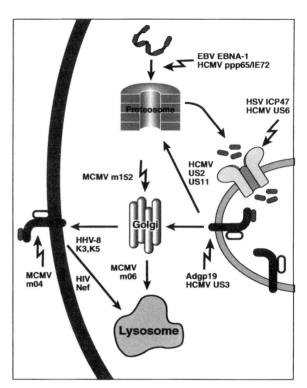

Figure 1. Viral inhibition of the MHC class I antigen presentation pathway.

INHIBITION OF ANTIGEN PRESENTATION TO CD8⁺ AND CD4⁺ T CELLS AND NATURAL KILLER CELLS

Inhibition of the MHC Class I Antigen Presentation Pathway

CD8$^+$ T cells are major players in the struggle between viruses and the host. CD8$^+$ T cells can recognize early stages of virus infection by scanning host cells for the presence of peptides derived from viral proteins and presented by the MHC class I antigen presentation pathway found in most cells. CD8$^+$ T cells can then destroy the virally infected cells, before virus particles are produced, or cause the secretion of lymphokines or cytokines to activate and enhance cellular defenses and to allow host cells to resist infection (Guidotti and Chisari, 2000). Viral and cellular proteins are degraded into antigenic peptides by the proteasome (Fig. 1). Peptides are transported into the lumen of the ER by the transporter associated with antigen presentation (TAP) (Fruh et al., 1999; Tortorella et al., 2000). Newly synthesized class I proteins bind the antigenic peptides and convey them to the cell surface for recognition by the T-cell receptors of CD8$^+$ T cells.

A number of virus families have evolved mechanisms to thwart recognition by CD8$^+$ T cells. This is especially true for herpesviruses and adenoviruses, viruses that establish persistent or latent infections

and which possess relatively large coding capacities (Johnson and Hill, 1998; Alcami and Koszinowski, 2000; Tortorella et al., 2000). For herpesviruses, reactivation from latency occurs in the face of robust, fully primed host immunity, and it appears that it is important to evade CD8$^+$ T cells, at least for a time, e.g., immediately after reactivation of latent herpesviruses, or in specific tissues, e.g., the nervous system (Johnson and Hill, 1998). These viruses often encode multiple inhibitors of the MHC class I antigen presentation pathway, and individual inhibitors of the MHC class I pathway may have important effects in some cell types yet may be less effective in other cells. Expression of higher levels of class I proteins after IFN upregulation nullifies the effects of some of these inhibitors (Goldsmith et al., 1998; Hengel et al., 2000). Thus, these inhibitors may act at specific times during the course of disease to provide the virus a window of opportunity, allowing it to spread to other hosts (Johnson and Hill, 1998). It appears that the generation or priming of CD8$^+$ T cells by professional antigen-presenting cells (APC), which may not be infected or which express high levels of class I, is infrequently blocked. However, specific cell types that serve as hosts for the virus may be invisible to the CD8$^+$ T cells that are present.

Viral proteins that avoid proteolysis or presentation

Virtually every stage of the well-characterized MHC class I antigen presentation pathway is obstructed by one or another animal virus (Fig. 1). The simplest evasion strategy is to alter dominant or well-recognized CD8$^+$ T-cell epitopes. There are examples of this with many viruses, including HIV, which can also express antagonistic peptides that prevent activation of groups of antiviral T cells, producing broader resistance (Bertoletti et al., 1994; Klenerman et al., 1994). EBV uses a mechanism similar to that used by certain long-lived cellular proteins, avoiding proteolysis and antigen presentation of a viral protein, EBNA-1. All EBV-associated malignancies express EBNA-1, yet the protein is not recognized by CD8$^+$ T cells, while other EBV latency-associated proteins, EBNA-2, EBNA-3, and EBNA-4, can be recognized (Levitskaya et al., 1997). A glycine-alanine repeat of variable length that is found internally in EBNA-1 transferred this resistance to EBNA-4. In a cell-free system, EBNA-4 and a Gly-Ala-deficient mutant of EBNA-1 were degraded by proteasomes whereas EBNA-1 was more resistant (Levitskaya et al., 1997). Similar repeats in the adenovirus (Ad) E1A proteins and the NF-κB1 precursor p105 may also regulate protein turnover (Levitskaya et al., 1997).

HCMV introduces a component of virus particles, pp65, into the host cytoplasm during virus entry. pp65 can effectively inhibit the presentation of the immediate-early (IE) transcription factor IE72 to CD8$^+$ T cells (Gilbert et al., 1996). pp65 has protein kinase activity, or there is kinase activity associated with the expression of pp65. Mutation of carboxy-terminal residues that contain a serine/threonine consensus domain abolished its ability to prevent IE72 presentation. Therefore, it appears that phosphorylation by pp65 or an associated kinase can alter the presentation of viral antigens by restricting access to the antigen presentation machinery.

Inhibitors of TAP

A substantial number of viruses block TAP-mediated peptide transport into the ER (Fig. 1). Since TAP is an essential enzyme in the class I pathway, it is reasonable to consider it the Achilles heel of this pathway. HSV encodes a 10-kDa cytoplasmic protein, ICP47, that is expressed before the vast majority of the other 80 HSV polypeptides and effectively inhibits presentation to anti-HSV cytotoxic T lymphocyes (CTL) (Johnson and Hill, 1998). ICP47 blocks TAP by binding to its cytoplasmic surface, at a site that overlaps the peptide binding site, blocking

peptide binding and destabilizing the TAP1-TAP2 heterodimer (Johnson and Hill, 1998; Lacaille and Androlewicz, 1998).

In a mouse model of HSV infection, an ICP47-negative HSV mutant replicated normally at the site of innoculation in the cornea, but there was markedly reduced disease in the nervous system days later (Goldsmith et al., 1998). However, if the mice were first depleted of CD8$^+$ T cells, the ICP47-negative mutant caused neuropathology similar to that caused by wild-type HSV. It was concluded that ICP47 can defend HSV against CD8$^+$ T cells in the mouse nervous system. These results must be considered with some caution because ICP47 inhibits the murine TAP relatively poorly, at least in mouse fibroblasts. It appears that ICP47 may be more effective in the nervous system, where components of the class I pathway are expressed at low levels. Even though mice are not the ideal model in which to test the effects of ICP47, these results illustrate a principle. The effects of a viral immune evasion protein can be restricted to a specific tissue type in vivo, where the ability to remain invisible to the immune system for a time is important. There is also evidence that the effects of ICP47 may be restricted to the earliest phases of disease, directly after reactivation, in human epithelial tissues (Johnson and Hill, 1998). In many cell types, including fibroblasts and epithelial cells, the effects of ICP47 are abolished by IFN-γ. In human lesions, the arrival of CD8$^+$ T cells lags behind that of CD4$^+$ T cells by 2 to 3 days, suggesting that CD8$^+$ T cells may be initially unable to recognize early stages of HSV disease (Johnson and Hill, 1998). With the appearance of other cells in lesions, e.g., natural killer (NK) and CD4$^+$ T cells, and IFN-γ, the effects of ICP47 are overcome.

HCMV expresses a membrane glycoprotein, US6, that also inhibits TAP. A soluble form of US6 lacking the cytoplasmic and membrane-spanning domains can inhibit TAP (Fruh et al., 1999; Alcami and Koszinowski, 2000; Tortorella et al., 2000). Thus, in contrast to ICP47, US6 interacts largely with luminal domains of TAP. Other herpesviruses also inhibit TAP (Ambagala et al., 2000; P. Jugovic and D. C. Johnson, unpublished data), as do AdV (Bennett et al., 1999), and it is likely that this is the case for other virus families, just as TAP is blocked in many tumors.

Viral proteins that bind to or mislocalize MHC class I proteins

There are several classes of viral proteins that interact with class I molecules directly or indirectly, restricting their ability to present peptides to CD8 T cells. Ad E3 gp19 binds to class I complexes, causing retention in the ER or recycling back to the ER from the Golgi (Tortorella et al., 2000). A short sequence in the C-terminal cytoplasmic domain of the gp19 including a dilysine motif, a classic ER retention or recycling motif, is responsible for localization to the ER. Ad gp19 also binds TAP, acting as a tapasin inhibitor and preventing MHC class I-TAP association (Bennett et al., 1999).

HCMV expresses a membrane glycoprotein, US3, that retains peptide-loaded class I molecules, but retention is by a mechanism different from that used by Ad gp19, since there is no recognizable ER retention motif in US3 (Fruh et al., 1999). Moreover, US3 is transported slowly from the ER to the *trans*-Golgi network (TGN) or lysosomes and is degraded, whereas class I proteins are largely localized to the ER in US3-expressing cells (K. Frueh, personal communication; R. Tomazin and D. C. Johnson, unpublished data). Either newly synthesized US3 can exchange with more mature US3 to retain class I molecules or there are long-term effects on the folding or posttranslational modification of class I molecules or interactions with chaperones. There are two related HCMV membrane glycoproteins, US2 and US11, encoded by genes adjacent to US3, which bind MHC class I heavy chains (HC) and cause their proteolysis (Tortorella et al., 2000). Studies of US2 and US11 have shed new light on the molecular details of degradation in the ER. Newly synthesized class I proteins bound by US2 or US11 are rapidly removed from the ER membrane, through the Sec61 proteinaceous pore, extruded into the cytoplasm, and degraded by proteasomes. It appears that US2 and US11 connect class I HC to a normal cellular pathway by which misfolded or aberrant ER-resident proteins are degraded and in some way accelerates this process (Johnson and Haigh, 2000). US3 has been described as an IE protein, whereas US2 is an early protein and is expressed after US3, at least in human fibroblasts. Therefore, it has been suggested that US3 may retain class I proteins that subsequently become more susceptible to the effects of US2 (Fruh et al., 1999). However, in other cell types, e.g., macrophages or endothelial cells, the order of expression of these proteins and other inhibitors may differ. Therefore, HCMV encodes at least four inhibitors of the class I pathway: US2, US3, US6, and US11. It is possible that individual glycoproteins function better in different cell types or with different class I alleles.

MCMV also encodes at least three glycoproteins that bind to class I proteins: m152 retains class I in the ER-Golgi intermediate compartment, m06 targets class I complexes to lysosomes for degradation, and m04 is found in the ER and on the cell surface (re-

viewed in Hengel et al., 1999; Alcami and Koszinowski, 2000; Tortorella et al., 2000). m152 appears similar to the HCMV US3 glycoprotein in that there is a transient interaction with class I molecules which remain in the ER-Golgi intermediate compartment, while m152 is eventually degraded in the endosomal-lysosomal compartment. An m152-MCMV mutant displayed reduced virus titers in the lungs and spleen, although normal titers were observed in β_2-microglobulin$^{-/-}$ or CD8 knockout mice (Hengel et al., 2000). Thus, m06 and m04 together could not totally compensate for m152 in the natural host. m04 is novel among these class I binding glycoproteins in that it reaches the cell surface without altering the transport of MHC class I (Tortorella et al., 2000). Moreover, m04 can collaborate with m152 to reduce recognition by CD8$^+$ T cells by binding class I alleles that are not efficiently bound by m152 (D. Cavanaugh, M. Gold, and A. Hill, unpublished data). Thus, as with the HCMV US2, US3, and US6 glycoproteins, there may be additive or synergistic effects of m04, m152, and m06 and differential effects on class I allelles or in specific cell types in vivo.

HIV expresses two proteins that downregulate MHC class I by different mechanisms (Fig. 1). Nef, a 206-amino-acid myristoylated protein, interrupts the normal recycling of class I molecules between the cell surface and endosomes, diverting the class I molecules from early endosomes to late endosomes and lysosomes for degradation (Piguet et al., 1999). Nef acts to connect class I proteins to AP1 or AP2 clathrin adapter complexes, and this involves a tyrosine-sorting motif in the cytoplasmic domain of class I. PACS1, a component of the TGN sorting machinery, is also essential for this mislocalization and acts through a cluster of acidic residues in Nef (Piguet et al., 2000). Nef affects HLA-A and HLA-B and protects cells from CD8$^+$ T cells, but, by contrast, HLA-C and HLA-E are not affected, and this selective downregulation allows HIV-infected cells to avoid lysis by NK cells (Cohen et al., 1999). HIV Vpu, a small integral membrane protein, destabilizes newly synthesized class I proteins in the ER without affecting peptide loading or transport to the cell surface (Kerkau et al., 1997; Piguet et al., 1999). The effects of Vpu on MHC class I molecules appear similar to its effects on CD4, which is ubiquitinated and degraded by proteasomes in the cytoplasm (Schubert et al., 1998). It is not clear whether Nef and Vpu work together, even synergistically, to inhibit class I-mediated presentation. However, it is likely that these viral proteins contribute substantially to the persistence of HIV in the face of vigorous CD8$^+$ T cells, and this may account, at least in part, for observations that Nef⁻ HIV and SIV strains are attenuated.

Inhibitions of NK Cell Recognition

NK cells are a population of lymphocytes that kill various targets including virus-infected and bacterially infected cells, parasites, and tumors without prior sensitization (Biron, 1999). NK cells also produce an important array of cytokines such as IFNs and TNF-α that curtail virus infection and attract professional antigen-presenting cells (Biron, 1999). NK cells lack T-cell receptors and instead use both activating and inhibitory cell surface receptors to recognize target cells (Lanier, 1998; Bakker et al., 2000; Moretta et al., 2000). Inhibitory receptors bind surface MHC class I proteins, delivering signals into the NK cells that inhibit target cell lysis or NK-cell triggering. Thus, virus-induced downregulation of MHC class I proteins is detected by a panel of different NK inhibitory receptors, and this provokes target cell lysis and cytokine production. These effects occur before priming and expansion of CD8⁺ T cells, and NK cells serve important functions in the early or innate antiviral immune response and in shaping adaptive responses.

The role of NK cells in virus disease is perhaps best illustrated by studies of human and animal herpesviruses. Humans lacking NK cells experience frequent and severe HSV and HCMV infections (Biron, 1999). In mice, MCMV infections are poorly contained by NK-deficient animals and transfer of NK cells confers protection (Bukowski et al., 1985). Moreover, cytokines such as IFN-γ, which are produced in large amounts by NK cells, have important implications for HSV disease, overcoming the effects of ICP47 and allowing cells to become recognized by CD8⁺ T cells (see above). The severity of the HSV lesions and the time to recrudescence are closely correlated with IFN-γ production at early stages. Since HSV, HCMV, and probably all herpesviruses severely downregulate MHC class I molecules, it seems highly likely that virus-infected cells would be targets for NK cells. This has been demonstrated in a limited fashion (Huard and Früh, 2000) but is probably more universal. However, herpesviruses also express proteins that confer resistance to NK cells.

MCMV, HCMV, and rat CMV all express MHC class I homologs that appear to act as decoys for NK-cell inhibitory receptors (Farrell et al., 2000). HCMV encodes a glycoprotein, UL18, that conferred resistance to NK cell lysis when transfected into MHC class I-deficient 721.221 cells (Reyburn et al., 1997). However, more recent studies have suggested that this story is more complex than was orig-

inally reported. UL18 has been difficult to detect both in HCMV-infected cells and on the surfaces of transfected cells (Reyburn et al., 1997). NK lysis of UL18-transfected cells was inhibited by a human C-type lectin-like NK inhibitory receptor, CD94 (Reyburn et al., 1997). Recent analysis indicated that CD94 recognizes HLA-E, which is not expressed at the cell surface in 721.221 cells (Farrell et al., 2000). HLE-E binds and presents signal sequences derived from nascent MHC class I proteins, and this might include that of UL18. In contrast to the earlier results, direct binding studies have demonstrated that UL18 interacts with leukocyte immunoglobulin-like receptor (Cosman et al., 1999). Binding of a UL18 fusion protein to various cells indicated a preference for LIR-1 rather than for CD94. Transfection of UL18 into various cells and use of an HCMV UL18⁻ mutant indicated that UL18 increased, rather than decreased, NK-cell susceptibility (Leong et al., 1998). It remains to be determined if NK cells or some other cells are inhibited by UL18 expression.

MCMV expresses an MHC class I homolog, m144, that differs from UL18 and class I HC in that there is a sizable deletion of the α-2 domain (Farrell et al., 2000). An MCMV m144⁻ mutant had reduced titers in the spleen, livers and lungs, but not in the salivary glands, and depletion experiments demonstrated a role for NK cells in clearance of the m144⁻ mutant. m144-expressing cells resisted NK cells (Farrell et al., 2000), but to date there is no definition of the receptors used to recognize m144. There is also evidence that the effects of m144 may extend beyond NK cells. The major in vivo effect of m144 in rejection of class I-deficient tumors was to regulate NK cell accumulation and activation in the peritoneum (Cretney et al., 1999). This suggested that other cells, perhaps monocytes/macrophages, were involved and that m144 may alter recognition by these cells. These mouse studies of m144⁻ MCMV remain the best evidence that herpesvirus class I decoys can act as effective inhibitors of NK cells; however, the molecular details of how these virus homologs function are still unclear.

A poxvirus, MCV expresses an MHC class I homolog that complexes with β_2-microglobulin (Senkevich and Moss, 1998). This MCV glycoprotein does not alter cell surface MHC class I. Since MCV shares with the beta-herpesviruses the ability to persist, it is interesting that these viruses both express class I homologs while other poxviruses, which do not persist, apparently do not express class I homologs.

HHV-8, a gammaherpesvirus involved in Kaposi's sarcoma, expresses two similar proteins, K3 and K5, which cause internalization of MHC class I proteins by mechanisms that are not well characterized (Coscoy and Ganem, 2000; Ishido et al., 2000b). K3 and K5 are especially interesting in that class I is downregulated at the cell surface yet K3 and K5 appear to be largely retained in the ER. K5 can also reduce NK cell-mediated lysis by downregulating the costimulatory molecules intercellular cell adhesion molecule 1 (ICAM-1) and B7-2 (Ishido et al., 2000a). Thus, HHV-8-infected cells with reduced levels of cell surface MHC class I would normally be sensitive to NK cells, but by reducing adhesion or costimulation, the cells are less sensitive to NK cells. This is a novel mechanism for evading lymphocytes and is likely to be common.

NK receptors may be found not only on NK cells but also on CD8$^+$ T cells. For example, a substantial fraction of human CD8$^+$ T cells express NK2GD, an activating receptor that interacts with a nonpolymorphic MHC class I-like protein, MIC-A (Bauer et al., 1999). MIC-A can be strongly upregulated after HCMV infection of human fibroblasts, and there is recent evidence that this allows CD8$^+$ T cells to better recognize HCMV-infected cells (Groh et al., 2001). Since the HCMV genes US2, US3, US6, and US11 will downregulate the MHC class I pathway, MIC-A appears to partially compensate, so that CD8$^+$ T cells can better recognize HCMV-infected target cells. Consistent with this, anti-MIC-A antibodies substantially reduced the recognition of HCMV-infected fibroblasts by anti-HCMV CD8$^+$ CTL. This illustrates an important principle, i.e., that cells respond to virus infection and damage to the class I pathway by upregulating costimulatory or adhesion molecules, thereby increasing recognition by lymphocytes. Based on previous observations, it is very likely that there will be a substantial class of virus inhibitors that can block costimulatory molecules such as ICAM-1, B7-2, and MIC-A.

Inhibition of the MHC Class II Antigen Presentation Pathway

Recognition of MHC class II proteins by CD4$^+$ T cells is a crucial component of antiviral responses. Class II proteins are normally restricted to a subset of APC (dendritic cells, macrophages, lymphocytes, thymic epithelium), but a number of other cells also express class II molecules, especially after stimulation with IFN-γ. Class II complexes consist of α and β transmembrane proteins and peptides of 11 to 20 amino acids (Pieters, 2000). These peptides are normally derived from exogenous or extracellular proteins taken up by endocytosis or phagocytosis, proteolyzed by cathepsins in acidic compartments, and then loaded onto the class II peptide binding pocket in place of CLIP, a fragment of the invariant chain, Ii (Fig. 2). This loading requires the action of DM, a nonpolymorphic class II-like polypeptide (Denzin et al., 1996). Once loaded, class II proteins move to the cell surface for presentation to the T-cell receptors of CD4+ T cells.

Induction of MHC class II genes

Expression of class II genes in a number of cell types, including endothelial and epithelial cells, is induced by cytokines. IFN-γ activates the JAK/STAT pathway, which induces transcription of the CIITA, the class II transactivator that turns on class II genes (Harton and Ting, 2000). Members of the herpesvirus and Ad families inhibit IFN-γ and IFN-α signaling pathways and block induction of CIITA and class II proteins. HCMV proteins block several steps in the IFN pathway, acting on Jak1 and p48 transcription factors needed for CIITA expression (Miller et al., 1999). This may be especially important in cells, e.g., endothelial cells, where induction of class II proteins from low basal states is important. MCMV blocks IFN signaling at a later step (Heise et al., 1998), and Ad E1A inhibits STAT1 and p48, inhibiting both IFN-γ and IFN-α signaling (Leonard and Sen, 1997).

Inhibition of the MHC class II pathway

The class II antigen presentation pathway is also a target for viruses. HCMV US2, a glycoprotein that causes proteasome-mediated degradation of class I HC, also targets class II-α chains for degradation (Tomazin et al., 1999). The effects of US2 on class II-α chains are somewhat different from those described for the class I HC. α chains remain in the ER membrane and are not translocated into the cytoplasm when the proteasome is blocked (Tomazin et al., 1999), whereas class I HC accumulate in a soluble, deglycosylated form (Tortorella et al., 2000). US2 not only causes degradation of class II DR-α chains but also causes destruction of DM-α. DM is an enzyme that is necessary for peptide loading and is expressed at relatively low levels compared with class I and II proteins. As such, DM represents an attractive target for US2. It is not clear what preferences US2 has for various substrates: class I HC, class II DR-α and DM-α. However, in cells that express all three proteins and that express class II proteins at relatively high levels, US2 expression effectively blocks the presentation of exogenously added proteins to CD4 T cells (Tomazin et al., 1999). Recently, the HCMV US3 glycoprotein that retains class I HC in the ER was found to mediate resistance to CD4 T

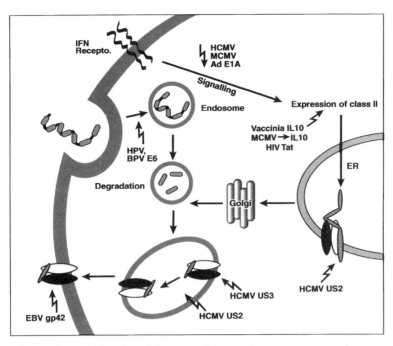

Figure 2. Viral inhibition of the MHC class II antigen presentation pathway.

cells and causes sodium dodecyl sulfate-unstable class II proteins to accumulate in cells (R. Tomazin, N. Hegde, and D. C. Johnson, unpublished data). This appears to be related to effects on Ii.

Inhibition of the MHC class II pathway by HCMV US2 and US3 apparently highlights an important and novel aspect of antiviral immune recognition, where it relates to MHC class II-presenting cells. Normally, "professional" APC (dendritic cells or macrophages) take up exogenous or extracellular antigens and present peptides derived from these antigens to CD4$^+$ T cells. However, US2 and US3 are expressed solely within HCMV-infected cells and would not be expected to affect the majority of APC, i.e., those that have not been infected by HCMV. However, monocytes/macrophages appear to be an important reservoir for HCMV, and endothelial cells can also be infected (Soderberg-Naucler et al., 1997). In either of these cells or other cells, US2 and US3 might be expected to inhibit the presentation of endogenous antigens, viral proteins that traffic into or through the class II-loading compartments. This is consistent with observations that HCMV glycoprotein gB recycles extensively into endosomal compartments in macrophages (Fish et al., 1998). Moreover, it is becoming well established that herpesviruses, at least alphaherpesviruses, target numerous structural components to the TGN and acquire their envelope there (reviewed in McMillan et al., 2001). By this hypothesis, HCMV destroys class II proteins, preventing the presentation of endogenous

antigens and escaping detection by CD4$^+$ T cells that can produce antiviral cytokines or act as CTL. It appears likely that other viruses that can similarly infect class II-expressing cells (macrophages, dendritic cells, B cells, and endothelial cells) will also express inhibitors of the MHC class II presentation pathway.

Inhibition of cell surface MHC class II

EBV produces a trimeric glycoprotein, consisting of gH, gL, and gp42, that binds to cell surface MHC class II during virus entry into B cells, and anti-gp42 antibodies inhibit infection (Li et al., 1997). A soluble form of gp42 bound to the β chain of HLA-DR, although there was not diminished surface MHC class II, and inhibition of MHC class II-induced proliferation of T cells was observed (Spriggs et al., 1996).

OBSTRUCTION OF CELL KILLING AND APOPTOSIS

T lymphocytes and NK cells restrict virus infections in large part by killing virus-infected cells. However, this process is often an indirect one, where contact with a target cells triggers programmed cell death (apoptosis) through cell surface receptors. Direct cell-to-cell contact between cytotoxic lymphocytes and virus-infected cells causes the release of pore-forming perforins and granzymes, delivery of

Fas ligand (FasL), or release of cytotoxic cytokines such as TNFs. These extracellular or cell surface events lead to signaling cascades involving cellular caspases and induction of programs that ultimately lead to cell death. The number and variety of viral inhibitors that target cell surface death receptors and the signal-transducing molecules in the cytoplasm are enormous. This relates to the fact that many intracellular events during the life cycle of viruses, such as replication of the viral genome, transcription, synthesis of viral proteins, and assembly, all induce or activate cellular apoptotic pathways. Thus, viruses have evolved extensive hardware to deal with the premature death of host cells, whether induced by virus replication, cytokines, or CTL. Since the list of inhibitors is extensive, we will concentrate on only a few examples and refer the reader to other, more comprehensive reviews (Barry and McFadden, 1998b; Wold et al., 1999; Tortorella et al., 2000).

TNF and FasL Receptors

As described in "Other Anticytokine Strategies" (above), poxviruses including rabbit MYX, VV, and CPV encode TNF receptor homologs that block TNF-mediated cell death (Barry and McFadden, 1998a). These receptor homologs are expressed both as secreted and as membrane-bound forms. Moreover, HCMV encodes a TNF receptor homolog that is retained intracellularly (Benedict et al., 1999).

Ad encode a panel of proteins, many in the E3 region, that inhibit TNF- and Fas-mediated apoptosis (Wold et al., 1999). The 10.4- and 14.5-kDa proteins induce endocytosis and lysosomal degradation of Fas, TNF, and nerve growth factor receptors. CTL that lack perforin are less able to lyse targets expressing the 10.4- and 14.5-kDa proteins. A third Ad E3 protein, the 6.7-kDa protein, participates in downregulation of death receptors (Benedict et al., in press). The 10.4- and 14.5-kDa proteins, along with the E3 14.7-kDa protein, can also prevent mobilization of phospholipase A_2, reducing the secretion of proinflammatory prostaglandins (Wold et al., 1999). Oligomerization of TNF or Fas receptors and activation of "death domains" transduce signals to caspases, triggering apoptosis. Herpesviruses such as HHV-8, HVS, and bovine herpesvirus 4, and a poxvirus, MCV, all prevent this signaling by inhibiting interactions between cytoplasmic domains of TNF or Fas receptors and downstream caspases (Tschopp et al., 1998).

Caspase Inhibitors

Caspases are members of a family of aspartate-specific cysteine proteases that act in a proteolytic cascade, a central component of the apoptotic signaling from TNF or Fas receptors (Deveraux et al., 1999). Caspase-3, caspase-6, and caspase-7, downstream components of this pathway, and caspase-8 and caspase-10, which interact with cell surface receptors, are all inhibited directly or indirectly by a variety of viral polypeptides (Earnshaw et al., 1999). The poxviruses VV, CPV, and MYX express CrmA proteins that block caspase-1 (ICE) and caspase-8, effectively blocking apoptosis, initiated by several different stimuli, including TNF, FasL, and granzyme B (Deveraux et al., 1999). Two insect viruses, baculovirus and *Autographica californica* nuclear polyhedrosis virus, also express caspase inhibitors (Miller, 1997). The Ad E3-encoded 14.7-kDa protein inhibits caspase-8, apparently through interactions with a number of cellular proteins including a small GTPase and dynein (Lukashok et al., 2000).

Regulation of Bcl-2

The Bcl-2 family members play critical roles in regulating downstream signaling from cell surface apoptosis receptors and programmed cell death. Bcl-2 inhibits the release of cytochrome *c* from the mitochondria, which causes activation of caspases. A number of viruses, including several members of the herpesvirus family, express Bcl-2 homologs which share heterodimerization and membrane pore-forming domains with Bcl-2 (Barry and McFadden, 1998a; Griffin and Hardwick, 1999; Wensing and Farrell, 2000). It is likely that these viral proteins can function, at least in part, at the mitochondrial membrane, as does cellular Bcl-2, and may also dimerize with cellular Bcl-2. EBV LMP-1 can upregulate the transcription of Bcl-2, along with other survival proteins. Thus, LMP-1 acts at several levels in apoptosis, also inhibiting signaling at the plasma membrane (Wensing and Farrell, 2000). Ad E1A-19K binds Bax, a protein that promotes apoptosis, and transcriptionally upregulates Bcl-2-related proteins (Kasof et al., 1999).

Inhibition of Cytotoxic Lymphocyte Killing

There are numerous mechanisms by which viruses inhibit apoptosis besides those described above. However, in most instances, it is not clear whether this inhibition provides resistance to the cytotoxic effects of lymphocytes or provides protection from apoptosis triggered intracellularly by virus replication. There are limited examples where inhibition of lymphocyte killing has been demonstrated and fewer still where a responsible viral protein has been identified. There is evidence that HSV can inhibit apoptosis in HL-60 cells and fibroblasts (Jerome et al., 1998). HSV US3 and US5 gene products confer resistance to Fas-mediated apoptosis, so that caspase-3 and caspase-8 are not activated by granzyme B (K. A. Jerome, Z. Cheng, M. R. Torres, S. Smith, J. R. Hofmeister, R. Fox, and L. Grey, *Proc. Abstr. Int. Herpesvirus Workshop*, abstr. 507, 2000). These results suggest that US3 and US5 may cause cells to resist CTL, but this is not well established to date. HSV can inactivate the cytolytic properties of IL-2-activated killer cells or NK cells as well as T lymphocytes (Johnson and Hill, 1998). Inactivation occurs only after direct contact between HSV-infected fibroblasts and the lymphocytes, not when the lymphocytes are incubated with high concentrations of cell-free virus. Analysis of a panel of virus mutants demonstrated that HSV spreads directly from an infected cell into the NK cells. It appears that either a cell surface receptor is occupied during direct contact with virus-infected cells or an HSV IE or early gene product is introduced into the lymphocytes, causing inhibition of function or apoptosis (Johnson and Hill, 1998; Raftery et al., 1999).

CONCLUDING REMARKS

Animal viruses have, in many cases, hijacked cellular proteins in order to defend themselves from the host immune responses. Proteins with some sequence similarity to cellular proteins of known function are quickly recognized in the genomes of viruses. However, there is also a substantial class of viral proteins that have clearly evolved from viral or cellular proteins and that function in quite different ways during the long coevolution with the host. For example, the HSV IgG receptor appears to have coevolved along with other viral glycoproteins, e.g., gD, that function as receptor binding proteins. Moreover, large DNA viruses such as HCMV and MCMV express 60 or more glycoproteins, few of which bear any homology to cellular proteins. It appears likely that many of these glycoproteins are involved in immune evasion or similar functions. In the future, there is much to learn from studies of viruses and their extensive collections of immune evasion proteins. As these studies continue, we expect that there will be examples where mechanisms of viral immune subterfuge cast light on poorly understood parameters of the immune response and new cellular pathways.

REFERENCES

Albini, A., R. Benelli, D. Giunciuglio, T. Cai, G. Mariani, S. Ferrini, and D. M. Noonan. 1998a. Identification of a novel domain of HIV tat involved in monocyte chemotaxis. *J. Biol. Chem.* 273:15895–15900.

Albini, A., S. Ferrini, R. Benelli, S. Sforzini, D. Giunciuglio, M. G. Aluigi, A. E. Proudfoot, S. Alouani, T. N. Wells, G. Mariani., et al. 1998b. HIV-1 Tat protein mimicry of chemokines. *Proc. Natl. Acad. Sci. USA* 95:13153–13158.

Alcami, A., and U. H. Koszinowski. 2000. Viral mechanisms of immune evasion. *Trends Microbiol.* 8:410–418.

Ambagala, A. P., S. Hinkley, and S. Srikumaran. 2000. An early pseudorabies viral protein downregulates MHC class I expression by inhibition of the transporter associated with antigen presentation (TAP). *J. Immunol.* 164:93–99.

Arvanitakis, L., E. Geras-Raaka, A. Varma, M. C. Gershengorn, and E. Cesarman. 1997. Human herpesvirus KSHV encodes a constitutively active G-protein-coupled receptor linked to cell proliferation. *Nature* 385:347–349.

Baggiolini, M., and P. Loetscher. 2000. Chemokines in inflammation and immunity. *Immunol. Today* 21:418–420.

Bakker, A. B., J. Wu, J. H. Phillips, and L. L. Lanier. 2000. NK cell activation: distinct stimulatory pathways counterbalancing inhibitory signals. *Hum. Immunol.* 61:18–27.

Barry, M., and G. McFadden. 1997. Virokines and viroceptors, p. 251–261. *In* D. G. Remick and J. S. Friedland (ed.), *Cytokines in Health and Disease.* Marcel Dekker, Inc., New York, N.Y.

Barry, M., and G. McFadden. 1998a. Apoptosis regulators from DNA viruses. *Curr. Opin. Immunol.* 10:422–430.

Barry, M., and G. McFadden. 1998b. Virus encoded cytokines and cytokine receptors. *Parasitology* 115:S89–S100.

Bauer, S., V. Groh, J. Wu, A. Steinle, J. H. Phillips, L. L. Lanier, and T. Spies. 1999. Activation of NK cells and T cells by NKG2D, a receptor for stress-inducible MICA. *Science* 285: 727–729.

Benedict, C. A., K. D. Butrovich, N. S. Lurain, J. Corbeil, I. Rooney, P. Schneider, J. Tschopp, and C. F. Ware. 1999. Cutting edge: a novel viral TNF receptor superfamily member in virulent strains of human cytomegalovirus, *J. Immunol.* 162: 6967–6970.

Benedict, C. A., P. S. Norris, T. I. Prigozy, J. L. Bodmer, J. A. Mahr, C. T. Garnett, F. Martinon, J. Tschopp, L. R. Gooding, and C. F. Ware. Three adenovirus E3 proteins cooperate to evade apoptosis by TRAIL receptor-1 and 2. *J. Biol. Chem.*, in press.

Bennett, E. M., J. R. Bennink, J. W. Yewdell, and F. M. Brodsky. 1999. Cutting edge: adenovirus E19 has two mechanisms for affecting class I MHC expression, *J. Immunol.* 162:5049–5052.

Bertoletti, A., A. Sette, F. V. Chisari, A. Penna, M. Levrero, M. De Carli, F. Fiaccadori, and C. Ferrari. 1994. Natural variants of cytotoxic epitopes are T-cell receptor antagonists for antiviral cytotoxic T cells. *Nature* 369:407–410.

Biron, C. 1998. Role of early cytokines, including alpha and beta interferons, in innate and adaptive immune responses to viral infection. *Semin. Immunol.* 10:383–390.

Biron, C. A. 1999. Initial and innate responses to viral infections—pattern setting in immunity or disease. *Curr. Opin. Microbiol.* 2:374–381.

Biron, C. A., K. B. Nguyen, G. C. Pien, L. P. Gousens, and T. P. Salazar-Mather. 1999. Natural killer cells in antiviral defense: function and regulation by innate cytokines. *Annu. Rev. Immunol.* 17:189–220.

Bodaghi, B., T. R. Jones, D. Zipeto, C. Vita, L. Sun, L. Laurent, F. Arenzana-Seisedos, J. L. Virelizier, and S. Michelson. 1998. Chemokine sequestration by viral chemoreceptors as a novel viral strategy: withdrawal of chemokines from the environment of cytomegalovirus-infected cells. *J. Exp. Med.* 188:855–866.

Born, T., L. A. Morrison, D. J. Esteban, T. VandenBos, L. G. Thebeau, N. Chen, M. K. Spriggs, J. E. Sims, and R. M. L.

Buller. 2000. A poxvirus protein that binds to and inactivates IL-18, and inhibits NK cell response. *J. Immunol.* **164:**3246–3254.

Boshoff, C., Y. Endo, P. D. Collins, Y. Takeuchi, J. D. Reeves, V. L. Schweickart, M. A. Siani, T. Sasaki, T. J. Williams, P. W. Gray, et al. 1997. Angiogenic and HIV-inhibitory functions of KSHV-encoded chemokines. *Science* **278:**290–294.

Bowie, A., E. Kiss-Toth, J. A. Symons, G. L. Smith, S. K. Dower, and L. A. J. O'Neill. 2000. A46R and A52R from vaccinia virus are antagonists of host IL-1 and toll-like receptor signaling. *Proc. Natl. Acad. Sci. USA* **97:**10162–10167.

Bukowski, J. F., J. F. Warner, G. Dennert, and R. M. Welsh. 1985. Adoptive transfer studies demonstrating the antiviral effect of natural killer cells in vivo. *J. Exp. Med.* **161:**40–52.

Burysek, L., W. S. Yeow, and P. M. Pitha. 1999. Unique properties of a second herpesvirus 8-encoded interferon regulatory factor (vIRF-2). *J. Hum. Virol.* **2:**19–32.

Cebulla, C. M., D. M. Miller, and D. D. Sedmak. 1999. Viral inhibition of interferon signal transduction. *Intervirology* **42:**325–330.

Cesarman, E., E. A. Mesri, and M. C. Gershengorn. 2000. Viral G-protein-coupled receptor and Kaposi's sarcoma: a model of paracrine neoplasia? *J. Exp. Med.* **191:**417–421.

Chapman, T. L., I. You, I. M. Joseph, P. J. Bjorkman, S. L. Morrison, and M. Raghavan. 1999. Characterization of the interaction between the herpes simplex virus I Fc receptor and immunoglobulin G. *J. Biol. Chem.* **274:**6911–6919.

Chirivi, R. G. S., G. Taraboletti, M. R. Bani, L. Barra, G. Piccinini, M. Giacca, F. Bussolino, and R. Giavazzi. 1999. Human immunodeficiency virus-1 (HIV-1)-Tat protein promotes migration of acquired immunodeficiency syndrome-related lymphoma cells and enhances their adhesion to endothelial cells. *Blood* **94:**1747–1754.

Clemens, M. J., and A. Elia. 1997. The double-stranded RNA-dependent protein kinase PKR: structure and function. *J. Interferon Cytokine Res.* **17:**503–524.

Cohen, G. B., R. T. Gandhi, D. M. Davis, O. Mandelboim, B. K. Chen, J. L. Strominger, and D. Baltimore. 1999. The selective downregulation of class I major histocompatibility complex proteins by HIV-1 protects HIV-infected cells from NK cells. *Immunity* **10:**661–671.

Corey, L., and P. G. Spear. 1986. Infections with herpes simplex viruses. *N. Engl. J. Med.* **314:**749–757.

Coscoy, L., and D. Ganem. 2000. Kaposi's sarcoma-associated herpesvirus encodes two proteins that block cell surface display of MHC class I chains by enhancing their endocytosis. *Proc. Natl. Acad. Sci. USA* **97:**8051–8056.

Cosman, D., N. Fanger, and L. Borges. 1999. Human cytomegalovirus MHC class I and inhibitory signalling receptors: more questions than answers. *Immunol. Rev.* **168:**177–185.

Cretney, E., M. A. Degli-Esposti, E. H. Densley, H. E. Farrell, N. J. Davis-Poynter, and M. J. Smyth. 1999. m144, a murine cytomegalovirus (MCMV)-encoded major histocompatibility complex class I homologue, confers tumor resistance to natural killer cell-mediated rejection. *J. Exp. Med.* **190:**435–444.

Cunnion, K. M. 1999. Tumor necrosis factor receptors encoded by poxviruses. *Mol. Genet. Metab.* **67:**278–282.

Dairaghi, D. J., D. R. Greaves, and T. J. Schall. 1998. Abduction of chemokine elements by herpesviruses. *Semin. Virol.* **8:**377–385.

Denzin, L. K., C. Hammond, and C. Cresswell. 1996. HLA-DM interacts with intermediates in HLA-DR maturation and a role for HLA-DM in stabilizing empty HLA-DR molecules. *J. Exp. Med.* **184:**2153–2165.

Deveraux, Q. L., H. R. Stennicke, G. S. Salvesen, and J. C. Reed. 1999. Endogenous inhibitors of caspases. *J. Clin. Immunol.* **19:**388–398.

DiMaio, D., C.-C. Lai, and O. Klein. 1998. Virocrine transformation: the intersection between viral transforming proteins and cellular signal transduction pathways. *Annu. Rev. Microbiol.* **52:**397–421.

Dingwell, K. S., C. R. Brunetti, R. L. Hendricks, Q. Tang, M. Tang, A. J. Rainbow, and D. C. Johnson. 1994. Herpes simplex virus glycoproteins E and I facilitate cell-to-cell spread in vivo and across junctions of cultured cells. *J. Virol.* **68:**834–845.

Dubin, G., I. Frank, and H. M. Friedman. 1990. Herpes simplex virus type 1 encodes two Fc receptors which have different binding characteristics for monomeric immunoglobulin G (IgG) and IgG complexes. *J. Virol.* **64:**2725–2731.

Earnshaw, W. C., L. M. Martins, and S. H. Kaufmann. 1999. Mammalian caspases: structure, activation, substrates, and functions during apoptosis. *Annu. Rev. Biochem.* **68:**383–424.

Fantuzzi, G., and C. A. Dinarello. 1999. Interleukin-18 and interleukin-1β: two cytokine substrates for ICE (caspase-1). *J. Clin. Immun.* **19:**1–11.

Farrell, H., M. Degli-Esposti, E. Densley, E. Cretney, M. Smyth, and N. Davis-Poynter. 2000. Cytomegalovirus MHC class I homologues and natural killer cells: an overview. *Microbes Infect.* **2:**521–532.

Favoreel, H. W., H. J. Nauwynck, P. Van Oostveldt, T. C. Mettenleiter, and M. B. Pensaert. 1997. Antibody-induced and cytoskeleton-mediated redistribution and shedding of viral glycoproteins, expressed on pseudorabies virus-infected cells. *J. Virol.* **71:**8254–8261.

Fish, K. N., C. Soderberg-Naucler, and J. A. Nelson. 1998. Steady-state plasma membrane expression of human cytomegalovirus gB is determined by the phosphorylation of state of ser$_{900}$. *J. Virol.* **72:**6657–6664.

Fleming, P., N. Davis-Poynter, M. Degli-Esposti, E. Densley, J. Papadimitriou, G. Shellam, and H. Farrell. 1999. The murine cytomegalovirus chemokine homolog, m131/129, is a determinant of viral pathogenicity. *J. Virol.* **73:**6800–6809.

Fodor, W. L., S. A. Rollins, S. Bianco-Caron, R. P. Rother, E. R. Guilmette, W. V. Burton, J. C. Albrecht, B. Fleckenstein, and S. P. Squinto. 1995. The complement control protein homolog of herpesvirus saimiri regulates serum complement by inhibiting C3 convertase activity. *J. Virol.* **69:**3889–3892.

Frank, I., and H. M. Friedman. 1989. A novel function of the herpes simplex virus type 1 Fc receptor: participation in bipolar bridging of antiviral immunoglobulin G. *J. Virol.* **63:**4479–4488.

Fruh, K., A. Gruhler, R. M. Krishna, and G. J. Schoenhals. 1999. A comparison of viral immune escape strategies targeting the MHC class I assembly pathway. *Immunol. Rev.* **168:**157–166.

Gale, M., and M. G. Katze. 1998. Molecular mechanisms of interferon resistance mediated by viral-directed inhibition of PKR, the interferon-induced protein kinase. *Phamacol. Ther.* **78:**29–46.

Gilbert, M. J., S. R. Riddell, B. Plachter, and P. D. Greenberg. 1996. Cytomegalovirus selectively blocks antigen processing and presentation of its immediate-early gene product. *Nature* **383:**720–722.

Goldsmith, K., W. Chen, D. C. Johnson, and R. L. Hendricks. 1998. ICP47 enhances herpes simplex virus neurovirulence by blocking the CD8[+] T cell response. *J. Exp. Med.* **187:**341–348.

Goodbourn, S., L. Didcock, and R. E. Randall. 2000. Interferons: cell signaling, immune modulation, antiviral response and virus countermeasures. *J. Gen. Virol.* **81:**2341–2364.

Graham, K. A., A. S. Lalani, J. L. Macen, T. L. Ness, M. Barry, L.-Y. Liu, A. Lucas, I. Clark-Lewis, R. W. Moyer, and G. McFadden. 1997. The T1/35kDa family of poxvirus secreted proteins bind chemokines and modulate leukocyte influx into virus infected tissues. *Virology* **229:**12–24.

Griffin, D. E., and J. M. Hardwick. 1999. Perspective: virus infections and the death of neurons. *Trends Microbiol.* 7:155–160.

Groh, V., R. Rhinehart, J. Randolph-Habecker, M. S. Topp, S. R. Riddell, and T. Spies. 2000. Costimulation of CD8$\alpha\beta$ T cells by NKG2D via engagement by MIC induced on virus-infected cells. *Nat. Immunol.* 2:255–260.

Guidotti, L. G., and F. V. Chisari. 2000. Cytokine-mediated control of viral infections. *Virology* 273:221–227.

Harton, J. A., and J. P. Ting. 2000. Class II transactivator: mastering the art of major histocompatibility complex expression. *Mol. Cell. Biol.* 20:6185–6194.

Heise, M. T., M. Connick, and H. W. Virgin III. 1998. Murine cytomegalovirus inhibits interferon gamma-induced antigen presentation to CD4 T cells by macrophages via regulation of expression of major histocompatibility complex class II-associated genes. *J. Exp. Med.* 187:1037–1046.

Hengel, H., U. Reusch, G. Geginat, R. Holtappels, T. Ruppert, E. Hellebrand, and U. H. Koszinowski. 2000. Macrophages escape inhibition of major histocompatibility complex class I-dependent antigen presentation by cytomegalovirus. *J. Virol.* 74:7861–7868.

Hengel, H., U. Reusch, A. Gutermann, H. Ziegler, S. Jonjic, P. Lucin, and U. H. Koszinowski. 1999. Cytomegaloviral control of MHC class I function in the mouse. *Immunol. Rev.* 168:167–176.

Huard, B., and K. Fruh. 2000. A role for MHC class I downregulation in NK cell lysis of herpes virus-infected cells. *Eur. J. Immunol.* 30:509–515.

Isaacs, S. N., G. J. Kotwal, R. McKenzie, M. M. Frank, and B. Moss. 1992. Vaccinia virus complement-control protein prevents antibody-dependent complement-enhanced neutralization of infectivity and contributes to virulence. *Proc. Natl. Acad. Sci. USA* 89:628–632.

Ishido, S., J. K. Choi, B. S. Lee, C. Wang, M. DeMaria, R. Johnson, G. B. Cohen, and J. U. Jung. 2000a. Inhibition of natural killer cell-mediated cytotoxicity by Kaposi's sarcoma-associated herpesvirus K5 protein. *Immunity* 13:365–374.

Ishido, S., C. Wang, B. S. Lee, G. B. Cohen, and J. U. Jung. 2000b. Downregulation of major histocompatibility complex class I molecules by Kaposi's sarcoma-associated herpesvirus K3 and K5 proteins. *J. Virol.* 74:5300–5309.

Janeway, C., and R. Medzhitov. 2000. Viral interference with IL-1 and Toll signaling. *Proc. Natl. Acad. Sci. USA* 97:10682–10683.

Jerome, K. R., J. F. Tait, D. M. Koelle, and L. Corey. 1998. Herpes simplex virus type 1 renders infected cells resistant to cytotoxic T-lymphocyte-induced apoptosis. *J. Virol.* 72:436–441.

Johnson, A. E., and N. G. Haigh. 2000. The ER translocon and retrotranslocation: is the shift into reverse manual or automatic? *Cell* 102:709–712.

Johnson, D. C., M. C. Frame, M. W. Ligas, A. M. Cross, and N. D. Stow. 1988. Herpes simplex virus immunoglobulin G Fc receptor activity depends on a complex of two viral glycoproteins, gE and gI. *J. Virol.* 62:1347–1354.

Johnson, D. C., and A. B. Hill. 1998. Herpesvirus evasion of the immune system. *Curr. Top. Microbiol. Immunol.* 232:149–177.

Jones, K. D., Y. Aoki, Y. Chang, P. S. Moore, R. Yarchoan, and G. Tosato. 1999. Involvement of interleukin-10 (IL-10) and viral IL-6 in the spontaneous growth of Kaposi's sarcoma herpesvirus-associated infected primary effusion lymphoma cells. *Blood* 94:2871–2879.

Kalvakolanu, D. V. 1999. Virus interception of cytokine-regulated pathways. *Trends Microbiol.* 7:166–171.

Kasof, G. M., L. Goyal, and E. White. 1999. Btf, a novel death-promoting transcriptional repressor that interacts with Bcl-2 related proteins. *Mol. Cell. Biol.* 19:4390–4404.

Kerkau, T., I. Bacik, J. R. Bennink, J. W. Yewdell, T. Hunig, A. Schimpl, and U. Schubert. 1997. The human immunodeficiency virus type 1 (HIV-1) Vpu protein interferes with an early step in the biosynthesis of major histocompatibility complex (MHC) class I molecules. *J. Exp. Med.* 185:1295–1305.

Kim, S.-H., M. Eisenstein, L. Reznikov, G. Fantuzzi, D. Novick, M. Rubinstein, and C. A. Dinarello. 2000. Structural requirements of six naturally occurring isoforms of the IL-18 binding protein to inhibit IL-18. *Proc. Natl. Acad. Sci. USA* 97:1190–1195.

Klenerman, P., S. Rowland-Jones, S. McAdam, J. Edwards, S. Daenke, D. Lalloo, B. Koppe, W. Rosenberg, D. Boyd, A. Edwards, et al. 1994. Cytotoxic T-cell activity antagonized by naturally occurring HIV-1 Gag variants. *Nature* 369:403–407.

Kotwal, G. J. 2000. Poxviral mimicry of complement and chemokine system components: what's the end game? *Immunol. Today* 21:242–248.

Kotwal, G. J., C. G. Miller, and D. E. Justus. 1998. The inflammation modulatory protein (IMP) of cowpox virus drastically diminishes the tissue damage by down-regulating cellular infiltration resulting from complement activation. *Mol. Cell. Biochem.* 185:39–46.

Krajcsi, P., and W. S. M. Wold. 1998. Viral proteins that regulate cellular signalling. *J. Gen. Virol.* 79:1323–1335.

Lacaille, V. G., and M. J. Androlewicz. 1998. Herpes simplex virus inhibitor ICP47 destabilizes the transporter associated with antigen processing (TAP) heterodimer. *J. Biol. Chem.* 273:17386–17390.

Lalani, A. S., J. Barrett, and G. McFadden. 2000. Modulating chemokines: More lessons from viruses. *Immunol. Today* 21:100–106.

Lalani, A. S., J. Masters, K. Graham, L. Liu, A. Lucas, and G. McFadden. 1999. The role of the myxoma virus soluble CC-chemokine inhibitor glycoprotein, M-T1, during myxoma virus pathogenesis. *Virology* 256:233–245.

Lalani, A. S., and G. McFadden. 1999. Evasion and exploitation of chemokines by viruses. *Cytokine Growth Factor Rev.* 10:219–233.

Lanier, L. L. 1998. NK cell receptors. *Annu. Rev. Immunol.* 16:359–393.

Lehner, T., J. M. Wilton, and E. J. Shillitoe. 1975. Immunological basis for latency, recurrences and putative oncogenicity of herpes simplex virus. *Lancet* ii:60–62.

Leib, D. A., M. A. Machalek, B. R. G. Williams, R. H. Silverman, and H. W. Virgin. 2000. Specific phenotypic restoration of an attenuated virus by knockout of a host resistance gene. *Proc. Natl. Acad. Sci. USA* 97:6097–6101.

Leonard, G. T., and G. C. Sen. 1997. Restoration of interferon responses of adenovirus E1A-expressing HT1080 cell lines by overexpression of p48 protein. *J. Virol.* 71:5095–5101.

Leong, C. C., T. L. Chapman, P. J. Bjorkman, D. Formankova, E. S. Mocarski, J. H. Phillips, and L. L. Lanier. 1998. Modulation of natural killer cell cytotoxicity in human cytomegalovirus infection: the role of endogenous class I major histocompatibility complex and a viral class I homolog. *J. Exp. Med.* 187:1681–1687.

Levitskaya, J., A. Sharipo, A. Leonchiks, A. Ciechanover, and M. G. Masucci. 1997. Inhibition of ubiquitin/proteasome-dependent protein degradation by the Gly-Ala repeat domain of the Epstein–Barr virus nuclear antigen 1. *Proc. Natl. Acad. Sci. USA* 94:12616–12621.

Li, M. T., H. Lee, J. Guo, F. Neipel, B. Fleckenstein, K. Ozato, and J. U. Jung. 1998. Kaposi's sarcoma-associated herpesvirus viral interferon regulatory factor. *J. Virol.* 72:5433–5440.

Li, Q., M. K. Spriggs, S. Kovats, S. M. Turk, M. R. Comeau, B. Nepom, and L. M. Hutt-Fletcher. 1997. Epstein-Barr virus uses

HLA class II as a cofactor for infection of B lymphocytes. *J. Virol.* 71:4657–4662.

Liu, L. Y., A. Lalani, E. Dai, B. Seet, C. Macauley, R. Singh, L. Fan, G. McFadden, and A. Lucas. 2000. The viral anti-inflammatory chemokine-binding protein M-T7 reduces intimal hyperplasia after vascular injury. *J. Clin. Investig.* 105:1613–1621.

Lubinski, J., L. Wang, D. Mastellos, A. Sahu, J. D. Lambris, and H. M. Friedman. 1999. In vivo role of complement-interacting domains of herpes simplex virus type 1 glycoprotein gC. *J. Exp. Med.* 190:1637–1646.

Lubyova, B., and P. M. Pitha. 2000. Characterization of a novel human herpesvirus 8-encoded protein, vIRF-3, that shows homology to viral and cellular interferon regulatory factors. *J. Virol.* 74:8194–8201.

Lukashok, S. A., L. Tarassishin, Y. Li, and M. S. Horwitz. 2000. An adenovirus inhibitor of tumor necrosis factor alpha-induced apoptosis complexes with dynein and a small GTPase. *J. Virol.* 74:4705–4709.

Lusso, P. 2000. Chemokines and viruses: the dearest enemies. *Virology* 273:228–240.

Macen, J. L., R. S. Garner, P. Y. Musy, M. A. Brooks, P. C. Turner, R. W. Moyer, G. McFadden, and R. C. Bleackley. 1996. Differential inhibition of the Fas- and granule-mediated cytolysis pathways by the orthopoxvirus cytokine response modifier A/SPI-2 and SPI-1 protein. *Proc. Natl. Acad. Sci. USA* 93:9108–9113.

Mahalingam, S., and G. Karupiah. 2000. Modulation of chemokines by poxvirus infections. *Curr. Opin. Immunol.* 12:409–412.

McFadden, G., A. Lalani, H. Everett, P. Nash, and X. Xu. 1998. Virus encoded-receptors for cytokines and chemokines. *Semin. Cell Dev. Biol.* 9:359–368.

McFadden, G., and P. M. Murphy. 2000. Host-related immunomodulators encoded by poxviruses and herpesviruses. *Curr. Opin. Microbiol.* 3:371–378.

McMillan, T. N., and D. C. Johnson. 2001. Cytoplasmic domain of herpes simplex virus gE causes accumulation in the *trans*-Golgi network, a site of virus envelopment and sorting of virions to cell junctions. *J. Virol.* 75:1928–1940.

Meinl, E., H. Fickenscher, M. Thome, J. Tschopp, and B. Fleckenstein. 1998. Anti-apoptotic strategies of lymphotropic viruses. *Immunol. Today* 19:474–479.

Miller, D. M., Y. Zhang, B. M. Rahill, W. J. Waldman, and D. D. Sedmak. 1999. Human cytomegalovirus inhibits IFN-alpha-stimulated antiviral and immunoregulatory responses by blocking multiple levels of IFN-alpha signal transduction. *J. Immunol.* 162:6107–6113.

Miller, L. K. 1997. Baculovirus interaction with host apoptotic pathways. *J. Cell. Physiol.* 173:178–182.

Miskin, J. E., C. C. Abrams, and L. K. Dixon. 2000. African swine fever virus protein A238L interacts with the cellular phosphatase calcineurin via a binding domain similar to that of NFAT. *J. Virol.* 74:9412–9420.

Miskin, J. E., C. C. Abrams, L. C. Goatley, and L. K. Dixon. 1998. A viral mechanism for inhibition of the cellular phosphatase calcineurin. *Science* 281:562–565.

Moretta, A., R. Biassoni, C. Bottino, M. C. Mingari, and L. Moretta. 2000. Natural cytotoxicity receptors that trigger human NK-cell-mediated cytolysis. *Immunol. Today* 21:228–234.

Mossman, K., P. Nation, J. Macen, M. Garbutt, A. Lucas, and G. McFadden. 1996. Myxoma virus M-T7, a secreted homolog of the interferon-γ receptor, is a critical virulence factor for the development of myxomatosis in European rabbits. *Virology* 215:17–30.

Murdoch, C., and A. Finn. 2000. Chemokine receptors and their role in inflammation and infectious disease. *Blood* 95:3032–3043.

Nash, P., J. Barrett, J.-X. Cao, S. Hota-Mitchell, A. S. Lalani, H. Everett, X.-M. Xu, J. Robichaud, S. Hnatiuk, C. Ainslie. et al. 1999. Immunomodulation by viruses: the myxoma virus story. *Immunol. Rev.* 168:103–120.

Neilan, J. G., Z. Lu, G. F. Kutish, L. Zsak, T. L. Lewis, and D. L. Rock. 1997. A conserved African swine fever virus IκB homolog, 5EL, is nonessential for growth *in vitro* and virulence in domestic swine. *Virology* 235:377–385.

Novick, D., S.-H. Kim, G. Fantuzzi, L. L. Reznikov, C. A. Dinarello, and M. Rubinstein. 1999. Interleukin-18 binding proteins: a novel modulator of the Th1 cytokine response. *Immunity* 10:127–136.

O'Brien, V. 1998. Viruses and apoptosis. *J. Gen. Virol.* 79:1833–1845.

Osborne, J., P. S. Moore, and Y. Chang. 1999. KSHV-encoded viral IL-6 activates multiple human IL-6 signaling pathways. *Hum. Immunol.* 60:921–927.

Parry, B. C., J. P. Simas, V. P. Smith, C. A. Stewart, A. C. Minson, S. Efstathiou, and A. Alcamí. 2000. A broad spectrum secreted chemokine binding protein encoded by a herpesvirus. *J. Exp. Med.* 191:573–578.

Pease, J. E., and P. M. Murphy. 1998. Microbial corruption of the chemokine system: An expanding paradigm. *Semin. Immunol.* 10:169–178.

Penfold, M. E., D. J. Dairaghi, G. M. Duke, N. Saederup, E. S. Mocarski, G. W. Kemble, and T. J. Schall. 1999. Cytomegalovirus encodes a potent alpha chemokine. *Proc. Natl. Acad. Sci. USA* 96:9839–9844.

Pickup, D. J. 1994. Poxviral modifiers of cytokine responses to infection. *Infect. Agents Dis.* 3:116–127.

Pieters, J. 2000. MHC class II-restricted antigen processing and presentation. *Adv. Immunol.* 75:159–208.

Piguet, V., O. Schwartz, S. Le Gall, and D. Trono. 1999. The downregulation of CD4 and MHC-I by primate lentiviruses: a paradigm for the modulation of cell surface receptors. *Immunol. Rev.* 168:51–63.

Piguet, V., L. Wan, C. Borel, A. Mangasarian, N. Demaurex, G. Thomas, and D. Trono. 2000. HIV-1 Nef protein binds to the cellular protein PACS-1 to downregulate class I major histocompatibility complexes. *Nat. Cell Biol.* 2:163–167.

Pitha, P. M., W. C. Au, W. Lowther, Y. T. Juang, S. L. Schafer, L. Burysek, J. Hiscott, and P. A. Moore. 1998. Role of the interferon regulatory factors (IRFs) in virus-mediated signaling and regulation of cell growth. *Biochimie* 80:651–658.

Raftery, M. J., C. K. Behrens, A. Muller, P. H. Krammer, H. Walczak, and G. Schonrich. 1999. Herpes simplex virus type 1 infection of activated cytotoxic T cells: induction of fratricide as a mechanism of viral immune evasion. *J. Exp. Med.* 190:1103–1114.

Reyburn, H. T., O. Mandelboim, M. Vales-Gomez, D. M. Davis, L. Pazmany, and J. L. Strominger. 1997. The class I MHC homologue of human cytomegalovirus inhibits attack by natural killer cells. *Nature* 386:514–517.

Roulston, A., R. C. Marcellus, and P. E. Branton. 1999. Viruses and apoptosis. *Annu. Rev. Microbiol.* 53:577–628.

Saederup, N., Y. C. Lin, D. J. Dairaghi, T. J. Schall, and E. S. Mocarski. 1999. Cytomegalovirus-encoded beta chemokine promotes monocyte-associated viremia in the host. *Proc. Natl. Acad. Sci. USA* 96:10881–10886.

Salazar-Mather, T., T. Hamilton, and C. Biron. 2000. A chemokine-to-cytokine cascade critical in antiviral defense. *J. Clin. Investig.* 105:985–993.

Saldanha, C. E., J. Lubinski, C. Martin, T. Nagashunmugam, L. Wang, H. van der Keyl, R. Tal-Singer, and H. M. Friedman. 2000. Herpes simplex virus type 1 glycoprotein E domains involved in virus spread and disease. *J. Virol.* **74**:6712–6719.

Schreiber, M., L. Sedger, and G. McFadden. 1997. Distinct domains of M-T2, the myxoma virus TNF receptor homolog, mediate extracellular TNF binding and intracellular apoptosis inhibition. *J. Virol.* **71**:2171–2181.

Schubert, U., L. C. Anton, I. Bacik, J. H. Cox, S. Bour, J. R. Bennink, M. Orlowski, K. Strebel, and J. W. Yewdell. 1998. CD4 glycoprotein degradation induced by human immunodeficiency virus type 1 Vpu protein requires the function of proteasomes and the ubiquitin-conjugating pathway. *J. Virol.* **72**:2280–2288.

Sears, A. E., B. S. McGwire, and B. Roizman. 1991. Infection of polarized MDCK cells with herpes simplex virus 1: two asymmetrically distributed cell receptors interact with different viral proteins. *Proc. Natl. Acad. Sci. USA* **88**:5087–5091.

Senkevich, T. G., and B. Moss. 1998. Domain structure, intracellular trafficking, and beta2-microglobulin binding of a major histocompatibility complex class I homolog encoded by molluscum contagiosum virus. *Virology* **250**:397–407.

Smith, G. L. 1999. Vaccinia virus immune evasion. *Immunol. Lett.* **65**:55–62.

Smith, G. L. 2000. Secreted poxvirus proteins that interact with the immune system, p. 491–507. *In* M. W. Cunningham and R. S. Fujinami (ed.), *Effects of Microbes on the Immune System.* Lippincott Williams & Wilkins, Phildelphia, Pa.

Smith, G. L., J. A. Symons, and A. Alcamí. 1998. Poxviruses: interfering with interferon. *Semin. Virol.* **8**:409–416.

Smith, K. J., J. Yeager, and H. Skelton. 1999. Molluscum contagiosum: its clinical histopathologic and immunohistochemical spectrum. *Int. J. Dermatol.* **38**:664–672.

Smith, V. P., N. A. Bryant, and A. Alcamí. 2000. Ectromelia, vaccinia and cowpox viruses encode secreted interleukin-18-binding proteins. *J. Gen. Virol.* **81**:1223–1230.

Soderberg-Naucler, C., K. N. Fish, and J. A. Nelson. 1997. Reactivation of latent human cytomegalovirus by allogeneic stimulation of blood cells from healthy donors. *Cell* **91**:119–126.

Spear, G. T., N. S. Lurain, C. J. Parker, M. Ghassemi, G. H. Payne, and M. Saifuddin. 1995. Host cell-derived complement control proteins CD55 and CD59 are incorporated into the virions of two unrelated enveloped viruses. Human T cell leukemia/lymphoma virus type I (HTLV-I) and human cytomegalovirus (HCMV). *J. Immunol.* **155**:4376–4381.

Spiller, O. B., B. P. Morgan, F. Tufaro, and D. V. Devine. 1996. Altered expression of host-encoded complement regulators on human cytomegalovirus-infected cells. *Eur. J. Immunol.* **26**:1532–1538.

Spriggs, M. K. 1996. One step ahead of the game: Viral immunomodulatory molecules. *Annu. Rev. Immunol.* **14**:101–131.

Spriggs, M. K., R. J. Armitage, M. R. Comeau, L. Strockbine, T. Farrah, B. Macduff, D. Ulrich, M. R. Alderson, J. Mullberg, and J. I. Cohen. 1996. The extracellular domain of the Epstein-Barr virus BZLF2 protein binds the HLA-DR beta chain and inhibits antigen presentation. *J. Virol.* **70**:5557–5563.

Stine, J. T., C. Wood, M. Hill, A. Epp, C. J. Raport, V. L. Schweickart, Y. Endo, T. Sasaki, G. Simmons, C. Boshoff, et al. 2000. KSHV-encoded CC chemokine vMIP-III is a CCR4 agonist, stimulates angiogenesis, and selectively chemoattracts TH2 cells. *Blood* **95**:1151–1157.

Stoiber, H., C. Pinter, A. G. Siccardi, A. Clivio, and M. P. Dierich. 1996. Efficient destruction of human immunodeficiency virus in human serum by inhibiting the protective action of complement factor H and decay accelerating factor (DAF, CD55). *J. Exp. Med.* **183**:307–310.

Stordeur, P., and M. Goldman. 1998. Interleukin-10 as a regulatory cytokine induced by cellular stress: molecular aspects. *Int. Rev. Immunol.* **16**:501–522.

Streblow, D. N., C. Soderberg-Naucler, J. Vieira, P. Smith, E. Wakabayashi, F. Ruchti, K. Mattison, Y. Altschuler, and J. A. Nelson. 1999. The human cytomegalovirus chemokine receptor US28 mediates vascular smooth muscle cell migration. *Cell* **99**:511–520.

Tomazin, R., J. Boname, N. R. Hegde, D. M. Lewinsohn, Y. Altschuler, T. R. Jones, P. Cresswell, J. A. Nelson, S. R. Riddell, and D. C. Johnson. 1999. Cytomegalovirus US2 destroys two components of the MHC class II pathway, preventing recognition by CD4+ T cells. *Nat. Med.* **5**:1039–1043.

Tortorella, D., B. E. Gewurz, M. H. Furman, D. J. Schust, and H. L. Ploegh. 2000. Viral subversion of the immune system. *Annu. Rev. Immunol.* **18**:861–926.

Tschopp, J., M. Irmler, and M. Thome. 1998. Inhibition of fas death signals by FLIPs. *Curr. Opin. Immunol.* **10**:552–558.

Turner, P. C., and R. W. Moyer. 1998. Control of apoptosis by poxviruses. *Semin. Virol.* **8**:453–469.

Tzahar, E., J. D. Moyer, H. Waterman, E. G. Barbacci, G. Levkowitz, M. Shelly, S. Strano, R. Pinkas-Kramarski, J. H. Pierce, G. C. Andrews, and Y. Yarden. 1998. Pathogenic poxviruses reveal viral strategies to exploit the ErbB signaling network. *EMBO J.* **17**:5948–5963.

van Berkel, V., J. Barrett, H. L. Tiffany, D. H. Fremont, P. M. Murphy, G. McFadden, S. H. Speck, and H. W. Virgin. 2000. Identification of a gammaherpesvirus selective chemokine binding protein that inhibits chemokine action. *J. Virol.* **74**:6741–6747.

Vanderplasschen, A., E. Mathew, M. Hollinshead, R. B. Sim, and G. L. Smith. 1998. Extracellular enveloped vaccinia virus is resistant to complement because of incorporation of host complement control proteins into its envelope. *Proc. Natl. Acad. Sci. USA* **95**:7544–7549.

Wan, X. Y., H. L. Wang, and J. Nicholas. 1999. Human herpesvirus 8 interleukin-6 (vIL-6) signals through gp130 but has structural acid receptor-binding properties distinct from those of human IL-6. *J. Virol.* **73**:8268–8278.

Wells, T. N. C., and T. W. Schwartz. 1998. Plagiarism of the host immune system: lessons about chemokine immunology from viruses. *Curr. Opin. Biotechnol.* **8**:741–748.

Wensing, B., and P. J. Farrell. 2000. Regulation of cell growth and death by Epstein-Barr virus. *Microbes Infect.* **2**:77–84.

Wold, W. S., K. Doronin, K. Toth, M. Kuppuswamy, D. L. Lichtenstein, and A. E. Tollefson. 1999. Immune responses to adenoviruses: viral evasion mechanisms and their implications for the clinic. *Curr. Opin. Immunol.* **11**:380–386.

Xiang, Y., and B. Moss. 1999a. Identification of human and mouse homologs of the MC51L-53L-54L family of secreted glycoproteins encoded by the molluscum contagiosum poxvirus. *Virology* **257**:297–302.

Xiang, Y., and B. Moss. 1999b. IL-18 binding and inhibition of interferon γ induction by human poxvirus-encoded proteins. *Proc. Natl. Acad. Sci. USA* **96**:11537–11542.

Xu, X., P. Nash, and G. McFadden. 2000. Myxoma virus expresses a TNF receptor homolog with two distinct functions. *Virus Genes* **21**:97–109.

Zhou, Q., and G. S. Salvesen. 2000. Viral caspase inhibitors CrmA and p35. *Apoptosis* **322**:143–154.

Zimring, J. C., S. Goodbourn, and M. K. Offermann. 1997. Human herpesvirus 8 encodes an interferon regulatory factor (IRF) homolog that represses IRF-1-mediated transcription. *J. Virol.* **72**:701–707.

Immunology of Infectious Diseases
Edited by S. H. E. Kaufmann, A. Sher, and R. Ahmed
© 2002 ASM Press, Washington, D.C.

Chapter 25

Immune Evasion by Parasites

JOHN M. MANSFIELD AND MARTIN OLIVIER

Parasites have evolved a variety of mechanisms to evade host immune recognition and elimination. Such evolution is a direct consequence of the fact that parasites must survive for prolonged periods in host tissues during their life cycle; this period must be sufficient for the organisms to replicate and develop into the life cycle stages necessary for successful transmission in nature. This chapter will critically examine two paradigms of parasite immune evasion during infection: one is a new theme emerging from a classic paradigm of surface antigen variation by extracellular parasites, and the other is a new paradigm of modified antigen recognition of intracellular parasites.

ANTIGENIC VARIATION

There are substantial structural as well as practical constraints on molecular variation by parasites. Antigenic variation is limited in that it must occur in concert with the maintenance of critical molecular structures that provide cellular integrity and permit functional molecular interactions with the parasite's environment. For organisms that are extracellular at any stage of their life cycle, all surface-exposed molecules are potential targets for host B-cell-mediated immunity, and these antigens, as well as other cellular constituents, are capable of triggering T-cell-mediated immune responses that can affect parasite survival in the extracellular environment. The problem for the parasite is to express reduced numbers of surface-exposed molecules, to permit selective or limited immune responses to target antigens that can accommodate molecular variation, and/or to couple limited antigenic variation with immune modulation that prevents immune targeting of all antigens. For parasites residing inside nucleated host cells, the release or secretion of any molecules intra- or extracellularly potentially can result in the immune targeting of infected cells by major histocompatibility complex (MHC) class I- and II-restricted effector T cells. The problem for these parasites is to control the accessibility of antigenic molecules and their peptide substituents to class I or class II antigen-processing pathways, to permit antigenic variation in noncritical cellular constituents that access these pathways, and/or to modulate host cell antigen processing or immune effector cell recognition of invariant and critical parasite molecules. As noted above, the problems for both extra- and intracellular parasites are exponentially more complex if potential immune target antigens serve as critical structural, metabolic, transport, or other essential invariant components of cells.

Antigenic variation occurs in several parasitic diseases (for recent reviews, see Allred [1998], Anderson [1998], Cross [1996], Damian [1997], Dea-Ayuela and Bolas-Fernandez [1999]; Donelson et al. [1998], Hommel [1997], Muller and Gottstein [1998], Nash [1997], Newbold [1999], and Ramasamy [1998]), although the mechanisms used by these parasites to promote variation are quite different and it is sometimes unclear whether the antigens involved represent substantially protective antigens. Arguably the most well-known example of immune evasion by parasites is antigenic variation by the African trypanosomes, which for nearly a century have provided the classical paradigm for microbial antigenic variation as a means of escaping host antibody (Ab)-mediated immunity (Mansfield, 1995). African trypanosomes have evolved a highly ordered monomolecular surface coat structure that covers the entire plasma membrane of the parasite (Color Plate 8);

John M. Mansfield • Department of Bacteriology, University of Wisconsin—Madison, Madison, WI 53706. **Martin Olivier** • Infectious Diseases Unit, CHUL, Laval University, Sainte-Foy, Quebec G1V 4G2, Canada.

this coat is composed of glycosylphosphatidylinositol (GPI)-anchored variant surface glycoprotein (VSG) homodimers that are identically oriented on the membrane and are so densely packed together that they prevent Ab from binding to subsurface epitopes of the VSG coat as well as to any plasma membrane determinants underlying it. Trypanosome growth in an infected host results in the generation of strong B-cell responses to exposed epitopes of the VSG coat, however. This host response results in the catastrophic elimination of trypanosomes expressing the relevant surface coat glycoprotein. Trypanosomes have evolved a successful mechanism for coping with host Ab responses by extensive antigenic variation of the VSG during infection (Vickerman and Luckins, 1969; Cross, 1975, 1990, 1996; Van der Ploeg et al., 1992; Borst and Rudenko, 1994; Borst et al., 1996). This variation occurs as the result of transcriptional activation of distinct VSG genes from among a large resident VSG gene family that may encompass up to 10^3 different members. VSG gene switching occurs spontaneously and at a relatively high frequency of 1 switch in 10^2 to 10^6 cells (Turner and Barry, 1989; Turner, 1997). Only one VSG gene is expressed at a time, however, and expressed VSG genes are transcribed from active chromosome telomeric expression sites; these sites normally generate large polycistronic transcripts that encompass a number of upstream expression site-associated genes as well as the telomeric VSG gene (Cross, 1990, 1996). There are several mechanisms that serve to duplicate and transpose copies of internal chromosome basic-copy VSG genes into telomeric sites or to transcriptionally activate existing copies of silent VSG genes already present in telomeric sites (Hoeijmakers et al., 1980; Borst et al., 1981; Borst and Cross, 1982; Cross, 1990, 1996; Navarro and Cross, 1996; Horn and Cross, 1997; Cross et al., 1998). Therefore, during each wave of trypanosome parasitemia, new antigenic variants constantly arise, and it is the Ab-mediated destruction of the predominant variant antigenic type (VAT) that leads to immune selection for one or more new VATs that have arisen within the previous population. This cycle of host VSG-specific Ab production and VAT elimination, coupled with changes in trypanosome VSG expression, occurs throughout infection until, at some point, the host dies without ever completely eliminating the organisms from the body.

T-cell-independent surface antigen recognition of the VSG coat structure represents one of the earliest events in the B-cell response to trypanosomes and is sufficient to control parasitemia (Mansfield et al., 1981; Reinitz and Mansfield, 1988, 1990; Mansfield, 1994; Schopf et al., 1998). This represents "an-tigen pattern" recognition and is similar to B-cell responses to viral capsid determinants; Ab is directed at exposed epitopes displayed as part of the three-dimensional architectural configuration of VSG molecules in the surface coat (Fig. 1). Classically, pattern recognition has been held to involve antigen-nonspecific receptors displayed primarily by cells other than B or T cells. However, it has been proposed by Zinkernagel (Bachmann and Zinkernagel, 1996; Zinkernagel, 2000) and others (Mansfield, 1994) that B cells also have the capacity to scan architectural surface structures of microbes for polymeric epitope patterns associated with an assemblage of identical unit molecules. This type of polymeric epitope recognition event is distinct from individual unit molecule epitope recognition by B cells, which requires T-cell help in generating a significant Ab response (Snapper et al., 1994, 1995a, 1995b; Snapper and Mond, 1996). The ability to stimulate T-independent B-cell responses in such an antigen pattern-specific manner is dependent on the homogeneity, orientation, density, and rigidity of molecules expressed within an exposed structure (Bachmann and Zinkernagel, 1996; Zinkernagel, 2000). In this regard, the trypanosome VSG coat represents an ideal B-cell-stimulatory surface structure. The dense packaging of identical VSG homodimers on the plasma membrane (10^7 molecules/cell), the internal rigidity of each VSG provided by long antiparallel A and B α-helices, and the orientation of each subunit VSG monomer in the coat with the hydrophilic folded N terminus displayed outward and the C terminus anchored to the plasma membrane by a GPI anchor all contribute to the repetitive antigen pattern recognized by B cells (Metcalf et al., 1987; Carrington et al., 1991; Blum et al., 1993).

It is clear that athymic nu/nu mice are able to make a rapid and substantial Ab response to the VSG surface determinants of intact trypanosomes during infection but, unlike wild-type mice, cannot respond to immunization with purified VSG molecules (Reinitz and Mansfield, 1990; Mansfield, 1994; Schopf et al., 1998). Thus, the surface of intact and viable trypanosomes displays intrinsic signals sufficient to induce a mature T-independent B-cell response; these signals include repetitive arrays of N-terminal amino acids that are displayed, at the architectural multiplex level but not at the level of single molecules (Fig. 1), as classical T-independent antigens. The nature of secondary signals required to generate a rapid T-independent B-cell response to VSG and the question whether distinct subsets of B cells are involved are unknown elements of the response. Overall, these types of findings reinforced the central role of B cells

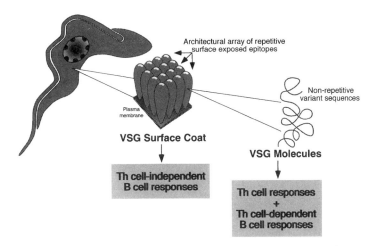

Figure 1. The trypanosome VSG coat presents a T-cell-independent surface "antigen pattern" that activates B cells. The three-dimensional or architectural array of exposed repetitive VSG epitopes is sufficient to activate B cells and produce a rapid immunoglobulin M response during infection in the absence of Th cells. Subsequent exposure of the immune system to VSG molecules liberated from the surface coat induces strong VSG-specific Th1-cell and T-dependent B-cell responses. Adapted from Mansfield (1994).

in variant-specific control of trypanosomes during infection.

However, a profound shift in this paradigm occurred as the result of new insights into the immunobiology of trypanosomiasis. The old central paradigm first began to unravel as the result of functional and genetic studies on the role of Ab in determining host resistance to experimental trypanosome infection. It was demonstrated using semiallogeneic bone marrow radiation chimera mice that control of parasitemia by Ab was not functionally linked to overall host resistance (De Gee and Mansfield, 1984). The central finding was that susceptible mice, which are genetically unable to make Abs to VSG surface coat determinants and to control parasitemias, were afforded a functional VSG-specific B-cell response after transplantation and reconstitution of the lymphoid system with *H-2*-compatible bone marrow cells from resistant mice (De Gee and Mansfield, 1984); this response was sufficient to eliminate trypanosomes from the blood in a variant-specific manner. However, despite Ab-mediated control of trypanosomes, the radiation chimera mice lived no longer than wild-type susceptible mice that could not make VSG-specific Ab or control the parasitemia (De Gee and Mansfield, 1984). Subsequently, classical genetic approaches with crosses between resistant and susceptible animals demonstrated that Ab-mediated control of parasitemia by itself was not genetically linked to the host resistance phenotype (De Gee et al., 1988). This work has been substantiated in other laboratories and by different approaches (Seed and Sechelski, 1989). Thus, although VSG-specific Abs provide a very important mechanism for controlling

trypanosome numbers in the blood, this event by itself is insufficient to provide a significant level of host resistance.

These seminal experiments laid the foundation for studies in which resistant and susceptible animals were examined for T-cell-mediated immune responses to trypanosome antigens. Th-cell responses to VSG previously had not been detected in animals infected with the African trypanosomes, despite evidence that such animals made T-dependent B-cell responses to VSG molecules (Reinitz and Mansfield, 1988, 1990) and that primary sequence variation was evident in buried subregions of VSG molecules making up the surface coat (see below) (Reinitz et al., 1992; Blum et al., 1993; Field and Boothroyd, 1996). The first direct evidence for VSG-specific Th-cell responses came from experimental studies with *Trypanosoma brucei rhodesiense* LouTat 1 infections of inbred mice (Schleifer et al., 1993; Schleifer and Mansfield, 1993; Mansfield, 1995; Hertz et al., 1998; Schopf et al., 1998; Hertz and Mansfield, 1999). T-cell populations derived from various tissues were tested for their ability to be activated following exposure to purified VSG in vitro. The results of these studies showed that VSG-specific T cells exhibited a degree of tissue-specific compartmentalization and did not proliferate in vitro in response to antigen but that they produced substantial cytokine responses when stimulated; the principal cytokines produced were gamma interferon (IFN-γ) and interleukin-2 (IL-2) but not IL-4 or IL-5. The cellular phenotype of VSG-responsive T cells was that of classical Th cells in that all cells were CD4 positive and expressed the CD3 α/β T-cell receptor membrane complex (Schleifer et al., 1993). Thus, VSG appeared to preferentially drive a polarized Th1-cell cytokine response during infection. Intrinsic molecular characteristics of the VSG did not induce mice to make this response, however, since VSG-specific T-cell lines derived from VSG-immunized but not infected mice displayed cytokine profiles characteristic of both Th1 and Th2 cells (Schleifer et al., 1993). Unusual features of the VSG-specific T-cell response were not only that it was somewhat tissue compartmentalized but also that products of IFN-γ-activated macrophages suppressed the proliferative but not the cytokine secretory responses of antigen-stimulated Th1 cells. Subsequently, it was demonstrated that IL-12, in conjunction with infection-associated inhibition of Th2-cell outgrowth, was responsible for induction of this polarized Th1-cell response (J. M. Mansfield et al., unpublished data). Parasite antigen-specific B-cell responses were also affected by Th1-cell cytokine responses in terms of immunoglobulin Ig isotype switch events of the T-dependent B-cell responses (Schopf et al., 1998; X.-J. Bi et al., unpublished data). Also, Th1 cells appeared to serve as the major source of IFN-γ that was linked to host resistance phenotype through macrophage activation events (De Gee et al., 1985; Hertz et al., 1998; Hertz and Mansfield, 1999; M. Imboden et al., unpublished data). Thus, these results revealed for the first time that Th1-cell and IFN-γ cytokine responses to VSG regulated a major component of host resistance to African trypanosomes. However, like B-cell responses to VSG, Th1-cell responses alone were insufficient to provide full resistance.

Sequence and structural analyses have revealed several additional and interesting facets of VSG structure that may be important in the context of host B- and Th-cell responses. First, VSG molecules are members of a protein superfamily, in which molecules of a specific class and type exhibit highly conserved secondary and tertiary structural features (Fig. 2) (Blum et al., 1993). This results in predictable folding patterns that ultimately permit VSG molecules to pack closely together on the membrane; newly expressed variant VSGs are also able to intercalate among existing molecules on the membrane during VSG switching events in a manner that does not disrupt the surface coat architecture to permit Ab access to membrane determinants beneath. An early comparison of the full-length protein sequence encoded by the *T. b. rhodesiense* LouTat 1 VSG gene to other full-length VSG molecules was made with the intention of predicting, based on the conserved secondary and tertiary structural features associated with trypanosome VSGs, which primary amino acid subsequences might be exposed on the VSG molecule

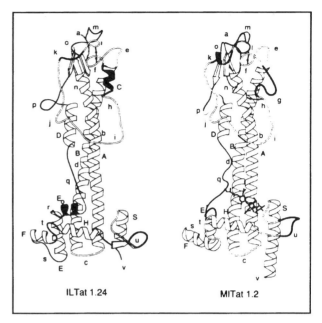

Figure 2. VSG molecules are members of a protein superfamily that exhibit a highly conserved structure. Two VSG molecules are shown that differ significantly in primary sequence but display conserved secondary and tertiary structural features; these structural features are retained among different molecules because VSGs contain highly conserved subsequences necessary for proper folding of the molecule. Highlighted in the figure are the minimal structural differences seen between these two VSGs, as well as other molecular landmarks (Blum et al., 1993). Reprinted from Blum et al. (1993) with permission of the publisher.

and surface coat (Reinitz et al., 1992). An unexpected finding was that in addition to amino acids conserved at specific sites to maintain the structural features of VSGs (Metcalf et al., 1987; Carrington et al., 1991; Reinitz et al., 1992; Blum et al., 1993), numerous hypervariable regions, or amino acid sequence-variable hot spots, were detected that appeared to be conserved at specific sites among different trypanosome VSG molecules (Reinitz et al., 1992). Some of these amino acid-hypervariable regions were predicted to be buried within the surface coat structure and therefore would not play a role in evasion of an Ab response to the surface coat. Wiley and coworkers subsequently published a study with newer crystal structure data in a broader sequence survey of VSG molecules related by class (the pattern of Cys residues in the N terminus) and type (sequence similarities within the C terminus) (Blum et al., 1993). Essentially the same finding was presented, i.e., that amino acid-hypervariable regions existed among different VSGs and that some of these were buried within the surface coat. Wiley and coworkers proposed that this represented evidence at the primary sequence level for antigenic variation within potential Th-cell epitope sites, and they made the formal hypothesis that antigenic variation by trypanosomes was done to evade host B- and T-cell responses. It was the subsequent publication of work on VSG-specific Th-cell responses (see above) that demonstrated the existence of VSG-specific T cells for the first time (Schleifer et al., 1993; Schleifer and Mansfield, 1993; Mansfield, 1994, 1995; Hertz et al., 1998; Schopf et al., 1998; Hertz and Mansfield, 1999).

Since evidence revealed that VSG specificity was inherent in the Th-cell response to VSG (e.g., no cross-reactivity between T-cell responses to the LouTat 1, LouTat 1.5, or other VSG molecules was displayed by *T. b. rhodesiense* [Schleifer et al., 1993]), this presented interesting implications both for the biological role of Th-cell responses during infection and for the sequence variation seen in VSGs. While the dense molecular packing of VSG homodimers on the trypanosome plasma membrane ultimately limits protective B-cell responses to exposed VSG residues, it also provides the parasites with a limited number of VSG subregions that can be varied at the primary sequence level to avoid elimination. A major question is how the parasite avoids stimulating Th-cell responses to highly conserved regions existing throughout the VSG molecule that preserve proper folding and membrane orientation. It follows that either all potential VSG peptides capable of being processed to associate with MHC class II determinants for presentation to Th cells are different among different VSG molecules expressed within a serodeme or T-cell recognition is somehow limited to discrete subregions within the molecule in which variation can take place.

To address these hypotheses, *T. b. rhodesiense* LouTat 1 VSG-specific T-cell lines and clones were examined for VSG sequence specificity (Mansfield et al., unpublished). Sequence algorithms used to predict T-cell epitope sites within proteins revealed that the LouTat 1 VSG molecule contains numerous potential T-cell epitope sites (amphipathic α-helices and Rothbard-Taylor sequences) throughout the entire molecule. Subsequently, purified VSG was proteolytically digested, the resultant peptides were segregated by high-pressure liquid chromatography, and the peptide fractions were examined for T-cell stimulation. Surprisingly, there was limited reactivity of T-cell lines and clones with these fractions. Experiments revealed that one high-pressure liquid chromatography fraction (containing two major and one minor defined peptides) appeared to stimulate a majority of T-cell clones and all of the T-cell lines. These peptides were subsequently purified and partially sequenced. The larger peptide encompassed a portion of the LouTat 1 VSG molecule that appeared to contain multiple Th-cell reactive sites (Asp85 to Trp134) while the others appeared to contain no, or minor, reactive sites. The immunodominant Asp85-to-Trp134 subsequence was localized within the internal B α-helix within the three-dimensional structure of LouTat 1 VSG (Color Plate 8; Fig. 2) and therefore is not exposed on the surface coat. The underlying reasons for this focusing of Th-cell reactive sites within one subregion of the VSG are not yet clear, but since T cells from animals with a different MHC II haplotype can also recognize an epitope(s) within the same LouTat 1 VSG subsequence (J. M. Mansfield, unpublished data), simple MHC II restriction is probably not a factor. Antigen processing is a more likely explanation for selective or limited recognition of VSG sequences. One can envision that conserved primary sequences and structural elements among different VSGs may promote similar unfolding of the molecules within the endosomal pathway and may control sequence-specific accessibility to proteolytic enzymes that generate MHC class II-binding peptides. Although discrete physical limits of individual epitope-specific sites within the immunodominant VSG subregion have not been mapped, this preliminary work provides the first functional evidence for limited reactivity of T cells to a buried subregion(s) of the VSG molecule and may provide a natural model for epitope dominance within complex protein antigens (Schneider and Sercarz, 1997; Moudgil et al., 1998; Sercarz, 1998).

Coincident with this functional VSG epitope-mapping study, a report from the Boothroyd laboratory appeared in which the *T. b. brucei* 117 VSG gene family was examined (Field and Boothroyd, 1996); these interrelated VSG family sequences exhibited predictable amino acid hypervariability within three well-defined regions when the molecules were aligned for comparison. These regions of hypervariability were better defined than similar regions identified in earlier studies (Reinitz et al., 1992; Blum et al., 1993) because the previous comparisons largely had been made among many different VSG molecules (e.g., not within a single VSG gene family). Like LouTat 1 VSG, the 117 VSG protein superfamily members are class A VSG molecules, and these VSGs contain a number of conserved residues that direct the molecules to fold in a similar pattern. Therefore, inspection of 117 VSG family hypervariability regions in comparison with the Th-cell epitope-mapping studies with LouTat 1 mentioned above revealed that hypervariable region I (HV-1), spanning amino acid residues 75 to 140, was predicted to be buried within the VSG molecule; this region overlapped exactly with the immunodominant Asp85-to-Trp134 region identified in the preliminary functional mapping study of the LouTat 1 molecule (Fig. 3). This finding has generated significant interest in the biological significance of antigenic variation in T-cell epitope sites buried within the VSG molecule.

This excitement is justified not only because T-cell reactivity seems to be limited to VSG HV-1 subsequences but also because it has been demonstrated that VSG-specific Th1-cell responses and IFN-γ production are critical components of host protection (Hertz et al., 1998; Hertz and Mansfield, 1999). Additional evidence that VSG-specific Th-cell responses contribute to host resistance has come from a recent unexpected finding (C. J. Hertz and J. M. Mansfield, unpublished data). In this work, C57BL/6-Igh-6 mice that lack mature B cells were infected with *T. b. rhodesiense* LouTat 1. After 1 week of infection, these B⁻ mice were drug cured with Berenil (without drug cure, the mice are unable, due to the lack of Ab control of parasitemia, to control high numbers of trypanosomes and are relatively susceptible). Subsequently, the mice were reinfected with the homologous VAT, LouTat 1, or a heterologous VAT, LouTat 1.5, which differs extensively in primary sequence as well as in the class and type of VSG (Reinitz et al., 1992; Schopf and Mansfield, 1998). All mice infected with the heterologous VAT died during the same period as the nonprimed B⁻ mice (15 to 20 days) and exhibited T-cell responses to VSG of the original VAT as well as weak responses to the new heterologous VAT. In contrast, all mice reinfected with LouTat 1 exhibited evidence of strong Th1-cell responses to LouTat 1 VSG due to prior exposure; even though the levels of trypanosomes expressing the LouTat 1 phenotype in the blood remained very high (e.g., no variant-specific Ab was present to select against trypanosome VATs), these animals survived for over 100 days. This is the first clear experiment to demonstrate that a strong Th1-cell

response, alone, can influence the resistance status of a trypanosome-infected animal, even in the complete absence of B-cell responses. Therefore, a direct test of the hypothesis that VSG subsurface T-cell epitopes within the HV-1 region induce host resistance may provide the first evidence that T-cell responses serve as a selective pressure for driving VSG sequence variation in regions other than those encoding surface-exposed epitopes accessible to Ab.

Overall, then, the original paradigm of VSG-specific B-cell-mediated immunity to African trypanosomes has evolved to include Th-cell responses to parasite antigens. The overall hypothesis that has emerged from experimental studies on resistance to trypanosomes is that animals with the highest level of resistance express two crucial components of an immune response to trypanosomes: (i) an early and strong B-cell response to the VSG surface coat controls parasitemia within the vascular compartment by promoting variant-specific immune clearance, and (ii) an early and strong parasite antigen-specific Th1-cell response, coupled with IFN-γ-dependent activation of macrophages, leads to parasite control within the extravascular tissue compartment. It follows that animals compromised, wholly or in part, in either arm of the immune response exhibit comparative susceptibility. It is equally clear that African trypanosomes employ several important mechanisms to avoid immune elimination. The primary mechanism involves a display of a highly ordered but variant surface coat structure that simultaneously protects the plasma membrane from Ab attack and permits Abs to bind only to relatively small exposed subregions of the VSG coat. A secondary mechanism involves restricting Th-cell responses to a highly variable internal subregion of the VSG. The end result is that primary sequence variation underlying antigenic variation only has to occur within defined exposed and buried hypervariable regions of the VSG; this permits the conservation of amino acid sequences elsewhere so that different VSG molecules can fold in similar secondary and tertiary structural patterns—patterns important for maintaining the surface coat structure throughout the course of infection.

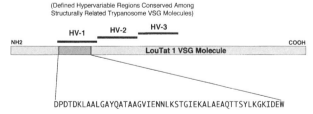

Figure 3. Th-cell-reactive sites are found within a buried hypervariable region conserved among VSG molecules. The relative placement of three different hypervariable (HV) regions found within trypanosome VSGs is shown (Field and Boothroyd, 1996). HV-2 and HV-3 are predicted to contain amino acids that would be exposed on the surface of the VSG coat, while HV-1 contains amino acids that are predicted to be buried within VSG molecules. The Th-cell-reactive subsequence shown for the LouTat 1 VSG lies within the predicted conserved HV-1 region.

MODULATION OF SIGNALING PATHWAYS

Some parasites reside intracellularly during infection and do not exhibit substantial antigenic variation. For these organisms, some of which reside in antigen-processing cells capable of triggering protective host T-cell responses to antigenic peptides displayed by MHC molecules, other mechanisms are employed to evade host immunity. In this section, the novel means by which *Leishmania* modulates intracellular signaling pathways of the infected cell to evade immunity are explored and evaluated.

Leishmania parasites infect host macrophage cells during their life cycle. Development of effective cell-mediated immune responses to these organisms requires that infected macrophages induce significant Th1 cell activation against leishmanial antigens (Locksley et al., 1987, 1991, 1995; Heinzel et al., 1988, 1989; Scott et al., 1989; Scott, 1990, 1991; Locksley and Scott, 1991; Reiner and Locksley, 1995; Scharton-Kersten and Scott, 1995; Fearon and Locksley, 1996). The subsequent type 1 cytokine response activates macrophages to become microbicidal effector cells (Belosevic et al., 1990; Mauel, 1990; Olivier et al., 1989a, 1989b; Murray et al., 1982, 1987; Olivier and Tanner, 1989). In this regard, IFN-γ has been recognized as the most potent activator of macrophage functions important for parasite control; IFN-γ ligation with the IFN-γ receptor leads to rapid activation of the JAK2-STAT1α signaling pathway (Leonard and O'Shea, 1998), which regulates the expression of key macrophage genes and proteins. The integrity of this type of signaling pathway is of paramount importance for host protection against *Leishmania*.

However, infection of macrophage with *Leishmania donovani* leads to the inhibition of many cellular functions including phagocytosis, IFN-γ-inducible MHC class II expression, IL-1 production, lipopolysaccharide (LPS)- and phorbol ester-mediated *c-fos* gene expression, and generation of oxygen radicals in response to the chemotactic peptide fMet-Leu-Phe (fMLP) or phorbol myristate acetate (Olivier, 1996). It has been demonstrated that Ca^{2+}- and protein kinase C (PKC)-dependent signaling is deficient in *L. donovani*-infected human monocytes (Olivier et al., 1992a, 1992b), and this was directly responsible for inhibition of several macrophage functions (Color Plate 9). One of the consequences of *L. donovani* infection was the induction of abnormal macrophage plasma membrane permeability to Ca^{2+}, leading to rapid and sustained elevation of the intracellular Ca^{2+} concentration ($[Ca2+]_i$) (Olivier et al., 1992a), possibly involving a capacitative mechanism maintained by persistent depletion of intracellular Ca^{2+} stores (Color Plate 10). The most abundant parasite surface molecule, lipophosphoglycan (LPG), and its structural substituents may be involved to some extent in this cellular process (Color Plate 10). Such Ca^{2+} mobilization also may have led to the activation of an inositol triphosphate (IP$_3$) phosphatase that can dephosphorylate and degrade the inositol phosphates (Kukita et al., 1986), thus explaining in part the low fMLP-

stimulated IP$_3$ activity measured in *L. donovani*-infected macrophages (Olivier et al., 1992a). On the other hand, such $[Ca^{2+}]_i$ elevation may have promoted the activation of Ca^{2+}-sensitive phosphoprotein phosphatases, such as the Ser/Thr phosphatase calcineurin (Klee et al., 1979) (Fig. 4), leading to the dephosphorylation and inactivation of several critical cellular proteins. In addition, it should be noted that other phosphatases, like phosphotyrosine phosphatases (PTP), endogenously produced by host cells in response to *Leishmania* infection (Blanchette et al., 1999) or produced by the pathogen, as reported for *Yersinia* infection, in which the PTP YopH is inducible by $[Ca^{2+}]_i$ present in infected cells, may cause dephosphorylation of tyrosyl residues of host cell proteins and interfere with signaling cascades (Blanchette et al., 1999; Bliska et al., 1991, 1993).

Phosphorylation of tyrosyl residues by phosphotyrosine kinases (PTK) is a primordial step in the regulation of many cellular events. A number of growth factors have been demonstrated to use tyrosine phosphorylation as a mechanism for transduction of an extracellular signal via their specific receptors (Hunter and Cooper, 1985). Tyrosine phosphorylation is a common event in the initiation of cell proliferation, but its role in signal transduction regulating the cellular functions of nonproliferative hematopoietic cells is also well documented (Dong et al., 1993a, 1993b; Glaser et al., 1993; Golden et al., 1986; Golden and Brugge, 1989; Green et al., 1992; Greenberg et al., 1993). With regard to PTP, it has been estimated that there are more than 500 genes coding for this phosphatase (Hooft van Huijsduijnen, 1998), and studies of the role of PTP and PTK in the regulation of various cellular functions are of great interest (Walton and Dixon, 1993; Fantl et al., 1993). Activation of macrophage functions such as generation of a respiratory burst in response to zym-

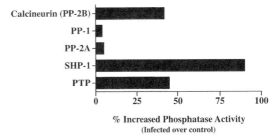

% Increased Phosphatase Activity
(Infected over control)

Figure 4. Induction of host cell phosphatases by *L. donovani* infection. The Ca^{2+}-dependent serine/threonine phosphatase PP-2B (calcineurin) activity is increased over the Ser/Thr phosphatase PP-1 and P-2A activities in *Leishmania*-infected macrophages. PTP activity is rapidly triggered by *Leishmania*, and, in particular, the PTP SHP-1 is recognized for its role as a negative signaling regulator in leukocytes.

osan (Green et al., 1992), phagocytosis via Fc receptors (Greenberg et al., 1993), tumoricidal activity induced by LPS and IFN-γ (Dong et al., 1993a), nitric oxide (NO) production in response to LPS and/or IFN-γ (Dong et al., 1993b; Olivier et al., 1998), regulation of eicosanoid biosynthesis (Glaser et al., 1993), and MHC class II expression following IFN-γ stimulation of 2C4 cells in somatic-cell genetic experiments (Watling et al., 1993) have all been shown to involve tyrosine phosphorylation-mediated signaling events.

Recently the importance of macrophage PTP in NO downregulation has been demonstrated (Olivier et al., 1998); inhibition of PTP with peroxovanadium (pV) compounds led to increased responsiveness to IFN-γ stimulation, which was reflected in increased NO production. A correlation between PTP inhibition in macrophages and enhancement of NO production was further supported by an increase in PTK activity and tyrosyl residue hyperphosphorylation (Olivier et al., 1998). It is clear that IFN-γ induces tyrosine phosphorylation-mediated cellular functions (Dong et al., 1993a, 1993b; Olivier et al., 1998), and there is strong evidence that this cytokine can specifically activate JAK2 kinase, a PTK, to achieve its effect (Hunter, 1993; Muller et al., 1993; Shuai et al., 1993; Silvennoinen et al., 1993; Watling et al., 1993). JAK2 kinase becomes rapidly phosphorylated following IFN-γ activation (Watling et al., 1993) and subsequently induces tyrosine phosphorylation of the latent cytoplasmic transcriptional activator STAT proteins (Shuai et al., 1993). This signaling pathway is altered in *L. donovani*-infected macrophages due to immediate PTP SHP-1 activation following the initial parasite-macrophage interaction (Blanchette et al., 1999) (Fig. 4; Color Plate 9). This finding permits a better understanding of how IFN-γ-inducible phagocyte functions (e.g., MHC class II expression and IL-12 generation) are inhibited by *Leishmania*. It is possible that the IFN-γ receptor may be differentially expressed in *Leishmania*-infected macrophages, and this might explain the cellular unresponsiveness to IFN-γ stimulation. However, contradictory observations, potentially due to the different types of macrophages studied or the use of inadequately differentiated cells (Reiner et al., 1988; Ray et al., 2000), render this interpretation uncertain. In fact, whereas IFN-γ-induced IL-12, inducible NO synthase (iNOS), and MHC class II expression are affected by *Leishmania* infection, the induction of MHC class I antigen presentation (Kima et al., 1987) and the expression of immunoproteasome subunits LMP-2, LMP-7, and MECL-1 mRNA in response to this cytokine are normal (unpublished data). These observations suggest that IFN-γ receptor generally is not affected in *Leishmania*-infected cells and further reinforce the notion that other signaling pathways are triggered in response to IFN-γ stimulation. Experiments performed in vitro and in vivo using viable motheaten mice deficient for PTP SHP-1 have firmly established that SHP-1 plays a pivotal role in *Leishmania*-induced macrophage dysfunction and the survival of this parasite within its host cell (G. Forget and M. Olivier, submitted for publication): the development of cutaneous leishmaniasis was completely abolished in the absence of SHP-1 and was coincident with the upregulation of inflammatory and NO-dependent protective mechanisms regulated in part by STAT1α-dependent signaling events.

Phosphorylation of proteins at their tyrosyl residues can result from increases in PTK activity, decreases in PTP activity, or a combination of the two. As described previously (Olivier et al., 1998), the use of PTP inhibitors coupled with direct measurements of PTK or PTP activities in cell preparations is a valuable tool for investigating whether the regulation of tyrosine phosphorylation following specific stimulation is PTK or PTP regulated. In macrophages, SHP-1 can be rapidly phosphorylated on its tyrosyl residues following stimulation with colony-stimulating factor 1 (CSF-1); this observation suggests that this PTP may be involved in early events of growth factor signal transduction (Yeung et al., 1992). SHP-1 contains two SH2 domains in its N-terminal region that may direct this unique PTP to tyrosine-phosphorylated proteins, thereby modulating PTK-related signal transduction (Shen et al., 1991). SHP-1 is expressed predominantly in hematopoietic cells and is thought to play a major role in functions regulated by tyrosine phosphorylation, with dephosphorylation acting as a signaling terminator (Matthews et al., 1992; Plutzky et al., 1992; Yi et al., 1992). As discussed above, the recent demonstration (Olivier et al., 1998) that macrophages pretreated with the pV compound bpV(phen) were more responsive to IFN-γ stimulation is consistent with previous observations concerning the use of PTP inhibitors to modulate tyrosyl phosphorylation-dependent mechanisms (Posner et al., 1994). pV treatments clearly render macrophages more responsive to extracellular stimuli; experiments performed with these compounds in vivo have revealed that modulation of PTP activities completely blocks the progression of murine visceral and cutaneous leishmaniasis (Olivier et al., 1998). NO was one of the key molecules modulated by pV treatment leading to the control of *Leishmania* infection (Matte et al., 2000). Collectively, these experiments have provided the first demonstration that inhibitors directed toward a signaling molecule can modulate the progression of an infection.

Activation of macrophage PTPs must involve signaling events that are rapidly induced following parasite attachment to the host cell membrane. For example, activation of the macrophage SHP-1 in response to CSF-1 is accompanied by tyrosine phosphorylation of the enzyme (Yeung et al., 1992). *Leishmania* can also induce tyrosine phosphorylation of macrophage SHP-1 (Blanchette et al., 1999). It is interesting that both macrophage Ca^{2+} influx and PTP activities are rapidly inducible by *Leishmania* infection and that the $[Ca^{2+}]_i$ of *L. donovani*-infected human monocytes was abnormally elevated (Olivier et al., 1992a) due to increased macrophage plasma membrane permeability for Ca^{2+}. This increase in macrophage Ca^{2+} influx was rapidly induced following the initial *Leishmania*-macrophage membrane interaction (Color Plate 10).

Internalization of *Leishmania*, coated or not with host opsonins such as Ab or C3b (Mosser and Edelson, 1984, 1985; Dominguez and Torano, 1999), is known to occur via specific macrophage receptors (i.e., FcγR, CR3, CR1, and mannose receptor) (Guy and Belosevic, 1993; reviewed by Russell and Talamas-Rohana [1989]). Recently, several reports have shown that specific ligation of macrophage receptors such as FcγR and CR3 leads to the inhibition of certain macrophage functions (Berger et al., 1997; Marth and Kelsall, 1997; Sutterwala et al., 1997). It has also been shown that CR3 ligation inhibits IFN-γ-induced phosphotyrosine phosphorylation of STAT1. In light of these aggregate observations, it is predictable that one or more of these ligand-receptor interactions are involved in *Leishmania*-induced host cell PTP activation.

As discussed above, there is supportive evidence for the hypothesis that SHP-1 is responsible for host cell tyrosyl residue dephosphorylation, JAK2 signaling alterations, and subsequent macrophage dysfunctions (Blanchette et al., 1999) (Color Plate 9). The central involvement of macrophage SHP-1 in these deactivating processes has been confirmed in experiments with immortalized bone marrow-derived macrophage (BMDM) cell lines from SHP-1-deficient motheaten (C3HeBFeJ *me/me*) and viable motheaten (C57BL/6J *me^v/me^v*) mice and from their respective littermates (C3HeB/FeJ *me/+* and C57BL/6J *me^v/+*) which are not deficient in SHP-1 (Kozlowski et al., 1993; G. Forget and M. Olivier, submitted for publication). Whereas SHP-1-mediated JAK2 alteration may result in the inability to tyrosyl phosphorylate STAT1α and consequently abolishes its nuclear translocation, it is possible that *L. donovani* infection has triggered other cellular mechanisms that affect

STAT1α proteolysis. Contrary to what was initially believed, i.e., that STAT1α alteration was caused solely by SHP-1, IFN-γ-inducible STAT1α translocation in SHP-1-deficient BMDM infected by *Leishmania* was not seen even if infected cells were capable of mounting a normal response to IFN-γ by secreting NO (J. Cauchard, G. Forget, and M. Olivier, Woods Hole ImmunoParasitology Meeting, 2000, abstr. 59). Observations that macrophage STAT1α protein was degraded in *Leishmania*-infected cells in comparison to uninfected macrophages led to the supposition that STAT1α degradation may be mediated by proteasome activation following *Leishmania* infection.

Proteasomes are known to modulate several transcriptional regulators, including Iκ /NF-κB activation (Chen et al., 1995), as well as STAT proteins (Yu and Burakoff, 1997). STAT1α inactivation following *Leishmania* infection could involve the participation of proteasome (26S [20S+PA700,11S]; responsible for ATP-dependent proteolysis) (reviewed by Rivett [1998]) and/or other proteolytic molecules (Color Plates 9 and 11). Using the proteasome antagonists Lactacystin and MG-132, it has been possible to block *Leishmania*-induced macrophage STAT1α proteolysis in a dose-dependent manner (unpublished data). A role for proteasome-mediated proteolysis involving ubiquitination in the regulation of the transcription factor STAT previously has been reported (Haspel et al., 1996; Darnell, 1997; Yu and Burakoff, 1997), but the participation of PTP such as SHP-1 in this control is still controversial (Haspel et al., 1996). The fact that SHP-1 is not responsible for *Leishmania*-induced STAT1α inactivation (Forget and Olivier, Woods Hole ImmunoParasitology Meeting, 2000) strongly suggests that SHP-1 is not involved in the regulation of this transcription factor. A new molecule acting negatively on STAT1 regulation has been recently described and named PIAS1 (for "protein inhibitor of activated STAT1") (Liu et al., 1998). PIAS1 specifically associates with STAT1 dimers, leading to their inactivation by an unknown mechanism. A possibility that this STAT1-inhibitory molecule is activated by *Leishmania* infection remains to be determined.

Whereas the 26S proteasome is involved in the degradation of regulatory proteins controlling various biological processes, the IFN-γ-inducible immunoproteasome formed by LMP-2, LMP-7, and MECL-1 subunits and activation of the 20S regulatory subunits PA28α,β is essential for appropriate peptide generation in the context of MHC class I antigen presentation (Rivett, 1998) (Color Plate 11). Presentation of antigen by the MHC class I-processing pathway occurs in *Leishmania*-infected cells (Kima et al., 1987), even though it was initially reported that MHC class I mRNA expression was abnormal (Reiner et al., 1987). Immunoproteasome modulation by IFN-γ is reflected in enhanced mRNA expression of the different subunits (Brown et al., 1991; Rivett, 1998; Stohwasser et al., 1997) in *Leishmania*-infected macrophages (Cauchard et al., abstract). It is noteworthy that infection was shown to affect the expression of some IFN-γ-inducible immunoproteasome subunits (i.e., LMP-2 and PA28α). Similarly, IFN-γ-inducible immunoproteasome subunits LMP-2, PA28α,β, and MECL-1 in *T. cruzi*-infected macrophages were shown to be strongly affected at the mRNA and protein levels (unpublished data) (Color Plate 11). Such alterations may be detrimental for immunoproteasome formation and thus may affect adequate peptide preparation in the context of MHC class I antigen presentation.

In summary, the protozoan parasite *Leishmania* has developed several powerful strategies to subvert the macrophage signaling system, and this consequently affects the development of protective immune responses to favor parasite survival. Other unicellular and multicellular parasites have evolved different means of desensitizing immune cells to avoid detection and destruction by the immune system; this involves altering signal transduction mechanisms driving the activation of T or B cells that are indispensable for host protection. For instance, the rodent filarial nematode *Acanthocheilonema viteae* secretes a phosphorylcholine-containing glycoprotein, termed ES-62, which desensitizes B and T lymphocytes to subsequent activation of several signaling pathways involving the PKC, Ras mitogen-activating protein kinase, and phosphoinositide-3-kinase (PI3K) (Harnett et al., 1999). A homologue of ES-62 exists in *Brugia malayi*, a human filarial nematode, at concentrations equivalent to those found in the bloodstream of infected humans; it is possible that such phosphorylcholine-containing molecules affect the signaling integrity of human lymphocytes. *Theileria annulata*-infected bovine leukocytes are transformed into proliferating metastatic tumors resembling a leukemia-like disease. This infection is a good example where the subversive mechanism by which the parasite favors its dissemination and pathogenesis involves the activation of specific signaling events. For instance, Chaussepied et al. (1998) have shown that uncontrolled leukocyte proliferation triggered by this infection was the consequence of constitutive AP-1 transcriptional activation involving upregulation of all members of Jun/Fos protein family, associated with permanent *Theileria*-induced JNK activation. Recent observations revealed that GPI-anchored surface proteins and related glycoconjuga-

tes of *Plasmodium*, *Trypanosoma*, and *Leishmania* differentially modulate the host immune response and may affect specific signaling pathways (Tachado et al., 1999). Whereas GPI purified from *Plasmodium* and *Trypanosoma* was shown to induce PTK- and PKC-dependent signaling events leading to NF-κB/rel-dependent IL-1, tumor necrosis factor alpha and iNOS gene expression, GPI substituents isolated from *L. mexicana* were capable of antagonizing PKC activity, leading to the inhibition of tumor necrosis factor alpha expression (Tachado et al., 1997). Similarly, the *Leishmania* surface molecule LPG has been extensively studied and reported to be a powerful inhibitor of PKC, leading to the inactivation of several macrophage functions regulated by this signaling pathway (Turco, 1999). Down-modulation of macrophage functions as the result of abnormal signaling also has been reported for macrophages that have engulfed malarial pigment hemozoin (Schwarzer and Arese, 1996; Schwarzer et al., 1998). *Toxoplasma gondii* infections cause host immune response downregulation and, in particular, CD4+ T-cell anergy. Expression of the immunosuppressive cytokine IL-10 may be responsible in part for this inactivation, but recent observations suggest that alterations in Ca^{2+} mobilization in T cells isolated from *Toxoplasma*-infected animals directly affect the translocation of the Ca^{2+}-dependent transcription factor NF-ATc that is required for T-cell proliferation (Haque et al., 1998).

SUMMARY

In overall summary, a number of parasites modulate antigen expression and/or the signaling pathways of the cells that they infect or interact with, effectively subverting or suppressing cellular mechanisms that affect parasite survival. A variety of molecular mechanisms underlie these antigen recognition and signaling abnormalities, and the challenge for immunologists is to determine how these events are triggered and what can be done to regulate them.

REFERENCES

Allred, D. R. 1998. Antigenic variation in *Babesia bovis*: how similar is it to that in *Plasmodium falciparum*? *Ann. Trop. Med. Parasitol.* **92**:461–472.

Anderson, R. M. 1998. Complex dynamic behaviours in the interaction between parasite population and the host's immune system. *Int. J. Parasitol.* **28**:551–566.

Bachmann, M. F., and R. Zinkernagel. 1996. The influence of virus structure on antibody responses and virus serotype formation. *Immunol. Today* **17**:553–558.

Belosevic, M., D. S. Findbloom, M. S. Meltzer, and C. A. Nacy. 1990. IL-2. A cofactor for induction of activated macrophage resistance to infection. *J. Immunol.* **145**:831–839.

Berger, S., R. Chandra, H. Ballo, R. Hildenbrand, and H. J. Stutte. 1997. Immune complexes are potent inhibitors of interleukin-12 secretion by human monocytes. *Eur. J. Immunol.* **27**:2994–3000.

Blanchette, J., N. Racette, K. A. Siminovitch, R. Faure, and M. Olivier. 1999. *Leishmania*-induced increases in activation of macrophage SHP-1 phosphatase are associated with impaired IFN-γ-triggered JAK2 activation. *Eur. J. Immunol.* **29**:3737–3744.

Bliska, J. B., J. E. Galan, and S. Falkow. 1993. Signal transduction in the mammalian cell during bacterial attachment and entry. *Cell* **73**:903–920.

Bliska, J. B., K. L. Guan, J. E. Dixon, and S. Falkow. 1991. Tyrosine phosphate hydrolysis of host proteins by an essential *Yersinia* virulence determinant. *Proc. Natl. Acad. Sci. USA* **88**:1187–1191.

Blum, J. L., J. A. Down, A. M. Gurnett, M. Carrington, M. J. Turner, and D. C. Wiley. 1993. A structural motif in the variant surface glycoproteins of *Trypanosoma brucei*. *Nature* **362**:603–609.

Borst, P., and G. A. Cross. 1982. Molecular basis for trypanosome antigenic variation. *Cell* **29**:291–303.

Borst, P., A. C. Frasch, A. Bernards, L. H. Van der Ploeg, J. H. Hoeijmakers, A. C. Arnberg, and G. A. Cross. 1981. DNA rearrangements involving the genes for variant antigens in *Trypanosoma brucei*. *Cold Spring Harbor Symp. Quant. Biol.* **2**:935–943.

Borst, P., and G. Rudenko. 1994. Antigenic variation in African trypanosomes. *Science* **264**:1872–1873.

Borst, P., G. Rudenko, M. C. Taylor, P. A. Blundell, F. Vanleeuwen, W. Bitter, M. Cross, and R. McCulloch. 1996. Antigenic variation In trypanosomes. *Arch. Med. Res.* **27**:379–388.

Brown, M. G., J. Driscoll, and J. J. Monaco. 1991. Structural and serological similarity of MHC-linked LMP and proteasome (multicatalytic proteinase) complexes. *Nature* **353**:355–357.

Carrington, M., N. Miller, M. Blum, I. Roditi, D. Wiley, and M. Turner. 1991. Variant specific glycoprotein of *Trypanosoma brucei* consists of two domains each having an independently conserved pattern of cysteine residues *J. Mol. Biol.* **221**:823–835.

Chaussepied, M., D. Lallemand, M. F. Moreau, R. Adamson, R. Hall, and G. Langsley. 1998. Upregulation of Jun and Fos family members and permanent JNK activity lead to constitutive AP-1 activation in *Theileria*-transformed leukocytes. *Mol. Biochem. Parasitol.* **94**:215–226.

Chen, Z., J. Hagler, V. J. Palombella, F. Melandri, D. Scherer, D. Ballard, and T. Maniatis. 1995. Signal-induced site-specific phosphorylation targets I kappa B alpha to the ubiquitin-proteasome pathway. *Genes Dev.* **9**:1586–1597.

Cross, G. 1990. Cellular and genetic aspects of antigenic variation in trypanosomes. *Annu. Rev. Immunol.* **8**:83–110.

Cross, G. A. 1975. Identification, purification and properties of clone-specific glycoprotein antigens constituting the surface coat of *Trypanosoma brucei*. *Parasitology* **71**:393–417.

Cross, G. A. 1996. Antigenic variation in trypanosomes: secrets surface slowly. *Bioessays* **18**:283–291.

Cross, G. A., L. E. Wirtz, and M. Navarro. 1998. Regulation of vsg expression site transcription and switching in *Trypanosoma brucei Mol. Biochem. Parasitol.* **91**:77–91.

Damian, R. T. 1997. Parasite immune evasion and exploitation: reflections and projections. *Parasitology* **115**:S169–S175.

Darnell, J. E. 1997. STATs and gene regulation. *Science* **277**:1630–1635.

Dea-Ayuela, M. A., and F. Bolas-Fernandez. 1999. *Trichinella* antigens: a review. *Vet. Res.* **30**:559–571.

De Gee, A. L., R. F. Levine, and J. M. Mansfield. 1988. Genetics of resistance to the African trypanosomes. VI. Heredity of resistance and variable surface glycoprotein-specific immune responses. *J. Immunol.* **140**:283–288.

De Gee, A. L., and J. M. Mansfield. 1984. Genetics of resistance to the African trypanosomes. IV. Resistance of radiation chimeras to *Trypanosoma rhodesiense* infection. *Cell. Immunol.* **87**:85–91.

De Gee, A. L., G. Sonnenfeld, and J. M. Mansfield. 1985. Genetics of resistance to the African trypanosomes. V. Qualitative and quantitative differences in interferon production among susceptible and resistant mouse strains. *J. Immunol.* **134**:2723–2726.

Dominguez, M., and A. Torano. 1999. Immune adherence-mediated opsonophagocytosis: the mechanism of *Leishmania* infection. *J. Exp. Med.* **189**:25–35.

Donelson, J. E., K. L. Hill, and N. M. El-Sayed. 1998. Multiple mechanisms of immune evasion by African trypanosomes. *Mol. Biochem. Parasitol.* **91**:51–66.

Dong, Z., C. A. O'Brian, and I. J. Fidler. 1993a. Activation of tumoricidal properties in macrophages by lipopolysaccharide requires protein-tyrosine kinase activity. *J. Leukoc. Biol.* **53**:53–60.

Dong, Z., X. Qi, K. Xie, and I. J. Fidler. 1993b. Protein tyrosine kinase inhibitors decrease induction of nitric oxide synthase activity in lipopolysaccharide-responsive and lipopolysaccharide-nonresponsive murine macrophages. *J. Immunol.* **151**:2717–2724.

Fantl, W. J., D. E. Johnson, and L. T. Williams. 1993. Signalling by receptor tyrosine kinases. *Annu. Rev. Biochem.* **62**:453–481.

Fearon, D. T., and R. M. Locksley. 1996. The instructive role of innate immunity in the acquired immune response. *Science* **272**:50–53.

Field, M. C., and J. C. Boothroyd. 1996. Sequence divergence in a family of variant surface glycoprotein genes from trypanosomes: coding region hypervariability and downstream recombinogenic repeats. *J. Mol. Evol.* **42**:500–511.

Glaser, K. B., A. Sung, J. Bauer, and B. M. Weichman. 1993. Regulation of eicosanoid biosynthesis in the macrophage. Involvement of protein tyrosine phosphorylation and modulation by selective protein tyrosine kinase inhibitors. *Biochem. Pharmacol.* **45**:711–721.

Golden, A., and J. S. Brugge. 1989. Thrombin treatment induces rapid changes in tyrosine phosphorylation in platelets. *Proc. Natl. Acad. Sci. USA* **86**:901–905.

Golden, A., S. P. Nemeth, and J. S. Brugge. 1986. Blood platelets express high levels of the pp60c-src-specific tyrosine kinase activity. *Proc. Natl. Acad. Sci. USA* **83**:852–856.

Green, S. P., J. A. Hamilton, and W. A. Phillips. 1992. Zymosan-triggered tyrosine phosphorylation in mouse bone-marrow-derived macrophages is enhanced by respiratory-burst priming agents. *Biochem. J.* **288**:427–432.

Greenberg, S., P. Chang, and S. C. Silverstein. 1993. Tyrosine phosphorylation of the gamma subunit of Fc gamma receptors, p72syk, and paxillin during Fc receptor-mediated phagocytosis in macrophages. *J. Biol. Chem.* **269**:3897–3902.

Guy, R. A., and M. Belosevic. 1993. Comparison of receptors required for entry of *Leishmania major* amastigotes into macrophages. *Infect. Immun.* **61**:1553–1558.

Haque, S., H. Dumon, A. Haque, and L. H. Kasper. 1998. Alteration of intracellular calcium flux and impairment of nuclear factor-AT translocation in T cells during acute *Toxoplasma gondii* infection in mice. *J. Immunol.* **161**:6812–6818.

Harnett, W., M. R. Deehan, K. M. Houston, and M. M. Harnett. 1999. Immunomodulatory properties of a phosphorylcholine-containing secreted filarial glycoprotein. *Parasite Immunol.* **21**: 601–608.

Haspel, R. L. M. Salditt-Georgieff, and J. E. Darnell. 1996. The rapid inactivation of nuclear tyrosine phosphorylated Stat1 depends upon a protein tyrosine phosphatase. *EMBO J.* **15**:6262–6268.

Heinzel, F. P., M. D. Sadick, B. J. Holaday, R. L. Coffman, and R. M. Locksley. 1989. Reciprocal expression of interferon gamma or interleukin 4 during the resolution or progression of murine leishmaniasis. Evidence for expansion of distinct helper T cell subsets. *J. Exp. Med.* **169**:59–72.

Heinzel, F. P., M. D. Sadick, and R. M. Locksley. 1988. *Leishmania major:* analysis of lymphocyte and macrophage cellular phenotypes during infection of susceptible and resistant mice. *Exp. Parasitol.* **65**:258–268.

Hertz, C. J., and J. M. Mansfield. 1999. IFN-gamma-dependent nitric oxide production is not linked to resistance in experimental African trypanosomiasis. *Cell. Immunol.* **192**:24–32.

Hertz, C. J., H. Filutowicz, and J. M. Mansfield. 1998. Resistance to the African trypanosomes is IFN-gamma dependent. *J. Immunol.* **161**:6775–6783.

Hoeijmakers, J. H., A. C. Frasch, A. Bernards, P. Borst, and G. A. Cross. 1980. Novel expression-linked copies of the genes for variant surface antigens in trypanosomes. *Nature* **284**:78–80.

Hommel, M. 1997. Modulation of host cell receptors: a mechanism for the survival of malaria parasites. *Parasitology* **115**:S45–S54.

Hooft van Huijsduijnen, R. 1998. Protein tyrosine phosphatases: counting the trees in the forest. *Gene* **225**:1–8.

Horn, D., and G. A. Cross. 1997. Analysis of *Trypanosoma brucei vsg* expression site switching in vitro. *Mol. Biochem. Parasitol.* **84**:189–201.

Hunter, T. 1993. Signal transduction. Cytokine connections. *Nature* **366**:114–116.

Hunter, T., and B. M. Sefton. 1980. Transforming gene product of Rous sarcoma virus phosphorylates tyrosine. *Proc. Natl. Acad. Sci. USA* **77**:1311–1315.

Hunter, T., and J. A. Cooper. 1985. Protein-tyrosine kinases. *Annu. Rev. Biochem.* **54**:897–930.

Kima, P. E., N. H. Ruddle, and D. McMahon-Pratt. 1987. Presentation via the class I pathway by *Leishmania amazonensis*-infected macrophages of an endogenous leishmanial antigen to CD8+ T cells. *J. Immunol.* **159**:1828–1834.

Klee, C. B., T. H. Crouch, and M. H. Krinks. 1979. Calcineurin: a calcium- and calmodulin-binding protein of the nervous system. *Proc. Natl. Acad. Sci. USA* **76**:6270–6273.

Kozlowski, M., I. Mlinaric-Rascan, G. S. Feng, R. Shen, T. Pawson, and K. A. Siminovitch. 1993. Expression and catalytic activity of the tyrosine phosphatase PTP1C is severely impaired in motheaten and viable motheaten mice. *J. Exp. Med.* **178**:2157–2163.

Kukita, M., M. Hirata, and T. Koga. 1986. Requirement of Ca2+ for the production and degradation of inositol 1,4,5-triphosphate in macrophages. *Biochim. Biophys. Acta* **885**:121–128.

Leonard, W. J., and J. J. O'Shea. 1998. JAKs and STATs: biological implications. *Annu. Rev. Immunol.* **16**:293–322.

Liu, B., J. Liao, X. Rao, S. A. Kushner, C. D. Chung, D. D. Chang, and K. Shuai. 1998. Inhibition of Stat1-mediated gene activation by PIAS1. *Proc. Natl. Acad. Sci. USA* **95**:10626–10631.

Locksley, R. M., F. P. Heinzel, B. J. Holaday, S. S. Mutha, S. L. Reiner, and M. D. Sadick. 1991. Induction of Th1 and Th2 CD4+ subsets during murine *Leishmania major* infection. *Res. Immunol.* **142**:28–32.

Locksley, R. M., F. P. Heinzel, M. D. Sadick, B. J. Holaday, and K. Gardner. 1987. Murine cutaneous leishmaniasis: susceptibil-

ity correlates with differential expansion of helper T-cell subsets. *Ann. Inst. Pasteur Immunol.* **138**:744–749.

Locksley, R. M., and P. Scott. 1991. Helper T-cell subsets in mouse leishmaniasis: induction, expansion and effector function. *Immunol. Today* **12**:A58–A61.

Locksley, R. M., A. E. Wakil, D. B. Corry, S. Pingel, M. Bix, and D. J. Fowell. 1995. The development of effector T cell subsets in murine *Leishmania major* infection. *Ciba Found. Symp.* **195**: 110–117.

Mansfield, J. M. 1994. T-cell responses to the trypanosome variant surface glycoprotein: a new paradigm? *Parasitol. Today* **10**:267–270.

Mansfield, J. M. 1995. Immunobiology of African trypanosomiasis: a revisionist view, p. 477–496. *In* J. C. Boothroyd and R. Komuniecki (ed.), *Molecular Approaches to Parasitology*. Wiley-Liss, New York, N.Y.

Mansfield, J. M., R. F. Levine, W. L. Dempsey, S. R. Wellhausen, and C. T. Hansen. 1981. Lymphocyte function in experimental African trypanosomiasis. IV. Immunosuppression and suppressor cells in the athymic nu/nu mouse. *Cell. Immunol.* **63**:210–215.

Marth, T., and B. L. Kelsall. 1997. Regulation of interleukin-12 by complement receptor 3 signaling. *J. Exp. Med.* **185**:1987–1995.

Matte, C., J.-F. Marquis, J. Blanchette, P. Gros, R. Faure, and M. Olivier. 2000. Peroxovanadium-mediated protection against murine leishmaniasis: role of the modulation of nitric oxide. *Eur. J. Immunol.* **30**:2555–2564.

Matthews, R. J., D. B. Bowne, E. Flores, and M. L. Thomas. 1992. Characterization of hematopoietic intracellular protein tyrosine phosphatases: description of a phosphatase containing an SH2 domain and another enriched in proline-, glutamic acid-, serine-, and threonine-rich sequences. *Mol. Cell. Biol.* **12**:2396–2405.

Mauel, J. 1990. Macrophage-parasite interactions in *Leishmania* infections. *J. Leukoc. Biol.* **47**:187–193.

Metcalf, P., M. Blum, D. Freymann, M. Turner, and D. C. Wiley. 1987. Two variant surface glycoproteins of *Trypanosoma brucei* of different sequence classes have similar 6 Å resolution X-ray structures *Nature* **325**:84–86.

Mosser, D. M., and P. J. Edelson. 1984. Activation of the alternative complement pathway by *Leishmania* promastigotes: parasite lysis and attachment to macrophages. *J. Immunol.* **132**: 1501–1505.

Mosser, D. M., and P. J. Edelson. 1985. The mouse macrophage receptor for C3bi (CR3) is a major mechanism in the phagocytosis of *Leishmania* promastigotes. *J. Immunol.* **135**:2785–2789.

Moudgil, K. D., E. E. Sercarz, and I. S. Grewal. 1998. Modulation of the immunogenicity of antigenic determinants by their flanking residues. *Immunol. Today* **19**:217–220.

Muller, M., J. Briscoe, C. Laxton, D. Guschin, A. Ziemiecki, O. Silvennoinen, A. G. Harpur, G. Barbieri, B. A. Witthuhn, C. Schindler, et al. 1993. The protein tyrosine kinase JAK1 complements defects in interferon-alpha/beta and -gamma signal transduction. *Nature* **366**:129–135.

Muller, N., and B. Gottstein. 1998. Antigenic variation and the murine immune response to *Giardia lamblia*. *Int. J. Parasitol.* **28**:1829–1839.

Murray, H. W., H. Masur, and J. S. Keithly. 1982. Cell-mediated immune response in experimental visceral leishmaniasis. I. Correlation between resistance to Leishmania donovani and lymphokine-generating capacity. *J. Immunol.* **129**:344–350.

Murray, H. W., J. J. Stern, K. Welte, B. Y. Rubin, S. M. Carriero, and C. F. Nathan. 1987. Experimental visceral leishmaniasis: production of interleukin 2 and interferon-gamma, tissue immune reaction, and response to treatment with interleukin 2 and interferon-gamma. *J. Immunol.* **138:**2290–2297.

Nash, T. E. 1997. Antigenic variation in *Giardia lamblia* and the host's immune response. *Philos. Trans. R. Soc. London Ser. B* **352:**1369–1375.

Navarro, M., and G. A. M. Cross. 1996. DNA rearrangements associated with multiple consecutive directed antigenic switches in *Trypanosoma brucei*. *Mol. Cell. Biol.* **16:**3615–3625.

Newbold, C. I. 1999. Antigenic variation in *Plasmodium falciparum:* mechanisms and consequences. *Curr. Opin. Microbiol.* **2:** 420–425.

Olivier, M. 1996. Modulation of host cell intracellular Ca^{2+}. *Parasitol. Today* **12:**145–150.

Olivier, M., K. G. Baimbridge, and N. E. Reiner. 1992a. Stimulus-response coupling in monocytes infected with *Leishmania*. Attenuation of calcium transients is related to defective agonist-induced accumulation of inositol phosphates. *J. Immunol.* **148:**1188–1196.

Olivier, M., S. Bertrand, and C. E. Tanner. 1989a. Killing of *Leishmania donovani* by activated liver macrophages from resistant and susceptible strains mice. *Int. J. Parasitol.* **19:**377–383.

Olivier, M., R. W. Brownsey, and N. E. Reiner. 1992b. Defective stimulus-response coupling in human monocytes infected with *Leishmania donovani* is associated with altered activation and translocation of protein kinase C. *Proc. Natl. Acad. Sci. USA* **89:** 7481–7485.

Olivier, M., C. Proulx, and C. E. Tanner. 1989b. Importance of lymphokines in the control of the multiplication and dispersion of *Leishmania donovani* within liver macrophages of resistant and susceptible mice. *J. Parasitol.* **75:**720–727.

Olivier, M., B. J. Romero-Gallo, C. Matte, J. Blanchette, B. I. Posner, M. J. Tremblay, and R. Faure. 1998. Modulation of interferon-gamma-induced macrophage activation by phosphotyrosine phosphatases inhibition. Effect on murine leishmaniasis progression. *J. Biol. Chem.* **273:**13944–13949.

Olivier, M., and C. Tanner. 1989. The effect of cyclosporin A in murine visceral leishmaniasis. *Trop. Med. Parasitol.* **40:**32–38.

Plutzky, J., B. B. Neel, and R. D. Rosenberg. 1992. Isolation of a src homology 2-containing tyrosine phosphatase. *Proc. Natl. Acad. Sci. USA* **89:**1123–1127.

Posner, B. I., R. Faure, J. W. Burgess, A. P. Bevan, D. Lachance, G. Zhang-Sun, J. B. Ng, D. A. Hall, B. S. Lum, and A. Shaver. 1994. Peroxovanadium compounds. A new class of potent phosphotyrosine phosphatase inhibitors which are insulin mimetics. *J. Biol. Chem.* **269:**4596–4604.

Ramasamy, R. 1998. Molecular basis for evasion of host immunity and pathogenesis in malaria. *Biochim. Biophys. Acta* **1406:**10–27.

Ray, M., A. A. Gam, R. A. Boykins, and R. T. Kenney. 2000. Inhibition of interferon-γ signaling by *Leishmania donovani*. *J. Infect. Dis.* **181:**1121–1128.

Reiner, N. E., W. Ng, T. Ma, and W. R. McMaster. 1988. Kinetics of gamma interferon binding and induction of major histocompatibility complex class II mRNA in Leishmania-infected macrophages. *Proc. Natl. Acad. Sci. USA* **85:**4330–4334.

Reiner, N. E., W. Ng, and W. R. McMaster. 1987. Parasite-accessory cell interactions in murine leishmaniasis. II. *Leishmania donovani* suppresses macrophage expression of class I and class II major histocompatibility complex gene products. *J. Immunol.* **138:**1926–1932.

Reiner, S. L., and R. M. Locksley. 1995. The regulation of immunity to *Leishmania major*. *Ann. Rev. Immunol.* **13:**151–177.

Reinitz, D. M., B. D. Aizenstein, and J. M. Mansfield. 1992. Variable and conserved structural elements of trypanosome variant surface glycoproteins. *Mol. Biochem. Parasitol.* **51:**119–132.

Reinitz, D. M., and J. M. Mansfield. 1988. Independent regulation of B cell responses to surface and subsurface epitopes of African trypanosome variable surface glycoproteins. *J. Immunol.* **141:** 620–626.

Reinitz, D. M., and J. M. Mansfield. 1990. T-cell-independent and T-cell-dependent B-cell responses to exposed variant surface glycoprotein epitopes in trypanosome-infected mice. *Infect. Immun.* **58:**2337–2342.

Rivett, A. J. 1998. Intracellular distribution of proteasomes. *Curr. Opin. Immunol.* **10:**110–114.

Roach, P. J. 1991. Multisite and hierarchal protein phosphorylation. *J. Biol. Chem.* **266:**14139–14142.

Russell, D. G., and P. Talamas-Rohana. 1989. *Leishmania* and the macrophage: a marriage of inconvenience. *Immunol. Today* **10:** 328–333.

Scharton-Kersten, T., and P. Scott. 1995. The role of the innate immune response in Th1 cell development following *Leishmania major* infection. *J. Leukoc. Biol.* **57:**515–522.

Schleifer, K. W., H. Filutowicz, L. R. Schopf, and J. M. Mansfield. 1993. Characterization of T helper cell responses to the trypanosome variant surface glycoprotein. *J. Immunol.* **150:**2910–2919.

Schleifer, K. W., and J. M. Mansfield. 1993. Suppressor macrophages in African trypanosomiasis inhibit T cell proliferative responses by nitric oxide and prostaglandins. *J. Immunol.* **151:** 5492–5503.

Schneider, S. C., and E. E. Sercarz. 1997. Antigen processing differences among APC. *Hum. Immunol.* **54:**148–158.

Schopf, L. R., H. Filutowicz, X. J. Bi, and J. M. Mansfield. 1998. Interleukin-4-dependent immunoglobulin G1 isotype switch in the presence of a polarized antigen-specific Th1-cell response to the trypanosome variant surface glycoprotein *Infect. Immun.* **66:**451–461.

Schopf, L. R., and J. M. Mansfield. 1998. Characterization of a relatively rare class B, type 2 trypanosome variant surface glycoprotein gene. *J. Parasitol.* **84:**284.

Schwarzer, E., M. Alessio, D. Ulliers, and P. Arese. 1998. Phagocytosis of the malarial pigment, hemozoin, impairs expression of major histocompatibility complex class II antigen, CD54, and CD11c in human monocytes. *Infect. Immun.* **66:**1601–1606.

Schwarzer, E., and P. Arese. 1996. Phagocytosis of malarial pigment hemozoin inhibits NADPH-oxidase activity in human monocyte-derived macrophages. *Biochim. Biophys. Acta* **1316:** 169–175.

Scott, P. 1990. T-cell subsets and T-cell antigens in protective immunity against experimental leishmaniasis. *Curr. Top. Microbiol. Immunol.* **155:**35–52.

Scott, P. 1991. Host and parasite factors regulating the development of CD4+ T-cell subsets in experimental cutaneous leishmaniasis. *Res. Immunol.* **142:**32–36.

Scott, P., E. Pearce, A. W. Cheever, R. L. Coffman, and A. Sher. 1989. Role of cytokines and CD4+ T-cell subsets in the regulation of parasite immunity and disease. *Immunol. Rev.* **112:** 161–182.

Seed, J. R., and J. B. Sechelski. 1989. African trypanosomes: inheritance of factors involved in resistance. *Exp. Parasitol.* **69:** 1–8.

Sercarz, E. E. 1998. Immune focusing vs diversification and their connection to immune regulation. *Immunol. Rev.* **164:**5–10.

Shen, S.-H., L. Bastien, B. I. Posner, and P. Chretien. 1991. A protein-tyrosine phosphatase with sequence similarity to the SH2 domain of the protein-tyrosine kinases. *Nature* **352:**736–739.

Shuai, K., G. R. Stark, I. M. Kerr, and J. E. Darnell. 1993. A single phosphotyrosine residue of Stat91 required for gene activation by interferon-gamma. *Science* **261:**1744–1746.

Silvennoinen, O., J. N. Ihle, J. Schlessinger, and D. E. Levy. 1993. Interferon-induced nuclear signalling by Jak protein tyrosine kinases. *Nature* **366:**583–585.

Snapper, C. M., M. R. Kehry, B. E. Castle, and J. J. Mond. 1995a. Multivalent, but not divalent, antigen receptor cross-linkers synergize with CD40 ligand for induction of Ig synthesis and class switching in normal murine B cells. A redefinition of the TI-2 vs T cell-dependent antigen dichotomy *J. Immunol.* **154:**1177–1187.

Snapper, C. M. and J. J. Mond. 1996. A model for induction of T cell-independent humoral immunity in response to polysaccharide antigens. *J. Immunol.* **157:**2229–2233.

Snapper, C. M., F. R. Rosas, L. Jin, C. Wortham, M. R. Kehry, and J. J. Mond. 1995b. Bacterial lipoproteins may substitute for cytokines in the humoral immune response to T cell-independent type II antigens. *J. Immunol.* **155:**5582–5589.

Snapper, C. M., H. Yamaguchi, M. A. Moorman, and J. J. Mond. 1994. An in vitro model for T cell-independent induction of humoral immunity. A requirement for NK cells. *J. Immunol.* **152:**4884–4892.

Stenger, S., N. Donhauser, H. Thüring, M. Röllinghoff, and C. Bogdan. 1996. Reactivation of latent leishmaniasis by inhibition of inducible nitric oxide synthase. *J. Exp. Med.* **183:**1501–1514.

Stohwasser, R., S. Standera, I. Peters, P. M. Kloetzel, and M. Groettrup. 1997. Molecular cloning of the mouse proteasome subunits MC14 and MECL-1: reciprocally regulated tissue expression of interferon-gamma-modulated proteasome subunits. *Eur. J. Immunol.* **27:**1182–1187.

Sutterwala, F. S., G. J. Noel, R. Clynes, and D. M. Mosser. 1997. Selective suppression of interleukin-12 induction after macrophage receptor ligation. *J. Exp. Med.* **185:**1977–1985.

Tachado, S. D., P. Gerold, R. Schwarz, S. Novakovic, M. McConville, and L. Schofield. 1997. Signal transduction in macrophages by glycosylphosphatidylinositols of *Plasmodium*, *Trypanosoma*, and *Leishmania*: activation of protein tyrosine kinases and protein kinase C by inositolglycan and diacylglycerol moieties. *Proc. Natl. Acad. Sci. USA* **94:**4022–4027.

Tachado, S. D., R. Mazhari-Tabrizi, and L. Schofield. 1999. Specificity in signal transduction among glycosylphosphatidyl-inositols of *Plasmodium falciparum*, *Trypanosoma brucei*, *Trypanosoma cruzi* and *Leishmania* spp. *Parasite Immunol.* **21:**609–617.

Turco, S. J. 1999. Adversarial relationship between the leishmania lipophosphoglycan and protein kinase C of host macrophages. *Parasite Immunol.* **21:**597–600.

Turner, C. M., and J. D. Barry. 1989. High frequency of antigenic variation in *Trypanosoma brucei rhodesiense* infections. *Parasitology* **1:**67–75.

Turner, C. M. R. 1997. The rate of antigenic variation in fly-transmitted and syringe-passaged infections of *Trypanosoma brucei*. *FEMS Microbiol. Lett.* **153:**227–231.

Van der Ploeg, L. H., K. Gottesdiener, and M. G. Lee. 1992. Antigenic variation in African trypanosomes. *Trends Genet.* **8:**452–457.

Vickerman, K., and A. G. Luckins. 1969. Localization of variable antigens in the surface coat of *Trypanosoma brucei* using ferritin conjugated antibody. *Nature* **224:**1125–1126.

Walton, K. M., and J. E. Dixon. 1993. Protein tyrosine phosphatases. *Annu. Rev. Biochem.* **62:**101–120.

Watling, D., D. Guschin, M. Muller, O. Silvennoinen, B. A. Witthuhn, F. W. Quelle, N. C. Rogers, C. Schindler, G. R. Stark, J. N. Ihle, et al. 1993. Complementation by the protein tyrosine kinase JAK2 of a mutant cell line defective in the interferon-gamma signal transduction pathway. *Nature* **366:**166–170.

Yeung, Y. G., K. L. Berg, F. J. Pixley, R. H. Angeletti, and E. R. Stanley. 1992. Protein tyrosine phosphatase-1C is rapidly phosphorylated in tyrosine in macrophages in response to colony stimulating factor-1. *J. Biol. Chem.* **267:**23447–23450.

Yi, T., J. L. Cleveland, and J. N. Ihle. 1992. Protein tyrosine phosphatase containing SH2 domains: characterization, preferential expression in hematopoietic cells, and localization to human chromosome 12p12-p13. *Mol. Cell. Biol.* **12:**836–846.

Yu, C. L., and S. J. Burakoff. 1997. Involvement of proteasomes in regulating Jak-STAT pathways upon interleukin-2 stimulation. *J. Biol. Chem.* **272:**14017–14020.

Zinkernagel, R. M. 2000. What is missing in immunology to understand immunity? *Nat. Immunol.* **1:**181–185.

VII. IMMUNOGENETICS

Immunology of Infectious Diseases
Edited by S. H. E. Kaufmann, A. Sher, and R. Ahmed
© 2002 ASM Press, Washington, D.C.

Chapter 26

Immunogenetics of the Host Response to Bacteria and Parasites in Humans

Laurent Abel and Jean-Laurent Casanova

A causative infectious agent (virus, bacterium, or parasite) is absolutely required but often not sufficient for the development of an infectious disease. This results in extensive variation in the response observed among individuals exposed to a given infectious agent, strongly suggesting that host factors play an important role in susceptibility or resistance to infections. Evidence for this variability is provided by the following observations: (i) for most infectious agents, a fraction of the subjects exposed never become infected; (ii) the level of infection (e.g., egg counts in infection by *Schistosoma mansoni*) often differs greatly among infected subjects; (iii) some infected subjects do not develop clinical disease; and (iv) clinical manifestations of disease (severity, time to onset, etc.) may differ greatly among symptomatic patients. Furthermore, this large interindividual variability generally contrasts with the high level of intraethnic and/or intrafamilial similarity.

The use of experimental animal models in which infection, environmental factors, and genetic background (gene knockout, natural mutants, and transgenic animals) can be controlled has demonstrated the profound influence of the genetic makeup of the host on resistance to infections (Wakelin and Blackwell, 1988; McLeod et al., 1995). In humans, two basic types of situation are observed. In certain rare infections, the family structure (e.g., consanguineous parents) or the familial relationships between infected subjects suggest simple Mendelian inheritance (monogenic). Although rare, a number of Mendelian syndromes of susceptibility to infectious agents have been described, notably the predisposition to infection by weakly virulent mycobacteria (Altare et al., 1998b). Mendelian resistance to some pathogens, such as *Plasmodium vivax* (Miller et al., 1976; Barn-

well et al., 1989), has also been described, and the molecular basis of the Duffy blood group system accounting for this resistance to *P. vivax* has been elucidated (Iwamoto et al., 1995; Tournamille et al., 1995). More commonly, the genetic predisposition is more complex (polygenic), as suggested by various lines of evidence (e.g., a higher frequency of the disease in monozygotic than in dizygotic twins and ethnic or familial aggregation for the disease under study). The distinction between these two categories is somewhat blurred because other genes may have a substantial impact on the clinical expression of a Mendelian predisposition and because polygenic susceptibility may primarily reflect the effect of a predominant gene often referred to as a major gene. Therefore, some aspects of the strategies for searching for the genetic factors in these two situations are specific and others are complementary. These aspects are summarized in Fig. 1 and described in the next two paragraphs.

The genetic etiology of human Mendelian disorders can be determined using several strategies. Positional cloning approaches are based on the genotyping of polymorphic chromosomal markers in a number of affected kindreds. This strategy requires a sufficient number of informative families, and genetic homogeneity is absolutely required. Linkage analysis (classical lod-score or homozygosity mapping) is usually the first step, although the identification of visible cytogenetic rearrangements can be very helpful for the mapping of the gene (Collins, 1995). Another strategy, known as the candidate gene approach, relies on the selection of genes based on studies in animal models or in vitro. The contribution of these candidate genes "by hypothesis" is tested by using functional arrays and/or mutation de-

Laurent Abel and Jean-Laurent Casanova • Laboratory of Human Genetics of Infectious Diseases, Necker Medical School, 75015 Paris, France.

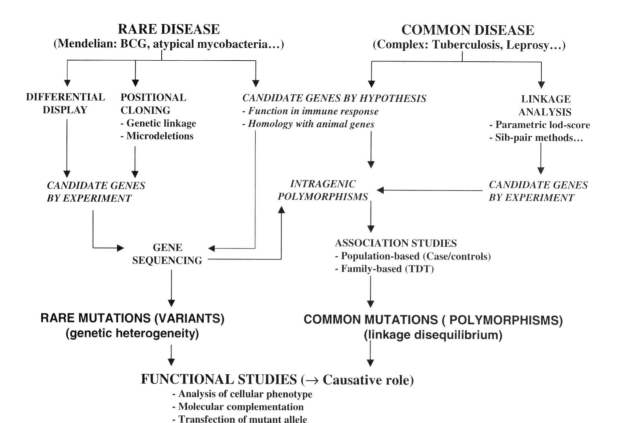

Figure 1. Summary of the methods and strategies used to identify the genes and genetic polymorphisms involved in human infectious diseases. The genetic etiology of rare Mendelian disorders can be determined by several strategies. Linkage analysis is usually the first step in the positional cloning approach, although the identification of visible cytogenetic rearrangements can be of great help in the mapping of the gene. Another strategy, known as the candidate gene approach ("by hypothesis"), involves the prior selection of genes (from animal models or in vitro experiments), which are then tested by functional arrays and/or mutation detection. Another promising strategy, which may be more fruitful in the future, is based on analysis of the differential expressions of genes in tissues from affected and healthy individuals. In common infectious diseases, linkage studies (model based or model free) are used to search for a chromosomal region that segregates nonrandomly with the infectious disease-related phenotype within families. The role of polymorphisms of candidate genes located within this candidate region is tested by population-based or family-based association studies. Candidate genes by hypothesis can also be chosen on the basis of their function or homology to animal loci. Evidence for an association should be validated by functional studies to determine whether the detected polymorphism modifies gene expression or the gene product in a manner that may affect susceptibility to the disease.

tection. Interestingly, these two strategies can be combined. For example, the isolation of *IFNGR1* as a Mendelian susceptibility gene was achieved by a genomewide positional cloning to identify a candidate region in which *IFNGR1* was tested as a candidate gene "by experiment" (Newport et al., 1996) and by a candidate gene approach in which *IFNGR1* was selected a candidate gene by hypothesis and positional cloning to test for linkage with *IFNGR1* by homozygosity mapping (Jouanguy et al., 1996). Another promising strategy, which may be more fruitful in the future, is based on analysis of the differential expressions of genes in tissues from affected and healthy individuals.

The role of genetic factors in common infectious diseases can be investigated by the analysis of several complementary traits (Abel and Dessein, 1998). These traits include clinical phenotypes, which are generally binary (i.e., affected or unaffected); biological phenotypes, such as measures of infection, which may be quantitative (e.g., fecal egg counts in schistosomiasis) or binary (seropositive/seronegative); and measures of the immune response (e.g., antibody levels, cytokine levels, and skin test response). The panel of phenotypes available for study for a given infectious disease facilitates investigation of the genetic control of various steps in the pathogenic process (Abel and Dessein, 1997). Specific methods of genetic epidemiology, combining epidemiological and genetic information, are used to determine the respective roles of genetic and environmental factors in the expression of phenotypes and to identify the principal genes involved (Khoury et al., 1993; Lander and Schork, 1994; Abel and Dessein, 1998). Epidemiological data include classical risk factors that may influence the trait under study (e.g., age and factors affecting exposure to the infectious agent). Genetic information includes the familial relationship between study subjects (e.g., collections of families) and the typing of genetic markers. Recent developments, such as the establishment of a genetic map of the human genome based on highly polymorphic markers (Dib et al., 1996) and the growing availability of single nucleotide polymorphisms located within candidate genes (Wang et al., 1998; Kruglyak, 1999), have led to the creation of tools essential for these genetic studies.

The ultimate goal of genetic epidemiology methods is to identify the genes (and the alleles of these genes) that significantly account for the phenotype of interest and to determine the possible interactions of these alleles with environmental factors. Numerous methods have been (and are being) developed, and they generally fall into two categories (Lander and Schork, 1994; Abel and Dessein, 1997, 1998): linkage analysis methods, which seek to locate a chromosomal region that segregates nonrandomly with the phenotype of interest within families, and association studies, which test for a statistically significant association between a specific genetic polymorphism and a phenotype within a population (Fig. 1). In human genetics of infectious diseases, linkage analyses are used to locate a chromosomal region that contains one or several genes of interest. Linkage studies can be used to explore the whole genome (genome screen), ensuring that all major loci involved in the control of a phenotype are identified and making it possible to discover new genes (and, consequently, new physiopathologic pathways). Linkage studies are classically divided into model-based and model-free approaches (Abel and Dessein, 1997; Ott, 1999). The model-based (or parametric) approach, corresponding to the classical lod-score method (Morton, 1955), is so called since it requires explicit specification of the phenotype and genotype model. The parameters of this model (allelic frequency, penetrance functions) are estimated by segregation analysis, taking into account the role of relevant environmental factors (such as those influencing the risk of infection). This strategy has been successfully used in schistosomiasis studies. The model-free (or nonparametric) approach is so called because specification of the phenotype and genotype model is not required. The most commonly used model-free approach is the sib-pair method, which has been used in studies of leprosy and malaria. Although these linkage studies can demonstrate the involvement of

a chromosomal region, they are not able to provide a fine mapping of the genes responsible for such complex phenotypes.

Association studies can then be used to investigate the role of polymorphisms (or alleles) of candidate genes located in the regions previously identified (candidate genes by experiment). Association studies can also be used as a first step by directly investigating the influence of candidate genes by hypothesis (e.g., genes that confer Mendelian predispositions to infectious diseases). Classical association studies are population-based case-control studies comparing the frequency of a given marker allele (or polymorphism) in unrelated affected individuals and unrelated unaffected controls (Khoury et al., 1993). Family-based association methods, such as the transmission disequilibrium test (Spielman et al., 1993), have recently been developed and avoid the possible control selection bias (e.g., due to a population admixture) of population-based studies. Optimal results for association studies are obtained using candidate gene approaches. However, interpretation of the results may be difficult because the power of such studies depends on several factors such as linkage disequilibrium between polymorphisms, polymorphism frequencies, and the prior probability that the true functional polymorphism belongs to the tested polymorphisms (Muller-Myhsok and Abel, 1997; Abel and Muller-Myhsok, 1998). In any case, the role of a given genetic polymorphism must be validated by functional studies, underlying the complementary nature of genetic epidemiology and molecular genetics.

There is no single optimal strategy for investigation of the genes involved in human infectious diseases, and the choice of a design for a particular study depends on several factors related to phenotype (e.g., nature and frequency), population, possibility of measuring environmental factors accurately, and known genetic background. Various infections have been studied in recent years. The following sections focus on the main findings obtained in studies of susceptibility or resistance to mycobacterial and certain parasitic infections.

MYCOBACTERIAL INFECTIONS

Tuberculosis and leprosy, the most common human mycobacterial diseases, are caused by *Mycobacterium tuberculosis* and *M. leprae*, respectively. Many other mycobacterial species are present in the environment and are denoted as nontuberculous mycobacteria (NTM). Like the live attenuated *M. bovis* BCG vaccine, they are generally less pathogenic than

M. tuberculosis and *M. leprae,* but they do cause a variety of infections. There is now clear evidence that the intrinsic virulence of mycobacterial species is not the sole factor determining clinical outcome, which depends to a large extent on the genetic background of the infected individual. Major advances have been made by genetic dissection of disseminated infections caused by poorly virulent mycobacteria such as NTM and BCG. In addition, many genetic epidemiology studies have shown that human genes play an important role in the expression of leprosy and tuberculosis, although the molecular basis of this genetic control remains largely unknown.

Disseminated Infections with Weakly Pathogenic Mycobacteria

In humans, BCG and NTM may cause severe infections in patients with hereditary immunodeficiency (World Health Organization, 1997). Such infections may also occur in apparently healthy individuals with no known immunodeficiency (Casanova et al., 1995, 1996; Levin et al., 1995; Frucht and Holland, 1996). Autosomal recessive transmission of this syndrome is generally observed (Casanova et al., 1996; McKusick, 1998). In some families, however, the segregation of the disease is autosomal dominant (Jouanguy et al., 1999b) or recessive and X-chromosome linked (Frucht and Holland, 1996). The clinical prognosis is variable and correlates strongly with the type of histopathological lesions observed, suggesting that the genetic defect is indeed heterogeneous (Emile et al., 1997). In the last 5 years, we and others have described extensively various types of causative mutations in four genes defining eight genetic diseases.

The first identified genetic determinant of the syndrome is a complete deficiency in the first chain of the gamma interferon (IFN-γ) receptor (IFN-γR1) (Jouanguy et al., 1996, 2000; Newport et al., 1996; Pierre-Audigier et al., 1997; Altare et al., 1998a; Holland et al., 1998; Roesler et al., 1999). All causative mutations are both null and recessive, but depending on the type of mutation, the receptor may or may not be expressed on the cell surface. The precise immunological cells responsible for infection are not known, because the IFN-γ receptor is ubiquitously expressed. Complete deficiencies in the IFN-γR1 chain are associated with the early onset of severe mycobacterial infection (Casanova et al., 1999). The granulomas are lepromatoid, often multibacillary, poorly defined, and poorly differentiated without giant cells. Curative treatment involves bone marrow transplantation because treatment with antibiotics does not ensure complete remission of infection and because IFN-γ is inefficient in the absence of a specific receptor.

A partial, as opposed to complete, recessive IFN-γR1 chain deficiency (Jouanguy et al., 1997) was found in two siblings. The functional defect is partial because high concentrations of IFN-γ may induce a cellular response. Other patients had partial dominant, but not recessive, deficiencies of the IFN-γR1 chain (Jouanguy et al., 1999b). The same mutation has arisen independently in 12 families, defining the first hot spot for small deletions in humans. This disease may arise in adults, and the granulomas are tuberculous, paucibacillary, well defined, and well differentiated with giant cells. Infections are treated with antibiotics and IFN-γ. Thus, there is a correlation between *IFNGR1* genotype, cellular phenotype (partial or complete defects), pathological phenotype (tuberculoid or lepromatoid granulomas), and clinical phenotype (good or poor prognosis) (Jouanguy et al., 1999b).

A patient with a recessive complete deficiency of the second chain of the IFN-γR (IFN-γR2) has been described (Dorman and Holland, 1998). The pathological and clinical phenotypes were severe, apparently similar to those of patients with a complete deficiency of the IFN-γR1 chain. Treatment of this condition also necessitates bone marrow transplantation. Another patient with a partial recessive defect in the IFN-γR2 chain has been reported (Doffinger et al., 2000). This mutation did not compromise the surface expression of the IFN-γR2 molecule and decreased, but did not completely abolish, the cellular response to IFN-γ. The patient displayed attenuated pathological and clinical phenotypes. Thus, there is also a strict correlation between the *IFNGR2* genotype and the cellular, pathological, and clinical phenotypes.

A recessive null mutation in the gene encoding the p40 subunit of interleukin-12 (IL-12) has been identified in a child (Altare et al., 1998c). IL-12 is a heterodimeric cytokine (p70, made up of p35 and p40) secreted by macrophages and dendritic cells. The lymphocytes of this patient produced only low levels of IFN-γ after in vitro stimulation. However, this involved a secondary defect in the production of IFN-γ, since it was complemented in a dose-dependent manner by exogenous IL-12. Recessive null mutations of the gene encoding the β1 chain of the IL-12 receptor (IL-12Rβ1) have been identified in other patients (Altare et al., 1998a; de Jong et al., 1998). The defect in IFN-γ secretion, which is dependent on IL-12, is responsible for mycobacterial infections, and the treatment of these infections is therefore based on IFN-γ administration. Residual immunity mediated by IFN-γ, which persists independently of IL-12, is responsible for the attenuated phenotype.

In total, mutations in four genes are responsible for eight genetic diseases, which result in a predisposition to severe infections with BCG and NTM (Altare et al., 1998b; Jouanguy et al., 1999a). Biologically, these studies suggest that the degree of IL-12-dependent IFN-γ-mediated immunity is the determining factor in the development of mycobacterial infections in humans. Clinically, they stress the importance of accurate molecular diagnosis of the underlying inherited disorder for the rational treatment of patients with mycobacterial disease.

Leprosy

Leprosy, caused by *M. leprae,* is a chronic mycobacterial disease, whose prevalence has markedly decreased in recent years (less than 1 million cases worldwide in 1998). However, its incidence remains stable, around 700,000 new cases per year (Jacobson and Krahenbuhl, 1999). The clinical expression of the disease results from the interaction between the bacillus and the host immune system (Sansonetti and Lagrange, 1981). Whereas most infected individuals develop an effective immunity with no clinical disease (Jacobson and Krahenbuhl, 1999), some develop a wide spectrum of disease that is correlated with the immunological response of the patient. At one extreme of this spectrum, tuberculoid leprosy patients show well-developed specific cellular responses and low *M. leprae* antibody levels, whereas at the other extreme, lepromatous leprosy patients have poorly developed specific cellular responses and high *M. leprae* antibody levels.

Many studies of familial aggregation, twin studies, and segregation analyses have clearly shown that leprosy susceptibility has a significant genetic component (reviewed by Abel et al. [1995]). In particular, a segregation analysis performed on Desirade Island in the French West Indies found evidence for a recessive major gene controlling susceptibility to leprosy per se (i.e., regardless of clinical subtype) (Abel and Demenais, 1988). Association studies between leprosy and HLA have provided other lines of evidence for the role of genetic factors in diseases caused by *M. leprae*. In tuberculoid leprosy, the most consistent results were obtained for *HLA-DR2* (reviewed by van Eden and de Vries [1984] and Ottenhoff and de Vries [1987]). Using HLA molecular typing, Zerva et al. (1996) refined these results by showing a positive association between Indian tuberculoid leprosy patients and alleles *DRB1*1501, DRB1*1502* (both of which are *DR2* alleles), and *DRB1*1404*. Lepromatous leprosy was found to be

associated with *HLA-DR3* in several studies (reviewed by van Eden and de Vries [1984] and Ottenhoff and de Vries [1987]). A number of sib-pair linkage analyses have also shown nonrandom segregation of parental HLA haplotypes in sets of children with tuberculoid leprosy and in siblings with lepromatous leprosy (reviewed by van Eden and de Vries [1984], van Eden et al. [1985], and Abel et al. [1995]). However, the random segregation of HLA haplotypes in all leprosy patients and in healthy siblings in multicase leprosy families suggests that HLA-linked factors are not involved in the susceptibility to leprosy per se.

The identification of the human gene *NRAMP1* (Cellier et al., 1994), a homologue of the mouse gene *Nramp1,* has provided an excellent candidate gene for the study of susceptibility to leprosy per se. In mice, a single nonconservative amino acid substitution in the *Nramp1* gene is associated with susceptibility to several intracellular pathogens including *M. lepraemurium,* the rodent-tropic equivalent of *M. leprae* (Malo et al., 1994; Govoni et al., 1996; Vidal et al., 1996). Functional studies have shown that the *Nramp1* gene plays an important role early in the macrophage activation pathway and has many pleiotropic effects on macrophage function (reviewed by Canonne-Hergaux et al. [1999]). A recent sib-pair study of human subjects in Vietnam showed significant linkage between leprosy per se and *NRAMP1* haplotypes corresponding to six intragenic variants of *NRAMP1* and four polymorphic flanking markers (Abel et al., 1998). This provided the first evidence that *NRAMP1* may be a leprosy susceptibility locus. Combined with the segregation analysis performed in the same population (Abel et al., 1995), this study suggested a genetic heterogeneity according to the ethnic origin of the families (Vietnamese or Chinese). Genetic heterogeneity may account, at least in part, for the results of two previous studies that failed to detect linkage between leprosy and distal chromosome 2q, on which *NRAMP1* is located (Shaw et al., 1993; Levee et al., 1994). In the same Vietnamese study, the *NRAMP1* region was also found to be linked with the in vivo Mitsuda reaction, measuring the delayed immune response to intradermally injected lepromin (Alcais et al., 2000). This is consistent with the view that *NRAMP1* may be involved in the development of immune responses to mycobacterial antigens with a putative role in the regulation of Th1/Th2 differentiation (Blackwell et al., 1999). There is an increasing body of evidence that tuberculoid leprosy (generally displaying positive Mitsuda reactions) is associated with a predominantly Th1-type response, whereas a more Th2-type response is observed in lepromatous leprosy (Yamamura et al., 1991; Misra et al., 1995).

A recent association study in India indicated that vitamin D receptor (*VDR*) genotypes may also influence this Th1/Th2 balance (Roy et al., 1999). In this study, the two alleles of a polymorphism at codon 352 of the *VDR* gene, denoted T and t (with t being the less frequent), were found to be positively associated with lepromatous and tuberculoid leprosy, respectively. This finding suggests that TT homozygotes tend to have a Th2-type immune response and that tt homozygotes have a Th1-type response. These results, and those for parasitic diseases, highlight the considerable value of identifying the genetic factors regulating the Th1/Th2 balance in response to foreign antigens.

Tuberculosis

Tuberculosis, a chronic mycobacterial disease caused by *M. tuberculosis,* affects about one third of the world's population and causes about 2 million deaths each year (Dye et al., 1999). As with leprosy, the disease probably results from complex interactions between *M. tuberculosis,* environmental factors, and host genes. Among the vast number of infected persons, only 8 million people (around 10% of infected individuals) actually develop the disease each year. The role of genetic factors in tuberculosis in humans was suggested on the basis of strong ethnic differences, in particular a higher prevalence of the disease among blacks than among Caucasians (Stead et al., 1990). Twin studies also showed the importance of host genes by showing differences in concordance rates between monozygotic (~60%) and dizygotic (~20%) twins (reviewed by Fine [1981]). Far fewer familial studies have been performed for tuberculosis than for leprosy. A recent segregation analysis in Brazil (Shaw et al., 1997) found evidence for a complex genetic model involving oligogenic inheritance. Weak linkage was observed with the *NRAMP1* region in this study, but so far, no definitive results of ongoing genome-wide linkage studies (Hill, 1998) have been reported.

Numerous association studies have been performed for tuberculosis and HLA alleles, and the most consistent results have been obtained for class II alleles (reviewed by Hill [1998] and Goldfeld et al. [1998]). An effect of polymorphisms located within the genes for the IL-1 receptor antagonist and IL-1β on delayed-type hypersensitivity and tuberculosis expression has been reported for a Hindu population (Wilkinson et al., 1999). Finally, a study in Gambia investigated the influence of *NRAMP1* polymorphisms (Bellamy et al., 1998). Four *NRAMP1* variants

were found to predispose subjects to tuberculosis, with a particularly high risk of disease for subjects who were heterozygous for the two variants located in intron 4 and the 3′ untranslated region of the gene (Bellamy et al., 1998). In the same population, the frequency of subjects homozygous for allele t of the *VDR* polymorphism (described above in the leprosy section) was lower for tuberculosis patients than for controls (Bellamy et al., 1999). In this context, it is interesting that a deficiency in 25-hydroxycholecalciferol was recently found to be associated with active tuberculosis in a population of Asian origin (Wilkinson et al., 2000).

PARASITIC INFECTIONS

With the exception of malaria, the involvement of host genes in susceptibility to human parasitic infections has not been readily accepted, probably because environmental factors (i.e., vectors and reservoirs) play an important role in transmission. It was also thought that the changing properties of parasites accounted for much of the heterogeneity observed among individuals in areas of endemic infection. However, this view has evolved in recent years, and there is now solid evidence that intrinsic resistance to parasitic infections may differ greatly among individuals. Host genetics may strongly influence the outcome of infection for major parasitic diseases such as schistosomiasis and leishmaniasis, as well as for malaria. In the two following sections, we will review the main findings observed in malaria and schistosomiasis during the last few years.

Malaria

Severe malaria clinical phenotype

Most genetic epidemiology studies of malaria have searched for genes involved in generating the severe clinical phenotype (e.g., cerebral malaria with coma or severe anemia due to *Plasmodium falciparum* infection). Since this phenotype is relatively rare, familial studies are extremely difficult; instead, population-based association studies have been performed comparing the frequency of candidate gene polymorphisms in severe malaria cases and various types of control subjects.

The existence of genetic polymorphisms in red blood cells affecting susceptibility to severe malaria was first suggested more than 40 years ago, based on the high frequency of alleles encoding mutant hemoglobin chains (e.g., sickle cell anemia) in areas where malaria was endemic (reviewed by Weatherall

[1987] and Nagel and Roth [1989]). Recent studies have also confirmed the protective effect against severe malaria of glucose-6-phosphate dehydrogenase deficiency in Africa (Ruwende et al., 1995), and that of α^+-thalassemia in children living in Papua New Guinea (Allen et al., 1997). However, despite the remarkable frequency of some inherited red blood cell polymorphisms in areas where malaria is endemic (Miller, 1994), none of the polymorphisms confers absolute resistance to *P. falciparum,* which has been a major killer for many years. Thus, although the genetic red blood cell variants have reached high allele frequencies in many populations, the degree of individual protection they afford may be small (Weatherall, 1987).

Apart from genetic red blood cell variants, the most highly studied polymorphisms for severe malaria are those located within the major histocompatibility complex (MHC). A case-control study in Gambia (Hill et al., 1991) reported a protective effect of *HLA-B53* (and, to a lesser degree, *HLA-DRB1*1302*), which was found at a lower frequency among patients with severe malaria (15.7%) than among various groups of controls (23 to 25%). However, the immunological mechanisms underlying this protection, which may be related to the activity of cytotoxic T cells against malaria liver-stage antigen epitopes (Hill et al., 1992), have been debated (Dieye et al., 1997). In addition, the protective role of *HLA-B53* was not confirmed in a population from Kenya (Hill, 1998). These conflicting results may result from an interaction between HLA type and polymorphisms in the malaria parasite (Udhayakumar et al., 1997; Gilbert et al., 1998). Two other studies with the same Gambian population examined polymorphisms within the promoter region of the tumor necrosis factor alpha (*TNF-α*) gene. An initial study analyzed the diallelic polymorphism $TNF_{-308G/-308A}$ and found a higher frequency of TNF_{-308A} homozygosity in patients with severe cerebral malaria (McGuire et al., 1994). After some debate (Goldfeld and Tsai, 1996), it was shown that the rare TNF_{-308A} allele functions to allow higher levels of transcription of the *TNF-α* gene than the more common TNF_{-308G} allele (Wilson et al., 1997). A second study investigated the role of two other single nucleotide polymorphisms $TNF_{-238G/-238A}$ and $TNF_{-376G/-376A}$. The rare TNF_{-376A} allele increases TNF production by recruiting the transcription factor OCT-1 (Knight et al., 1999), but the functional role of TNF_{-238A} has not been established. Multivariate analysis of these polymorphisms in the Gambian population showed that TNF_{-376A} was associated with an increased risk of cerebral malaria whereas TNF_{-238A} had no effect and TNF_{-308A} (for homozygous subjects) had a bor-

derline significant effect (Knight et al., 1999). A similar analysis in a population from Kenya provided results that were more difficult to interpret, with a protective effect of TNF_{-238A} that appeared to be counterbalanced by a deleterious effect of TNF_{-376A} (due to complete linkage disequilibrium, the TNF_{-376A} allele is always associated with TNF_{-238A}). Furthermore, no effect of TNF_{-308A} was observed in the Kenyan population. In conclusion, polymorphisms in the *TNF-α* promoter appear to be potentially interesting, but further studies in other populations are needed to refine their effect.

Malaria biological phenotypes

A second group of genetic epidemiology studies in malaria have focused on factors involved in the control of quantitative phenotypes, in which either the intensity of infection or the immune response to the parasite is measured. Considerable evidence, including recent experimental results (Foote et al., 1997; Fortin et al., 1997), suggests that genetic factors (referred to as quantitative trait loci) are involved in the regulation of these phenotypes. For example, an elegant study in Burkina Faso demonstrated clear interethnic differences in infection rates, febrile malaria episodes, and antibody response to a major *Plasmodium* surface protein that could not be accounted for by differences in malaria protective measures, sociocultural factors, exposure to environmental factors, or known genetic factors of resistance (Modiano et al., 1996). Strong evidence for the role of genetic factors in regulation of the immune response to plasmodial antigens was also provided by twin studies in which humoral and cellular responses were more concordant within monozygotic than within dizygotic pairs (Sjoberg et al., 1992). Furthermore, comparison of dizygotic pairs showed that genes lying both within and outside the MHC regulate these immune responses, with a greater contribution from the non-MHC genes (Jepson et al., 1997).

Segregation analyses on malaria infection levels have been performed in populations from Cameroon and Burkina Faso. Infection levels were assessed by multiple measurements of *P. falciparum* parasitemia, and the data were adjusted for factors known to influence parasitemia, such as season, area of residence, and age of the subject. An initial study indicated that a recessive major gene controlled blood parasite levels (Abel et al., 1992), but two subsequent reports found evidence of a more complex genetic mechanism (Garcia et al., 1998a; Rihet et al., 1998a). These discrepant results may be due to differences in the host, the parasite, and vectorial transmission. However, all studies showed sibling correlation and the dramatic effect of age, with children being much more heavily infected than adults. Therefore, two further linkage analyses were conducted using sib-pair methods. The first analysis (Garcia et al., 1998b), performed in a small sample from Cameroon, provided suggestive evidence of linkage with the 5q31-q33 region, an area previously shown to be linked to *Schistosoma mansoni* infection levels (Marquet et al., 1996). The second sib-pair study, performed in a larger sample from Burkina Faso, confirmed the linkage of *P. falciparum* infection levels to chromosome 5q31-q33 (Rihet et al., 1998b). This region contains several candidate genes implicated in the regulation of the immune responses to *Plasmodium* species and in malaria pathogenesis, such as those coding for IL-4, IL-12, and IFN regulatory factor.

Schistosomiasis

Levels of *Schistosoma mansoni* infection

Model-based approaches have been particularly successful in the search for susceptibility genes for human schistosomiasis. In a first step, segregation analysis in a Brazilian population showed that the intensity of infection by *S. mansoni* was controlled by a major gene (Abel et al., 1991). This gene, referred to as *SM1*, accounts for 66% of the residual variance after other risk factor effects (water contact levels, age, and gender) are taken into account. Under this major gene model, about 3% of the population are homozygous and are predisposed to very high infection levels, 68% are homozygous and are resistant, and 29% are heterozygous and have an intermediate level of resistance. The second phase of this study was the mapping of this gene by parametric linkage analysis, using the model estimated from segregation analysis. A genome-wide search was carried out, and *SM1* was mapped to human chromosome 5q31-q33 (Marquet et al., 1996, 1999), a genetic region containing a cluster of Th2-related cytokine genes such as those encoding IL-4, IL-5, and IL-9. More recently, a study of a Senegalese population confirmed the presence of a locus influencing *S. mansoni* infection levels on chromosome 5q31-q33 (Muller-Myhsok et al., 1997). In addition, this region has been linked with loci related to immunoglobulin E and eosinophilia production (i.e., a locus regulating IgE levels [Marsh et al., 1994; Meyers et al., 1994]), a locus controlling bronchial hyperresponsiveness in asthma [Postma et al., 1995], and a locus involved in familial hypereosinophilia [Rioux et al., 1998]).

Other data strongly support the view that differences in human susceptibility to schistosomiasis are influenced by polymorphisms in a gene controlling T-lymphocyte subset differentiation. Human resistance to schistosomiasis is regulated by lymphokines characteristic of Th2 subsets (Couissinier-Paris and Dessein, 1995). Resistant *SM1* homozygotes mount a Th2 response to schistosomes, whereas susceptible *SM1* homozygotes mount a Th1 response (Rodrigues et al., 1999). In addition, a segregation analysis of the Brazilian population mentioned above showed that IL-5 levels are also under the control of a major gene (Rodrigues et al., 1996). This raises the possibility that this major gene plays a critical role in resistance, a view consistent with the known role of IL-5 in defense against schistosome infections. A recent association study also suggested that polymorphisms within the IL-4 locus may be involved in the regulation of Th1/Th2 differentiation in the immune response to mycobacterial antigens (Blackwell et al., 1997). Association studies investigating the role of polymorphisms within candidate genes in the 5q31-q33 region in human schistosomiasis are under way.

Severe hepatic fibrosis due to *Schistosoma mansoni*

Another trait of interest in schistosomiasis is hepatic periportal fibrosis, which occurs in 2 to 10% of persons infected by *S. mansoni* in regions of endemic infection such as Sudan. The reason why only a fraction of infected individuals develop severe disease is not known, and several observations suggest that inherited factors may play a role in the development of fibrosis (Mohamed-Ali et al., 1999). A segregation analysis in pedigrees from a Sudanese village (Dessein et al., 1999) provided evidence for a codominant major gene controlling the development of severe hepatic fibrosis and portal hypertension. The frequency of allele D, which predisposes to advanced periportal fibrosis, was estimated to be 0.16. The penetrance reached 50% after 9, 14, and 19 years of residence in the area for DD males, DD females, and Dd heterozygous males, respectively. For other subjects, penetrance remained below 2% after 20 years of exposure. Using this phenotype-genotype model, a parametric linkage analysis performed with four candidate regions (including the 5q31-q33 region) showed that this major locus mapped to chromosome 6q22-q23 and was closely linked to the *IFNGR1* gene, encoding the ligand-binding chain for the receptor of the strongly antifibrogenic cytokine IFN-γ (Dessein et al., 1999). Therefore, infection levels and advanced hepatic fibrosis in human schistosomiasis are controlled by different loci, and polymorphisms within the *IFNGR1* gene may determine the development of severe hepatic disease due to *S. mansoni* infection. These results also suggest that the *IFNGR1* gene is a strong candidate for the control of fibrosis observed in other diseases.

CONCLUSION

Essential tools for identifying the genes and alleles that influence the development of human infectious diseases have been developed recently. These tools include genetic epidemiology methods, a dense human genetic map, and a growing number of candidate genes identified on the basis of their function or location (through linkage results or homology to mouse resistance loci). Progress in the genetic dissection of infectious diseases will also come from the complementary analysis of the various biological and clinical phenotypes associated with a given infectious agent. There is now strong evidence that genetic factors are involved in most infectious diseases, but the molecular basis of genetic susceptibility and resistance remains largely unknown for most diseases. It is likely that several different genes and several functional polymorphisms within the same gene influence the outcome of many infectious agents. This results in complex methodological problems due to interaction and linkage disequilibrium between intragenic variants, as already suggested by studies of the *TNF-α* gene in cerebral malaria (Knight et al., 1999). This tremendous challenge will require new analytic strategies. We cannot yet fully appreciate the way in which genetic information will modify our approach to the prevention and treatment of infectious diseases. However, the identification of susceptibility or resistance genes in malaria, schistosomiasis, and mycobacterial infections has already opened new avenues for understanding pathogenic mechanisms, screening genetically predisposed subjects, designing vaccines, and developing novel drugs.

REFERENCES

Abel, L., M. Cot, L. Mulder, P. Carnevale, and J. Feingold. 1992. Segregation analysis detects a major gene controlling blood infection levels in human malaria. *Am. J. Hum. Genet.* **50:**1308–1317.

Abel, L., and F. Demenais. 1988. Detection of major genes for susceptibility to leprosy and its subtypes in a Caribbean island: Desirade Island. *Am. J. Hum. Genet.* **42:**256–266.

Abel, L., F. Demenais, A. Prata, A. E. Souza, and A. Dessein. 1991. Evidence for the segregation of a major gene in human susceptibility/resistance to infection by *Schistosoma mansoni*. *Am. J. Hum. Genet.* **48:**959–970.

Abel, L., and A. J. Dessein. 1997. The impact of host genetics on susceptibility to human infectious diseases. *Curr. Opin. Immunol.* **9:**509–516.

Abel, L., and A. J. Dessein. 1998. Genetic epidemiology of infectious diseases in humans: design of population-based studies. *Emerg. Infect. Dis.* **4:**593–603.

Abel, L., V. D. Lap, J. Oberti, N. V. Thuc, V. V. Cua, M. Guilloud-Bataille, E. Schurr, and P. H. Lagrange. 1995. Complex segregation analysis of leprosy in southern Vietnam. *Genet. Epidemiol.* **12:**63–82.

Abel, L., and B. Muller-Myhsok. 1998. Maximum-likelihood expression of the transmission/disequilibrium test and power considerations. *Am. J. Hum. Genet.* **63:**664–667.

Abel, L., F. O. Sanchez, J. Oberti, N. V. Thuc, L. V. Hoa, V. D. Lap, E. Skamene, P. H. Lagrange, and E. Schurr. 1998. Susceptibility to leprosy is linked to the human NRAMP1 gene. *J. Infect. Dis.* **177:**133–145.

Alcais, A., F. O. Sanchez, N. V. Thuc, V. D. Lap, J. Oberti, P. H. Lagrange, E. Schurr, and L. Abel. 2000. Granulomatous reaction to intradermal injection of lepromin (Mitsuda reaction) is linked to the human NRAMP1 gene in Vietnamese leprosy sibships. *J. Infect. Dis.* **181:**302–308.

Allen, S. J., A. O'Donnell, N. D. Alexander, M. P. Alpers, T. E. A. Peto, J. B. Clegg, and D. J. Weatherall. 1997. Alpha⁺-Thalassemia protects children against disease caused by other infections as well as malaria. *Proc. Natl. Acad. Sci. USA* **94:**14736–14741.

Altare, F., A. Durandy, D. Lammas, J. F. Emile, S. Lamhamedi, F. Le Deist, P. Drysdale, E. Jouanguy, R. Doffinger, F. Bernaudin, O. Jeppsson, J. A. Gollob, E. Meinl, A. W. Segal, A. Fischer, D. Kumararatne, and J. L. Casanova. 1998a. Impairment of mycobacterial immunity in human interleukin-12 receptor deficiency. *Science* **280:**1432–1435.

Altare, F., E. Jouanguy, S. Lamhamedi, R. Doffinger, A. Fischer, and J. L. Casanova. 1998b. Mendelian susceptibility to mycobacterial infection in man. *Curr. Opin. Immunol.* **10:**413–417.

Altare, F., D. Lammas, P. Revy, E. Jouanguy, R. Doffinger, S. Lamhamedi, P. Drysdale, D. Scheel-Toellner, J. Girdlestone, P. Darbyshire, M. Wadhwa, H. Dockrell, M. Salmon, A. Fischer, A. Durandy, J. L. Casanova, and D. S. Kumararatne. 1998c. Inherited interleukin 12 deficiency in a child with bacille Calmette-Guerin and *Salmonella enteritidis* disseminated infection. *J. Clin. Investig.* **102:**2035–2040.

Barnwell, J. W., M. E. Nichols, and P. Rubinstein. 1989. In vitro evaluation of the role of the Duffy blood group in erythrocyte invasion by *Plasmodium vivax*. *J. Exp. Med.* **169:**1795–1802.

Bellamy, R., C. Ruwende, T. Corrah, K. P. McAdam, M. Thursz, H. C. Whittle, and A. V. Hill. 1999. Tuberculosis and chronic hepatitis B virus infection in Africans and variation in the vitamin D receptor gene. *J. Infect. Dis.* **179:**721–724.

Bellamy, R., C. Ruwende, T. Corrah, K. P. McAdam, H. C. Whittle, and A. V. Hill. 1998. Variations in the NRAMP1 gene and susceptibility to tuberculosis in West Africans. *N. Engl. J. Med.* **338:**640–644.

Blackwell, J. M., G. F. Black, C. S. Peacock, E. N. Miller, D. Sibthorpe, D. Gnananandha, J. J. Shaw, F. Silveira, Z. Lins-Lainson, F. Ramos, A. Collins, and M. A. Shaw. 1997. Immunogenetics of leishmanial and mycobacterial infections: the Belem Family Study. *Philos. Trans. R. Soc. London Ser. B* **352:**1331–1345.

Blackwell, J. M., G. F. Black, C. Sharples, S. S. Soo, C. S. Peacock, and N. Miller. 1999. Roles of Nramp1, HLA, and a gene(s) in allelic association with IL-4, in determining T helper subset differentiation. *Microbes Infect.* **1:**95–102.

Canonne-Hergaux, F., S. Gruenheid, G. Govoni, and P. Gros. 1999. The Nramp1 protein and its role in resistance to infection and macrophage function. *Proc. Assoc. Am. Physicians* **111**:283–289.

Casanova, J. L., S. Blanche, J. F. Emile, E. Jouanguy, S. Lamhamedi, F. Altare, J. L. Stephan, F. Bernaudin, P. Bordigoni, D. Turck, A. Lachaux, M. Albertini, A. Bourrillon, J. P. Dommergues, M. A. Pocidalo, F. Le Deist, J. L. Gaillard, C. Griscelli, and A. Fischer. 1996. Idiopathic disseminated bacillus Calmette-Guerin infection: a French national retrospective study. *Pediatrics* **98**:774–778.

Casanova, J. L., E. Jouanguy, S. Lamhamedi, S. Blanche, and A. Fischer. 1995. Immunological conditions of children with BCG disseminated infection. *Lancet* **346**:581.

Casanova, J. L., M. Newport, A. Fischer, and M. Levin. 1999. Inherited interferon gamma receptor deficiency, p. 209–221. *In* H. D. Ochs, E. Smith, and J. Puck (ed.), *Primary Immunodeficiency Diseases: a Molecular and Genetic Approach*. Oxford University Press, New York, N.Y.

Cellier, M., G. Govoni, S. Vidal, T. Kwan, N. Groulx, J. Liu, F. Sanchez, E. Skamene, E. Schurr, and P. Gros. 1994. Human natural resistance-associated macrophage protein: cDNA cloning, chromosomal mapping, genomic organization, and tissue-specific expression. *J. Exp. Med.* **180**:1741–1752.

Collins, F. S. 1995. Positional cloning moves from perditional to traditional. *Nat. Genet.* **9**:347–350.

Couissinier-Paris, P., and A. J. Dessein. 1995. *Schistosoma*-specific helper T cell clones from subjects resistant to infection by *Schistosoma mansoni* are Th0/2. *Eur. J. Immunol.* **25**:2295–2302.

de Jong, R., F. Altare, I. A. Haagen, D. G. Elferink, T. Boer, P. J. van Breda Vriesman, P. J. Kabel, J. M. Draaisma, J. T. van Dissel, F. P. Kroon, J. L. Casanova, and T. H. Ottenhoff. 1998. Severe mycobacterial and *Salmonella* infections in interleukin-12 receptor-deficient patients. *Science* **280**:1435–1438.

Dessein, A. J., D. Hillaire, N. E. Elwali, S. Marquet, Q. Mohamed-Ali, A. Mirghani, S. Henri, A. A. Abdelhameed, O. K. Saeed, M. M. Magzoub, and L. Abel. 1999. Severe hepatic fibrosis in *Schistosoma mansoni* infection is controlled by a major locus that is closely linked to the interferon-gamma receptor gene. *Am. J. Hum. Genet.* **65**:709–721.

Dib, C., S. Faure, C. Fizames, D. Samson, N. Drouot, A. Vignal, P. Millasseau, S. Marc, J. Hazan, E. Seboun, M. Lathrop, G. Gyapay, J. Morissette, and J. Weissenbach. 1996. A comprehensive genetic map of the human genome based on 5,264 microsatellites. *Nature* **380**:152–154.

Dieye, A., C. Rogier, J. F. Trape, J. L. Sarthou, and P. Druilhe. 1997. HLA class I-associated resistance to severe malaria: a parasitological re-assessment. *Parasitol. Today* **13**:48–49.

Doffinger, R., E. Jouanguy, S. Dupuis, M. C. Fondaneche, J. L. Stephan, J. F. Emile, S. Lamhamedi-Cherradi, F. Altare, A. Pallier, G. Barcenas-Morales, E. Meinl, C. Krause, S. Pestka, R. D. Schreiber, F. Novelli, and J. L. Casanova. 2000. Partial interferon-gamma receptor signaling chain deficiency in a patient with bacille Calmette-Guerin and *Mycobacterium abscessus* infection. *J. Infect. Dis.* **181**:379–384.

Dorman, S. E., and S. M. Holland. 1998. Mutation in the signal-transducing chain of the interferon-gamma receptor and susceptibility to mycobacterial infection. *J. Clin. Investig.* **101**:2364–2369.

Dye, C., S. Scheele, P. Dolin, V. Pathania, and M. C. Raviglione. 1999. Consensus statement. Global burden of tuberculosis: estimated incidence, prevalence, and mortality by country. WHO Global Surveillance and Monitoring Project. *JAMA* **282**:677–686.

Emile, J. F., N. Patey, F. Altare, S. Lamhamedi, E. Jouanguy, F. Boman, J. Quillard, M. Lecomte-Houcke, O. Verola, J. F. Mousnier, F. Dijoud, S. Blanche, A. Fischer, N. Brousse, and J. L. Casanova. 1997. Correlation of granuloma structure with

clinical outcome defines two types of idiopathic disseminated BCG infection. *J. Pathol.* **181**:25–30.

Fine, P. E. 1981. Immunogenetics of susceptibility to leprosy, tuberculosis, and leishmaniasis. An epidemiological perspective. *Int. J. Lepr. Other Mycobact. Dis.* **49**:437–454.

Foote, S. J., R. A. Burt, T. M. Baldwin, A. Presente, A. W. Roberts, Y. L. Laural, A. M. Lew, and V. M. Marshall. 1997. Mouse loci for malaria-induced mortality and the control of parasitaemia. *Nat. Genet.* **17**:380–381.

Fortin, A., A. Belouchi, M. F. Tam, L. Cardon, E. Skamene, M. M. Stevenson, and P. Gros. 1997. Genetic control of blood parasitaemia in mouse malaria maps to chromosome 8. *Nat. Genet.* **17**:382–383.

Frucht, D. M., and S. M. Holland. 1996. Defective monocyte costimulation for IFN-gamma production in familial disseminated *Mycobacterium avium* complex infection: abnormal IL-12 regulation. *J. Immunol.* **157**:411–416.

Garcia, A., M. Cot, J. P. Chippaux, S. Ranque, J. Feingold, F. Demenais, and L. Abel. 1998a. Genetic control of blood infection levels in human malaria: evidence for a complex genetic model. *Am. J. Trop. Med. Hyg.* **58**:480–488.

Garcia, A., S. Marquet, B. Bucheton, D. Hillaire, M. Cot, N. Fievet, A. J. Dessein, and L. Abel. 1998b. Linkage analysis of blood *Plasmodium falciparum* levels: interest of the 5q31-q33 chromosome region. *Am. J. Trop. Med. Hyg.* **58**:705–709.

Gilbert, S. C., M. Plebanski, S. Gupta, J. Morris, M. Cox, M. Aidoo, D. Kwiatkowski, B. M. Greenwood, H. C. Whittle, and A. V. Hill. 1998. Association of malaria parasite population structure, HLA, and immunological antagonism. *Science* **279**:1173–1177.

Goldfeld, A. E., J. C. Delgado, S. Thim, M. V. Bozon, A. M. Uglialoro, D. Turbay, C. Cohen, and E. J. Yunis. 1998. Association of an HLA-DQ allele with clinical tuberculosis. *JAMA* **279**:226–228.

Goldfeld, A. E., and E. Y. Tsai. 1996. TNF-alpha and genetic susceptibility to parasitic disease. *Exp. Parasitol.* **84**:300–303.

Govoni, G., S. Vidal, S. Gauthier, E. Skamene, D. Malo, and P. Gros. 1996. The Bcg/Ity/Lsh locus: genetic transfer of resistance to infections in C57BL/6J mice transgenic for the Nramp1 Gly169 allele. *Infect. Immun.* **64**:2923–2929.

Hill, A. V. 1998. The immunogenetics of human infectious diseases. *Annu. Rev. Immunol.* **16**:593–617.

Hill, A. V., C. E. Allsopp, D. Kwiatkowski, N. M. Anstey, P. Twumasi, P. A. Rowe, S. Bennett, D. Brewster, A. J. McMichael, and B. M. Greenwood. 1991. Common west African HLA antigens are associated with protection from severe malaria. *Nature* **352**:595–600.

Hill, A. V., J. Elvin, A. C. Willis, M. Aidoo, C. E. Allsopp, F. M. Gotch, X. M. Gao, M. Takiguchi, B. M. Greenwood, A. R. Townsend, A. J. McMichael, and H. C. Whittle. 1992. Molecular analysis of the association of HLA-B53 and resistance to severe malaria. *Nature* **360**:434–439.

Holland, S. M., S. E. Dorman, A. Kwon, I. F. Pitha-Rowe, D. M. Frucht, S. M. Gerstberger, G. J. Noel, P. Vesterhus, M. R. Brown, and T. A. Fleisher. 1998. Abnormal regulation of interferon-gamma, interleukin-12, and tumor necrosis factor-alpha in human interferon-gamma receptor 1 deficiency. *J. Infect. Dis.* **178**:1095–1104.

Iwamoto, S., T. Omi, E. Kajii, and S. Ikemoto. 1995. Genomic organization of the glycoprotein D gene: Duffy blood group Fya/Fyb alloantigen system is associated with a polymorphism at the 44-amino acid residue. *Blood* **85**:622–626.

Jacobson, R. R., and J. L. Krahenbuhl. 1999. Leprosy. *Lancet* **353**:655–660.

Jepson, A., W. Banya, F. Sisay-Joof, M. Hassan-King, C. Nunes, S. Bennett, and H. Whittle. 1997. Quantification of the relative contribution of major histocompatibility complex (MHC) and non-MHC genes to human immune responses to foreign antigens. *Infect. Immun.* 65:872–876.

Jouanguy, E., F. Altare, S. Lamhamedi, P. Revy, J. F. Emile, M. Newport, M. Levin, S. Blanche, E. Seboun, A. Fischer, and J. L. Casanova. 1996. Interferon-gamma-receptor deficiency in an infant with fatal bacille Calmette-Guerin infection. *N. Engl. J. Med.* 335:1956–1961.

Jouanguy, E., R. Doffinger, S. Dupuis, A. Pallier, F. Altare, and J. L. Casanova. 1999a. IL-12 and IFN-gamma in host defense against mycobacteria and salmonella in mice and men. *Curr. Opin. Immunol.* 11:346–351.

Jouanguy, E., S. Dupuis, A. Pallier, R. Doffinger, M. C. Fondaneche, C. Fieschi, S. Lamhamedi-Cherradi, F. Altare, J. F. Emile, P. Lutz, P. Bordigoni, H. Cokugras, N. Akcakaya, J. Landman-Parker, J. Donnadieu, Y. Camcioglu, and J. L. Casanova. 2000. In a novel form of IFN-gamma receptor 1 deficiency, cell surface receptors fail to bind IFN-gamma. *J. Clin. Investig.* 105:1429–1436.

Jouanguy, E., S. Lamhamedi-Cherradi, F. Altare, M. C. Fondaneche, D. Tuerlinckx, S. Blanche, J. F. Emile, J. L. Gaillard, R. Schreiber, M. Levin, A. Fischer, C. Hivroz, and J. L. Casanova. 1997. Partial interferon-gamma receptor 1 deficiency in a child with tuberculoid bacillus Calmette-Guerin infection and a sibling with clinical tuberculosis. *J. Clin. Investig.* 100:2658–2664.

Jouanguy, E., S. Lamhamedi-Cherradi, D. Lammas, S. E. Dorman, M. C. Fondaneche, S. Dupuis, R. Doffinger, F. Altare, J. Girdlestone, J. F. Emile, H. Ducoulombier, D. Edgar, J. Clarke, V. A. Oxelius, M. Brai, V. Novelli, K. Heyne, A. Fischer, S. M. Holland, D. S. Kumararatne, R. D. Schreiber, and J. L. Casanova. 1999b. A human *IFNGR1* small deletion hotspot associated with dominant susceptibility to mycobacterial infection. *Nat. Genet.* 21:370–378.

Khoury, M. J., T. H. Beaty, and B. H. Cohen. 1993. Fundamentals of genetic epidemiology. *Monogr. Epidemiol. Biostat.* 19:1–448.

Knight, J. C., I. Udalova, A. V. Hill, B. M. Greenwood, N. Peshu, K. Marsh, and D. Kwiatkowski. 1999. A polymorphism that affects OCT-1 binding to the TNF promoter region is associated with severe malaria. *Nat. Genet.* 22:145–150.

Kruglyak, L. 1999. Prospects for whole-genome linkage disequilibrium mapping of common disease genes. *Nat. Genet.* 22:139–144.

Lander, E. S., and N. J. Schork. 1994. Genetic dissection of complex traits. *Science* 265:2037–2048.

Levee, G., J. Liu, B. Gicquel, S. Chanteau, and E. Schurr. 1994. Genetic control of susceptibility to leprosy in French Polynesia; no evidence for linkage with markers on telomeric human chromosome 2. *Int. J. Lepr. Other Mycobact. Dis.* 62:499–511.

Levin, M., M. J. Newport, S. D'Souza, P. Kalabalikis, I. N. Brown, H. M. Lenicker, P. V. Agius, E. G. Davies, A. Thrasher, N. Klein, and J. M. Blackwell. 1995. Familial disseminated atypical mycobacterial infection in childhood: a human mycobacterial susceptibility gene? *Lancet* 345:79–83.

Malo, D., K. Vogan, S. Vidal, J. Hu, M. Cellier, E. Schurr, A. Fuks, N. Bumstead, K. Morgan, and P. Gros. 1994. Haplotype mapping and sequence analysis of the mouse Nramp gene predict susceptibility to infection with intracellular parasites. *Genomics* 23:51–61.

Marquet, S., L. Abel, D. Hillaire, and A. Dessein. 1999. Full results of the genome-wide scan which localises a locus controlling the intensity of infection by *Schistosoma mansoni* on chromosome 5q31-q33. *Eur. J. Hum. Genet.* 7:88–97.

Marquet, S., L. Abel, D. Hillaire, H. Dessein, J. Kalil, J. Feingold, J. Weissenbach, and A. J. Dessein. 1996. Genetic localization of

a locus controlling the intensity of infection by *Schistosoma mansoni* on chromosome 5q31-q33. *Nat. Genet.* 14:181–184.

Marsh, D. G., J. D. Neely, D. R. Breazeale, B. Ghosh, L. R. Freidhoff, E. Ehrlich-Kautzky, C. Schou, G. Krishnaswamy, and T. H. Beaty. 1994. Linkage analysis of IL4 and other chromosome 5q31.1 markers and total serum immunoglobulin E concentrations. *Science* 264:1152–1156.

McGuire, W., A. V. Hill, C. E. Allsopp, B. M. Greenwood, and D. Kwiatkowski. 1994. Variation in the TNF-alpha promoter region associated with susceptibility to cerebral malaria. *Nature* 371:508–510.

McKusick, V. A. 1998. *Mendelian Inheritance in Man.* Johns Hopkins University Press, Baltimore, Md.

McLeod, R., E. Buschman, L. D. Arbuckle, and E. Skamene. 1995. Immunogenetics in the analysis of resistance to intracellular pathogens. *Curr. Opin. Immunol.* 7:539–552.

Meyers, D. A., D. S. Postma, C. I. Panhuysen, J. Xu, P. J. Amelung, R. C. Levitt, and E. R. Bleecker. 1994. Evidence for a locus regulating total serum IgE levels mapping to chromosome 5. *Genomics* 23:464–470.

Miller, L. H. 1994. Impact of malaria on genetic polymorphism and genetic diseases in Africans and African Americans. *Proc. Natl. Acad. Sci. USA* 91:2415–2419.

Miller, L. H., S. J. Mason, D. F. Clyde, and M. H. McGinniss. 1976. The resistance factor to *Plasmodium vivax* in blacks. The Duffy-blood-group genotype, FyFy. *N. Engl. J. Med.* 295:302–304.

Misra, N., A. Murtaza, B. Walker, N. P. Narayan, R. S. Misra, V. Ramesh, S. Singh, M. J. Colston, and I. Nath. 1995. Cytokine profile of circulating T cells of leprosy patients reflects both indiscriminate and polarized T-helper subsets: T-helper phenotype is stable and uninfluenced by related antigens of *Mycobacterium leprae*. *Immunology* 86:97–103.

Modiano, D., V. Petrarca, B. S. Sirima, I. Nebie, D. Diallo, F. Esposito, and M. Coluzzi. 1996. Different response to *Plasmodium falciparum* malaria in west African sympatric ethnic groups. *Proc. Natl. Acad. Sci. USA* 93:13206–13211.

Mohamed-Ali, Q., N. E. Elwali, A. A. Abdelhameed, A. Mergani, S. Rahoud, K. E. Elagib, O. K. Saeed, L. Abel, M. M. Magzoub, and A. J. Dessein. 1999. Susceptibility to periportal (Symmers) fibrosis in human *Schistosoma mansoni* infections: evidence that intensity and duration of infection, gender, and inherited factors are critical in disease progression. *J. Infect. Dis.* 180:1298–1306.

Morton, N. E. 1955. Sequential tests for the detection of linkage. *Am. J. Hum. Genet.* 7:277–318.

Muller-Myhsok, B., and L. Abel. 1997. Genetic analysis of complex diseases. *Science* 275:1328–1329.

Muller-Myhsok, B., F. F. Stelma, F. Guisse-Sow, B. Muntau, T. Thye, G. D. Burchard, B. Gryseels, and R. D. Horstmann. 1997. Further evidence suggesting the presence of a locus, on human chromosome 5q31-q33, influencing the intensity of infection with *Schistosoma mansoni*. *Am. J. Hum. Genet.* 61:452–454.

Nagel, R. L., and E. F. Roth, Jr. 1989. Malaria and red cell genetic defects. *Blood* 74:1213–1221.

Newport, M. J., C. M. Huxley, S. Huston, C. M. Hawrylowicz, B. A. Oostra, R. Williamson, and M. Levin. 1996. A mutation in the interferon-gamma-receptor gene and susceptibility to mycobacterial infection. *N. Engl. J. Med.* 335:1941–1949.

Ott, J. 1999. *Analysis of Human Genetic Linkage.* Johns Hopkins University Press, Baltimore, Md.

Ottenhoff, T. H., and R. R. de Vries. 1987. HLA class II immune response and suppression genes in leprosy. *Int. J. Lepr. Other Mycobact. Dis.* 55:521–534.

Pierre-Audigier, C., E. Jouanguy, S. Lamhamedi, F. Altare, J. Rauzier, V. Vincent, D. Canioni, J. F. Emile, A. Fischer, S. Blanche,

J. L. Gaillard, and J. L. Casanova. 1997. Fatal disseminated *Mycobacterium smegmatis* infection in a child with inherited interferon gamma receptor deficiency. *Clin. Infect. Dis.* 24:982–984.

Postma, D. S., E. R. Bleecker, P. J. Amelung, K. J. Holroyd, J. Xu, C. I. Panhuysen, D. A. Meyers, and R. C. Levitt. 1995. Genetic susceptibility to asthma—bronchial hyperresponsiveness coinherited with a major gene for atopy. *N. Engl. J. Med.* 333:894–900.

Rihet, P., L. Abel, Y. Traore, T. Traore-Leroux, C. Aucan, and F. Fumoux. 1998a. Human malaria: segregation analysis of blood infection levels in a suburban area and a rural area in Burkina Faso. *Genet. Epidemiol.* 15:435–450.

Rihet, P., Y. Traore, L. Abel, C. Aucan, T. Traore-Leroux, and F. Fumoux. 1998b. Malaria in humans: *Plasmodium falciparum* blood infection levels are linked to chromosome 5q31-q33. *Am. J. Hum. Genet.* 63:498–505.

Rioux, J. D., V. A. Stone, M. J. Daly, M. Cargill, T. Green, H. Nguyen, T. Nutman, P. A. Zimmerman, M. A. Tucker, T. Hudson, A. M. Goldstein, E. Lander, and A. Y. Lin. 1998. Familial eosinophilia maps to the cytokine gene cluster on human chromosomal region 5q31-q33. *Am. J. Hum. Genet.* 63:1086–1094.

Rodrigues, V., Jr., L. Abel, K. Piper, and A. J. Dessein. 1996. Segregation analysis indicates a major gene in the control of interleukine-5 production in humans infected with *Schistosoma mansoni. Am. J. Hum. Genet.* 59:453–461.

Rodrigues, V., Jr., K. Piper, P. Couissinier-Paris, O. Bacelar, H. Dessein, and A. J. Dessein. 1999. Genetic control of schistosome infections by the SM1 locus of the 5q31-q33 region is linked to differentiation of type 2 helper T lymphocytes. *Infect. Immun.* 67:4689–4692.

Roesler, J., B. Kofink, J. Wendisch, S. Heyden, D. Paul, W. Friedrich, J. L. Casanova, W. Leupold, M. Gahr, and A. Rosen-Wolff. 1999. Listeria monocytogenes and recurrent mycobacterial infections in a child with complete interferon-gamma-receptor (IFNγR1) deficiency: mutational analysis and evaluation of therapeutic options. *Exp. Hematol.* 27:1368–1374.

Roy, S., A. Frodsham, B. Saha, S. K. Hazra, C. G. Mascie-Taylor, and A. V. Hill. 1999. Association of vitamin D receptor genotype with leprosy type. *J. Infect. Dis.* 179:187–191.

Ruwende, C., S. C. Khoo, R. W. Snow, S. N. Yates, D. Kwiatkowski, S. Gupta, P. Warn, C. E. Allsopp, S. C. Gilbert, N. Peschu, C. I. Newbold, B. M. Greenwood, K. Marsh, and A. V. S. Hill. 1995. Natural selection of hemi- and heterozygotes for G6PD deficiency in Africa by resistance to severe malaria. *Nature* 376:246–249.

Sansonetti, P., and P. H. Lagrange. 1981. The immunology of leprosy: speculations on the leprosy spectrum. *Rev. Infect. Dis.* 3:422–469.

Shaw, M. A., S. Atkinson, H. Dockrell, R. Hussain, Z. Lins-Lainson, J. Shaw, F. Ramos, F. Silveira, S. Q. Mehdi, F. Kaukab, S. Khaliq, T. Chiang, and J. Blackwell. 1993. An RFLP map for 2q33-q37 from multicase mycobacterial and leishmanial disease families: no evidence for an Lsh/Ity/Bcg gene homologue influencing susceptibility to leprosy. *Ann. Hum. Genet.* 57:251–271.

Shaw, M. A., A. Collins, C. S. Peacock, E. N. Miller, G. F. Black, D. Sibthorpe, Z. Lins-Lainson, J. J. Shaw, F. Ramos, F. Silveira, and J. M. Blackwell. 1997. Evidence that genetic susceptibility to *Mycobacterium tuberculosis* in a Brazilian population is under oligogenic control: linkage study of the candidate genes NRAMP1 and TNFA. *Tubercle Lung Dis.* 78:35–45.

Sjoberg, K., J. P. Lepers, L. Raharimalala, A. Larsson, O. Olerup, N. T. Marbiah, M. Troye-Blomberg, and P. Perlmann. 1992. Genetic regulation of human anti-malarial antibodies in twins. *Proc. Natl. Acad. Sci. USA* 89:2101–2104.

Spielman, R. S., R. E. McGinnis, and W. J. Ewens. 1993. Transmission test for linkage disequilibrium: the insulin gene region and insulin-dependent diabetes mellitus (IDDM). *Am. J. Hum. Genet.* 52:506–516.

Stead, W. W., J. W. Senner, W. T. Reddick, and J. P. Lofgren. 1990. Racial differences in susceptibility to infection by *Mycobacterium tuberculosis. N. Engl. J. Med.* 322:422–427.

Tournamille, C., Y. Colin, J. P. Cartron, and C. Le Van Kim. 1995. Disruption of a GATA motif in the Duffy gene promoter abolishes erythroid gene expression in Duffy-negative individuals. *Nat. Genet.* 10:224–228.

Udhayakumar, V., J. M. Ongecha, Y. P. Shi, M. Aidoo, A. S. Orago, A. J. Oloo, W. A. Hawley, B. L. Nahlen, S. L. Hoffman, W. R. Weiss, and A. A. Lal. 1997. Cytotoxic T cell reactivity and HLA-B35 binding of the variant *Plasmodium falciparum* circumsporozoite protein CD8+ CTL epitope in naturally exposed Kenyan adults. *Eur. J. Immunol.* 27:1952–1957.

van Eden, W., and R. R. P. de Vries. 1984. HLA and leprosy: a reevaluation. *Lepr. Rev.* 55:89–104.

van Eden, W., N. M. Gonzalez, R. R. de Vries, J. Convit, and J. J. van Rood. 1985. HLA-linked control of predisposition to lepromatous leprosy. *J. Infect. Dis.* 151:9–14.

Vidal, S. M., E. Pinner, P. Lepage, S. Gauthier, and P. Gros. 1996. Natural resistance to intracellular infections: Nramp1 encodes a membrane phosphoglycoprotein absent in macrophages from susceptible (Nramp1 D169) mouse strains. *J. Immunol.* 157:3559–3568.

Wakelin, D., and J. M. Blackwell. 1988. *Genetics of Resistance to Bacterial and Parasitic Infection.* Taylor & Francis, London, United Kingdom.

Wang, D. G., J. B. Fan, C. J. Siao, A. Berno, P. Young, R. Sapolsky, G. Ghandour, N. Perkins, E. Winchester, J. Spencer, L. Kruglyak, L. Stein, L. Hsie, T. Topaloglou, E. Hubbell, E. Robinson, M. Mittmann, M. S. Morris, N. Shen, D. Kilburn, J. Rioux, C. Nusbaum, S. Rozen, T. J. Hudson, R. Lipshutz, M. Chee, and E. S. Lander. 1998. Large-scale identification, mapping, and genotyping of single-nucleotide polymorphisms in the human genome. *Science* 280:1077–1082.

Weatherall, D. J. 1987. Common genetic disorders of the red cell and the "malaria hypothesis." *Ann. Trop. Med. Parasitol.* 81:539–548.

Wilkinson, R. J., M. Llewelyn, Z. Toossi, P. Patel, G. Pasvol, A. Lalvani, D. Wright, M. Latif, and R. N. Davidson. 2000. Influence of vitamin D deficiency and vitamin D receptor polymorphisms on tuberculosis among Gujarati Asians in west London: a case-control study. *Lancet* 355:618–621.

Wilkinson, R. J., P. Patel, M. Llewelyn, C. S. Hirsch, G. Pasvol, G. Snounou, R. N. Davidson, and Z. Toossi. 1999. Influence of polymorphism in the genes for the interleukin (IL)-1 receptor antagonist and IL-1beta on tuberculosis. *J. Exp. Med.* 189:1863–1874.

Wilson, A. G., J. A. Symons, T. L. McDowell, H. O. McDevitt, and G. W. Duff. 1997. Effects of a polymorphism in the human tumor necrosis factor alpha promoter on transcriptional activation. *Proc. Natl. Acad. Sci. USA* 94:3195–3199.

World Health Organization. 1997. Primary immunodeficiency diseases. Report of a WHO scientific group. *Clin. Exp. Immunol.* 109(Suppl. 1):1–28.

Yamamura, M., K. Uyemura, R. J. Deans, K. Weinberg, T. H. Rea, B. R. Bloom, and R. L. Modlin. 1991. Defining protective responses to pathogens: cytokine profiles in leprosy lesions. *Science* 254:277–279.

Zerva, L., B. Cizman, N. K. Mehra, S. K. Alahari, R. Murali, C. M. Zmijewski, M. Kamoun, and D. S. Monos. 1996. Arginine at positions 13 or 70-71 in pocket 4 of HLA-DRB1 alleles is associated with susceptibility to tuberculoid leprosy. *J. Exp. Med.* 183:829–836.

Immunology of Infectious Diseases
Edited by S. H. E. Kaufmann, A. Sher, and R. Ahmed
© 2002 ASM Press, Washington, D.C.

Chapter 27

Immunogenetics of the Host Response to Bacteria in Mice

PHILIPPE GROS AND ERWIN SCHURR

Inbred strains of mice have been used extensively as an experimental model to study the physiopathology and host response to infection with human bacterial pathogens. A genetic approach to the study of interstrain differences in susceptibility to infection has led to the mapping of major loci affecting initial susceptibility, progression, and outcome of infection. Several such loci have now been isolated by positional cloning, and the characterization of the encoded proteins has provided new insight into the molecular basis of antimicrobial defenses of the host including those expressed by macrophages and T and B lymphocytes. More recently, the advent of novel analytical tools and high-density marker maps of the mouse genome have allowed the analysis of multigenic control of susceptibility by quantitative trait locus mapping in genomewide scans. New chromosomal regions associated with susceptibility and identified in the mouse can be readily tested in humans for a parallel role in areas where the disease is endemic, in either association or linkage studies. This chapter presents an overview of the specific mouse loci identified as playing a key role in susceptibility to infection with human bacterial pathogens.

MYCOBACTERIUM SPECIES

Studies in mouse infection models have identified a genetic control for susceptibility to infection with both highly virulent human strains of *Mycobacterium tuberculosis* and less pathogenic mycobacteria such as *M. bovis* BCG, *M. avium,* and *M. intracellulare.* The most extensively studied genetic model is *M. bovis* BCG. Inbred mouse strains infected intravenously with low doses (10^4 CFU) of *M. bovis* are either permissive or completely nonpermissive for

bacterial replication in the spleen and liver during the first 3 weeks of infection (Gros et al., 1981). Segregation analysis in informative crosses indicates that resistance to infection is dominant and is controlled by a single autosomal gene, designated *Bcg* (Gros et al., 1981). Studies with inbred and congenic strains showed that *Bcg* regulates the replication of a number of other mycobacterial species in the host, such as *M. avium* (Stokes et al., 1986; De Chastellier et al., 1993), *M. intracellulare* (Gotto et al., 1989), *M. smegmatis* (Denis et al., 1990), and *M. lepraemurium* (Brown et al., 1982; Skamene et al., 1984). Early mapping studies positioned *Bcg* on the proximal part of mouse chromosome 1 (Skamene et al., 1982), either very tightly linked or identical to two other host resistance loci, *Ity* (Plant and Glynn, 1976) and *Lsh* (Bradley et al., 1979), that control early replication of *Salmonella enterica* serovar Typhimurium and *Leishmania donovani* in the host in a very similar fashion. Thus, it was proposed that the *Bcg/Ity/Lsh* locus may play a major role in host resistance to infection with intracellular parasites (Skamene et al., 1982).

Additional studies in vivo with mutant strains of mice (Gros et al., 1983), as well as studies in vitro with an explanted cell population, showed that *Bcg/Ity/Lsh* is phenotypically expressed by macrophages and affects the ability of these cells to control intracellular microbial replication (Lissner et al., 1983; Crocker et al., 1984; Stach et al., 1984; Stokes et al., 1986; Denis et al., 1990; Arias et al., 1997). Indeed, in permissive *Bcg*^{s} strains such as C57BL/6J and BALB/c, mycobacteria can block phagolysosomal fusion, while in *Bcg*^{r} strains such as A/J, DBA/2J, and C3H/HeJ, there is complete phagosome maturation and bactericidal activity (De Chastellier et al., 1993). A positional cloning approach based on high reso-

Philippe Gros • Centre for the Study of Host Resistance, Department of Biochemistry, McGill University, Montréal, Québec H3G 1Y6, Canada.   **Erwin Schurr** • Centre for the Study of Host Resistance, Departments of Medicine and Human Genetics, McGill University, and McGill University Health Centre Research Institute—Montréal General Hospital, Montréal, Québec, H3G 1A4, Canada.

lution genetic (Schurr et al., 1989, Malo et al., 1993a), physical (Malo et al., 1993b) and transcriptional (Vidal et al., 1993) mapping was used to identify *Bcg*. In the minimal physical interval of *Bcg*, a gene was identified that is expressed exclusively in the spleen and liver and was enriched in macrophages derived from them. The protein encoded by this mRNA (natural resistance-associated macrophage protein 1 [Nramp1]) is predicted to be an integral membrane protein with many features of an ion transporter or channel, including 12 transmembrane (TM) domains, charged residues in TM domains, and a consensus transport motif (Vidal et al., 1993).

Sequence analyses with 27 inbred strains indicated that susceptibility to infection in *Bcg^s* strains is associated with a glycine-to-aspartate substitution in predicted TM4 of the protein (Malo et al., 1994). The replacement of a small neutral residue (Gly) by a bulkier residue with a charged side chain (Asp) is nonconservative and thermodynamically disfavored in the hydrophobic environment of the lipid bilayer. Creation of a null *Nramp1* mutant by homologous recombination in embryonal stem cells has confirmed that *Nramp1* and *Bcg/Ity/Lsh* are indeed allelic, since *Nramp1^{-/-}* mice created on a 129sv background (*Bcg^r*) become susceptible to infection with *M. bovis*, *M. avium*, *S. enterica* serovar Typhimurium, and *L. donovani* (Vidal et al., 1995a). In addition, mutant mice bearing one or two null alleles at *Nramp1* were as susceptible to infection as were their *Nramp1^{Asp169}* counterparts, suggesting that the G169D mutation causes a complete loss of function at *Nramp1*. Finally, the transfer of a wild-type allele of *Nramp1*(G169) onto a mutant *Nramp1^{Asp169}* allele of C57BL/6J mice was shown to restore resistance to infection with the above-mentioned organisms in transgenic mice (Govoni et al., 1996). Likewise, introduction and overexpression of a wild-type copy of the *Nramp1* cDNA (*Nramp1^{G169}*) in RAW macrophages (*Nramp1^{D169}*) eliminates the permissiveness of these cells to replication of *S. enterica* serovar Typhimurium (Govoni et al., 1999). Together, these results establish that *Nramp1* is indeed *Bcg/Ity/Lsh*.

The human *NRAMP1* homolog was cloned, mapped to the long arm of chromosome 2, and sequenced in its totality (Cellier et al., 1996; Marquet et al., 2000). *NRAMP1* mRNA is expressed in the spleen and liver but is more abundant in the lungs and is most abundant in peripheral blood leukocytes. In primary cells, human *NRAMP1* mRNA is specifically expressed in monocytes, alveolar macrophages, and, at very high levels, granulocytes. Maturation of monocytes into macrophages in vitro or in vivo is associated with increased *NRAMP1* mRNA expression. Myeloid cell-specific expression of *NRAMP1* in the monocytic and granulocytic pathways was also verified using the HL-60 model cell line differentiated with dimethyl sulfoxide or phorbol myristate acetate (Cellier et al., 1997). These results suggest that *NRAMP1* may play a functional role in the bactericidal activity of neutrophils as well as macrophages.

The role of *NRAMP1* in host defenses against clinically relevant strains of *M. tuberculosis* and *M. leprae* was addressed in genetic studies in humans from areas of endemic tuberculosis (The Gambia) and leprosy (South Vietnam) infection, using informative markers derived from the *NRAMP1* gene region (Liu et al., 1995; Buu et al., 1995; Searle and Blackwell, 1999). In the first study, the distribution of four *NRAMP1* alleles was determined in 410 adults with smear-positive pulmonary tuberculosis and in 410 ethnically matched healthy controls. A strong association between disease and two specific allelic variants at *NRAMP1* was found (odds ratio, 4.09; 95% confidence interval, 1.86 to 9.12; chi-square, 14.58; $P < 0.001$) (Bellamy et al., 1998). In a second study, segregation analyses were conducted on 285 Vietnamese and 117 Chinese families with leprosy in southern Vietnam. There was evidence for a codominant major gene in the Vietnamese families but no evidence for a major gene in the Chinese families (Abel et al., 1995). Interestingly, evidence for linkage to *NRAMP1* was stronger in the Vietnamese families alone for both intragenic *NRAMP1* ($P < 0.05$) and extended *NRAMP1* ($P < 0.02$) haplotypes (Abel et al., 1998). The authors concluded that genetic variations at *NRAMP1* affect susceptibility to tuberculosis and leprosy in humans. In a follow-up study to the analysis of leprosy susceptibility, Alcais et al. (2000) found that the *NRAMP1* gene was highly significantly linked to the extent of the specific in vivo anti-*M. leprae* granulomatous response in Vietnamese families. Such linkage was independent of the leprosy disease status of individual family members and, in the case of leprosy patients, of the subtype of leprosy. These results clearly show that a link exists between *NRAMP1* alleles and specific acquired immune responses.

A first glimpse of the *NRAMP1* gene environment interaction was obtained in a recent genetic study of a tuberculosis outbreak in an extended Canadian Aboriginal family (Greenwood et al., in press). Due to a relatively detailed knowledge of exposure histories, it was possible to perform a parametric linkage analysis of *NRAMP1* with tuberculosis susceptibility, employing four well-defined liability classes. This model-based analysis detected a strong effect of a dominant risk allele (relative risk, 10) on clinically defined tuberculosis. Multilocus analysis placed the risk allele in or very close to *NRAMP1*, with a lod score of 4.2, i.e., the odds in favor of linkage were >15,000:1. Interestingly, if the same family was analyzed in a nonparametric fashion, i.e. without taking advantage of the known genetic and clinicoepidemiological information, no evidence for linkage of tuberculosis susceptibility to *NRAMP1* was obtained. This result illustrates one of the major difficulties faced when moving from candidate genes in animal models to human populations. Even major genetic effects may go undetected if underlying gene-environment interactions are not taken into consideration.

In the mouse, *Nramp1* mRNA is expressed in primary macrophages and in macrophage cell lines RAW and J774, and its expression can be further stimulated by bacterial lipopolysaccharide (LPS) and gamma interferon or by inflammatory stimuli in vivo (Govoni et al., 1997). Immunoblotting and immunoprecipitation studies with specific polyclonal antisera show that Nramp1 is an integral membrane protein extensively modified by phosphorylation and glycosylation in macrophages to a final 100- to 120-kDa mature protein (Vidal et al., 1996). In *Bcg*^{s} macrophages, no mature protein is detected, suggesting that the G169D mutation affects protein maturation, with possible targeting for degradation (Vidal et al., 1996). In colocalization studies with primary macrophages, the Nramp1 protein was found not to be expressed in the plasma membrane but, rather, to be localized in the late endosomal-lysosomal, Lamp1-positive compartment (Gruenheid et al., 1997). Double-immunofluorescence and confocal microscopy in intact cells and biochemical studies of purified phagosomes containing latex particles demonstrated that on phagocytosis, Nramp1 is rapidly recruited and remains associated with the membrane of the phagosome, with kinetics similar to those seen for Lamp1 and distinct from those of Rab7 (Gruenheid et al., 1997). The association of Nramp1 with bacterial phagosomes was also studied in RAW macrophages (defective *Nramp1*^{D169} allele) transfected with the functional *Nramp1* cDNA (*Nramp1*^{G169}) fused to a c-Myc epitope tag. Immunofluorescence and confocal microscopy showed that within 30 min of phagocytosis, Nramp1–cMyc is recruited to the membrane of phagosomes containing either *S. enterica* serovar Typhimurium or *Yersinia enterocolitica* (Govoni et al., 1999). Thus, Nramp1 is an integral membrane protein with possible transport function that is rapidly recruited to the membrane of phagosomes containing either inert particles or live bacteria, where it may affect bacterial replication.

The effects of Nramp1 acquisition on biochemical composition, maturation, and bactericidal activity of the phagosome were investigated. Microfluorescence ratio imaging of 129sv (+/+) and *Nramp1*$^{-/-}$ primary macrophages was used to measure the pH of individual phagosomes containing either live or dead *M. bovis* (Hackam et al., 1998). The pH of phagosomes containing live *M. bovis* was significantly lower in +/+ macrophages than in *Nramp1*$^{-/-}$ cells (pH 5.5 ± 0.06 versus 6.6 ± 0.05; [$P < 0.005$]). The enhanced acidification could not be accounted for by differences in proton consumption during dismutation of superoxide, phagosomal buffering power, counterion conductance, or the rate of proton "leak." Rather, following ingestion of live *M. bovis*, 129sv cells exhibited increased concanamycin-sensitive H$^+$ pumping across the phagosomal membrane, associated with enhanced recruitment of vacuolar-ATPase-positive endosomes and/or lysosomes. The effect of Nramp1 on pH was seen only with live *M. bovis* and not in phagosomes containing dead *M. bovis* or latex beads (Hackam et al., 1998). Similar observations were made in RAW macrophages expressing a transfected, epitope-tagged Nramp1 protein (Govoni et al., 1999). The functional consequence of targeting Nramp1 to the *M. avium* phagosome (Trudeau Institute Mycobacterial Collection 724) was recently studied by electron microscopy: there was a 10-fold difference in CFU counts recovered from infected bone marrow macrophages from *Nramp1*$^{-/-}$ (10^5 CFU) compared to +/+ cells (10^4 CFU). This increased bacteriostatic activity of Nramp1$^{+/+}$ cells was associated with increased acidification and increased fusion to secondary lysosomes (C. De Chastellier and P. Gros, unpublished data). Together, these studies indicate that Nramp1 targeting to the membrane of bacterial phagosomes results in decreased bacterial viability and is concomitant with increased bactericidal or bacteriostatic activity of the macrophage.

Insight into the biochemical mechanism and transport substrate of Nramp proteins has come from studies of Nramp homologs of phylogenetically distant species, including complementation experiments with model organisms. It has recently become evident that Nramp defines a large superfamily of membrane proteins with members in vertebrates, insects, plants, yeasts, and bacteria (Cellier et al., 1995, 1996). A second *Nramp* gene, *Nramp2*, was identified in mice and humans (Vidal et al., 1995b; Gruenheid et al., 1995); *Nramp2* mRNA encodes a protein highly similar to Nramp1 (78% identity over the hydrophobic core), which, as opposed to its phagocyte-specific Nramp1 counterpart, is expressed in most tissues and cell types analyzed (Gruenheid et al.,

1995; Gunshin et al., 1997). Recently, *Nramp2* was found mutated (G185R) in two animal models of iron deficiency, the *mk* mouse (Fleming et al., 1997) and the *Belgrade* rat (Fleming et al., 1998). Both animals showed very severe microcytic anemia, with impaired intestinal iron uptake and deficient iron metabolism in peripheral tissues (Russell et al., 1970; Farcich and Morgan, 1992) that could not be corrected by oral or intravenous administration of iron (reviewed by Andrews, [1999]). Independently, *Nramp2* (divalent cation transporter 1) was reisolated by expression cloning in *Xenopus* oocytes, where it was shown to transport a number of divalent cations such as Fe^{2+}, Zn^{2+}, and Mn^{2+} in a pH-dependent and electrogenic fashion (Gunshin et al., 1997). Using isoform-specific antisera, we have shown that Nramp2 is expressed at low levels throughout the small intestine and that dietary iron starvation results in a dramatic up-regulation of Nramp2 isoform I in the proximal portion of the duodenum only. Immunostaining showed that Nramp2 is expressed in the absorptive epithelium of the mucosa and is very intensely expressed at the brush border of the apical pole of the enterocytes, strongly suggesting that Nramp2 indeed functions in transferrin-independent iron uptake at the brush border (Canonne-Hergaux et al., 1999). Immunoblotting experiments also showed that Nramp2 is present in a number of cell types and is coexpressed with Nramp1 in primary macrophages and macrophage cell lines (Gruenheid et al., 1999). Subcellular localization studies by immunofluorescence microscopy indicate that while Nramp1 is expressed in the lysosomal compartment only, Nramp2 is absent from lysosomes but is expressed in recycling endosomes and at the plasma membrane, colocalizing with transferrin (Gruenheid et al., 1999). Together, these results suggest that Nramp2 not only can transport Fe^{2+} in intestinal mucosa, but also may play a key role in the metabolism of transferrin-bound iron in peripheral tissues by transporting free iron across the endosomal membrane and into the cytoplasm on acidification of this compartment. Conserved transport function in the Nramp superfamily (see below), together with distinct subcellular localization of the two Nramp proteins, suggests that Nramp1 and Nramp2 may carry out the same function but at different subcellular sites.

The yeast *Nramp* homolog, *Smf1* (40% identity), functions as a manganese and iron transporter, and *smf1*-null mutants cannot grow on EGTA-containing medium (Supek et al., 1996; Chen et al., 1999). It was recently shown that transfection and overexpression of *Nramp2*, but not *Nramp1* or *Nramp2* mutant variants, in yeast *smf1* mutants could complement the hypersensitivity to EGTA and susceptibility to alkaline pH (pH 7.9) phenotypes of this *smf1* mutant. Since Mn^{2+} was the only divalent cation suppressing *Nramp2* complementation, these results suggested that like Smf1, Nramp2 can transport Mn^{2+} in yeast (Pinner et al., 1997). Mutations in the *Drosophila Nramp* homolog, *Malvolio*, cause a defect in taste discrimination (Rodrigues et al., 1995) that can be suppressed by growing the mutant flies on medium supplemented with Mn^{2+} and Fe^{2+} (Orgad et al., 1998). Expression of a human *NRAMP1* transgene under control of the hsp70 promoter in *Malvolio* transgenic flies can complement the taste defect in the flies in a fashion similar to that of dietary metal (D'Sousa et al., 1999). These findings suggest that human *NRAMP1* can act on Mn^{2+} and Fe^{2+} in flies. Finally, bacterial genome-sequencing projects have identified *Nramp* homologs in many bacterial species (35 to 40% identity). We have functionally characterized (Makui et al., 2000) an *Nramp* homolog from *Escherichia coli* K-12 (the *mntH* gene). Elimination of *mntH* impaired the survival of a metal-dependent mutant strain, *hflB1*(Ts). Transport assays in cells overexpressing *mntH* on a null background show that the protein can transport $^{55}Fe^{2+}$ and $^{54}Mn^{2+}$ in a temperature-, time-, and proton-dependent manner (Makui et al., 2000).

The fact that divalent cation transport is common to Nramp homologs from bacteria to mammals implies that Nramp1 is also a divalent cation transporter. Sequestration of iron and other divalent metals away from the internalized microbe could explain the advantage of macrophages possessing functional *Nramp1*. Divalent metals are essential for survival of all organisms, including bacteria. Divalent cations are also essential cofactors for bacterial superoxide dismutase and catalase, enzymes that neutralize some of the antimicrobial actions of the phagolysosome (Paramchuk et al., 1997) and that may thus enhance intracellular microbial survival (Lundrigan et al., 1997). Additionally, transcriptional regulators such as the iron-dependent *iroA* and *fur* of *Salmonella* and *fur* and *ideR* of mycobacteria, lead to the downstream regulation of multiple pathways in response to divalent cation availability. This suggests that differences in divalent-cation concentrations within the phagosome may lead to differential expression of virulence factors of the pathogen as well. The presence of functional Nramp homologs in gram-negative bacteria and mycobacteria (Makui et al., 2000; Agranoff et al., 1999) suggests the intriguing possibility that bacterial and mammalian Nramp proteins may compete for the same divalent cations in the phagosomal space.

Genetic Factors in Susceptibility to Virulent *M. tuberculosis*

It is well documented in the literature that inbred strains of laboratory mice differ dramatically in their susceptibility to infection with virulent *M. tuberculosis* (Pierce et al., 1947; Lynch et al., 1965; Nikonenko et al., 1985; Musa et al., 1987; Medina and North, 1998). There are, however, differences in the relative resistance and susceptibility ranking of common laboratory mouse strains that could relate to different sizes of the infectious inoculum, different routes of infection, possible divergence of mouse strains bred for extended periods at separate locations, use of specific-pathogen-free mice versus animals kept in conventional facilities, or use of different susceptibility phenotypes.

An important role of both class I and class II restricted T cells as mediators of resistance to tuberculosis has been clearly established in the mouse (Orme and McMurray, 1995; Flynn et al., 1992). Likewise, a strong influence of *H2* haplotypes on granuloma formation and dissemination of *M. tuberculosis* has been reported (Brett and Ivanyi, 1990; Brett et al., 1992). In terms of mortality, $I\text{-}A^b/D^b$ allele combinations are associated with reduced survival times (susceptibility) while $I\text{-}A^k/D^d$ combinations are associated with increased survival times (Apt et al., 1993). The identification of protective or susceptible *H2* haplotypes or specific major histocompatibility complex alleles that control bacterial loads in infected organs has been less conclusive. However, the $H2^f$ haplotype seems to be associated with an inability of its carriers to benefit from BCG vaccination (Apt et al., 1993). To identify non-*H2* genes that are important for the anti-*M. tuberculosis* host response, several gene deletion mouse strains have been generated and tested for increased susceptibility to *M. tuberculosis*. For example, following this strategy, gamma interferon (Flynn et al., 1993), tumor necrosis factor alpha (Flynn et al., 1995), and nitric oxide (MacMicking et al., 1997) were identified as important effector molecules of the anti-*M. tuberculosis* response. A reasonable expectation would be that more subtle allelic changes in these proven effector molecules would result in a slightly modulated biological activity that, in turn, would correlate with the known tuberculosis susceptibility spectrum of mouse strains. Presently, such alleles have not been discovered among laboratory mice, possibly as a consequence of the limited genetic diversity represented in inbred mouse strains.

A second strategy to identify allelic variants that contribute to the variable tuberculosis susceptibility of inbred strains is to identify strains that are located at opposite ends of the susceptibility spectrum and then to perform genetic crosses between these strains. The genetic analysis of such crosses clearly shows that tuberculosis susceptibility of laboratory mice manifests itself as a quantitative trait that is under the control of multiple genes (Kramnik et al., 1998; Lavebratt et al., 1999). Such traits cannot be analyzed by classical Mendelian methods. However, the advent of new and powerful analytical tools (Darvasi et al., 1993; Jansen, 1993) and the availability of high-density genomewide marker maps have made it possible to link quantitative trait loci (QTL) with high reliability to specific chromosomal regions. Employing methods of quantitative genetic analysis, Kramnik et al. (1998) localized a tuberculosis susceptibility gene to mouse chromosome 1 in a panel of almost 400 F_2 mice derived from C57BL/6J and C3HeB/FeJ progenitor strains. This locus, which is associated with very short survival times, is located approximately 15 centimorgans (cM) distal of the *Nramp1* gene. The two loci are probably different, since the allele which confers short survival times (susceptibility) is derived from the C3H strain, which carries an *Nramp1*-resistant allele. In a second study, Lavebratt et al. (1999) performed a genomewide QTL analysis in a panel of (A/Sn × I/St)F_1 × I/St backcross animals. Using loss of body weight as a measure of tuberculosis severity, these authors identified two QTL, on chromosomes 3 and 9, in female mice. Additional suggestive linkages were identified on four different chromosomes in both females and males. The molecular identity has not been identified for any of the detected tuberculosis susceptibility loci.

As discussed above, among human populations the *NRAMP1* gene has been found associated (Bellamy et al., 1998) or linked (Greenwood et al., in press) with tuberculosis susceptibility in vastly different epidemiological settings and ethnic groups. By contrast, the role of the *Nramp1* gene in modulating tuberculosis susceptibility in mice is not clear. Although *Nramp1^r* mice consistently showed decreased survival times in a strain survey (Medina and North, 1998), a recent study of *M. tuberculosis* susceptibility employing *Nramp1$^{-/-}$* gene deletion strains and their progenitors found little evidence for a role of Nramp1 in tuberculosis susceptibility. Although these experiments do not rule out a role of *Nramp1* in modulating tuberculosis susceptibility in mice with different genetic backgrounds, the results seem at apparent odds with the demonstrated contribution of *NRAMP1* to tuberculosis susceptibility among humans. There are several possible explanations for these divergent observations. First, only one isolate of *M. tuberculosis* (H37Rv) was used in the

$Nramp1^{-/-}$ mouse experiments. It is possible that a role of $Nramp1$ would be more pronounced if fresh human *M. tuberculosis* isolates had been used for infection. Second, the tissue distribution and tissue-specific expression levels of Nramp1 differ between human and mice. It is possible that divergent Nramp1 expression may have important consequences in the context of natural infection and pathogenesis. Finally, it is possible that infection of laboratory mice with *M. tuberculosis* is not a good model of human tuberculosis. In contrast to humans, *M. tuberculosis* is not a natural pathogen of laboratory mice, and the resulting disease, despite its strong lung pathology, differs in several important aspects from the human disease. In this context, it has been suggested that infection of laboratory mice with *M. microti,* the vole bacillus, may represent a better model of human tuberculosis. Clearly, development of a mouse model that best reflects the human disease, including latency of infection, is a high priority of present tuberculosis research.

S. ENTERICA SEROVAR TYPHIMURIUM

Inbred strains of mice vary considerably in their level of innate resistance and susceptibility to infection with *S. enterica* serovar Typhimurium, as well as in their cellular responsiveness to serovar Typhimurium products (endotoxin). One of the major regulators of serovar Typhimurium in the murine host is the $Nramp1/Ity$ locus discussed above. Indeed, mice bearing naturally occurring ($Nramp1^{D169}$) or experimentally induced ($Nramp1^{-/-}$) mutations at $Nramp1$ are extremely susceptible to intravenous or subcutaneous infection with low doses of serovar Typhimurium (10^3 CFU), with uncontrolled bacterial replication in the spleen and liver of susceptible mice leading to uniform death within 4 to 5 days of infection (Vidal et al., 1995a; Govoni et al., 1999). However, $Nramp1$ is only one of several loci that affect serovar Typhimurium replication. Indeed, although mouse strains bearing a wild-type $Nramp1^{G169}$ allele have a clear advantage over $Nramp1^{D169}$ mutant strains early in the infection, a wide spectrum of infection can develop in the latter phase of infection in $Nramp1^{G169}$ animals (DBA/2J, C3H/He, A/J, and CBA), ranging from complete cure and recovery to lethal disease with different survival times (Plant and Glynn, 1974). Early studies with $H2$ congenic mouse strains showed that major histocompatibility complex-associated genes play a key role in regulating microbial replication and extent of disease in the non-early phase of serovar Typhimurium in $Nramp1^{G169}$ mouse strains. More

recently, a genetic approach has been initiated to identify additional genes playing an important role in susceptibility to serovar Typhimurium infection, starting with the mapping of modulators of $Nramp1$ action. Despite bearing an $Nramp1^{G169}$ allele, the wild mouse strain *Mus molossinus* (MOLF/E) is susceptible to serovar Typhimurium infection, as measured by survival to an intravenous challenge. Sequence analysis of $Nramp1$ in MOLF/E failed to identify deleterious mutations in $Nramp1,$ and expression studies by Northern blotting indicated similar levels of $Nramp1$ mRNA expression in MOLF/E mice compared to other inbred strains. An F_2 cross was generated between C57BL/6J and MOLF/E, and a genomewide scan was performed to map genes (QTL mapping) that affect survival time in an $Nramp1$-independent fashion (Sebastiani et al., 1998). The *Salmonella* resistance phenotype in this cross was linked to a newly mapped region on chromosome 11 (maximum lod score of 7.0 with $D11Mit5$), and a susceptibility locus was mapped on mouse chromosome 1 (maximum lod score of 4.8 with $D1Mit100$) approximately 25 cM distal to $Nramp1$ (Sebastiani et al., 1998). The host cell populations expressing the genetic advantage and disadvantage at these loci, as well as the genes responsible for the noted effects, have yet to be identified.

LPS is an abundant glycolipid of the outer membrane of gram-negative bacteria, which can provoke a generalized proinflammatory response in the infected host (Raetz et al., 1991). This inflammatory response can dramatically alter the ultimate outcome of the infection and is itself under genetic control of the Lps locus (Qureshi et al., 1999). Variation in the inflammatory response in inbred strains after challenge with purified LPS was noted 40 years ago (Heppner and Weiss, 1965). Of particular interest was the C3H/HeJ mouse strain, which was noted to be innately resistant to lethal challenge with LPS and was generally hyporesponsive to LPS in vitro, as measured by determining the polyclonal mitogenic response of B cells (Sultzer, 1968; reviewed by Rosenstreich [1985]). A second mouse strain, C57BL/10ScN, was also identified as hyporesponsive to LPS by the same criteria (McAdam and Ryan, 1978). Studies with informative populations of segregating animals generated by mating of high and low responders to LPS indicated that hyporesponsiveness in C3H/HeJ mice was controlled by a single locus, designated $Lps,$ with two alleles in inbred strains, Lps^n (normal, wild type), and Lps^d (defective, C3H/HeJ) (reviewed by Vogel [1999]). Lps appeared to control several aspects of the B-cell response to endotoxin, including in vivo susceptibility to toxic doses, mitogenic response in B cells, and antibody response to LPS. The Lps^d allele also impairs LPS-mediated macrophage activation, as measured by lymphokine production, oxidative burst, stimulation of phagocytosis, and survival of infection with gram-negative bacteria such as serovar Typhimurium and *Klebsiella pneumoniae*. Indeed, C3H/HeJ mice are extremely susceptible to serovar Typhimurium infection (50% lethal dose, <2 organisms), even though they bear a wild-type allele at *Nramp1* (Malo et al., 1994). At the molecular level, the mutant phenotype of C3H/HeJ mice has been attributed to defective recognition of the lipid A moiety of LPS by lymphocytes and macrophages. *Lps* was initially mapped to mouse chromosome 4 by cosegregation analysis in BXH recombinant inbred strains (Watson et al., 1977, 1978), and subsequently a 1-cM *Lps* interval was delineated (Qureshi et al., 1996; Poltorak et al., 1998). *Lps* was recently identified by positional cloning, as the Toll-like receptor 4 gene (*Tlr4*) (Poltorak et al., 1998a; Qureshi et al., 1999b). The Tlr4 protein is an 835-amino-acid polypeptide with an extracellular domain containing 22 leucine-rich repeat motifs connected by a single transmembrane domain to an intracellular signaling domain with homology to the interleukin-1 (IL-1) receptor. C3H/HeJ mice show a single H712P substitution in the signaling domain, while C57BL/10ScCr mice express no *Tlr4* RNA due to a homozygous deletion of the locus. Mammalian Toll-like receptors constitute a family of five homologous genes (in humans) that have been highly conserved in invertebrates and plants (Rock et al., 1998). In *Drosophila*, Toll was initially identified as an IL-1 receptor triggering activation of the NF-κB pathway and, ultimately, gene transcription. A connection between Toll function and susceptibility to infection in the fly was established by the observation that *Toll* mutants are susceptible to overwhelming fungal infections (Lemaitre et al., 1996). Stable expression of an activated version of the human Toll homolog (TLR4) activated NF-κB and stimulated the transcriptional activation of several inflammatory cytokines, including IL-1, IL-6, and IL-8 (Medzhitov et al., 1997). However, gene-targeting experiments showed that *Tlr4*-deficient mice have severe defects in macrophage and B-lymphocyte responses to LPS (Hoshino et al., 1999). On the other hand, transfection studies have shown that *Tlr4* expression in human embryonic kidney cells confers responsiveness to LPS as measured by NF-κB-dependent reporter gene expression, while the H712P variant of C3H/HeJ cannot do so in the same assay. These findings suggest that Tlr4 functions as an LPS cell surface receptor in macrophages and B lymphocytes and plays a key role in pattern recognition of microbial surfaces by these cells. Parallel studies of human TLR2 in similar assay systems have shown that TLR2 can also function as a receptor for LPS, allowing NF-κB-mediated transcriptional activation of cytokine genes (Yang et al., 1998; Kirschning et al., 1998). Specifically, it has been shown that microbial lipoproteins mediate IL-12, reactive oxygen intermediates, and nitric oxide production by human macrophages via Toll-like receptors (Aliprantis et al., 1999). Moreover, human TLR2-mediated interaction with microbial lipoprotein induced apoptosis of epithelial cells (Aliprantis et al., 1999). Thus, the study of the *Lps* mutation has allowed the identification of a novel group of membrane receptors and signaling molecules that play a key role in macrophage activation and resistance to infections.

LEGIONELLA PNEUMOPHILA

Legionella pneumophila is a facultative intracellular bacterium that can cause an acute form of pneumonia called Legionnaires' disease in humans. *L. pneumophila* enters macrophages through a unique "coiling-phagocytosis" mechanism and replicates within maturation-defective phagosomes, which do not fuse to endosomes or lysosomes (reviewed by Yamamoto [1994]). Successful intracellular survival and replication of *L. pneumophila* appear to involve modulation of host macrophage apoptosis. *L. pneumophila* induces apoptosis during infection of permissive human macrophages and in alveolar epithelial cell lines (Muller et al., 1996; Gao and Kwaik, 1999a). *L. pneumophila*-induced apoptosis occurs within 1 to 2 h of infection, can take place in the absence of intracellular replication, and can also be induced by extracellular bacteria. Induction of apoptosis in *L. pneumophila*-infected macrophages is mediated by activation of caspase 3 (Gao and Kwaik, 1999a, 1999b) and does not require a functional tumor necrosis factor alpha pathway (Hagele et al., 1998). Avirulent *L. pneumophila* mutants cannot induce either apoptosis or caspase 3 activation, and specific inhibition of caspase 3 activity can block both *L. pneumophila*-induced apoptosis and cytopathogenicity (Gao and Kwaik, 1999b).

In contrast to their human and guinea pig counterparts, mouse macrophages are not permissive to *L. pneumophila* replication even though the bacteria still rapidly inhibit phagosome-lysosome fusion soon after phagocytosis (reviewed by Yamamoto [1994]). The A/J strain is an exception, however, since A/J inflammatory peritoneal macrophages are highly permissive to *L. pneumophila* replication in vitro, resulting in a 1,000-fold increase in the number of viable bacteria during a 72-h infection, compared to macrophages from nonpermissive mouse strains such as C57BL/6J, C3H, and DBA/2J (Yamamoto et al., 1988; Yoshida et al., 1991). Linkage studies have indicated that a single autosomal, recessive gene designated *Lgn1* (Yoshida et al., 1991) determines macrophage permissiveness to intracellular replication of *L. pneumophila*. *Lgn1* maps to the distal mouse chromosome 13 (Dietrich et al., 1995; Scharf et al., 1996; Beckers et al., 1997), within a genetic interval of 0.3 cM, defined distally by the genetic marker *D13Die3* and proximally by *D13Die6/D13Die26*. Physical mapping studies and assembly of a cloned contig of BAC and YAC clones for the region suggest a minimal physical interval for *Lgn1* of approximately 350 kb (Diez et al., 1997; Endrizzi et al., 1999). The murine chromosome 13 *Lgn1* region is syntenic with the spinal muscular atrophy (*SMA*) locus on human chromosome 5, which includes the survival motor neuron (*SMN*) gene and the neuronal apoptosis inhibitory protein (*NAIP*) gene (Lefebvre et al., 1995; Roy et al., 1995). NAIP protein inhibits the apoptosis of neurons and other cell types both in vitro and in vivo (Liston et al., 1996; Xu et al., 1997). In addition, NAIP inhibits the proapoptotic cysteine proteases known as caspases; in particular, caspases 3 and 7 interact with NAIP (A. MacKenzie, personal communication). The mouse *Lgn1* locus includes the *Smn* gene as well as six copies of the *Naip* gene, and at least three of the *Naip* copies (*Naip1, Naip2,* and *Naip3*) encode full-length mRNA and possibly functional proteins (Yaraghi et al., 1998; Huang et al., 1999).

A possible link between *Lgn1, Naip,* and macrophage function was recently investigated (Diez et al., 2000). RNA expression studies show that *Naip* (mostly copy 2) mRNA transcripts are expressed in macrophage-rich tissues, such as spleen, lung, and liver, and are abundant in primary macrophages. Immunoblotting and immunoprecipitation analyses identify Naip protein expression in mouse macrophages and in macrophage cell lines RAW 264.7 and J774A. Interestingly, macrophages from permissive A/J mice express significantly less Naip protein than do their counterparts from nonpermissive C57BL/6J mice. Naip protein expression is increased following phagocytic events. Naip protein levels during infection with either virulent or avirulent strains of *L. pneumophila* increase during the first 6 h postinfection and remain elevated during the 48-h observation period. This enhanced expression is also observed in macrophages infected with *S. enterica* serovar Typhimurium. Likewise, an increase in Naip protein levels in macrophages is observed 24 h after phagocytosis of latex beads (Diez et al., 2000). Thus, the genetic mapping data, the known function of Naip,

and the role proposed for apoptosis in *L. pneumophila* infection, together with the expression of Naip protein detected in cells phenotypically expressing the genetic difference at *Lgn1* and the modulation of Naip protein expression observed in macrophages during phagocytosis of inert particles or live bacteria, combine to make Naip an attractive candidate for *Lgn1*. In such a model, successful infection of macrophages by *L. pneumophila* is dependent on the induction of apoptosis. In mouse macrophages, constitutive or inducible Naip expression may play a protective role by preventing the induction of apoptosis. This Naip-mediated inhibition of *L. pneumophila* replication would be lost in A/J cells by a loss-of-function mutation.

OTHER BACTERIAL INFECTIONS

Compared to the above examples, less is known about the genetic control of susceptibility to other bacterial infections. An early paper suggested that *Nramp1^r* macrophages were superior to their *Nramp1^s* counterparts in the extracellular killing of *Escherichia coli, Staphylococcus aureus,* and *Corynebacterium diphtheriae* (Lissner et al., 1985). In addition, a small number of phenotypically defined "resistance" and "susceptibility" alleles for bacterial infections have been mapped in the mouse genome. For example, bacterial proliferation following intraperitoneal injection of mice with *Listeria monocytogenes* is controlled by a phenotypically defined biallelic locus termed *Lsr1* (Cheers et al., 1980). Resistance, which is dominant over susceptibility, is characterized by an increased recruitment of inflammatory macrophages and neutrophils to the site of infection. *Lsr1* is closely linked to but distinct from *Hc*, which controls the level of C5 protein (Gervais et al., 1984). Interestingly, the strain distribution pattern of *Lsr1* is completely concordant with the one for *Ack*, a single locus controlling susceptibility to *Corynebacterium kutscheri* (Hirst and Wallace, 1976), suggesting a possible identity of *Ack* to *Lsr1*. The level of the C5 component of complement and the *Hc* gene have also been implicated in resistance or susceptibility to infection with the Sterne vaccine strain of *Bacillus anthracis*. Using backcross, F$_2$, or recombinant inbred mice, resistance to *B. anthracis* was highly significantly linked to production of C5 protein, although the modulating effect of an additional unknown gene(s) was noted (Welkos and Friedlander, 1988). The multigenic nature of *B. anthracis* susceptibility is even more evident if virulent strains are used for infection. In this case, inbred strains represent a spectrum of survival times postinfection, showing clear evidence for multigenic control of susceptibility (Welkos et al., 1986). A relatively well studied model is the genetic control of *Rickettsia tsutsugamushi* infection (Groves et al., 1980). The phenotypically defined *Ric^r* and *Ric^s* alleles correspond to different forms of the secreted phosphoprotein (*Spp1*) locus. *Spp1* was shown to be identical to the early T-lymphocyte activation gene, *Eta-1* (Patarca et al., 1989). Eta-1 is synthesized and secreted during the early stage of T-cell activation and mediates macrophage activation via its binding to high-affinity Eta-1 receptors on the surface of macrophages (Singh et al., 1990). Finally, corneal susceptibility to infection with *Pseudomonas aeruginosa* has been postulated to be under the control of two distinct single genes in C57BL/6 and BALB/c mice (Berk et al., 1981). However, a formal genetic proof for this postulated model of genetic control has not been provided.

CONCLUSION

What can be concluded from this vast amount of genetic and phenotypic information? It seems likely that for most bacterial pathogens, differences in susceptibility among inbred strains can be detected if the experimental conditions of infection are adjusted appropriately. It also seems that in the past, researchers were more likely to accept and pursue a genetic hypothesis if the analyzed phenotype followed classical Mendelian segregation. With the advent of improved analytical and experimental tools for the analysis of quantitative traits, this restriction is rapidly becoming obsolete. Hence, it seems likely that the number of described susceptibility and resistance loci for divergent bacterial infections in the mouse will increase dramatically over the coming years.

REFERENCES

Abel, L.,V. D. Lap, J. Oberti, N. Y. Thuc, V. V. Cua, M. Guillod-Bataille, E. Schurr, and P. Lagrange. 1995. Complex segregation analysis of leprosy in Southern Vietnam. *Genet. Epidemiol.* **12:** 63–70.

Abel, L., F. O. Sanchez, J. Oberti, N. V. Thuc, L. V. Hoa, V. D. Lap, E. Skamene, P. H. Lagrange, and E. Schurr. 1998. Susceptibility to leprosy is linked to the human *NRAMP1* gene. *J. Infect. Dis.* **177:**133–145.

Agranoff, D., I. M. Monahan, J. A. Mangan, P. D. Butcher, and S. Krishna. 1999. *Mycobacterium tuberculosis* expresses a novel pH-dependent divalent cation transporter belonging to the Nramp family *J. Exp. Med.* **190:**717–724.

Alcais, A., F. O. Sanchez, N. Y. Thuc, V. D. Lap, J. Oberti, P. H. Lagrange, E. Schurr, and L. Abel. 2000. Granulomatous reaction to intradermal injection of lepromin (Mitsuda reaction) is

linked to the human *NRAMP1* gene in Vietnamese leprosy sibships. *J. Infect. Dis.* **181:**302– 308.

Aliprantis, A. O., R. B. Yang, M. R. Mark, S. Suggett, B. Devaux, J. D. Radolf, G. R. Klimpel, P. Godowski, and A. Zychlinsky. 1999. Cell activation and apoptosis by bacterial lipoproteins through toll-like receptor 2. *Science* **285:**736–739.

Andrews, N. C. 1999. Disorders of iron metabolism. *N. Engl. J. Med.* **341:**1986–1995.

Apt, A. S., V. G. Avdienko, B. V. Nikonenko, I. B. Kramnik, A. M. Moroz, and E. Skamene. 1993. Distinct H-2 complex control of mortality, and immune responses to tuberculosis infection in virgin and BCG-vaccinated mice. *Clin. Exp. Immunol.* **94:**322–329.

Arias, M., M. Rojas, J. Zabaleta, S. C. Rodriguez, L. Paris, L. F. Barrera, and L. F. Garcia. 1997. Inhibition of virulent *M. tuberculosis* by *Bcg^r* and *Bcg^s* macrophages correlates with nitric oxide production. *J. Infect. Dis.* **176:**1552–1560.

Beckers, M.-C., E. Ernst, E. Diez, C. Morissette, F. Gervais, K. Hunter, D. Housman, S.-I. Yoshida, E. Skamene, and P. Gros. 1997. High-resolution linkage map of mouse chromosome 13 in the vicinity of the host resistance locus *Lgn1*. *Genomics* **39:** 254–263.

Bellamy, R., C. Ruwende, T. Corrah, K. P. McAdam, H. C. Whittle, and A. V. Hill. 1998. Variations in the NRAMP1 gene and susceptibility to tuberculosis in West Africans. *N. Engl. J. Med.* **338:**640–644.

Berk, R. S., K. Beisel, and L. D. Hazlett. 1981. Genetic studies of murine corneal response to *Pseudomonas aeruginosa*. *Infect. Immun.* **34:**1–5.

Bradley D. J., B. A. Taylor, J. Blackwell, E. P. Evans, and J. Freeman. 1979. Regulation of *Leishmania* populations within the host. III. Mapping of the locus controlling susceptibility to visceral leishmaniasis in the mouse. *Clin. Exp. Immunol.* **37:**7–14.

Brett, S. J., and J. Ivanyi. 1990. Genetic influences on the immune repertoire following tuberculosis infection in mice. *Immunology* **71:**113–119.

Brett, S. J., J. M. Orrell, J. Swanson-Beck, and J. Ivanyi. 1992. Influence of H2 genes on growth of *Mycobacterium tuberculosis* in the lungs of chronically infected mice. *Immunology* **76:**129–132.

Brown, I. N., A. A. Glynn, and J. Plant. 1982. Inbred mouse strain resistance to *Mycobacterium lepraemurium* follows the *Ity/Lsh* pattern. *Immunology* **47:**149–156.

Buu, N. T., M. Cellier, P. Gros, and E. Schurr. 1995. Identification of a highly polymorphic length variant in the 3′ UTR of *NRAMP1*. *Immunogenetics* **42:**428–429.

Canonne-Hergaux, F., S. Gruenheid, P. Ponka, and P. Gros. 1999. Cellular and sub-cellular localization of the Nramp2 iron transporter in the intestinal brush border and regulation by iron. *Blood* **93:**4406–4417.

Cellier, M., A. Belouchi, and P. Gros. 1996. Resistance to intracellular infections: comparative genome of NRAMP. *Trends Genet.* **12:**201–204.

Cellier, M., G. Govoni, S. Vidal, N. Groulx, J. Liu, F. Sanchez, E. Skamene, E. Schurr, and P. Gros. 1994. The human *NRAMP* gene: cDNA cloning, chromosomal mapping, genomic organization and tissue specific expression. *J. Exp. Med.* **180:**1741–1752.

Cellier, M., G. Prive, A. Belouchi, T. Kwan, V. Rodrigues, W. Chia, and P. Gros. 1995. The natural resistance associated macrophage protein (Nramp) defines a new family of membrane proteins conserved throughout evolution. *Proc. Natl. Acad. Sci. USA* **92:**10089–10094.

Cellier, M., C. Shustik, W. Dalton, E. Rich, J. Hu, D. Malo, E. Schurr, and P. Gros. 1997. The human *NRAMP1* gene as a marker of professional primary phagocytes: studies in blood cells and in induced HL-60 promyelocytic leukemia. *J. Leukoc. Biol.* **61:**96–105.

Cheers, C., I. F. C. McKenzie, T. E. Mandel, and Y. Y. Chan. 1980. A single gene controlling natural resistance to murine listeriosis, p. 141–147. *In* E. Skamene, P. A. L. Kongshavn, and M. Landy (ed.), *Genetic Control of Natural Resistance to Infection and Malignancy.* Academic Press, Inc., New York, N.Y.

Chen, X.-Z., J.-B. Peng, A. Cohen, H. Nelson, N. Nelson, and M. Hediger. 1999. Yeast SMF1 mediates H^+-coupled iron uptake with concomitant uncoupled cation currents. *J. Biol. Chem.* **274:** 35089–35094.

Crocker, P. R., J. M. Blackwell, and D. J. Bradley. 1984. Expression of the natural resistance gene *Lsh* in resident liver macrophages. *Infect. Immun.* **43:**1033–1040.

Darvasi, A., A. Weinreb, V. Minke, J. I. Weller, and M. Soller. 1993. Detecting marker QTL linkage and estimating QTL gene effects and map location using a saturated genetic map. *Genetics* **134:**943–951.

De Chastellier, C., C. Frehel, C. Offreso, and E. Skamene. 1993. Implication of phagosome-lysosome fusion in restriction of *Mycobacterium avium* growth in bone marrow macrophages from genetically resistant mice. *Infect. Immun.* **61:**3775–3784.

Denis, M., A. Forget, M. Pelletier, F. Gervais, and E. Skamene. 1990. Killing of *Mycobacterium smegmatis* by macrophages from genetically susceptible and resistant mice. *J. Leukoc. Biol.* **47:**25–30.

Dietrich, W. F., D. M. Damron, R. R. Isberg, E. S. Lander, and M. S. Swanson. 1995. *Lgn1,* a gene that determines susceptibility to *Legionella pneumophila,* maps to mouse chromosome 13. *Genomics* **26:**443–450.

Diez, E., M.-C. Beckers, E. Ernst, C. J. DiDonato, L. R. Simard, C. Morissette, F. Gervais, S.-I. Yoshida, and P. Gros. 1997. Genetic and physical mapping of the mouse host resistance locus Lgn1. *Mamm. Genome* **8:**682–685.

Diez, E., Z. Yaraghi, A. MacKenzie, and P. Gros. 2000. The apoptosis inhibitor protein NAIP: constitutive and inducible expression in macrophages, and candidacy for the host resistance locus *Lgn1. J. Immunol.* **164:**1470–1477.

D'Sousa, J., P. W. Cheah, P. Gros, W. Chia, and V. Rodrigues. 1999. Functional complementation of the *malvolio* mutation in the taste pathway of *Drosophila* by the human natural resistance-associated macrophage protein 1 (NRAMP-1). *J. Exp. Biol.* **202:**1909–1915.

Endrizzi, M., S. Huang, J. M. Scharf, A. R. Kelter, B. Wirth, L. M. Kunkel, W. Miller, and W. F. Dietrich. 1999. Comparative sequence analysis of the mouse and human *Lgn1*/SMA interval. *Genomics* **60:**137–151.

Farcich, E. A., and E. H. Morgan. 1992. Diminished iron acquisition by cells and tissues of Belgrade laboratory rats. *Am. J. Physiol.* **262:**R220.

Fleming, M. D., M. A. Romano, M. A. Su, L. M. Garrick, M. D. Garrick, and N. C. Andrews. 1998. Nramp2 is mutated in the anemic Belgrade (b) rat: evidence of a role for Nramp2 in endosomal iron transport. *Proc. Natl. Acad. Sci. USA* **95:**1148–1153.

Fleming, M. D., C. C. Trenor III, M. A. Su, D. Foernzler, D. R. Beier, W. F. Dietrich, and N. C. Andrews. 1997. Microcytic anaemia mice have a mutation in Nramp2, a candidate iron transporter gene. *Nat. Genet.* **16:**383–386.

Flynn, J. L., J. Chan, K. J. Triebold, D. K. Dalton, T. A. Stewart, and B. R. Bloom. 1993. An essential role for interferon gamma in resistance to *Mycobacterium tuberculosis* infection. *J. Exp. Med.* **178:**2249–2254.

Flynn, J. L., M. M. Goldstein, J. Chan, K. Pfeffer, C. J. Lowenstein, R. Schreiber, T. W. Mak, and B. R. Bloom. 1995. Tumor necrosis factor alpha is required in the protective immune re-

sponse against *Mycobacterium tuberculosis* in mice. *Immunity* **2:**561–572.

Flynn, J. L., M. M. Goldstein, K. J. Triebold, B. Koller, and B. R. Bloom. 1992. Major histocompatibility complex class I-restricted T cells are required for resistance to *Mycobacterium tuberculosis* infection. *Proc. Natl. Acad. Sci. USA* **89:**12013–12017.

Gao, L. Y., and Y. A. Kwaik. 1999a. Apoptosis in macrophages and alveolar epithelial cells during early stages of infection by *Legionella pneumophila* and its role in cytopathogenicity. *Infect. Immun.* **67:**862–870.

Gao, L.-Y., and Y. A. Kwaik. 1999b. Activation of caspase 3 during *Legionella pneumophila*-induced apoptosis. *Infect. Immun.* **67:**4886–4894.

Gervais, F., M. M. Stevenson, and E. Skamene. 1984. Genetic control of resistance to *Listeria monocytogenes*:regulation of leukocyte inflammatory responses by the Hc locus. *J. Immunol.* **132:**2078–2083.

Gotto, Y., E. Buschman, and E. Skamene. 1989. Regulation of host resistance to *Mycobacterium intracellulare in vivo* and *in vitro* by the *Bcg* gene. *Immunogenetics* **30:**218–221.

Govoni, G., F. Canonne-Hergaux, C. G. Pfeifer, S. Marcus, S. Mills, D. Hackam, S. Grinstein, D. Malo, B. Finlay, and P. Gros. 1999. Functional expression of Nramp1 in vitro after transfection into the murine macrophage line RAW264.7. *Infect. Immun.* **67:**2225–2232.

Govoni, G., S. Gauthier, N. N. Iscove, and P. Gros. 1997. Cell specific and inducible *Nramp1* gene expression in macrophages *in vitro* and *in vivo J. Leukoc. Biol.* **62:**277–286.

Govoni, G., S. Vidal, S. Gauthier, E. Skamene, D. Malo, and P. Gros. 1996. The *Bcg/Ity/Lsh* locus: genetic transfer of resistance to infections in C57BL/6J mice transgenic for the *Nramp1*^{Gly169} allele. *Infect. Immun.* **64:**2923–2929.

Greenwood, C. M. T., T. M. Fujiwara, L. Boothroyd, A. Fanning, M. Miller, E. Schurr, and K. Morgan. 2000. Genetic epidemiology of tuberculosis susceptibility and analysis of linkage to chromosome 2q35 near *NRAMP1* in a large Aboriginal Canadian family. *Am. J. Hum. Genet.* **67:**405–416.

Gros, P., E. Skamene, and A. Forget. 1981. Genetic control of natural resistance to *Mycobacterium bovis* (BCG) in mice. *J. Immunol.* **127:**2417–2422.

Gros, P., E. Skamene, and A. Forget. 1983. Cellular mechanisms of genetically-controlled host resistance to *Mycobacterium bovis* (BCG). *J. Immunol.* **131:**1966–1973.

Groves, M. G., D. L. Rosenstreich, B. A. Taylor, and J. V. Osterman. 1980. Host defenses in experimental scrub typhus: mapping the gene that controls natural resistance in mice. *J. Immunol.* **125:**1395–1399.

Gruenheid, S., F. Canonne-Hergaux, S. Gauthier, D. J. Hackam, S. Grinstein, and P. Gros. 1999. The iron transport protein Nramp2 is an integral membrane protein that co-localizes with transferrin in recycling endosomes. *J. Exp. Med.* **189:**831–841.

Gruenheid, S., M. Cellier, S. Vidal, and P. Gros. 1995. Identification and characterization of a second mouse *Nramp* gene. *Genomics* **25:**514–525.

Gruenheid, S., E. Pinner, M. Desjardins, and P. Gros. 1997. Natural resistance to infection with intracellular parasites: the Nramp1 protein is recruited to the membrane of the phagosome. *J. Exp. Med.* **185:**717–730.

Gunshin, H., B. Mackenzie, U. V. Berger, Y. Gunshin, M. F. Romero, W. F. Boron, S. Nussberger, J. L. Gollan, and M. A. Hediger. 1997. Cloning and characterization of a mammalian proton-coupled metal-ion transporter. *Nature* **388:**482–488.

Hackam, D. J., O. D. Rotstein, W.-J. Zhang, S. Gruenheid, P. Gros, and S. Grinstein 1998. Host resistance to intracellular infections: mutation at *Nramp1* impair phagosomal acidification. *J. Exp. Med.* **188**:351–364.

Hagele, S., J. Hacker, and B. C. Brand. 1998. *Legionella pneumophila* kills human phagocytes but not protozoan host cells by inducing apoptotic cell death. *FEMS Microbiol. Lett.* **169**:51–58.

Heppner, G,. and D. W. Weiss. 1965. High susceptibility of strain A mice to endotoxin and endotoxin-red blood cell mixtures *J. Bacteriol.* **90**:696–703.

Hirst, R. G., and M. E. Wallace. 1976. Inherited resistance to *Corynebacterium kutscheri* in mice. *Infect. Immun.* **14**:475–482.

Hoshino, K., O. Takeuchi, T. Kawai, H. Sanjo, T. Ogawa, Y. Takeda, K. Takeda, and S. Akira. 1999. Toll-like receptor 4 (TLR4)-deficient mice are hyporesponsive to lipopolysaccharide: evidence for TLR4 as the Lps gene product *J. Immunol.* **162**:3749–3752.

Huang, S., J. M. Sharf, J. D. Growney, M. G. Endrizzi, and W. F. Dietrich. 1999. The mouse *Naip* gene cluster on chromosome 13 encodes several distinct fucntional transcripts. *Mamm. Genome* **10**:1032–1035.

Jansen, R. C. 1993. Interval mapping of multiple quantitative trait loci. *Genetics* **135**:205–211.

Kirschning, C. J., H. Wesche, T. M. Ayres, and M. Rothe. 1998. Human Toll-like receptor 2 confers responsiveness to bacterial lipopolysaccharide. *J. Exp. Med.* **188**:2091–2097.

Kramnik, I., P. Demant, and B. R. Bloom. 1998. Susceptibility to tuberculosis as a complex genetic trait: analysis using recombinant congenic strains of mice, p. 120–137. *In* D. J. Chadwick and G. Cardew (ed.), *Genetics of Tuberculosis.* Novartis Foundation Symposium 217. John Wiley & Sons, Inc., Chichester, United Kingdom.

Lavebratt, C., A. Apt, B. V. Nikonenko, M. Schalling, and E. Schurr. 1999. Severity of tuberculosis is linked to distal chromosome 3 and proximal chromosome 9. *J. Infect. Dis.* **180**:150–155.

Lefebvre, S., L. Burglen, S. Reboullet, O. Clermont, P. Burlet, L. Viollet, B. Benichou, C. Cruaud, P. Millasseau, M. Zeviani, D. Le Paslier, J. Frezal, D. Cohen, J. Weissenbach, A. Munnich, and J. Melki. 1995. Identification and characterization of a spinal muscular atrophy-determining gene. *Cell* **80**:155–165.

Lemaitre, B., E. Nicolas, L. Michaud, J.-M. Reichhart, and J. A. Hoffman. 1996. The dorsoventral regulatory gene cassette *spatzle/Toll/cactus* controls the potent anti-fungal response in *Drosophila* adults. *Cell* **86**:973–983.

Lissner, C. R., R. N. Swanson, and A. D. O'Brien. 1983. Genetic control of the innate resistance of mice to *Salmonella typhimurium:* expression of the *Ity* gene in peritoneal and splenic macrophages isolated *in vitro. J. Immunol.* **131**:3006–3013.

Lissner, C. R., D. L. Weinstein, and A. D. O'Brien. 1985. Mouse chromosome 1 Ity locus regulates microbicidal activity of isolated peritoneal macrophages against a diverse group of intracellular and extracellular bacteria. *J. Immunol.* **135**:544–547.

Liston, P., N. Roy, K. Tamai, C. Lefebvre, S. Baird, G. Cherton-Horvat, R. Farahani, M. McLean, J.-E. Ikeda, A. MacKenzie, and R. G. Korneluk. 1996. Suppression of apoptosis in mammalian cells by Naip and a related family of IAP genes. *Nature* **379**:349–353.

Liu, J., M. T. Fujiwara, N. T. Buu, F. Sanchez, M. Cellier, A. Paradis, D. Frappier, P. Gros, E. Skamene, K. Morgan, and E. Schurr. 1995. Identification of polymorphisms and sequence variants in the human natural resistance-associated macrophage protein (*NRAMP*) gene, a candidate gene for susceptibility to tuberculosis. *Am. J. Hum. Genet.* **56**:845–853.

Lundrigan, M. D., J. E. Arceneaux, W. Zhu, and B. R. Byers. 1997. Enhanced hydrogen peroxide sensitivity and altered stress protein expression in iron-starved *Mycobacterium smegmatis. Biometals* **10**:215–225.

Lynch, C. J., C. H. Pierce-Chase, and R. Dubos. 1965. A genetic study of susceptibility to experimental tuberculosis in mice infected with mammalian tubercle bacilli. *J. Exp. Med.* **121**:1051–1070.

MacMicking, J. D., R. J. North, R. LaCourse, J. S. Mudgett, S. K. Shah, and C. F. Nathan. 1997. Identification of nitric oxide synthase as a protective locus against tuberculosis. *Proc. Natl. Acad. Sci. USA* **94**:5243–5248.

Makui, H., E. Roig, S. T. Cole, J. D. Helmann, P. Gros, and M. Cellier. 2000. Identification of *Escherichia coli* K-12 *Nramp* (*mntH*) as a selective divalent metal ion transporter. *Mol. Microbiol.* **35**:1065–1078.

Malo, D., S. Vidal, J. Lieman, D. C. Ward, and P. Gros. 1993b. Physical delineation of the minimal chromosomal segment encompassing the host resistance locus *Bcg. Genomics* **17**:667–675.

Malo, D., S. Vidal, E. Skamene, and P. Gros. 1993a. High resolution linkage map in the vicinity of the host resistance locus *Bcg* on mouse chromosome 1. *Genomics* **16**:655–663.

Malo, D., K. Vogan, S. Vidal, J. Hu, M. Cellier, A. Schurr, A. Fuks, K. Morgan, and P. Gros. 1994. Haplotype mapping and sequence analysis of the mouse *Nramp* gene predict susceptibility to infection with intracellular parasites. *Genomics* **23**:51–61.

Marquet, S., P. Lepage, T. Hudson, J. M. Musser, and E. Schurr. 2000. Complete nucleotide sequence and genomic structure of the human *NRAMP1* gene region on human chromosome region 2q35. *Mamm. Genome* **11**:755–762.

McAdam, K. W., and J. L. Ryan. 1978. C57BL/10CR mice: nonresponders to activation by the lipid A moiety of bacterial lipopolysaccharide. *J. Immunol.* **120**:249–253.

Medina, E., and R. J. North. 1998. Resistance ranking of some common inbred mouse strains to *Mycobacterium tuberculosis* and relationship to major histocompatibility haplotype and *Nramp1* genotype. *Immunology* **93**:270–274.

Medzhitov, R., P. Preston-Hurlburt, and C. A. Janeway, Jr. 1997. A human homologue of the *Drosophila* Toll protein signals activation of adaptive immunity. *Nature* **388**:394–397.

Muller, A., J. Hacker, and B. C. Brand. 1996. Evidence for apoptosis of human macrophage-like HL-60 cells by *Legionella pneumophila* infection. *Infect. Immun.* **64**:4900–4906.

Musa, S. A., Y. Kim, R. Hashim, G. Wang, C. Dimmer, and D. W. Smith. 1987. Response of inbred mice to aerosol challenge with *Mycobacterium tuberculosis. Infect. Immun.* **55**:1862–1866.

Nikonenko, B. V., A. S. Apt, A. M. Moroz, and M. M. Averbakh. 1985. Genetic analysis of susceptibility of mice to H37Rv tuberculosis infection: sensitivity versus relative resistance, p. 291–298. *In* E. Skamene (ed.), *Genetic Control of Host Resistance to Infection and Malignancy.* Alan R. Liss, New York, N.Y.

North, R. J., R. LaCourse, L. Ryan, and P. Gros. 1999. Consequence of *Nramp1* deletion to *Mycobacterium tuberculosis* infection in mice. *Infect. Immun.* **67**:5811–5814.

Orgad, S., H. Nelson, D. Segal, and N. Nelson. 1998. Metal ions suppress the abnormal taste behavior of the *Drosophila* mutant *malvolio. J. Exp. Biol.* **201**:115–120.

Orme, I. M., and D. N. McMurray. 1995. The immune response to tuberculosis in animal models, p. 269–280. *In* W. N. Rom, S. M. Garay, and S Little (ed.), *Tuberculosis.* Little, Brown, and Co., Boston, Mass.

Paramchuck, W. J., S. O. Ismail, A. Bhatia, and L. Gedamu. 1997. Cloning, characterization and overexpression of two iron superoxide dismutase cDNAs from *Leishmania chagasi:* role in pathogenesis. *Mol. Biochem. Parasitol.* **90**:203–221.

Patarca, R., G. J. Freeman, R. P. Singh, F. Y. Wei, T. Durfee, F. Blattner, D. C. Regnier, C. A. Kozak, B. A. Mock, and H. C.

Morse III. 1989. Structural and functional studies of the early T lymphocyte activation 1 (*Eta-1*) gene. Definition of a novel T cell-dependent response associated with genetic resistance to bacterial infection. *J. Exp. Med.* 170:145–161.

Pierce, C. R., J. Dubos, and G. Middlebrook. 1947. Infection of mice with mammalian tubercle bacilli grown in Tween-albumin liquid medium. *J. Exp. Med.* 86:159–165.

Pinner, E., S. Gruenheid, M. Raymond, and P. Gros. 1997. Functional complementation of the yeast divalent cation transporter family SMF by a member of the mammalian natural resistance associated macrophage family, Nramp2. *J. Biol. Chem.* 272:28933–28938.

Plant, J., and A. A. Glynn. 1974. Natural resistance to *Salmonella* infection, delayed hypersensitivity and Ir genes in different strains of mice. *Nature* 248:345–348.

Plant, J., and A. A. Glynn. 1976. Genetics of resistance with *Salmonella typhimurium* in mice. *J. Infect. Dis.* 133:72–78.

Poltorak, A., X. He, I. Smirnova, M. Y. Liu, C. V. Huffel, X. Du, D. Birdwell, E. Alejos, M. Silva, C. Galanos, M. Freudenberg, P. Ricciardi-Castagnoli, B. Layton, and B. Beutler. 1998a. Defective LPS signaling in C3H/HeJ and C57BL/10ScCr mice: mutations in *Tlr4* gene. *Science* 282:2085–2088.

Poltorak, A., I. Smirnova, X. He, M. Y. Liu, C. Van Huffel, O. McNally, D. Birdwell, E. Alejos, M. Silva, X. Du, P. Thompson, E. K. Chan, J. Ledesma, B. Roe, S. Clifton, S. N. Vogel, and B. Beutler. 1998b. Genetic and physical mapping of the *Lps* locus: identification of the toll-4 receptor as a candidate gene in the critical region. *Blood Cells Mol. Dis.* 24:340–355.

Qureshi, S. T., P. Gros, and D. Malo. 1999a. Host resistance to infection: genetic control of lipopolysaccharide responsiveness by TOLL-like receptor genes. *Trends Genet.* 15:291–294.

Qureshi, S. T., L. Larivière, G. Leveque, S. Clermont, K. Moore, P. Gros, and D. Malo. 1999b. Endotoxin-tolerant mice have mutations in Toll-like receptor 4 (*Tlr4*). *J. Exp. Med.* 189:615–625.

Qureshi, S. T., L. Larivière, G. Sebastiani, S. Clermont, E. Skamene, P. Gros, and D. Malo. 1996. A high-resolution map in the chromosomal region surrounding the *Lps* locus. *Genomics* 31:283–294.

Raetz, C. R. H., R. J. Ulevitch, S. D. Wright, C. H. Sibley, A. Ding, and C. Nathan. 1991. Gram-negative endotoxin: an extraordinary lipid with profound effects on eukaryotic signal transduction. *FASEB J.* 5:2652–2660.

Rock, F., G. Hardiman, J. C. Timans, R. A. Kastelein, and J. F. Bazan. 1998. A family of human receptors structurally related to *Drosophila* Toll. *Proc. Natl. Acad. Sci. USA* 95:588–593.

Rodrigues, V., P. Y. Cheah, K. Ray, and W. Chia. 1995. *malvolio*, the *Drosophila* homologue of mouse NRAMP-1(*Bcg*), is expressed in macrophages and in the nervous system and is required for normal taste behavior. *EMBO J.* 14:3007–3020.

Rosenstreich, D. L. 1985. Genetic control of the endotoxin response: C3H/HeJ mice, p. 82–122. *In* L. J. Berry, (ed.), *Handbook of Endotoxin*, vol. 3, Elsevier Biomedical Press, New York, N.Y.

Roy, N., M. S. Mahadevan, M. D. McLean, G. Shutler, Z. Yaraghi, R. Farahani, S. Baird, A. Besner-Johnston, C. Lefebvre, X. Kang, M. Salih, K. Tamai, X. Guan, P. Ioannou, T. Crawford, P. J. de Jong, L. Surh, J.-E. Ikeda, R. G. Korneluk, and A. MacKenzie. 1995. The gene for neuronal apoptosis inhibitory protein is partially deleted in individuals with spinal muscular atrophy. *Cell* 80:167–178.

Russell, E. S., D. J. Nash, S. E. Bernstein, E. L. Kent, E. C. McFarland, S. M. Matthews, and M. S. Norwood. 1970. Characterization and genetic studies of microcytic anemia in house mouse. *Blood* 35:838–850.

Scharf, J. M., D. Damron, A. Frisella, S. Bruno, A. H. Beggs, L. M. Kunkel, and W. F. Dietrich. 1996. The mouse region syntenic for human spinal muscular atrophy lies within the Lgn1 critical interval and contains copies of Naip exon 5. *Genomics* 38:405–417.

Schurr, E., A. Forget, E. Skamene, and P. Gros. 1989. Identification and mapping of a linkage group overlapping the host resistance *Bcg* gene on mouse chromosome 1. *J. Immunol.* 142:4507–4514.

Searle, S., and J. M. Blackwell. 1999. Evidence for a functional repeat polymorphism in the promoter of the human NRAMP1 gene that correlates with autoimmune versus infectious disease susceptibility. *J. Med. Genet.* 36:295–299.

Sebastiani, G., L. Olien, S. Gauthier, E. Skamene, K. Morgan, P. Gros, and D. Malo. 1998. Mapping of genetic modulators of natural resistance to infection with *Salmonella typhimurium* in mice. *Genomics* 47:180–186.

Singh, R. P., R. Patarca, J. Schwartz, P. Singh, and H. Cantor. 1990. Definition of a specific interaction between the early T lymphocyte activation 1 (Eta-1) protein and murine macrophages in vitro and its effect upon macrophages in vivo. *J. Exp. Med.* 171:1931–1942.

Skamene, E., P. Gros, A. Forget, P. A. L. Kongshavn, C. St. Charles, and B. A. Taylor. 1982. Genetic regulation of resistance to intracellular pathogens. *Nature* 297:506–509.

Skamene, E., P. Gros, A. Forget, P. J. Patel, and M. Nesbitt. 1984. Regulation of resistance to leprosy by chromosome 1 locus in the mouse. *Immunogenetics* 19:117–120.

Stach, J. L., P. Gros, A. Forget, and E. Skamene. 1984. Phenotypic expression of genetically controlled natural resistance to *Mycobacterium bovis* (BCG). *J. Immunol.* 132:888–892.

Stokes, R. W., I. Orme, and F. M. Collins. 1986. Role of mononuclear phagocytes in expression of resistance and susceptibility to *Mycobacterium avium* infections in mice. *Infect. Immun.* 54:811–819.

Sultzer, B. M. 1968. Genetic control of leukocyte responses to endotoxin. *Nature* 219:1253–1254.

Supek, F., L. Supekova, H. Nelson, and N. Nelson. 1996. A yeast manganese transporter related to the macrophage protein involved in conferring resistance to mycobacteria. *Proc. Natl. Acad. Sci. USA* 93:5105–5110.

Vidal, S., A. M. Belouchi, M. Cellier, B. Beatty, and P. Gros. 1995b. Cloning and characterization of a second human *NRAMP* gene on chromosome 12q13. *Mamm. Genome* 6:224–230.

Vidal, S., E. Pinner, S. Gauthier, P. Lepage, and P. Gros. 1996. Nramp1 is an integral membrane phosphoglycoprotein absent from macrophages of inbred mouse strains susceptible to infection with intracellular parasites. *J. Immunol.* 157:3559–3568.

Vidal., S., M. Tremblay, G. Govoni, G. Sebastiani, D. Malo, M. Olivier, E. Skamene, S. Jothy, and P. Gros. 1995a. The *Ity/Lsh/Bcg* locus: natural resistance to infection with intracellular parasites is abrogated by disruption of the *Nramp1* gene. *J. Exp. Med.* 182:655–666.

Vidal, S. M., D. Malo, K. Vogan, E. Skamene, and P. Gros. 1993. Natural resistance to infection with intracellular parasites: isolation of a candidate for *Bcg*. *Cell* 73:469–486.

Vogel, S. N. 1999. Genetic regulation of endotoxin responsiveness: the *Lps* gene revisited, p. 127–142. *In* H. Brade, D. C. Morrison, S. Opal, and S. N. Vogel (ed.), *Endotoxin in Health and Disease*. Marcel Dekker, Inc., New York, N.Y.

Watson, J., K. Kelly, M. Lergen, and B. A. Taylor. 1978. The genetic mapping of a defective LPS response gene in C3H/HeJ mice. *J. Immunol.* 120:422–424.

Watson, J., R. Riblet, and B. A. Taylor. 1977. The response of recombinant inbred strains of mice to bacterial lipopolysaccharides. *J. Immunol.* 118:2088–2093.

Welkos, S. L., and A. M. Friedlander. 1988. Pathogenesis and genetic control of resistance to the Sterne strain of *Bacillus anthracis*. *Microb. Pathog.* 4:53–69.

Welkos, S. L., T. J. Keener, and P. H. Gibbs. 1986. Differences in susceptibility of inbred mice to *Bacillus anthracis*. *Infect. Immun.* 51:795–800.

Xu, D. G., S. J. Crocker, J.-P. Doucet, M. St. Jean, K. Tamai, A. Hakim, J.-E. Ikeda, P. Liston, C. S. Thompson, R. G. Korneluk, A. MacKenzie, and G. S. Robertson. 1997. Elevation of neuronal expression of NAIP reduces ischemic damage in the hippocampus. *Nat. Med.* 3:997–1004.

Yamamoto, Y., T. W. Klein, and H. Friedman. 1994. *Legionella* and macrophages. *Immunol. Ser.* 60:329–348.

Yamamoto, Y., T. W. Klein, C. A. Newton, R. Widen, and H. Friedman. 1988. Growth of *Legionella pneumophila* in thioglycolate-elicited peritoneal macrophages from A/J mice. *Infect. Immun.* 56:370–375.

Yang, R. B., M. R. Mark, A. Gray, A. Huang, M. H. Xie, M. Zhang, A. Goddard, W. I. Wood, A. L. Gurney, and P. J. Godowski. 1998. Toll-like receptor-2 mediates lipopolysaccharide-induced cellular signalling. *Nature* 395:284–288.

Yaraghi, Z, R. G. Korneluk, and A. MacKenzie. 1998. Cloning and characterization of the multiple murine homologues of NAIP (neuronal apoptosis inhibitory protein). *Genomics* 51:107–113.

Yoshida, S.-I., Y. Goto, Y. Mizuguchi, K. Nomoto, and E. Skamene. 1991. Genetic control of natural resistance in mouse macrophages regulating intracellular *Legionella pneumophila* replication in vitro. *Infect. Immun.* 59:428–432.

Immunology of Infectious Diseases
Edited by S. H. E. Kaufmann, A. Sher, and R. Ahmed
© 2002 ASM Press, Washington, D.C.

Chapter 28

Immunogenetics of the Host Response to Viral Infections

MICHEL BRAHIC, CHARLES M. BANGHAM, GABRIEL GACHELIN, AND
JEAN-FRANÇOIS BUREAU

Variations in the susceptibility of laboratory animals, particularly inbred mouse strains, to infectious agents are well known. Although it is a matter of common observation that not everybody reacts to the same infectious agent in the same way, our understanding of the immunogenetics of infectious diseases in humans is much less advanced. However, this is a fast-moving field that takes advantage of new approaches in human genetics and will soon benefit from the sequencing of the human genome (Hill, 1998).

The existence of genetic factors of susceptibility is suggested by familial clustering, a property usually expressed as the λ_S factor. This is the increase in risk for a sibling of a patient compared to the risk for the general population. Since siblings frequently share their environment, λ_S for infectious diseases somewhat overestimates the importance of genetic factors of susceptibility. However, studying twins and adoptees can help cancel the effect of shared environment, as exemplified by a study of susceptibility to the hepatitis B virus (HBV) carrier state in the Chinese population (Lin et al., 1989). In natural populations, it is obviously difficult to control for the degree of exposure to a virus. Furthermore, it is important to consider that infections can remain subclinical and that genes responsible for susceptibility to infection should be distinguished from those responsible for susceptibility to clinical disease. In most cases, susceptibility to infection can be demonstrated, even retrospectively, by serology surveys. The distinction between infection and disease is, of course, more easily studied in animal models, such as the chronic murine neurological disease due to Theiler's virus, which will be discussed below.

As illustrated in this chapter, the genetic control of infections is usually multigenic. Most of the current work in the field is aimed at locating and identifying the genes involved. This can be done by two main approaches. The first, association studies, involves making a list of candidate genes, such as the genes of the major histocompatibility complex (MHC), which can be chosen based on what is known about the pathogenesis of the infection and also on analogies to animal models. Testing for association requires a well-matched control group, a requirement which can be difficult to fulfill in human studies, especially with urban, ethnically heterogeneous populations. New approaches, which require that both parents of patients be available, have been designed to overcome this difficulty (Flanders and Khoury, 1996). In experimental murine infections, the association is sought in the progeny of a classical cross, such as a backcross or an F_2 cross. Association studies are very powerful in confirming or ruling out the presence of a susceptibility gene in the region genetically linked to the candidate gene. Obviously, their ability to uncover "new" susceptibility loci is limited. However, new high-throughput techniques and the detailed genetic and physical maps available for the genomes of humans and mice make it possible to perform genome-wide surveys of association with anonymous markers, such as microsatellites. In principle, the second technique, genome-wide linkage analysis, should identify susceptibility loci anywhere on the genome, provided that their effects are sufficiently pronounced. Collecting samples and analyzing them for linkage analysis is labor intensive: a large number of families must be iden-

Michel Brahic and Jean-François Bureau • Unité des Virus Lents, CNRS URA 1930, Institut Pasteur, 28, rue du Dr Roux, 75724 Paris Cedex 15, France. **Charles M. Bangham** • Department of Immunology, Imperial College School of Medicine at St Mary's, Norfolk Place, London W2 1PG, United Kingdom. **Gabriel Gachelin** • Unité de Biologie Moléculaire du Gène, Institut Pasteur, 28, rue du Dr Roux, 75724 Paris Cedex 15, France.

tified, and two or more affected siblings and their parents have to be analyzed. Since it is sometimes difficult to classify unaffected members as resistant or unexposed to the agent, an alternative approach involves studying allele-sharing in pairs of affected siblings (Risch, 1990). There are two ways of analyzing genetic linkage. In the so-called nonparametric methods, no assumption is made regarding the mode of inheritance of the trait. In parametric studies, on the other hand, a model for the mode of inheritance of the trait has to be established from segregation analysis of the pedigrees. Nonparametric methods are considered safer, but they require a larger number of families with affected sib pairs. The fast advances in the human—and mouse—genome projects are having a major impact on these studies, chiefly by providing lists of candidate genes in regions identified by linkage analysis.

In this chapter, we will briefly review the main steps of the adaptive immune responses and discuss the consequences of genetic polymorphism for the susceptibility to viral infections; we will then review recent important results obtained with particular viral infections of mice and of humans; and we will conclude with some general remarks on the consequences of these studies for both our fundamental understanding of viral pathogenesis and practical applications to human medicine.

GENETIC CONTROL OF THE ADAPTIVE IMMUNE RESPONSE TO VIRUSES, WITH AN EMPHASIS ON THE ROLE OF THE MHC

Studies of the host responses to viruses have been dominated by those dealing with the role of the adaptive immune responses: specific antibody secretion, the production of cytotoxic $CD8^+$ T cells, and, to a lesser extent, the production of $CD4^+$ T cells. This should not minimize the role of the innate responses, which is particularly well illustrated for interferon by the phenotype of mouse strains in which components of this system have been genetically inactivated (Fiette et al., 1995; Müller et al., 1994).

The adaptive immune response is initiated by the presentation of viral peptide epitopes to the immune system by MHC class I and class II molecules. Recognition of MHC class I-peptide complexes by the T-cell receptor (TCR) of $CD8^+$ T cells leads to their activation, proliferation, and acquisition of the ability to kill infected cells. MHC class II-peptide complexes are recognized by the TCR of $CD4^+$ T cells. The activation of these cells triggers regulatory mechanisms which orient the immune response. Fi-

nally, specific memory cells segregate out of the activated T cells after the burst of cell proliferation.

The basic MHC class I pathway is active in nearly all nucleated cells (Rock and Goldberg, 1999). Briefly, newly synthesized viral proteins are degraded in the cytoplasm by proteasomes and the resulting peptides are injected into the endoplasmic reticulum (ER) by the TAP peptide transporters. After further trimming in the ER, the proper peptides bind to MHC class I molecules in the lumen of the ER and the complexes mature in the Golgi apparatus and migrate to the cell surface. The basic MHC class II pathway is active only in specialized antigen-presenting cells such as dendritic cells, macrophages, and B cells. In this case, proteins or particles taken from extracellular fluids are degraded within endosomes, where they meet MHC class II molecules protected by an invariant chain. The invariant chain is dislodged and replaced by an antigenic peptide, and the resulting complex migrates to the cell surface (Cresswell, 1994). This oversimplified view of antigenic presentation is shown as a diagram in Fig. 1. One should keep in mind that there is leakage of the class I pathway into the class II pathway and vice versa and that monomorphic class I molecules may present nonpeptidic antigens.

One might expect that polymorphism in any of the many components of this complex machinery could result in alterations of the specific immune response and therefore in changes in susceptibility to viral infections (Fig. 1). However, the effects of subtle polymorphism on susceptibility remain largely unexplored. In natural populations, including human populations, studies have dealt mainly with "clearcut" phenotypes, such as the complete absence of one pathway (e.g., the rare cases of children deficient in class I or class II pathways or the *nude*, *scid*, and *beige* mouse mutants). In the laboratory mouse, the roles of individual components of the class I and class II pathways have been studied by inactivating the corresponding genes. The results are more ambiguous than expected and point to the existence of large overlaps of the defense mechanisms selected during evolution. For example, mice devoid of class I molecules are not significantly more sensitive than wild-type mice to several viral infections (Ojcius et al., 1994). On the other hand, inactivation of the class II pathway has much more profound effects.

Class I and class II molecules are highly polymorphic. The complete sequencing of the MHC locus of several animals and of humans has shown that alleles of class I and class II genes differ by short stretches of coding DNA which have been involved in multiple gene conversion events (Ohta, 1999). During these events, segments of genes are trans-

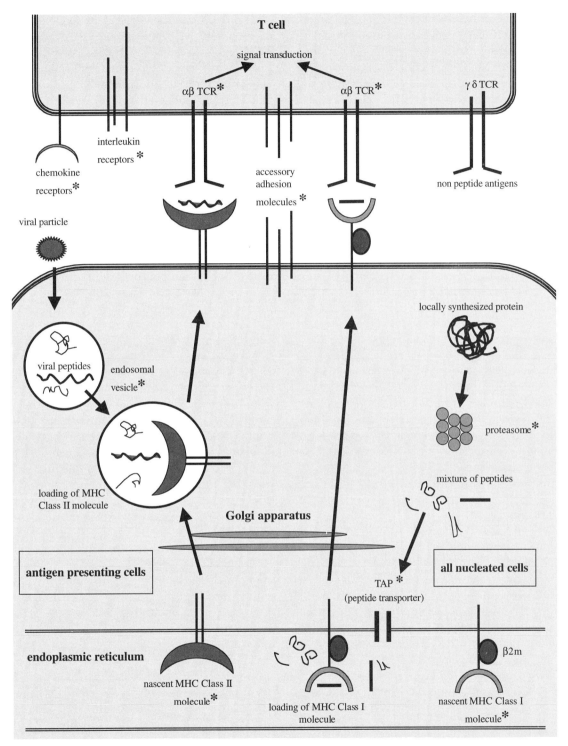

Figure 1. Summary of antigen presentation by the MHC class I and class II pathways. The class I pathway, present in all nucleated cells, is illustrated on the right, and the class II pathway, which is specific to antigen-presenting cells, is illustrated on the left. The T cell is at the top, and the presenting cell at the bottom. The asterisks denote the steps in the pathways of antigen processing and presentation in which host polymorphism might influence the specificity or efficiency of immune recognition. Polymorphism in the proteases involved in these pathways (i.e., the proteasomal, cytoplasmic, and endosomal proteases) might affect the repertoire of peptides generated from viral proteins.

ferred from a donor gene to a highly homologous but nonallelic recipient gene. In mice and humans, gene conversions and point mutations have generated hundreds of MHC class I and class II molecules, with differences located mainly in the peptide binding groove. This non-Mendelian unequal recombination has generated in individual mice variable numbers of genes and pseudogenes because of the deletion or duplication of whole genomic regions. This has not been observed in humans, probably because of the recent genetic bottleneck associated with the emergence of *Homo sapiens sapiens*. The peptides bound to the grooves of class I and class II molecules obey precise rules: they are 8 to 10 amino acids long (class I molecules) or 14 to 16 amino acids long (class II molecules). Anchor residues are located at precise positions, mainly at the termini for class I bound peptides and at three or four locations along the chain for class II bound peptides. The other amino acids can be diverse (Rammensee et al., 1995).

Extensive polymorphism of class I and class II molecules, the number of alleles, and their heterozygosity account for the ability to mount efficient immune responses against a large variety of infectious agents. Nevertheless, the modulation of the immune response to viruses by the MHC haplotype is well documented for mice and other laboratory animals, as will be described below. The *dm1* mutation illustrates the effect of gene conversion on susceptibility to lymphocytic choriomeningitis virus and to Theiler's virus. Finally the evidence is mounting for an association, in humans, of a given class I allele and resistance to human T-cell leukemia virus type 1 (HTLV-1)-associated disorders.

The MHC molecule-peptide complexes are recognized by TCR through the antigen recognition site of the β chain named the CDR3b region and the diversity region of the α chain. The diversity of the TCR CDR3 regions is enormous, large enough to account for the recognition of any MHC-peptide complex. Such diversity explains why naturally occurring deletions in the *Tcrb* locus of some mouse strains, such as the SJL/J strain, have no effect, or only minor effects, on the immune responses to viruses.

Besides recognition of the MHC molecule-peptide complex by the TCR, activation of the T cell requires accessory molecules such as the CD4, CD8, LFA1, and intercellular cell adhesion molecule (ICAM) proteins. Several natural polymorphisms, or the absence of accessory molecules, have been described which result in modest to severe deficiencies of the adaptive immune responses to viral infections.

Finally, it should be noted that some specialized TCR and T-cell populations link the MHC to the innate immune system. These cells may detect gly-

colipids presented by MHC class I CD1 molecules (Porcelli and Modlin, 1999), control the activity of NK cells (Qa1 molecules), or control chemoattraction (H2-M3 molecules). Also, the human γδ TCR recognizes, in the absence of presentation by class I or class II molecules, phosphoantigens or alkylamines produced during viral or microbial infection (Bonneville and Fournié, 1999).

VIRAL INFECTIONS OF THE MOUSE

Mx

The *Mx* genes and their protein products constitute one of the best-characterized systems of genetically regulated control of viral infections (Haller et al., 1998). In the early 1960s, Lindenmann (1962) made the chance observation that the A2G mouse strain was resistant to large doses of influenza virus that were lethal to other laboratory mouse strains. This led to the demonstration that resistance was inherited as a dominant trait which was mapped to a single gene, *Mx1*, on chromosome 16 (Reeves et al., 1988). Importantly, the effect of the *Mx1* gene on resistance was not mediated by the adaptive immune responses but was dependent on alpha/beta interferon. The *Mx1* gene covers more than 55 kb of genomic DNA and consists of 14 exons. The gene is defective in the majority of standard laboratory mouse strains because of either a deletion or a point mutation causing premature termination of translation (Staeheli et al., 1988). The exceptions are the A2G and SL/NiA strains, which possess the functional *Mx*+ allele, as do eight strains derived from wild mice of different geographical origins (Jin et al., 1998). Interestingly, the *Mx*+ and *Mx*− alleles occur at about the same frequency in outbred wild-mouse populations (Haller et al., 1987). The presence of the *Mx*+ allele in wild mice suggests that the Mx protein plays a role in resistance to the viruses to which these mice are exposed. Since influenza virus is not a natural pathogen of the mouse, other viruses must be concerned. One of them could be Thogoto virus, a tick-borne orthomyxovirus which is extremely sensitive to the effect of Mx (Haller et al., 1995). Since the *Mx*+ allele is dominant, roughly 75% of wild mice are resistant to orthomyxoviruses. The reason for the selection of the *Mx*− allele in wild-mouse populations is unclear. It suggests that there must be a price to pay to be resistant to orthomyxoviruses infections.

The mouse genome contains another *Mx* gene, *Mx2*, which is closely linked to *Mx1*. The two genes show a high degree of sequence similarity. *Mx2* is defective in most laboratory mouse strains but not in wild mice (Staeheli and Sutcliffe, 1988). The Mx2 protein of feral strains does not cause resistance to influenza virus but, instead, causes resistance to vesicular stomatitis virus.

The human genome contains two Mx related genes, *MxA* and *MxB,* which are close to each other on chromosome 21, in a region which is syntenic to that of mouse chromosome 16 bearing the *Mx1* and *Mx2* genes (Staeheli and Haller, 1985). The MxA protein has antiviral activity against a broad range of human RNA viruses, including influenza and Thogoto viruses but also bunyaviruses, phleboviruses, and hantaviruses. At present, there is no evidence for the existence of functional polymorphisms in the *MxA* or *MxB* gene.

The mechanism of the antiviral activity of the Mx proteins is now broadly understood. Mx proteins are induced by alpha/beta interferon and restrict viral replication. Therefore, they contribute to the sequestration of the infection to limited foci surrounding the initially infected cells. Their role in pathogenesis is in recovery from, rather than prevention of, the infection. This is well illustrated with influenza in mice. *Mx1*[+] animals do get infected and show symptoms. However, they recover, whereas *Mx1*[-] animals die.

Early on in these studies it was recognized that following induction by interferon, the Mx1 protein of mouse is translocated to the nucleus, where it interferes with primary transcription of the influenza virus nucleocapsid. Surprisingly, the human MxA protein remains in the cytoplasm and blocks influenza virus replication at a posttranscriptional step. Interestingly, a chimeric MxA with a nuclear localization signal will be translocated to the nucleus and will restrict influenza virus replication there.

The Mx proteins belong to the dynamin superfamily of GTPases. These large GTPases have an N-terminal regulatory domain which binds GTP and a C-terminal effector domain containing a leucine zipper. GTP-bound dynamins are known to self-assemble around intracellular membrane invaginations and to play a role in endocytosis and intracellular vesicle transport. Both GTP binding activity and the leucine zipper are essential for antiviral activity, as shown by site-directed mutagenesis. On GTP binding, the MxA protein forms aggregates with a helicoidal structure. It has been postulated for some time that Mx proteins restrict viral replication by wrapping around helical viral structures such as the nucleocapsids of negative strand RNA viruses. There is now direct evidence that GTP-bound MxA interacts with the nucleocapsid of Thogoto virus, thereby

blocking its nuclear import (Kochs and Haller, 1999a, 1999b).

The Friend Virus Complex

The genetic control of murine retroviral infections has been studied extensively with Friend virus (FV) (Chesebro et al., 1990; Hasenkrug and Chesebro, 1997). FV is a complex made of spleen focus-forming virus, a replication-defective virus, and Friend murine leukemia virus (F-MuLV), a replication-competent helper virus. In adult mice, binding of the viral gp55 env protein to the erythropoietin receptor (Epor) causes polyclonal proliferation of immature erythroblasts, leading rapidly to acute splenomegaly. Subsequently, proviral integration at the *ets* oncogene locus and inactivation of the p53 tumor suppressor gene result in malignant erythroleukemia (Moreau-Gachelin et al., 1988; Paul et al., 1991). Inbred mouse strains vary in their susceptibility to FV-induced leukemia, an observation which led to the identification of several host genes which control the disease. These genes can be divided into two categories according to their mechanism of action. The first group consists of genes which interfere with virus replication; the second consists of genes which enhance the immune response to FV and bring about the clearance of an already established infection. What follows is a summary of the salient features of some of these loci or genes.

Fv-1

In vivo, *Fv-1* affects the magnitude of the proliferative response to FV, as measured by the spleen focus assay. In mouse cells grown in vitro, it controls the replication of helper MuLV, as well as that of most MuLVs. Two alleles were originally defined, *Fv-1*[n] and *Fv-1*[b], according to cell permissiveness to MuLV. Strains of MuLV, in turn, are classified as N-tropic if they replicate best in *Fv-1*[n] cells and B-tropic if they replicate best in *Fv-1*[b] cells. Heterozygous *Fv-1*[nb] cells are resistant to both types of viruses, indicating that resistance is dominant. *Fv-1 n* and *b* alleles are present at roughly the same frequency among inbred laboratory mouse strains (Jolicoeur, 1979). Interestingly, most wild mice from areas other than Europe and Japan, the areas from which the "old inbred" laboratory mouse strains were derived, carry new *Fv-1* alleles and do not restrict MuLV replication (Kozak, 1985).

The fact that *Fv-1* restriction manifests itself in vitro implies that the locus acts directly on viral replication. Different approaches indicated that *Fv-1* acts after virus entry but prior to provirus integration and that its target is the p30 viral capsid protein (Stoye, 1998). These observations are congruent since p30 is part of the subviral complex on which reverse transcription takes place and since it participates in nuclear import and integration. The *Fv-1* gene has been cloned recently. It consists of a single exon related to the *gag* gene of the MuERV-L family of murine endogenous retroviruses, a family unrelated to MuLV. The *n* and *b* alleles differ by a deletion and two point mutations. The current hypothesis is that the *Fv-1* gene acts on the incoming virus as a dominant negative mutation (Best et al., 1996). Although the *Fv-1* open reading frame appears to be present in all subspecies of *Mus musculus*, *Fv-1* alleles which restrict MuLV replication are present in some of them only (Kozak, 1985). Therefore, it is possible that the *Fv-1* gene acquired resistant alleles under selective pressure from infection by exogenous MuLV retroviruses.

Fv-2

Unlike *Fv-1*, *Fv-2* is specific to FV. The resistant allele is recessive, but *Fv-2^rr^* mice are totally resistant to FV-induced leukemia. Most inbred laboratory mouse strains are *Fv-2^ss^*. *Fv-2* does not restrict virus replication in target cells. Rather, it determines whether erythroblasts proliferate in response to the viral *env* product, gp55. As a result, the *Fv-2^s^* allele has an indirect effect on the viral load by increasing the number of viral target cells in the animal (Weiss et al., 1982). The *Fv-2* gene has been identified recently (Persons et al., 1999). It codes for Stk, a receptor tyrosine kinase which is probably part of the Epor complex. *Fv-2^ss^* mice express a truncated form of Stk (Sf-stk), which lacks the extracellular domain of the protein but retains the transmembrane and intracellular tyrosine kinase domains. Sf-stk is expressed from an alternative promoter which is mutated, and inactive, in *Fv-2^rr^* strains. These results suggest that the extracellular domain of Stk prevents the binding of gp55 to Epor, thereby making mice resistant to leukemogenesis. Conversely, binding of gp55 to Epor in *Fv-2^s^* mice is made possible by the truncation in Sf-stk.

Fv-4

The *Fv-4* locus was described independently in an outbred mouse strain in Japan and in a wild-mouse population near Lake Casitas, Calif. (The locus was originally called *Akvr-1* by the group working with mice from Lake Casitas.) The resistant allele, *Fv-4^r^*, is dominant and restricts viral replication in target cells. The distribution of *r* and *s* alleles

in the Lake Casitas mice paralleled the frequency of MuLV-associated disorders (Best et al., 1997; Gardner et al., 1991). Unlike *Fv-4^ss^* cells, *Fv-4^rr^* cells express at their surface a gp70 molecule related to the envelope glycoprotein of ecotropic retroviruses. It was suggested that the *Fv-4^r^* gene restricts FV replication by a so-called viral interference phenomenon whereby the expression of an *env* gene in target cells makes them resistant to a related exogenous retrovirus. This hypothesis was confirmed by the cloning of *Fv-4*. The gene consists of a truncated endogenous MuLV provirus coding for a complete *env* gene (Ikeda and Sugimura, 1989). It is absent in mice with the *s* haplotype. Therefore, *Fv-4* must have been acquired recently in the history of *M. musculus*, following germ line infection by an ecotropic murine retrovirus. (Incidentally, the distribution of the *Fv-4* gene has helped in tracing the migrations of *M. musculus* subspecies.) *Fv-4* is a remarkable example of adaptive exploitation of the acquisition of endogenous retroviral sequences. Acquisition of the truncated provirus did not cause disease but provided a selective advantage in populations exposed to ecotropic retroviruses. On the other hand, there is probably a price to be paid for carrying *Fv-4*, since the *s* allele persists in the Lake Casitas population, including in homozygous *ss* individuals. In fact, it looks as if the gene persists in balance with the leukemia-causing retrovirus.

H-2

The MHC, together with the *Rfv-3* locus described below, has a strong effect on recovery from FV infection and splenomegaly. Specific class I and class II alleles, which correlate with the intensity of the virus-specific cytotoxic T-cell (CTL), T-helper cell, and antibody responses, are required for recovery. The MHC H-2D region has a strong influence through its role in the antiviral CTL response. The *H-2A* and *H-2E* MHC class II genes are also important. The effect of *H-2A* is linked to viral antigen presentation to CD4^+^ T cells and to the help provided to both virus-specific antibody and CTL responses. The model illustrates the complexity of the genetic control of nonoverlapping immune functions required to clear a retroviral infection (Hasenkrug and Chesebro, 1997).

Rfv-3

The antibody response plays an important role in recovery from FV infection. *Rfv-3* is a non-MHC locus which has a strong effect on FV-specific neutralizing antibodies. Because of low antibody levels,

Rfv-3^{ss} mice have mortality rates of 90% or greater, even if they bear the resistant *H-2^{bb}* haplotype. The mechanism through which the locus affects antibody production is still unknown. *Rfv-3* has been mapped recently to a 1-centimorgan (cM) region of chromosome 15 which contains several candidate genes, including *Il2rb* (interleukin 2 receptor beta), *Il3rb1* (interleukin-3 receptor beta 1), and *Pdgfb* (platelet-derived growth factor beta) (Super et al., 1999). As with the other loci mentioned above, the identification of *Rfv-3* should pave the way to determining its mechanism of action.

Theiler's Virus

Theiler's murine encephalomyelitis virus causes an early acute encephalomyelitis followed by a persistent low-grade infection of the spinal cord white matter with chronic inflammation and primary demyelination. This late disease is being studied as a model of multiple sclerosis (Brahic and Bureau, 1998; Monteyne et al., 1997). Inbred mouse strains vary greatly in their susceptibility to persistent infection and the accompanying disease, although all of them are susceptible to the early encephalomyelitis. Susceptibility to persistence of the infection is multigenic, with the MHC having a major effect.

H-2D region of the MHC

Early studies indicated that the MHC has a strong effect on susceptibility to the demyelinating disease and that, within the MHC, the H-2D region plays the major role (Clatch et al., 1985; Rodriguez et al., 1986). This role was subsequently linked to an effect on the susceptibility to persistence of the infection (Bureau et al., 1992). MHC haplotypes fall into three classes: *q*, which confers a high level of susceptibility, *b*, which confers resistance in a dominant fashion, and *d*, *k*, and *s*, which are associated with intermediate levels of susceptibility. Genetic studies eventually demonstrated that the *H-2D* gene itself was responsible: *H-2^q* FVB mice transgenic for the *H-2D^b* gene become resistant (Azoulay et al., 1994; Rodriguez and David, 1995). Conversely, *H-2^b* mice that are *H-2D* gene knockouts become susceptible (Azoulay-Cayla et al., 2000) and mutations in the *H-2D^b* gene modify susceptibility (Lipton et al., 1995). The effect of the class I *H-2D* gene is most probably due to its role in the antiviral CTL response. Indeed, the resistant *H-2^b* C57BL/6 strain mounts a fast, *H-2D^b*-restricted response to an immunodominant viral epitope. Large numbers of virus-specific CTL precursors are present in the spleens of these mice. In contrast, the response of the sus-

ceptible *H-2^s* SJL/J strain is much slower and weaker (Dethlefs et al., 1997).

Non-H-2 genes

Several non-*H-2* loci have been implicated in susceptibility to persistent infection. The *Tcrb* locus, which codes for the V$_\beta$ chains of the TCR, was an obvious candidate since it is partially deleted in the susceptible SJL/J strain. Although the evidence in favor of the presence of a susceptibility gene in the region is strong, the gene is probably not *Tcrb* (Monteyne et al., 1997). The existence of non-*H-2* susceptibility genes is illustrated by a comparison of the SJL/J and B10.S strains. Both bear the same *H-2^s* haplotype, but the former is more susceptible than the latter (Monteyne et al., 1997). A complete genome scan of a backcross between the SJL/J and the B10.S strains gave good evidence for linkage with the *Ifng* locus (Bureau et al., 1993; Monteyne et al., 1997). Although gamma interferon has a major effect in preventing viral persistence, the *Ifng* gene was excluded from a list of candidate genes in a study of a panel of congenic mice. Instead, the region seems to contain at least two susceptibility genes which have not been characterized yet (Bihl et al., 1999; Monteyne et al., 1999). Complete genome scans have been used in two other *H-2* identical crosses to map loci (on chromosome 14) responsible for susceptibility to demyelination and (on chromosome 11) for susceptibility to clinical disease (Aubagnac et al., 1999; Bureau et al., 1998).

Flaviviruses

Flaviviruses cause fatal encephalitis in the majority of laboratory mouse strains. The study of genetic control of the resistance and susceptibility of mice to flaviviruses goes back to the work of Sawyer and Lloyd and that of Webster in the 1930s (Shellam et al., Sangster, 1998). In the 1950s, Sabin (1952) showed that resistance was transmitted as a single dominant autosomal allele, later called *Flv^r*, and 13 years later, resistant congenic inbred mouse strains were developed by Groschel and Koprowski (1965). Interestingly, *Flv^r* confers resistance to every member of the flavivirus family which has been tested, including yellow fever virus, dengue virus, and Japanese encephalitis virus, but not to any of the more than 12 nonflaviviruses tested. Resistance is not immune mediated and can be observed and studied in mouse cells in culture, including in splenic or peritoneal macrophages. The mechanism of resistance is not yet understood. The roles of the interferon system and of the production by the infected cells of defective interfering particles have been investigated thoroughly. In particular, biochemical studies showed that *Flv^r* cells generate more defective interfering particles in vitro than susceptible ones do and that they produce less viral genomic RNA and more defective viral RNA (Brinton, 1983). However, defective viral RNA could not be demonstrated in the brains of resistant mice (Urosevic et al., 1997). Four cellular proteins which bind the 3' extremity of the minus-strand RNA of West Nile virus have been identified. Although the same RNA-bound proteins were present in resistant and susceptible C3H sublines, the half-life of one of the RNA-protein complex was three times shorter in the susceptible subline, suggesting that one of these proteins could be responsible for the resistant phenotype (Shi et al., 1996). The *Flv* locus has been mapped with respect to other markers on chromosome 5 (Sangster et al., 1994), and the localization has been refined to a 0.45-cM interval by using several backcrosses.

HUMAN VIRAL INFECTIONS

Human Immunodeficiency Virus Type 1

From the beginning of the human immunodeficiency virus type 1 (HIV-1) epidemic, it has been clear that the rate of progression of disease varies widely among infected people. There have been many studies of the association of the HLA genotype with different aspects of HIV-1 infection (Itescu et al., 1992; Jeannet et al., 1989; Kaslow et al., 1990; Klein et al., 1994; Scorza-Smeraldi et al., 1986). Many of the results were inconclusive because of inadequate sample sizes. However, two consistent relationships have emerged: rapid progression to AIDS and/or a rapid decline in the $CD4^+$ T-cell count is associated with both HLA-B35 (Carrington et al., 1999; Itescu et al., 1992; Klein et al., 1994; Sahmoud et al., 1993; Scorza-Smeraldi et al., 1986) and the common haplotype HLA-A1, B8, Cw7, DR3 (Carrington et al., 1999; Kaslow et al., 1996; Kaslow et al., 1990; McNeil et al., 1996).

Why these genotypes appear to confer dominant susceptibility is not understood. The function of HLA molecules is to present peptides to the immune system for recognition by T cells, and indeed both the CTL response (McMichael and Phillips, 1997) and the helper T-cell response (Kalams et al., 1999) play an important part in controlling the rate of HIV-1 disease progression. One would therefore expect to find associations either with dominant resistance ("high-responder alleles") or recessive susceptibility ("low-responder alleles"). The failure

to detect resistance alleles might occur because individuals differ in the dominant HIV-1 antigen to which their T cells respond. In contrast, most people infected with the retrovirus HTLV-1 mount a strong CTL response to the Tax protein, and dominant protection is associated with the class I allele HLA-A2 (Jeffery et al., 1999) (see below).

The situation has been clarified by an important paper by Carrington et al. (1999). These authors analyzed the data from several large cohorts of HIV-1-infected people and reached two clear conclusions. First, the survival time in HIV-1 infection was positively correlated with the degree of heterozygosity at class I HLA loci. Second, they confirmed previous reports that HLA-B35 was associated with a poor prognosis in HIV-1 infection. The protection associated with HLA class I heterozygosity accords with the view that class I-restricted CTLs play a significant role in limiting the virus load (McMichael and Phillips, 1997). The more diverse repertoire of viral peptides that are presented by heterozygotes leads to a broader and therefore more effective CTL response to the virus.

In a study of French long-term nonprogressors and progressors with HIV-1 infection, Magierowska et al. (1999) found that four HLA alleles appeared to have independent protective effects: HLA-A3, HLA-B14, HLA-B17, and HLA-DR7. If an HIV-1-infected person carries three or four of these alleles, his or her odds of being a long-term nonprogressor are increased by a factor of approximately 50.

There are suggestions that disease progression can accelerate when HIV-1 escapes from surveillance by HLA-B27-restricted $CD8^+$ T cells (Goulder et al., 1997). In support of this interpretation, Magierowska et al. (1999) showed that if an HIV-1-infected individual carries the HLA-B27 allele but lacks HLA-DR6, his or her odds of being a long-term nonprogressor are about 50 times greater than those of infected people with other HLA genotypes.

A small proportion of exposed individuals appear to be resistant to HIV-1 infection. In some cases this might be due to an efficient CTL response to the virus (Rowland-Jones et al., 1995). However, in 1996 it became clear that the chemokine receptor CCR5 also acts as a coreceptor for HIV-1 and that individuals who were homozygous for a 32-bp deletion were highly resistant to HIV-1 infection (Liu et al., 1996; Sampson et al., 1996), although this protection was not absolute (Biti et al., 1997). Heterozygosity for this 32-bp deletion is also associated with a prolonged survival of about 2 years in HIV-1-infected people but does not appear to prevent infection (see Michael [1999] for a review). The population frequency of the 32-bp deletion declines from northern Europe (1 to 3% homozygotes) to the south, and it may have arisen about 700 years ago as a single event in Europe (Libert et al., 1998; Stephens et al., 1998). This has given rise to the interesting hypothesis that the deletion might give protection against another infectious disease, such as bubonic plague (Libert et al., 1998; Stephens et al., 1998). In addition to the 32-bp deletion in CCR5, there are at least 10 polymorphisms in the CCR5 promoter, of which two, CCR5P1 and CCR5P4, are present in all racial groups: homozygotes for CCR5P1 progress more rapidly to disease in the absence of other protective alleles of chemokine receptors or chemokines (Martin et al., 1998; McDermott et al., 1998).

The other major coreceptor for HIV-1, CXCR4, seems to lack polymorphisms, possibly because it is the sole receptor for the vital chemokine SDF1. However, a polymorphism in the SDF1 gene (Gly801Ala) was associated with delayed progression to disease (Winkler et al., 1998), although two studies have obtained the opposite result (Mummidi et al., 1998; van Rij et al., 1998).

The influence on disease progression of polymorphisms in the minor coreceptors for HIV-1, CCR2B, and CCR3 is less clear. The CCR2B Val64Ile polymorphism does appear to confer weak protection against progression of disease but not against infection (Smith et al., 1997).

By analyzing the genotypes at loci encoding HLA, chemokines, and chemokine receptors, Magierowska et al. (1999) showed that the protective effects of the different loci were independent. A multivariate logistic regression model, based on these genotypes, was able to classify correctly 70% of long-term nonprogressors and 81% of progressors. This result emphasizes the important role played by the host genotype in determining the course of infections by viruses such as HIV-1.

Human T-Cell Leukemia Virus Type 1

Most people infected with HTLV-1 become asymptomatic lifelong carriers of the virus. About 2% develop a chronic inflammatory disease, and another 2% die of a refractory T-cell leukemia/lymphoma. The best-recognized inflammatory disease is HTLV-1-associated myelopathy/tropical spastic paraparesis (HAM/TSP), in which there is multifocal inflammation in the central nervous system, especially in the spinal cord, which causes paralysis of the legs. The inflammatory conditions are associated with a high provirus load of HTLV-1, about 10 copies per 100 peripheral blood mononuclear cells; however, even healthy carriers have 0.1 to 1 copy per 100 peripheral blood mononuclear cells (Nagai et al., 1998). In

most viral infections, whether acute or chronic, different individuals frequently mount a dominant T-cell response to different antigens of the virus. An unusual feature of the host response to HTLV-1 is the dominant recognition of a single viral antigen, Tax, in most individuals (Bangham et al., 1999; Jacobson et al., 1990; Kannagi et al., 1991; Parker et al., 1992). It is therefore not surprising that HTLV-1 provides the clearest example in humans where dominant protection against a viral disease is associated with a class I HLA allele. In the prefecture of Kagoshima in southern Japan, where the virus infects about 8% of adults, possession of the HLA-A*02 allele is associated with a 2-fold reduction in the risk of the disease HAM/TSP and a 3.5-fold reduction in the provirus load (Jeffery et al., 1999). The presence of the HLA-A*02 allele in approximately 50% of the population prevents about 28% of potential cases of HAM/TSP in the Kagoshima prefecture (Jeffery et al., 1999). The three commonest subtypes of HLA-A*02 in Kagoshima, A*0201, A*0206, and A*0207, each independently appears to confer protection in HTLV-1 infection, although the repertoires of peptides that bind to each respective subtype differ somewhat (K. Jeffery et al., unpublished data). More recent evidence indicates that another class I allele, HLA-Cw08, is also associated with a reduction in provirus load and in the risk of HAM/TSP (Jeffery et al., 2000). The effect seems to be independent of that of A*02: the presence of these two class I alleles prevents nearly 40% of potential HAM/TSP cases in Kagoshima.

While certain class I alleles are associated with protection, the DR1 (DRB1*0101) allele confers susceptibility to HAM/TSP (Usuku et al., 1988, 1990), especially in the absence of the protective effect associated with HLA-A*02 (Jeffery et al., 1999). As with the dominant susceptibility effects of certain HLA phenotypes in HIV-1 infection (see above), the mechanism of the DR1-associated susceptibility to HAM/TSP is not known.

Hepatitis B Virus

Infection with hepatitis B virus (HBV) is frequently followed by lifelong persistence of the virus, especially if infection occurs during childhood. Persistent HBV is associated with an increased risk of hepatocellular carcinoma and is largely responsible for the maintenance of endemicity of the virus in many populations. In 1942, more than 45,000 U.S. military personnel were vaccinated against yellow fever with a vaccine accidentally contaminated with HBV. A total of 914 cases of hepatitis were recorded, of which 580 were mild, 301 were moderate, and 33 were severe (Sawyer et al., 1944). More recently, the concordance rate for chronic HBV carriage in China was found to be 50% in monozygotic twins, while dizygotic twins and nontwinned siblings had a concordance rate of 20% (Lin et al., 1989). This gives a powerful indication of the influence of host genotype on the course of HBV infection.

In a large study in West Africa, Thursz et al. (1995) found that the class II MHC allele DRB1*1302 was associated with clearance of HBV in both children and adults. The class II gene DRB1*1301 also appeared to protect, but a definitive conclusion could not be reached in this study. However, a subsequent study (Hohler et al., 1997) confirmed the protective effect of both DRB1*1301 and DRB1*1302. HLA-DR2 was associated with HBV clearance and HLA-DR7 was associated with persistence in a smaller study (Almarri and Batchelor, 1994).

While heterozygosity at class I HLA loci is associated with a better prognosis in HIV-1 infection (Carrington et al., 1999), heterozygosity at class II loci is associated with prevention of chronic carriage of HBV (Thursz et al., 1997). This is consistent with the finding (Ferrari et al., 1990) that chronic HBV carriers make a weaker helper T-cell response to the virus than do those with acute hepatitis.

A stronger class I-restricted CTL response to HBV is found in patients with acute HBV-induced hepatitis (Bertoletti et al., 1991) than in those who develop chronic HBV carriage (Chisari and Ferrari, 1995). However, the role of the class I HLA loci in influencing the outcome of HBV infection is less clear. In the survey carried out in The Gambia (Thursz et al., 1995), the class I alleles HLA-B50 and HLA-Cw1 appeared to increase the likelihood of persistent HBV carriage, but the data were not conclusive. Other studies have suggested associations between HLA-B15 and chronic HBV carriage (Giani et al., 1979) and between HLA-B35 and moderate to severe chronic hepatitis (Mota et al., 1987); however, further data are again needed to confirm or refute these effects.

The molecular mechanism by which certain class II alleles confer protection against chronic HBV carriage is not known. The class II-restricted helper T cell usually acts in virus infections by helping the CTL response and the antibody response; the lack of difference in anti-HBV antibody titers between DRB1*1302-positive and -negative individuals suggests that the protective effect of class II alleles is more likely to be exerted either via the CTL response or by a direct protective effect of the helper T cell. If the CTL response plays a significant part in protection, one might expect to observe a protective ef-

fect of certain class I HLA alleles, as is seen in HTLV-1 infection (see above). The failure to observe such clear protective effects might result from the greater degree of polymorphism at class I loci and the dominant recognition of different viral antigens by different individuals. However, a direct protective effect of class II-restricted cells, perhaps exerted by cytokines, has not been excluded.

An association has also been described between persistence of HBV and a functionally deficient variant of mannose binding protein (Thomas et al., 1996), but this was not confirmed in larger studies (Mead et al., 1997; Summerfield et al., 1997). Homozygosity for the allele of the vitamin D receptor associated with osteoporosis is associated with clearance of HBV (Bellamy et al., 1999). Polymorphisms in certain liver enzymes may affect the risk of progression to hepatocellular carcinoma in chronic HBV infection (McGlynn et al., 1995).

Hepatitis C Virus

Hepatitis C virus (HCV) is emerging as an increasingly important cause of cirrhosis, liver failure, and (less commonly) liver carcinoma. As in HBV infection, HCV-associated diseases are associated with persistent viral replication.

Kuzushita et al. (1998) reported HLA haplotypes associated with either protection against (HLA-B44-DRB1*1302-DQB1*0604) or susceptibility to (HLA-B54-DRB1*0405-DQB1*0401) HCV-associated diseases. However, these results need confirmation in larger studies.

A common polymorphism in the haptoglobin gene (Hp1-1) is associated with chronic HCV infection: the relative risk for homozygotes is approximately 1.6 (Louagie et al., 1996). The reason for this association is not understood. Patients with persistent HCV often have high levels of the cytokine interleukin-10 (IL-10) in the circulation. Edwards-Smith et al. (1999) found a positive association between the presence of a high IL-10-producer polymorphism and a poor response to alpha interferon treatment: the authors suggested that such patients might benefit from treatments that are designed to enhance a Th1 response to the virus.

Epstein-Barr Virus

If the CTL response to a virus is important in reducing virus load, persistence, and the risk of virus-induced disease, a variant virus that escapes a common class I HLA allele might have a significant survival advantage in the population. A possible example of this was observed in Papua New Guinea by de Campos-Lima et al. (1993) in a population where HLA-A11 is highly prevalent. A variant of Epstein-Barr virus (EBV) was found in which a single amino acid substitution (Lys424Thr) abrogated the recognition of a dominant A11-restricted CTL epitope. The same group (de Campos-Lima et al., 1993) subsequently found substitutions in two different residues in the same epitopes among EBV isolates from southern Chinese populations in whom HLA-A11 is again frequent. They also identified substitutions in the next most dominant HLA-A11-restricted epitope. Burrows et al. (1996) questioned the interpretation that the variant EBV had become established in these populations as a result of the putative CTL escape mutations, because they found identical amino acid residues in EBV isolates from other populations of Papua New Guinea in whom HLA-A11 is less frequent. However, the relative size of the populations concerned and the frequency of contact between them were not clear.

EBV is also associated with a heterogeneous group of posttransplantation lymphoproliferative disorders (PT-LPDs) in immunosuppressed transplant recipients. Cesarman et al. (1998) identified mutations in the Bcl-6 gene in 44% of patients with PT-LPDs. The Bcl-6 protein is a transcriptional repressor, expressed in the nucleus of mature B cells and CD4$^+$ T cells in germinal centers. It has not been established whether common polymorphisms in Bcl-6, as opposed to rare mutations, can affect the course of EBV infection.

Human Papillomaviruses

It is now established that certain types of human papillomavirus (HPV) are the cause of most cervical carcinomas and cervical intraepithelial neoplasias. These malignancies are commoner in immunosuppressed people (Kiviat et al., 1990; Vermund et al., 1991), which suggests that immune surveillance, as in EBV, restricts the oncogenicity of these viruses. Apple et al. (1994) found that two class II HLA haplotypes were associated with cervical carcinoma (DRB1*1501-DQB1*0602 and DRB1*0407-DQB1*0302), while DR13-associated haplotypes seemed to be protective.

A statistical test of heterogeneity indicated a significantly different distribution of class II HLA haplotypes in patients with HPV16-positive severe dysplasia or carcinoma in situ and those with milder degrees of dysplasia (Apple et al., 1994). The study confirmed the previously described susceptibility haplotypes mentioned above. However, no such differences in the distribution of HLA genotypes were observed in patients infected with other HPV types.

Bontkes et al. (1998) found a significant association between HLA-B*44 and clinical progression of the tumor during follow-up, but the statistical significance did not survive correction for multiple tests. In this study, the class II allele HLA-DRB1*07 was commoner in patients infected with HPV16 than in those with other HPV types; again, further studies are needed to confirm this finding.

The susceptibility to certain HPV-associated diseases is also affected by non-MHC loci. Epidermodysplasia verruciformis is a rare skin disorder which results from genetically determined susceptibility to a group of HPV strains, including the oncogenic HPV5. Ramoz et al. (1999, 2000) have carried out a genome-wide linkage search with microsatellite markers in three consanguineous families whose members suffer from epidermodysplasia verruciformis. They have mapped two susceptibility loci, on chromosomes 2p21-24 and 17q25. The latter was mapped to a 1-cM region containing a susceptibility locus for psoriasis. However, the responsible genes have not yet been identified.

Other Viruses

Piyasirisilp et al. (1999) found a small increase in the frequency of two class II HLA genes, DRB1*0901 and DRB1*0301, among Thai patients with autoimmune encephalitis induced by Semple rabies vaccine; the frequency of DQB1*0301 was decreased in these patients.

Hayney et al. (1996, 1997) observed an association between measles vaccine nonresponders and both HLA-DRB1*07 (Hayney et al., 1996) and homozygosity at position 665 in the TAP2 gene, which encodes part of the transporter associated with antigen presentation (Hayney et al., 1997). In the same study, HLA-DRB1*13 was found to be significantly commoner in hyperresponders to a vaccine than in nonresponders.

CONCLUSIONS

The forces that select and maintain the remarkable degree of genetic polymorphism observed in animal genomes are only beginning to be understood. Until the mid-1980s, it was often suggested that MHC genes were subjected to genetic drift in the absence of selection. However, Haldane (1949) had suggested that infectious diseases might exert strong selection on the population and so might account for much of the observed polymorphism. The elucidation of the function of MHC molecules in presenting antigens for recognition by the immune system

(Bjorkman et al., 1987; Townsend et al., 1986; Zinkernagel and Doherty, 1974) made it clear that these molecules are indeed in the front line of defense against infectious pathogens, and so the MHC genes cannot escape the selection imposed by such organisms. These considerations have two corollaries. First, we should expect the MHC genes to select variants—escape mutants—of the pathogen that escape recognition and destruction by the host immune system. Conversely, we should also expect that certain pathogens will exert significant selection on the frequency of MHC alleles. However, evidence for these propositions has been hard to find in natural populations. This difficulty is likely to be due to the complexity of the host genetic systems involved, especially the MHC, and the multiplicity of pathogens that infect the population.

For many years the only good evidence that an infectious disease exerted significant genetic selection on the human population came from studies of sickle cell disease (Allison, 1964), in which heterozygotes for the mutant hemoglobin molecule carry a lower risk of death from malaria. However, more examples have recently been described in which the genetic composition of a natural population significantly influences the outcome of an infectious disease, notably malaria (Hill et al., 1991), AIDS (Carrington et al., 1999), and HTLV-1-associated diseases (Jeffery et al., 1999).

Evidence for selection of immune escape mutants of viruses in natural infections has also been hard to obtain, but it now seems clear that persistent viruses, particularly RNA viruses, are subject to important immune selection in vivo (Evans et al., 1999; Goulder et al., 1997; Niewiesk et al., 1994; Phillips et al., 1991; Price et al., 1997). There are also suggestions that DNA viruses such as EBV can coevolve with human populations (de Campos-Lima et al., 1993), but this remains a matter for debate.

The enormous disparity between the reproductive rates of pathogens—especially viruses—and their hosts not only has influenced the evolution of the highly flexible vertebrate immune system (Hughes and Hughes, 1995; Vogel et al., 1999), but also may have played the decisive role in the evolution and maintenance of sexual reproduction (Hamilton et al., 1990). The high costs and indirect consequences of such adaptations may become evident only after the impact of infections has been lessened by many years of the use of vaccines and antibiotics.

A better comprehension of the genetic control of virus infections will help us understand not only how we have evolved but also what we can and cannot achieve with antiviral drugs and vaccines.

REFERENCES

Allison, A. C. 1964. Polymorphism and natural selection in human populations. *Cold Spring Harbor Symp. Quant. Biol.* **29**:137–149.

Almarri, A., and J. Batchelor. 1994. HLA and hepatitis B infection. *Lancet* **344**:1194–1195.

Apple, R. J., H. A. Erlich, W. Klitz, M. M. Manos, T. M. Becker, and C. M. Wheeler. 1994. HLA DR-DQ associations with cervical carcinoma show papillomavirus-type specificity. *Nat. Genet.* **6**:157–162.

Aubagnac, S., M. Brahic, and J.-F. Bureau. 1999. Viral load and a locus on chromosome 11 affect the late clinical disease caused by Theiler's virus. *J. Virol.* **73**:7965–7971.

Azoulay, A., M. Brahic, and J.-F. Bureau. 1994. FVB mice transgenic for the *H-2D^b* gene become resistant to persistent infection by Theiler's virus. *J. Virol.* **68**:4049–4052.

Azoulay-Cayla, A., S. Dethlefs, B. Pérarnau, E. L. Larsson-Sciard, F. A. Lemonnier, M. Brahic, and J.-F. Bureau. 2000. *H-2D^{b−/−}* mice are susceptible to persistent infection by Theiler's virus. *J. Virol.* **74**:5470–5476.

Bangham, C. R., S. E. Hall, K. J. Jeffery, A. M. Vine, A. Witkover, M. A. Nowak, D. Wodarz, K. Usuku, and M. Osame. 1999. Genetic control and dynamics of the cellular immune response to the human T-cell leukaemia virus, HTLV-I. *Philos. Trans. R. Soc. London Ser. B* **354**:691–700.

Bellamy, R., C. Ruwende, T. Corrah, K. McAdam, M. Thursz, H. Whittle, and A. Hill. 1999. Tuberculosis and chronic hepatitis B virus infection in Africans and variation in the vitamin D receptor gene. *J. Infect. Dis.* **179**:721–724.

Bertoletti, A., C. Ferrari, F. Fiaccadori, A. Penna, R. Margolskee, H. Schlicht, P. Fowler, S. Guilhot, and F. Chisari. 1991. HLA class I restricted human cytotoxic T cells recognize endogenously synthesized hepatitis B virus nucleocapsid antigen. *Proc. Natl. Acad. Sci. USA* **88**:10445–10449.

Best, S., P. Le Tissier, G. Towers, and J. P. Stoye. 1996. Positional cloning of the mouse retrovirus restriction gene *Fv1*. *Nature* **382**:826–829.

Best, S., P. R. Le Tissier, and J. P. Stoye. 1997. Endogenous retroviruses and the evolution of resistance to retroviral infection. *Trends Microbiol.* **5**:313–318.

Bihl, F., M. Brahic, and J.-F. Bureau. 1999. Two loci, *Tmevp2* and *Tmevp3*, located on the telomeric region of chromosome 10, control the persistence of Theiler's virus in the central nervous system. *Genetics* **152**:385–392.

Biti, R., R. Ffrench, J. Young, B. Bennetts, G. Stewart, and T. Liang. 1997. HIV-1 infection in an individual homozygous for the CCR5 deletion allele. *Nat. Med.* **3**:252–253.

Bjorkman, P. J., M. A. Saper, B. Samraoui, W. S. Bennett, J. L. Strominger, and D. C. Wiley. 1987. Structure of the human class I histocompatibility antigen HLA-A2. *Nature* **329**:506.

Bonneville, M., and J. J. Fournié. 1999. γδ T lymphocytes, a link between immunity and homeostasis? *Microbes Infect.* **1**:173.

Bontkes, H. J., M. van Duin, T. D. de Gruijl, M. F. Duggan-Keen, J. M. Walboomers, M. J. Stukart, R. H. Verheijen, T. j. Helmerhorst, C. J. Meijer, R. J. Scheper, F. R. Stevens, P. A. Dyer, P. Sinnott, and P. L. Stern. 1998. HPV 16 infection and progression of cervical intra-epithelial neoplasia: analysis of HLA polymorphism and HPV 16 E6 sequence variants. *Int. J. Cancer* **78**:166–171.

Brahic, M., and J.-F. Bureau. 1998. Genetics of susceptibility to Theiler's virus infection. *Bioessays* **20**:627–633.

Brinton, M. A. 1983. Analysis of extracellular West Nile virus particles produced by cell cultures from genetically resistant and susceptible mice indicates enhanced amplification of defective interfering particles by resistant cultures. *J. Virol.* **46**:860–870.

Bureau, J.-F., K. M. Drescher, L. R. Pease, T. Vikoren, M. Delcroix, L. Zoecklein, M. Brahic, and M. Rodriguez. 1998. Chromosome 14 contains determinants that regulate susceptibility to Theiler's virus-induced demyelination in the mouse. *Genetics* **148**:1941–1949.

Bureau, J.-F., X. Montagutelli, F. Bihl, S. Lefebvre, J.-L. Guénet, and M. Brahic. 1993. Mapping loci influencing the persistence of Theiler's virus in the murine central nervous system. *Nat. Genet.* **5**:87–91.

Bureau, J.-F., X. Montagutelli, S. Lefebvre, J.-L. Guénet, M. Pla, and M. Brahic. 1992. The interaction of two groups of murine genes determines the persistence of Theiler's virus in the central nervous system. *J. Virol.* **66**:4698–4704.

Burrows, J., S. Burrows, L. Poulsen, T. Sculley, D. Moss, and R. Khanna. 1996. Unusually high frequency of Epstein-Barr virus genetic variants in Papua New Guinea that can escape cytotoxic T-cell recognition: implications for virus evolution. *J. Virol.* **70**:2490–2496.

Carrington, M., G. W. Nelson, M. P. Martin, T. Kissner, D. Vlahov, J. J. Goedert, R. Kaslow, S. Buchbinder, K. Hoots, and S. J. O'Brien. 1999. HLA and HIV-1: heterozygote advantage and B*35-Cw*04 disadvantage. *Science* **283**:1748–1752.

Cesarman, E., A. Chadburn, Y. Liu, A. Migliazza, R. Dalla-Favera, and D. Knowles. 1998. BCL-6 gene mutations in post-transplantation lymphoproliferative disorders predict response to therapy and clinical outcome. *Blood* **92**:2294–2302.

Chesebro, B., M. Miyazawa, and W. J. Britt. 1990. Host genetic control of spontaneous and induced immunity to friend murine retrovirus infection. *Annu. Rev. Immunol.* **8**:477–499.

Chisari, F. and C. Ferrari. 1995. Hepatitis B virus immunopathogenesis. *Annu. Rev. Immunol.* **13**:29–60.

Clatch, R. J., R. W. Melvold, S. D. Miller, and H. L. Lipton. 1985. Theiler's murine encephalomyelitis virus (TMEV) induced demyelinating disease in mice is influenced by the H-2D region: correlation with TMEV specific delayed-type hypersensitivity. *J. Immunol.* **135**:1408–1413.

Cresswell, P. 1994. Assembly, transport, and function of MHC class II molecules. *Annu. Rev. Immunol.* **12**:259–293.

de Campos-Lima, P.-O., R. Gavioli, Q.-J. Zhang, L. Wallace, R. Dolcetti, M. Rowe, A. Rickinson, and M. Masucci. 1993. HLA-A11 epitope loss isolates of Epstein-Barr virus from a highly A11+ population. *Science* **260**:98–100.

Dethlefs, S., M. Brahic, and E. L. Larsson-Sciard. 1997. An early, abundant cytotoxic T-lymphocyte response against Theiler's virus is critical for preventing viral persistence. *J. Virol.* **71**:8875–8878.

Edwards-Smith, C., J. Jonsson, D. Purdie, A. Bansal, C. Shorthouse, and E. Powell. 1999. Interleukin-10 promoter polymorphism predicts initial response of chronic hepatitis C to interferon alfa. *Hepatology* **30**:526–530.

Evans, D. T., D. H. O'Connor, P. Jing, J. L. Dzuris, J. Sidney, J. da Silva, T. M. Allen, H. Horton, J. E. Venham, R. A. Rudersdorf, T. Vogel, C. D. Pauza, R. E. Bontrop, R. DeMars, A. Sette, A. L. Hughes, and D. I. Watkins. 1999. Virus-specific cytotoxic T-lymphocyte responses select for amino-acid variation in simian immunodeficiency virus Env and Nef. *Nat. Med.* **5**:1270–1276.

Ferrari, A. C., H. N. Seuanez, S. M. Hanash, and G. F. Atweh. 1990. A gene that encodes for a leukemia-associated phosphoprotein (p18) maps to chromosome bands 1p35-36.1. *Genes, Chromosomes Cancer* **2**:125–129.

Fiette, L., C. Aubert, U. Müller, S. Huang, M. Aguet, M. Brahic, and J.-F. Bureau. 1995. Theiler's virus infection of 129Sv mice

that lack the interferon α/β or interferon γ receptors. *J. Exp. Med.* **181**:2069–2076.

Flanders, W. D., and M. J. Khoury. 1996. Analysis of case parental control studies: method for the study of associations between disease and genetic markers. *Am. J. Epidemiol.* **144**:696–703.

Gardner, M. B., C. A. Kozak, and S. J. O'Brien. 1991. The Lake Casitas wild mouse: evolving genetic resistance to retroviral disease. *Trends Genet.* **7**:22–27.

Giani, G., M. Chiaramonte, C. Pasini, U. Fagiolo, and R. Naccarato. 1979. Hepatitis B surface antigenaemia and HLA antigens. *N. Engl. J. Med.* **300**:1056.

Goulder, P., R. Phillips, R. Colbert, S. McAdam, G. Ogg, M. Nowak, P. Giangrande, G. Luzzi, B. Morgan, A. Edwards, A. McMichael, and S. Rowland-Jones. 1997. Late escape from an immunodominant cytotoxic T-lymphocyte response associated with progression to AIDS. *Nat. Med.* **3**:212–217.

Groschel, D., and H. Koprowski. 1965. Development of a virus-resistant inbred mouse strain for the study of innate resistance to Arbo B viruses. *Arch. Gesamte Virusforsch* **17**:379–391.

Haldane, J. B. S. 1949. Disease and evolution. *Ric. Sci.* **19**(Suppl.): 68–76.

Haller, O., M. Acklin, and P. Staeheli. 1987. Influenza virus resistance of wild mice: wild-type and mutant Mx alleles occur at comparable frequencies. *J. Interferon Res.* **7**:647–656.

Haller, O., M. Frese, and G. Kochs. 1998. Mx proteins: mediators of innate resistance to RNA viruses. *Rev. Sci. Tech. Off. Int. Epizool.* **17**:220–230.

Haller, O., M. Frese, D. Rost, P. A. Nutall, and G. Kochs. 1995. Tick-borne Thogoto virus infection in mice is inhibited by orthomyxovirus resistance gene product. *J. Virol.* **69**:2596–2601.

Hamilton, W. D., R. Axelrod, and R. Tanese. 1990. Sexual reproduction as an adaptation to resist parasites. *Proc. Natl. Acad. Sci. USA* **87**:3566–3573.

Hasenkrug, K. J., and B. Chesebro. 1997. Immunity to retroviral infection: the friend virus model. *Proc. Natl. Acad. Sci. USA* **94**: 7811–7816.

Hayney, M., G. Poland, P. Dimanlig, D. Schaid, R. Jacobson, and J. Lipsky. 1997. Polymorphisms of the TAP2 gene may influence antibody response to live measles vaccine virus. *Vaccine* **15**:3–6.

Hayney, M., G. Poland, R. Jacobson, D. Schaid, and J. Lipsky. 1996. The influence of the HLA-DRB1*13 allele on measles vaccine response. *J. Investig. Med.* **44**:261–263.

Hill, A. V., C. E. Allsopp, D. Kwiatkowski, N. M. Anstey, P. Twumasi, P. A. Rowe, S. Bennett, D. Brewster, A. J. McMichael, and B. M. Greenwood. 1991. Common west African HLA antigens are associated with protection from severe malaria. *Nature* **352**:595–600.

Hill, A. V. S. 1998. The immunogenetics of human infectious diseases. *Annu. Rev. Immunol.* **16**:593–617.

Hohler, T., G. Gerken, A. Notghi, R. Lubjuhn, H. Taheri, U. Protzer, H. Lohr, P. Schneider, K. Meyer zum Buschenfelde, and C. Rittner. 1997. HLA-DRBl*1301 and *1302 protect against chronic hepatitis B. *J. Hepatol.* **26**:503–507.

Hughes, A. L., and M. K. Hughes. 1995. Natural selection on the peptide-binding regions of major histocompatibility complex molecules. *Immunogenetics* **42**:233–243.

Ikeda, H., and H. Sugimura. 1989. Fv-4 resistance gene: a truncated endogenous murine leukemia virus with ecotropic interference properties. *J. Virol.* **63**:5405–5412.

Itescu, S., U. Mathur Wagh, M. L. Skovron, L. J. Brancato, M. Marmor, J. A. Zeleniuch, and R. Winchester. 1992. HLA-B35 is associated with accelerated progression to AIDS. *J. Acquired Immune Defic. Syndr.* **5**:37–45.

Jacobson, S., H. Shida, D. McFarlin, A. Fauci, and S. Koenig. 1990. Circulating CD8+ cytotoxic T lymphocytes specific for

HTLV-I pX in patients with HTLV-I associated neurological disease. *Nature* 348:245–248.

Jeannet, M., R. Sztajzel, N. Carpentier, B. Hirschel, and J. M. Tiercy. 1989. HLA antigens are risk factors for development of AIDS. *J. Acquired Immune Defic. Syndr.* 2:28–32.

Jeffery, K., K. Usuku, S. Hall, W. Matsumoto, G. Taylor, J. Procter, M. Bunce, G. Ogg, K. Welsh, J. Weber, A. Lloyd, M. Nowak, M. Nagai, D. Kodama, S. Izumo, M. Osame, and C. Bangham. 1999. HLA alleles determine human T-lymphotropic virus-I (HTLV-I) proviral load and the risk of HTLV-I-associated myelopathy. *Proc. Natl. Acad. Sci. USA* 96:3848–3853.

Jeffery, K., A. A. Siddiqui, M. Bunce, A. L. Lloyd, A. M. Vine, A. D. Witkoven, S. Izumo, K. Usuku, K. I. Welsh, M. Osame, and C. R. Bangham. 2000. The influence of HLA class I alleles and heterozygosity on the outcome of human T cell lymphotropic virus type I infection. *J. Immunol.* 12:7278–7284.

Jin, H. K., T. Yamashita, K. Ochiai, O. Haller, and T. Watanabe. 1998. Characterization and expression of the *Mx1* gene in wild mouse species. *Biochem. Genet.* 36:311–322.

Jolicoeur, P. 1979. The Fv-1 gene of the mouse and its control of murine leukemia virus replication. *Curr. Top. Microbiol. Immunol.* 86:67–122.

Kalams, S., S. Buchbinder, E. Rosenberg, J. Billingsley, D. Colbert, N. Jones, A. Shea, A. Trocha, and B. Walker. 1999. Association between virus-specific cytotoxic T-lymphocyte and helper responses in human immunodeficiency virus type 1 infection. *J. Virol.* 73:6715–6720.

Kannagi, M., S. Harada, I. Maruyama, H. Inoko, H. Igarashi, G. Kumashima, S. Sato, and M. Morita. 1991. Predominant recognition of human T cell leukemia virus type I (HTLV-I) pX gene products by human CD8+ cytotoxic T cells directed against HTLV-I-infected cells. *Int. Immunol.* 3:761–767.

Kaslow, R. A., M. Carrington, R. Apple, L. Park, A. Munoz, A. J. Saah, J. J. Goedert, C. Winkler, S. J. O'Brien, C. Rinaldo, R. Detels, W. Blattner, J. Phair, H. Erlich, and D. L. Mann. 1996. Influence of combinations of human major histocompatibility complex genes on the course of HIV-1 infection. *Nat. Med.* 2:405–411.

Kaslow, R. A., R. Duquesnoy, M. VanRaden, L. Kingsley, M. Marrari, H. Friedman, S. Su, A. J. Saah, R. Detels, J. Phair, and C. Rinaldo. 1990. Al, Cw7, B8, DR3 HLA antigen combination associated with rapid decline of T helper lymphocytes in HIV-I infection. *Lancet* 335:927–930.

Kiviat, N., A. Rompalo, R. Bowden, D. Galloway, K. K. Holmes, L. Corey, P. L. Roberts, and W. E. Stamm. 1990. Anal human papillomavirus infection among human immunodeficiency virus-seropositive and -seronegative men. *J. Infect. Dis.* 162:358–361.

Klein, M. R., I. P. Keet, J. D'Amaro, R. J. Bende, A. Hekman, B. Mesman, M. Koot, L. P. de Waal, R. A. Coutinho, and F. Miedema. 1994. Associations between HLA frequencies and pathogenic features of human immunodeficiency virus type I infection in seroconverters from the Amsterdam cohort of homosexual men. *J. Infect. Dis.* 169:1244–1259.

Kochs, G., and O. Haller. 1999a. GTP-bound human MxA protein interacts with the nucleocapsids of Thogoto virus (Orthomyxoviridae). *J. Biol. Chem.* 274:4370–4376.

Kochs, G., and O. Haller. 1999b. Interferon-induced human MxA GTPase blocks nuclear import of Thogoto virus nucleocapsids. *Proc. Natl. Acad. Sci. USA* 96:2082–2086.

Kozak, C. A. 1985. Analysis of wild-derived mice for Fv-1 and Fv-2 murine leukemia virus restriction loci: a novel wild mouse Fv-1 allele responsible for lack of host range restriction. *J. Virol.* 55:281–285.

Kuzushita, N., N. Hayashi, T. Moribe, K. Katayama, T. Kanto, S. Nakatani, T. Kaneshige, T. Tatsumi, A. Ito, K. Mochizuki,

Y. Sasaki, A. Kasahara, and M. Hori. 1998. Influence of HLA haplotypes on the clinical courses of individuals infected with hepatitis C virus. *Hepatology* 27:240–244.

Libert, F., P. Cochaux, G. Beckman, M. Samson, M. Aksenova, A. Cao, A. Czeizel, M. Claustres, C. de la Rua, M. Ferrari, C. Ferrec, G. Glover, B. Grinde, S. Güran, V. Kucinskas, J. Lavinha, B. Mercier, G. Ogur, L. Peltonen, C. Rosatelli, M. Schwartz, V. Spitsyn, L. Timar, L. Beckman, M. Parmentier, and G. Vassart. 1998. The deltaccr5 mutation conferring protection against HIV-1 in Caucasian populations has a single and recent origin in Northeastern Europe. *Hum. Mol. Genet.* 7:399–406.

Lin, T., C. Chen, M. Wu, C. Yang, J. Chen, C. Lin, T. Kwang, S. Hsu, S. Lin, and L. Hsu. 1989. Hepatitis B virus markers in Chinese twins. *Anticancer Res.* 9:737–741.

Lindenmann, J. 1962. Resistance of mice to mouse adapted influenza A virus. *Virology* 16:203–204.

Lipton, H. L., R. Melvold, S. D. Miller, and M. C. Dal Canto. 1995. Mutation of a major histocompatibility class I locus, H-2D, leads to an increased virus burden and disease susceptibility in Theiler's virus-induced demyelinating disease. *J. Neurovirol.* 1:138–144.

Liu, R., W. Paxton, S. Choe, D. Ceradini, S. Martin, R. Horuk, M. MacDonald, H. Stuhlmann, R. Koup, and N. Landau. 1996. Homozygous defect in HIV-1 coreceptor accounts for resistance of some multiply-exposed individuals to HIV-1 infection. *Cell* 86:367–377.

Louagie, H., J. Brouwer, J. Delanghe, M. De Buyzere, and G. Leroux-Roels. 1996. Haptoglobin polymorphism and chronic hepatitis C. *J. Hepatol.* 25:10–14.

Magierowska, M., I. Theodorou, P. Debre, F. Sanson, B. Autran, Y. Riviere, D. Charron, and D. Costagliola. 1999. Combined genotypes of CCR5, CCR2, SDF1, and HLA genes can predict the long-term nonprogressor status in human immunodeficiency virus-1-infected individuals. *Blood* 93:936–941.

Martin, M., M. Dean, M. Smith, C. Winkler, B. Gerrard, N. Michael, B. Lee, R. Dams, J. Margolick, S. Buchbinder, J. J. Goedert, T. R. O'Brien, M. W. Hilgartner, D. Vlahov, S. J. O'Brien, and M. Carrington. 1998. Genetic acceleration of AIDS progression by a promoter variant of CCR5. *Science* 282:1907–1911.

McDermott, D., P. Zimmerman, F. Guignard, C. Kleeberger, S. Leitman, and P. Murphy. 1998. CCR5 promoter polymorphism and HIV-1 disease progression. Multicenter AIDS Cohort Study (MACS). *Lancet* 352:866–870.

McGlynn, K., E. Rosvold, E. Lustbader, Y. Hu, M. Clapper, T. Zhou, C. Wild, X. Xia, A. Baffoe Bonnie, D. Ofori Adjei, G. C. Chen, W. T. London, F. M. Shen, and K. H. Buetow. 1995. Susceptibility to hepatocellular carcinoma is associated with genetic variation in the enzymatic detoxification of aflatoxin B1. *Proc. Natl. Acad. Sci. USA* 92:2384–2387.

McMichael, A., and R. Phillips. 1997. Escape of human immunodeficiency virus from immune control. *Annu. Rev. Immunol.* 15:271–296.

McNeil, A. J., P. L. Yap, S. M. Gore, R. P. Brettle, M. McColl, R. Wyld, S. Davidson, R. Weightman, A. M. Richardson, and J. R. Robertson. 1996. Association of HLA types A1 B8 DR3 and B27 with rapid and slow progression of HIV disease. *Q. J. Med.* 89:177–185.

Mead, R., D. Jack, M. Pembrey, L. Tyfield, and M. Turner. 1997. Mannose binding lectin alleles in a prospectively recruited UK population. *Lancet* 349:1669–1670.

Michael, N. 1999. Host genetic influences on HIV-1 pathogenesis. *Curr. Opin. Immunol.* 11:466–474.

Monteyne, P., F. Bihl, F. Levillayer, M. Brahic, and J.-F. Bureau. 1999. The Th1/Th2 balance does not account for the difference of susceptibility of mouse strains to Theiler's virus persistent infection. *J. Immunol.* **162**:7330–7334.

Monteyne, P., J.-F. Bureau, and M. Brahic. 1997. The infection of mouse by Theiler's virus: from genetics to immunology. *Immunol. Rev.* **159**:163–176.

Moreau-Gachelin, F., A. Tavitian, and P. Tambourin. 1988. Spi-1 is a putative oncogene in virally induced murine erythroleukaemias. *Nature* **331**:277–280.

Mota, A., R. Fainboim, R. Terg, and L. Fainboim. 1987. Association of chronic active hepatitis and HLA-B35 in patients with hepatitis B virus. *Tissue Antigen* **30**:238–240.

Müller, U., U. Steinhoff, L. F. L. Reis, S. Hemmi, J. Pavlovic, R. M. Zinkernagel, and M. Aguet. 1994. Functional role of type I and type II interferons in antiviral defense. *Science* **264**:1918–1921.

Mummidi, S., S. Ahuja, E. Gonzalez, S. Anderson, E. Santiago, K. Stephan, F. Craig, P. O'Connell, V. Tryon, R. A. Clark, M. J. Dolan, and S. Ahuja. 1998. Genealogy of the CCR5 locus and chemokine system gene variants associated with altered rates of HIV-1 disease progression. *Nat. Med.* **4**:786–793.

Nagai, M., K. Usuku, W. Matsumoto, D. Kodama, N. Takenouchi, T. Moritoyo, S. Hashiguchi, M. Ichinose, C. R. M. Bangham, S. Izumo, and M. Osame. 1998. Analysis of HTLV-I proviral load in 202 HAM/TSP patients and 243 asymptomatic HTLV-I carriers: high proviral load strongly predisposes to HAM/TSP. *J. Neurovirol.* **4**:586–593.

Niewiesk, S., S. Daenke, C. E. Parker, G. Taylor, J. Weber, S. Nightingale, and C. R. Bangham. 1994. The transactivator gene of human T-cell leukemia virus type I is more variable within and between healthy carriers than patients with tropical spastic paraparesis. *J. Virol.* **68**:6778–6781.

Ohta, T. 1999. Effect of gene conversion on polymorphic patterns at major histocompatibility complex loci. *Immunol. Rev.* **167**:319–325.

Ojcius, D. M., C. Delarbre, P. Kourilsky, and G. Gachelin. 1994. Major histocompatibility complex class I molecules and resistance against intracellular pathogens. *Crit. Rev. Immunol.* **14**:193–220.

Parker, C., S. Daenke, S. Nightingale, and C. Bangham. 1992. Activated HTLV-I specific cytotoxic T cells are found in healthy seropositives as well as patients with tropical spastic paraparesis. *Virology* **188**:628–636.

Paul, R., S. Schuetze, S. L. Kozak, C. A. Kozak, and D. Kabat. 1991. The Sfpi-1 proviral integration site of Friend erythroleukemia encodes the ets-related transcription factor Pu.1. *J. Virol.* **65**:464–467.

Persons, D. A., R. F. Paulson, M. R. Loyd, M. T. Herley, S. M. Bodner, A. Bernstein, P. H. Correll, and P. A. Ney. 1999. Fv2 encodes a truncated form of the Stk receptor tyrosine kinase. *Nat. Genet.* **23**:159–165.

Phillips, R. E., S. Rowland-Jones, D. F. Nixon, F. M. Gotch, J. P. Edwards, A. O. Ogunlesi, J. G. Elvin, J. A. Rothbard, C. R. Bangham, C. R. Rizza, and A. J. McMichael. 1991. Human immunodeficiency virus genetic variation that can escape cytotoxic T cell recognition. *Nature* **354**:453–459.

Piyasirisilp, S., B. Schmeckpeper, D. Chandanayingyong, T. Hemachudha, and D. Griffin. 1999. Association of HLA and T-cell receptor gene polymorphisms with Semple rabies vaccine-induced autoimmune encephalomyelitis. *Ann. Neurol.* **45**:595–600.

Porcelli, S. A., and R. L. Modlin. 1999. The CD1 system: antigen-presenting molecules for T cell recognition of lipids and glycolipids. *Annu. Rev. Immunol.* **17**:297–329.

Price, D. A., P. J. Goulder, P. Klenerman, A. K. Sewell, P. J. Easterbrook, M. Troop, C. R. Bangham, and R. E. Phillips. 1997. Positive selection of HIV-1 cytotoxic T lymphocyte escape var-

iants during primary infection. *Proc. Natl. Acad. Sci. USA* **94**:1890–1895.

Rammensee, H. G., T. Friede, and S. Stevanoviic. 1995. MHC ligands and peptide motifs: first listing. *Immunogenetics* **41**:178–228.

Ramoz, N., L. A. Rueda, B. Bouadjar, M. Favre, and G. Orth. 1999. A susceptibility locus for epidermodysplasia verruciformis, an abnormal predisposition to infection with the oncogenic human papillomavirus type 5, maps to chromosome 17qter in a region containing a psoriasis locus. *J. Investig. Dermatol.* **112**:259–263.

Ramoz, N., A. Taieb, L. A. Rueda, L. S. Montoya, B. Bouadjar, M. Favre, and G. Orth. 2000. Evidence for a non-allelic heterogeneity of epidermodysplasia verruciformis with two susceptibility loci mapped to chromosome regions 2p21-p24 and 17q25. *J. Investig. Dermatol.* **114**:1148–1153.

Reeves, R. H., B. F. O'Hara, W. J. Pavan, J. D. Gearhart, and O. Haller. 1988. Genetic mapping of the Mx influenza virus-resistance gene within the region of mouse chromosome 16 that is homologous to human chromosome 21. *J. Virol.* **62**:4372–4375.

Risch, N. 1990. Linkage strategies for genetically complex traits. II. The power of affected relative pairs. *Am. J. Hum. Genet.* **46**:229–241.

Rock, K. L., and A. L. Goldberg. 1999. Degradation of cell proteins and the generation of MHC class I-presented peptides. *Annu. Rev. Immunol.* **17**:739–779.

Rodriguez, M., and C. S. David. 1995. *H-2D*^{d} transgene suppresses Theiler's virus-induced demyelination in susceptible strains of mice. *J. Neurovirol.* **1**:111–117.

Rodriguez, M., J. L. Leibowitz, and C. S. David. 1986. Susceptibility to Theiler's virus-induced demyelination. Mapping of the gene within the *H-2D* region. *J. Exp. Med.* **163**:620–631.

Rowland-Jones, S., J. Sutton, K. Ariyoshi, T. Dong, F. Gotch, S. McAdam, D. Whitby, S. Sabally, A. Gallimore, T. Corrah, M. Takiguchi, T. Schultz, A. McMichael, and H. Whittle. 1995. HIV-specific cytotoxic T-cells in HIV-exposed but uninfected Gambian women. *Nat. Med.* **1**:59–64.

Sabin, A.B. 1952. Genetic, hormonal and age factors in natural resistance to certain viruses. *Ann. N. Y. Acad. Sci.* **54**:936–944.

Sahmoud, T., Y. Laurian, C. Gazengel, Y. Sultan, C. Gautreau, and D. Costagliola. 1993. Progression to AIDS in French haemophiliacs: association with HLA B35. *AIDS* **7**:497–500.

Sampson, M., F. Libert, B. Doranz, J. Rucker, C. Liesnard, C.-M. Farber, S. Saragosti, C. Lapoumeroulie, J. Cognaux, C. Forceille, et al. 1996. Resistance to HIV-1 infection in Caucasian individuals bearing mutant alleles of the CCR-5 chemokine receptor gene. *Nature* **382**:722–725.

Sangster, M. Y., N. Urosevic, J. P. Mansfield, J. S. Mackenzie, and G. R. Shellam. 1994. Mapping the Flv locus controlling resistance to flaviviruses on mouse chromosome 5. *J. Virol.* **68**:448–452.

Sawyer, W., K. Meyer, M. Eaton, J. Bauer, P. Putnam, and F. Schwentker. 1944. Jaundice in army personnel in the western region of the United States and its relation to vaccination against yellow fever. *Am. J. Hyg.* **39**:337–440.

Scorza-Smeraldi, R., G. Fabio, A. Lazzarin, N. B. Eisera, M. Moroni, and C. Zanussi. 1986. HLA associated susceptibility to acquired immunodeficiency syndrome in Italian patients with human immunodeficiency virus infection. *Lancet* **ii**:1187–1189.

Shellam, G. R., M. Y. Sangster, and N. Urosevic. 1998. Genetic control of host resistance to flavivirus infection in animals. *Rev. Sci. Tech.* **17**:231–248.

Shi, P. Y., W. Li, and M. A. Brinton. 1996. Cell proteins bind specifically to West Nile virus minus-strand 3' stem-loop RNA. *J. Virol.* **70**:6278–6287.

Smith, M., M. Dean, M. Carrington, C. Winkler, G. Huttley, D. Lomb, J. Goedert, T. O'Brien, L. Jacobsen, R. Kaslow, S. Buchbinder, E. Vittinghoff, D. Vlahov, K. Hoots, M. W. Hilgartner, and S. J. O'Brien. 1997. Contrasting genetic influence of CCR2 and CCR5 variants on HlV-1 infection and disease progression. Haemophilia Growth and Development Study (HGDS), Multicenter AIDS Cohort Study, Multicenter Hemophilia Cohort Study (MHCS), San Francisco City Cohort, ALIVE Study. *Science* 277:959–965.

Staeheli, P., R. Grob, E. Meier, J. G. Sucliffe, and O. Haller. 1988. Influenza virus-susceptible mice carry *Mx* genes with a large deletion or a nonsense mutation. *Mol. Cell. Biol.* 8:4518–4523.

Staeheli, P., and O. Haller. 1985. Interferon-induced human protein with homology to protein Mx of influenza virus resistant mice. *Mol. Cell. Biol.* 5:2150–2153.

Staeheli, P., and J. G. Sutcliffe. 1988. Identification of a second interferon-regulated murine Mx gene. *Mol. Cell. Biol.* 8:4524–4528.

Stephens, J., D. Reich, D. Goldstein, H. Shin, M. Smith, M. Carrington, C. Winkler, G. Huttley, R. Allikmets, L. Schriml, B. Gerrard, M. Malasky, M. D. Ramos, S. Morlot, M. Tzetis, C. Oddoux, F. S. di Giovine, G. Nasioulas, D. Chandler, M. Aseev, M. Hanson, L. Kalaydjieva, D. Glavac, P. Gasparini, D. Kanavakis, M. Claustres, M. Kambouris, H. Ostrer, G. Duff, V. Baranov, H. Sibul, A. Metspalu, D. Goldman, N. Martin, D. Duffy, J. Schmidtke, X. Estivill, S. J. O'Brien, and M. Dean. 1998. Dating the origin of the CCR5-A32 AIDS-resistance allele by the coalescence of haplotypes. *Am. J. Hum. Genet.* 62:1507–1515.

Stoye, J. P. 1998. Fv1, the mouse retrovirus resistance gene. *Rev. Sci. Tech.* 17:269–277.

Summerfield, J., M. Sumiya, M. Levin, and M. Turner. 1997. Association of mutations in mannose binding protein gene with childhood infection in consecutive hospital series. *Br. Med. J.* 314:1229–1232.

Super, H. J., K. J. Hasenkrug, S. Simmons, D. M. Brooks, R. Konzek, K. D. Sarge, R. I. Morimoto, N. A. Jenkins, D. J. Gilbert, N. G. Copeland, W. Frankel, and B. Chesebro. 1999. Fine mapping of the friend retrovirus resistance gene, *Rfv3*, on mouse chromosome 15. *J. Virol.* 73:7848–7852.

Thomas, H., G. Foster, M. Sumiya, D. Mcintosh, D. Jack, M. Turner, and M. Summerfield. 1996. Mutation of gene of mannose binding protein associated with chronic hepatitis B viral infection. *Lancet* 348:1417–1419.

Thursz, M., D. Kwiatkowski, C. Allsopp, B. Greenwood, H. Thomas, and A. Hill. 1995. Association between an MHC class II allele and clearance of hepatitis B virus in the Gambia. *N. Engl. J. Med.* 332:1065–1069.

Thursz, M., H. Thomas, B. Greenwood, and A. Hill. 1997. Heterozygote advantage for HLA class II type in hepatitis B virus infection. *Nat. Genet.* 17:11–12.

Townsend, A. R. M., J. Rothbard, F. M. Gotch, G. Bahadur, D. Wraith, and J. McMichael. 1986. The epitopes of influenza nucleoprotein recognized by cytotoxic T lymphocytes can be defined with short synthetic peptides. *Cell* 44:959–968.

Urosevic, N., M. van Maanen, J. P. Mansfield, J. S. Mackenzie, and G. R. Shellam. 1997. Molecular characterization of virus-specific RNA produced in the brains of flavivirus-susceptible and -resistant mice after challenge with Murray Valley encephalitis virus. *J. Gen. Virol.* 78:23–29.

Usuku, K., M. Nishizawa, K. Matsuki, K. Tokunaga, K. Takahashi, N. Eiraku, M. Suehara, T. Juji, M. Osame, and T. Tabira. 1990. Association of a particular amino acid sequence of the HLA-DR beta1 chain with HTLV-I-associated myelopathy. *Eur. J. Immunol.* 20:1603–1606.

Usuku, K., S. Sonoda, M. Osame, S. Yashiki, K. Takahashi, T. Sawada, M. Matsumoto, M. Tara, K. Tsuji, and A. Igata. 1988. HLA haplotype-linked high immune responsiveness against HTLV-I in HTLV-I-associated myelopathy: comparison with adult T-cell leukemia/lymphoma. *Ann. Neurol.* 23(Suppl.):S143–S150.

van Rij, R., S. Broersen, J. Goudsmit, R. Coutinho, and H. Scuitemaker. 1998. The role of a stromal cell-derived factor-1 chemokine gene variant in the clinical course of HIV-1 infection. *AIDS* 12:F85–F90.

Vermund, S., K. Kelley, R. Klein, A. R. Feingold, K. Schreiber, G. Munk, and R. D. Burk. 1991. High risk of human papillomavirus infection and cervical squamous intraepithelial lesions among women with symptomatic human immunodeficiency virus infection. *Am. J. Obstet. Gynecol.* 165:392–400.

Vogel, T. U., D. T. Evans, J. A. Urvater, D. H. O'Connor, A. L. Hughes, and D. I. Watkins. 1999. Major histocompatibility complex class I genes in primates: co-evolution with pathogens. *Immunol. Rev.* 167:327–337.

Weiss, R., N. Teich, H. Varmus, and J. Coffin (ed.). 1982. *RNA Tumor Viruses*, p. 871–874. Cold Spring Harbor Laboratory, Cold Spring Harbor, N.Y.

Winkler, C., W. Modi, M. Smith, G. Nelson, X. Wu, M. Carrington, M. Dean, T. Honjo, K. Tashiro, D. Yabe, S. Buchbinder, E. Vittinghoff, J. J. Goedert, T. R. O'Brien, L. P. Jacobson, R. Detels, S. Donfield, A. Willoughby, E. Gomperts, D. Vlahov, J. Phair, and S. J. O'Brien. 1998. Genetic restriction of AIDS pathogenesis by an SDF-1 chemokine gene variant. ALIVE Study, Hemophilia Growth and Development Study (HGDS), Multicenter AIDS Cohort Study (MACS), Multicenter Hemophilia Cohort Study (MHCS), San Francisco City Cohort (SFCC). *Science* 279:389–393.

Zinkernagel, R. M., and P. C. Doherty. 1974. Restriction of in vitro T cell-mediated cytotoxicity in lymphocytic choriomeningitis within a syngeneic or semiallogeneic system. *Nature* 248:701–702.

VIII. IMMUNE INTERVENTION

Immunology of Infectious Diseases
Edited by S. H. E. Kaufmann, A. Sher, and R. Ahmed
© 2002 ASM Press, Washington, D.C.

Chapter 29

Immune Intervention in Tuberculosis

Douglas B. Young and Brian D. Robertson

RATIONALE FOR IMMUNE INTERVENTION IN TUBERCULOSIS

It is estimated that as much as one third of the world's population is currently "infected" with *Mycobacterium tuberculosis* (Kochi, 1991). This statistic is based on evidence of an immune response (delayed-type hypersensitivity) to intradermal injection of a mixture of *M. tuberculosis* antigens. While the prognostic value of a positive skin test can be debated, it seems likely that it is indicative of an infection that has progressed at least to a stage which engages the attention of the immune system. Anecdotal evidence of the onset of active tuberculosis many years after initial exposure, together with postmortem detection of viable organisms in quiescent lesions, demonstrates that the infection can persist over many years in the absence of clinical symptoms, although the percentage of skin test-positive individuals actually harboring live bacilli is unknown (Fine and Small, 1999). It is abundantly clear, however, that the global incidence of around 8 million cases of tuberculosis per year represents only a small fraction of the estimated 2 billion "infected" population (Dye et al., 1999). Most people are able to cope with *M. tuberculosis* infection and show no obvious harmful effects; on average, around 1 in 10 of the infected population will go on to develop disease at some stage in their life. At an individual level, a variety of factors can markedly alter this susceptibility. As with most infectious diseases, poor nutrition and high stress are associated with an increased incidence of tuberculosis (Dubos and Dubos, 1952). Comparison of the incidence of disease in identical and nonidentical twins demonstrates involvement of a genetic element (Comstock, 1978), while a high male-to-female ratio and relative resistance in preadolescent

age groups attest to endocrine influences (Dubos and Dubos, 1952). Finally, the direct influence of the immune response is dramatically illustrated by the 5 to 10% annual risk of disease in individuals who are coinfected with *M. tuberculosis* and human immunodeficiency virus (HIV) (Hopewell, 1992).

Thus, *M. tuberculosis* infection progresses to disease at a frequency that is low and dependent on the genetic background and physiology of the infected individual. Enhancing the resistance of infected individuals—and specifically, boosting their immune response—would seem to offer a compelling rationale as a strategy for control of tuberculosis. It is probably useful to note from the outset that this is not identical to the rationale that led Edward Jenner to experiment with smallpox vaccination. In contrast to smallpox, individuals who recover from tuberculosis are not necessarily immune to a second infection; in fact, the majority of cases of pulmonary tuberculosis arise in individuals who appear to have been able to control the primary infection (Fine and Small, 1999). Regardless of the theoretical attraction of immune intervention in tuberculosis and although *M. bovis* BCG provides a mainstay of global vaccination campaigns, current efforts in tuberculosis control are almost exclusively directed toward implementation of antimicrobial therapy (Kochi, 1991). The aim of this chapter is to review the prospects for changing this situation by developing improved immune interventions. First, it is useful to summarize briefly the checkered history of immune intervention in tuberculosis.

ROBERT KOCH AND TUBERCULIN

Following his definitive demonstration of *M. tuberculosis* as the etiologic agent of human tubercu-

Douglas B. Young and Brian D. Robertson • Department of Infectious Diseases and Microbiology, Faculty of Medicine, Imperial College, London W2 1PG, United Kingdom.

losis at the end of the 19th century (Koch, 1882), Robert Koch was well aware of the potential for immune intervention in control of the disease. In August 1890, he delivered a speech to the Tenth International Congress of Medicine in Berlin in which he described a preparation that, when injected into guinea pigs, could protect against subsequent challenge with tuberculosis as well as curing existing disease. The announcement triggered a massive public response; however, within less than a year, a review of its use in over 2,000 patients provided no clear evidence of any beneficial effect (Brock, 1988). Koch's vaccine, "tuberculin," consisted of antigens present in concentrated supernatant from an *M. tuberculosis* culture; in a more refined form, it provides the basis for the current skin test reagent.

Tuberculin provided an early lesson in the pitfalls of tuberculosis vaccine development. Mycobacterial extracts are certainly capable of inducing a strong immune response, but this cannot be equated with resistance to disease. Injection of tuberculin carried unpleasant side effects. During experimentation on himself, Koch experienced "pain in the joints, languor, a tendency to cough and difficulty in breathing . . followed by . . very severe rigour . . then nausea, vomiting, and a rise in temperature" (Brock, 1988). However, the extent of longer-term clinical damage to patients involved in the tuberculin trials is hard to assess in the absence of any controlled studies. The tuberculin story provided a strong disincentive for subunit vaccine development.

ALBERT CALMETTE AND ATTENUATED VACCINES

Experiments on rabbits in his sanatorium at Saranac Lake led Edward Trudeau to note in 1905 that while "dead bacteria increase, though to a very slight degree, the animal's resistance to subsequent inoculation . . . . the living attenuated bacillus gives a stronger degree of immunity than the same bacillus killed by heat" (Dubos and Dubos, 1952). The concept that bacterial viability held the key to induction of protective immunity was tenaciously pursued by Albert Calmette and Camille Guérin, working at the Institut Pasteur, initially in Lille and later in Paris. Starting in 1908 with a virulent isolate of *M. bovis*, they carried out a series of subcultures over 13 years, using a glycerin-bile-potato medium. The resulting culture, termed bacille Calmette Guérin (BCG), had lost its ability to cause disease in calves and guinea pigs and was first applied as a human vaccine by oral administration to the child of a tuberculous mother in 1921 (Calmette, 1927). Subsequent evaluation of

the efficacy of BCG eschewed reliance on statistical method but, with the exception of a disastrous experimental contamination with virulent *M. tuberculosis* in Lübeck in 1929, suggested it to be both safe and beneficial (Dormandy, 1999). Endorsement by the League of Nations and fear of a resurgence in tuberculosis at the end of the Second World War encouraged the widespread adoption of BCG vaccination in Europe. A more complex picture emerged when BCG was tested in randomized controlled trials (adopted as the standard methodology in the 1950s following successful application to evaluation of streptomycin therapy). BCG was found to confer a high degree of protection in some trials—in Medical Research Council trials carried out in the United Kingdom, the incidence of tuberculosis in the vaccinated group was reduced by almost 80% in comparison to the control group—while having an overall efficacy close to zero in other trials (most notably in South India) (Bloom and Fine, 1994). Variations between trials reflect differences in the ability of BCG to protect against the predominant adult form of pulmonary tuberculosis. BCG has consistently shown significant protective efficacy against the disseminated forms of tuberculosis that are a major cause of childhood mortality (Colditz et al., 1995), justifying its inclusion in the World Health Organization Expanded Programme for Immunization. BCG also confers protection against leprosy, caused by the related pathogen *M. leprae* (Karonga Prevention Trial Group, 1996).

The reasons for the variations in efficacy have been widely discussed (Bloom and Fine, 1994; Fine, 1995). Analysis of BCG efficacy in immigrant groups points to geographical rather than genetic factors, and there is a notable trend toward reduced efficacy in trials carried out close to the equator (Colditz et al., 1994). A possible explanation is that saprophytic mycobacteria, which are more common in the environment and water supply in warmer climates, may influence the results of the trials (Bloom and Fine, 1994). This could occur if exposure to environmental mycobacteria has the effect of reversing immunological benefits conferred by BCG vaccination or simply if the environmental mycobacteria reproduce the effect of BCG, effectively equilibrating responses in control and trial groups (Palmer and Long, 1966). An alternative hypothesis to account for the variations in trial results is based on a recent genomic analysis of BCG. Using the genome of *M. tuberculosis* H37Rv as a blueprint, it has been possible to identify genetic regions that are missing from the various contemporary substrains of the original BCG vaccine (Behr et al., 1999; Gordon et al., 1999; Mahairas et al., 1996). In addition to regions absent from all *M.*

bovis isolates, five regions encompassing 38 open reading frames were found to have been deleted from some or all BCG substrains. By a process of forensic genomics, a chronology for the occurrence of the different deletions could be drawn up (Behr et al., 1999). While the potential contribution of the deleted genes to the virulence and immunogenicity of *M. tuberculosis* is not yet clear, it is possible that the sequential loss of genes during subculture of BCG substrains has been accompanied by a parallel decline in their protective ability (Behr and Small, 1997).

BCG provides some hard lessons for would-be developers of new tuberculosis vaccines. On the positive side, it vindicates the concept of vaccination as an approach to tuberculosis control. While precise numbers are hard to obtain, it seems reasonable to extrapolate that BCG has saved the lives of millions of potential victims of childhood tuberculosis. On the other hand, do the BCG trial results imply that any new vaccine will have to be evaluated in costly randomized control trials in every country for which its use is proposed? Is it possible to move forward with any kind of rational development of new vaccines in the absence of an understanding of the mechanisms underlying the observed variations in BCG efficacy?

IMMUNE MECHANISMS IN TUBERCULOSIS

The difficulty in understanding the varying results of the BCG trials is a consequence of the difficulty in understanding the fundamental mechanisms of protective immunity to tuberculosis. While we can measure many different aspects of the immune response to mycobacterial infection, we have yet to identify any single parameter, or combination of parameters, that can provide a reliable correlate of resistance or susceptibility to tuberculosis. It would seem that every weapon in the extensive immunological arsenal is brought into play in the battle against tuberculosis. These are given detailed consideration elsewhere in this volume, and a brief summary will suffice in the present chapter.

Experimental infections of gene knockout mice, together with clinical studies of rare genetic defects in humans, identify the cycle of interleukin-12 (IL-12), gamma interferon (IFN-γ), and activated macrophages as the cornerstone of protective immunity (Altare et al., 1998; Cooper et al., 1997; Flynn et al., 1993; Newport et al., 1996). While *M. tuberculosis* is well adapted to survival within macrophages, this ability is significantly reduced in cells that have been activated by IFN-γ and tumor necrosis factor alpha (TNF-α) (Chan and Kaufmann, 1994). TNF-α is produced by macrophages themselves, together with IL-

12, as a result of triggering of cell surface receptors by components of the mycobacterial cell wall. IFN-γ can be supplied by the innate immune system (by natural killer cells, for example) or as a result of acquired immunity. The T-helper 1 (Th1) phenotype of CD4$^+$ T cells induced in the presence of IL-12 is a major source of IFN-γ, and much of the effort directed toward vaccine development is based on priming of this particular subset of cells. Although essential, CD4$^+$ T cells are not on their own sufficient for optimal resistance to tuberculosis, at least in the mouse model, where CD8$^+$ T cells are also required (Flynn et al., 1992; Sousa et al., 2000) and may provide an additional source of IFN-γ (Tascon et al., 1998). Alternatively, their cytotoxic function may be important, either by directly killing intracellular mycobacteria (Stenger et al., 1997) or by releasing them for uptake by activated macrophages (Kaufmann, 1988). Two other T-cell subsets recognize nonprotein antigens derived from mycobacteria. These are T cells expressing an antigen-specific receptor composed of γ and δ chains, which respond to phosphorylated ligands (Constant et al., 1994), and CD1-restricted T cells that recognize glycolipid antigens (Moody et al., 1997; Sieling et al., 1995). Again, these T-cell subsets have the potential to influence the course of mycobacterial infection by cytokine-mediated or cytolytic mechanisms. Finally, mycobacteria provide a potent signal for antibody production. While the thick cell wall and intracellular location of mycobacteria would seem to render them resistant to direct damage by antibody and complement, opsonizing antibodies may influence the course of their interaction with phagocytic cells in vivo (Teitelbaum et al., 1998).

Notwithstanding its complexity, the immune response to mycobacterial infection is not particularly efficient. Mycobacteria are robust organisms, and the mechanisms that are effective in killing them—activated macrophages, toxic radicals, and cell lysis—are also liable to cause damage to surrounding host tissues (Dannenberg and Rook, 1994). The general compromise for the host is that after an initial aggressive immune response, the site of infection is isolated in the form of a granuloma, which suffices to contain, although perhaps not always eliminate, the remaining viable organisms. Protective immunity can be envisaged as a judicious combination of a rapid response to the initial infection, avoidance of excessive tissue damage, and maintenance of the ability to mount a secondary response to any subsequent escape of mycobacteria from the granuloma. Factors that determine the effectiveness of the response are likely to include the type and number of the various T-cell subsets, as well as the kinetics of their recruitment and activation (Chan and Kaufmann, 1994). From the microbial perspective, the challenge is to weather the initial response, leaving a pool of persisting viable organisms capable of exploiting subsequent opportunities for multiplication and transmission to a new host. It is important to note that the most efficient transmission occurs after the breakdown of infected lung tissues, a process which is largely dependent on the action of the immune response (Dannenberg and Rook, 1994). The immune response is therefore something of a necessary evil as far as the mycobacterium is concerned; a non-immunogenic *M. tuberculosis* might gain short-term benefit in an extended period of unopposed replication but would ultimately pay for this by reduced transmissibility.

SCOPE FOR IMPROVED
IMMUNE INTERVENTIONS

In considering the prospects for development of improved immune interventions in tuberculosis, it is useful to focus on three distinct phases of the disease. The ideal intervention would involve a vaccine that could be delivered prior to exposure to *M. tuberculosis* and would ensure complete killing of the bacteria during any subsequent infection. A second target would be to boost immunity in individuals who have controlled the initial infection but remain susceptible to reactivation or reinfection. Finally, immunotherapy—the nemesis of Robert Koch—merits reevaluation, particularly in the context of multidrug-resistant disease. The scope for design of new interventions has been widened dramatically by recent advances in the field of bacterial genomics. The genome sequence is available for two *M. tuberculosis* isolates (Cole et al., 1998) (http://www.tigr.org), and genome projects are well advanced for an *M. bovis* isolate and for BCG Pasteur (http://www.sanger.ac.uk). These sequences contain detailed information on all of the ~4,000 protein antigens that might be considered for inclusion in subunit vaccine candidates. Meanwhile, advances in mycobacterial genetics now permit the construction of mutant strains, either by deletion of selected genes or by random insertion of transposons throughout the genome (Bardarov et al., 1997; Pelicic et al., 1997). These new tools set the stage for targeted reenactments of the experiments of Koch and Calmette.

ENHANCING THE INITIAL RESPONSE
TO INFECTION

Classically, vaccination involves specific priming of the immune system to make a more effective sec-

ondary response during the first encounter with the pathogen. In experimental-animal models, BCG vaccination conforms to this paradigm. In naïve animals, the population of *M. tuberculosis* increases for several weeks after infection before being brought under the control of the immune response. This period is significantly reduced in BCG-vaccinated animals, resulting in a decreased number of viable mycobacteria progressing to the chronic phase of the infection, reduced spread from the lungs to other organs, and a corresponding increase in survival (McMurray, 1994; Orme and Collins, 1994). These experimental findings are consistent with the ability of BCG to protect against disseminated forms of tuberculosis in humans. Is it possible to enhance this initial response still further? In particular, is it possible to establish an immune response that results in killing of all of the infecting mycobacteria?

New Vaccine Candidates

A broad range of new vaccine candidates have been screened for their ability to protect against subsequent challenge with *M. tuberculosis* in mouse and guinea pig models. Advances have been made in two areas. First, it has been possible to modify BCG in a way that further attenuates its ability to cause sustained, progressive infection without apparently compromising its protective efficacy. It was shown that in contrast to wild-type BCG, a mutant strain that requires an exogenous supply of leucine for growth is unable to cause disease in immunocompromised SCID mice (Guleria et al., 1996). While BCG has a distinguished record of safe use in humans, it can cause disease in individuals carrying rare genetic polymorphisms (Jouanguy et al., 1996) and there is concern about potential future risks in populations with extensive HIV-related immunodeficiency. The development of safer BCG strains may help to address these concerns. The second area of progress has been in reproducing the protective effect of BCG by using nonliving subunit vaccines. Notable successes have been achieved by immunization with proteins harvested from *M. tuberculosis* culture filtrates (Andersen, 1994; Baldwin et al., 1998; Horwitz et al., 1995) and by using the technique of nucleic acid vaccination. Nucleic acid vaccination has focused mainly on the use of genes encoding secreted antigens—in particular, members of the antigen 85 complex of mycolyl transferases (Huygen et al., 1996)—although protection has also been reported using genes encoding conserved heat shock proteins, such as Hsp60, localized mainly to the bacterial cytoplasm (Tascon et al., 1996). In the Hsp60 studies (which involved intravenous challenge rather than direct aerosol delivery to the lungs), adoptive-transfer experiments suggested that protection is mediated predominantly by IFN-γ-secreting CD8$^+$ T cells (Tascon et al., 1998). Vaccination with defined antigenic subunits has an important advantage over vaccination with BCG in being compatible with continued use of skin testing as a diagnostic tool. In the United States (where BCG vaccination is not used), a positive tuberculin skin test is considered an indicator for prophylactic drug treatment. Difficulties in distinguishing a skin test response induced by BCG vaccination from that induced by infection with *M. tuberculosis* limits the utility of this approach in other countries. Replacement of BCG by a subunit vaccine might be considered to have diagnostic advantages even in the absence of any actual immunological benefit.

Better than BCG?

New candidate vaccines are equal to BCG in terms of their ability to reduce the bacterial load during the initial phase of infection in the mouse model; typically a reduction of around 10-fold is observed in comparison to an identical challenge in unvaccinated animals (Andersen, 1994; Huygen et al., 1996). So far, however, there is no experimental evidence of any vaccine capable of reducing the bacterial load significantly beyond the level obtained with BCG. Perhaps this is an impossible goal? Perhaps maintenance of a sufficiently intense immune response for long enough to ensure complete sterilization of the *M. tuberculosis* challenge would in itself directly threaten host survival? The level of protection conferred by previous exposure to *M. tuberculosis* itself (with subsequent treatment-based elimination of the infection) is similar to that obtained with BCG. The rationale for imagining that we might do better is that the natural immune response to *M. tuberculosis*, even in those who survive the primary infection, may be suboptimal. Given a life-style that is heavily dependent on the host immune response, it would be surprising if *M. tuberculosis* had not evolved means of turning this response to its advantage. The complex "natural" immune response to infection may therefore contain elements that have been selected on the basis of microbial survival as well as those selected by host survival. By understanding this response, it may be possible to specifically amplify elements that are particularly beneficial to the host.

From the perspective of protective immunity, speed would seem to be of the essence in the initial stages of *M. tuberculosis* infection (in contrast, speed does not seem to have been at a premium during evolution of the agonizingly slow-growing mycobacterial pathogens). Early activation of macrophages to cope with a localized infection involving only a few mycobacteria is less likely to entail tissue damage than a later response to more extensive infection. Also, at least in vitro, there is evidence that macrophages that have been infected with *M. tuberculosis* for several days become compromised in their ability to respond to activation signals and to present antigens (Hmama et al., 1998; Pancholi et al., 1993). The current focus on secreted antigens as vaccine targets is based on the rationale that these may be among the first antigens to be displayed on the surface of infected cells and may therefore be associated with early T-cell recognition. By looking closely at these early stages of infection, is it possible to gain any further clues for vaccine optimization?

Mycobacteria provide a potent signal to the innate immune system, with cell wall components triggering scavenger and Toll-like receptors on the cell surface, activating NF-κB transduction pathways leading to secretion of IL-12 and proinflammatory cytokines (Brightbill et al., 1999; Chatterjee et al., 1992; Means et al., 1999). While mannose capping of lipoarabinomannan may reduce this somewhat in the case of slow-growing mycobacteria (Roache et al., 1993), there is no evidence that the pathogens have evolved means for significant downregulation of the overall initial inflammatory response. There is evidence of interference with early events inside phagocytic cells, however. Maturation of the mycobacterial phagosome, in terms of acidification and fusion with bacteriocidal lysosomal vesicles, occurs only very slowly after infection with the live pathogens (Deretic and Fratti, 1999). In part, this may reflect the hydrophobic nature of the mycobacterial cell wall, although the dependence on viability is indicative of an active contribution from the microbe itself. Since processing of antigens for recognition by CD4$^+$ T cells (the major histocompatibility complex MHC class II presentation pathway) relies on delivery of proteins to acidic compartments (Watts, 1997), phagosomal arrest is likely to have implications for the kinetics of the T-cell response to live mycobacterial infection. The delay in triggering the T-cell response may provide an important advantage to the pathogen, and shortening the delay might therefore represent a useful vaccine target. Can antigen presentation occur in advance of phagosome maturation? Lipid components are exported from the immature mycobacterial phagosome and may provide an early target for CD1-restricted T cells (Beatty et al., 2000; Schaible et al., 2000; Sugita et al., 1999). Lipoproteins also escape from the phagosome (O. Neyrolles and D. Young, unpublished observations) and might gain access to both class I and class II processing pathways. Finally, permeabilization of the phagosome membrane may facilitate the release of mycobacterial proteins into the cytoplasm of the infected cell, making them available for class I presentation (Mazzaccaro et al., 1996; Teitelbaum et al., 1999). These early responses may represent only a minor component in relation to the dominant responses occurring after phagosome maturation; boosting them might result in a response that is more effective than that seen during natural infection.

BEING PERSISTENT AND TAKING SECOND CHANCES

While BCG vaccination would seem to be at least partially effective in helping to control the initial infection, the results of the clinical trials demonstrate that it is unreliable as a stimulus of later responses to reactivation or reinfection. In the light of conventional vaccinology, it seems paradoxical that an immune response which is effective against primary infection should be less effective against secondary challenge. Is the immune response induced by BCG ineffective against mycobacteria that have been present in the body for a long period? This might be the case if there is a radical change in the antigen profile of the persistent bacilli, for example. It is clear that mycobacteria undergo a process at least of metabolic adaptation during chronic infection in the mouse model (Höner Zu Bentrup et al., 1999; Wallace, 1961), and bacterial genomics, along with associated microarray and proteomic tools (Behr et al., 1999; Jungblut et al., 1999; Wilson et al., 1999), provides a powerful new opportunity to study the in vivo phenotype of *M. tuberculosis*. Alternatively, does the immune response induced by BCG wane over time? This might occur if memory cells induced by the initial vaccination decay or are actively depleted and are not replaced. The definition and subsequent quantification of memory T-cell pools represent an important area of research in cellular immunology. Significant progress has been made in the accurate assessment of antigen-specific CD8+ T-cell populations in viral infection, for example (Ogg and McMichael, 1998), and application of analogous quantitative approaches to mycobacterial immunity is of high priority.

In the meantime, vaccination capable of conferring reliable protection against reactivation and reinfection in addition to disseminated primary disease would obviously be of immense public health benefit. One possible approach to this goal involves modification of the primary vaccine in a way that results in

establishment of a more extensive memory pool, perhaps including additional T-cell subsets recognizing antigens specific to mycobacterial phenotypes predominant in vivo. It is relatively straightforward to supplement BCG with additional antigen-encoding genes (e.g., Snewin et al., 2000), and introduction of an active hemolysin provides a strategy for enhancement of its ability to prime CD8+ T cells (Hess et al., 1998). An alternative approach would be to consider a second vaccination, delivered at a time closer to that of the onset of clinical tuberculosis in the late teens. While this second strategy is attractive from a logistic point of view, it would necessarily include immunization after initial exposure to the pathogen, a very different immunological paradigm from that of most conventional vaccine programs. In this section, we will focus on discussion of this second, postexposure, strategy.

Postexposure Vaccination

Assuming continuation of the current global program of neonatal BCG vaccination, the target population for postexposure vaccination would all have received BCG and would include three groups: those who have remained unexposed to *M. tuberculosis,* those who have been exposed but were able to eliminate subsequent infection with *M. tuberculosis,* and those who are currently infected with viable *M. tuberculosis* in some subclinical form. What are the prospects for a vaccine that would reinforce the immune response in the first two groups and help either to contain or to eliminate the infection in the third group?

An obvious strategy is simply to repeat the BCG vaccination. Although this has been applied as a standard procedure in some countries, there is little evidence to demonstrate its efficacy. In fact, the single randomized controlled study to address the question of repeat BCG vaccination (carried out in Malawi) failed to demonstrate any benefit (Karonga Prevention Trial Group, 1996). A second large trial is under way in Brazil. An alternative strategy would be to present the immune system with a novel stimulus, in the form of different antigens or of antigens presented in a different immunological context. Proteins present in *M. tuberculosis* but absent from the original BCG vaccination represent an attractive set of candidates for this approach. From comparative genomics, we know of approximately 100 *M. tuberculosis* genes that are not present in BCG vaccine strains (Behr et al., 1999; Gordon et al., 1999). As noted above, these represent a combination of genes absent from the parent *M. bovis,* along with genes lost during subculture of BCG. At least one of these proteins, a low-molecular-weight secreted protein referred to as ESAT6, is prominent in the natural immune response to *M. tuberculosis* infection (Sorensen et al., 1995), and it seems likely that others could provide additional immune targets.

The selection of mycobacterial antigens for testing as subunit vaccine candidates has been the subject of prolonged if inconclusive debate (Andersen and Brennan, 1994; Snewin et al., 2000). One approach to this question has been to identify proteins eliciting a strong recall response following infection with *M. tuberculosis* in mice or in healthy tuberculin-positive humans (Alderson et al., 2000; Andersen et al., 1992). Interestingly, when the genes encoding these dominant antigens are compared among different clinical isolates of *M. tuberculosis,* they are found to be identical (Musser et al., 2000). This is in contrast to genes encoding targets of a protective immune response in other pathogens, which are characteristically subject to antigenic variation (Robertson and Meyer, 1992) as a result of the selection of mutations that confer reduced immune recognition. Although the comparatively recent evolutionary origin of *M. tuberculosis* is reflected in a very high degree of overall genetic identity among current isolates (Sreevatsan et al., 1997), variations do emerge rapidly in response to selective pressure exerted by antimicrobial drugs (Blanchard, 1996; Heym et al., 1996). The lack of variation in the antigen-encoding genes identified so far implies that in contrast to the drug targets, they are not subject to selective pressure from the immune system. If these antigens are targets of a protective immune response, why do we not see any evolutionary imprint of this? Does the presence of multiple antigens occupy the immune system to such an extent that variation of one particular antigen offers insufficient advantage to warrant selection? This sounds reasonable, although it would seem to contradict the observation that, at least in mice, effective vaccination can be targeted to a single antigen (Huygen et al., 1996; Tascon et al., 1996). Some caution must be exercised, however, in considering the extent to which murine infections will model human immune responses that may have evolved during prolonged intimate interactions with *M. tuberculosis.* Alternatively, perhaps we have yet to identify the genuine protective antigens. Approximately 10% of the coding capacity of the *M. tuberculosis* genome is taken up by two protein families—the PE and PPE families—that have no known function but exhibit a degree of strain variation (Cole et al., 1998). Is it possible that these families are targets of some as yet unidentified form of immune pressure? One of the PPE proteins has been identified as the target of a CD4$^+$ T-cell response (Dillon et al., 1999), and two

PE-PGRS genes have been identified among those which are upregulated during infection of macrophages with *M. marinum* (Ramakrishnan et al., 2000). It is intriguing that repetitive sequences occurring within these proteins are reminiscent of motifs characteristic of variable antigens found in parasites (Deitsch et al., 1997). Finally, perhaps the absence of antigenic variation confers some positive benefit for the mycobacteria. As discussed above, *M. tuberculosis* relies on immune-mediated tissue damage for efficient transmission; could it be that the prominent targets of the natural immune response are a reflection of this microbial agenda?

When considering targets for postexposure vaccination, it may be useful to look for antigens that feature less prominently in the natural response to infection. Obviously, target antigens have to be presented during natural infection in some form that makes them visible to the immune system, but amplification of responses to subdominant determinants might provide an interesting approach to the restimulation of the immune response during postexposure vaccination. Similarly, in considering the type of immune activities that might usefully be induced by postexposure vaccination, there may be advantages in looking at T-cell subsets that are poorly represented during natural infection rather than reproducing existing responses.

Although most preexposure vaccine testing in animal models includes consideration of the effect of vaccination on bacterial load, pathology, and survival during the chronic phase of the infection, there has been little experimental analysis of postexposure vaccine strategies. In large part, this reflects the absence of any accepted standard model of postexposure vaccination. Following challenge with a low to moderate dose of *M. tuberculosis,* the initial acute phase of infection in most inbred mouse strains is followed by a chronic phase lasting weeks or months, during which the bacterial load in infected organs remains constant (Orme and Collins, 1994). This provides a relatively straightforward model for mycobacterial persistence, although, in human terms, it is difficult to say whether this would be considered a subclinical latent infection or the early stages of active disease. It was recently reported that immunization with Hsp60 in the form of a nucleic acid vaccine resulted in a decrease in bacterial load during this chronic phase (Lowrie et al., 1999). A similar effect was also achieved when Hsp60 was replaced by IL-12, and it is hard to disentangle the relative contributions of innate and acquired immune responses. The same study also reported an effect of nucleic acid vaccination in a second, more complex model of mycobacterial persistence (Lowrie et al., 1999). Generally referred to as the Cornell model (in recognition of the important contribution of McDermott and McCune, working at Cornell University in the 1950s and 1960s), this involves infection of mice with *M. tuberculosis,* followed by near complete antimicrobial therapy. Subsequent treatment with immunosuppressive steroids results in reactivation of the infection in some mice (McCune et al., 1966). In contrast to BCG, vaccination with Hsp60 DNA in the post-therapy phase was found to prevent reactivation, suggesting that immune-mediated clearance of the residual low-level infection had occurred (Lowrie et al., 1999). While encouraging from the perspective of postexposure immunomodulation, these findings are in conflict with the views of other researchers (Turner et al., 2000), and it will be important to determine the extent to which they are dependent on specific features of the particular model used in these studies. It may also be argued that, particularly in the Cornell model, this type of experiment is more informative in the context of immunotherapy, i.e., treatment of active disease, than of immunoprophylaxis.

IMMUNOTHERAPY—KOCH REVISITED

The striking effectiveness of drugs in the treatment of tuberculosis led to abandonment of concepts of immunotherapy popular in the first half of the 20th century. However, two circumstances have promoted some renewal of interest in this area. First, an important practical limitation in current tuberculosis therapy is the need for a consistent supply and intake of drugs over a period of at least 6 months. Although in most cases the symptoms of disease and the transmission of live bacteria are eliminated within a few weeks, prolonged treatment is required to complete the clearance of persistent organisms that would otherwise trigger relapse. Why can we not use drugs to eliminate the bulk of the mycobacteria and then rely on the immune system to cope with persisters? A plausible explanation is that the immune system is actively damaged by the process of tuberculosis. While it might be interesting (although ethically unthinkable) to study patients who spontaneously recover from active tuberculosis, low levels of IFN-γ production in response to mycobacterial antigens in patients undergoing treatment suggests that disease is associated with a relative suppression in immunity compared to that in healthy tuberculin-positive controls (Hirsch et al., 1999a). The mechanisms underlying this effect are unclear. Important factors might include the production of cytokines that suppress Th1-mediated responses (transforming growth factor

β, for example) or the loss of lymphocytes via apoptosis (Hirsch et al., 1999b). Perhaps reversal of this suppression by immunotherapy would assist in recovery. The second impetus for immunotherapy is supplied by the inexorable rise in multidrug-resistant (MDR) strains of *M. tuberculosis* (Pablos-Mendez et al., 1998). Will the erosion of our major antimycobacterial weapon force us to fall back on the immune response?

In addition to the work with experimental models described above, clinical trials have been carried out to assess the effectiveness of a novel immunotherapy as an adjunct to drug treatment of tuberculosis. This involved injection of an autoclaved preparation of *M. vaccae* (Stanford et al., 1990). *M. vaccae* is a nonpathogenic soil organism which, like all mycobacteria, provides a potent signal for induction of IL-12. Use of *M. vaccae* as an adjuvant or challenge with *M. vaccae* on its own tends to bias the immune response toward the Th1 phenotype. If active tuberculosis involves an imbalance in favor of a Th2 response, immunotherapy with *M. vaccae* may prove beneficial. There is some limited evidence to support this concept in a murine model (Rook and Hernandez-Pando, 1996), although an inherent bias toward a strong Th1 dominance would seem to be a fundamental characteristic of the immune response to mycobacteria. *M. vaccae* was initially tested in a series of clinical trials which generated encouraging results but which were open to criticism in terms of methodology (Corlan et al., 1997; Onyebujoh et al., 1995). More recently, a rigorously controlled trial was carried out in South Africa (Durban Immunotherapy Group, 1999). The trial was designed to evaluate whether administration of *M. vaccae* immunotherapy in combination with optimal drug treatment would enhance the rate of reduction in bacterial load, as assessed by sputum analysis. The results of the trial were clear: *M. vaccae* was without deleterious side effects, but immunotherapy had no effect on sputum clearance. A second *M. vaccae* trial carried out in Uganda was slightly more encouraging (Johnson et al., 2000), and a trial to assess longer-term benefits is under way in Tanzania.

Does this once again prove the ineffectiveness of immunotherapy? Clearly, the immune system cannot begin to compete with drugs in dealing with active tuberculosis at a stage when mycobacteria are replicating freely in diseased lung tissues. However, neither the tuberculin experience nor the *M. vaccae* trials rule out a potential role for immunotherapy in shortening treatment. Ultimately, this will have to be tested in trials which involve the delivery of shortened chemotherapy regimens. The methodological and ethical framework of such trials and the question whether they should employ *M. vaccae* or some other vaccine candidate deserve to be the subject of active debate.

Direct cytokine-based modulation of immunological activities in tuberculosis represents a second important aspect of immunotherapy. Can cytokines be used to augment antimycobacterial activity and/or to reduce immunopathology? There is a compelling case for evaluation of cytokine therapy in patients infected with MDR tuberculosis. Limited trials have been carried out using IL-2 (Johnson et al., 1997). So far, it has been shown that the treatment is safe, although further studies are required to assess any beneficial effect. Efforts to reduce pathology have focused on TNF-α. TNF-α is required for optimal macrophage activation, but at higher concentrations it contributes to the tissue necrosis and wasting characteristic of tuberculosis. After its withdrawal as a general analgesic, thalidomide continued to be used for treatment of reactional episodes associated with pain and nerve damage in patients with leprosy. It now seems clear that the effectiveness of such treatment is due to the ability of thalidomide to reduce the expression of TNF-α, probably by causing a reduction in mRNA half-life (Moreira et al., 1993). The potential benefit of thalidomide treatment in acute tuberculosis is currently being evaluated in clinical trials (Tramontana et al., 1995). In addition to a possible reduction in tissue damage due to tuberculosis itself, a reduction in the level of TNF-α might have an important impact on interactions between *M. tuberculosis* and HIV (Bekker et al., 2000). Enhanced HIV replication in TNF-α-activated cells may contribute to accelerated progression to AIDS in coinfected individuals; thalidomide may reduce such progression and thereby increase survival.

MOVING VACCINES INTO HUMANS

Laboratory models provide a powerful means of developing strategies for immune intervention in tuberculosis, but species-specific differences in the response to mycobacterial infection preclude direct extrapolation of vaccination successes (and failures) from small animals to humans. Clinical trials will be central to progress in vaccine development. For the three intervention targets discussed above—preexposure, postexposure, and immunotherapy—there is an inverse correlation between the feasibility of clinical trials and the solidity of the immunological foundation. As illustrated by the experience with *M. vaccae,* immunotherapy trials can be carried out with relatively minor amendments to current treatment regimens. A postexposure vaccine directed toward a

young-adult group in a high-incidence area could conceivably be evaluated in a relatively short-term trial over a few years. In contrast, evaluation of protection against adult tuberculosis by preexposure vaccination would entail neonatal delivery and a 20-year time frame if conducted in an area of endemic infection. If the new vaccine was to be compared to BCG, consideration would also have to be given to the question of withdrawing BCG coverage from part of the trial group, perhaps increasing their risk of potentially fatal childhood tuberculosis. To give a realistic prospect for introduction of new tuberculosis vaccines within the first half of the 21st century, it seems likely that some pragmatism will be required in balancing the immunological rationale and clinical goals of future vaccine trials. There would be obvious attractions in trial formats which would allow simultaneous assessment of more than one form of intervention: trials comparing responses in exposed and unexposed individuals within a heterogeneous test population, for example.

Should we be concerned about the evolution of resistance to vaccine-induced immunity? So far, this has not occurred for the vaccines currently in use against other infections, but there are a number of possible explanations for this (McLean, 1999). It could be that current vaccines function optimally and are cross-reactive enough to prevent the emergence of competitive resistant strains. However, models predict that in any event this would take a very long time to happen, so it may be too early to be sure. Another explanation is that current vaccine coverage is so low that resistant strains have no competitive advantage, although for current vaccines such as measles-mumps-rubella and diphtheria-pertussis-tetanus this seems unlikely. This last point is of particular relevance to vaccines that target specific groups, such as meningococcal meningitis and hepatitis B, and that could include a post-tuberculosis-exposure vaccine. Indeed, this may be a way of avoiding the emergence of vaccine-resistant strains in the future, since they will always remain competitively inferior. Consequently, a subunit vaccine consisting of *M. tuberculosis* antigens is probably most suitable in the first instance for at-risk groups such as tuberculosis-contacts and HIV-positive patients. This would also allow the necessary data to be acquired to determine whether a global vaccination program was appropriate.

CONCLUDING REMARKS

Even though the outcome of infection with *M. tuberculosis* is critically dependent on the immune response, a century of effort to control the disease by vaccination has yielded only modest success. Advances in mycobacterial genomics and cellular immunology now provide a wide new range of opportunities for tuberculosis vaccine development. In this chapter we have attempted to highlight some of these opportunities, focusing in particular on the thesis that in spite of the success of the classical vaccine paradigm in other diseases, consideration of immune interventions in tuberculosis should be broadened beyond the concept of mimicking the natural infection in advance of encounter with the pathogen. The natural immune response to *M. tuberculosis* may well have been shaped as much by the evolutionary needs of the microbe as by those of the host. Rather than simply trying to reproduce natural immunity, we should try and understand its mechanisms and search for strategies to augment its shortcomings.

REFERENCES

Alderson, M. R., T. Bement, C. H. Day, L. Zhu, D. Molesh, Y. A. W. Skeiky, R. Coler, D. M. Lewinsohn, S. G. Reed, and D. C. Dillon. 2000. Expression cloning of an immunodominant family of *Mycobacterium tuberculosis* antigens using human CD4⁺ T cells. *J. Exp. Med.* 191:551–559.

Altare, F., A. Durandy, D. Lammas, J. F. Emile, S. Lamhamedi, F. Le Deist, P. Drysdale, E. Jouanguy, R. Doffinger, F. Bernaudin, O. Jeppsson, J. A. Gollob, E. Meinl, A. W. Segal, A. Fischer, D. Kumararatne, and J. L. Casanova. 1998. Impairment of mycobacterial immunity in human interleukin-12 receptor deficiency. *Science* 280:1432–1435.

Andersen, A. B., and P. Brennan. 1994. Proteins and antigens of *Mycobacterium tuberculosis*, p. 307–332. *In* B. R. Bloom (ed.), *Tuberculosis: Protection, Pathogenesis, and Control.* American Society for Microbiology, Washington, D.C.

Andersen, P. 1994. Effective vaccination of mice against *Mycobacterium tuberculosis* infection with a soluble mixture of secreted mycobacterial proteins. *Infect. Immun.* 62:2536–2544.

Andersen, P., D. Askgaard, A. Gottschau, J. Bennedsen, S. Nagai, and I. Heron. 1992. Identification of immunodominant antigens during infection with *Mycobacterium tuberculosis*. *Scand. J. Immunol.* 36:823–831.

Baldwin, S. L., C. D'Souza, A. D. Roberts, B. P. Kelly, A. A. Frank, M. A. Lui, J. B. Ulmer, K. Huygen, D. M. McMurray, and I. M. Orme. 1998. Evaluation of new vaccines in the mouse and guinea pig model of tuberculosis. *Infect. Immun.* 66:2951–2959.

Bardarov, S., J. Kriakov, C. Carriere, S. Yu, C. Vaamonde, R. A. McAdam, B. R. Bloom, G. F. Hatfull, and W. R. Jacobs, Jr. 1997. Conditionally replicating mycobacteriophages: a system for transposon delivery to *Mycobacterium tuberculosis*. *Proc. Natl. Acad. Sci. USA* 94:10961–10966.

Beatty, W., E. Rhoades, H.-J. Ullrich, D. Chatterjee, J. Heuser, and D. Russell. 2000. Trafficking and release of mycobacterial lipids from infected macrophages. *Traffic* 1:235–247.

Behr, M. A., and P. M. Small. 1997. Has BCG attenuated to impotence? *Nature* 389:133–134.

Behr, M. A., M. A. Wilson, W. P. Gill, H. Salamon, G. K. Schoolnik, S. Rane, and P. M. Small. 1999. Comparative genomics of BCG vaccines by whole-genome DNA microarray. *Science* 284:1520–1523.

Bekker, L. G., P. Haslett, G. Maartens, L. Steyn, and G. Kaplan. 2000. Thalidomide-induced antigen-specific immune stimulation in patients with human immunodeficiency virus type 1 and tuberculosis. *J. Infect. Dis.* 181:954–965.

Blanchard, J. S. 1996. Molecular mechanisms of drug resistance in *Mycobacterium tuberculosis*. *Annu. Rev. Biochem.* 65:215–239.

Bloom, B. R., and P. E. M. Fine. 1994. The BCG experience: implications for future vaccines against tuberculosis, p. 531–558. *In* B. R. Bloom (ed.), *Tuberculosis: Protection, Pathogenesis, and Control.* American Society for Microbiology, Washington, D.C.

Brightbill, H. D., D. H. Libraty, S. R. Krutzik, R. B. Yang, J. T. Belisle, J. R. Bleharski, M. Maitland, M. V. Norgard, S. E. Plevy, S. T. Smale, P. J. Brennan, B. R. Bloom, P. J. Godowski, and R. L. Modlin. 1999. Host defense mechanisms triggered by microbial lipoproteins through toll-like receptors. *Science* 285:732–736.

Brock, T. D. 1988. *Robert Koch. A Life in Medicine and Bacteriology.* Springer Velag, New York, N.Y.

Calmette, A. 1927. *La Vaccination Preventive contra la Tuberculosis.* Madison et Cie, Paris, France.

Chan, J., and S. H. E. Kaufmann. 1994. Immune mechanisms of protection, p. 389–415. *In* B. R. Bloom (ed), *Tuberculosis: Protection, Pathogenesis, and Control.* American Society for Microbiology, Washington, D.C.

Chatterjee, D., A. D. Roberts, K. Lowell, P. J. Brennan, and I. M. Orme. 1992. Structural basis of capacity of lipoarabinomannan to induce secretion of tumor necrosis factor. *Infect. Immun.* 60:1249–1253.

Colditz, G. A., C. S. Berkey, F. Mosteller, T. F. Brewer, M. E. Wilson, E. Burdick, and H. V. Fineberg. 1995. The efficacy of bacillus Calmette-Guerin vaccination of newborns and infants in the prevention of tuberculosis: meta-analyses of the published literature. *Pediatrics* 96:29–35.

Colditz, G. A., T. F. Brewer, C. S. Berkey, M. E. Wilson, E. Burdick, H. V. Fineberg, and F. Mosteller. 1994. Efficacy of BCG vaccine in the prevention of tuberculosis. Meta-analysis of the published literature. *JAMA* 271:698–702.

Cole, S., R. Brosch, J. Parkhill, T. Garnier, C. Churcher, D. Harris, S. Gordon, K. Eiglmeier, S. Gas, C. E. Barry III, F. Tekaia, K. Badcock, D. Basham, D. Brown, T. Chillingworth, R. Connor, R. Davies, K. Devlin, T. Feltwell, S. Gentles, N. Hamlin, S. Holroyd, T. Hornsby, K. Jagels, and B. Barrell. 1998. Deciphering the biology of *Mycobacterium tuberculosis* from the complete genome sequence. *Nature* 393:537–544.

Comstock, G. W. 1978. Tuberculosis in twins: a reanalysis of the Prophit survey. *Am. Rev. Respir. Dis.* 117:621–624.

Constant, P., F. Davodeau, M. A. Peyrat, Y. Poquet, G. Puzo, M. Bonneville, and J. J. Fournie. 1994. Stimulation of human gamma delta T cells by nonpeptidic mycobacterial ligands. *Science* 264:267–270.

Cooper, A. M., J. Magram, J. Ferrante, and I. M. Orme. 1997. Interleukin 12 (IL-12) is crucial to the development of protective immunity in mice intravenously infected with *Mycobacterium tuberculosis*. *J. Exp. Med.* 186:39–45.

Corlan, E., C. Marica, C. Macavei, J. L. Stanford, and C. A. Stanford. 1997. Immunotherapy with *Mycobacterium vaccae* in the treatment of tuberculosis in Romania. 2. Chronic or relapsed disease. *Respir. Med.* 91:21–29.

Dannenberg, A. M., and G. A. W. Rook. 1994. Pathogenesis of pulmonary tuberculosis: an interplay of tissue-damaging and macrophage-activating immune responses—dual mechanisms that control bacillary multiplication, p. 459–483. *In* B. R. Bloom (ed.), *Tuberculosis: Protection, Pathogenesis, and Control.* American Society for Microbiology, Washington, D.C.

Deitsch, K. W., E. R. Moxon, and T. E. Wellems. 1997. Shared themes of antigenic variation and virulence in bacterial, protozoal, and fungal infections. *Microbiol. Mol. Biol. Rev.* **61:**281–293.

Deretic, V., and R. A. Fratti. 1999. *Mycobacterium tuberculosis* phagosome. *Mol. Microbiol.* **31:**1603–1609.

Dillon, D. C., M. R. Alderson, C. H. Day, D. M. Lewinsohn, R. Coler, T. Bement, A. Campos-Neto, Y. A. Skeiky, I. M. Orme, A. Roberts, S. Steen, W. Dalemans, R. Badaro, and S. G. Reed. 1999. Molecular characterization and human T-cell responses to a member of a novel *Mycobacterium tuberculosis* mtb39 gene family. *Infect. Immun.* **67:**2941–2950.

Dormandy, T. 1999. *The White Death. A History of Tuberculosis.* Hambledon Press, London, United Kingdom.

Dubos, R., and J. Dubos. 1952. *The White Plague. Tuberculosis, Man, and Society.* Rutgers University Press, New Brunswick, N.J.

Durban Immunotherapy Group. 1999. Immunotherapy with *Mycobacterium vaccae* in patients with newly diagnosed pulmonary tuberculosis: a randomised controlled trial. *Lancet* **354:**116–119.

Dye, C., S. Scheele, P. Dolin, V. Pathania, and M. C. Raviglione. 1999. Global burden of tuberculosis. Estimated incidence, prevalence, and mortality by country. *JAMA* **282:**677–686.

Fine, P. E. M. 1995. Variation in protection by BCG: implications of and for heterologous immunity. *Lancet* **346:**1339–1345.

Fine, P. E. M., and P. M. Small. 1999. Exogenous reinfection in tuberculosis (editorial). *N. Engl. J. Med.* **341:**1226–1227.

Flynn, J., J. Chan, K. Triebold, D. Dalton, T. Stewart, and B. R. Bloom. 1993. An essential role for interferon gamma in resistance to *Mycobacterium tuberculosis* infection. *J. Exp. Med.* **178:**2249–2254.

Flynn, J., M. Goldstein, K. Triebold, B. Koller, and B. R. Bloom. 1992. Major histocompatibility complex class I-restricted T cells are required for resistance to *Mycobacterium tuberculosis* infection. *Proc. Natl. Acad. Sci. USA* **89:**12013–12017.

Gordon, S. V., R. Brosch, A. Billault, T. Garnier, K. Eiglmeier, and S. T. Cole. 1999. Identification of variable regions in the genomes of tubercle bacilli using bacterial artificial chromosome arrays. *Mol. Microbiol.* **32:**643–655.

Guleria, I., R. Teitelbaum, R. A. McAdam, G. Kalpana, W. R. Jacobs, Jr., and B. R. Bloom. 1996. Auxotrophic vaccines for tuberculosis. *Nat. Med.* **2:**334–337.

Hess, J., D. Miko, A. Catic, V. Lehmensiek, D. G. Russell, and S. H. E. Kaufmann. 1998. *Mycobacterium bovis* Bacille Calmette-Guerin strains secreting listeriolysin of *Listeria monocytogenes. Proc. Natl. Acad. Sci. USA* **95:**5299–5304.

Heym, B., W. Philipp, and S. T. Cole. 1996. Mechanisms of drug resistance in *Mycobacterium tuberculosis. Curr. Top. Microbiol. Immunol.* **215:**49–69.

Hirsch, C. S., Z. Toossi, C. Othieno, J. L. Johnson, S. K. Schwander, S. Robertson, R. S. Wallis, K. Edmonds, A. Okwera, R. Mugerwa, P. Peters, and J. J. Ellner. 1999a. Depressed T-cell interferon-gamma responses in pulmonary tuberculosis: analysis of underlying mechanisms and modulation with therapy. *J. Infect. Dis.* **180:**2069–2073.

Hirsch, C. S., Z. Toossi, G. Vanham, J. L. Johnson, P. Peters, A. Okwera, R. Mugerwa, P. Mugyenyi, and J. J. Ellner. 1999b. Apoptosis and T cell hyporesponsiveness in pulmonary tuberculosis. *J. Infect. Dis.* **179:**945–953.

Hmama, Z., R. Gabathuler, W. A. Jefferies, G. de Jong, and N. E. Reiner. 1998. Attenuation of HLA-DR expression by mononuclear phagocytes infected with *Mycobacterium tuberculosis* is related to intracellular sequestration of immature class II heterodimers. *J. Immunol.* **161:**4882–4893.

Höner Zu Bentrup, K., A. Miczak, D. L. Swenson, and D. G. Russell. 1999. Characterization of activity and expression of isocitrate lyase in *Mycobacterium avium* and *Mycobacterium tuberculosis. J. Bacteriol.* **181:**7161–7167.

Hopewell, P. C. 1992. Impact of human immunodeficiency virus infection on the epidemiology, clinical features, management and control of tuberculosis. *Clin. Infect. Dis.* **18:**540–546.

Horwitz, M. A., B. W. Lee, B. J. Dillon, and G. Harth. 1995. Protective immunity against tuberculosis induced by vaccination with major extracellular proteins of *Mycobacterium tuberculosis. Proc. Natl. Acad. Sci. USA* **92:**1530–1534.

Huygen, K., J. Content, O. Denis, D. L. Montgomery, A. M. Yawman, R. R. Deck, C. M. DeWitt, I. M. Orme, S. Baldwin, C. D'Souza, A. Drowart, E. Lozes, P. Vandenbussche, J. P. Van Vooren, M. A. Liu, and J. B. Ulmer. 1996. Immunogenicity and protective efficacy of a tuberculosis DNA vaccine. *Nat. Med.* **2:**893–898.

Johnson, B. J., L. G. Bekker, R. Rickman, S. Brown, M. Lesser, S. Ress, P. Willcox, L. Steyn, and G. Kaplan. 1997. rhuIL-2 adjunctive therapy in multidrug resistant tuberculosis: a comparison of two treatment regimens and placebo. *Tubercle Lung Dis.* **78:**195–203.

Johnson, J. L., R. M. Kamya, A. Okwera, A. M. Loughlin, S. Nyole, D. L. Hom, R. S. Wallis, C. S. Hirsch, K. Wolski, J. Foulds, R. D. Mugerwa, and J. J. Ellner. 2000. Randomized controlled trial of *Mycobacterium vaccae* immunotherapy in non-human immunodeficiency virus-infected Ugandan adults with newly diagnosed pulmonary tuberculosis. The Uganda-Case Western Reserve University Research Collaboration. *J. Infect. Dis.* **181:**1304–1312.

Jouanguy, E., F. Altare, S. Lamhamedi, P. Revy, J. F. Emile, M. Newport, M. Levin, S. Blanche, E. Seboun, A. Fischer, and J. L. Casanova. 1996. Interferon-gamma-receptor deficiency in an infant with fatal bacille Calmette-Guerin infection. *N. Engl. J. Med.* **335:**1956–1961.

Jungblut, P. R., U. E. Schaible, H. J. Mollenkopf, U. Zimny Arndt, B. Raupach, J. Mattow, P. Halada, S. Lamer, K. Hagens, and S. H. E. Kaufmann. 1999. Comparative proteome analysis of *Mycobacterium tuberculosis* and *Mycobacterium bovis* BCG strains: towards functional genomics of microbial pathogens. *Mol. Microbiol.* **33:**1103–1117.

Karonga Prevention Trial Group. 1996. Randomised controlled trial of single BCG, repeated BCG, or combined BCG and killed *Mycobacterium leprae* vaccine for prevention of leprosy and tuberculosis in Malawi. *Lancet* **348:**17–24.

Kaufmann, S. H. E. 1988. CD8+ T lymphocytes in intracellular microbial infections. *Immunol. Today* **9:**168–174.

Koch, R. 1882. Die aetiologie der Tuberculose. *Berl. Klin. Wochenschr.* **19:**221–230.

Kochi, A. 1991. The global tuberculosis situation and the new control strategy of the World Health Organization. *Tubercle* **72:**1–6.

Lowrie, D. B., R. E. Tascon, V. L. D. Bonato, V. M. F. Lima, L. H. Faccioli, E. Stavropoulos, M. J. Colston, R. G. Hewinson, K. Moelling, and C. L. Silva. 1999. Therapy of tuberculosis in mice by DNA vaccination. *Nature* **400:**269–271.

Mahairas, G. G., P. J. Sabo, M. J. Hickey, D. C. Singh, and C. K. Stover. 1996. Molecular analysis of genetic differences between *Mycobacterium bovis* BCG and virulent *M. bovis. J. Bacteriol.* **178:**1274–1282.

Mazzaccaro, R., M. Gedde, E. Jensen, H. van Santen, H. Ploegh, K. Rock, and B. R. Bloom. 1996. Major histocompatibility class I presentation of soluble antigen facilitated by *Mycobacterium tuberculosis* infection. *Proc. Natl. Acad. Sci. USA* **93**:11786–11791.

McCune, R. M., F. M. Feldman, H. P. Lambert, and W. Mc-Dermott. 1966. Microbial persistence. I. The capacity of tubercle bacilli top survive sterilization in mouse tissues. *J. Exp. Med.* **123**:445–468.

McLean, A. 1999. Development and use of vaccines against evolving pathogens: vaccine design, p. 138–151. In S. C. Stearns (ed.), *Evolution in Health and Disease.* Oxford University Press, Oxford, United Kingdom.

McMurray, D. N. 1994. Guinea pig model of tuberculosis, p. 135–148. *In* B. R. Bloom (ed.), *Tuberculosis: Protection, Pathogenesis, and Control.* American Society for Microbiology, Washington, D.C.

Means, T. K., S. Wang, E. Lien, A. Yoshimura, D. T. Golenbock, and M. J. Fenton. 1999. Human Toll-like receptors mediate cellular activation by *Mycobacterium tuberculosis. J. Immunol.* **163**:3920–3927.

Moody, D. B., B. B. Reinhold, M. R. Guy, E. M. Beckman, D. E. Frederique, S. T. Furlong, S. Ye, V. N. Reinhold, P. A. Sieling, R. L. Modlin, G. S. Besra, and S. A. Porcelli. 1997. Structural requirements for glycolipid antigen recognition by CD1b-restricted T cells. *Science* **278**:283–286.

Moreira, A. L., E. P. Sampaio, A. Zmuidzinas, P. Frindt, K. A. Smith, and G. Kaplan. 1993. Thalidomide exerts its inhibitory action on tumor necrosis factor alpha by enhancing mRNA degradation. *J. Exp. Med.* **177**:1675–1680.

Musser, J. M., A. Amin, and S. Ramaswamy. 2000. Negligible genetic diversity of *Mycobacterium tuberculosis* host immune system targets: evidence of limited selective pressure. *Genetics* **155**:7–16.

Newport, M. J., C. M. Huxley, S. Huston, C. M. Hawrylowicz, B. A. Oostra, R. Williamson, and M. Levin. 1996. A mutation in the interferon-gamma-receptor gene and susceptibility to mycobacterial infection. *N. Engl. J. Med.* **335**:1941–1949.

Ogg, G. S., and A. J. McMichael. 1998. HLA-peptide tetrameric complexes. *Curr. Opin. Immunol.* **10**:393–396.

Onyebujoh, P. C., T. Abdulmumini, S. Robinson, G. A. Rook, and J. L. Stanford. 1995. Immunotherapy with *Mycobacterium vaccae* as an addition to chemotherapy for the treatment of pulmonary tuberculosis under difficult conditions in Africa. *Respir. Med.* **89**:199–207.

Orme, I. M., and F. M. Collins. 1994. Mouse model of tuberculosis, p. 113–134. *In* B. R. Bloom (ed.), *Tuberculosis: Protection, Pathogenesis, and Control.* American Society for Microbiology, Washington, D.C.

Pablos-Mendez, A., M. Raviglione, A. Laszlo, N. Binkin, H. Rieder, F. Bustreo, D. Cohn, C. Lambregts-van Weezenbeek, S. Kim, P. Chaulet, and P. Nunn. 1998. Global surveillance for antituberculosis-drug resistance, 1994–1997. World Health Organization—International Union against Tuberculosis and Lung Disease Working Group on Anti-Tuberculosis Drug Resistance Surveillance. *N. Engl. J. Med.* **338**:1641–1649.

Palmer, C. E., and M. W. Long. 1966. Effects of infection with atypical mycobacteria on BCG vaccination and tuberculosis. *Am. Rev. Respir. Dis.* **94**:553–568.

Pancholi, P., A. Mirza, N. Bhardwaj, and R. M. Steinman. 1993. Sequestration from immune CD4$^+$ T cells of mycobacteria growing in human macrophages. *Science* **260**:984–986.

Pelicic, V., M. Jackson, J. M. Reyrat, W. R. Jacobs, Jr., B. Gicquel, and C. Guilhot. 1997. Efficient allelic exchange and transposon mutagenesis in *Mycobacterium tuberculosis. Proc. Natl. Acad. Sci. USA* **94**:10955–10960.

Ramakrishnan, L., N. A. Federspiel, and S. Falkow. 2000. Granuloma-specific expression of mycobacterium virulence proteins from the glycine-rich PE-PGRS family. *Science* **288**:1436–1439.

Roache, T. I., C. H. Barton, D. Chatterjee, and J. M. Blackwell. 1993. Macrophage activation: lipoarabinomannan from avirulent and virulent strains of *Mycobacterium tuberculosis* differentially induces the early genes c-fos, KC, JE, and tumour necrosis factor-alpha. *J. Immunol.* **150**:1886–1896.

Robertson, B. D., and T. F. Meyer. 1992. Genetic variation in pathogenic bacteria. *Trends Genet.* **8**:422–427.

Rook, G. A., and R. Hernandez-Pando. 1996. The pathogenesis of tuberculosis. *Annu. Rev. Microbiol.* **50**:259–284.

Schaible, U. E., K. Hagens, K. Fischer, H. L. Collins, and S. H. E. Kaufmann. 2000. Intersection of group 1 CD1 molecules and mycobacteria in different intracellular compartments of dendritic cells. *J. Immunol.* **164**:4843–4852.

Sieling, P. A., D. Chatterjee, S. A. Porcelli, T. I. Prigozy, R. J. Mazzaccaro, T. Soriano, B. R. Bloom, M. B. Brenner, M. Kronenberg, P. J. Brennan, and R. L. Modlin. 1995. CD1-restricted T cell recognition of microbial lipoglycan antigens. *Science* **269**:227–230.

Snewin, V., G. Stewart, and D. Young. 2000. Genetic strategies for vaccine development, p. 279–296. *In* G. F. Hatfull and W. R. Jacobs, Jr. (ed.), *Molecular Genetics of Mycobacteria.* American Society for Microbiology, Washington, D.C.

Sorensen, A. L., S. Nagai, G. Houen, P. Andersen, and A. B. Andersen. 1995. Purification and characterization of a low-molecular-mass T-cell antigen secreted by *Mycobacterium tuberculosis. Infect. Immun.* **63**:1710–1717.

Sousa, A. O., R. J. Mazzaccaro, R. G. Russell, F. K. Lee, O. C. Turner, S. Hong, L. Van Kaer, and B. R. Bloom. 2000. Relative contributions of distinct MHC class I-dependent cell populations in protection to tuberculosis infection in mice. *Proc. Natl. Acad. Sci. USA* **97**:4204–4208.

Sreevatsan, S., X. Pan, K. E. Stockbauer, N. D. Connell, B. N. Kreiswirth, T. S. Whittam, and J. M. Musser. 1997. Restricted structural gene polymorphism in the *Mycobacterium tuberculosis* complex indicates evolutionarily recent global dissemination. *Proc. Natl. Acad. Sci. USA* **94**:9869–9874.

Stanford, J. L., G. A. Rook, G. M. Bahr, Y. Dowlati, R. Ganapati, K. Ghazi Saidi, S. Lucas, G. Ramu, P. Torres, H. Minh Ly, and N. Anstey. 1990. *Mycobacterium vaccae* in immunoprophylaxis and immunotherapy of leprosy and tuberculosis. *Vaccine* **8**:525–530.

Stenger, S., R. J. Mazzaccaro, K. Uyemura, S. Cho, P. F. Barnes, J. P. Rosat, A. Sette, M. B. Brenner, S. A. Porcelli, B. R. Bloom, and R. L. Modlin. 1997. Differential effects of cytolytic T cell subsets on intracellular infection. *Science* **276**:1684–1687.

Sugita, M., E. P. Grant, E. van Donselaar, V. W. Hsu, R. A. Rogers, P. J. Peters, and M. B. Brenner. 1999. Separate pathways for antigen presentation by CD1 molecules. *Immunity* **11**:743–752.

Tascon, R. E., M. J. Colston, S. Ragno, E. Stavropoulos, D. Gregory, and D. B. Lowrie. 1996. Vaccination against tuberculosis by DNA injection. *Nat. Med.* **2**:888–892.

Tascon, R. E., E. Stavropoulos, K. V. Lukacs, and M. J. Colston. 1998. Protection against *Mycobacterium tuberculosis* infection by CD8$^+$ T cells requires the production of gamma interferon. *Infect. Immun.* **66**:830–834.

Teitelbaum, R., M. Cammer, M. L. Maitland, N. E. Freitag, J. Condeelis, and B. R. Bloom. 1999. Mycobacterial infection of macrophages results in membrane-permeable phagosomes. *Proc. Natl. Acad. Sci. USA* **96**:15190–15195.

Teitelbaum, R., A. Glatman-Freedman, B. Chen, J. B. Robbins, E. Unanue, A. Casadevall, and B. R. Bloom. 1998. A mAb recognizing a surface antigen of *Mycobacterium tuberculosis* enhances host survival. *Proc. Natl. Acad. Sci. USA* **95:**15688–15693.

Tramontana, J. M., U. Utaipat, A. Molloy, P. Akarasewi, M. Burroughs, S. Makonkawkeyoon, B. Johnson, J. D. Klausner, W. Rom, and G. Kaplan. 1995. Thalidomide treatment reduces tumor necrosis factor alpha production and enhances weight gain in patients with pulmonary tuberculosis. *Mol. Med.* **1:**384–397.

Turner, O. C., A. D. Roberts, A. A. Frank, S. W. Phalen, D. M. McMurray, J. Content, O. Denis, S. D'Souza, A. Tanghe, K. Huygen, and I. M. Orme. 2000. Lack of protection in mice and necrotizing pneumonia with bronchiolitis in guinea pigs immu-

nized with vaccines directed against the hsp60 molecule of *Mycobacterium tuberculosis. Infect. Immun.* **68:**3674–3679.

Wallace, J. G. 1961. The heat resistance of tubercle in the lungs of infected mice. *Am. Rev. Respir. Dis.* **83:**866–871.

Watts, C. 1997. Capture and processing of exogenous antigens for presentation on MHC molecules. *Annu. Rev. Immunol.* **15:**821–850.

Wilson, M., J. DeRisi, H. H. Kristensen, P. Imboden, S. Rane, P. O. Brown, and G. K. Schoolnik. 1999. Exploring drug-induced alterations in gene expression in *Mycobacterium tuberculosis* by microarray hybridization. *Proc. Natl. Acad. Sci. USA* **96:**12833–12838.

Immunology of Infectious Diseases
Edited by S. H. E. Kaufmann, A. Sher, and R. Ahmed
© 2002 ASM Press, Washington, D.C.

Chapter 30

Immune Intervention in AIDS

GUIDO SILVESTRI AND MARK B. FEINBERG

INTRODUCTION

General Concepts

AIDS was first recognized in 1981 as an unprecedented constellation of opportunistic infections appearing in individuals with no known predisposition for immune system dysfunction (Durack, 1981). From the earliest reports, it was appreciated that the central feature of AIDS was a progressive and ultimately profound depletion of the CD4$^+$ T-lymphocyte populations, which play essential regulatory roles in enabling diverse immune effector functions (Fauci, 1988). The etiologic agents of AIDS, retroviruses known as human immunodeficiency virus types 1 and 2 (HIV-1 and HIV-2), originated in chimpanzees (*Pan troglodytes*) and sooty mangabey monkeys (*Cercocebus atys*), respectively (Gao et al., 1999; Hahn et al., 2000). Both HIV-1 and HIV-2 infections can lead to AIDS, although HIV-1 does so more rapidly and more reproducibly and now represents the most prevalent cause of AIDS worldwide (Hahn et al., 2000). Although AIDS was originally rare, unexpected, and puzzling, our appreciation of its complexities and impact has grown tremendously over the last 20 years. Whereas it was once an unexplained acquired immune deficiency represented by only a handful of cases of *Pneumocystis carinii* pneumonia and aggressive Kaposi's sarcoma, it is now known to be the greatest pandemic of modern times. An estimated 36 million individuals are currently infected worldwide, and the spread of HIV infection continues at an alarming rate, with over 16,000 new infections occurring each day (UNAIDS, 2000). HIV causes a persistent infection that, once established, cannot be cleared by host immune responses and that also appears to be refractory to clearance by seemingly potent antiviral

therapies. Although the time between initial HIV infection and progression to AIDS averages between 7 and 10 years, it is estimated that in the absence of effective therapy, HIV-1 infection will result in progressive immune deficiency, AIDS, and death in 98% or more of all infected individuals (Collaborative Group, 2000). As such, it is likely to be one of the most virulent virus infections affecting human populations. While substantial uncertainties remain about key aspects of the pathogenesis of AIDS, more is now known about the virology and immunology of HIV infection than about any other viral disease of humans. In the 20 years since the first descriptions of AIDS, the etiologic agent has been identified and its genetic composition has been characterized in great detail (Frankel and Young, 1998). The nature of the constituent proteins of HIV has been described, and three-dimensional crystal structures for most of these proteins have been solved (Frankel and Young, 1998). Fundamental aspects of the HIV replication cycle have been elucidated, and important insights into the complex ways in which the virus interacts with host target cells have been gained (Cohen et al., 1997). The natural history of HIV disease has been defined in substantial detail, and effective antiviral therapies have been developed that enable infected individuals to live longer and healthier lives. However, despite this impressive degree of progress, there remains a tremendous need for the development of new therapeutic interventions to ameliorate HIV disease. Since AIDS is fundamentally a disease of the immune system, substantial interest has been aroused by the possibility of manipulation of host immune responses to HIV infection as a way of delaying, preventing, or reversing the immune system damage that follows HIV infection. This chapter will review concepts and strategies that are being consid-

Guido Silvestri and Mark B. Feinberg • Departments of Medicine and of Microbiology and Immunology, Emory University School of Medicine and Emory Vaccine Research Center, Atlanta, GA 30329.

ered for the development of effective immune interventions for the treatment of HIV disease (Table 1).

Infection with HIV typically leads to progressive depletion of CD4$^+$ T lymphocytes from peripheral blood and lymphoid organs, ultimately resulting in a state of profound immunodeficiency characterized by susceptibility to a wide variety of (but, interestingly, not all) types of opportunistic infections and neoplasms (Fauci, 1988). The same CD4 cell surface molecule that plays an essential role in helper/inducer T-cell antigen recognition, through interactions with major histocompatibility complex (MHC) class II molecules on antigen-presenting cells, also serves as the initial cell surface protein that interacts with the HIV envelope surface glycoprotein gp120 (Dalgleish et al., 1984). As such, HIV infection is targeted to cell populations that express CD4 on their cell surfaces, including helper/inducer T cells and macrophages. In addition to their expression of the CD4 cell surface protein, HIV infection is focused to CD4$^+$ T cells and macrophages by virtue of their expression of specific chemokine receptors (CCR5 and CXCR4) that serve as essential coreceptors for HIV entry into target cells (Moore et al., 1997; Berger et al., 1999). The susceptibility of target cells to HIV infection and the amount of virus they produce following infection are also enhanced by activation of CD4$^+$ T cells, an effect that is operative at multiple levels including activation of coreceptor expression, enhanced efficiency of the process of reverse transcription, increased facility of nuclear transport of newly reverse-transcribed HIV genomes, and augmented NF-κB-mediated transcriptional activity of

Table 1. Mechanisms of immune evasion by HIV

1. Inherently high error rate of the HIV reverse transcriptase and great predisposition for genetic recombination, collectively leading to continuous generation of viral variants that can escape host immune responses

2. Early deletion of activated HIV-specific CD4$^+$ T cells as preferential targets of HIV replication, leading to loss of virus-specific CD4$^+$ T-cell help and potentially predisposing to compromised virus-specific CD8$^+$ T-cell responses through deletion or anergy

3. Ability of HIV to establish an "immunologically invisible" state of latency in resting CD4$^+$ T cells wherein the provirus is maintained but not expressed

4. Down modulation of HLA class I molecules by the HIV *nef* gene product, potentially compromising the ability of infected cells to be recognized and killed by anti-HIV CTLs

5. Conformational structure and extensive glycosylation of the HIV gp120 surface envelope protein leading to limited ability of the host antibody response to neutralize HIV infectivity

integrated HIV proviruses (Stevenson et al., 1995). It is not known why CD4 was "chosen" as the primary virus receptor in the course of evolution of the progenitors of HIV in the original nonhuman primate hosts for the infection. However, this evolutionary choice has determined that HIV infection will lead to immune system pathology rather than some other type of disease. While it is well established that the primary target cells for HIV infection in vivo are CD4$^+$ T cells and that AIDS is ultimately a syndrome of CD4$^+$ T-cell deficiency, it is still not completely understood how HIV infection induces the progressive failure of the immune system seen in AIDS patients. Three major areas of controversy now exist regarding the immunopathogenesis of HIV disease: (i) the relative importance of directly HIV-mediated killing of CD4$^+$ T cells versus the loss of uninfected CD4$^+$ T cells due to indirect "bystander" effects resulting from the generalized state of aberrant immune system activation seen in HIV-infected individuals; (ii) the relative contribution of HIV-induced peripheral destruction of CD4$^+$ T cells versus compromise of the proper regenerative capacity of the CD4$^+$ T-cell compartment; and (iii) the beneficial and/or potentially detrimental effects of the different arms of the anti-HIV immune response in determining the ultimate clinical outcome of HIV infection (Fig. 1).

It is likely that the development of effective immune-based interventions for the treatment of HIV infection will be greatly facilitated by an improved understanding of the fundamental mechanisms of the immunopathogenesis of AIDS. However, it is also likely that well-designed studies of immune interventions can be used to probe and thereby elucidate key host-virus interactions that underlie the processes governing the numerical and functional compromise of CD4$^+$ T-cell populations seen in HIV-infected persons. In both respects, immune interventions for AIDS therapy are at a very preliminary stage of development; nonetheless, this area of research offers substantial promise for future progress.

Is Direct HIV-Mediated Killing of CD4$^+$ T Cells Sufficient To Explain AIDS?

In HIV-infected individuals, the level of viremia is directly associated with rates of CD4$^+$ T-cell decline and clinical progression to AIDS and death (Mellors et al., 1997). Virus replication is most readily and most accurately assessed by quantitative determination of levels of HIV genomic RNA present in virus particles in the plasma fraction of a peripheral blood specimen (so-called virus load assays)

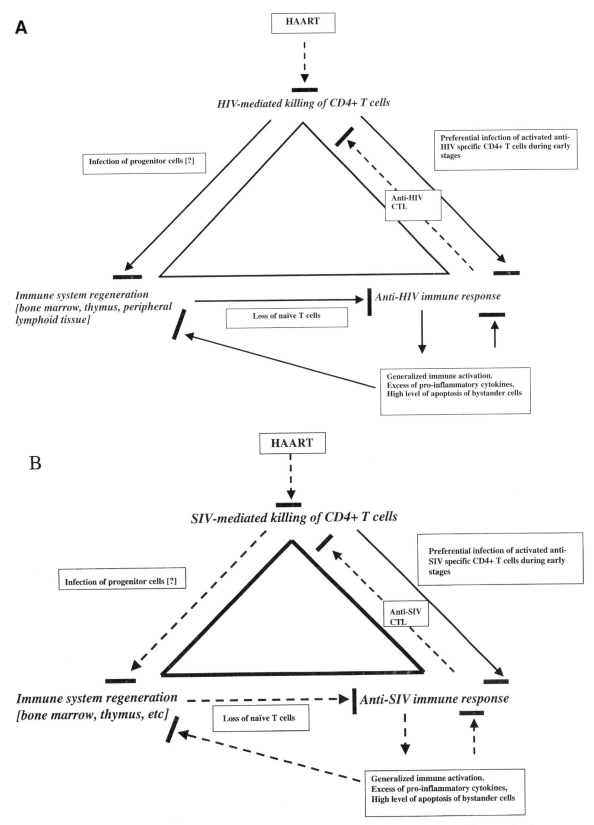

Figure 1. Immunopathogenesis of HIV infection (A) in humans and SIV infection (B) in a natural host species (sooty mangabeys). Straight lines represent specific pathogenic mechanisms contributing to disease progression in chronically infected individuals. Dotted-bar lines represent physiologic (CTL) or therapeutic (HAART) events opposing the progression of the infection toward chronic immunodeficiency and AIDS. Dotted lines in panel B represent immunopathologic mechanisms of disease that are absent in the nonpathogenic chronic SIV infection of sooty mangabeys.

(Saag et al., 1996). Within 6 to 12 months of initial HIV infection, virus replication as measured by plasma HIV RNA levels often stabilizes around a so-called steady-state set point (Daar et al., 1991; Clark et al., 1991; Pontesilli et al., 1997). While terms such as "steady-state set point" imply a rather static process of HIV infection, important studies that measured the turnover rates of virus in circulation and the longevity of HIV-infected cells indicate that, on the contrary, HIV infection in vivo is a remarkably dynamic process (Wei et al., 1995; Ho et al., 1995). In particular, infected cells appear to turn over with a half-life of ~1.25 days, probably the result of direct cytopathic effects of HIV infection and within a time frame only slightly longer than the single cycle of HIV infection in a target cell (Wei et al., 1995; Ho et al., 1995; Perelson et al., 1996). Approximately 99% of the virus found in the plasma of infected individuals is estimated to have been produced from cells that were infected within the past 1 to 2 days, indicating that HIV infection in vivo is sustained by an active process of de novo infection of susceptible target cells (Wei et al., 1995; Ho et al., 1995). Drugs that inhibit HIV replication can block new rounds of virus replication and thereby spare previously uninfected cells from virus infection and destruction. As a result, the use of potent antiretroviral therapies is associated with major immunological and virological effects, including increases in CD4$^+$ T-cell counts and a substantial decline in virus replication, which are often followed by substantial laboratory evidence of immunologic recovery and, most importantly, by clinical improvement and improved survival rates (Powderly et al., 1998).

Set point levels of virus replication can vary substantially between different individuals, and values that are established early in infection are highly predictive of subsequent rates of HIV disease progression (Mellors et al., 1997). The determinants of viral load set points are incompletely understood at present. HIV-specific CD4 and CD8 T-cell response levels are reported to be inversely correlated with virus replication levels, suggesting that efficacy of the host immune response is an important variable (Walker et al., 1998). However, precise definition of the role of the cellular immune responses in the determination of ongoing set-point levels of HIV replication has been complicated by both technical and biological issues. For example, the extent to which the reported inverse association between specific cellular immune responses and relative containment of viremia is the cause or consequence of the observed immune system preservation is unknown. Furthermore, the use of different assay methods to quantitate HIV-specific CD4$^+$ and CD8$^+$ T-cell responses has led to apparently conflicting results for the relationship between specific cellular responses and in vivo control of HIV replication. While assessment of HIV-specific CD4$^+$ T-cell responses by standard antigen-specific proliferative responses in culture clearly shows an inverse association (Rosenberg et al., 1997), measurement of HIV-specific CD4$^+$ T-cell responses by flow cytometric determination of HIV antigen-induced intracellular cytokine (e.g., gamma interferon) production by CD4$^+$ T cells fails to demonstrate a clear association between cellular responses and viremia in many HIV-infected individuals (Pitcher et al., 1999). More recently, measurement of HIV-specific CD8$^+$ T-cell responses by intracellular cytokine production assays has disclosed high-level HIV-specific CD8$^+$ T-cell responses in patients with chronic low-level viremia as well as in those with high levels of viremia (Gea-Banacloche et al., 2000). Such evidence indicating that different individuals with similar levels of HIV-specific CD8$^+$ T cells assessed by available immune function assays can have substantially different levels of plasma viremia suggests that HIV-specific immune responses may differ in important qualitative and quantitative ways (Gea-Banacloche et al., 2000). If this suggestion is validated in future studies, it would be of substantial theoretical and practical importance. Unfortunately, however, none of the assays available to quantitate HIV-specific cellular immune responses appears able to reveal clearly how such qualitative differences in salutary effector function may determine the ultimate in vivo efficacy of the host cellular immune response.

Of the relevant antiviral cellular immune responses, particular attention has been focused on the CD8$^+$ cytotoxic T-lymphocyte (CTL) responses. The high viremia of primary HIV infection declines with the emergence of the antiviral CTL response, and during the chronic phase of infection, virus replication is inversely related to the host CD8 CTL responses (Ogg et al., 1998; Walker et al., 1998). In experimental models of AIDS, transient depletion of CD8$^+$ T cells in rhesus macaques by using anti-CD8 monoclonal antibodies leads to substantial transient increases in simian immunodeficiency virus (SIV) replication (Schmitz et al., 1999; Jin et al., 1999; Metzner et al., 2000); if this occurs during primary infection, it can result in chronic high-level viremia and accelerated disease progression (Schmitz et al., 1999; Jin et al., 1999; Metzner et al., 2000). However, although important, the antiviral role of HIV-specific CTLs is clearly not sufficient to protect against disease development, since the vast majority of HIV-infected individuals will progress to AIDS within 10 years of the primary infection unless effective antiretroviral therapy is initiated. The persistence of HIV infection despite active anti-HIV CD8 CTL responses is believed to be the cumulative manifestation of a number of simultaneously operative viral strategies for evasion of host immune responses. Mechanisms of virus evasion of host immune responses (Table 2) include immune escape resulting from the constantly evolving genetic diversity of HIV populations present in infected persons; the conformation of the gp120 surface envelope protein, which makes virus infection refractory to neutralization by the host antibody response; down modulation of class I HLA molecules by the viral *nef* gene product; and the ability of HIV to establish an immunologically "invisible" latent state of infection in target cells (reviewed by Kamp et al. [2000]). Furthermore, since HIV infection is known to be facilitated by immune activation of CD4$^+$ T-cell targets, HIV-specific CD4$^+$ T cells may be preferentially infected and lost. Indeed, HIV-specific CD4$^+$ T-cell responses appear to be lost early in the course of HIV infection. Importantly, while initiation of highly active antiretroviral therapy (HAART) during the first weeks of primary HIV infection appears able to protect HIV-specific CD4$^+$ T-cell responses from being acutely deleted or anergized, these responses do not return once HAART is initiated during the chronic phase of the infection (Rosenberg et al., 1997; Oxenius et al., 2000). Since CD4$^+$ T cells play critical roles in the induction and maintenance of CD8$^+$ T-cell responses, loss of HIV-specific CD4$^+$ T-cell responses may limit the magnitude and duration of effective HIV-specific CTL responses through the induction of clonal deletion or anergy of HIV-specific CD8$^+$ T-cell populations (Kalams and Walker, 1998; Zajac et al., 1998). Thus, the "classical" model of the immunopathogenesis of AIDS is summarized by the vicious cycle between HIV replication, loss of helper CD4$^+$ T cells, decline of CTL responses, further increases of HIV replication, accelerated destruction of CD4$^+$ T-cell populations, and so on.

Although the direct cytopathic effect of HIV is a well-established phenomenon, the classical model of AIDS pathogenesis has been challenged by a large body of evidence indicating that HIV infection is also associated with major losses of uninfected T lymphocytes of both the CD4$^+$ and CD8$^+$ T-cell lineages (Haase, 1999). Losses of uninfected CD4$^+$ and CD8$^+$ T cells are thought to result primarily from abnormally prevalent activation-induced programmed cell death (apoptosis), which in turn appears to be associated with chronic high levels of host immune activation (Badley et al., 2000). According to recent estimates, more uninfected CD4$^+$ T cells die of apoptosis in HIV-infected persons than are lost due to the direct cytopathic effects of virus infection (Haase, 1999). Perhaps not surprisingly, elevated levels of immune activation and lymphocyte apoptosis are associated with increased risk of disease progression (Gougeon et al., 1996). Other potential pathogenic consequences of the chronic immune activation extant in HIV-infected individuals include perturbations of the function of key lymphoid organs such as the bone marrow, thymus, and lymph nodes (see below), all of which potentially contribute to the overall immune dysfunction of AIDS patients. Thus, HIV-mediated disease is not simply the result of viral factors alone but, rather, results from a complex balance between direct impact of the virus infection and the host response to infection. This conclusion supports the concept that manipulation of host factors, if they can be developed, might be of substantial potential benefit to the clinical management of HIV-infected individuals.

Is AIDS a "Lympholytic" Disease, a "Lymphoaplastic" Disease, or Both?

As mentioned above, a highly controversial issue in AIDS pathogenesis is the extent to which CD4 depletion is the result of an increased rate of lymphocyte destruction or a decreased rate of lymphocyte production. The observation that HIV viremia is maintained by continuous rounds of viral infection and destruction of virus-infected cells led to the formulation of a model in which active HIV replication induces CD4$^+$ T-cell destruction at a very high rate ($>10^9$ cells/day), resulting in the exhaustion of the host capacity for lymphocyte regeneration and, ultimately, in the collapse of the immune system (Ho et al., 1995; Wei et al., 1995; Perelson et al., 1996). In

Table 2. Immune interventions in HIV-infected individuals

1. Enhancement of the anti-HIV immune responses
   - Therapeutic vaccination (recombinant Env proteins, inactivated virus preparation, DNA vaccines, viral vectors)
   - Structured treatment interruptions (STI)

2. Adoptive transfer of CTLs, with or without prior genetic manipulation

3. Cytokine-based interventions
   - IL-2
   - Others (IL-12, CD40L + IL12, IL-7, GM-CSF, IFNs)

4. Expansion ex vivo and reinfusion of HIV-resistant (CCR5-negative) CD4$^+$ cells

5. Immunosuppressive agents
   - Cyclosporin A
   - Others (steroids, pentoxyphilline, thalidomide, and mycophenolate)

contrast, others have suggested that CD4⁺ T-cell depletion results primarily from the inability of the infected host to replace CD4⁺ T cells lost to virus infection rather than from excess CD4⁺ T-cell destruction alone (Hellerstein et al., 1999). In this latter model, a key factor would be the extent of direct or indirect HIV-induced interference with the proper generative function of bone marrow, thymus, and peripheral sites of lymphocyte proliferation and differentiation. Destruction of proper lymph node structures during the course of HIV infection, as well as the prevailing increased propensity for lymphocyte apoptosis, may lead to progressive compromise of peripheral T-cell expansion (Pantaleo and Fauci, 1995; Haase, 1999). Progressively severe suppression of bone marrow function, resulting in neutropenia, thrombocytopenia, and total lymphopenia, may contribute to the exhaustion of the CD4⁺ T-cell regenerative capacity by limiting the production of prethymic T-lymphocyte progenitors (Moses et al., 1998). Observed decreases in the levels of recent thymic emigrants in HIV-infected humans, as measured by quantitative assessment of T-cell receptor excision circles within CD4 and CD8 T-cell populations, suggest that HIV infection results in either a decreased thymic production of naive T cells or an increased proliferative drain on the pool of naive cells (due to pressure to maintain total T-cell homeostasis and/or due to the prevailing generalized state of immune activation), or both (Douek et al., 1998; Hazenberg et al., 2000). In addition to the compromised production of naive T cells, the regenerative capacity of the mature peripheral T-cell pool, as well as the ability of peripheral T cells to generate effective immune responses, is believed to be impaired as a result of progressive damage to lymph node architecture that accrues with advancing HIV disease. Overall, there is compelling evidence that HIV infection results in a significant compromise of the regenerative capacity of the lymphoid compartment. This conclusion provides the theoretical foundation for immune-based interventions aimed at restoring this regenerative capability. This goal could be pursued either by providing specific cytokines or growth factors or by counterpoising the suppressive effects on bone marrow, thymus, and lymph node function that are the indirect result of excessive, HIV-induced immune activation.

The Good and Bad of Anti-HIV Immune Responses

Among HIV-infected humans, rare individuals have been described who have survived long-term (>20-year) HIV infection without substantial compromise in total CD4 T-cell numbers (long-term nonprogressors [LTNPs]). Studies of such LTNPs, who are believed to represent 2% or less of all infected persons, have demonstrated that they maintain very low chromic viremia and active anti-HIV CD4 and CD8 cellular immune responses (Pantaleo et al., 1995; Cao et al., 1995; Harrer et al., 1996; Rosenberg et al., 1997). In this situation, the lack of disease appears to be correlated with the presence of strong immune responses acting to keep HIV replication in check. Unfortunately, in most HIV-infected individuals, the cellular antiviral immune response is unable to achieve adequate control of HIV replication. Furthermore, the maintenance of active but incompletely effective antiviral immune responses also appears to induce a constellation of negative effects through induction of chronic immune activation that may compromise host regenerative functions acting to restore the CD4⁺ T cells lost to the direct cytopathic effects of HIV infection (Cohen et al., 1997). As described above, the level of CD8⁺ T-cell activation in HIV-infected individuals is as strong a predictor of disease progression as is the plasma viral load, and in the late stages of the disease it is even more predictive of subsequent immune deterioration than is the plasma viral load (Giorgi et al., 1999). On initiation of HAART, ongoing virus replication falls precipitously, but so do the HIV-specific cellular immune responses, and the generalized state of host immune activation similarly resolves. Thus, it seems that both the antigen-specific immune responses and the attendant generalized immune activation are driven by ongoing virus replication that is being actively chased but never adequately controlled by the host immune responses. While it might be hoped that cellular immune responses would provide an effective adjunct to HAART in facilitating the clearance of the persistent reservoir of HIV infection, the association between falling viremia and decreasing host immune responses probably limits any beneficial role that immune responses might play in accomplishing this goal. Coincident with declining viremia and immune activation induced by HAART, CD4 T-cell counts rise in many treated individuals, but they rarely attain normal levels and sometimes hardly increase at all (Powderly et al., 1998). Increased CD4 T-cell counts reflect the cumulative result of a number of beneficial processes including sparing of uninfected CD4⁺ T cells from direct destruction by HIV infection and amelioration of the impairment of lymphocyte regeneration due to lower levels of chronic immune activation (Hellerstein et al., 1999). The extent to which restoration of CD4⁺ T-cell populations is achieved in HAART-treated patients varies substantially among individuals and probably depends on a number of important variables including the degree of virus suppression, the residual structural and functional integrity of essential immune regenerative compartments, and the extent to which damage inflicted by untreated HIV infection can be reversed.

Interestingly, the nonhuman primate species that are natural hosts of SIV do not develop AIDS despite high chronic virus replication and limited host antiviral cellular immune responses (Rey-Cuille et al., 1998; G. Silvestri, unpublished data; R. Grant, unpublished data). Thus, the natural host species, which have harbored these viruses for tens of thousands of years or more, seem to have evolved strategies for dealing with chronic infection by a cytopathic virus wherein preservation of health is not dependent on the presence of strong anti-SIV cellular immune responses. A typical example is the nonpathogenic SIV infection in sooty mangabey monkeys, in which near-normal levels of $CD4^+$ T cells are maintained despite high viremia, low CTL activity, and the short in vivo life span of infected $CD4^+$ cells (Silvestri, unpublished; Grant, unpublished). In contrast, in HIV-infected LTNPs, $CD4^+$ T-cell homeostasis appears to be maintained by minimization of HIV replication through strong antiviral CD4 and CD8 responses (Pantaleo et al., 1995; Cao et al., 1995; Harrer et al., 1996; Rosenberg et al., 1997). An additional important feature of the host virus equilibrium in LTNPs is their ability to effectively control HIV replication without showing substantially increased generalized immune activation and lymphocyte apoptosis (Pantaleo et al., 1995; Cao et al., 1995; Harrer et al., 1996; Rosenberg et al., 1997). In marked contrast, $CD4^+$ T-cell populations in SIV-infected sooty mangabeys appear to be maintained by a preserved regenerative capacity of the immune system and the lack of negative effects related to the immune activation (Fig. 2). Thus, it appears that lentivirus infection can be tolerated successfully by the host when a very strong, focused, and effective immune response leads to effective control of virus replication. Alternatively, immunologic "ignorance" of the infection and the consequent diminution of the processes leading to indirect loss of uninfected lymphocytes and preservation of compensatory mechanisms for $CD4^+$ T-cell generation allow the host to readily replace the cells killed by the direct cytopathic consequences of virus infection. Between these two extremes are found active but incompletely effective cellular immune responses that fail to substantially contain virus replication and create a milieu in which the host antiviral immune responses, through inadvertent induction of substantial bystander damage wherein uninfected cells are destroyed and host immune regenerative mechanisms are impaired, are in-

effective. In such circumstances, the host antiviral immune response may ultimately prove to be more destructive than protective. Models of HIV disease that envision the immunopathologic consequences of the host antiviral response have been championed by Zinkernagel and colleagues and have been developed by analogy to lymphocytic choriomeningitis virus infection of mice (Zinkernagel and Hengartner, 1994). Lymphocytic choriomeningitis virus is a noncytopathic virus that causes disease only when active virus replication occurs in the setting of chronic but incompletely effective cellular antiviral immune responses. In contrast, HIV, being a cytopathic virus, results in infections where $CD4^+$ T-cell depletion is the cumulative result of both the direct cytopathic consequences of infection and the indirect immunopathologic consequences of the host response. In this circumstance, immune-based interventions can be envisioned in two distinct ways. On the one hand, it may be beneficial to augment the magnitude and effectiveness of the cellular antiviral immune response so that it is possible to achieve more potent and durable control of HIV replication. Alternatively, or in addition, it may be useful to manipulate the system in order to avoid the deleterious indirect effects of active but only partially effective immune responses, through the targeted use of immunosuppression strategies. An important challenge for future research efforts will be to discover ways of modulating the host immune response so its beneficial aspects are enhanced without simultaneously increasing its deleterious aspects. Similarly, any attempt to use immunosuppression as an approach to abrogation of the deleterious indirect consequences of HIV infection will need to be done in a way that does not also compromise the beneficial aspects of immune-mediated control of HIV replication.

Why Do We Need Immune-Based Therapies for AIDS?

HIV replication can be effectively inhibited by targeting specific phases of the virus life cycle with combinations of potent antiviral drugs. This is commonly achieved in HIV-infected patients with drugs that inhibit essential HIV-specific enzymes, such as the viral reverse transcriptase and protease. A growing number of these compounds have been used in combination to treat HIV-infected patients and have been clearly shown to be efficacious in reducing HIV viremia, increasing CD4 counts, slowing progression to AIDS, and substantially reducing AIDS-associated morbidity and mortality (Powderly et al., 1998). However, available anti-HIV treatment options suffer from important limitations, including (i) the

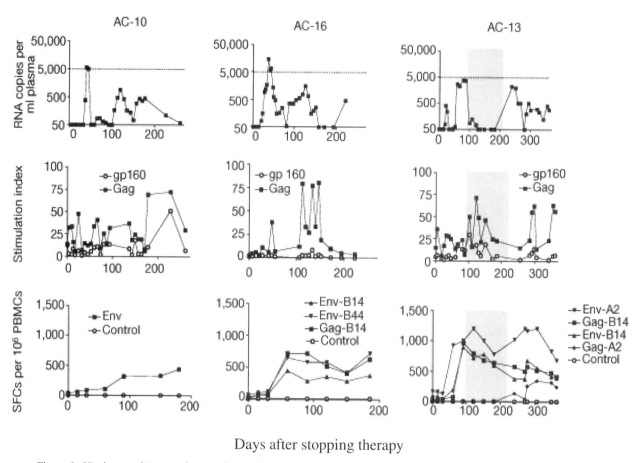

Days after stopping therapy

Figure 2. Virology and immunology in three subjects who controlled viremia after the first treatment interruption. In all three, the plasma viral load rose but then dropped, remaining consistently below 5,000 copies of HIV-1 RNA per ml (top row). Gag-specific T-helper-cell responses were maintained in all three subjects (middle row). CTL responses increased significantly from baseline values and are shown as responses to individual CTL epitopes with HLA restriction (bottom row). CTL responses were confirmed by cloning and testing in cytolytic assays. The shaded area indicates antiviral therapy reinitiated for subject 3, despite not meeting protocol indication for retreatment. Reprinted from Rosenberg et al. (2000) with permission of the publisher.

emergence of multi-drug-resistant HIV strains as a result of past unsuccessful treatment or poor adherence to the complicated antiretroviral treatment regimens and the increasing evidence of transmission of drug-resistant HIV variants to newly infected individuals; (ii) the need for long-term, probably lifelong, therapy with both known and unknown drug-related toxicities; and (iii) the high cost of therapy, which makes most of these drugs unaffordable in resource-poor countries where over 95% of all HIV-infected people live (UNAIDS, 2000).

In addition to the numerous practical challenges confronting the use of HAART in clinical practice, there are important biologic issues that limit its ultimate success. First, although HAART is able to decrease HIV replication to below the detection limits of sensitive plasma HIV RNA assays (<50 copies/ml), recent evidence indicates that ongoing virus replication is not completely inhibited. It is not yet

known whether replication during HAART is the result of anatomic sanctuaries where antiviral drugs do not adequately penetrate, of activation of HIV expression from latently infected cells, or of the difficulty in inhibiting the transmission of HIV between cells in close proximity (Grossman et al., 1999). Second, the availability of potent antiretroviral drugs has focused attention on the reservoir of latently infected CD4$^+$ cells that could not be cleared by antiviral drugs or by otherwise effective immune responses (Pierson et al., 1998). Recent estimates suggest that the turnover of the reservoir of latently infected CD4$^+$ T cells is so slow as to make ultimate pharmacologic eradication of the infection implausible (Finzi et al., 1999). However, the recognition that HIV replication continues at low level even in individuals effectively treated with HAART makes interpretation of the estimates of the latent reservoir problematic, since it is not possible to distinguish between long-lived latently infected cells and cells that were recently infected as a result of ongoing low-level virus production. As such, it remains to be seen whether new pharmacologic or immunologic strategies might be derived that could accelerate the clearance of HIV-infected cells and, hopefully, lead to eventual eradication of the infection.

Furthermore, it is still unclear to what extent the immune reconstitution induced by anti-HIV drug regimens is associated with an actual recovery of the overall immune function in patients who have previously experienced a major CD4$^+$ T-cell depletion (Connors et al., 1997). Even in the most desirable scenario, wherein complete suppression of HIV replication and numerical recovery of CD4$^+$ T-cell counts to near-normal levels is achieved, interventions that facilitate healing an injured or perhaps just "scarred" CD4 T-cell repertoire may be beneficial. As a whole, these considerations suggest that immune-based intervention strategies may provide important innovations for optimizing the clinical management of HIV-infected individuals.

IMMUNE INTERVENTION FOR AIDS

General Concepts

Immune interventions for AIDS can be summarized as belonging to one of several categories: (i) interventions designed to enhance the anti-HIV immune responses to achieve better control of virus replication; (ii) interventions designed to numerically and functionally restore CD4$^+$ T-cell populations; (iii) interventions designed to make CD4$^+$ T cells resistant to HIV infection; and (iv) interventions designed to suppress the deleterious effects of the HIV-induced generalized immune activation.

Enhancing the Anti-HIV Immune Response

Evidence that HIV-specific immune responses play important roles in determining the set-point levels of HIV replication and that these immune responses are impaired in most HIV-infected patients provides a strong rationale for interventions aimed at increasing antiviral immunity in HIV-infected persons. However, the extent to which HIV-specific immune responses can be restored or newly engendered in individuals chronically infected with HIV is not clear. Studies of patients undergoing HAART have suggested that the overall recovery of the immune function, especially in the CD4$^+$ T-helper cell compartment, that follows viremia-induced suppression is less effective in restoring T-helper responses to

HIV antigens (Komanduri et al., 1998; Appay et al., 2000) than to antigens directed towards other pathogens (e.g., cytomegalovirus). The most likely explanation for this phenomenon is that because of their activation state, many HIV-specific CD4$^+$ T-helper cells may be preferentially targeted for virus replication and consequently killed early in the course of an infection. Nonetheless, the observation that naive T-cell numbers can also be increased to various degrees after initiation of HAART suggests that new HIV-specific CD4$^+$ T-cell clones might be generated de novo in individuals with a history of longer-term HIV infection (Silvestri et al., 1998; Hengel et al., 1999; Douek et al., 1998; McCune et al., 2000). These observations underscore the importance of HAART and/or more direct immune interventions during acute HIV infection as important tools to avoid the early deletion of HIV-specific CD4$^+$ T cells and therefore to more effectively preserve anti-HIV T-helper responses (Rosenberg et al., 1997; Oxenius et al., 2000; Malhotra et al., 2000).

The anti-HIV immune response could theoretically be enhanced in HIV-infected persons by two types of strategies: those based on the administration of HIV antigens to accomplish so-called therapeutic vaccination (such as recombinant or natural proteins, and DNA vaccines or recombinant expression vectors that encode HIV antigens) and those based on direct manipulation of one or more components of the host immune system.

Therapeutic vaccination

The idea of therapeutic vaccination of HIV-infected individuals dates back to the early years of the AIDS epidemic, and clinical trials aimed at augmenting anti-HIV cellular immune responses in infected patients by immunization with the recombinant HIV envelope glycoproteins gp120 and gp160 were first performed in the early 1990s (Redfield et al., 1991). These early trials were predicated on the belief that neutralizing-antibody responses might play an important role in controlling the magnitude of HIV replication in vivo—a tenet that is now believed to be inaccurate. Despite some promising preliminary unpublished reports, these trials failed to demonstrate any clinical benefit in the management of HIV-infection (Birx et al., 2000; Goebel et al., 1999; Lambert et al., 1998; Sandstrom and Wahren, 1999; Tsoukas et al., 1998; Wright et al., 1999; reviewed by Peters [2000]). It is likely that several important factors were responsible for these failures. First, all of these early trials were performed in the pre-HAART era, and it is therefore likely that immune responses would be attenuated in the face of untreated HIV replication (Fogelman et al., 2000). In the event that antigen-specific immune responses could be elicited by vaccination in this setting, it is likely that antigen-specific CD4$^+$ T cells activated in response to immunization would be preferentially targeted for HIV infection and deletion. Second, in the absence of effective containment of virus replication, the vast majority of viral antigens present in an infected host would be those produced endogenously by HIV-infected cells, and the amount of antigen presented to the immune system in the form of the therapeutic vaccine would quantitatively pale in comparison. Third, the immunogens used were composed of recombinant proteins whose structures did not recapitulate, let alone improve upon, those of the naturally occurring HIV proteins. Even if they had presented more natural conformations, it is known that the native HIV envelope protein is a poor immunogen for raising potent and broadly reactive neutralizing antibodies (Wyatt and Sodroski, 1998). Given all of these considerations, it is in retrospect not surprising that the clinical trials conducted to date using various recombinant HIV *env* proteins have been notably unsuccessful (Birx et al., 2000; Goebel et al., 1999; Lambert et al., 1998; Peters, 2000; Sandstrom and Wahren, 1999; Tsoukas et al., 1998; Wright et al., 1999).

In a related approach originally championed by Jonas Salk, therapeutic immunization studies have involved preparations of inactivated whole-virus particles (formulated in incomplete Freund's adjuvant) (Remune) prepared from an HIV isolate from Zaire, which are relatively depleted of *env* proteins during the course of purification (Moss et al., 1998). Early studies of this approach were performed before effective combination antiretroviral therapies were available, and they showed inconsistent effects on surrogate markers and no evidence for reduction in plasma HIV RNA levels (Churdboonkart et al., 1998). More recently, this immunogen was studied in a large placebo-controlled trial involving HIV-infected patients whose CD4$^+$ T-cell counts were between 300 and 549/mm^3 and who were receiving stable or no concomitant antiretroviral therapy. The study participants were immunized every 12 weeks for a total of 13 immunizations. Patients receiving the active vaccine appeared to have increased HIV-specific T-helper responses to the specific immunogen administered compared to those receiving the placebo. However, no clinical benefit in terms of HIV RNA levels, CD4 percentages, or HIV progression-free survival was observed relative to results achieved by antiretroviral therapy alone (Kahn et al., 2000; F. T. Valentine, V. DeGruttola,

and the Rumune 816 Study Team, *6th Conf. Retroviruses Opportunistic Infect.*, abstr. 346, 1999).

The negative trial results obtained to date using recombinant viral proteins or inactivated virion preparations may reflect the nature of the specific immunogens used. However, most if not all therapeutic vaccination studies conducted with HIV-infected patients and immunogens consisting of recombinant or natural (e.g., virion-derived) HIV proteins will probably suffer from a number of inherent limitations. First, while these immunogens might be able to elicit CD4$^+$ and humoral immune responses via MHC class II pathways of antigen presentation, they are not expected to raise strong HIV-specific CD8 T-cell responses, which require processing and presentation through MHC class I pathways. Second, unless the immunogen used has particularly favorable or unique antigenic properties that distinguish it from the endogenously produced HIV proteins, it is unclear how it can be expected to beneficially augment host antiviral immune responses.

Therapeutic vaccines based on DNA vaccines and recombinant viral vectors that encode HIV antigens could provide a more effective way to elicit HIV-specific CD4 and CD8 cellular immune responses in HIV-infected patients. Given the increasing recognition of the importance of CD4 and CD8 T-cell responses in controlling HIV infection, elicitation of high-level cellular antiviral immune responses is an important goal for future therapeutic-vaccination strategies. To date, the results of a number of uncontrolled clinical trials of therapeutic vaccination regimens employing DNA vaccines that express HIV antigens to immunize HIV-infected patients have been reported (reviewed by Fomsgaard [1999]). In all trials reported to date, DNA vaccines have been safe and well tolerated. However, the magnitude of the immune responses raised in HIV-infected persons by DNA vaccines alone has been disappointing so far, whether or not HAART was used concurrently. Wahren and colleagues studied immunization of a small number of patients with DNA constructs expressing HIV Tat, Rev, and Nef proteins (Calarota et al., 1998, 1999) and reported some increase in proliferative responses to and CTL reactivity with the inserted antigens when the patients were also treated with HAART. Weiner and colleagues have used DNA vaccines that express Env and Rev (MacGregor et al., 1998; Boyer et al., 1999) and reported CTL responses to the encoded Env in a small percentage of treated patients, some of whom also had evidence of CTL activity prior to immunization. A number of studies are now investigating attenuated recombinant poxvirus vectors (primarily the avipoxvirus vector ALVAC-HIV-vCP1452, which expresses envelope, Gag, Pol, and Nef antigens), but no results have yet been reported. However, given that similar avipoxvirus vectors have demonstrated disappointingly weak immunogenicity even in HIV-uninfected volunteers, it remains to be seen whether sufficiently strong cellular immune responses will be raised in HIV-infected individuals.

Both the initial DNA vectors and the avipoxvirus recombinant viruses used in early studies of therapeutic immunization are substantially less immunogenic than the DNA and recombinant viral expression vectors that are now available. Furthermore, initial studies used single modalities of expression systems for HIV antigens, whereas it has recently been shown that so-called prime-boost approaches raise the highest virus-specific immune responses in uninfected hosts. Recent studies of prophylactic DNA vaccine in macaque models of SIV infection have shown that DNA vaccines, in combination with cytokines (e.g., interleukin-2 [IL-2]) or followed by boosting with recombinant viral vectors (e.g., an attenuated strain of vaccinia virus known as modified vaccinia Ankara), can induce potent anti-HIV CD4$^+$ and CD8$^+$ T-cell responses and enable substantial control of SIV viremia following experimental challenge with virulent virus strains (Barouch et al., 2000; Amara et al., 2001). Analogous, highly immunogenic combinations of DNA vaccines and recombinant viral vectors that express HIV antigens are now being studied in phase I clinical trials in humans. Combination approaches involving vaccination with immunogenic vaccines in the setting of HAART, and potentially used in association with other immune interventions, deserve careful evaluation in the clinical management of HIV-infected patients.

While the development of more immunogenic vaccine modalities will probably be essential before progress can be made in the development of effective therapeutic vaccination approaches, this strategy, at least as currently envisioned, also suffers from important inherent limitations. Specifically, the vaccines to be used will almost always be derived from molecular clones or virus isolates, and these genotypes are thus likely to be quite divergent from the endogenous viral sequences actually present in the infected person. Therefore, even if active vaccination is able to raise appreciable immune responses to the immunogen used, these responses may bear little relevance to the extensively diverse resident HIV quasi-species. As a result, unless substantial cellular immune responses to antigenic determinants that are well conserved among diverse HIV isolates can be raised, vaccine-elicited immune responses will be unlikely to translate into clinical benefit for the immunized patient.

It is likely that clear assessment of the potential benefit of therapeutic immunization strategies must await the availability of more potent and biologically relevant immunogens, as well as the conduct of well-designed and appropriately controlled clinical trials. Fortunately, as described above, substantial recent progress has been reported in the development of novel immunogens and immunization strategies that can raise strong cellular immune responses in preclinical models. Should these new approaches prove equally immunogenic in ongoing phase I clinical trials in healthy HIV-negative volunteers, their evaluation in HIV-infected patients taking HAART will be highly informative. Such studies will help provide direct evidence of how and to what extent a period of untreated HIV replication early in infection can affect an individual's subsequent ability to mount relevant antiviral immune responses following HAART therapy and therapeutic vaccination. Importantly, carefully designed studies using the informative and quantitative immunologic and virologic assays now available result in a clear assessment of the potential immunologic and clinical benefits of this overall approach.

Structured treatment interruptions

Institution of HAART induces suppression of virus replication, increases in CD4 number and function, and declines in the number of circulating HIV-specific CD4$^+$ and CD8$^+$ T cells (Pitcher et al., 1999; Ogg et al., 1999; Mollet et al., 2000). However, our understanding of how HAART actually influences anti-HIV cellular immune responses in vivo is complicated by the fact that measurable anti-HIV responses appear to be dependent on levels of circulating HIV antigens (Ogg et al., 1999). In the majority of HIV-infected patients, interruption of HAART results in a rapid rebound of viral replication and the resurgent virus population typically remains sensitive to the antiviral drugs initially used on reinitiation of therapy. Based on these observations, several investigators have developed HAART protocols in which so-called structured treatment interruptions (STIs) are scheduled with the goal of providing "natural booster" vaccinations of patients with their own virus. Theoretically, this strategy represents a substantial improvement over therapeutic vaccination protocols in which the triggering antigen is genetically distinct from the HIV quasi-species that constitute the reservoir of infection in a given individual.

In an important recent study, HIV-infected patients who were identified during their primary HIV infection syndrome (and prior to seroconversion) were promptly treated with HAART (Rosenberg et al., 2000). Following at least 8 months with undetectable levels of virus in plasma (<50 copies/ml), patients underwent a series of treatment interruptions to assess the levels of viremia reached after withdrawal of drug therapy. HAART was restarted when their plasma HIV RNA levels remained above 5,000 copies/ml on three separate occasions or rose above 50,000 copies on at least one occasion. Interestingly, a number of treated patients achieved apparent immunologic control of HIV replication following such STIs, with an increasing number gaining improved control with additional cycles of STI. Prolonged follow-up of these patients indicated that STIs led to improved anti-HIV immune responses, including preserved CD4$^+$ T-helper responses and augmented CD8$^+$ CTL responses. Thus, it appears that apparently stable containment of HIV replication can be achieved, in at least some patients, who are treated during primary HIV infection and then undergo carefully monitored STIs (Rosenberg et al., 2000). It is important to note that this study was not conducted in a randomized, placebo-controlled fashion, and, indeed, it would probably be difficult if not impossible to do so. However, the proportion of STI-treated patients who attained high-level control of HIV replication in the absence of therapy was substantially higher than would have been expected from available data from large natural history studies. Interestingly, similar studies have been performed with acutely SIV-infected macaques, leading to the observations that HAART plus STIs during acute infection improves antiviral immune responses and enables better control of viremia (Lori et al., 2000; Hel et al., 2000). One such study also suggested that combinations of STIs with administration of an SIV vaccine may be a useful strategy to explore in HIV-infected humans (Lori et al., 2000; Hel et al., 2000). That congruent results have been obtained in both humans and animal models may enable the accelerated development of even more effective treatment strategies and help illuminate the mechanisms by which improved host immune control is achieved by early treatment used in concert with subsequent STIs.

While the work of Rosenberg, Walker, and colleagues had provided provocative evidence that the host-virus equilibrium can be favorably altered in HIV infection by early intervention with HAART therapy during primary infection, only a small percentage of infected individuals are actually diagnosed during this stage of their infections and are thus able to benefit from this treatment approach. The challenge, then, is to see whether host immune responses can also be boosted by some version of STIs during the chronic phase of the infection. Unfortunately, in

a study designed to assess the ability of STIs to boost anti-HIV cellular immune responses in individuals chronically infected with HIV, STIs failed to result in significantly improved HIV-specific cellular immune responses in the 11 HIV-infected patients with a CD4 count of >400 (Carcelain et al., 2001). A number of similar uncontrolled studies of STIs with chronically infected individuals have been conducted, and although some investigators have suggested a modest impact of STIs in this setting (Ruiz et al., 2000), the bulk of the evidence suggested that little if any benefit was obtained. Further, the true impact of STIs in chronic HIV infection will require the conduct of well-designed clinical trials that include appropriate control groups.

Taken as a whole, these results suggest that STI may be a very effective approach to control HIV replication in the relatively rare individuals who are identified during primary infection and treated promptly with HAART. However, STI-based strategies as currently pursued appear to be unlikely to yield any significant immunologic or clinical benefit to the vast majority of HIV-infected individuals, who are diagnosed some substantial time following their primary HIV infection. However, the provocative results obtained in studies where STIs followed the early initiation of antiviral treatment during primary infection suggest that the host-virus equilibrium can be favorably altered through focused virologic and immunologic interventions that are based on our expanding understanding of essential interactions between HIV and the immune system. It is now essential to define the biologic variables that determine why STIs initiated in individuals who were treated with HAART during primary infections appear to work while similar STIs initiated during chronic infection appear to fail. It will also be important to learn more about the immune effector mechanisms responsible for improved host control over virus replication. The window period during which HAART must be instituted to result in any benefit from STIs needs to be established, although preliminary evidence suggests that treatment prior to seroconversion may be necessary. Further, while the transient episodes of virus replication occurring during the periods when treatment is interrupted do not appear to harm the individuals undergoing STIs, it will be important to determine how these replication peaks may influence, and potentially increase, the size of the reservoir of cells latently infected with HIV. Guided by information obtained from such studies, new approaches that include STIs may ultimately be devised that can be of benefit in the treatment of individuals with chronic HIV infection. Progress in this area will probably also depend on the identification of novel immunologic interventions that successfully restore and amplify the host immune responses that are spared by HAART during primary infection but are lost in most infected persons in the transition from acute to chronic HIV infection. Perhaps if STIs are imaginatively performed in association with manipulation of the levels of virus replication with HAART and the use of more potent methods to modulate the host antiviral immune response (such as the administration of specific cytokines, manipulation of relevant costimulatory signals, and expansion and activation of critical dendritic cells), beneficial immune responses might be generated by STIs (or therapeutic vaccinations [see below]) even during chronic HIV infection. Carefully designed clinical trial protocols are necessary to determine whether HIV-specific immune responses can be enhanced and clinical benefit can be realized in individuals chronically infected with HIV.

Adoptive transfer of cytotoxic T lymphocytes

As discussed above, substantial evidence has been presented indicating the importance of host HIV-specific CTL responses in controlling the extent of HIV replication in vivo. As a consequence, numerous therapeutic approaches aimed at increasing the anti-HIV CTL activity have been explored. Development of a strong CTL activity requires a number of factors, including effective antigen presentation, appropriate costimulatory interactions between T cells and antigen-presenting cells, and the provision of a $CD4^+$ T-cell-mediated helper effect, which consists mainly of generation of an appropriate cytokine milieu (Harty et al., 2000). In addition, cytokines such as IL-2, IL-12, gamma interferon (IFN-γ), and IL-15 play important roles in the generation and/or maintenance of high CTL activity. Among costimulatory molecules, CD28 appears to be critical in generating the primary CTL immune response while molecules such as ICOS, a member of the CD28 family of receptors, and 4-1BB and LIGHT, two members of the TNF-R family of receptors, are probably more important for maintaining high levels of CTL activity over time (Whitmire and Ahmed, 2000).

Direct reinfusion of ex vivo-expanded anti-HIV CD8 clones represents the main approach used to date to attempt to increase the levels of anti-HIV CTL responses in vivo. However, this approach has yet to be shown to have clinical benefit. In an early pilot study, a Nef-specific CTL clone was expanded ex vivo with recombinant IL-2 (rIL-2) and then infused into the original patient (Koenig et al., 1995). However, rather than lowering virus replication fol-

lowing CTL infusion, the infusion had the opposite effect and acceleration of disease progression was seen. Given the monospecificity of the clone used and the lack of CD4 T-cell help probably extant in vivo, it is not surprising that this treatment was unsuccessful. However, evidence of immune escape was observed with a proportion (~20%) of viral sequences with altered sequences in the Nef CTL epitope. Given the selection of variant viruses from among the highly diverse quasi-species present in vivo by any monospecific selection pressure, whether immunologic or pharmacologic, these data do support the suggestion that the transfused clone exerted at least some antiviral effect in vivo (Koenig et al., 1995). Greenberg and colleagues have demonstrated the in vivo antiviral effects and clinical benefits of transferred CTL clones in the treatment of cytomegalovirus and Epstein-Barr virus infection arising in individuals with other types of acquired immune deficiency states such as allogeneic bone marrow stem cell transplants (Greenberg and Riddell, 1999). These investigators have extended these studies to include transfer of HIV-specific $CD8^+$ T-cell clones (Brodie, 1999; Brodie, 2000). Modification of HIV-specific clones by retroviral transduction with marker genes (e.g., the *neo* resistance gene) has made it possible for Riddell and colleagues to monitor the fate of antigen-specific CTL clones following reinfusion in vivo (Brodie et al., 1999, 2000). The infusion of 10^9 CTLs/m^2 transiently yielded frequencies of 1 to 40% of peripheral blood $CD8^+$ T cells, but these levels declined precipitously in the ensuing 3 to 4 days. While transiently increased HIV-specific cytolytic activity and transiently decreased numbers of HIV-infected cells in the peripheral blood were observed, no changes were noted in the levels of plasma HIV RNA, which is believed to be the most accurate measure of overall HIV replication in vivo. To broaden the spectrum of antiviral reactivity exerted by this approach to adoptive CTL-based anti-HIV therapy, Lieberman et al. (1997) infused HIV-infected patients with multiple ex vivo-expanded CTL clones. The approach proved to be safe, but only short-term decreases in the number of circulating HIV-infected cells and only transient increases in CD4 counts were observed. Interestingly, as in the studies of Riddell and colleagues, no significant changes in virus replication were observed in this study when assessed by measurements of the plasma HIV RNA level. Thus, it remains to be determined whether any of the reported changes in the levels of HIV-infected cells circulating in the peripheral blood following CTL infusions truly reflect changes in total-body levels of HIV replication or merely the redistribution of specific $CD4^+$ T-cell populations.

The results of the CTL transfer studies conducted to date indicate that one of the major challenges for adoptive immunotherapy approaches using CTL clones is the fate of ex vivo-expanded cells following reinfusion into the patient. According to recent studies, reinfused cells tend to rapidly migrate to lymph nodes (Brodie et al., 2000) where they appear to be able to colocalize with HIV-1-infected cells in tissues and induce a short-term reduction in the number of circulating HIV-infected CD4$^+$ T cells (Brodie et al., 1999). However, the overall in vivo half-life of reinfused CTLs appears to be very short. A recent study by Tan et al. (1999) monitored the fate of reinfused HIV-specific CTLs by HLA class I tetramer staining to identify the infused CTL clone and found that over 90% of HIV antigen-specific cells had undergone apoptosis within 2 days of reinfusion. The short life span of transferred CTL clones in vivo may derive from their withdrawal from the tissue culture conditions used to propagate them or the relative deficiency of appropriate CD4$^+$ T-cell help available in the HIV-infected recipient. In addition to these short-term effects limiting the persistence of transferred CTL clones, Riddell et al. (1996) noted that even HIV-infected individuals can readily mount CTL responses to selectable marker genes (e.g., *neo*) transduced into CTL clones, which probably leads to the accelerated clearance of the infused clones. In addition, in CTL transfer experiments with SCID/Hu mice, it was observed that transfused CTLs could also be lost following encounter with virus-infected cells (McKinney et al., 1999). However, the mechanism of the observed deletion and its relevance to the in vivo circumstance of CTL transfer in humans is unclear (McKinney et al., 1999). Although there are some conceptual problems with this approach, such as the lack of in vivo help, they might be circumvented by simultaneous IL-2 (or other cytokine) administration or the simultaneous infusion of relevant CD4$^+$ T helper cells. However, it is unlikely that adoptive transfer of CTL clones will ever play an important role in the clinical management of HIV-infected patients. The main factors that will probably limit the widespread utility of such adoptive immunotherapy strategies are the rapid emergence of viral escape mutants when effective but monospecific CTLs are transferred (if the CTL clone actually mediates an antiviral effect in vivo) and the substantial practical difficulties involved in applying this method to a large number of HIV-infected patients.

Ex vivo genetic manipulation of CTL

More recently, a novel approach has been pursued to modify ex vivo the antigen specificity of CD8$^+$ T cells so that they recognize HIV-infected target cells regardless of their original T-cell receptor (TCR)-determined capacity for antigen recognition. In this strategy, isolated CD8$^+$ T cells are transduced via ex vivo gene transfer with a genetically engineered chimeric receptor, expanded in vitro, and finally reinfused into HIV-infected individuals from whom the original CD8 T cells were derived (Walker et al., 2000; Mitsuyasu et al., 2000). The chimeric receptor contained the extracellular portion of human CD4 fused with the intracellular signaling domain of CD3 zeta chain. On binding of HIV gp120 (expressed on the surface of an HIV-infected target cell) to CD4, the chimeric receptor (expressed by the genetically modified CTL) would be expected to trigger an effector response that could result in increased anti-HIV CTL activity and production of cytokines such as IFN-γ. The theoretical advantages of this approach include possible broad redirection of the antigenic specificity of many CD8$^+$ T cells toward HIV-infected cells, as well as potential for circumvention of the barriers of HLA restriction. In addition, since the ability to bind CD4 is common to all HIV isolates of otherwise widely diverse genotypes and is a requisite function in the virus life cycle, this strategy would not be expected to be subject to limitations imposed by the genetic diversity of resident HIV quasi-species and would also be less likely to be subject to escape from the effector CTL population through antigenic variation. In the study by Walker et al., syngeneic CD8 T cells from an HIV-uninfected monozygotic twin were transduced in vitro with the CD4/CD3-zeta chain chimeric receptor-encoding retroviral vector and then reinfused into the HIV-infected twin. The same approach was studied by Mitsuyasu et al. (2000), who treated 24 HIV-infected with 2×10^{10} to 3×10^{10} autologous CD4/CD3-zeta-modified CD4$^+$ and CD8$^+$ T cells, administered with or without simultaneous IL-2 infusion. Interestingly, both groups demonstrated that sustained in vivo survival of transduced cells could be achieved, especially when modified CD8$^+$ T cells were reinfused along with similarly modified syngeneic CD4$^+$ T cells and a 2-week ex vivo costimulation with anti-CD3 and anti-CD28 antibodies was performed (Mitsuyasu et al., 2000). Unfortunately, no decrease of HIV plasma viremia was observed in either trial. However, Mitsuyasu et al. (2000) found that modified T cells appeared to be able to traffic to the rectal mucosa, where a decrease in rectal tissue–associated HIV replication was seen; the significance of this decrease remains unclear.

In principle, such modified CD8$^+$ T cells might exert a strong anti-HIV effect in vivo. However, it is not known to what extent the signal transduced through the CD4/CD3-zeta chain receptor recapitulates the physiologic signals transduced by natural T-cell receptor signaling pathways or appropriately activates important immune effector functions. Likewise, since complex and incompletely understood regulatory mechanisms are known to maintain the homeostatic balance of T-cell populations of defined antigenic specificity, it remains to be determined how the population dynamics of such "polyspecific" T cells might be regulated. The possibility of triggering an autoimmune-like reaction on binding of the re-infused cells to the physiologic CD4 ligand (i.e., class II molecules on the surface of B cells, macrophages, etc.) also needs to be considered. Furthermore, it is known that the extracellular domains of CD4 that are included in these chimeric receptors are sufficient to enable HIV infection of target cells that express them (Golding et al., 1993). Thus, the modified CTLs might themselves be potential new targets for HIV infection and therefore might be rapidly lost after in vivo administration in patients with high HIV replication.

Immune enhancement by cytokines

Immune enhancement by cytokines appears to be a more approachable and potentially more broadly applicable strategy. Among the so-called type 1 cytokines, IL-2 has been the most extensively studied in clinical trials (Blankson et al., 2000). Since most of the attention paid to IL-2 as a potential therapy in HIV-infected individuals relates to its function as a CD4$^+$ T-cell growth factor, its role in anti-HIV therapy will be discussed at length in the following section. IL-12, perhaps the most important cytokine for promotion of Th1 differentiation and cellular immune responses, has also been proposed as a potential anti-HIV therapy. Despite some promising preliminary results indicating that IL-12 can increase anti-HIV immune reactivity in vitro (Nagy-Agren and Cooney, 1999; Belyakov et al., 1998; McFarland et al., 1998), r-IL-12 failed to induce clinically relevant improvement in immune responses after infusion into AIDS patients with fungal infections (Harrison and Levitz, 1996). Furthermore, short-term IL-12 treatment did not induce any change in immunological and virological parameters in rhesus monkeys infected with SIV (Watanabe et al., 1998). In all, additional studies are needed to better define the potential role of IL-12 therapy in the clinical management of AIDS patients and whether its benefit varies at different stages of HIV disease. The extent to which CTL numbers and functions are autonomously maintained in vivo or depend on some form of non-cytokine CD4$^+$ T-cell-mediated helper activity re-

mains unclear. To try to increase this CD4-mediated effect, a combined approach using CD40 ligand trimer (CD40LT) and IL-12 has been proposed (Dybul et al., 2000). Interestingly, ex vivo exposure of peripheral blood lymphocytes obtained from HIV-infected patients to combinations of CD40L and IL-12 ex vivo has been reported to increase both HIV p24-specific CD4$^+$ T-cell responses and IFN-γ production. This observation implies that at least some of the decreased HIV-specific CD4$^+$ T-cell responses measured in specimens from HIV-infected people may reflect anergy rather than complete deletion of the potential antiviral response in vivo.

At present, clear evidence indicating that cytokines other than IL-2 may play a major role in the clinical management of HIV-infected patients is still lacking (Mastroianni et al., 2000; Skowron et al., 1999). However, it is possible that cytokines such as IL-12, granulocyte-macrophage colony-stimulating factor, and others might be an important component of combination protocols in which HAART with STI will be coupled with interventions aimed at directly increasing the immune responses directed against the autologous virus.

Restoring CD4$^+$ T-Lymphocyte Populations

Since AIDS is characterized by progressive diminution of CD4$^+$ T-cell numbers, there is a clear rationale for interventions aimed at increasing the overall pool of CD4$^+$ T cells. Among potential growth factors acting on CD4$^+$ T cells in vivo, IL-2 has stimulated the greatest interest as a potential therapy for HIV infection. IL-2 is perhaps the best-characterized autocrine and paracrine proliferation factor for T lymphocytes, and its effect on T cells primed by antigenic stimuli is well known (Lanzavecchia et al., 1999). Primary T-cell activation results in IL-2 production and expression of IL-2 receptor alpha chain (IL-2R alpha-chain or CD25). On binding to its receptor, IL-2 induces activation of the Janus kinase system (JAK), with phosphorylation and nuclear localization of the STAT-5 transcription factor, and ultimately induces activation of the cell cycle machinery (Nelson and Willerford, 1998). Interestingly, the effect of IL-2 on lymphocytes is phase dependent, since the strong proliferation induced after primary immune response is somehow counteracted by a proapoptotic effect of IL-2 on T lymphocytes that takes place later in the activation cycle. Consistent with this latter function, IL-2$^{-/-}$ mice have a typical phenotype characterized by abnormal T-cell proliferation in vitro and autoimmune disease. Despite this dichotomy in the role of IL-2 on T-cell activation, numerous studies with uninfected humans have shown that rIL-2 administration results in marked increases in peripheral CD4$^+$ T-cell counts (Yamaguchi et al., 1988; Kaplan et al., 1991; Ardizzoni et al., 1994). Clearly, this is a highly desirable effect in clinical settings where patients suffer from progressive depletion of this lymphocyte subpopulation. Furthermore, the rationale for the use of IL-2 in AIDS patients is also supported by the idea that rIL-2 administration might potentially induce a desirable functional activation of anti-HIV CTL, which could help augment the host cellular immune response to the virus (Chia et al., 1994; Zou et al., 1999). However, this effect would be only transient unless a sufficient number of anti-HIV specific CD4$^+$ T-helper cells were eventually able to provide ongoing and appropriately coordinated IL-2 production once therapy was discontinued, and it may also depend on the level of HIV antigens that are extant in vivo. Finally, another potential rationale for the use of IL-2 in HIV-infected patients comes from the observation that in vitro IL-2 administration reduces the cell cycle abnormalities that have been observed in lymphocytes from HIV-infected patients (Piedimonte et al., 1999; Cannavo et al., 2001; Paiardini et al., in press).

The first clinical trials of rIL-2 in HIV-infected patients were carried out in the early 1990s. In these trials, IL-2 was used at various doses and via various routes of administration, as well as in combination with a variety of different antiretroviral drug regimens. The initial studies were plagued by frequent toxicity, probably related to the high doses of IL-2 used. These studies were followed by alternative protocols of IL-2 administration using either lower or intermittent doses, which were better tolerated. Intermittent courses of intravenous administration of IL-2 produced a substantial and sustained increase in CD4 T-cell counts without a substantial increase of HIV viremia in HIV patients with more than 200 CD4$^+$ T cells/mm^3 (Kovacs et al., 1995, 1996). Protocols based on intermittent subcutaneous (s.c.) administration of rIL-2 in the outpatient setting also resulted in an increase in the number of CD4$^+$ T cells, most notably when the dose was increased to 15×10^6 IU per day, with only transient increases seen in plasma viremia (Davey et al., 1997, 1999; Losso et al., 2000). In a recent study by the same group (Davey et al., 2000), s.c. addition of IL-2 to HAART was reported to be beneficial in terms of the overall decrease in viral load achieved. It is of interest that in most reports, the effect of IL-2 on CD4$^+$ T-cell counts was found to be directly correlated with the baseline CD4$^+$ T-cell count, suggesting that the presence of a relatively preserved infrastructure for maintenance of lymphocyte homeostasis may be im-

portant for determining the degree of the response induced by exogenous IL-2 administration. However, in a recent study, daily s.c. rIL-2 administration was also found to improve several immunological parameters in HIV-infected patients with a CD4$^+$ T-cell count lower than 250/mm^3 (Arno et al., 1999). Taken as a whole, these results indicate that IL-2 may ultimately prove to be an effective tool in the clinical management of HIV-infected patients with relatively high CD4$^+$ T-cell counts when used in combination with conventional HAART.

An important question regarding IL-2 treatment, as well as any therapy which induces an increase in CD4$^+$ T-cell counts in AIDS patients, is whether this increase corresponds to a real and clinically meaningful improvement of the host immune function. Specifically, does the newly expanded pool of CD4$^+$ T cells merely represent the product of the peripheral expansion of the few clones that were spared by the HIV-induced depletion prior to initiation of IL-2 therapy or does it represent a true expansion of the overall T-cell repertoire? Further, to what extent does the IL-2-expanded pool of CD4$^+$ T cells possess full functional capacity? The practical implications of these questions, with respect to the risk of development of opportunistic infections and disease progression, are of obvious importance. However, despite numerous studies performed over the past few years, the issue is still unresolved. The regeneration of a wider diversity in the TCR repertoire is dependent on the overall function of the regenerative lymphocyte compartment, which includes the bone marrow, thymus, and integrity of homeostatic mechanisms governing levels of peripheral naive T cells. In an attempt to address these important issues, a study by Connors et al. (1997) showed that the disruptions of the TCR repertoire induced by HIV infection did not appear to be promptly reversed by HAART with or without the addition of rIL-2. However, a positive effect of IL-2 therapy on increasing the relative levels of naive CD4$^+$ T cells and on increasing their ability to produce cytokines has been described by others (De Paoli et al., 1997).

When planning the first trials of rIL-2 in HIV-infected patients, researchers had to confront some potentially adverse consequences of IL-2 therapy. Given the known positive influence of immune activation on the susceptibility of CD4$^+$ T cells to HIV infection, concern was raised that IL-2-induced activation of CD4$^+$ T cells might lead to increased HIV replication in treated patients. This effect might potentially result in an overall increase of HIV replication by promoting increases in the numbers of uninfected CD4$^+$ T cells that are susceptible to HIV infection, as well as the potential for reactivation of

HIV quasi-species present as latent proviruses in resting, infected CD4$^+$ T cells. Although transient increases in plasma HIV viremia have been observed in some patients, they appear not to be associated with sustained increases in HIV replication or in the expression of previously silent quasi-species or drug-resistant HIV variants (Kovacs et al., 2000). Interestingly, the same authors did not observe increased HIV viremia in a number of patients whose CD4$^+$ T cells showed an IL-2-induced up regulation of CCR5, the most common HIV coreceptor (Weissmann et al., 2000). The potential activating effect of IL-2 on virus replication in CD4$^+$ T cells has been proposed as a strategy for flushing out of nonreplicating proviruses from latently infected T cells. A pilot protocol in which classical HAART was alternated with short-term IL-2 administration suggested that combined HAART plus IL-2 treatment reduced the level of replication-competent virus in the blood and the lymph nodes in some HIV-infected individuals (Chun et al., 1999). However, given recent indications that HIV replication continues at low levels even during HAART, it appears unlikely that any currently available modality of therapy will be able to lead to complete virus eradication.

Despite these promising results in terms of safety, improvement in CD4$^+$ T-cell count, and control of HIV viremia, clinical end-point trials are necessary to determine whether rIL-2 therapy for HIV-infected patients will, in fact, translate into improved clinical outcomes. In this regard, a recent pooled analysis of three randomized trials that started before 1995 and involved a total of 155 patients showed only a nonsignificant trend toward improved clinical outcome (Emery et al., 2000). The ultimate answer to these compelling questions will await the results of a large, ongoing phase III trial of IL-2 plus HAART versus HAART alone that is now being conducted with HIV-infected patients with CD4 counts of >300/mm^3 (Evaluation of Subcutaneous Proleukin in a Randomized International Trial [ESPRIT]).

Making CD4$^+$ Cells Resistant to HIV

It is conceivable that the progression of HIV disease could be substantially slowed if methods could be developed to make CD4$^+$ T cells unable to support HIV replication. Recent progress in understanding the interaction between HIV and host cells has defined a number of potential targets for interventions aimed at artificially inducing a state of resistance to HIV infection. In particular, attention has been focused on the cell surface molecules that serve as receptors (CD4) and coreceptors (CCR5) for HIV

binding to and entry into target cells. It is well established that HIV entry into CD4$^+$ T cells, an absolute requirement for replication, involves sequential binding of the HIV Env protein to CD4 and one of the chemokine receptors, such as CCR5 or CXCR4. While expression of CD4 is constitutive, the presence of chemokine receptors on the surface of T cells can be modulated in various ways. Of interest, individuals lacking CCR5 appear to be resistant to HIV infection and CD4$^+$ T cells are difficult to infect in culture if down regulation of CCR5 is artificially induced ex vivo (Samson et al., 1996; Carroll et al., 1997). Expression of the CCR5 mRNA transcripts is substantially reduced when CD4$^+$ T cells are activated in vitro with immobilized antibodies directed against CD3 and CD28, so that this method can be used to expand CD4$^+$ T cells ex vivo and make them more resistant to HIV infection (Carroll et al., 1997). This effect is specific for the CCR5 coreceptor, since expression of the CXCR4 gene is not altered under the same experimental conditions and confers a state of resistance to infection with CCR5-tropic strains of HIV in vitro. It was proposed that these CD4 lymphocytes expanded in this manner and relatively resistant to HIV infection could then be reinfused to generate a stable population of lymphocytes that would survive the HIV-mediated damage. Although of basic interest, these approaches are subject to several intrinsic problems. First, it is not clear how durable the down modulation of CCR5 gene expression will be on CD4$^+$ T cells following infusion in vivo, but there is no a priori reason to believe that it represents a stable phenotype. Reexpression of CCR5 in vivo would clearly abrogate any acquired resistance to HIV infection. Second, it is unclear how the ex vivo manipulation will affect the in vivo half-life of reinfused cells. Indeed, it has been found that ex vivo activation of lymphocyte results in short postreinfusion survival, probably as a result of overexpression of apoptosis-inducing receptors such as CD95/Fas (Tan et al., 1999). Third, HIV can use several coreceptors other than CCR5 to gain entry into CD4$^+$ T cells, and the outgrowth in infected persons of HIV variants that use the CXCR4 chemokine receptor for entry is known to be associated with higher rates of CD4 T-cell decline. More recently, the same investigators studied the role of CTLA4 expression on the in vitro susceptibility of CD4$^+$ T cells to HIV infection. CTLA4 engagement was found to counteract the antiviral effect of anti-CD28 stimulation, and the ratio of CTLA4 to CD28 binding appeared to determine the susceptibility to infection (Riley et al., 2000). Interestingly, blocking CTLA4-mediated signaling with an antagonist anti-CTLA4 antibody decreased the susceptibility of activated

CD4$^+$ T cells to HIV replication, thus prompting the authors to discuss a possible therapeutic role of antagonist anti-CTLA4 antibodies associated with anti-CD28 stimulation in the treatment of HIV infection.

A variety of gene therapy-based approaches have also been conceived as potential immune interventions for HIV infection (reviewed by Pomerantz and Trono [1995]). The common goal of all of the proposed approaches is to induce a condition of resistance in CD4$^+$ T cells to HIV infection and/or replication through transduction of interfering genes. The potentially inhibitory transgenes investigated include those encoding dominant negative versions of HIV gene products that interfere in *trans* with the function of the natural gene product, RNA-based inhibitors based on decoy variants of the *trans*-activation response element essential for Tat function or the Rev response element essential for Rev function, ribozymes engineered to cleave specific sites in the HIV genome, and intracellular antibodies or modified chemokines intended to block HIV gene product or cellular coreceptor function (reviewed by Amado et al. [1999]). While many of these approaches have been studied in tissue culture models, few gene therapy strategies have yet to be tested in clinical trials in humans. Studies performed by Nabel and colleagues (Ranga et al., 1998) have shown that a state of HIV resistance can be induced in tissue culture models by transduction of a modified HIV gene, Rev M10, delivered by a retroviral vector consisting of the Moloney murine leukemia virus. Rev M10 acts as a dominant negative inhibitor of Rev function and thereby antagonizes an essential regulatory function in the HIV life cycle. Interestingly, in a pilot clinical trial of this strategy, polyclonal CD4$^+$ T cells modified ex vivo with the Rev M10 transgene could be detected for an average of 6 months in the blood of three HIV-positive patients following reinfusion in vivo, apparently surviving longer than unprotected cells (Ranga et al., 1998). Although these gene transfer-based approaches are interesting and creative, they all carry severe inherent limitations, including the need for stem cell modification and preserved thymic function to enable transgene introduction into the important naive cell compartment of the T-cell repertoire, the inefficiency of current gene transduction techniques, and the unsolved problem of near-complete transcriptional extinction of transgene expression soon after in vivo transfer. Furthermore, from a practical point of view, these approaches will probably be difficult to implement in the clinical setting of substantial numbers of HIV-infected patients.

Back to the Paradox: Should We Treat HIV Patients with Immunosuppression?

As discussed above, the paradigm that AIDS is simply the result of the direct HIV-induced depletion of CD4$^+$ T cells has been challenged by a number of observations. As a result, it is now apparent that the pathogenesis of HIV disease is at least partly related to the negative effects of abnormal chronic immune activation. This aberrant chronic activation has been associated with a number of factors, including excessive amounts of proinflammatory cytokines and the induction of pronounced abnormalities in lymphocyte phenotype and function (Gougeon et al., 1996; Muro-Cacho et al., 1995; Cohen et al., 1997; Giorgi et al., 1999). As a result, excessive apoptotic death of uninfected lymphocytes is seen in HIV-infected persons and a consequent major interference with the normal function of lymphoid organs and bone marrow is generated. Thus, favorable manipulation of this inadvertently "wrong" immune response may therefore prove to be beneficial in HIV-infected patients, most notably in that subset of HIV-infected patients for whom suppression of HIV viremia is not followed by a prompt down regulation of the overall markers of immune activation.

In this context, numerous immunosuppressive agents have been proposed as potential therapy for HIV infection, including steroids, cyclosporin, mycophenolate, and anti-tumor necrosis factor alpha drugs such as pentoxiphylline and thalidomide (reviewed by Ravot et al. [1999]). An immunomodulatory effect in the context of HIV infection could potentially be achieved with non-immunophyllin-dependent agents such as steroids. In one clinical study, a sustained increased in CD4 counts without changes in HIV viremia was observed in a cohort of 44 HIV-infected patients treated with prednisolone only for 1 year (Andrieu et al., 1995). While these results were provocative, no longer-term follow-up studies of this approach have been reported.

Interestingly, more powerful immunosuppressive agents such as cyclosporin A (CyA) and mycophenolate have, in addition to their role in modulating host immune function, direct inhibitory effects on HIV replication or possess the ability to potentiate the antiviral action of nucleoside analog reverse transcriptase inhibitors commonly included in HAART regimens. The multiple effects thus complicate the interpretation of the potential role, as well as the mechanism of beneficial action, of these immunosuppressive agents. CyA has been well characterized as an effective antirejection drug, and its mechanism of action has recently been shown to be based on inhibition of the cyclophilin-dependent calcineurin phosphatase and blockade of the nuclear factor of activated T cells (NFAT) nuclear translocation (Crabtree, 1999). Interestingly, CyA also has a direct anti-HIV effect due to its binding to cyclophilin and consequent disruption of the interaction between cyclophilin and the HIV Gag protein that is required for HIV replication (Thali et al., 1994; Franke and Luban, 1996). The antiviral effect of CyA mediated through association with HIV Gag can be dissociated from its immunosuppressive action, and nonimmunosuppressive analogues of CyA, such as SDZ NIM81, also have anti-HIV effects in vitro (Bartz et al., 1995; Billich et al., 1995). More recently, however, it was shown that activation of NFAT, the final target of the immunosuppressive effect of CyA, is important for making $CD4^+$ T cells permissive for HIV infection (Kinoshita et al., 1998). This finding suggests that even the intrinsically immunosuppressive action of CyA may have the potential for an anti-HIV effect. As a result of these findings, CyA has been used in HIV patients, but unfortunately it did not appear to have any significant impact in terms of clinical outcome, immunological function, and levels of viral replication in vivo (Levy et al., 1995). Another recently introduced immunomodulatory agent, mycophenolate, has also been demonstrated to have a dual antiviral function, by virtue of its depletion of intracellular levels of guanosine nucleotides that are necessary to act as substrates for enabling both antigen-activated lymphocyte proliferation and HIV replication. When administered to HIV-infected patients, mycophenolate seems to synergize with more classical anti-HIV drugs (Margolis et al., 1999), as well as reduce the overall rates of T-cell turnover, probably by provoking apoptosis in activated $CD4^+$ T cells (Chapuis et al., 2000). In all, while definitive evidence supporting the clinical utility of immunosuppressive agents in the management of HIV-infected individuals is still lacking, it seems that at least for selected subclasses of HIV-infected patients, a rationale remains for conducting additional well-designed clinical trials in which immunomodulatory strategies are used in combination with standard HAART regimens.

FUTURE DIRECTIONS

The rapidly expanding understanding of the basic immunology and pathogenesis of HIV infection suggests that immune interventions will probably play an important role in the clinical management of HIV disease in the future. Complex approaches, in which HAART will be combined with immune interventions such as cytokine-based therapy and/or manipulation of costimulatory pathways of T-cell activation and/or activation of antigen-presenting cells, may prove very useful in subsets of HIV-infected patients. For example, the recent elucidation of the role of different costimulatory pathways in activation and maintenance of specific CD4 and CD8 T-cell responses will permit the design of new approaches in which focused immunologic manipulations can be used to augment anti-HIV immune responses in vivo. Dendritic cells (DC), the most potent antigen-presenting cells in vivo, have also been suggested to be numerically and functionally deficient during HIV infection, and evaluation of immune interventions aimed at improving the function of DC will be important in the context of HIV infection. For example, administration of cytokines such as GM-CSF and FMS-like tyrosine kinase 3 (FLT-3) ligand may augment DC numbers and promote effective DC maturation and might thereby contribute to the generation of a more effective anti-HIV immune response. Furthermore, cytokines such as IL-2, IL-7, IL-12, IL-15, and GM-CSF, to name just a few, all have the potential to improve anti-HIV responses in vivo when administered to patients undergoing HAART with or without STIs. Promising evidence from recent prophylactic vaccine studies with nonhuman primates and STI studies with humans clearly suggested that the host immune response can be manipulated to favorably alter the course of HIV infection. With the expanding repertoire of rational approaches to the modulation of immune responses in vivo and substantially improved methods to study and quantitate HIV-specific immune responses (e.g., enzyme-linked immunospot assay, flow cytometric determination of intracellular cytokine production, and MHC tetramer methods), as well as to assess the regenerative potential of T-cell populations (e.g., T-cell receptor excision circle assays and TCR spectratyping), that are now available, the field of immune-based therapies of HIV infection appears poised to enter a highly productive and informative phase. Clinical trials combining direct anti-HIV drugs with immune interventions can now be designed, with the ultimate complementary goals of improving the health and well-being of HIV-infected individuals and better understanding the pathogenesis of HIV infection.

REFERENCES

Amado, R. G., R. T. Mitsuyasu, and J. A. Zack. 1999. Gene therapy for the treatment of AIDS: animal models and human clinical experience. *Front. Biosci.* 4:D468–D475.

Amara, R. R., F. Villinger, J. D. Altman, S. L. Lydy, S. P. O'Neil, S. I. Staprans, D. C. Montefiori, Y. Xu, J. G. Herndon, L. S.

Wyatt, M. A. Candido, N. L. Kozyr, P. L. Earl, J. M. Smith, H.-L. Ma, B. D. Grimm, M. L. Hulsey, J. Miller, H. M. McClure, J. M. McNicholl, B. Moss, and H. L. Robinson. 2001. Control of mucosal challenge and prevention of AIDS by a multiprotein DNA/MVA vaccine. *Science* 292:69–74.

Andrieu, J. M., W. Lu, and R. Levy. 1995. Sustained increases in CD4 cell counts in asymptomatic human immunodeficiency virus type 1-seropositive patients treated with prednisolone for 1 year. *J. Infect. Dis.* 17:523–530.

Appay, V., D. F. Nixon, S. M. Donahoe, G. M. Gillespie, T. Dong, A. King, G. S. Ogg, H. M. Spiegel, C. Conlon, C. A. Spina, D. V. Havlir, D. D. Richman, A. Waters, P. Easterbrook, A. J. McMichael, and S. L. Rowland-Jones. 2000. HIV-specific CD8(+) T cells produce antiviral cytokines but are impaired in cytolytic function. *J. Exp. Med.* 192:63–75.

Ardizzoni, A., M. Bonavia, M. Viale, E. Baldini, A. Mereu, A. Verna, S. Ferrini, A. Cinquegrana, S. Molinari, and G. L. Mariani. 1994. Biologic and clinical effects of continuous infusion interleukin-2 in patients with non-small cell lung cancer. *Cancer* 73:1353–1360.

Arno, A., L. Ruiz, M. Juan, A. Jou, C. Balague, M. K. Zayat, S. Marfil, J. Martinez-Picado, M. A. Martinez, J. Romeu, R. Pujol-Borrell, C. Lane, and B. Clotet. 1999. Efficacy of low-dose subcutaneous interleukin-2 to treat advanced human immunodeficiency virus type 1 in persons with ≤250/μl CD4 T cells and undetectable plasma virus load. *J. Infect. Dis.* 180:56–60.

Badley, A. D., A. A. Pilon, A. Landay, and D. H. Lynch. 2000. Mechanisms of HIV-associated lymphocyte apoptosis. *Blood* 96:2951–2964.

Barouch, D. H., S. Santra, J. E. Schmitz, M. J. Kuroda, T. M. Fu, W. Wagner, M. Bilska, A. Craiu, X. X. Zheng, G. R. Krivulka, K. Beaudry, M. A. Lifton, C. E. Nickerson, W. L. Trigona, K. Punt, D. C. Freed, L. Guan, S. Dubey, D. Casimiro, A. Simon, M. E. Davies, M. Chastain, T. B. Strom, R. S. Gelman, D. C. Montefiori, and M. G. Lewis. 2000. Control of viremia and prevention of clinical AIDS in rhesus monkeys by cytokine-augmented DNA vaccination. *Science* 290:486–492.

Bartz, S. R., E. Hohenwalter, M. K. Hu, D. H. Rich, and M. Malkovsky. 1995. Inhibition of human immunodeficiency virus replication by nonimmunosuppressive analogs of cyclosporin A. *Proc. Natl. Acad. Sci. USA* 92:5381–5385.

Belyakov, I. M., J. D. Ahlers, B. Y. Brandwein, P. Earl, B. L. Kelsall, B. Moss, W. Strober, and J. A. Berzofsky. 1998. The importance of local mucosal HIV-specific CD8(+) cytotoxic T lymphocytes for resistance to mucosal viral transmission in mice and enhancement of resistance by local administration of IL-12. *J. Clin. Invest.* 102:2072–2081.

Berger, E. A., P. M. Murphy, and J. M. Farber. 1999. Chemokine receptors as HIV-1 coreceptors: roles in viral entry, tropism, and disease. *Annu. Rev. Immunol.* 17:657–700.

Billich, A., F. Hammerschmid, P. Peichl, R. Wenger, G. Zenke, V. Quesniaux, and B. Rosenwirth. 1995. Mode of action of SDZ NIM 811, a nonimmunosuppressive cyclosporin A analog with activity against human immunodeficiency virus (HIV) type 1: interference with HIV protein-cyclophilin A interactions. *J. Virol.* 69:2451–2461.

Birx, D. L., L. D. Loomis-Price, N. Aronson, J. Brundage, C. Davis, L. Dayton, R. P. Garner, F. Gordin, D. Henry, W. Holloway, T. Kerkering, R. Luskin-Hawk, J. McNeil, N. Michael, P. Foster Pierce, D. Poretz, S. Ratto-Kim, P. Renzullo, N. Ruiz, K. V. Sitz, G. Smith, C. Tacket, M. Thompson, E. Tramont, B. Yangco, R. Yarrish, and R. R. Redfield. 2000. Efficacy testing of recombinant HIV gp160 as a therapeutic vaccine in early-stage HIV-1 infected volunteers. rgp160 phase II vaccine investigators. *J. Infect. Dis.* 181:881–889.

Blankson, J. N., D. Finzi, T. C. Pierson, B. P. Sabundayo, K. Chadwick, J. B. Margolick, T. C. Quinn, and R. F. Siliciano. 2000. Biphasic decay of latently infected CD4+ T cells in acute human immunodeficiency virus type 1 infection. *J. Infect. Dis.* 182:1636–1642.

Boyer, J. D., M. A. Chattergoon, K. E. Ugen, A. Shah, M. Bennett, A. Cohen, S. Nyland, K. E. Lacy, M. L. Bagarazzi, T. J. Higgins, Y. Baine, R. B. Ciccarelli, R. S. Ginsberg, R. R. MacGregor, and D. B. Weiner. 1999. Enhancement of cellular immune response in HIV-1 seropositive individuals: a DNA-based trial. *Clin. Immunol.* 90:100–107.

Brodie, S. J., D. A. Lewinsohn, B. K. Patterson, D. Jiyamapa, J. Krieger, L. Corey, P. D. Greenberg, and S. D. Riddell. 1999. In vivo migration and function of transferred HIV-1 specific cytotoxic T cells. *Nat. Med.* 5:34–41.

Brodie, S. J., B. K. Patterson, D. A. Lewinsohn, K. Diem, D. Spach, P. D. Greenberg, S. D. Riddell, and L. Corey. 2000. HIV-specific cytotoxic T lymphocytes traffic to lymph nodes and localize at sites of HIV replication and cell death. *J. Clin. Investig.* 105:1407–1417.

Calarota, S., G. Bratt, S. Nordlund, J. Hinkula, A. C. Leandersson, E. Sandstrom, and B. Wahren. 1998. Cellular cytotoxic response induced by DNA vaccination in HIV-1-infected patients. *Lancet* 351:1320–1325.

Calarota, S. A., A. C. Leandersson, G. Bratt, J. Hinkula, D. M. Klinman, K. J. Weinhold, E. Sandstrom, and B. Wahren. 1999. Immune responses in asymptomatic HIV-1-infected patients after HIV-DNA immunization followed by highly active antiretroviral treatment. *J. Immunol.* 163:2330–2338.

Cannavo, G., M. Paiardini, D. Galati, B. Cervasi, M. Montroni, D. Guetard, G. DeVico, R. Ientile, I. Picerno, M. Magnani, G. Silvestri, and G. Piedimonte. 2001. Abnormal intracellular kinetics of cell cycle dependent proteins during HIV-infection: a novel biological link between immune activation, accelerated T cell turnover and high level of apoptosis. *Blood* 97:6.

Cao, Y., L. Qin, L. Zhang, J. Safrit, and D. D. Ho. 1995. Virologic and immunologic characterization of long-term survivors of human immunodeficiency virus type 1 infection. *N. Engl. J. Med.* 332:201–208.

Carcelain, G., R. Tubiana, A. Samri, V. Calvez, C. Delaugeree, H. Agut, C. Kathama, and B. Autran. 2001. Transient mobilization of human immunodeficiency virus (HIV)-specific CD4 T-helper cells fails to control viral rebounds during intermittent antiretroviral therapy in chronic HIV type-1 infection. *J. Virol.* 75:234–241.

Carroll, R. G., J. L. Riley, B. L. Levine, Y. Feng, S. Kaushal, D. W. Ritchey, W. Bernstein, O. S. Weislow, C. R. Brown, E. A. Berger, C. H. June, and D. C. St. Louis. 1997. Differential regulation of HIV-1 fusion cofactor expression by CD28 costimulation of CD4+ T cells. *Science* 276:273–276.

Chapuis, A. G., G. P. Rizzardi, C. D'Agostino, A. Attinger, C. Knabenhans, S. Fleury, H. Acha-Orbea, and G. Pantaleo. 2000. Effects of mycophenolic acid on human immunodeficiency virus infection in vitro and in vivo. *Nat. Med.* 6:762–768.

Chia, W. K., E. Nisbet-Brown, X. Li, I. Salit, S. Joshi, and S. E. Read. 1994. Lack of correlation between phenotype activation markers of CD8 lymphocytes and cytotoxic T lymphocyte (CTL) function in HIV-1 infection: evidence for rescue with rIL-2. *Viral Immunol.* 7:81–95.

Chun, T. W., D. Engel, S. B. Mizell, C. W. Hallahan, M. Fischette, S. Park, R. T. Davey Jr, M. Dybul, J. A. Kovacs, J. Metcalf, J. M. Mican, M. M. Berrey, L. Corey, H. C. Lane, and A. S. Fauci. 1999. Effect of IL-2 on the pool of latently infected, resting CD4+ T cells in HIV-1-infected patients receiving highly active anti-retroviral therapy. *Nat. Med.* 5:651–655.

Churdboonchart, V., R. B. Moss, W. Sirawaraporn, B. Smutharaks, R. Sutthent, F. C. Jensen, P. Vacharak, J. Grimes, G. Theofan, and D. J. Carlo. 1998. Effect of HIV-specific immune-based therapy in subjects infected with HIV-1 subtype E in Thailand. *AIDS* **12**:1521–1527.

Clark, S. J., M. S. Saag, W. D. Decker, S. Campbell-Hill, J. L. Roberson, P. J. Veldkamp, J. C. Kappes, B. H. Hahn, and G. M. Shaw. 1991. High titers of cytopathic virus in plasma of patients with symptomatic primary HIV-1 infection. *N. Engl. J. Med.* **324**:954–960.

Cohen, O. J., A. Kinter, and A. S. Fauci. 1997. Host factors in the pathogenesis of HIV disease. *Immunol. Rev.* **159**:31–48.

Collaborative Group on AIDS Incubation and HIV Survival. 2000. Time from HIV-1 seroconversion to AIDS and death before widespread use of highly-active antiretroviral therapy: a collaborative reanalysis. Collaborative Group on AIDS Incubation and HIV Survival including the CASCADE EU Concerted Action. Concerted Action on SeroConversion to AIDS and Death in Europe. *Lancet* **355**:1131–1137.

Connors, M., J. A. Kovacs, S. Krevat, J. C. Gea-Banacloche, M. C. Sneller, M. Flanigan, J. A. Metcalf, R. E. Walker, J. Falloon, M. Baseler, I. Feuerstein, H. Masur, and H. C. Lane. 1997. HIV infection induces changes in CD4+ T-cell phenotype and depletions within the CD4+ T-cell repertoire that are not immediately restored by antiviral or immune-based therapies. *Nat. Med.* **3**:533–540.

Crabtree, G. R. 1999. Generic signals and specific outcomes: signaling through Ca2+, calcineurin, and NF-AT. *Cell* **96**:611–614.

Daar, E. S., T. Moudgil, R. D. Meyer, and D. D. Ho. 1991. Transient high levels of viremia in patients with primary human immunodeficiency virus type 1 infection. *N. Engl. J. Med.* **324**:961–964.

Dalgleish, A. G., P. C. Beverley, P. R. Clapham, D. H. Crawford, M. F. Greaves, and R. A. Weiss. 1984. The CD4 (T4) antigen is an essential component of the receptor for the AIDS retrovirus. *Nature* **312**:763–767.

Davey, R. T., Jr., D. G. Chaitt, J. M. Albert, S. C. Piscitelli, J. A. Kovacs, R. E. Walker, J. Falloon, M. A. Polis, J. A. Metcalf, H. Masur, R. Dewar, M. Baseler, G. Fyfe, M. A. Giedlin, and H. C. Lane. 1999. A randomized trial of high- versus low-dose subcutaneous interleukin-2 outpatient therapy for early human immunodeficiency virus type 1 infection. *J. Infect. Dis.* **179**:849–858.

Davey, R. T., Jr., D. G. Chaitt, S. C. Piscitelli, M. Wells, J. A. Kovacs, R. E. Walker, J. Falloon, M. A. Polis, J. A. Metcalf, H. Masur, G. Fyfe, and H. C. Lane. 1997. Subcutaneous administration of interleukin-2 in human immunodeficiency virus type 1-infected persons. *J. Infect. Dis.* **175**:781–789.

Davey, R. T., Jr., R. L. Murphy, F. M. Graziano, S. L. Boswell, A. T. Pavia, M. Cancio, J. P. Nadler, D. G. Chaitt, R. L. Dewar, D. K. Sahner, A. M. Duliege, W. B. Capra, W. P. Leong, M. A. Giedlin, H. C. Lane, and J. O. Kahn. 2000. Immunologic and virologic effects of subcutaneous interleukin 2 in combination with antiretroviral therapy: a randomized controlled trial. *JAMA* **284**:183–189.

De Paoli, P., S. Zanussi, C. Simonelli, M. T. Bortolin, M. D'Andrea, C. Crepaldi, R. Talamini, M. Comar, M. Giacca, and U. Tirelli. 1997. Effects of subcutaneous interleukin-2 therapy on CD4 subsets and in vitro cytokine production in HIV+ subjects. *J. Clin. Immunol.* **100**:2737–2743.

Douek, D. C., R. D. McFarland, P. H. Keiser, E. A. Gage, J. M. Massey, B. F. Haynes, M. A. Polis, A. T. Haase, M. B. Feinberg, J. L. Sullivan, B. D. Jamieson, J. A. Zack, L. J. Picker, and R. A. Koup. 1998. Changes in thymic function with age and during the treatment of HIV infection. *Nature* **396**:690–695.

Durack, D. T. 1981. Opportunistic infections and Kaposi's sarcoma in homosexual men. *N. Engl. J. Med.* **305**:1465–1467.

Dybul, M., G. Mercier, M. Belson, C. W. Hallahan, S. Liu, C. Perry, B. Herpin, L. Ehler, R. T. Davey, J. A. Metcalf, J. M. Mican, R. A. Seder, and A. S. Fauci. 2000. CD40 ligand trimer and IL-12 enhance peripheral blood mononuclear cells and CD4+ T cell proliferation and production of IFN-gamma in response to p24 antigen in HIV-infected individuals: potential contribution of anergy to HIV-specific unresponsiveness. *J. Immunol.* **165**:1685–1691.

Emery, S., W. B. Capra, D. A. Cooper, R. T. Mitsuyasu, J. A. Kovacs, P. Vig, M. Smolskis, L. D. Saravolatz, H. C. Lane, G. A. Fyfe, and P. T. Curtin. 2000. Pooled analysis of 3 randomized, controlled trials of interleukin-2 therapy in adult human immunodeficiency virus type 1 disease. *J. Infect. Dis.* **182**:428–434.

Fauci, A. S. 1988. The human immunodeficiency virus: infectivity and mechanisms of pathogenesis. *Science* **239**:617–622.

Finzi, D., J. Blankson, J. D. Siliciano, J. B. Margolick, K. Chadwick, T. Pierson, K. Smith, J. Lisziewicz, F. Lori, C. Flexner, T. C. Quinn, R. E. Chaisson, E. Rosenberg, B. Walker, S. Gange, J. Gallant, and R. F. Siliciano. 1999. Latent infection of CD4+ T cells provides a mechanism for lifelong persistence of HIV-1, even in patients on effective combination therapy. *Nat. Med.* **5**:512–517.

Fogelman, I., V. Davey, H. D. Ochs, M. Elashoff, M. B. Feinberg, J. Mican, J. P. Siegel, M. Sneller, and H. C. Lane III. 2000. Evaluation of CD4+ T cell function in vivo in HIV-infected patients as measured by bacteriophage phiX174 immunization. *J. Infect. Dis.* **182**:435–441.

Fomsgaard, A. 1999. HIV-1 DNA vaccines. *Immunol. Lett.* **65**:127–131.

Franke, E. K., and J. Luban. 1996. Inhibition of HIV-1 replication by cyclosporine A or related compounds correlates with the ability to disrupt the Gag-cyclophilin A interaction. *Virology* **222**:279–282.

Frankel, A. D., and J. A. Young. 1998. HIV-1: fifteen proteins and an RNA. *Annu. Rev. Biochem.* **67**:1–25.

Gao, F., E. Bailes, D. L. Robertson, Y. Chen, C. M. Rodenburg, S. F. Michael, L. B. Cummins, L. O. Arthur, M. Peters, G. M. Shaw, P. M. Sharp, and B. H. Hahn. 1999. Origin of HIV-1 in the chimpanzee *Pan troglodytes troglodytes*. *Nature* **397**:436–441.

Gea-Banacloche, J. C., S. A. Migueles, L. Martino, W. L. Shupert, A. C. McNeil, M. S. Sabbaghian, L. Ehler, C. Prussin, R. Stevens, L. Lambert, J. Altman, C. W. Hallahan, J. C. de Quiros, and M. Connors. 2000. Maintenance of large numbers of virus-specific CD8+ T cells in HIV-infected progressors and long-term nonprogressors. *J. Immunol.* **165**:1082–1092.

Giorgi J. V., L. E. Hultin, J. A. McKeating, T. D. Johnson, B. Owens, L. P. Jacobson, R. Shih, J. Lewis, D. J. Wiley, J. P. Phair, S. M. Wolinsky, and R. Detels. 1999. Shorter survival in advanced HIV-1 infection is more closely associated with T lymphocyte activation than with plasma virus burden or virus chemokine co-receptor usage. *J. Infect. Dis.* **179**:859–870.

Goebel, F. D., J. W. Manhalter, R. B. Belshe, M. M. Eibl, P. J. Grob, V. de Gruttola, P. D. Griffiths, V. Erfle, M. Kunschack, and W. Engl. 1999. Recombinant gp160 as a therapeutic vaccine for HIV-infection: results of a large randomized, controlled trial. European Multinational IMMUNO AIDS vaccine study group. *AIDS* **13**:1461–1468.

Golding, H., R. Blumenthal, J. Manischewitz, D. R. Littman, and D. S. Dimitrov. 1993. Cell fusion mediated by interaction of a hybrid CD4. CD8 molecule with the human immunodeficiency virus type 1 envelope glycoprotein does occur after a long lag time. *J. Virol.* **67**:6469–6475.

Gougeon, M. L., H. Lecoeur, A. Dulioust, M. G. Enouf, M. Crouvoiser, C. Goujard, T. Debord, and L. Montagnier. 1996. Programmed cell death in peripheral lymphocytes from HIV-infected persons: increased susceptibility to apoptosis of CD4 and CD8 T cells correlates with lymphocyte activation and with disease progression. *J. Immunol.* **156:**3509–3520.

Greenberg, P. D., and S. D. Riddell. 1999. Deficient cellular immunity-finding and fixing the defects. *Science* **285:**546–561.

Grossman, Z., M. Polis, M. B. Feinberg, Z. Grossman, I. Levi, S. Jankelevich, R. Yarchoan, J. Boon, F. de Wolf, J. M. Lange, J. Goudsmit, D. S. Dimitrov, and W. E. Paul. 1999. Ongoing HIV dissemination during HAART. *Nat. Med.* **5:**1099–1104.

Haase, A. T. 1999. Population biology of HIV-1 infection: viral and CD4+ T cell demographics and dynamics in lymphatic tissues. *Annu. Rev. Immunol.* **17:**625–656.

Hahn, B. H., G. M. Shaw, K. M. De Cock, and P. M. Sharp. 2000. AIDS as a zoonosis: scientific and public health implications. *Science* **287:**607–614.

Harrer, T., E. Harrer, S. A. Kalams, T. Elbeik, S. I. Staprans, M. B. Feinberg, Y. Cao, D. D. Ho, T. Yilma, A. M. Caliendo, R. P. Johnson, S. P. Buchbinder, and B. D. Walker. 1996. Strong cytotoxic T cell and weak neutralizing antibody responses in a subset of persons with stable nonprogressing HIV type 1 infection. *AIDS Res. Hum. Retroviruses* **12:**585–592.

Harrison, T. S., and S. M. Levitz. 1996. Role of IL-12 in peripheral blood mononuclear cell responses to fungi in persons with and without HIV infection. *J. Immunol.* **156:**4492–4497.

Harty, J. T., A. R. Tvinnereim, and D. W. White. 2000. CD8+ T cell effector mechanisms in resistance to infection. *Annu. Rev. Immunol.* **18:**275–308.

Hazenberg, M. D., S. A. Otto, J. W. Cohen Stuart, M. C. Verschuren, J. C. Borleffs, C. A. Boucher, R. A. Coutinho, J. M. Lange, T. F. Rinke de Wit, A. Tsegaye, J. J. van Dongen, D. Hamann, R. J. de Boer, and F. Miedema. 2000. Increased cell division but not thymic dysfunction rapidly affects the T-cell receptor excision circle content of the naive T cell population in HIV-1 infection. *Nat. Med.* **6:**1036–1042.

Hel, Z., D. Venzon, M. Poudyal, W. P. Tsai, L. Giuliani, R. Woodward, C. Chougnet, G. Shearer, J. D. Altman, D. Watkins, N. Bischofberger, A. Abimiku, P. Markham, J. Tartaglia, and G. Franchini. 2000. Viremia control following antiretroviral treatment and therapeutic immunization during primary SIV$_{251}$ infection of macaques. *Nat. Med.* **6:**1140–1146.

Hellerstein, M., M. B. Hanley, D. Cesar, S. Siler, C. Papageorgopoulos, E. Wieder, D. Schmidt, R. Hoh, R. Neese, D. Macallan, S. Deeks, and J. M. McCune. 1999. Directly measured kinetics of circulating T lymphocytes in normal and HIV-1-infected humans. *Nat. Med.* **5:**83–89.

Hengel, R. L., B. M. Jones, M. S. Kennedy, M. R. Hubbard, and J. S. McDougal. 1999. Lymphocyte kinetics and precursor frequency-dependent recovery of CD4(+)CD45RA(+)CD62L(+) naive T cells following triple-drug therapy for HIV type 1 infection. *AIDS Res. Hum. Retroviruses* **15:**435–443.

Ho, D. D., A. U. Neumann, A. S. Perelson, W. Chen, J. M. Leonard, and M. Markowitz. 1995. Rapid turnover of plasma virions and CD4 lymphocytes in HIV-1 infection. *Nature* **373:**123–126.

Jin, X., D. E. Bauer, S. E. Tuttleton, S. Lewin, A. Gettie, J. Blanchard, C. E. Irwin, J. T. Safrit, J. Mittler, L. Weinberger, L. G. Kostrikis, L. Zhang, A. S. Perelson, and D. D. Ho. 1999. Dramatic rise in plasma viremia after CD8(+) T cell depletion in simian immunodeficiency virus-infected macaques. *J. Exp. Med.* **189:**991–998.

Kahn, J. O., D. W. Cherng, K. Mayer, H. Murray, and S. Lagakos, for the 806 Investigator Team. 2000. Evaluation of HIV-1 immunogen, and immunologic modifier, administered to patients infected with HIV having 300 to 549 × 10^6/L CD4 cell counts. *JAMA* **284:**2193–2202.

Kalams, S. A., and B. D. Walker. 1998. The critical need for CD4 help in maintaining effective cytotoxic T lymphocyte responses. *J. Exp. Med.* **188:**2199–2204.

Kamp, W., B. M. Berk, C. J. Visser, and H. S. Nottet. 2000. Mechanisms of HIV-1 to escape from the host immune surveillance. *Eur. J. Clin. Investig.* **30:**740–746.

Kaplan, G., W. J. Britton, G. E. Hancock, W. J. Theuvenet, K. A. Smith, C. K. Job, P. W. Roche, A. Molloy, R. Burkhardt, and J. Barker. 1991. The systemic influence of recombinant interleukin 2 on the manifestations of lepromatous leprosy. *J. Exp. Med.* **173:**993–1006.

Kinoshita, S., B. K. Chen, H. Kaneshima, and G. P. Nolan. 1998. Host control of HIV-1 parasitism in T cells by the nuclear factor of activated T cells. *Cell* **95:**595–604.

Koenig, S., A. J. Conley, Y. A. Brewah, G. M. Jones, S. Leath, L. J. Boots, V. Davey, G. Pantaleo, J. F. Demarest, C. Carter, et al. 1995. Transfer of HIV-1-specific cytotoxic T lymphocytes to an AIDS patient leads to selection for mutant HIV variants and subsequent disease progression. *Nat. Med.* **1:**330–336.

Komanduri, K. V., M. N. Viswanathan, E. D. Wieder, D. K. Schmidt, B. M. Bredt, M. A. Jacobson, and J. M. McCune. 1998. Restoration of cytomegalovirus-specific CD4+ T-lymphocyte responses after ganciclovir and highly active antiretroviral therapy in individuals infected with HIV-1. *Nat. Med.* **4:**953–956.

Kovacs, J. A., M. Baseler, R. J. Dewar, S. Vogel, R. T. Davey, Jr., J. Falloon, M. A. Polis, R. E. Walker, R. Stevens, N. P. Salzman, et al. 1995. Increases in CD4 T lymphocytes with intermittent courses of interleukin-2 in patients with human immunodeficiency virus infection. A preliminary study. *N. Engl. J. Med.* **332:**567–575.

Kovacs, J. A., H. Imamichi, S. Vogel, J. A. Metcalf, R. L. Dewar, M. Baseler, R. Stevens, J. Adelsberger, L. Lambert, R. T. Davey, Jr., R. E. Walker, J. Falloon, M. A. Polis, H. Masur, and H. C. Lane. 2000. Effects of intermittent interleukin-2 therapy on plasma and tissue human immunodeficiency virus levels and quasispecies expression. *J. Infect. Dis.* **182:**1063–1069.

Kovacs, J. A., S. Vogel, J. M. Albert, J. Falloon, R. T. Davey, Jr., R. E. Walker, M. A. Polis, K. Spooner, J. A. Metcalf, M. Baseler, G. Fyfe, and H. C. Lane. 1996. Controlled trial of interleukin-2 infusions in patients infected with the human immunodeficiency virus. *N. Engl. J. Med.* **335:**1350–1356.

Lambert, J. S., J. McNamara, S. L. Katz, T. Fenton, M. Kang, T. C. VanCott, R. Livingston, E. Hawkins, J. Moye, W. Borkowsky, D. Johnson, R. Yogev, A. M. Duliege, D. Francis, A. Gershon, D. Wara, N. Martin, M. Levin, G. McSherry, and G. Smith. 1998. Safety and immunogenicity of HIV-recombinant envelope vaccines in HIV-infected infants and children. NIH-sponsored pediatric AIDS clinical trials group (ACTG-218). *AIDS Res. Hum. Retroviruses* **19:**451–461.

Lanzavecchia, A., G. Lezzi, and A. Viola. 1999. From TCR engagement to T cell activation: a kinetic view of T cell behavior. *Cell* **96:**1–4.

Levy, R., J. P. Jais, J. M. Tourani, P. Even, and J. M. Andrieu. 1995. Long-term follow-up of HIV positive asymptomatic patients having received cyclosporin A. *Adv. Exp. Med. Biol.* **374:**229–234.

Lieberman, J., P. R. Skolink, G. R. Parkerson, J. A. Fabry, B. Landry, J. Bethel, and J. Kagan. 1997. Safety of autologous, ex vivo expanded HIV-1 specific cytotoxic T-lymphocyte infusion in HIV-1 infected patients. *Blood* **90:**2196–2206.

Lori, F., M. G. Lewis, J. Xu, G. Varga, D. E. Zinn, C. Crabbs, W. Wagner, J. Greenhouse, P. Silvera, J. Valley-Ogunro, C.

Tinelli, and J. Lisziewicz. 2000. Control of SIV rebound through structured treatment interruptions during early infection. *Science* 290:1591–1593.

Losso, M. H., W. H. Belloso, S. Emery, J. A. Benetucci, P. E. Cahn, M. C. Lasala, G. Lopardo, H. Salomon, M. Saracco, E. Nelson, M. G. Law, R. T. Davey, M. C. Allende, and H. C. Lane. 2000. A randomized, controlled, phase II trial comparing escalating doses of subcutaneous interleukin-2 plus antiretrovirals versus antiretrovirals alone in human immunodeficiency virus-infected patients with CD4+ cell counts ≥350/mm³. *J. Infect. Dis.* 181:1614–1621.

MacGregor, R. R., J. D. Boyer, K. E. Ugen, K. E. Lacy, S. J. Gluckman, M. L. Bagarazzi, M. A. Chattergoon, Y. Baine, T. J. Higgins, R. B. Ciccarelli, L. R. Coney, R. S. Ginsberg, and D. B. Weiner. 1998. First human trial of a DNA-based vaccine for treatment of human immunodeficiency virus type 1 infection: safety and host response. *J. Infect. Dis.* 178:92–100.

Malhotra, U., M. M. Berrey, Y. Huang, J. Markee, D. J. Brown, S. Ap, L. Musey, T. Schacker, L. Corey, and M. J. McElrath. 2000. Effect of combination antiretroviral therapy on T-cell immunity in acute human immunodeficiency virus type 1 infection. *J. Infect. Dis.* 181:121–131.

Margolis, D., A. Heredia, J. Gaywee, D. Oldach, G. Drusano, and R. Redfield. 1999. Abacavir and mycophenolic acid, an inhibitor of inosine monophosphate dehydrogenase, have profound and synergistic anti-HIV activity. *J. Acquired Immune Defic. Syndr.* 21:362–370.

Mastroianni, C. M., G. d'Ettorre, G. Forcina, M. Lichtner, F. Mengoni, C. D'Agostino, A. Corpolongo, A. P. Massetti, and V. Vullo. 2000. Interleukin-15 enhances neutrophil functional activity in patients with human immunodeficiency virus infection. *Blood* 96:1979–1984.

McCune, J. M., M. B. Hanley, D. Cesar, R. Halvorsen, R. Hoh, D. Schmidt, E. Wieder, S. Deeks, S. Siler, R. Neese, and M. Hellerstein. 2000. Factors influencing T-cell turnover in HIV-1-seropositive patients. *J. Clin. Investig.* 105:R1–R8.

McFarland, E. J., P. A. Harding, S. McWhinney, R. T. Schooley, and D. R. Kuritzkes. 1998. In vitro effects of IL-12 on HIV-specific CTL lines from HIV-infected children. *J. Immunol.* 161:513–519.

McKinney, D. M., D. A. Lewinsohn, S. R. Riddell, P. D. Greenberg, and D. E. Moisier. 1999. The antiviral activity of HIV-specific CD8+ CTL clones is limited by elimination due to encounter with HIV-infected targets. *J. Immunol.* 163:861–867.

Mellors, J. W., A. Munoz, J. V. Giorgi, J. B. Margolick, C. J. Tassoni, P. Gupta, L. A. Kingsley, J. A. Todd, A. J. Saah, R. Detels, J. P. Phair, and C. R. Rinaldo, Jr. 1997. Plasma viral load and CD4+ lymphocytes as prognostic markers of HIV-1 infection. *Ann. Intern. Med.* 126:946–954.

Metzner, K. J., X. Jin, F. V. Lee, A. Gettie, D. E. Bauer, M. Di Mascio, A. S. Perelson, P. A. Marx, D. D. Ho, L. G. Kostrikis, and R. I. Connor. 2000. Effects of in vivo CD8(+) T cell depletion on virus replication in rhesus macaques immunized with a live, attenuated simian immunodeficiency virus vaccine. *J. Exp. Med.* 191:1921–1931.

Mitsuyasu, R. T., P. A. Anton, S. G. Deeks, D. T. Scadden, E. Connick, M. T. Downs, A. Bakker, M. R. Roberts, C. H. June, S. Jalali, A. A. Lin, R. Pennathur-Das, and K. M. Hege. 2000. Prolonged survival and tissue trafficking following adoptive transfer of CD4zeta gene-modified autologous CD4(+) and CD8(+) T cells in human immunodeficiency virus-infected subjects. *Blood* 96:785–793.

Mollet, L., T. S. Li, A. Samri, C. Tournay, R. Tubiana, V. Calvez, P. Debre, C. Katlama, and B. Autran. 2000. Dynamics of HIV-specific CD8+ T lymphocytes with changes in viral load. The RESTIM and COMET Study Groups. *J. Immunol.* 165:1692–1704.

Moore, J. P., A. Trkola, and T. Dragic. 1997. Co-receptors for HIV-1 entry. *Curr. Opin. Immunol.* 9:551–562.

Moses, A., J. Nelson, and G. C. Bagby. 1998. The influence of human immunodeficiency virus-1 on hematopoiesis. *Blood* 91:1479–1495.

Moss, R. B., W. K. Giermakowska, J. R. Savary, G. Theofan, A. E. Daigle, S. P. Richieri, F. C. Jensen, and D. J. Carlo. 1998. A primer on HIV type 1-specific immune function and REMUNE. *AIDS Res. Hum. Retroviruses* 14:S167–S175.

Muro-Cacho, C. A., G. Pantaleo, and A. S. Fauci. 1995. Analysis of apoptosis in lymph nodes of HIV-infected persons. Intensity of apoptosis correlates with the general state of activation of the lymphoid tissue and not with stage of disease or viral burden. *J. Immunol.* 154:5555–5566.

Nagy-Agren, S. E., and E. L. Cooney. 1999. Interleukin-12 enhancement of antigen-specific lymphocyte proliferation correlates with stage of human immunodeficiency virus infection. *J. Infect. Dis.* 179:493–496.

Nelson, B. H., and D. M. Willerford. 1998. Biology of the interleukin-2 receptor. *Adv. Immunol.* 70:1–81.

Ogg, G. S., X. Jin, S. Bonhoeffer, P. R. Dunbar, M. A. Nowak, S. Monard, J. P. Segal, Y. Cao, S. L. Rowland-Jones, A. Cerundolo, A. Hurley, M. Markowitz, D. D. Ho, D. F. Nixon, and A. J. McMichael. 1998. Quantitation of HIV-1-specific cytotoxic T lymphocytes and plasma load of viral RNA. *Science* 279:2103–2106.

Ogg, G. S., X. Jin, S. Bonhoeffer, P. Moss, M. A. Nowak, S. Monard, J. P. Segal, Y. Cao, S. L. Rowland-Jones, A. Hurley, M. Markowitz, D. D. Ho, A. J. McMichael, and D. F. Nixon. 1999a. Decay kinetics of human immunodeficiency virus-specific effector cytotoxic T lymphocytes after combination antiretroviral therapy. *J. Virol.* 73:797–800.

Ogg, G. S., S. Kostense, M. R. Klein, S. Jurriaans, D. Hamann, A. J. McMichael, and F. Miedema. 1999b. Longitudinal phenotypic analysis of human immunodeficiency virus type 1-specific cytotoxic T lymphocytes: correlation with disease progression. *J. Virol.* 73:9153–9160.

Oxenius, A., D. A. Price, P. J. Easterbrook, C. A. O'Callaghan, A. D. Kelleher, J. A. Whelan, G. Sontag, A. K. Sewell, and R. E. Phillips. 2000. Early highly active antiretroviral therapy for acute HIV-1 infection preserves immune function of CD8+ and CD4+ T lymphocytes. *Proc. Natl. Acad. Sci. USA* 97:3382–3387.

Paiardini, M., D. Galati, B. Cervasi, G. Cannavo, L. Galluzzi, M. Montroni, D. Guetard, M. Magnani, G. Piedimonte, and G. Silvestri. Exogenous interleukin-2 administration corrects the cell cycle perturbation of lymphocytes from human immunodeficiency virus-infected individuals. *J. Virol.*, in press.

Pantaleo, G., and A. S. Fauci. 1995. New concepts in the immunopathogenesis of HIV infection. *Annu. Rev. Immunol.* 13:487–512.

Pantaleo, G., S. Menzo, M. Vaccarezza, C. Graziosi, O. J. Cohen, J. F. Demarest, D. Montefiori, J. M. Orenstein, C. Fox, L. K. Schrager, and A. S. Fauci. 1995. Studies in subjects with long-term nonprogressive human immunodeficiency virus infection. *N. Engl. J. Med.* 332:209–216.

Perelson, A. S., A. U. Neumann, M. Markowitz, J. M. Leonard, and D. D. Ho. 1996. HIV-1 dynamics in vivo: virion clearance rate, infected cell life-span, and viral generation time. *Science* 271:1582–1586.

Peters, B. S. 2000. HIV immunotherapeutic vaccines. *Antiviral Chem. Chemother.* 11:311–320.

Piedimonte, G., D. Corsi, M. Paiardini, G. Cannavo, R. Ientile, I. Picerno, M. Montroni, G. Silvestri, and M. Magnani. 1999. Unscheduled cyclin B expression and p34 cdc2 activation in T lymphocytes from HIV-infected patients. *AIDS* 13:1159–1165.

Pierson T., J. McArthur, and R. F. Siliciano. 1998. Reservoirs for HIV-1: mechanisms for viral persistence in the presence of antiviral immune responses and antiretroviral therapy. *Annu. Rev. Immunol.* 18:665–708.

Pitcher, C. J., C. Quittner, D. M. Peterson, M. Connors, R. A. Koup, V. C. Maino, and L. J. Picker. 1999. HIV-1-specific CD4+ T cells are detectable in most individuals with active HIV-1 infection, but decline with prolonged viral suppression. *Nat. Med.* 5:518–525.

Pomerantz, R. J., and D. Trono. 1995. Genetic therapies for HIV infections: promise for the future. *AIDS* 9:985–993.

Pontesilli, O., M. R. Klein, S. R. Kerkhof-Garde, N. G. Pakker, F. de Wolf, H. Schuitemaker, and F. Miedema. 1997. Kinetics of immune functions and virus replication during HIV-1 infection. *Immunol. Lett.* 57:125–130.

Powderly, W. G., A. Landay, and M. M. Lederman. 1998. Recovery of the immune system with antiretroviral therapy: the end of opportunism? *JAMA* 280:72–77.

Ranga, U., C. Woffendin, S. Verma, L. Xu, C. H. June, D. K. Bishop, and G. J. Nabel. 1998. Enhanced T cell engraftment after retroviral delivery of an antiviral gene in HIV-infected individuals. *Proc. Natl. Acad. Sci. USA* 95:1201–1206.

Ravot, E., J. Lisziewicz, and F. Lori. 1999. New uses for old drugs in HIV infection: the role of hydroxyurea, cyclosporin and thalidomide. *Drugs* 58:953–963.

Redfield, R. R., D. L. Birx, N. Ketter, E. Tramont, V. Polonis, C. Davis, J. F. Brundage, G. Smith, S. Johnson, and A. Fowler. 1991. A phase 1 evaluation of the safety and immunogenicity of vaccination with recombinant gp160 in patients with early HIV-infection. *N. Engl. J. Med.* 324:1677–1684.

Rey-Cuille, M. A., J. L. Berthier, M. C. Bomsel-Demontoy, Y. Chaduc, L. Montagnier, A. G. Hovanessian, and L. A. Chakrabarti. 1998. Simian immunodeficiency virus replicates to high levels in sooty mangabeys without inducing disease. *J. Virol.* 72:3872–3886.

Riddell, S. R., M. Elliott, D. A. Lewinsohn, M. J. Gilbert, L. Wilson, S. A. Manley, S. D. Lupton, R. W. Overell, T. C. Reynolds, L. Corey, and P. D. Greenberg. 1996. T-cell mediated rejection of gene-modified HIV-specific cytotoxic T lymphocytes in HIV-infected patients. *Nat. Med.* 2:216–223.

Riley, J. L., K. Schlienger, P. J. Blair, B. Carreno, N. Craighead, D. Kim, R. G. Carroll, and C. H. June. 2000. Modulation of susceptibility to HIV-1 infection by the cytotoxic T lymphocyte antigen 4 costimulatory molecule. *J. Exp. Med.* 191:1987–1997.

Rosenberg, E. S., M. Altfeld, S. H. Poon, M. N. Phillips, B. M. Wilkes, R. L. Elridge, G. K. Robbins, R. T. D'Aquila, P. J. R. Goulder, and B. D. Walker. 2000. Immune control of HIV-1 after early treatment of acute infection. *Nature* 407:523–526.

Rosenberg, E. S., J. M. Billingsley, A. M. Caliendo, S. L. Boswell, P. E. Sax, S. A. Kalams, and B. D. Walker. 1997. Vigorous HIV-1 specific CD4+ T cell responses associated with control of viremia. *Science* 278:1447–1450.

Ruiz, L., J. Martinez-Picado, J. Romeu, R. Paredes, M. K. Zayat, S. Marfil, E. Negredo, G. Sirera, C. Tural, and B. Clotet. 2000. Structured treatment interruption in chronically HIV-1 infected patients after long-term viral suppression. *AIDS* 14:397–403.

Saag, M. S., M. Holodniy, D. R. Kuritzkes, W. A. O'Brien, R. Coombs, M. E. Poscher, D. M. Jacobsen, G. M. Shaw, D. D. Richman, and P. A. Volberding. 1996. HIV viral load markers in clinical practice. *Nat. Med.* 2:625–629.

Samson, M., F. Libert, B. J. Doranz, J. Rucker, C. Liesnard, C. M. Farber, S. Saragosti, C. Lapoumeroulis, J. Cognaux, C. For-

ceille, G. Muyldermans, C. Verhofstede, G. Burtonboy, M. Georges, T. Imai, S. Rana, Y. Yi, R. J. Smyth, R. G. Collman, R. W. Doms, G. Vassart, and M. Parmentier. 1996. Resistance to HIV-1 infection in caucasian individuals bearing mutant alleles of the CCR-5 chemokine receptor gene. *Nature* 382:722–725.

Sandstrom, E., and B. Wahren. 1999. Therapeutic immunisation with rgp160 in HIV-1 infection: a randomised double-blind placebo-controlled trial. Nordic VAC-40 study group. *Lancet* 353:1735–1742.

Schmitz, J. E., M. J. Kuroda, S. Santra, V. G. Sasseville, M. A. Simon, M. A. Lifton, P. Racz, K. Tenner-Racz, M. Dalesandro, B. J. Scallon, J. Ghrayeb, M. A. Forman, D. C. Montefiori, E. P. Rieber, N. L. Letvin, and K. A. Reimann. 1999. Control of viremia in simian immunodeficiency virus infection by CD8+ lymphocytes. *Science* 283:857–860.

Silvestri, G., C. Munoz-Calleja, P. Bagnarelli, G. Piedimonte, M. Clementi, and M. Montroni. 1998. Early increase of CD4+ CD45RA+ and CD4+ CD95- cells with conserved repertoire induced by anti-retroviral therapy in HIV-infected patients. *Clin. Exp. Immunol.* 111:3–11.

Skowron, G., D. Stein, G. Drusano, K. Melbourne, J. Bilello, D. Mikolich, K. Rana, J. M. Agosti, A. Mongillo, J. Whitmore, and M. J. Gilbert. 1999. The safety and efficacy of granulocyte-macrophage colony-stimulating factor (Sargramostim) added to indinavir- or ritonavir-based antiretroviral therapy: a randomized double-blind, placebo-controlled trial. *J. Infect. Dis.* 180:1064–1071.

Stevenson, M., B. Brichacek, N. Heinzinger, S. Swindells, S. Pirruccello, E. Janoff, and M. Emerman. 1995. Molecular basis of cell cycle dependent HIV-1 replication. Implications for control of virus burden. *Adv. Exp. Med. Biol.* 374:33–45.

Tan, R., X. Xu, G. S. Ogg, P. Hansasuta, T. Dong, T. Rostron, G. Luzzi, C. P. Conlon, G. R. Screaton, A. J. McMichael, and S. Rowland-Jones. 1999. Rapid death of adoptively transferred T cells in acquired immunodeficiency syndrome. *Blood* 93:1506–1510.

Thali, M., A. Bukovsky, E. Kondo, B. Rosenwirth, C. T. Walsh, J. Sodroski, and H. G. Gottlinger. 1994. Functional association of cyclophilin A with HIV-1 virions. *Nature* 372:363–365.

Tsoukas C. M., J. Raboud, N. F. Bernard, J. S. Montaner, M. J. Gill, A. Rachlis, I. W. Fong, W. Schlech, O. Djurdjev, J. Freedman, R. Thomas, R. Iafreniere, M. A. Weinberg, S. Cassol, M. O'Shaughnessy, J. Todd, F. Volvovitz, and G. E. Smith. 1998. Active immunization of patients with HIV infection: a study of the effect of VaxSyn, a recombinant HIV envelope subunit vaccine, on progression of immunodeficiency. *AIDS Res. Hum. Retroviruses* 14:483–490.

UNAIDS/WHO Joint United Nations Programme on HIV/AIDS. 2000. *AIDS Epidemic Update: December 2000.* United Nations, Geneva, Switzerland.

Walker, B. D., E. S. Rosenberg, C. M. Hay, N. Basgoz, and O. O. Yang. 1998. Immune control of HIV-1 replication. *Adv. Exp. Med. Biol.* 452:159–167.

Walker, R. E., C. M. Bechtel, V. Natarajan, M. Baseler, K. M. Hege, J. A. Metcalf, R. Stevens, A. Hazen, R. M. Blaese, C. C. Chen, S. F. Leitman, J. Palensky, J. Wittes, R. T. Davey, Jr., J. Falloon, M. A. Polis, J. A. Kovacs, D. F. Broad, B. L. Levine, M. R. Roberts, H. Masur, and H. C. Lane. 2000. Long-term in vivo survival of receptor-modified syngeneic T cells in patients with human immunodeficiency virus infection. *Blood* 96:467–474.

Watanabe, N., J. P. Sypek, S. Mittler, K. A. Reimann, P. Flores-Villanueva, G. Voss, C. I. Lord, and N. L. Letvin. 1998. Administration of recombinant human interleukin 12 to chronically SIVmac-infected rhesus monkeys. *AIDS Res. Hum. Retroviruses* **14:**393–399.

Wei, X., S. K. Ghosh, M. E. Taylor, V. A. Johnson, E. A. Emini, P. Deutsch, J. D. Lifson, S. Bonhoeffer, M. A. Nowak, B. H. Hahn, and G. M. Shaw. 1995. Viral dynamics in human immunodeficiency virus type 1 infection. *Nature* **373:**117–122.

Weissman, D., M. Dybul, M. B. Daucher, R. T. Davey, Jr., R. E. Walker, and J. A. Kovacs. 2000. Interleukin-2 up-regulates expression of the human immunodeficiency virus fusion coreceptor CCR5 by CD4+ lymphocytes in vivo. *J. Infect. Dis.* **181:**933–938.

Whitmire, J. K., and R. Ahmed. 2000. Costimulation in antiviral immunity: differential requirements for CD4(+) and CD8(+) T cell responses. *Curr. Opin. Immunol.* **12:**448–455.

Wright, P. F., J. S. Lambert, G. J. Gorse, R. H. Hsieh, M. J. McElrath K. Weinhold, D. W. Wara, E. L. Anderson, M. C. Keefer, S. Jackson, L. J. Wagner, D. P. Francis, P. E. Fast, and J. McNamara. 1999. Immunization with envelope MN rgp120 vaccine in HIV-infected pregnant women. *J. Infect. Dis.* **180:**1080–1088.

Wyatt, R., and J. Sodroski. 1998. The HIV-1 envelope glycoproteins: fusogens, antigens, and immunogens. *Science* **280:**1884–1888.

Yamaguchi, S., M. Onji, H. Kondoh, H. Miyaoka, and Y. Ohta. 1988. Immunologic effects on peripheral lymphoid cells from patients with chronic hepatitis type B during administration of recombinant interleukin 2. *Clin. Exp. Immunol.* **74:**1–6.

Zajac, A. J., J. N. Blattman, K. Murali-Krishna, D. J. Sourdive, M. Suresh, J. D. Altman, and R. Ahmed. 1998. Viral immune evasion due to persistence of activated T cells without effector function. *J. Exp. Med.* **188:**2205–2213.

Zinkernagel, R. M., and H. Hengartner. 1994. T-cell-mediated immunopathology versus direct cytolysis by virus: implications for HIV and AIDS. *Immunol. Today* **15:**262–268.

Zou, W., A. Foussat, C. Capitant, I. Durand-Gasselin, L. Bouchet, P. Galanaud, Y. Levy, and D. Emilie. 1999. Acute activation of CD8+ T lymphocytes in interleukin-2-treated HIV-infected patients. ANRS-048 IL-2 Study Group. Agence Nationale de Recherches sur le SIDA. *J. Acquired Immune Defic. Syndr.* **22:**31–38.

INDEX

env gene, 426, 462
Eosinophil(s), parasitic infection, 117–118
Eosinophilia, 402
Epidermodysplasia verruciformis, 431
Epidermophyton, 26, 29
Epitope spreading, 273
EPS, *see* Exopolysaccharide
Epstein-Barr virus, 89, 143, 145–146, 150, 170, 185,
    260, 271, 274–275, 282, 289, 307–309, 311,
    314, 318, 364, 367, 371–372
    immunogenetics of host response, 430–431
Equine herpesvirus 2, 363
Erythema nodosum, 283
Erythroleukemia, 425
Erythrophagocytosis, 301
Erythropoietin receptor, 425
ES-62 protein, 388
ESAT6 protein, 445
Escherichia coli, 196, 414
    enteroinvasive, 200
    enteropathogenic, 9–10
Esp proteins, 10
Eta-1 gene, 153, 415
Evolution
    host defense system, 67–76
    host immune response and microbial pathogenesis, 167
Exfoliative toxin, 7
Exogenic allergic alveolitis, 283–284
Exopolysaccharide (EPS), 346, 348
Exotoxin, 214–215
Exotoxin A, 6
Experimental autoimmune encephalomyelitis (EAE), 271–
    273
Extracellular bacteria, 5–12, 213–215

F-actin, 82
Factor H, 112–113, 360
Factor I, 112
FAE, *see* Follicle-associated epithelium
Farmer's lung, 284
Fas-FasL system, 211, 254, 260, 371–372
Fc receptor, 33, 81, 95, 185, 213–214, 239, 258, 282,
    358, 386
    Fcγ, 81, 83, 100, 256, 387
Feline immunodeficiency virus, 314
Feline leukemia virus, 314
Fibronectin, 32
Fibrosis, 293, 297
Ficolins, 96
Filariasis, 43–44
Flavivirus, 427–428
Flv gene, 427–428
fMet-Leu-Phe (fMLP), 385
Follicle-associated epithelium (FAE), 191–196
Follicular dendritic cells, 179, 184–185, 191, 199, 312,
    321
Food poisoning, 272
Foot-and-mouth disease virus, 307, 309, 311
Friend virus complex, 425–427
Fungal infection/disease, *see also* Mycosis

acquired immunity, 223–234
    association with B-cell deficiency, 225
    association with T-cell disorders, 224–225
    cell-mediated immunity, 229
    granulomatous inflammation, 227
    humoral immunity, 228–229
    immune evasion, 33–34
    innate immunity, 127–138
    invasion of host cells, 32–33
    latent, 227–228
    mouse models, 229–230
    passive immunization, 228
    subversion of host immune defenses, 33–34
    Th1 response, 227
    vaccines, 225–227
Fungi, 25–37
    adherence to host tissue, 31–32
    biology, 25–28
    cell structure, 27–28
    dimorphism, 26–27, 34–35, 223
    metabolism and nutritional requirements, 28
    morphology and morphogenesis, 26–27
    pathogenicity, 31
    reproduction, 28
    taxonomy, 26
    virulence, 31, 133–134
Fusarium, 30–31
Fv-1 gene, 425–426
Fv-2 gene, 426
Fv-4 gene, 426

gag gene, 426
Galactosylceramide, 197
Gallbladder, *S. enterica*, 342
GALT, 312
Gamma interferon, *see* Interferon gamma
Ganglioside antibodies, 275
Gastrointestinal tract
    nematodes, *see* Nematodes, gastrointestinal
    virus entry, 311–312
gB glycoprotein, 371
gC protein, 359
Gcp protein, 8
gE protein, 358
Gene conversion, 422–423
Gene duplication, 70, 73
Gene therapy, for AIDS, 470
Genetic epidemiology, 396–397
Genetic polymorphisms, 397, 422
Genetic predisposition, 395–419
Genital warts, 322
Genome duplication, 69–70
Genomic catastrophism, 69–70
Germinal center, 179, 185, 191
gI protein, 358
Giardia lamblia, 39
Glomerulonephritis, poststreptococcal, 218, 271, 276,
    283
β-Glucan receptor, 128
Glucose monomycolate, 211